# ACCESS TO
# Health

15E

Rebecca J. Donatelle

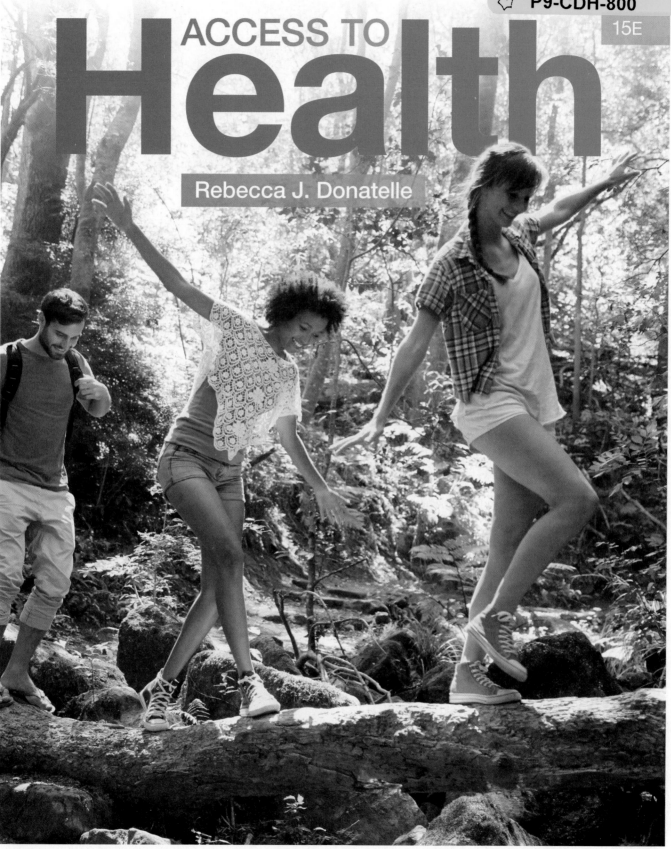

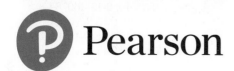

Pearson

Courseware Portfolio Manager: Michelle Yglecias
Content Producer: Deepti Agarwal
Managing Producer: Nancy Tabor
Courseware Director, Content Development: Barbara Yien
Development Editors: Nedah Rose, Nic Albert
Courseware Editorial Assistant: Nicole Constantine
Rich Media Content Producer: Timothy Hainley
Mastering Content Developer, Science: Lorna Perkins
Full-Service Vendor: SPi Global
Copyeditor: Laura Patchkofsky
Art Coordinator: Morgan Eawald, Lachina Publishing Services
Design Manager: Mark Ong
Interior Designer: tani hasegawa
Cover Designer: tani hasegawa
Rights & Permissions Project Manager: Matt Perry, Cenveo Publishing Services
Rights & Permissions Management: Ben Ferrini
Photo Researcher: Danny Meldung, Photo Affairs, Inc.
Manufacturing Buyer: Stacey Weinberger, LSC Communications
Executive Marketing Manager: Neena Bali
Senior Field Marketing Manager: Mary Salzman

Cover Photo Credit: Monkey Business Images / Shutterstock

Library of Congress Cataloging-in-Publication Data

Names: Donatelle, Rebecca J., 1950- author.
Title: Access to health / Rebecca J. Donatelle.
Description: 15e. | San Francisco, CA: Pearson Education, [2018] | Includes
    bibliographical references and index.
Identifiers: LCCN 2016048691| ISBN 9780134516257 (student edition) | ISBN
    0134516257 (student edition) | ISBN 9780134607849 (instructor's review
    copy) | ISBN 0134607848 (instructor's review Copy)
Subjects: | MESH: Attitude to Health | Health Behavior | Exercise | Popular
    Works
Classification: LCC RA776 | NLM W 85 | DDC 613—dc23 LC record
available at https://lccn.loc.gov/2016048691

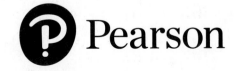
Pearson

ISBN 10: 0-13-451625-7
(Student edition)
ISBN 13: 978-0-13-451625-7
(Student edition)
ISBN 10: 0-13-460784-8
(Instructor's Review Copy)
ISBN 13: 978-0-13-460784-9
(Instructor's Review Copy)

# BRIEF CONTENTS

# CONTENTS

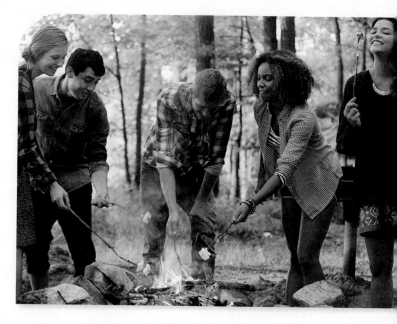

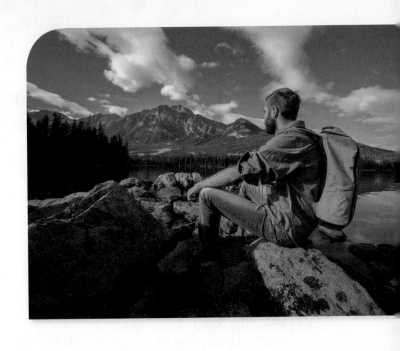

# FOCUS **ON** Cultivating Your Spiritual Health   51

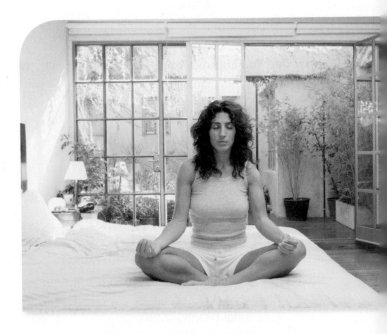

## 3 Managing Stress and Coping with Life's Challenges  63

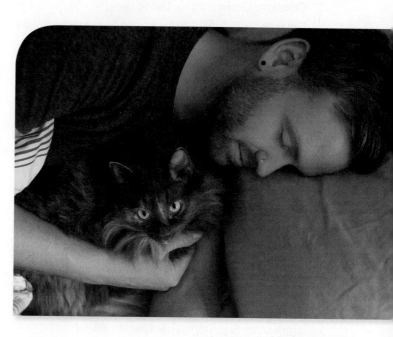

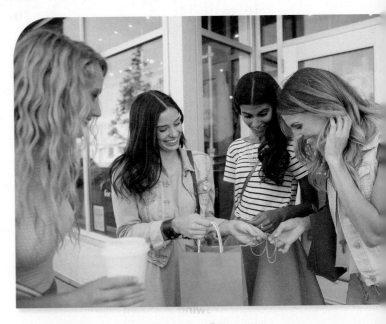

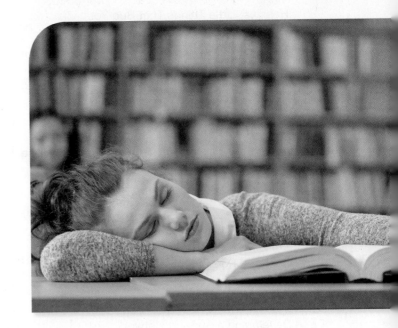

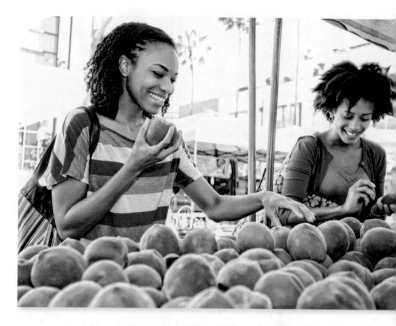

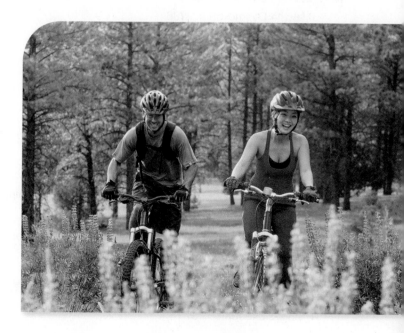

## FOCUS **ON**   Enhancing Your Body Image   176

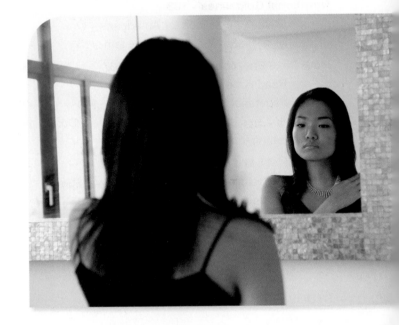

## 7   Improving Your Personal Fitness   189

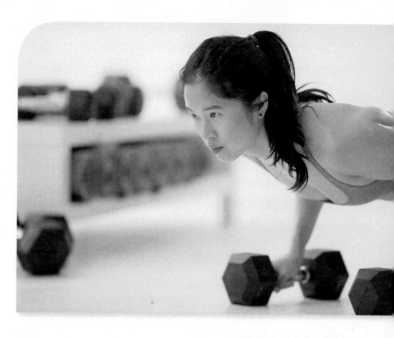

PART THREE | Creating Healthy and Caring Relationships

## 8 Connecting and Communicating in the Modern World   218

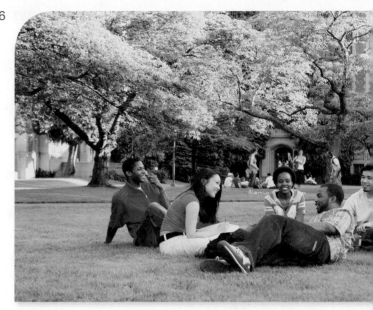

# 9   Understanding Your Sexuality   239

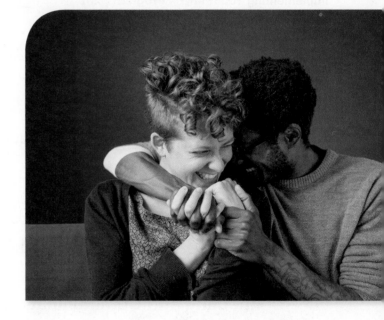

# 10   Considering Your Reproductive Choices   262

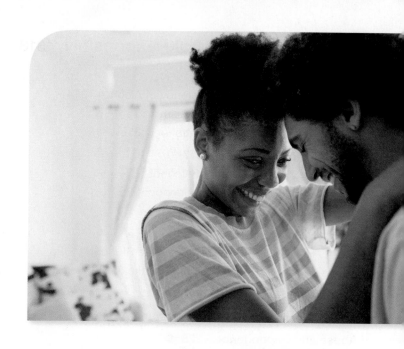

## PART FOUR | Avoiding Risks from Harmful Habits

## FOCUS ON Recognizing and Avoiding Addiction   299

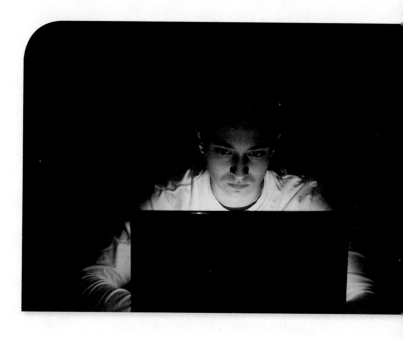

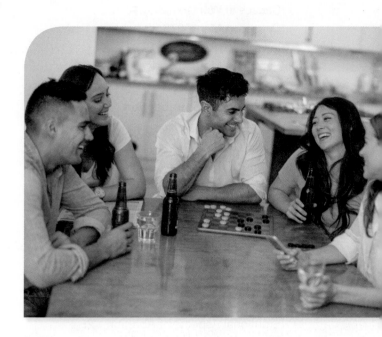

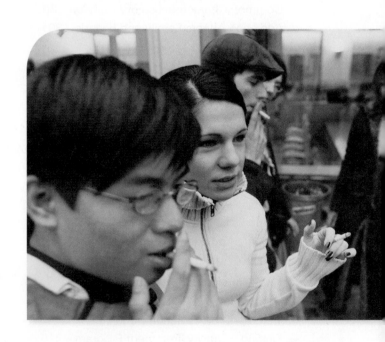

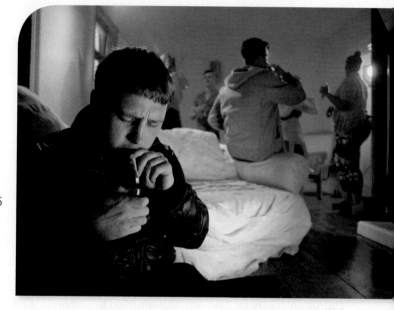

# 14 Protecting against Infectious Diseases 385

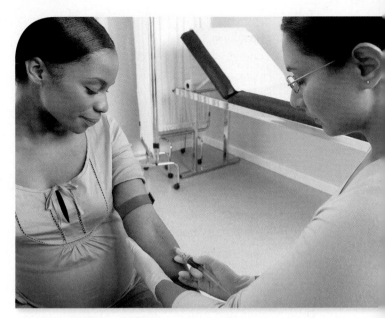

# 15 Protecting against Sexually Transmitted Infections 406

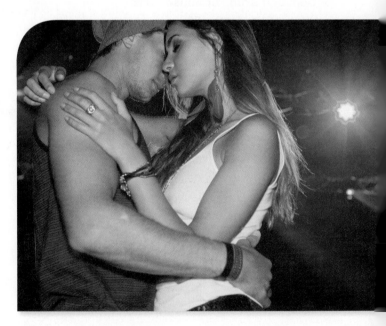

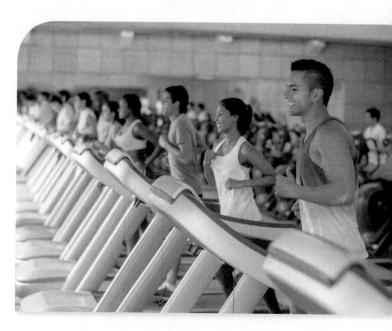
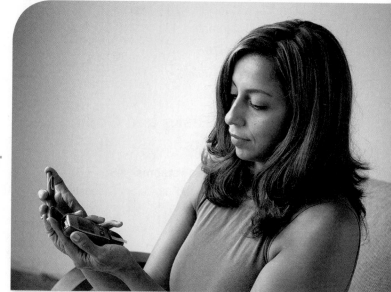

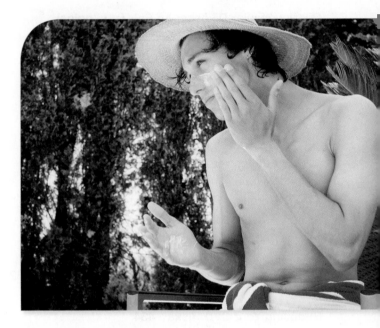

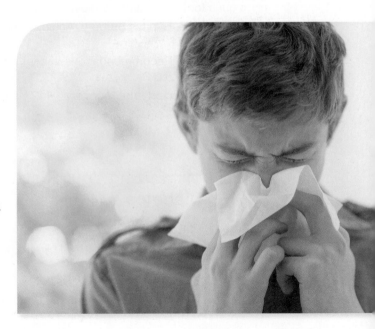

PART SIX │ Facing Life's Challenges

**19** Making Smart Health Care Choices   502

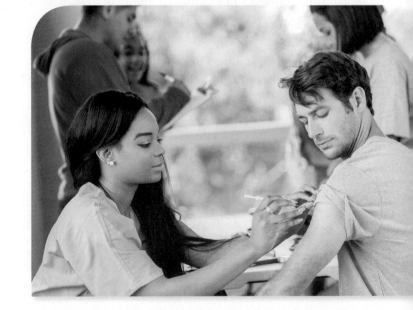

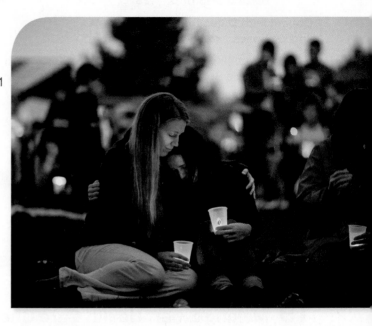

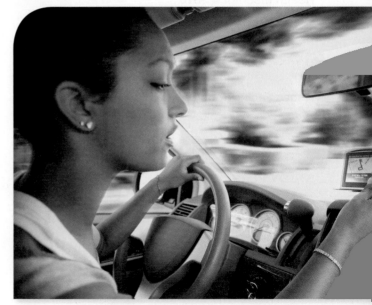

# 21   Preserving and Protecting Your Environment   562

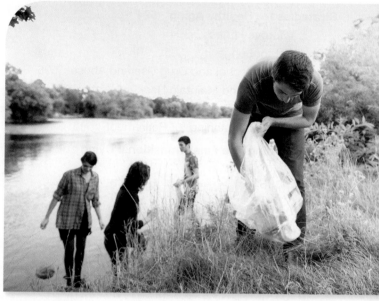

# 22   Preparing for Aging, Death, and Dying   586

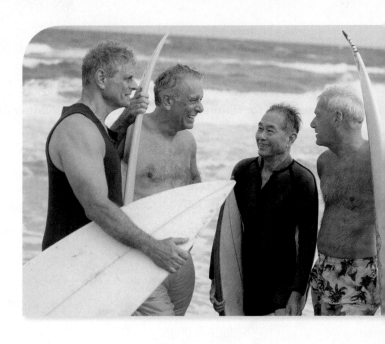

# FEATURE BOXES

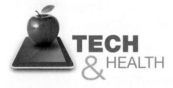
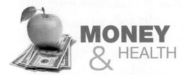

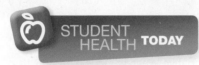

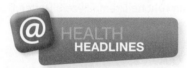

## HEALTH IN A DIVERSE WORLD

# ASSESS YOURSELF

The Assess Yourself activities are available online at **MasteringHealth**. Go to the **MasteringHealth** Study Area to find the chapter you want in the drop-down menu, and there you will see the Assess Yourself activities. Print them or save the PDF to your computer.

# PREFACE

**G**ot Health? If you are like most people, "health" is a subliminal message that is constantly playing in the back of your mind. When you sit down for dinner and think about whether you should eat that bacon cheeseburger, the health tape is playing. When you ride the elevator instead of walking up the stairs, it is there, gently nudging you to do the right thing and find the stairway. Whether it be the latest news headline or the latest app that pops up on your mobile device giving you tips about diet, exercise, stress, or sleep—it is hard to avoid those healthy messages. Even Pokemon has morphed into a way to get your daily exercise! Seemingly, with all that media bombardment and expert advice, getting healthy and staying healthy would be easy and we'd be the healthiest nation on Earth! Yet, soaring rates of obesity, increases in mental health issues, rapidly rising violence rates, skyrocketing cases of drug abuse, and evidence of devastating effects of human-influenced climate change all indicate that we are not doing better when it comes to health. In fact, even though we spend the most on health care of any nation, even though we pride ourselves on promoting health and well-being and provide amazing opportunities for people to change behaviors and get healthy, too many of us are not heeding those messages. "Just Do It" falls on deaf ears for the vast majority. Why? The answer to this is multifaceted. For many, the issues and information seem complex and contradictory and the pleasures of continuing certain behaviors trump the effort needed to be healthy. Others lack the resources and supports necessary to change. Still others don't believe they are at risk, don't trust the "system," and/or don't have the knowledge necessary to make choices that will promote health and prevent disease. Whether by geography, genetics, or social environment, some face overwhelming risks. The facts are clear. Getting healthy and staying healthy are challenges for most of us. There is no quick fix. It takes recognition of risks, knowledge, and motivation to make positive health changes. The good news is that no matter where you are right now in terms of health, you can make the changes that will work for you and enhance your chance for a healthy future. You can also serve as an agent for change within your family, your social networks, and in your community. That opportunity starts now.

My goal in writing *Access to Health* is to provide students with just what that title says: access to health information and to their own health potential. This book provides the most scientifically valid information available to help students be smarter in their health decision making, more positively involved in their personal health, and more active as advocates for healthy changes in their communities. Change isn't something that just happens. Let's face it—if it were easy to lose weight, maintain a healthy diet, manage stress, and exercise regularly, we wouldn't have one of the costliest and overburdened health care systems. However, the good news is that governmental agencies, communities, schools, and increasing numbers of individuals are taking steps (both small and large) to enhance, preserve, and protect our health. The key is to know where to look for accurate information, which information you can trust, and how to use the information to make the best choices for you and others. In short, it takes knowledge, preparation, and effort; therefore, this book places emphasis on empowering students to identify their health risks, create plans for reducing those risks, and make healthy lifestyle changes part of their daily routines.

*Access to Health* is designed to help students quickly grasp the information presented and understand its relevance to their own lives and the lives of others. Exciting revisions have been made to the art and design of the book in this new edition, with the purpose of capturing students' interest, engaging them in the subject matter, helping them find the most reliable resources available, and assisting them in weighing their options as they face health challenges today and in the future. In addition, there are six Focus On chapters that delve into areas of health that are of practical importance to college students but are not always given sufficient coverage in typical personal health texts. These Focus On chapters spotlight financial health, spiritual health, body image, addiction, diabetes, and unintentional injury.

Looking back to the time when I taught my first Personal Health course as a teaching assistant in graduate school and remembering the years of teaching countless numbers of students in classes like this, I am amazed that we are now in the 15th edition of *Access to Health*. Over the years, this text has morphed considerably, as we have focused on meeting the needs of an increasingly savvy student population facing increasingly challenging health threats. As I look back at all of the efforts by so many health and publishing professionals, I am filled with overwhelming gratitude for the many contributions that have helped make this book one of the most successful in the field. With each edition of the text, I have listened to the thoughtful suggestions of instructors and students using the book, as well as to the feedback from my own students in keeping the book relevant, timely, interesting, and accessible. I hope that this edition's rich foundation of scientifically valid information, its wealth of technological tools and resources, and its thought-provoking features will stimulate you to share my enthusiasm for personal health and to become actively engaged in behaviors that will lead to better health for all.

# NEW TO THIS EDITION

*Access to Health,* 15th edition, maintains many features that the text has become known for, while incorporating several major revisions and exciting new features. The most noteworthy changes to the text as a whole include:

- **New! Why Should I Care?** Introductory statements help focus students' attention on the importance and relevance of information in the chapter to them and to society as a whole.
- **New! Interactive Behavior Change Activities – Which Path Would You Take?** Allow students to explore various health choices through an engaging, interactive, low-stakes, and anonymous experience. These choose-your-own-adventure-style activities show students the possible consequences of various choices they make today on their future health; these activities are accessible via QR code from the book and made assignable in MasteringHealth with follow-up questions.
- **New! Order of chapters in the Table of Contents** To meet instructor requests for chapter ordering that better fits the sequence in which instructors typically teach the course. As such, nutrition, healthy weight, and physical fitness chapters now follow directly after the psychological health, stress, and sleep chapters. Instructors asked and we responded!
- **New! Chapter 4: Improving Your Sleep** Has been expanded from a Focus On chapter to a full chapter to more thoroughly examine the connections between sleep and stress, sleep and nutrition, and more.
- **New! Making Changes Today** Feature provides students with tools and techniques for making changes to their health today and during their lifetime.
- **New! *ABC News* Videos** Bring health to life and spark discussion with up-to-date hot topics from 2012 to 2016. MasteringHealth activities tied to the videos include multiple-choice questions that provide wrong-answer feedback to redirect students to the correct answer.
- **New! eText 2.0** Complete with embedded ABC News videos and Health Video Tutors; eText 2.0 is mobile friendly and ADA accessible.
  - Now available on smartphones and tablets.
  - Seamlessly integrated videos.
  - Accessible (screen-reader ready).
  - Configurable reading settings, including sizable type and night reading mode.
  - Instructor and student note taking, highlighting, bookmarking, and search.
- **Updated Learning Outcomes** At the beginning of each chapter, corresponding chapter headings to emphasize essential information, and navigational tools to help students measure their progress toward specific learning goals. These learning outcomes help students and instructors assess outcomes deemed most important.
- **Updated end-of-chapter Study Plan** Summarizes key points of the chapter and provides review questions and critical thinking questions to check understanding, all

specifically tied to the chapter's learning outcomes. This carefully planned approach is designed to allow students to drill down to the essential information and critically assess why these outcomes are so important.

## Chapter-by-Chapter Revisions

*Access to Health,* 15th edition, has been updated line by line to provide students with the most scientifically valid, comprehensive, and current information from well-designed professional sources. We painstakingly review studies, compare conflicting results, and provide a balanced and thorough overview of each topic as well as an overview of areas needing further study. Health research is dynamic and ever-changing and we strive to be as up-to-date as possible as we go to press. In addition, we have enhanced and reorganized portions of the text to improve the flow of topics, provided more thought-provoking scenarios and added, updated, and improved all figures, tables, feature boxes, and photos to enhance the learning experience. The following is a chapter-by-chapter listing of some of the many "other" noteworthy changes, updates, and additions.

### Chapter 1

- Updated information on health-related impediments to academic performance
- Updated information on student health and its relevance for today's students
- Updated material on factors that limit life expectancy by age, race, sex, and more
- Updated information on risks for young adults and priorities for change
- Updated information on costs of obesity and how your behaviors influence others both directly and indirectly
- New, more skills-focused **Making Changes Today** feature
- Expanded discussion of intellectual health
- Added material on epigenetics
- Updated material on health care reform and implications for college students
- Updated Health in a Diverse World box on health disparities

### Chapter 2

- Updated info on **Growing Problem of Mental Health on American Campuses**
- New coverage of emotional intelligence and why it is important
- Added coverage of family, community, and social supports
- Expanded discussion of positive psychology and PERMA
- Updated discussion of the role of happiness in overall health and well-being
- Updated statistics throughout, with particular emphasis on college student mental health issues, contributors, and consequences, including suicide and other outcomes
- New, skills-focused **Making Changes Today** feature on enhancing psychological health

## Chapter 2A

- Updated overview of latest research demonstrating the importance of spiritual health in overall health and well-being
- Updated material on characteristics that distinguish religion and spirituality and the importance of each in overall health and well-being
- Updated research on how millennials view spirituality and religion and the importance of each in their lives
- Updated material on the relationship between spirituality and academic performance
- Updated material on the relationship between spiritual well-being and physical health

## Chapter 3

- Updated research supporting the importance of stress in overall health, particularly as a factor in sleep, chronic and infectious disease, and overall mental health
- New figure indicating the importance of stress on various ages and stages of life
- Updated figure on physical symptoms of stress based on the latest science
- Updated section on the sources of stress in America, at-risk populations, and negative consequences
- Updated coverage of role of oxytocin in returning body to homeostasis
- Expanded coverage of the transactional model of stress and coping, minority stress and its implications for diverse populations, and the Yerkes-Dodson law of arousal
- Expanded coverage of the role of finances in stressful outcomes, particularly for college students
- Expanded section on strategies that individuals can take to reduce stress in their lives, including emphasis on mindfulness and journaling, as well as apps for helping to control stress reactions
- New section on the role of "self-compassion" in one's approach to stress and how "cutting yourself some slack" in your pursuit of excellence can dramatically influence stress levels

## Chapter 3A

- New explanation and revised figure on the role of the Health-Income Gradient on overall health outcomes
- Updated research/statistics focusing on how GDP per capita influences life expectancy at birth
- New figure on how families cut costs to make college more affordable
- New information on social capital, what it is, and how it can have a significant role in determining health
- New info on correlation between health insurance coverage and health
- Expanded discussion of SES and health
- Updated coverage or average college costs, as well as federal programs and tax credits to help offset costs of higher education
- Expanded discussion of wise credit card use

## Chapter 4

- Expanded coverage on the importance of sleep in overall health and why sleep is particularly challenging and important for college students
- New figure on the parts of the brain involved in sleep
- Expanded discussion of the problem of sleep deprivation in America and updated research on the various components of a good night's sleep
- Expanded and updated coverage of sleep issues on campus, factors that contribute to sleep deprivation, and possible consequences for students
- Expanded discussion of unique sleep needs of individuals throughout life
- New material on the unique aspects of the "short sleeper" and possible genetic aspects of circadian rhythm and sleep debt
- Updated material on sleep apnea, risks for untreated sleep apnea, and new options for treatment
- Expanded material on "sleep hygiene" and actions you can take to ensure a good night's sleep
- New info on reported sleep aids, what works and what doesn't, and associated risks

## Chapter 5

- Updated figure on caloric intake for various populations, and discussion of risks and new dietary challenges
- Updated info on essential nutrients, current evidence for dietary recommendations, and determining fact from fiction when it comes to nutrition
- Expanded coverage of dehydration and the importance of water in overall health
- Updated info on fat intake recommendations and the latest on healthy fats versus others
- New discussion of healthful eating patterns and new dietary recommendations
- New info on supplement labelling, what consumers need to know, and recent labelling changes to aid consumers in sound nutritional choices
- Enhanced skills-based info on how college students can eat healthily when on a budget and when there may be limitations in eating well in college
- Expanded coverage on the increasing prevalence of food-borne illnesses, new threats, and steps you can take to prevent infection

## Chapter 6

- Completely revised and updated research and statistics on the "globesity" epidemic as well as the growing threat of overweight/obesity in the United States by age, race, gender, socioeconomic status, and other factors
- New map showing trends in U.S. obesity as well as current prevalence by state
- Update of research supporting the potential threat of obesity and overweight, from increased risk for chronic disease, to increased risk of infectious disease, sexual

dysfunction issues, and stigma and social issues for the obese in America
- New figure and specific information focused on the 10 most obese and least obese countries of the world
- New research and updated material on childhood obesity as a predictor of future adult obesity
- New coverage of specific risk factors for obesity, including genetic, hormonal, and environmental factors in obesity development and maintenance
- New coverage of thrifty and spendthrift metabolism and how metabolism can influence obesity development

## Chapter 6A

- Updated statistics on prevalence of dissatisfaction with appearance and body dysmorphic behaviors
- Updated info on childhood dieting behavior and predictors of later life patterns
- Expanded info on Social Media and how it influences abnormal fixation on appearance
- Expanded coverage of disordered eating and the new obsession with food called orthorexia nervosa
- New coverage of Health At Every Size philosophy
- Expanded coverage of controversial questions of whether you can be fat and healthy

## Chapter 7

- Update on exercise in America, how we are doing in terms of meeting the exercise guidelines, and updated research and statistics on the benefits of exercise
- Updated figure on calories burned by exercise type
- New figure on the benefits of exercise on cognitive function and whether regular exercise can help your performance on exams
- Updated tables on popular fitness equipment
- New material on negative health outcomes of sitting for extended periods
- New material on peak bone mass and lifestyle factors— where you are now and what can you expect in terms of bone density
- Expanded discussion of strategies for losing weight, gaining weight, and overall improved weight management

## Chapter 8

- Updated research and trends in relationships in the United States, including marriage, cohabitation, singlehood, lesbian and gay relationships, and other options
- Expanded coverage of the trend toward remaining single and later-life marriage
- Updated info on the importance of healthy relationships and the effects of social isolation on physical health
- Expanded coverage of same-sex relationships, gay marriage laws, and issues of discrimination
- Enhanced coverage of the role of communication in the digital age and the effect of modern technology on relationships

- Enhanced coverage of strategies for improving communication and staying safe while interacting online
- Updated coverage of relationship failure and coping with conflict

## Chapter 9

- Expanded discussion of transgender and gender expression, current issues, and emerging policies
- Updated information on sexual prejudice
- Updated discussion of sexual dysfunction
- New information on desire and arousal disorders
- New coverage of the CERTS model for healthy sexuality
- Updated coverage of the health benefits and risks of sexual behavior
- Updated discussion of disability and sexual relationships

## Chapter 10

- Updated research and statistics on pregnancy in America
- New information on pregnancy and the Zika virus
- Updated information on contraceptive types and their advantages/disadvantages and risks/benefits
- New **Pop Quiz** questions
- Updated discussion on decision making and factors in reproductive choices
- New coverage of cycle tracking and reproductive health apps
- New coverage of enhancing men's involvement in reproductive choices
- Updated information on contraceptives in the developing world
- Updated information on communicating with a partner about contraceptive choices

## Chapter 10A

- Updated statistics and research on addictions, particularly newer addictions related to media and mobile devices and the urge to stay connected
- Updated information on gambling addiction
- Expanded coverage of Internet addiction and compulsive use of mobile devices
- Updated stats on the costs of addiction
- New, skills-based **Making Changes Today** box on what to do if you or a friend has a problem
- Updated coverage of treatment programs for addiction, their effectiveness, and factors to consider when seeking help

## Chapter 11

- Updated stats on alcohol use
- Updated stats on the prevalence of negative consequences associated with college drinking
- Updated info on driving fatalities among drivers with BACs above the legal limit
- Updated stats on binge drinking
- Coverage of new FDA approved "hangover cures"
- Updated stats on alcohol and sexual assault, rape, and dating violence

- More on alcohol and cancer and alcohol's impact on the immune system
- New section on alcohol inhalation
- New section on functional alcoholism
- Updated info on alcohol and costs to society

## Chapter 12

- Updated stats on prevalence of smoking among college students
- Updated coverage of advertising and education around smoking and cessation
- Expanded coverage of why people smoke
- Updated Health in a **Diverse World** box on fighting the tobacco epidemic
- New information on e-cigarettes

## Chapter 13

- Updated caffeine content comparison among popular products
- Updated info on benefits and hazards of caffeine use
- Updated stats on college marijuana use as well as legalization
- Updated information on stimulants
- Updated coverage of bath salts
- New information on costs of the drug war

## Chapter 14

- Expanded coverage and updated statistics of current, emerging, and resurging infectious diseases, risk factors, and strategies for prevention
- Updated adult immunization schedule with a focus on college students
- New figure on how antibiotic resistance occurs and spreads
- New coverage of the impact of the Zika virus and emerging threats from bacterial, viral, and other pathogenic diseases
- Expanded coverage of climate change and the likelihood of disease proliferation
- Expanded coverage of toxic chemicals and the immune system
- Updated coverage of vaccinations, particularly those of importance to college students, their effectiveness, and the validity of controversial stances on vaccinations

## Chapter 15

- New research and statistics on STI prevalence, risk factors, prevention, and treatment
- Updated figure on signs and symptoms of STIs
- New figure on rates of new HIV diagnoses and most affected populations
- Updated, skills-based **Making Changes Today** box on safe sex
- New information on prevention strategies for persons at high risk of HIV infection
- Updated stats on prevalence of a variety of STIs

## Chapter 16

- New statistics on CVD trends; current rates based on age, race, and sex; and key risk factors
- New information on how we are doing in terms of meeting the Ideal healthy heart measures in the United States
- New discussion of disparities in CVD by age, race, and gender
- New section on sudden cardiac death
- Updates on the social, emotional, and economic burden of CVD on individuals and families
- New comparisons of CVD rates in developed and developing countries
- New information on the SPRINT trial and its influence on new blood pressure treatment recommendations
- New information on using the ankle-brachial index for diagnosis of PAD
- New treatments for blockages caused by clots and other problems
- Update on MetS prevalence, risk factors, and prevention strategies
- Update of current research and statistics on stroke
- New material on potential impact of new Dietary Guidelines on CVD risk
- Update and expansion of newest strategies for reducing CVD rates and the diagnosis and treatment of CVD
- New update on use of aspirin for CVD risk reduction
- New information on emotional aspects of CVD survival for individuals and families
- New theory that bacteria in the gut may be more important than fat in the diet in predicting and treating CVD
- Update of strategies or actions to be initiated when a heart attack or stroke occurs
- Updated figure on major cardiovascular disease death rates by state
- Updated stats on the breakdown of deaths attributable to certain cardiovascular diseases
- Updated **Making Changes Today** box on what to do when a heart attack hits
- Updated info on blood pressure classification
- Updated info on changing fat and cholesterol intake recommendations

## Chapter 16A

- Updated figure on blood glucose levels in prediabetes and untreated diabetes to include A1C levels
- Updated stats on prevalence of prediabetes and diabetes in the U.S.
- New information on genetic predisposition to diabetes
- Updated statistics on medical costs of diabetes and related illness
- New, skills-based **Making Changes Today** box on reducing risks for diabetes

## Chapter 17

- New research and statistics in every section of chapter highlighting trends and current issues

- Updated data on 5-year survival cancer rates by site and race
- Updated data on leading sites of new cancer cases and deaths
- Expanded coverage of types of ALL and CLL leukemia prevalence, risks, prevention, and treatment
- Expanded coverage and updated stats on skin cancer risks, prevalence, and prevention
- Updated info on alcohol and cancer risks
- New information on "other" cancers that are related to HPV infections, particularly among young adults

## Chapter 18

- New **Why Should I Care**? focuses attention on the current and future relevance to chronic disease
- New information on the staggering social and economic impact of chronic diseases in the United States
- Updated stats on college students with chronic conditions
- New figure on asthma prevalence by age, sex, and race/ethnicity in the United States
- New figure on lost workdays by medical cause
- New information on asthma, allergies, and food sensitivity
- New information on repetitive motion disorders and new technology that increases risks
- Expanded coverage of ulcerative colitis and inflammatory bowel disease
- Updated info on anaphylaxis and anaphylactic shock
- Expanded coverage of neurological disorders

## Chapter 19

- New data and research on complementary and integrative medicine, who uses these health care options, and emerging trends
- New figure on types of complementary health approaches
- New, more skills-based **Making Changes Today** box on complementary health approaches and self-care
- Expanded information on the Affordable Care Act and complementary and integrative medicine
- More information on selecting doctors and nonmedical providers

## Chapter 20

- New data and statistics on crime contributors and risks by age, race, and gender
- Updated data and figure on changing crime rates, trends, types of crime, and risks
- Updated figure on homicide by type of weapon in the United States
- Updated information on substance use and crime
- Updated homicide statistics and discussions of gun violence and gun policies
- Expanded coverage of intimate partner violence
- New and expanded legal definition of what constitutes rape, as well as updated coverage of rape on campus
- Updated stats on campus hazing, sexual harassment, and other key violence issues

## Chapter 20A

- Updated information on prevalence of unintentional injury with particular emphasis on young, college-age adults
- Updated stats around injuries and fatalities related to motor vehicle crashes
- Updated information on marijuana and driving
- Expanded info on aggressive driving and vehicle safety issues, use of mobile devices while driving (texting, etc.)
- Updated information on injuries related to skiing, skateboarding, and snowboarding
- Updated stats around common home unintentional injuries
- New information on disaster preparedness
- More skills-based **Making Changes Today** box on avoiding motor vehicle injuries

## Chapter 21

- New **Why Should I Care**? focusing on current and future threats of unchecked population growth, increasing demand for scarce resources and potential future threats
- New data and statistics on global population trends, threats, and impact on climate change
- Updated figure of world population estimates
- Updated figure on world energy consumption by fuel type
- New figure on major energy sources and percent share of total U.S. electricity generation
- Updated information on what is in American trash and how we squander resources, such as food resources
- Expanded coverage of fracking and potential threats to the environment
- New and expanded coverage of alternative energy sources—how we are doing and how we compare to other countries of the world
- New **Health Headlines** box on the Flint Water Crisis and how archaic infrastructure in the United States contributes to health risks

## Chapter 22

- Updated information on successful aging and how to have vibrant and healthy later years
- Updated stats and projections on number of Americans age 65 and older
- Updated information on living arrangements of Americans age 65 and older
- Updated stats around organ donation and patients needing/receiving transplants
- Updated, more skills-based **Making Changes Today** box on how to talk to loved ones when someone dies
- New information on complicated grief
- New information on millennials and financial planning for future health and well-being

# TEXT FEATURES AND LEARNING AIDS

*Access to Health,* 15th Edition, includes the following special features, all of which have been revised and improved upon for this edition:

- Numbered learning outcomes at the beginning of each chapter are tied to each major chapter section, helping students navigate each chapter and measure their progress against specific learning goals and helping instructors assess the key information and skills students are meant to take away from each chapter.
- **What Do You Think?** critical thinking questions within the chapter prompt students to reflect on personal and societal issues relating to the material they have just learned.
- **Why Should I Care?** feature now opens every chapter and leads students to recognize the relevance of health issues and the upcoming chapter content to their own lives in the here and now.
- **Did You Know?** figures call attention to statistics that are relevant to the lives of college students in a fun and informative format.
- **Assess Yourself callouts at the end of every chapter** direct students to online self-assessment worksheets in MasteringHealth where they can assess their current health behaviors in order to better set goals and follow-through on behavior change.
- **Making Changes Today** boxes give students specific strategies for making lasting changes to their health behaviors.
- **Tech & Health** boxes cover key new technology innovations, from medical tests to calorie-counting smartphone apps and other devices that can help students stay healthy.
- **Student Health Today** boxes offer current data and information about health trends specific to college students, including potential risks and safety issues that affect students' lives.
- **Health Headlines** boxes highlight new discoveries and research, as well as interesting trends in the fields of public and personal health.
- **Health in a Diverse World** boxes expand discussion of health topics to diverse groups within the United States and around the world, as well as spurring discussion about key disparity issues facing many populations.
- **Money & Health** boxes cover health topics from the financial perspective, discussing everything from how to lessen money stress during school to how something like a plastic bag tax at the grocery store might impact behavior.
- A **running glossary** in the margins defines terms where students first encounter them, emphasizing and supporting understanding of material.
- **QR codes and media callout boxes** indicate when podcasts, videos, and assessments are available online in MasteringHealth for use with the book.
- The end-of-chapter **Study Plans** help students target their studying and master key chapter concepts by explicitly tying the chapter learning outcomes to the **Summary** points that

wrap up chapter content, the **Pop Quiz** multiple-choice questions and **Think About It!** discussion questions that encourage students to evaluate and apply new information, and the **Accessing Your Health on the Internet** sections offer more opportunities to explore areas of interest.
- The **appendices** at the end of the book include practical information on providing emergency care and a table of nutritive values for selected foods and fast foods.
- A **Behavior Change Contract** for students to fill out is included in the back of the book.

# SUPPLEMENTARY MATERIALS

Available with *Access to Health,* Fifteenth Edition, is a comprehensive set of ancillary materials designed to enhance learning and to facilitate teaching.

## Instructor Supplements

- **MasteringHealth with Pearson eText 2.0** MasteringHealth is an online homework, tutorial, and assessment product designed to improve results by helping students quickly master concepts. Students will benefit from self-paced tutorials that feature immediate wrong answer feedback and hints that emulate the office-hour experience to help keep them on track. With a wide range of interactive, engaging, and assignable activities, students will be encouraged to actively learn and retain tough course concepts:
  - **Before class**, assign adaptive Dynamic Study Modules and reading assignments from the eText with Reading Quizzes to ensure that students come prepared to class, having done the reading.
  - **During class**, Learning Catalytics, a "bring your own device" student engagement, assessment and classroom intelligence system, allows students to use their smartphone, tablet, or laptop to respond to questions in class. With Learning Catalytics, you can assess students in real-time using open ended question formats to uncover student misconceptions and adjust lectures accordingly.
  - **After class** assign, an array of assignments such as Which Path Would You Take activities, ABC Videos, Video Tutors, Behavior Change Videos, and much more. Students receive wrong-answer feedback personalized to their answers, which will help them get back on track.
  For more information on MasteringHealth, please visit www.masteringhealth.com
- **Video Tutors, *ABC News* Health and Wellness Lecture Launcher Videos, and Behavior Change Videos.** Twenty-seven brief video tutors accessible via QR codes in the text, plus 60 *ABC News* videos, each 5 to 10 minutes long, and ten whiteboard-style behavior change videos help instructors stimulate critical discussion in the classroom. Videos are provided already linked within Power-Point lectures and are available separately in large-screen format with optional closed captioning through MasteringHealth.

- ***Instructor Resource and Support Manual***. Easier to use than a typical instructor's manual, this key guide provides a step-by-step visual walk-through of all the resources available to you for preparing your lectures. Also included are tips and strategies for new instructors, sample syllabi, and suggestions for integrating MasteringHealth into your classroom activities and homework assignments.
- ***Teaching with Student Learning Outcomes***. This feature provides essays from 11 instructors who teach using student learning outcomes. They share goals and suggestions for developing good learning outcomes and give tips and suggestions for how to teach personal health in this manner.
- ***Teaching with Web 2.0***. From Facebook to Twitter and blogs, students are interacting with technology constantly. This handbook gives tips on how to incorporate technology in your course.
- ***Test Bank***. The Test Bank incorporates Bloom's Taxonomy, or the Higher Order of Learning, to help instructors create exams that encourage students to think analytically and critically, rather than simply to regurgitate information.
- ***Great Ideas! Active Ways to Teach Health & Wellness***. This manual provides ideas for classroom activities related to specific health and wellness topics, as well as suggestions for activities that can be adapted to various topics and class sizes.

## Student Supplements

- **MasteringHealth Student Study Area** also provides students with self-study material like access to the eText 2.0, practice quizzes, flashcards, videos, MP3s, and much more to help them get the best grade in your course at their own pace.

- **Dynamic Study Modules in MasteringHealth** assess students' performance and activity in real time. They use data and analytics that personalize content to target students' particular strengths and weaknesses. And, because we know students are always on the go, Dynamic Study Modules can be accessed from any computer, tablet, or smartphone.
- ***Behavior Change Log Book and Wellness Journal***. This assessment tool helps students track daily exercise and nutritional intake and create a long-term nutrition and fitness prescription plan. It includes behavior change contracts and topics for journal-based activities.
- ***Eat Right! Healthy Eating in College and Beyond***. This handy, full-color booklet provides students with practical guidelines, tips, shopper's guides, and recipes that turn healthy eating principles into blueprints for action. Topics include healthy eating in the cafeteria, dorm room, and fast-food restaurants; planning meals on a budget; weight management; vegetarian alternatives; and how alcohol affects health.
- ***Live Right! Beating Stress in College and Beyond***. This booklet gives students useful tips for coping with a variety of life's challenges both during college and for the rest of their lives. Topics include sleep, managing finances, time management, coping with academic pressure, relationships, and a closer look at advertised products that promise to make our lives better.
- **Digital 5-Step Pedometer**. Take strides to better health with this pedometer, which measures steps, distance (miles), activity time, and calories and provides a time clock.
- **MyDietAnalysis** (www.mydietanalysis.com). Powered by ESHA Research, Inc., MyDietAnalysis features a database of nearly 20,000 foods and multiple reports. It allows students to track their diet and activity using up to three profiles and to generate and submit reports electronically.

# ACKNOWLEDGMENTS

It is hard for me to believe that *Access to Health* is in its fifteenth edition and that this one may be the best one yet! Since its inception, the personal health textbook market has undergone remarkable changes. Whereas the text remains the foundation and springboard for information, the ability to communicate with students through the Internet and a wide range of other media and devices such as smartphones and tablets provides textbook authors and publishers entirely new and exciting ways of teaching, sharing information, motivating students to become actively engaged in the learning experience, and covering up-to-the-minute health topics in every class. Today's text offers opportunities for student engagement and thought-provoking exercises that do more than test basic factual data. *Access to Health* is also designed to help students understand complex issues surrounding health so they can make better decisions related to health care and behaviors.

To maximize student learning, we sought input from faculty members and experts in technology and e-learning—those who work with students daily and who understand how to engage today's learners with written and visual content. We also interviewed students and asked them about how they used technology in their learning and incorporated their recommendations in our student-centered approach.

Producing a text that students actually want to pick up and read—one that they find interesting and that encourages critical thinking and learning—is no small task. In fact, in addition to having an author and contributors with the professional training and expertise in the scientific foundations of the health field, it takes a small army of publishing professionals and media specialists who take the basic information and make it come alive for the reader. Each step in planning, developing, and marketing a high-quality textbook and supplemental materials requires a tremendous amount of work from many skilled and dedicated professionals. I often think how fortunate I have been to work with the many gifted and talented professionals who make up the Pearson family. Upon reflection, there have been so many names and faces along the way—from people who have carried a tremendous amount of responsibility from beginning to end to those who have quietly worked behind the scenes on special tasks, in many cases, to make *Access to Health* a resounding success from the first edition to this one. I owe each of them tremendous gratitude, for without their efforts, this book may have languished on the shelves along the way. From my perspective, Pearson personnel personify key aspects of what it takes to be successful in the publishing world: (1) skill and competence; (2) drive and motivation; (3) creativity and commitment to excellence; (4) a vibrant, youthful, and enthusiastic approach; and

(5) personalities that motivate an author to continually strive to produce market-leading texts.

In particular, I am indebted to my new Content Producer, Deepti Agarwal, who took over the reins with this edition of *Access to Health* and never missed a beat in ensuring that the project kept on schedule and continued to reflect excellent editorial skills. Deepti was able to juggle numerous responsibilities and organizational tasks, provide thoughtful recommendations, and problem-solve along the way to keep the team on task and working to provide a final manuscript on a tight schedule—all the while gently nudging the author, who has a slight tendency to want to add more and more in a limited space! In short, Deepti did a fantastic job in making this edition continue as a leading text in the field. In addition to Deepti, I am thankful to Kari Hopperstead and Nedah Rose, development editors, who continued working with us to refine and develop a newer, cutting-edge edition. Their history with the project allowed them to make excellent recommendations for revisions and incorporate new information seamlessly into each chapter. Their creative suggestions helped maintain continuity and excellence in the final product. Consistent with Pearson's team approach to publishing, so many people work with these projects over the years, and their collective memory, edition to edition, makes for a fantastic author/editor interaction.

In short, Deepti, Kari, and Nedah were part of the "dream team" that allowed the author and contributors to focus on the task at hand—using their knowledge to provide scientifically valid information about health. Thank you, all. I would also like to thank Nic Albert for his behind-the-scenes work as developmental editor on our chapters as we submitted our revisions. Having worked with Nic on several projects, I am thankful for his skill in focusing material, worrying the details in manuscript development, and helping keep the book on target. Laura Specht Patchkofsky played a key role in refining material, synthesizing my long narratives, and keeping the text clean and concise for students.

I also wish to give profound thanks to Susan Malloy, Content Producer, for her continued oversight, careful management, and wise decision making. Without Susan's dedicated support behind the scenes, this project would not have been possible. Susan is a great resource, a committed professional, and a huge part of the glue that helps keep the experience a success. Although many acquisitions editors play a more detached role in project management and development, I was fortunate in being able to work with a hands-on and enthusiastic editor on this edition. Much appreciation and many thanks go to senior acquisitions editor Michelle Yglecias.

Whether traveling to assist with adoptions, dealing with issues that inevitably arise in a changing health marketplace, or securing necessary resources to stay on top of a competitive field, Michelle has been key to the success of my books and the health list at the Pearson publishing enterprise. A tireless worker, an enthusiastic advocate for authors and her staff, Michelle has been a driving force in moving the *Access to Health* series into the twenty-first century of technologically savvy textbooks. Clearly, she "gets it" when it comes to keeping a steady hand on the pulse of the personal health market and what instructors are looking for and what students need. Although these individuals were key contributors to the finished work, there were many other people who worked on this revision of *Access to Health*. In particular, I would like to thank Patty Donovan of SPi Global who put everything together to make a polished finished product. Patty worked wonders in giving the book an exciting and fresh new look, both inside and out. Editorial Assistant Nicole Constantine gets major kudos for supporting the editorial team, as does Timothy Hainley, Senior Content Producer, who developed a comprehensive MasteringHealth program. Additional thanks go to the rest of the team at Pearson, especially Design Manager Mark Ong, Rights and Permissions Manager Ben Ferrini, and Director of Content Development Barbara Yien. A special thank you to Barbara for her steady hand and oversight of this project and her commitment to producing a quality text!

The editorial and production teams are critical to a book's success, but I would be remiss if I didn't thank another key group who ultimately help determine a book's success: the textbook representative and sales group and their leaders, Executive Product Marketing Manager Neena Bali and Field Marketing Manager Mary Salzman. Neena and Mary talk with faculty daily and provide the editorial and author teams with helpful advice and many good ideas. In keeping with my overall experiences with Pearson, the members of the marketing and sales staff are among the best of the best. I am very lucky to have them working with me on this project with each book, I appreciate their time, skill, and dedication even more! This is truly a great group of publishing professionals. Thank you to every one of you!

# CONTRIBUTORS TO THE FIFTEENTH EDITION

Many colleagues, students, and staff members have provided the feedback, reviews, extra time, assistance, and encouragement that have helped me meet the rigorous demands of publishing this book over the years. Whether acting as reviewers, generating new ideas, providing expert commentary, or revising chapters, each of these professionals has added his or her skills to our collective endeavor. I would like to thank other key contributors to chapters in this edition. As always, I would like to give particular thanks to Dr. Patricia Ketcham, who has helped with the *Access to Health* series since its beginnings. As

past president of the American College Health Association, former Associate Director of Health Promotion in Student Health Services at Oregon State University, and current Evaluation Specialist at Western Oregon University, Pat provides a current and unique perspective on key campus challenges and the innovative ways in which campuses are responding to a wide range of student health issues. Although she has been instrumental in the development and updating of several different chapters over the years, for this edition she used her skills in careful revisions of Chapter 2, "Promoting and Preserving Your Psychologial Health"; "Focus On: Recognizing and Avoiding Addiction"; Chapter 11, "Drinking Alcohol Responsibly"; Chapter 12, "Ending Tobacco Use"; Chapter 13, "Avoiding Drug Misuse and Abuse"; and Chapter 22, "Preparing for Aging, Death, and Dying".

Dr. Erica Taylor, associate professor in the Department of Public and Allied Health Sciences at Delaware State University, used her extensive background in exercise science and kinesiology to prepare an excellent update and revision for Chapter 7, "Improving Your Personal Fitness." Dr. Susan Dobie, Associate Professor in the Department of Health, Physical Education and Leisure Sciences at the University of Northern Iowa, has worked with our team for several recent editions, providing several outstanding chapter revisions. Susan utilized her expertise in the health promotion and health behavior areas to revise "Focus On: Enhancing Your Body Image"; Chapter 8, "Connecting and Communicating in the Modern World"; Chapter 9, "Understanding Your Sexuality"; and Chapter 10, "Considering Your Reproductive Choices." As an educator, mentor, and researcher, Dr. Dobie provided detailed, cutting-edge information in an interesting and well-written update designed to engage students and provide thought-provoking learning experiences.

Special thanks to Dr. Disa Cornish, assistant professor in the Department of Health Promotion and Education at Northern Iowa University, for her timely, thorough, and thoughtful revision of the "Focus On: Cultivating Your Spiritual Health," an area gaining increasing interest among millennials today.

Finally, Laura Bonazzoli, development editor and author, provided a thorough and timely revision of Chapter 1, "Accessing Your Health"; "Focus On: Improving Your Financial Health"; Chapter 5, "Nutrition: Eating for a Healthier You"; Chapter 19, "Making Smart Health Care Choices"; and "Focus On: Reducing Your Risk of Unintentional Injury." As per usual, Laura has done an outstanding job in revising chapters with the latest/greatest scientifically accurate information in a straightforward and thoughtful manner designed to motivate students.

The above contributors were brought on because of their history of working with college students, and their vital, enthusiastic approach to student learning. Importantly, they are all experts in subject-matter content and have proven academic training and research background in related fields. Thank you to each of you for your help in making this edition of *Access to Health* one of the best yet!

# REVIEWERS FOR THE FIFTEENTH EDITION

With each new edition of *Access to Health*, we have built on the combined expertise of many colleagues throughout the country who are dedicated to the education and healthy behavioral changes of students. I thank the many reviewers of the past 14 editions of *Access to Health* who have made such valuable contributions. I want you, the instructors who have used and reviewed the book over the years, to know that I am grateful for your support and guidance. You are an essential resource for knowing how to best stimulate students to learn, grow, and tackle the health challenges that lie ahead of them.

For the fifteenth edition, reviewers who have helped us continue this tradition of excellence include:

Aaron Fried, Glendale Community College
Chris Harman, California University of PA
Christine Foster, Western Michigan University
Lamia Scherzinger, Miami University
Melissa Mesman, Kennesaw State University
Nikki Bonanni, Ithaca College
Peter DiLorenzo, Camden County College
Richard Scheidt, Fresno City College

## Which Path Would You Take? Writers and Reviewers

Kathy Munoz, Humboldt State University
Michele Lomonaco, The Citadel
Brent Heidorn, University of West Georgia
Joshua Tarbay, Tarrant County College–Northwest Campus
Kelly Droege, Training and Organizational Development Business Partner, RESOLUTE Forest Products, Montreal, Canada
Dina Hayduk, Kutztown University
Susan Roberts-Dobie, University of Northern Iowa
Trevor Burns, Daytona State College
Carole Sloan, Henry Ford College
Karla Rues, Ozarks Technical Community College

## Contributors to Instructor Supplements and MasteringHealth

Karla Rues, Ozarks Technical Community College;
Brenda Moore, Ozarks Technical Community College;
Nicki Bonanni, Ithaca College; Laura Bonazzoli; Nic Albert;
Pardess Mitchell, Harper College;
Melanie Healy from University of Wisconsin La Crosse

Many thanks to all!
Rebecca J. Donatelle, PhD

# Changing Behavior Today
# for a Better Tomorrow

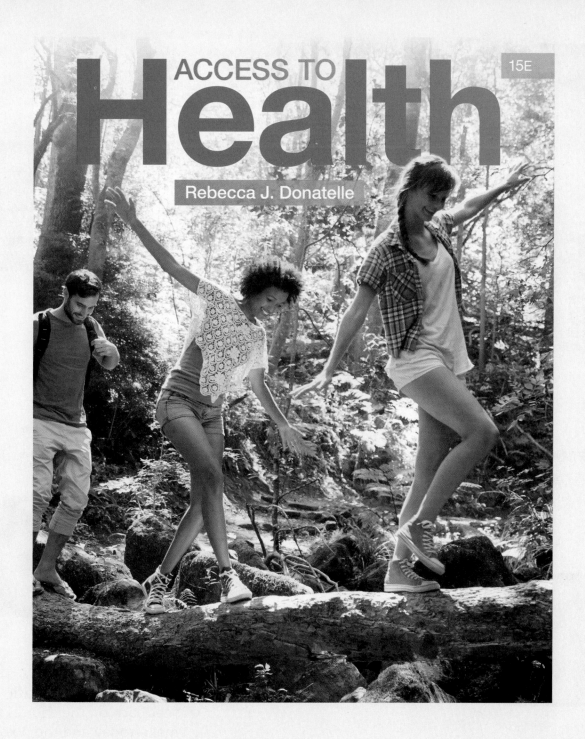

ACCESS TO
# Health

15E

Rebecca J. Donatelle

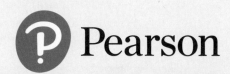

Pearson

# Focusing on Choices Today for Better Health

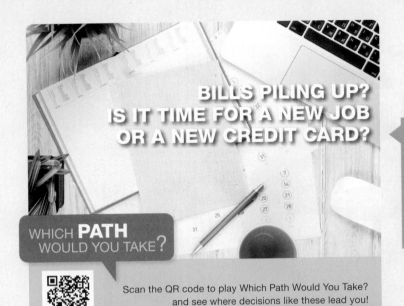

**BILLS PILING UP? IS IT TIME FOR A NEW JOB OR A NEW CREDIT CARD?**

WHICH **PATH** WOULD YOU TAKE?

Scan the QR code to play Which Path Would You Take? and see where decisions like these lead you!

**NEW! Interactive Behavior Change Activities—Which Path Would You Take?** By scanning QR codes with their mobile devices, students gain access to an exploration of various health choices through an engaging, interactive, low-stakes, and anonymous experience.

**Which Path Would You Take?** cover topics such as alcohol, smoking, nutrition, and fitness.

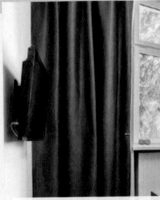

As a student, you have many financial responsibilities. You have to pay for food, rent, textbooks, clothes, your cell phone, and other bills. Sometimes there isn't enough to go around. It's the beginning of the semester, and you have to pay for rent and books. You're stressed. What should you do?

Pay the rent and do without the books. There is no middle ground here, and I need a roof over my head. Rent it is.

Consider my options. I can take on a roommate and buy the more cost-effective e-book or get the book from the reserve shelf in the library. Making the choice to scale back would cut my rent and book costs in half.

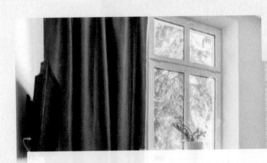

Consider "downshifting" or taking a step back. Perhaps, there are some unnecessary expenses you can cut out of your life. Doing so could help with your finances and your stress level.

continue

Students receive specific feedback on the choices they make today and the possible consequences on their future health.

# Outcomes Tomorrow

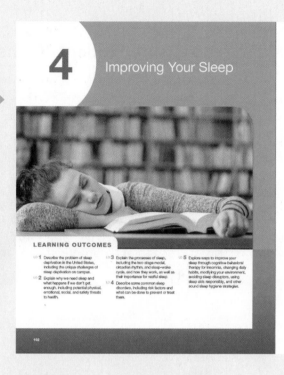

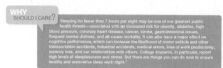

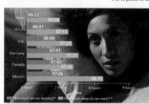

## MAKING **CHANGES** TODAY

### Shake Your Salt Habit

Take simple steps today to reduce your sodium intake:

- When buying packaged foods, choose low-sodium or sodium-free products.

- At the movies, order popcorn without salt.

- Use kosher salt—it has 25 percent less sodium than regular table salt.

- Avoid adding salt to foods during cooking or at the table; instead, try using fresh or dried herbs and spices to season foods.

**WHY** SHOULD I CARE?

A poor-quality diet is a major risk factor for three of the top five causes of death: heart disease, cancer, and stroke. The food and beverage choices you make now can have both immediate and long-term effects on your health.

# Continuous Learning
## Before, During, and After Class

## BEFORE CLASS

### Mobile Media and Reading Assignments Ensure Students Come to Class Prepared

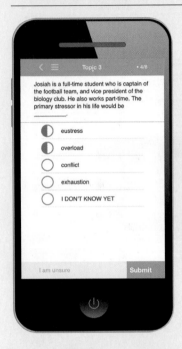

**UPDATED!** **Dynamic Study Modules** help students study effectively by continuously assessing student performance and providing practice in areas where students struggle the most. Each Dynamic Study Module, accessed by computer, smartphone, or tablet, promotes fast learning and long-term retention.

**NEW!** **Interactive eText 2.0** gives students access to the text whenever they can access the internet. eText features include:

- Now available on smartphones and tablets
- Seamlessly integrated videos and other rich media
- Accessible (screen-reader ready)
- Configurable reading settings, including resizable type and night reading mode
- Instructor and student note-taking, highlighting, bookmarking, and search
- Now available for offline use via the Pearson eText 2.0 app

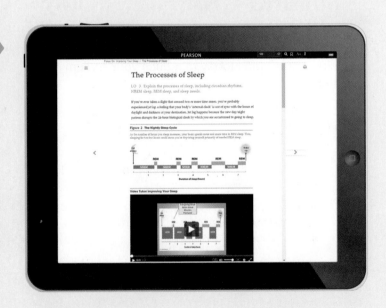

### Pre-Lecture Reading Quizzes are easy to customize and assign

**NEW!** Reading Questions ensure that students complete the assigned reading before class and stay on track with reading assignments. Reading Questions are 100% mobile ready and can be completed by students on mobile devices.

# with MasteringHealth™

## DURING CLASS

### Engage students with Learning Catalytics

Learning Catalytics, a "bring your own device" student engagement, assessment, and classroom intelligence system, allows students to use their smartphone, tablet, or laptop to respond to questions in class.

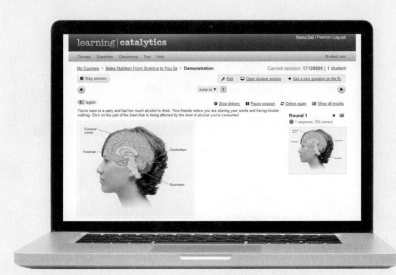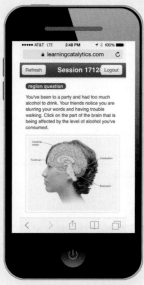

## AFTER CLASS

### MasteringHealth Delivers Automatically Graded Health and Fitness Activities

**NEW! Interactive Behavior Change Activities—Which Path Would You Take?**
Have students explore various health choices through an engaging, interactive, low-stakes, and anonymous experience. These activities show students the possible consequences of various choices they make today on their future health.
These activities are assignable in Mastering with follow-up questions.

# Continuous Learning
# Before, During, and After Class

## AFTER CLASS

### Easy-to-Assign, Customize, Media-Rich, and Automatically Graded Assignments

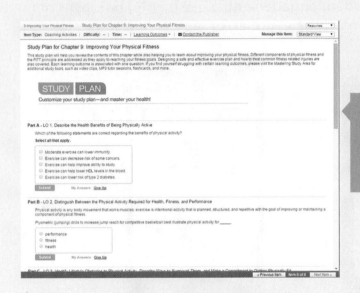

**UPDATED! Study Plans** tie all end-of-chapter material to specific numbered Learning Outcomes and Mastering assets. Assignable Study Plan items contain at least one multiple choice question per Learning Outcome and wrong-answer feedback.

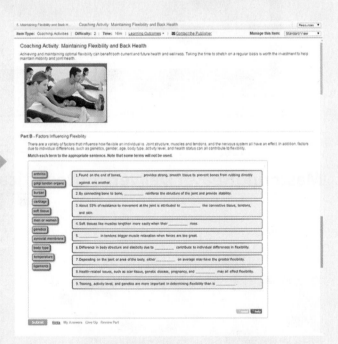

**HALLMARK! Coaching Activities** guide students through key health and fitness concepts with interactive mini-lessons that provide hints and feedback.

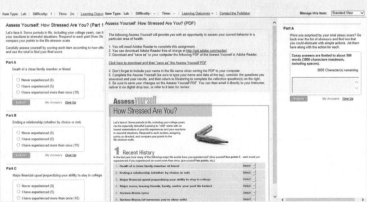

**HALLMARK! Assess Yourself Worksheets** are available as auto-graded, assignable assessments within **MasteringHealth**.

# with MasteringHealth™

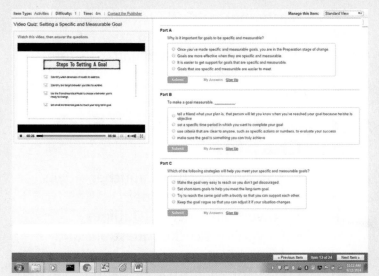

**Behavior Change Videos** are concise whiteboard-style videos that help students with the steps of behavior change, covering topics such as setting SMART goals, identifying and overcoming barriers to change, planning realistic timelines, and more. Additional videos review key fitness concepts such as determining target heart rate range for exercise. All videos include assessment activities and are assignable in **MasteringHealth**.

**NEW! ABC News Videos** bring health to life and spark discussion with up-to-date hot topics from 2012–2015. Activities tied to the videos include multiple choice questions that provide wrong-answer feedback to redirect students to the correct answer.

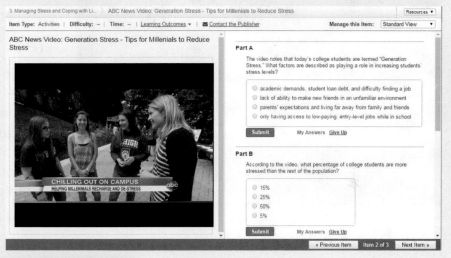

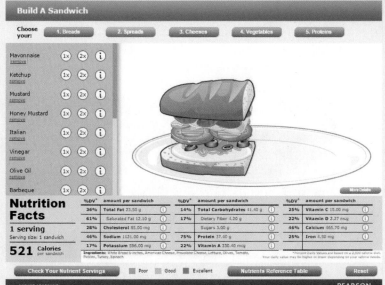

**UPDATED! NutriTools Coaching Activities** in the nutrition chapter allow students to combine and experiment with different food options and learn firsthand how to build healthier meals.

# Resources for YOU, the Instructor

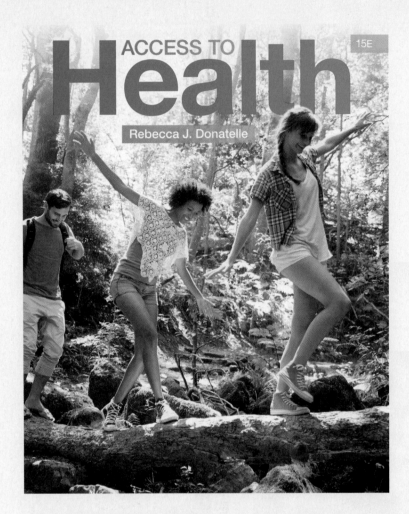

**ACCESS TO Health**
15E
Rebecca J. Donatelle

**MasteringHealth™** provides you with everything you need to prep for your course and deliver a dynamic lecture, in one convenient place. Resources include:

## Media Assets for Each Chapter

- *ABC News* Lecture Launcher videos
- Behavior Change videos
- PowerPoint Lecture Outlines
- PowerPoint clicker questions and Jeopardy-style quiz show questions
- Files for all illustrations and tables and selected photos from the text

## Test Bank

- Test Bank in Microsoft Word, PDF, and RTF formats
- Computerized Test Bank, which includes all the questions from the printed test bank in a format that allows you to easily and intuitively build exams and quizzes.

## Teaching Resources

- Instructor Resource and Support Manual in Microsoft Word and PDF formats
- Teaching with Student Learning Outcomes
- Teaching with Web 2.0
- Learning Catalytics: Getting Started
- Getting Started with **MasteringHealth**

## Student Supplements

- Take Charge of Your Health Worksheets
- Behavior Change Log Book and Wellness Journal
- Eat Right!
- Live Right!
- Food Composition Table

**Measuring Student Learning Outcomes?**
All of the MasteringHealth assignable content is tagged to book content and to Bloom's Taxonomy. You also have the ability to add your own learning outcomes, helping you track student performance against your learning outcomes. You can view class performance against the specified learning outcomes and share those results quickly and easily by exporting to a spreadsheet.

# 1 Accessing Your Health

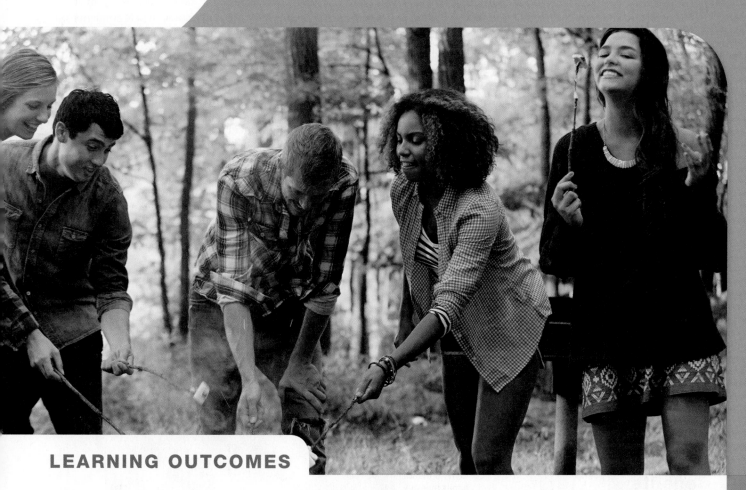

## LEARNING OUTCOMES

**LO 1** Describe the immediate and long-term rewards of healthy behaviors and the effects that your health choices may have on others.

**LO 2** Compare and contrast the medical model of health and the public health model, and discuss the six dimensions of health.

**LO 3** Identify modifiable and nonmodifiable personal and social factors that influence your health; discuss the importance of a global perspective on health; and explain how gender, racial, economic, and cultural factors influence health disparities.

**LO 4** Compare and contrast the health belief model, the social-cognitive model, and the transtheoretical model of behavior change, and explain how you might use them in making a specific behavior change.

**LO 5** Identify your own current risk behaviors, the factors that influence those behaviors, and the strategies you can use to change them.

G ot health? That may sound like a simple question, but it isn't. Health is a process, not something we just "get." People who are healthy in their 50s, 60s, and beyond aren't just lucky or the beneficiaries of hardy genes. Most have set the stage for good health by making it a priority in their early years. Whether the coming decades are filled with good health, productive careers, special relationships, and fulfillment of life goals is influenced by the health choices you make—beginning right now.

## LO 1 | WHY HEALTH, WHY NOW?

Describe the immediate and long-term rewards of healthy behaviors and the effects that your health choices may have on others.

Every day, the media remind us of health challenges facing the world, the nation—maybe even your campus or community. You might want to ignore these issues, but you can't. In the twenty-first century, your health is connected to the health of people with whom you directly interact, as well as to people you've never met, and to the well-being of your local environment, as well as the entire planet. Let's take a look at how.

## Choose Health Now for Immediate Benefits

Almost everyone knows that overeating leads to weight gain or that smoking causes lung cancer. But other choices you make every day may influence your well-being in ways you're not aware of. For instance, did you know that scientific research is increasingly finding that the amount of sleep you get each night can influence your weight, your susceptibility to chronic diseases, your ability to ward off colds, your mental health, your social interactions, and your driving? What's more, inadequate sleep

is one of the most commonly reported impediments to academic success (**FIGURE 1.1**). Similarly, drinking alcohol reduces your academic performance and sharply increases your risk of unintentional injuries—not only motor vehicle accidents, but also falls, burns, and drownings. This is especially significant because, for people between the ages of 15 and 44, unintentional injury—whether related to drowsiness, alcohol use, or any other factor—is the leading cause of death (**TABLE 1.1**).

It isn't an exaggeration to say that healthy choices have immediate benefits. When you're well nourished, fit, rested, and free from the influence of nicotine, alcohol, and other drugs, you're more likely to avoid illness, succeed in school, maintain supportive relationships, participate in meaningful work and community activities, and enjoy your leisure time.

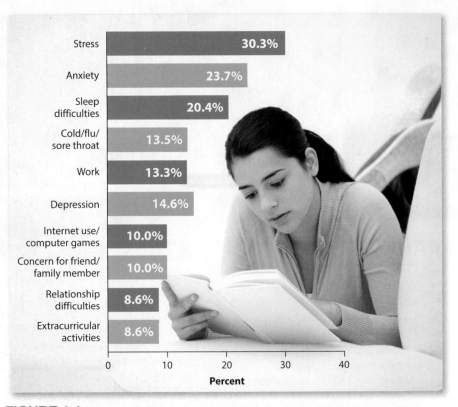

| | Percent |
|---|---|
| Stress | 30.3% |
| Anxiety | 23.7% |
| Sleep difficulties | 20.4% |
| Cold/flu/sore throat | 13.5% |
| Work | 13.3% |
| Depression | 14.6% |
| Internet use/computer games | 10.0% |
| Concern for friend/family member | 10.0% |
| Relationship difficulties | 8.6% |
| Extracurricular activities | 8.6% |

**FIGURE 1.1** **Top Ten Reported Impediments to Academic Performance—Past 12 Months** In a recent survey by the National College Health Association, students indicated that stress, anxiety, poor sleep, and other factors had prevented them from performing at their academic best.

**Source:** Data are from American College Health Association, *American College Health Association—National College Health Assessment II (ACHA-NCHA II) Reference Group Data Report, Fall 2015* (Baltimore, MD: ACHA, 2016).

## TABLE 1.1 | Leading Causes of Death in the United States, 2012, Overall and by Age Group (15 and older)

| All Ages | Number of Deaths |
|---|---|
| Diseases of the heart | 599,711 |
| Malignant neoplasms (cancer) | 582,623 |
| Chronic lower respiratory diseases | 143,489 |
| Cerebrovascular diseases (stroke) | 128,546 |
| Accidents (unintentional injuries) | 127,792 |
| **Aged 15–24** | |
| Accidents (unintentional injuries) | 11,908 |
| Suicide | 4,872 |
| Assault (homicide) | 4,614 |
| Malignant neoplasms (cancer) | 1,574 |
| Diseases of the heart | 956 |
| **Aged 25–44** | |
| Accidents (unintentional injuries) | 30,885 |
| Malignant neoplasms (cancer) | 15,011 |
| Diseases of the heart | 13,720 |
| Suicide | 12,974 |
| Assault (homicide) | 7,047 |
| **Aged 45–64** | |
| Malignant neoplasms (cancer) | 161,158 |
| Diseases of the heart | 106,493 |
| Accidents (unintentional injuries) | 36,216 |
| Chronic liver disease and cirrhosis | 20,107 |
| Chronic lower respiratory diseases | 19,745 |
| **Aged 65+** | |
| Diseases of the heart | 477,840 |
| Malignant neoplasms (cancer) | 403,497 |
| Chronic lower respiratory diseases | 122,375 |
| Cerebrovascular diseases | 109,127 |
| Alzheimer's disease | 82,690 |

**Source:** Data from S. L. Murphy, K. D. Kochanek, J. Xu, and M. Heron, "Deaths: Final Data for 2012, Table 10," *National Vital Statistics Reports* 63, no. 9 (August 2015), www.cdc.gov/nchs/data/nvsr/nvsr63/nvsr63_09.pdf.

## Choose Health Now for Long-Term Rewards

Successful aging starts now. The choices you make today are like seeds: Planting good seeds means you're more likely to enjoy the fruits of a longer and healthier life. In contrast, poor choices increase the likelihood of a shorter life, as well as a lower quality of life.

**Personal Choices Influence Your Life Expectancy** According to current **mortality** rates and death statistics—which reflect the proportion of deaths within a population—the average **life expectancy** at birth in the United States is projected to be 78.8 years for a child born in 2014.[1] In other words, we can expect that American infants born today will live to an average age of over 78 years, much longer than the 47-year life expectancy for people born in the early 1900s.

That's because life expectancy a century ago was largely determined by our susceptibility to infectious disease. In 1900, over 30 percent of all deaths occurred among children younger than 5 years old, and the leading cause of death was infection.[2] Even among adults, infectious diseases such as tuberculosis and pneumonia were the leading causes of death, and widespread epidemics of infectious diseases such as influenza crossed national boundaries to kill millions.

# 78.8 YEARS

is the **LIFE EXPECTANCY** in the United States.

With the development of vaccines and antibiotics, life expectancy increased dramatically as premature deaths from infectious diseases decreased. As a result, the leading cause of death shifted to **chronic diseases** such as heart disease, cerebrovascular disease (which leads to strokes), cancer, and chronic lower respiratory diseases. At the same time, advances in diagnostic technologies, heart and brain surgery, and radiation and other cancer treatments, as well as new medications, continued the trend of increasing life expectancy into the twenty-first century.

Unfortunately, life expectancy in the United States is several years below that of many other nations. Factors contributing to premature mortality and thus limiting U.S. life expectancy include tobacco and alcohol abuse, obesity, emerging infectious diseases, and drug overdose, which is now the leading cause of accidental death.[3] Access to health care, social inequality, and poverty are also part of the complex, multifactorial influences on our life expectancy.[4] For more, see **Health Headlines** on page 4.

**mortality** The proportion of deaths to population.

**life expectancy** Expected number of years of life remaining at a given age, such as at birth.

**chronic disease** A disease that typically begins slowly, progresses, and persists, with a variety of signs and symptoms that can be treated but not cured by medication.

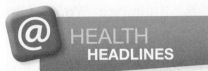

# AMERICA
## *Shorter Lives, Poorer Health*

In 2013, the Institute of Medicine (IOM), part of the National Academy of Sciences, published a report comparing health and longevity in the United States to that of 16 "peer" countries—high-income democracies including Canada, Australia, Japan, and 13 countries in western Europe. Its sobering finding was that, for decades, Americans have been dying at earlier ages than people in peer countries, and experiencing poorer health at all life stages, from birth through older adulthood.

An intriguing aspect of the findings is that Americans' reduced longevity reverses after age 75; that is, an American who lives to age 75 can actually expect to live longer than a 75-year-old from a peer country. This advantage is thought to be due to lower cancer death rates as well as better management of blood pressure and blood lipids, two factors in heart disease. Our reduced longevity overall, therefore, must be due to factors affecting us earlier in life. For example, the United States has a higher infant mortality rate than that of the peer countries. We also have a higher rate of homicides and accidental injury deaths, especially drug-related deaths, which are more common in young or middle adulthood. Americans also have higher rates of HIV/AIDS, obesity, and diabetes, conditions that reduce the likelihood that people will ever reach age 75.

The IOM report identifies four general factors for our high rates of life-threatening diseases and injuries:

- **Our troubled health care system.** Americans are more likely to be uninsured and underinsured
- **Our unequal society.** The United States has a high level of poverty and income inequality, as well as lower levels of social services.
- **Our car culture.** The infrastructure in communities throughout the United States tends to be designed for driving rather than for walking or cycling, discouraging physical activity.
- **Our poor behaviors.** Although our rates of smoking are lower, we're more likely to abuse drugs, use firearms, drive while intoxicated, and fail to wear a safety belt. We also consume the most calories per person.

If citizens of 16 peer countries can enjoy better health and longer lives, Americans can as well. Get involved by supporting increased access to health care and social services and pedestrian-friendly community redevelopment. As you learn about health-promoting behaviors in this text, be sure to put them into practice.

**Source:** Institute of Medicine, "U.S. Health in International Perspective: Shorter Lives, Poorer Health," January 2013, www.iom.edu/~/media/Files/Report%20Files/2013/US-Health-International-Perspective/USHealth_Intl_PerspectiveRB.pdf.

---

**Personal Choices Influence Your *Healthy Life Expectancy*** Another benefit of healthful choices is that they increase your **healthy life expectancy**, that is, the number of years remaining at a given age without disability, chronic pain, or significant illness. One dimension of healthy life expectancy is **health-related quality of life** (HRQoL), a concept that goes beyond mortality rates and life expectancy and focuses on the impact health status has on physical, mental, emotional, and social function. Closely related to this is *well-being*, which assesses the positive aspects of a person's life, such as positive emotions and life satisfaction.[5]

## Your Health Is Linked to Societal Health

Our personal health choices affect the lives of others. For example, as we have said, overeating and inadequate physical activity contribute to obesity. But obesity isn't a problem only for the individual. Along with its associated health problems, obesity burdens the U.S. health care system and the U.S. economy overall. According to the Centers for Disease Control and Prevention (CDC), the medical

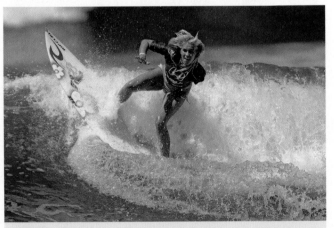

What is meant by *quality of life*? Hawaiian surfer Bethany Hamilton lost her arm in a shark attack while surfing at age 13, but that hasn't prevented her from achieving her goals as a professional surfer.

**healthy life expectancy** Expected number of years of full health remaining at a given age, such as at birth.

**health-related quality of life** Assessment of impact of health status—including elements of physical, mental, emotional, and social function—on overall quality of life.

costs of obesity in the United States are nearly $150 billion each year.[6] In addition, obesity costs the public *indirectly*. These indirect costs include reduced tax revenues because of income lost from absenteeism and premature death, increased disability payments because of an inability to remain in the workforce, and increased health insurance rates as claims rise for treatment of obesity itself as well as its associated diseases.

Smoking, excessive alcohol consumption, and illegal and prescription drug abuse also place an economic burden on our communities and society. Moreover, these behaviors burden caregivers who make financial, social, and emotional sacrifices to take care of those disabled by diseases.

At the root of the concern that individual health choices cost society is an ethical question causing considerable debate: To what extent should the public be held accountable for an individual's unhealthy choices? Should we require individuals to somehow pay for their poor choices? Of course, in some cases, we already do. We tax cigarettes and alcohol, and in 2015, Berkeley, California, became the first U.S. city to tax sweetened soft drinks, which have been blamed for rising obesity rates. On the other side of the debate are those who argue that smoking and drinking are addictions that require treatment, not punishment, and that obesity is a multifactorial disorder, with heredity, sociocultural factors, the food environment, public policy, and individual choices all contributing. Are behaviors that influence health always entirely within our control? Before we explore these questions further, it's essential to understand what health actually is.

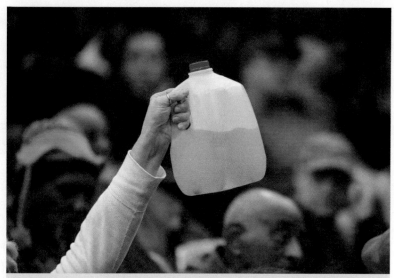

Negative health events can be caused by people's interaction with the physical environment. High levels of lead in the tap water in Flint, Michigan, have made water in the city largely undrinkable and put the health and wellness of many children and families at risk.

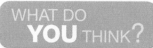

## WHAT DO YOU THINK?

■ In 2015, senators in Puerto Rico introduced legislation proposing to fine parents if their obese children failed to lose weight. Would you support such a law? Why or why not?

■ Since we tax cigarettes, is it reasonable to tax high-calorie sugary drinks? A so-called "soda tax" failed in New York City and San Francisco, but passed in Berkeley. Where do you stand, and why?

## LO 2 | WHAT IS HEALTH?

Compare and contrast the medical model of health and the public health model, and discuss the six dimensions of health.

For some, the word **health** simply means the antithesis of sickness. To others, it means fitness, wellness, or well-being—an increasingly enlightened way of viewing health that has taken shape over time. As our collective understanding of illness has improved, so has our ability to understand the many nuances of health.

## Models of Health

Over the centuries, different ideals—or models—of human health have dominated. Our current model of health has broadened from a focus on the individual physical body to an understanding of health as a reflection not only of ourselves, but also of our communities.

**Medical Model** Prior to the twentieth century, perceptions of health were dominated by the **medical model**, in which health status focused primarily on the individual and his or her tissues and organs. The surest way to improve health was to cure the individual's disease, either with medication to treat the disease-causing agent or through surgery to remove the diseased body part. Thus, government resources focused on initiatives that led to treatment, rather than prevention, of disease.

**Public Health Model** Not until the early decades of the 1900s did researchers begin to recognize that entire populations of poor people, particularly those living in certain locations, were victims of environmental factors over which they had little control: polluted water and air, a low-quality diet, poor housing, and unsafe work settings. As a result, researchers began to focus on an **ecological** or **public health model**, which views diseases and other negative health events as a result of an individual's interaction with his or her social and physical environment.

Recognition of the public health model enabled health officials to move to control contaminants in water, for example, by building adequate sewers, and to control burning and other forms of air pollution. In the early 1900s, colleges began offering courses in health and hygiene. Over time, public health officials began to recognize and address many other forces affecting human health, including hazardous work conditions; air, soil, and water pollution; negative influences

**health** The ever-changing process of achieving individual potential in the physical, social, emotional, intellectual, spiritual, and environmental dimensions.

**medical model** A view of health in which health status focuses primarily on the individual and a biological or diseased-organ perspective.

**ecological or public health model** A view of health in which diseases and other negative health events are seen as a result of an individual's interaction with his or her social and physical environment.

**disease prevention** Actions or behaviors designed to keep people from getting sick.

**health promotion** The combined educational, organizational, procedural, environmental, social, and financial supports that help individuals and groups reduce negative health behaviors and promote positive change.

**risk behaviors** Actions that increase susceptibility to negative health outcomes.

**wellness** The achievement of the highest level of health possible in each of several dimensions.

in the home and social environment; abuse of drugs and alcohol; stress; unsafe behavior; diet; sedentary lifestyle; and cost, quality, and access to health care.

By the 1940s progressive thinkers began calling for policies, programs, and services to improve individual health and that of the population as a whole—shifting focus from treatment of individual illness to **disease prevention**. For example, childhood vaccination programs reduced the incidence and severity of infectious disease; installation of safety features such as seat belts and airbags in motor vehicles reduced traffic injuries and fatalities; and laws governing occupational safety reduced injuries to and deaths of American workers. In 1947 at an international conference focusing on global health issues, the World Health Organization (WHO) proposed a new definition of health: "Health is the state of complete physical, mental, and social well-being, not just the absence of disease or infirmity."[7] This new definition definitively rejected the old medical model.

The public health model also began to emphasize **health promotion**—policies and programs that promote behaviors known to support good health. Health-promotion programs identify people who are engaging in **risk behaviors** (those that increase susceptibility to negative health outcomes) and motivate them to change their actions by improving their knowledge, attitudes, and skills. Numerous public policies and services, technological advances, and individual actions have worked to improve our overall health status greatly in the past 100 years. **FIGURE 1.2** lists the 10 greatest public health achievements of the twentieth century.

## Wellness and the Dimensions of Health

In 1968, biologist, environmentalist, and philosopher René Dubos proposed an even broader definition of health. In his Pulitzer Prize–winning book, *So Human an Animal*, Dubos defined health as "a quality of life, involving social, emotional, mental, spiritual, and

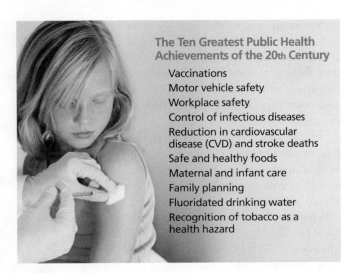

The Ten Greatest Public Health Achievements of the 20th Century

Vaccinations
Motor vehicle safety
Workplace safety
Control of infectious diseases
Reduction in cardiovascular disease (CVD) and stroke deaths
Safe and healthy foods
Maternal and infant care
Family planning
Fluoridated drinking water
Recognition of tobacco as a health hazard

**FIGURE 1.2** The Ten Greatest Public Health Achievements of the Twentieth Century

**Source:** Adapted from Centers for Disease Control and Prevention, "Ten Great Public Health Achievements in the 20th Century," April 26, 2013, www.cdc.gov/about/history/tengpha.htm.

biological fitness on the part of the individual, which results from adaptations to the environment."[8] This concept of adaptability, or the ability to cope successfully with life's ups and downs, became a key element in our overall understanding of health.

Later, the concept of **wellness** enlarged Dubos's definition of health by recognizing levels—or gradations—of health (**FIGURE 1.3**). To achieve *high-level wellness*, a person must move progressively higher on a continuum of positive health indicators. Those unable to achieve these levels may slip into illness, premature disability, or death.

Today, the words *health* and *wellness* are often used interchangeably to mean the dynamic, ever-changing process of

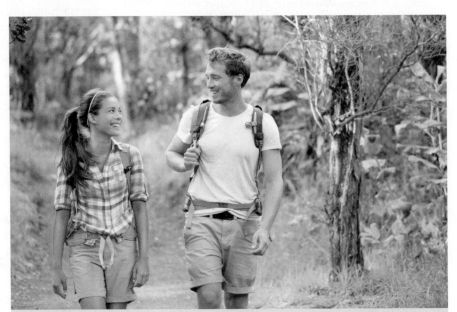

Today, health and wellness mean taking a positive, proactive attitude toward life and living it to the fullest.

| Irreversible disability and/or death | Chronic illness | Signs of illness | Signs of health/ wellness | Improved health/ wellness | Optimal wellness/ well-being |
|---|---|---|---|---|---|

▲
Neutral
point

**FIGURE 1.3** The Wellness Continuum

trying to achieve one's potential in each of six interrelated dimensions (**FIGURE 1.4**):

- **Physical health.** Physical health includes features like the shape and size of your body, how responsive and acute your senses are, and your body's ability to function at optimum levels with adequate sleep and rest, nutrition, and physical activity. It also includes your ability to avoid, manage, or heal from injury or illness, cope with challenges, and maintain equilibrium in the face of adversity. More recent definitions of physical health encompass a person's ability to perform *activities of daily living* (*ADLs*), or those activities that are essential to function normally in society—including things like getting up out of a chair, bathing and dressing yourself, cooking meals, and getting around without assistance.
- **Social health.** The ability to have a broad social network and maintain satisfying interpersonal relationships with friends, family members, and partners is a key part of overall wellness. Successfully interacting and communicating with others, adapting to various social situations, and other daily behaviors are all part of social health.
- **Intellectual health.** The ability to think clearly, reason objectively, analyze critically, and use brainpower effectively

to meet life's challenges are all part of this dimension. It involves being open minded and nonjudgmental, having a thirst for knowledge and information, being culturally competent and multiculturally aware, and acknowledging that there are often no simple answers to life's questions. In short, it means being aware and informed, and using that awareness and knowledge to create a better life for yourself and others.

- **Emotional health.** This is the feeling component—being able to express emotions when appropriate, and to control them when not. It also includes emotional intelligence, which is the ability to identify and manage emotional responses in positive ways. Self-esteem, self-confidence, trust, and love are all part of emotional health.
- **Spiritual health.** This dimension involves creating and expressing meaning and purpose in your life. This may include believing in a supreme being or following a particular religion's rules and customs, or simply feeling that you are part of a greater spectrum of existence. The capacities to contemplate life's experiences and to care about and respect all living things are aspects of spiritual health.
- **Environmental health.** This dimension entails understanding how the health of the environments in which you live, work, and play can positively or negatively affect you; protecting yourself from hazards in your own environment; and working to preserve, protect, and improve environmental conditions for everyone.

Achieving wellness means attaining the optimal level of well-being for your unique limitations and strengths. For example, a disabled person may function at his or her optimal level of physical and intellectual performance; enjoy satisfying relationships; and be engaged in environmental concerns. In contrast, a person who spends hours lifting weights to perfect the size and shape of each muscle, but pays little attention to others, may lack social or emotional health. The perspective we need is *holistic*, emphasizing the balanced integration of mind, body, and spirit.

## LO 3 | **WHAT** INFLUENCES YOUR HEALTH?

Identify modifiable and nonmodifiable personal and social factors that influence your health; discuss the importance of a global perspective on health; and explain how gender, racial, economic, and cultural factors influence health disparities.

If you're lucky, aspects of your world conspire to promote your health: Everyone in your family is slender and fit; there are locally grown, organic fruits and vegetables for sale at the neighborhood farmer's market; and a new bike trail opens along the river (and you have a bike!). If you're

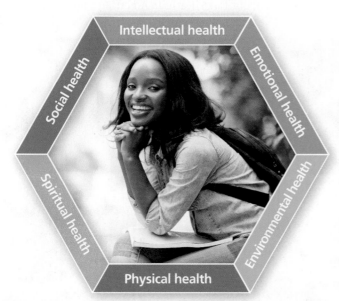

**FIGURE 1.4 The Dimensions of Health** When all dimensions are balanced and well developed, they support your active, thriving lifestyle.

Intellectual health · Emotional health · Environmental health · Physical health · Spiritual health · Social health

→ VIDEO TUTOR
Dimensions of Health

**determinants of health** The range of personal, social, economic, and environmental factors that influence health status.

**health disparities** Differences in the incidence, prevalence, mortality, and burden of diseases and other health conditions among specific population groups.

not so lucky, aspects of your life make getting and staying healthy much more challenging. Everyone in your family is overweight; your peers urge you to keep up with their drinking; there are only cigarettes, alcohol, and junk food for sale at the corner market; and you wouldn't dare walk or ride alongside the river for fear of being mugged. In short, seemingly personal choices aren't always totally within an individual's control.

Public health experts refer to the factors that influence health as **determinants of health**, a term the U.S. Surgeon General defines as "the range of personal, social, economic, and environmental factors that influence health status."[9] The Surgeon General's health promotion plan, called *Healthy People*, has been published every 10 years since 1990 with the goal of improving the quality and increasing the years of life for all Americans. The overarching goals set out by the newest version, *Healthy People 2020*, are as follows:

- Attain high-quality, longer lives free of preventable diseases.
- Achieve health equity, eliminate disparities, and improve health of all groups.
- Create social and physical environments that promote good health for all.
- Promote quality of life, healthy development, and healthy behaviors across all life stages.

*Healthy People 2020* classifies health determinants into five categories: individual behavior, biology and genetics, social factors, policymaking, and health services (FIGURE 1.5). It also includes strong language about reducing **health disparities** that exist between populations based on racial or ethnic background, income and education, and many other factors. See the **Health in a Diverse World** box for more information on health disparities.

## Individual Behavior

Individual behaviors can help you attain, maintain, or regain good health, or they can lead to deteriorating health and premature disease. Because most behaviors are within your power to change, health experts refer to them as *modifiable determinants*. Modifiable determinants significantly influence your risk for chronic disease—responsible for 7 out of 10 deaths.[10] Incredibly, just four modifiable determinants are responsible for most chronic disease (FIGURE 1.6). These are:[11]

- **Lack of physical activity.** Low levels of physical activity contribute to over 200,000 deaths in the United States annually.[12]

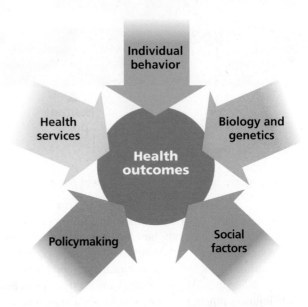

**FIGURE 1.5** *Healthy People 2020* Determinants of Health The determinants of health often overlap with one another. Collectively, they impact the health of individuals and communities.

- **Poor nutrition.** Diets low in whole foods like fruits, vegetables, nuts, and seeds, but high in sodium, processed meats, and *trans* fats are associated with the greatest burden of disease.[13]
- **Excessive alcohol consumption.** Alcohol causes 88,000 deaths in adults annually through cardiovascular disease, liver disease, cancer, and other diseases, as well as motor vehicle accidents and violence.[14]
- **Tobacco use.** Tobacco smoking and the cancer, high blood pressure, and respiratory disease it causes are responsible for about 1 in 5 deaths in American adults.[15]

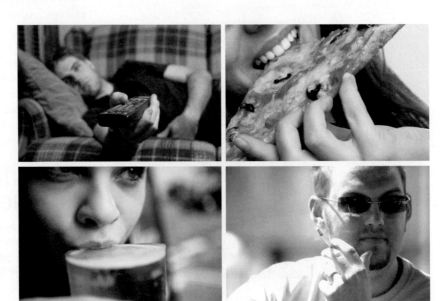

**FIGURE 1.6** Four Leading Causes of Chronic Disease in the United States Lack of physical activity, poor nutrition, excessive alcohol consumption, and tobacco use—all modifiable health determinants—are the four most significant factors leading to chronic disease among Americans today.

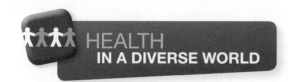

**HEALTH IN A DIVERSE WORLD**

# THE PUZZLE OF HEALTH DISPARITIES

Among the factors that can affect an individual's ability to achieve and maintain optimal health, race and ethnicity are prominent. Research indicates dramatic health disparities among African Americans in particular. For example, African Americans have higher rates of hypertension (high blood pressure)—41 percent versus 27 to 29 percent for Hispanic and white Americans, and die of heart disease at a rate of 141 per 100,000 versus 87 for Hispanic Americans and 118 for white Americans. African Americans also have the highest rates of lung cancer, colorectal cancer, prostate cancer, pancreatic cancer, and all cancers combined. African Americans experience the highest rate of preterm births as well—17 percent, versus 11 to 12 percent for Hispanic and white Americans.

Disparities in educational attainment and income are thought to contribute to—but not entirely explain—disparities in health. In 2014, the level of educational attainment among Americans was highest among Asian and white Americans: 97 and 96 percent, respectively, had a high school diploma and 61 and 41 percent had at least a bachelor's degree. On average, higher educational attainment is reflected in higher income: Americans who lack a high school diploma earn, on average, $6,000 less annually than those with a high school diploma, who themselves earn about $19,000 less than those with a bachelor's degree. Therefore it's not surprising that Asian and white Americans have the highest median income: about $67,000 annually for Asian Americans and about $58,000 for

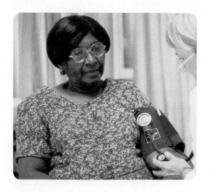

Income affects access to quality health services, such as blood pressure screenings, which in turn influences a population's burden of disease.

white Americans. Their poverty level is also lowest—about 10 percent.

Among African Americans, the educational attainment figures drop: 92 percent graduate from high school, but only 22 percent obtain at least a bachelor's degree. Median income is just $35,000 annually, and 27 percent of African Americans live in poverty.

On average, lower-income Americans experience increased rates of illness and premature death; a study involving over 3,000 United States counties found that low-income Americans had an average mortality rate of 491 per 100,000, whereas high-income Americans had an average mortality rate of 351 per 100,000. These disparities occur in part because reduced income means reduced ability to pay for quality health insurance, health care, medications and supplies, nutritious food, and quality housing. In addition, persistent financial stress is thought to increase

risk-taking behaviors such as smoking, binge drinking, and binge eating.

We noted that differences in educational attainment and income don't entirely explain disparities in health. Consider, for example, that the figures for educational attainment among Hispanic Americans are even lower than those for African Americans: just 75 percent graduate from high school, and only 15 percent have at least a bachelor's degree. Moreover, the median income of Hispanic Americans—$41,000 annually—is only slightly higher than that of African Americans, and their poverty level—24 percent—is only slightly lower. Nevertheless, Hispanic Americans do not experience the same level and variety of health disparities seen among African Americans. Clearly, more research into the role of genetics and biology, stress, discrimination, environmental factors, and other determinants of health is required if we are to increase our understanding of health disparities in the United States.

**Sources:** Data from Centers for Disease Control and Prevention, "CDC Health Disparities and Inequalities Report—United States, 2013," *Morbidity and Mortality Weekly Report* 62, Supplement 3 (November 22, 2013): 1–187, Available at www.cdc.gov/mmwr/preview/ind2013_su.html#HealthDisparities2013; National Center for Education Statistics, "Fast Facts," *The Condition of Education 2015* (NCES 2015-144). Available at https://nces.ed.gov/fastfacts/display.asp?id=77; C. DeNavas-Walt and B. D. Proctor, "Income and Poverty in the United States: 2013," U.S. Census Bureau, September 2014, Available at https://www.census.gov/content/dam/Census/library/publications/2014/demo/p60-249.pdf; E. R. Cheng and D. A. Kindig, "Disparities in Premature Mortality Between High- and Low-Income US Counties," *Preventing Chronic Disease* 9 (2012): 110120.

On the flip side, a recent study tracking more than 2,100 young adults (aged 18 to 30) found that those who maintained a healthful body weight, ate a nourishing diet, engaged in physical activity, and did not smoke were about twice as likely to maintain normal blood pressure and other indicators of cardiovascular health 25 years later as compared to those who did not practice these behaviors.[16]

In addition to these leading causes of chronic disease, other modifiable determinants wreak havoc on the lives of Americans, and lead to increased burdens on families, law enforcement, and our health care system. For example, the use of potentially

addictive prescription medications and illegal drugs among Americans is rising. In particular, prescriptions for opioid pain relievers quadrupled between 1999 and 2014, and overdoses of these drugs tripled. Between 2000 and 2014, nearly half a million Americans died from drug overdoses, more than the number killed by motor vehicle accidents.[17] Epidemic increases in mental health problems, increases in violent crime,

**SEE IT! VIDEOS**

What can one person do to fight childhood hunger? Watch **Viola Davis Fights to End Child Hunger**, available on MasteringHealth.™

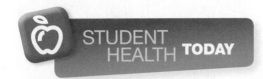
# OPTIMAL WELLNESS OR CHRONIC ILLNESS *What Will Your Future Bring?*

Every 2 years, American athletes gather to compete in the Senior Games. In the summer of 2015, gold medalists Brenda Matthews won the 200-meter dash in 33 seconds—at age 66—and Don Phillips ran the 400-meter dash in a minute and 42 seconds—at age 84! How do these athletes stay so fit when the majority of older Americans struggle with overweight and chronic disease? And what will your future bring?

Although imprecise, research into healthy aging has identified five modifiable factors that appear to most strongly influence your chances of living a longer and healthier life:

- **Diet.** A landmark report by the U.S. Burden of Disease Collaborators found that, since smoking rates have declined, dietary factors—such as high intake of processed meats and low intake of fruits and vegetables—contribute to the greatest reductions in life expectancy and healthy life expectancy in the United States. (See Chapter 5.)

- **Smoking.** Smokers have an average life expectancy more than 10 years shorter than people who don't smoke. (See Chapter 12.)
- **Physical activity.** An overwhelming number of studies indicate that an active life is a longer life. A recent analysis of studies involving more than 660,000 people found that, compared to inactive people, those who performed at least 75 minutes of vigorous or 150 minutes of moderate physical activity each week had a 31% reduced risk of death. (See Chapter 7.)
- **Body weight.** The role of body weight as an independent factor in life expectancy is the subject of a great deal of controversy. Population research suggests that, compared with people who are normal weight, those who are underweight or severely obese lose an average of over 5 years of healthy life expectancy. (See Chapter 6.)
- **Alcohol consumption.** Excessive alcohol use is involved in 31 percent of

all traffic-related deaths, which killed more than 10,000 Americans in 2013. Alcohol is also a risk factor for burns, drownings, homicides, suicides, several cancers, heart disease, and liver disease. (See Chapter 11.)

**Sources:** U.S. Burden of Disease Collaborators, "The State of U.S. Health, 1990–2010: Burden of Diseases, Injuries, and Risk Factors," *Journal of the American Medical Association* 310, no. 6 (2013): 591–606; P. Jha et al., "21st Century Hazards of Smoking and Benefits of Cessation in the United States," *New England Journal of Medicine* 368 (2013): 341–50; H. Arem et al., "Leisure Time Physical Activity and Mortality: A Detailed Pooled Analysis of the Dose–Response Relationship," *JAMA Internal Medicine* 175, no. 6 (2015), 959–67; H. Jia, M. M. Zack, and W. W. Thompson, "Population-Based Estimates of Decreases in Quality-Adjusted Life Expectancy Associated with Unhealthy Body Mass Index," *Public Health Reports* 131, no. 1 (2016): 177–84; U.S. Centers for Disease Control and Prevention, "Impaired Driving: Get the Facts," November 24, 2015, www.cdc.gov/motorvehiclesafety/impaired_driving/impaired-drv_factsheet.html.

increasing issues with climate change, and superbug increases are issues that are modifiable with individual behavior change as well as systemwide changes in policies and programs.

Still other modifiable determinants include use of alcohol, caffeine, over-the-counter medications, and dietary supplements; sexual behaviors and use of contraceptives; sleep habits; and handwashing and other simple infection-control measures. We explore these and many other behaviors in later chapters. Our actions, now and in the future, can make a huge difference.

For more on how today's choices affect how long you live, and how long you live *well*, check out the **Student Health Today** box on this page.

## Biology and Genetics

Biological and genetic determinants are things you can't typically change or modify. Health experts frequently refer to these factors as *nonmodifiable determinants*. Genetically inherited traits are important nonmodifiable determinants. They include genetic disorders such as sickle-cell disease, hemophilia, and cystic fibrosis, as well as predispositions to certain conditions—such as allergies and asthma, cardiovascular disease, diabetes, and certain cancers—that are linked to specific gene variants. Although we cannot influence the structure of our genes, the emerging field of *epigenetics* is increasingly linking aspects of our diet, physical activity, and other behavioral

choices to our cells' ability to use our genes to build proteins that influence our health. In the future, research into epigenetics might help us gain more control over our genetic inheritance.

Nonmodifiable determinants also refer to certain innate characteristics, such as your age, race, ethnicity, metabolic rate, and body structure. Your sex is a key biological determinant: As compared to men, women have an increased risk for low bone density and autoimmune diseases (in which the body attacks its own cells), whereas young and middle-aged men have an increased risk for heart disease compared to young and middle-aged women. Your own history of illness and injury also classifies as biology; for instance, if you had a serious knee injury in high school, it may cause pain with walking and exercise, which in turn may predispose you to weight gain.

## Social Factors

Social factors include both the social and physical conditions in the environment in which people are born or live. Exposure to crime, violence, mass media, technology, and poverty, as well as availability of healthful foods, transportation, living wages, social support, and educational or job opportunities, are all examples. Physical conditions include the natural environment; good lighting, trees, or benches; safety of community buildings, homes, schools, and workplaces; and whether workers are exposed to unsafe conditions, such as toxic chemicals, occupational hazards, or physical barriers, exposure to which can present problems, particularly for people with disabilities or those living in persistent poverty.

**Economic Factors** Even in affluent nations such as the United States, people who are in lower socioeconomic brackets on average have substantially shorter life expectancies and more illnesses than do people who are wealthy. For example, residents of an affluent county in the southeastern United States can expect to live, on average, 12 to 14 years longer than residents of a poor county a few hundred miles away.[18] As a student, you're also likely to face economic challenges. In a recent survey, nearly 34 percent of college students reported that in the past year their finances had been "very difficult to handle."[19] Economic disadvantages exert their effects on human health within nearly all domains of life, including:

- Lacking access to quality education from early childhood through adulthood
- Living in poor housing with potential exposure to asbestos, lead, dust mites, rodents and other pests, inadequate sanitation, unsafe drinking water, and high levels of crime
- Being unable to pay for nourishing food, warm clothes, and sturdy shoes; heat and other utilities; medications and medical supplies; transportation; and counseling services, fitness classes, and other wellness measures.[22]

**The Built Environment** As the name implies, the *built environment* includes anything created or modified by human beings, including buildings, roads, recreation areas, transportation systems, electric transmission lines, and communications cables.

Researchers in public health have increasingly been promoting changes to the built environment that can improve the health of community members.[20] These include, for example, increased construction of sidewalks, "open streets" free of motor traffic, and bike paths, as well as public transit systems to which commuters typically walk or bike.[21] Some communities are enticing supermarkets to open in inner-city neighborhoods to increase residents' access to fresh fruits and vegetables.[22]

**Pollutants and Infectious Agents** Physical conditions also include the quality of the air we breathe, our land, our water, and our foods. Exposure to toxins, radiation, and infectious agents via the environment can cause widespread harm within a region and, with the rise of global travel and commerce, affect the health of people around the world. Recent outbreaks of the Ebola and Zika viruses, for example, are grim reminders of the need for a proactive international response for disease prevention and climate change.

## Access to Quality Health Services

The health of individuals and communities is also determined by access to quality health care, including not only services for physical and mental health, but also accurate and

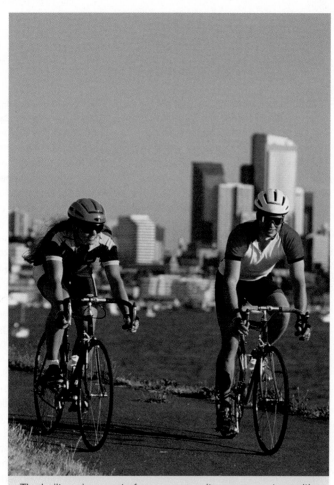

The built environment of your community can promote positive health behaviors. Wide bike paths and major thoroughfares closed to automobile traffic encourage residents to incorporate healthy physical activity into their daily lives.

relevant health information and products such as eyeglasses, medical supplies, and medications. Although the numbers of uninsured Americans fell by nearly 9 million people in 2014, the first year of enrollment under the 2010 Affordable Care Act (ACA), about 33 million are estimated to remain uninsured.[23] Nearly 8 million of these are young Americans, aged 19 to 34, and 13 million are people living in states that failed to accept federal funding to expand Medicaid (health insurance for low-income Americans).[24] Moreover, 30% of Americans who purchased plans in the ACA marketplace reported that they still lacked confidence that, if they became ill, they would be able to afford the care they needed.[25] Both individuals without health insurance and those with a high-deductible plan say they delay care. A survey conducted in the fall

# 33 MILLION
Americans are currently **WITHOUT HEALTH INSURANCE.**

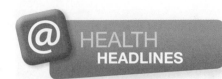
# NATIONAL HEALTH CARE REFORM

The United States saw four major political movements supporting national health insurance during the past century, but none succeeded. The Obama administration put health care reform at the top of its domestic agenda, and in March 2010, Congress passed the Patient Protection and Affordable Care Act (ACA) to provide a means for all Americans to obtain affordable health care and to encourage more Americans to seek preventive care and adopt wellness behaviors. The legislation expanded Medicaid eligibility to include more low-income Americans, provided tax credits to small businesses to help them pay for coverage for their employees, and opened an online "marketplace" in which consumers could compare insurance plans and apply for tax credits to offset the costs of care.

Young adults, aged 19 to 34, benefited most from ACA, with uninsured rates declining from 28 to 18 percent in this group. A key ACA provision allows parents to keep young adults on their existing insurance policies through age 26 if they do not have access to coverage through an employer. Because of this, more than 3 million additional 19- to 25-year-olds now have health insurance. In addition, because individuals can no longer be denied coverage for a preexisting condition, the 1 in 6 young adults who have a chronic illness such as cancer, diabetes, or asthma now are guaranteed coverage.

One of the most contentious aspects of the ACA is the so-called individual mandate: All Americans are required to carry health insurance or pay an annual penalty if they fail to do so. The individual mandate is necessary to push young, healthy Americans into the insurance pool and thereby dilute the cost of care overall. Incidentally, coverage under your college's student health plan typically qualifies under the health care law. Although opponents argued that compelling individuals to purchase health insurance was an overreach by the federal government, in June 2012, the U.S. Supreme Court ruled that Congress could enact the ACA under its authority to raise and collect taxes.

Another provision of the ACA requires insurers to cover certain preventive screenings such as blood pressure screenings for all adults and cervical cancer screenings for women; recommended vaccinations; approved contraceptives; smoking cessation programs for smokers; and many other services. Other provisions ban or place restrictions on certain insurance industry practices such as:

- Insurers are not allowed to cancel coverage because the insured made an honest mistake on his or her application.
- Insurers have to publicly justify rate hikes of 10 percent or more and must spend at least 80 percent of premiums on health care as opposed to administration, marketing, etc.
- New health insurance plans cannot impose annual or lifetime coverage limits.

You can find more information and updates on health care reform at www.healthcare.gov.

**Sources:** United States Department of Health and Human Services, "Affordable Care Act: About the Law," August 2015, www.hhs.gov/healthcare/about-the-law; S. Collins, P. Rasmussen, and M. Doty, "Gaining Ground: America's Health Insurance Coverage and Access to Care After the Affordable Care Act's First Open Enrollment Period-2014," Accessed March 2016, www.commonwealthfund.org/publications/issue-briefs/2014/jul/health-coverage-access-aca.

---

of 2014 found that 40% of Americans with a high-deductible plan had delayed needed care because of the deductible.[26]

In addition to the uninsured is the problem of the millions of "underinsured"—those who have some coverage, but not enough. These individuals cannot afford to pay the difference between what their insurance covers and what their providers and medications cost. Therefore, like the uninsured, they tend to delay care or try other cost-saving measures such as taking only half of the prescribed dose of their medications.

## Policymaking

Public policies and interventions can have a powerful and positive effect on the health of individuals and communities. Examples include policies banning tobacco sale to minors or smoking in public places, laws mandating seatbelt use in motor vehicles and helmets for bikes and motorcycles, policies that require you be vaccinated before enrolling in classes, and laws that ban cell phone use while driving. Health policies serve a key role in protecting public health and motivating individuals and communities to change, particularly when there are rewards and penalties for sticking to the policies.

Access to health services is also affected by policymaking—including health insurance legislation. As just noted, implementation of the 2010 ACA has begun to increase Americans' access to quality care. The ACA is discussed in the **Health Headlines** box on this page.

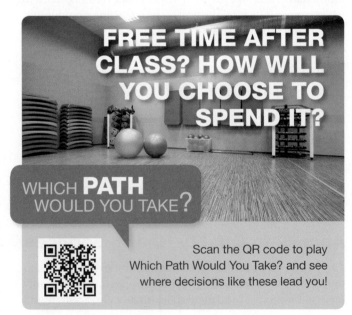

FREE TIME AFTER CLASS? HOW WILL YOU CHOOSE TO SPEND IT?

WHICH **PATH** WOULD YOU TAKE?

Scan the QR code to play Which Path Would You Take? and see where decisions like these lead you!

## LO 4 | HOW DOES BEHAVIOR CHANGE OCCUR?

Compare and contrast the health belief model, the social-cognitive model, and the transtheoretical model of behavior change, and explain how you might use them in making a specific behavior change.

While many factors influence your health status, you have the most control over factors in just one category: your individual behaviors. Over the years, social scientists and public health researchers have developed a variety of models to illustrate how individual behavior change occurs. We explore three of those here.

### Health Belief Model

We often assume that when rational people realize their behaviors put them at risk, they will change those behaviors and reduce that risk. However, it doesn't work that way for many of us. Consider the number of health professionals who smoke, consume junk food, and act in other unhealthy ways. They surely know better, but their "knowing" is disconnected from their "doing." One classic model of behavior change proposes that our beliefs may help to explain why this occurs.

A **belief** is an appraisal of the relationship between some object, action, or idea (e.g., smoking) and some attribute of that object, action, or idea (e.g., "Smoking is expensive, dirty, and causes cancer" or "Smoking is sociable and relaxing"). Psychologists studying the relationship between beliefs and health behaviors have determined that although beliefs may subtly influence behavior, they may or may not cause people to behave differently. In the 1950s, social psychologist Irwin M. Rosenstock and colleagues developed a classic theory, the **health belief model (HBM)**, to show when beliefs affect behavior change.[27] The HBM holds that several factors must support a belief before change is likely:

- **Perceived seriousness of the health problem.** The more serious the perceived effects are, the more likely it is that action will be taken.
- **Perceived susceptibility to the health problem.** People who perceive themselves at high risk are more likely to take preventive action.
- **Perceived benefits.** People are more likely to take action if they believe that this action will benefit them.
- **Perceived barriers.** Even if a recommended action is perceived to be effective, the individual may believe it is too expensive, difficult, inconvenient, or time-consuming. These perceived barriers must be overcome or acknowledged as less important than the perceived benefits.
- **Cues to action.** A person who is reminded or alerted about a potential health problem—by anything from early symptoms to an e-mail from a health care provider—is more likely to take action.

People follow the HBM every day. Take the example of smoking. Older people are likely to know smokers who have developed serious heart or lung disease and are thus more likely to

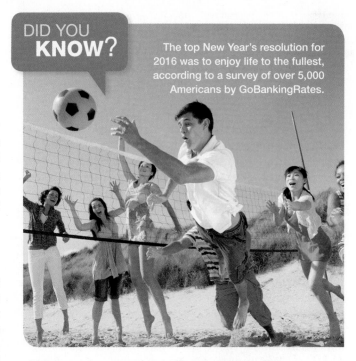

perceive tobacco as a threat to their health than are teenagers. The greater the perceived threat of health problems caused by smoking, the greater the chance a person will avoid it.

However, many chronic smokers know the risks, yet continue to smoke. Why? According to Rosenstock, some people do not believe they are susceptible to a severe problem—they act as though they are immune to it—and are unlikely to change their behavior. They also may feel that the immediate pleasure outweighs the long-range cost.

### Social-Cognitive Model

The **social-cognitive model (SCM)** developed from the work of several researchers over decades, but it is most closely associated with the work of psychologist Albert Bandura.[28] Fundamentally, the model proposes that three factors interact in a reciprocal fashion to promote and motivate change. These are the social environment in which we live, our thoughts or cognition (including our values, perceptions, beliefs, expectations, and sense of self-efficacy), and our behaviors. We change our behavior in part by observing models in our environments—from childhood to the present moment—reflecting on our observations, and regulating ourselves accordingly.

For instance, if we observe a family member successfully quitting smoking, we are more apt to believe we can do it, too. In addition, when we succeed in changing ourselves, we change our thoughts about ourselves, and this in turn may promote further behavior change. For instance, after we've successfully quit smoking, we may feel empowered to increase our

> **belief** Appraisal of the relationship between some object, action, or idea and some attribute of that object, action, or idea.
>
> **health belief model (HBM)** Model for explaining how beliefs may influence behaviors.
>
> **social-cognitive model (SCM)** Model of behavior change emphasizing the role of social factors and thought processes (cognition) in behavior change.

**transtheoretical model** Model of behavior change that identifies six distinct stages people go through in altering behavior patterns; also called the *stages-of-change model.*

level of physical activity. Moreover, as we change ourselves, we become a model for others to observe. Thus, we are not just products of our environments, but producers.

The SCM is often used to design health promotion programs. For example, one public health program engaged overweight and obese men in a program of goal setting, reward setting, journaling, and social support to improve their eating and activity patterns.[29] Another recent study designed according to the SCM increased condom use in participants who viewed a video of someone modeling self-efficacy and consideration of partner expectations.[30]

## Transtheoretical Model

Why do so many New Year's resolutions fail before Valentine's Day? According to Drs. James Prochaska and Carlos DiClemente, it's because most of us aren't really prepared to take action. Their research indicates that behavior changes usually do not succeed if they start with the change itself. Instead, we must go through a series of stages to adequately prepare ourselves for that eventual change.[31] According to Prochaska and DiClemente's **transtheoretical model** of behavior change (also called the *stages-of-change model*), our chances of keeping those New Year's resolutions will be greatly enhanced if we have proper reinforcement and help during each of the following stages:

1. **Precontemplation.** People in the precontemplation stage have no current intention of changing. They may have tried to change a behavior before and given up, or they may be in denial and unaware of any problem.

2. **Contemplation.** In this phase, people recognize that they have a problem and begin to contemplate the need to change. Despite this acknowledgment, people can languish in this stage for years, realizing that they have a problem but lacking the time or energy to make the change.

3. **Preparation.** Most people at this point are close to taking action. They've thought about what they might do and may even have come up with a plan.

4. **Action.** In this stage, people begin to follow their action plans. Those who have prepared for change appropriately and made a plan of action are more ready for action than are those who have given it little thought.

5. **Maintenance.** During the maintenance stage, a person continues the actions begun in the action stage and works toward making these changes a permanent part of his or her life. In this stage, it is important to be aware of the potential for relapses and to develop strategies for dealing with such challenges.

6. **Termination.** By this point, the behavior is so ingrained that constant vigilance may be unnecessary. The new behavior has become an essential part of daily living.

We don't necessarily go through these stages sequentially. They may overlap, or we may shuttle back and forth from one to another—say, contemplation to preparation, then back to contemplation—for a while before we become truly

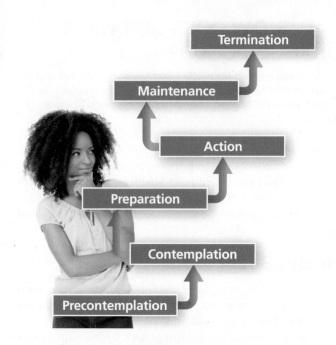

**FIGURE 1.7 Transtheoretical Model** People don't move through the transtheoretical model stages in sequence. We may make progress in more than one stage at one time, or we may shuttle back and forth from one to another—say, contemplation to preparation, then back to contemplation—before we succeed in making a change.

committed to making the change (**FIGURE 1.7**). Still, it's useful to recognize "where we are" with a change, so that we can consider the appropriate strategies to move us forward.

## LO 5 | HOW CAN YOU IMPROVE YOUR HEALTH BEHAVIORS?

Identify your own current risk behaviors, the factors that influence those behaviors, and the strategies you can use to change them.

Clearly, change is not always easy and multiple factors may converge to hinder your progress. To successfully change a behavior, you need to see change not as a singular *event* but instead as a *process* by which you substitute positive patterns for new ones—a process that requires preparation, has several stages, and takes time to occur. The following four-step plan integrates ideas from each of the above behavior change models into a simple guide to help you move forward.

## Step One: Increase Your Awareness

Before you can decide what you might want to change, you need to learn what researchers know about the behaviors that contribute to and detract from your health. Each

**SEE IT! VIDEOS**
How can you change your habits and stick with it? Watch **New Year's Resolutions**, available on MasteringHealth.™

chapter in this book provides a foundation of information focused on these factors. Check out the Table of Contents at the front of the book to locate chapters with the information you're looking for.

This is also a good time to take stock of the health determinants in your life: What aspects of your biology and behavior support your health, and which are obstacles to overcome? What elements of your social and physical environment could you tap into to help you change, and what elements might hold you back? Making a list of the health determinants that affect you—both positively and negatively—should greatly increase your understanding of what you might want to change and what you might need to do to make that change happen.

## Step Two: Contemplate Change

Once you've increased your awareness of the behaviors that contribute to wellness and the health determinants affecting you, you may find yourself contemplating change. In this stage, the following strategies may be helpful.

### Examine Your Current Health Habits and Patterns

Do you routinely stop at Dunkin' Donuts for breakfast? Smoke when you're feeling stressed? Party too much on the weekends? Get to bed way past 2:00 A.M.? When considering behavior you may want to change, ask yourself the following:

- How long has this behavior existed, and how frequently do I do it?
- How serious are the long- and short-term consequences of the habit or pattern?
- What are some of your reasons for continuing this problematic behavior?
- What kinds of situations trigger the behavior?
- Are other people involved in this behavior? If so, how?

Health behaviors involve elements of personal choice, but they are also influenced by other determinants. Some are *predisposing factors*—for instance, if your parents smoke, you're more likely to start smoking than someone whose parents don't smoke.

Some are *enabling factors*—for example, peers who smoke enable one another's smoking. Identifying the factors that encourage or discourage a habit is part of contemplating behavior change.

Various *reinforcing factors* can support or undermine your effort to change. If you decide to stop smoking, but your family and friends all smoke, then you may lose your resolve. In such cases, it can be helpful to employ the social-cognitive model

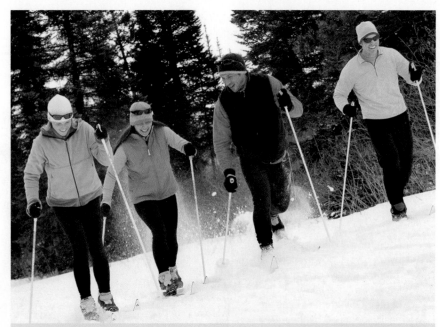

Many people find it easiest to stay motivated by planning small incremental changes, working toward a goal, and rewarding themselves along the way. Friends can also help you stay motivated by modeling healthy behaviors, offering support, joining you in your change efforts, and providing reinforcement.

and deliberately change aspects of your social environment. For instance, you could spend more time with nonsmoking friends to give yourself a chance to observe people modeling the positive behavior you want to emulate.

### Identify a Target Behavior

To clarify your thinking about the various behaviors you might like to target, ask yourself these questions:

- **What do I want?** Is your ultimate goal to lose weight? To exercise more? To reduce stress? To have a lasting relationship? You need a clear picture of your target outcome.
- **Which change is the greatest priority at this time?** Rather than saying, "I need to eat less *and* start exercising," identify one specific behavior that contributes significantly to your greatest problem, and tackle that first.
- **Why is this important to me?** Think through why you want to change. Are you doing it because of your health? To improve your academic performance? To look better? To win someone else's approval? It's best to target a behavior because it's right for you rather than because you think it will help you win others' approval.

### Learn More about the Target Behavior

Once you've clarified exactly what behavior you'd like to change, you're ready to learn more about that behavior. This text will help, and this is a great time to learn how to gain access to accurate and reliable health information on the Internet (see the **Tech & Health** box on page 16).

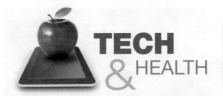

# TECH & HEALTH | SURFING FOR THE LATEST IN HEALTH

The Internet can be a wonderful resource for quickly finding answers to your questions, but it can also be a source of much *misinformation*. To ensure that the sites you visit are reliable and trustworthy, follow these tips.

- Look for websites sponsored by an official government agency, a university or college, or a hospital/medical center. Government sites are easily identified by their *.gov* extensions, college and university sites typically have *.edu* extensions, and many hospitals have an *.org* extension (e.g., the Mayo Clinic's website is www.mayoclinic.org). Major philanthropic foundations, such as the Robert Wood Johnson Foundation, the Kellogg Foundation, and others, often provide information about selected health topics. In addition, national nonprofit organizations, such as the American Heart Association and the American Cancer Society, are often good, authoritative sources of information. Foundations and nonprofits usually have URLs ending with an *.org* extension.
- Search for well-established, professionally peer-reviewed journals such as the *New England Journal of Medicine*

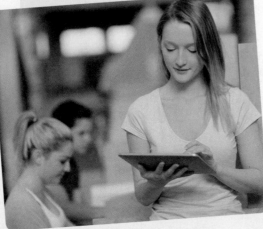

**Find reliable health information at your fingertips!**

(http://content.nejm.org) or the *Journal of the American Medical Association* (*JAMA*; http://jama.ama-assn.org). Although some of these sites require a fee for access, you can often locate concise abstracts and information that can help you conduct a search. Your college may make these journals available to students for no cost.
- Consult the Centers for Disease Control and Prevention (www.cdc.gov) for consumer news, updates, and alerts.
- For a global perspective on health issues, visit the World Health Organization website (www.who.int/en).

- Other sites offering reliable health information include:

  For College Women: www.4collegewomen.org
  Young Men's Health: www.youngmenshealthsite.org
  MedlinePlus: www.nlm.nih.gov/medlineplus
  Go Ask Alice!: www.goaskalice.columbia.edu

- The nonprofit health care accrediting organization Utilization Accreditation Review Commission (URAC; www.urac.org) has devised more than 50 criteria that health sites must satisfy to display its seal. Look for the "URAC Accredited Health Web Site" seal on websites you visit.
- Finally, gather information from two or more reliable sources to see whether facts and figures are consistent. Avoid websites that try to sell you something, whether products like dietary supplements or services such as medical testing. When in doubt, check with your own health care provider, health education professor, or state health division website.

---

**motivation** A social, cognitive, and emotional force that directs human behavior.

As you conduct your research, don't limit your focus to the behavior and its health effects. Learn all you can about aspects of your world that might support or pose obstacles to your success. For instance, let's say you decide you want to meditate for 15 minutes a day. Are there others in your dorm or neighborhood who might be interested in meditating with you? What about classes or a meditation group? On the other hand, do you live in a super-noisy dorm? Are you afraid your friends might think meditating is weird? In short, learn everything you can about your target behavior now, and you'll be better prepared for change.

**Assess Your Motivation and Your Readiness to Change** Wanting to change is an essential prerequisite of the change process, but to achieve change, you need more than desire. You need real **motivation**, which isn't just a feeling, but a social and cognitive force that directs your behavior. To understand what goes into motivation, let's return for a moment to two models of change discussed earlier: the health belief model and the social-cognitive model.

Remember that, according to the HBM, your beliefs affect your ability to change. For example, when reaching for another cigarette, smokers sometimes tell themselves, "I'll stop tomorrow," or "They'll have a cure for lung cancer before I get it."

These beliefs allow them to continue what they're doing. To put it another way, they dampen motivation. As you contemplate change, consider whether your beliefs are likely to motivate you to achieve lasting change. Ask yourself the following:

- Do you believe that your current pattern could lead to a serious problem? The more severe the consequences are, the more motivated you'll be to change the behavior. For example, smoking can cause cancer, emphysema, and other deadly diseases. The fear of developing those diseases can help you stop smoking. But what if cancer and emphysema were just words to you? In that case, you could research the tissue destruction, pain, loss of function, and emotional suffering they cause. Doing so might increase your motivation: In Canada, a law requires that graphic images of gangrenous limbs, diseased organs, and chests sawed open for autopsy cover at least half of cigarette packages. Researchers estimate that this graphic labeling has reduced smoking rates in Canada by 2.9 to 4.7 percent, cutting the total number of smokers by at least one-eighth.[32]
- Do you believe that you are personally likely to experience the consequences of your behavior? For example, losing a loved one to lung cancer could motivate you to work harder to stop smoking. If you can't convince yourself that your behavior will affect you personally, try employing the social-cognitive model to help change your beliefs and gain some motivation. For instance, you could interview people struggling with the consequences of the behavior you want to change. Ask them what their life is like, and if, when they were engaging in the behavior, they believed that it would harm them. Your health care provider may be able to put you in touch with patients who would be happy to support your behavior change plan in this way. And don't ignore the motivating potential of positive role models.

Even though motivation is powerful, by itself it's not enough to achieve change. Motivation has to be combined with common sense, commitment, and a realistic understanding of how best to move from point A to point B. *Readiness* is the state of being that precedes behavior change. People who are ready to change possess the knowledge, skills, and external and internal resources that make change possible.

## Develop Self-Efficacy
One of the most important factors influencing health status is **self-efficacy**, an individual's belief that he or she is capable of achieving certain goals or of performing at a level that may influence events in life. In general, people who exhibit high self-efficacy approach challenges confident that they can succeed. In turn, they may be more motivated to change and more likely to succeed. Prior success will lead to expectations of success in the future. In short, take small steps, experience success, and build on it!

Conversely, someone with low self-efficacy may give up easily or never even try to change a behavior. These people may have failed before, and when the going gets tough, they are more likely to revert to old patterns of behavior. A number of methods for developing self-efficacy follow.

## Cultivate an Internal Locus of Control
The conviction that you have the power and ability to change is a powerful motivator. People who have a strong *internal* **locus of control** believe that they have power over their own actions. They are more driven by their own thoughts and are more likely to state their opinions and be true to their own beliefs. In contrast, people who believe that external circumstances largely control their situation have an *external* locus of control. They may easily succumb to feelings of anxiety and disempowerment and give up. For example, a recent study among cancer patients found that, compared to those with a high internal locus of control, people with an external locus of control were more likely to perceive their cancer as a threat they felt unable to manage, and to respond with depression to their diagnosis.[33]

Having an internal or external locus of control can vary according to circumstance. For instance, someone who learns that diabetes runs in his family may resign himself to facing the disease one day instead of taking an active role in modifying his lifestyle to minimize his risk of developing diabetes. On this front, he would be demonstrating an external locus of control. However, the same individual might exhibit an internal locus of control when resisting a friend's pressure to smoke.

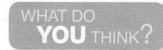

**WHAT DO YOU THINK?**

Do you have an internal or an external locus of control?

- Can you think of some friends whom you would describe as more internally or externally controlled?
- How do people with the different views deal with similar situations?

## Step Three: Prepare for Change

You've contemplated change for long enough! Now it's time to set a realistic goal, anticipate barriers, reach out to others, and commit. Here's how.

## Set SMART Goals
Unsuccessful goals are vague and open-ended: for instance, "Get into shape by exercising more." In contrast, SMART goals are:

- **Specific.** "Attend a Tuesday/Thursday aerobics class at the YMCA."
- **Measurable.** "Reduce my alcohol intake on Saturday nights from three drinks to two."
- **Action oriented.** "Volunteer at the animal shelter on Friday afternoons."
- **Realistic.** "Increase my daily walk from 15 to 20 minutes."
- **Time oriented.** "Stay in my strength-training class for the full 10-week session, then reassess."

Knowing that your SMART goals are attainable—that you can achieve them within the

**self-efficacy** Belief in one's ability to perform a task successfully.

**locus of control** The location, *external* (outside oneself) or *internal* (within oneself), that an individual perceives as the source and underlying cause of events in his or her life.

current circumstances of your life—increases your motivation. This, in turn, leads to a better chance of success and to a greater sense of self-efficacy—which can motivate you to succeed even more.

**Use Shaping** A stepwise process of making a series of small changes known as **shaping** can help you achieve your goal. Suppose you want to start jogging 3 miles every other day, but right now you get tired after half a mile. Shaping would dictate a process of slow, progressive steps, such as walking 1 hour every other day at a relaxed pace for the first week; at a faster pace the second week; and speeding up to a slow jog the third week.

Regardless of the change you plan, remember that current habits didn't develop overnight, and they won't change overnight, either. Start slowly to avoid hurting yourself. Master one small step before moving on to the next. Be flexible and willing to change the original plan if it proves too uncomfortable.

**Anticipate Barriers to Change** Recognizing possible stumbling blocks in advance will help you prepare fully for change. In addition to negative social determinants, aspects of the built environment, or lack of adequate health care, a few general barriers to change include:

- **Overambitious goals.** Remember the advice to set realistic goals? Even with the strongest motivation, overambitious goals can derail change. Habits are best changed one small step at a time.
- **Self-defeating beliefs and attitudes.** As the health belief model explains, believing you're too immune to the consequences of a bad habit can keep you from making a solid commitment to change. Likewise, thinking you are helpless to change your habits can also undermine efforts.
- **Failure to accurately assess your current state of wellness.** You might assume that you will be able to walk 2 miles to campus each morning, for example, only to discover that you're winded after 1 mile. Make sure that the planned change is realistic for *you*.
- **Lack of support and guidance.** If you want to cut down on your drinking, socializing with peers who drink heavily

To reach your behavior change goals, you need to take things one step at a time.

may be a powerful barrier to that change. To succeed, you need to recognize and limit interactions with people in your life who might oppose your decision to change.

- **Emotions that sabotage your efforts and sap your will.** Sometimes the best-laid plans go awry because you're having a bad day or are fighting with someone. Emotional reactions to life's challenges are normal, but don't let them derail your efforts to change. If you're experiencing severe psychological distress, seek counseling to help you address the underlying issues before trying to change other aspects of your health.

**Enlist Others as Change Agents** The social-cognitive model recognizes the importance of our social contacts in successful change. Most of us are highly influenced by the approval or disapproval (real or imagined) of others. In addition, **modeling**, or learning from role models, is a key component of the social-cognitive model of change. Observing a friend who is a good conversationalist, for example, can help you improve your communication skills. Change agents commonly include the following:

- **Family members.** From the time of your birth, your parents and other family members have influenced your food choices, activity patterns, and many other behaviors and values. Positive family units provide care and protection, are dedicated to the development of all family members, and work together to solve problems. If loving family members are not available to support your efforts to change, you'll need to turn to friends and professionals.
- **Friends.** As you leave childhood behind, your friends increasingly influence your behaviors. If your friends offer encouragement, or even express interest in joining with you in the behavior change, you are more likely to remain motivated. Thus, friends who share your personal values can greatly support your behavior change.
- **Professionals.** Consider enlisting support from professionals such as your health or PE instructor, coach, or health care provider. As appropriate, consider the counseling services offered on campus, as well as community services such as smoking cessation programs, support groups, and your local YMCA.

**Sign a Contract** It's time to get it in writing! A formal *behavior change contract* serves many powerful purposes. It functions as a promise to yourself and as an organized plan

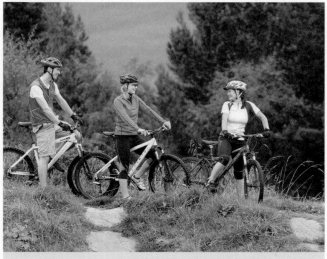

How do other people influence my health behaviors?

that lays out your goals, start and end dates, daily actions, and any barriers you anticipate. It's also a place to brainstorm strategies, list sources of support, and remind yourself of the benefits of sticking with the program. To get started, fill out the **Behavior Change Contract** at the back of this book. **FIGURE 1.8** shows an example of a completed contract.

## Step Four: Take Action to Change

As you begin to put your plan into action, the following behavior change strategies can help.

**Behavior Change Contract**

My behavior change will be:
To snack less on junk food and more on healthy foods.

My long-term goal for this behavior change is:
Eat junk food snacks no more than once a week

These are three obstacles to change (things that I am currently doing or situations that contribute to this behavior or make it harder to change):
1. The grocery store is closed by the time I come home from school.
2. I get hungry between classes, and the vending machines only carry candy bars.
3. It's easier to order pizza or other snacks than to make a snack at home.

The strategies I will use to overcome these obstacles are:
1. I'll leave early for school once a week so I can stock up on healthy snacks in the morning.
2. I'll bring a piece of fruit or other healthy snack to eat between classes.
3. I'll learn some easy recipes for snacks to make at home.

Resources I will use to help me change this behavior include:
a friend/partner/relative: my roommates. I'll ask them to buy healthier snacks instead of chips when they do the shopping.
a school-based resource: The dining hall. I'll ask the manager to provide healthy foods we can take to eat between classes.
a community-based resource: The library. I'll check out some cookbooks to find easy snack ideas.
a book or reputable website: The USDA nutrient database at www.ars.usda.gov. I'll use this site to make sure the foods I select are healthy choices.

In order to make my goal more attainable, I have devised these short-term goals:
short-term goal Eat a healthy snack 3 times per week    target date September 15    reward new CD
short-term goal Learn to make a healthy snack    target date October 15    reward concert tickets
short-term goal Eat a healthy snack 5 times per week    target date November 15    reward new shoes

When I make the long-term behavior change described above, my reward will be:
ski lift tickets for winter break    target date: December 15

I intend to make the behavior change described above. I will use the strategies and rewards to achieve the goals that will contribute to a healthy behavior change.

Signed: Elizabeth King    Witness: Susan Bauer

**FIGURE 1.8 Example of a Completed Behavior Change Contract**
A blank version is included in the back of the book for you to fill out.

**Visualize New Behavior** Athletes and artists often use a technique known as **imagined rehearsal** to reach their goals. Careful mental and verbal rehearsal of how you intend to act will help you anticipate problems and greatly improve your chances of success.

**Learn to "Counter"** **Countering** means substituting a desired behavior for an undesirable one. If you want to stop eating junk food, for example, compile a list of substitute foods and places to get them and have this ready before your mouth starts to water at the smell of a burger and fries.

**Control the Situation** Any behavior has both antecedents and consequences. *Antecedents* are the aspects of the situation that come beforehand; these cue or stimulate a person to act in certain ways. *Consequences*—the results of behavior—affect whether a person will repeat that action. Both antecedents and consequences can be physical events, thoughts, emotions, or the actions of other people.

Once you recognize the antecedents of a given behavior, you can employ **situational inducement** to modify those that are working against you—you can seek settings, people, and circumstances that support your efforts to change, as well as avoid those likely to derail your change.

**Change Your Self-Talk** There is a close connection between what people say to themselves, known as **self-talk**, and how they feel. According to psychologist Albert Ellis, most emotional problems and related behaviors stem from irrational statements that people make to themselves when events in their lives are different from what they would like them to be.[34]

For example, suppose that after doing poorly on a test you say to yourself, "I can't believe I flunked that easy exam. I'm so stupid." Now change this irrational, negative self-talk into rational, positive statements about what is really going on: "I really didn't study enough for that exam. I'm certainly not stupid; I just need to prepare better for the next test." Rational self-talk will help you recover more quickly from disappointment and take positive steps to correct the situation.

Another technique for changing self-talk is to practice blocking and stopping. For example, suppose you are preoccupied with thoughts of your ex-partner, who has recently left you for someone else. You can block those thoughts by focusing on the actions

**imagined rehearsal** Practicing, through mental imagery, to become better able to perform a task in actuality.

**countering** Substituting a desired behavior for an undesirable one.

**situational inducement** Attempts to influence a behavior through situations and occasions that are structured to exert control over that behavior.

**self-talk** The customary manner of thinking and talking to yourself, which can affect your self-image.

you're taking right now to help you move forward. The nearby Making Changes Today box offers more strategies for changing self-talk.

**Reward Yourself** Another way to promote positive behavior change is to reward yourself for it. This is called **positive reinforcement**. Each of us is motivated by different reinforcers, which may motivate or incentivize us to change. Common reinforcers include:

- *Consumable reinforcers* are edible items, such as your favorite snack.
- *Activity reinforcers* are opportunities to do something enjoyable, such as going on a hike or taking a trip.
- *Manipulative reinforcers* are incentives such as the promise of a better grade for doing an extra-credit project.
- *Possessional reinforcers* are tangible rewards, such as a new electronic gadget.
- *Social reinforcers* are signs of appreciation, approval, or love, such as affectionate hugs and praise.

## WHAT DO YOU THINK?

What type of reinforcers would most likely get you to change a behavior: money, praise, or recognition from someone?

- Why would it motivate you?
- Can you think of options to reinforce behavior changes?

The difficulty with employing positive reinforcement often lies in determining which incentive will be most effective. Your reinforcers may initially come from others (*extrinsic* rewards), but as you see positive changes in yourself, you will begin to reward and reinforce yourself (*intrinsic* rewards).

Keep in mind that reinforcers should immediately follow a behavior, but beware of overkill. If you reward yourself with a movie every time you go jogging, this reinforcer will soon lose its power. It would be better to give yourself this reward after, say, a full week of adherence to your jogging program.

**Journal** Writing personal experiences, interpretations, and results in a journal, notebook, or blog is an important skill for behavior change. You can log your daily activities, monitor your progress, record how you feel about it, and note ideas for improvement.

**Deal with Relapse** **Relapse** is often defined as a return of symptoms in a person thought to have been successfully treated for a serious disease. But relapse can also be defined as a return to a previous pattern of negative behavior (drinking, binge eating, etc.) after a period of time successfully avoiding that behavior. For example, an estimated 40 to 60 percent of people recovering from a substance abuse disorder suffer a relapse.[35] It doesn't mean that your program of change is a failure; behavior change is a process, and setbacks are part of learning to change.

**positive reinforcement** Presenting something positive following a behavior that is being reinforced.

**relapse** A return to a previous pattern of negative behavior after a period of time successfully avoiding that behavior.

## MAKING CHANGES TODAY

### Challenge the Thoughts That Sabotage Change

Are any of the following thoughts holding you back? If so, challenge them with the strategies below:

- **"I don't have enough time!"** Chart your hourly activities for 1 day. What are your highest priorities and what can you eliminate? Plan to make time for a healthy change next week.

- **"I'm too stressed!"** Assess your major stressors right now. List those you can control and those you can change or avoid. Then identify two things you enjoy that can help you reduce stress now.

- **"I'm worried about what others may think."** Ask yourself how much others influence your decisions about drinking, sex, eating habits, and the like. What is most important to you? What actions can you take to act in line with these values?

- **"I don't think I can do it."** Just because you haven't done something before doesn't mean you can't do it now. To develop some confidence, take baby steps and break tasks into small segments of time.

- **"I can't break this habit!"** Habits are difficult to break, but not impossible. What triggers your behavior? List ways you can avoid these triggers. Ask for support from friends and family.

A few simple strategies can help you get back on track after a relapse. First, figure out what went wrong. Every relapse begins with a slip—a one-time mistake.[36] What triggered that slip, and how can you modify your personal choices or the aspects of your environment that contributed to it? Second, use countering: If you've been overeating ever since your relationship ended, identify and choose other behaviors that comfort you. Third, a relapse might be telling you that you need some assistance with making this change; consider getting some professional help.

## Let's Get Started!

After you acquire the skills to support successful behavior change, you're ready to apply those skills to your target behavior. Place your behavior change contract where you will see it every day and where you can refer to it as you work through the chapters in this text. Consider it a visual reminder that change doesn't "just happen." Reviewing your contract helps you to stay alert to potential problems, consider your alternatives, and stick to your goals under pressure.

# STUDY **PLAN**

Customize your study plan—and master your health!—in the Study Area of **MasteringHealth**.

## ASSESS YOURSELF

**How healthy are you?** Want to find out?
Take the **How Healthy Are You?** assessment available on

**MasteringHealth.**™

## CHAPTER **REVIEW**

To hear an MP3 Tutor Session, scan here or visit the Study Area in **MasteringHealth**.

### LO 1 | Why Health, Why Now?

- Choosing good health has immediate benefits, such as reducing the risk of injury and illnesses and improving academic performance; long-term rewards, such as disease prevention, longevity, and improved quality of life; and societal and global benefits, such as reducing the global disease burden.
- For the U.S. population as a whole, the leading causes of death are heart disease, cancer, and chronic lower respiratory diseases. In the 15- to 24-year-old age group, the leading causes are unintentional injuries, suicide, and homicide.
- The average life expectancy at birth in the United States is 78.8 years. This has increased greatly over the past century; however, unhealthy behaviors related to chronic disease may prevent further increases in total life expectancy and cause a reduction in *healthy* life expectancy.

### LO 2 | What Is Health?

- The definition of *health* has changed over time. The medical model focused on treating disease, whereas the current ecological or public health model focuses on factors contributing to health, disease prevention, and health promotion.
- Health can be seen as existing on a continuum and encompassing the dynamic process of fulfilling one's potential in the physical, social, intellectual, emotional, spiritual, and environmental dimensions of life. Wellness means achieving the highest level of health possible in each of the health dimensions.

### LO 3 | What Influences Your Health?

- Health is influenced by factors called *determinants*. The Surgeon General's health promotion plan, *Healthy People*, classifies determinants as individual behavior, biology and genetics, social factors, policy-making, and health services. Disparities in health among different groups contribute to increased risks.

### LO 4 | How Does Behavior Change Occur?

- Models of behavior change include the health belief model, the social-cognitive model, and the transtheoretical (stages-of-change) model. A person can increase the chance of successfully changing a health-related behavior by viewing change as a process involving several steps and components.

### LO 5 | How Can You Improve Your Health Behaviors?

- When contemplating a behavior change, it is helpful to examine current habits; learn about a target behavior; and assess motivation and readiness to change. Developing self-efficacy and an internal locus of control are essential for maintaining motivation. When preparing to change, it is helpful to set SMART goals that employ shaping; anticipate barriers to change; enlist the help and support of others; and sign a behavior change contract. When taking action to change, it is helpful to visualize new behavior; practice countering; control the situation; change self-talk; reward oneself; and keep a log, blog, or journal.

## POP **QUIZ**

Visit **MasteringHealth** to personalize your study plan with Chapter Review Quizzes and Dynamic Study Modules.

### LO 1 | Why Health, Why Now?

1. What term is used to describe the expected number of years of full health remaining at a given age, such as at birth?
   a. Healthy lifespan
   b. Healthy life expectancy
   c. Health-related quality of life
   d. Wellness

## LO 2 | What Is Health?

2. Everyday tasks, such as walking up the stairs or tying your shoes, are known as
   a. dimensions of health.
   b. healthy life tasks.
   c. physical determinants.
   d. activities of daily living.

3. Janice describes herself as confident and trusting, and she displays both high self-esteem and high self-efficacy. The dimension of health this relates to is the
   a. social dimension.
   b. emotional dimension.
   c. spiritual dimension.
   d. intellectual dimension.

## LO 3 | What Influences Your Health?

4. *Healthy People 2020* is a(n)
   a. blueprint for improving the quality and years of life for all Americans.
   b. projection for life expectancy rates in the United States in the year 2020.
   c. international plan for achieving health priorities for the environment by the year 2020.
   d. set of health-related goals that states must achieve in order to receive federal funding for health care.

## LO 4 | How Does Behavior Change Occur?

5. The social-cognitive model of behavior change suggests that
   a. understanding the seriousness of and our susceptibility to a health problem motivates change.
   b. contemplation is an essential step to adequately prepare ourselves for change.
   c. behavior change usually does not succeed if it begins with action.
   d. the environment in which we live—from childhood to the present—influences change.

6. According to the transtheoretical model of behavior change, which of the following occurs during the preparation stage?
   a. The person recognizes that a health problem exists.
   b. The person identifies steps they might take to improve their health.
   c. The person takes initial actions toward a goal.
   d. The person works to maintain positive changes.

## LO 5 | How Can You Improve Your Health Behaviors?

7. Suppose you want to lose 20 pounds. To reach your goal, you take small steps. You start by joining a support group and counting calories. After 2 weeks, you begin an exercise program and gradually build up to your desired fitness level. What behavior change strategy are you using?
   a. Shaping
   b. Visualization
   c. Modeling
   d. Reinforcement

8. After Kirk and Tammy pay their bills, they reward themselves by watching TV together. The type of positive reinforcement that motivates them to pay their bills is a(n)
   a. activity reinforcer.
   b. consumable reinforcer.
   c. manipulative reinforcer.
   d. possessional reinforcer.

9. Jake is exhibiting *self-efficacy* when he
   a. believes that he is solely responsible for his shoulder injury.
   b. is doubtful that his injured shoulder will ever allow him to bench-press 125 pounds.
   c. believes that he can and will be able to heal from his shoulder injury and bench-press 125 pounds within 1 year.
   d. believes that he does not possess personal control over this situation.

10. The aspects of a situation that cue or stimulate a person to act in certain ways are called
    a. situational reinforcers
    b. antecedents.
    c. consequences.
    d. cues to action.

*Answers to the Pop Quiz can be found on page A-1. If you answered a question incorrectly, review the section identified by the Learning Outcome. For even more study tools, visit* **MasteringHealth**.

# THINK ABOUT IT!

## LO 1 | Why Health, Why Now?

1. How healthy is the U.S. population today? What factors influence today's disparities in health?

## LO 2 | What Is Health?

2. How are the words *health* and *wellness* similar? What, if any, are important distinctions between these terms? What is health promotion? Disease prevention?

## LO 3 | What Influences Your Health?

3. What are some of the health disparities existing in the United States today? Why do you think these differences exist? What policies do you think would most effectively address or eliminate health disparities?

## LO 4 | How Does Behavior Change Occur?

4. What is the health belief model? How may this model be working when a young woman decides to smoke her first cigarette? Her last cigarette?

## LO 5 | How Can You Improve Your Health Behaviors?

5. Using our four-step plan for behavior change, discuss how you might act

as a change agent to help a friend stop smoking. Why is it important that your friend be ready to change before trying to change?

## ACCESS YOUR HEALTH ON THE INTERNET

Visit **MasteringHealth** for links to the websites and RSS feeds.

The following websites explore further topics and issues related to personal health.

**CDC Wonder.** This is a clearinghouse for comprehensive information from the Centers for Disease Control and Prevention (CDC), including special reports, guidelines, and access to national health data. **http://wonder.cdc.gov**

**Mayo Clinic.** This reputable resource for specific information about health topics, diseases, and treatment options is provided by the staff of the Mayo Clinic. It is easy to navigate and is consumer friendly. **www.mayoclinic.org**

**National Center for Health Statistics.** This resource contains links to key reports; national survey information; information on mortality by age, race, gender, and geographic location; and other important information about health status in the United States. **www.cdc.gov/nchs**

**Health Finder.** This is an excellent resource for consumer information about health. **www.healthfinder.gov**

**World Health Organization.** This resource provides global information on the current state of health around the world, such as illness and disease statistics, trends, and illness outbreak alerts. **www.who.int/en**

# 2

# Promoting and Preserving Your Psychological Health

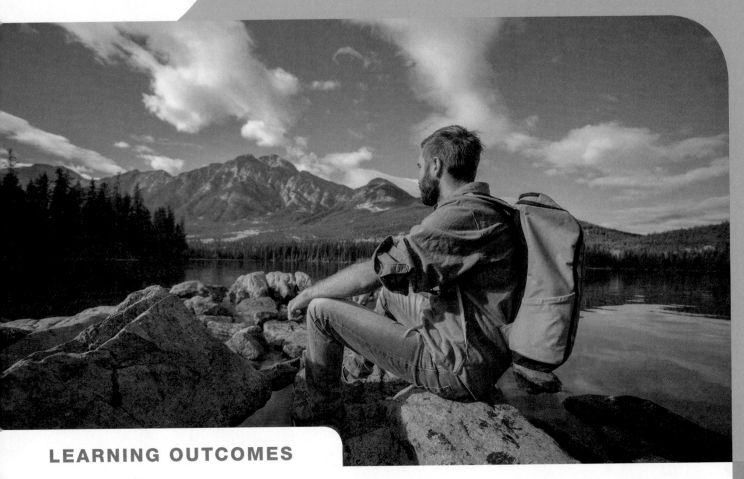

## LEARNING OUTCOMES

LO **1** Define each of the four components of psychological health, and identify the basic traits shared by psychologically healthy people.

LO **2** Discuss the roles of self-efficacy and self-esteem, emotional intelligence, personality, maturity, and happiness in psychological well-being.

LO **3** Describe and differentiate psychological disorders, including mood disorders, anxiety disorders, obsessive–compulsive disorders, posttraumatic stress disorder, personality disorders, and schizophrenia, and explain their causes and treatments.

LO **4** Discuss risk factors and possible warning signs of suicide, as well as actions that can be taken to help a person contemplating suicide.

LO **5** Explain the different types of treatment options and professional services available to those experiencing mental health problems.

Most students describe their college years as among the best of their lives, but they may also find the pressure of grades, finances, and relationships, along with the struggle to find themselves, to be extraordinarily difficult. Psychological distress caused by relationship issues, family concerns, academic competition, and adjusting to college life is common. Experts believe that the anxiety-inducing campus environment is a major contributor to poor health decisions such as high levels of alcohol consumption, sleeplessness, and overeating. These, in turn, can affect academic success and overall health.

Fortunately, humans possess **resiliency**, a trait that enables us to cope, adapt, and thrive, regardless of life's challenges. How we feel and think about ourselves, those around us, and our environment can tell us a lot about our psychological health.

## LO 1 | WHAT IS PSYCHOLOGICAL HEALTH?

Define each of the four components of psychological health, and identify the basic traits shared by psychologically healthy people.

Psychological health is the sum of how we think, feel, relate, and exist in our day-to-day lives. Our thoughts, perceptions, emotions, motivations, interpersonal relationships, and behaviors are a product of our experiences and the skills we have developed to meet life's challenges. **Psychological health** includes mental, emotional, social, and spiritual dimensions (FIGURE 2.1).

Most experts identify several basic elements psychologically healthy people regularly display:

- **They feel good about themselves.** They are not typically overwhelmed by fear, love, anger, jealousy, guilt, or worry. They know who they are, have a realistic sense of their capabilities, and respect themselves even though they realize they aren't perfect.
- **They feel comfortable with other people, respect others, and have compassion.** They enjoy satisfying and lasting personal relationships and do not take advantage of others or allow others to take advantage of them. They accept that there are others whose needs are greater than their own and take responsibility for fellow human beings. They can give love, consider others' interests, take time to help others, and respect personal differences.

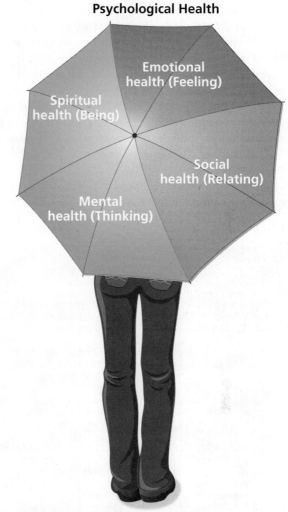

**Psychological Health**

Emotional health (Feeling)

Spiritual health (Being)

Social health (Relating)

Mental health (Thinking)

**FIGURE 2.1 Psychological Health** Psychological health is a complex interaction of the mental, emotional, social, and spiritual dimensions of health. Possessing strength and resiliency in these dimensions can maintain your overall well-being and help you weather the storms of life.

- **They are "self-compassionate."** Kind and understanding of their own imperfections and weaknesses, they acknowledge their "humanness." They are mindful of the problems in life and work to be the best that they can be, given their limitations and things they can't control. They are not self-absorbed, narcissistic, or overly critical of themselves.[1]

**resiliency** The ability to adapt to change and stressful events in healthy and flexible ways.

**psychological health** The mental, emotional, social, and spiritual dimensions of health.

- **They control tension and anxiety.** They recognize the underlying causes and symptoms of stress and anxiety in their lives and consciously avoid irrational thoughts, hostility, excessive excuse making, and blaming others for their problems. They use resources and learn skills to control reactions to stressful situations.

- **They meet the demands of life.** They try to solve problems as they arise, accept responsibility, and plan ahead. They set realistic goals, think for themselves, and make independent decisions. Acknowledging that change is inevitable, they welcome new experiences.

- **They curb hate and guilt.** They acknowledge and combat tendencies to respond with anger, thoughtlessness, selfishness, vengefulness, or feelings of inadequacy. They do not try to knock others aside to get ahead, but rather reach out to help others.

- **They maintain a positive outlook.** They approach each day with a presumption that things will go well. They look to the future with enthusiasm rather than dread. Having fun and making time for themselves are integral parts of their lives.

- **They value diversity.** They do not feel threatened by those of a different gender, religion, sexual orientation, race, ethnicity, age, or political party. They are nonjudgmental and do not force their beliefs and values on others.

- **They appreciate and respect the world around them.** They take time to enjoy their surroundings, are conscious of their place in the universe, and act responsibly to preserve their environment.

In sum, psychologically healthy people possess emotional, mental, social, and spiritual resiliency. Resilient individuals have the ability to overcome challenges from minor disappointments to major tragedies and the typical life obstacles we often face. They usually respond to challenges and frustrations in appropriate ways, despite occasional slips (see **FIGURE 2.2**). When they do slip, they recognize it, are kind to themselves rather than engaging in endless self-recrimination, and take action to rectify the situation.

Psychologists have long argued that before we can achieve any of the above characteristics of psychological health, we must meet certain basic human needs. In the 1960s, human

| Psychologically unhealthy | | | Psychologically healthy |
|---|---|---|---|
| No zest for life; pessimistic/cynical most of the time; spiritually down | Shows poorer coping than most, often overwhelmed by circumstances | Works to improve in all areas, recognizes strengths and weaknesses | Possesses zest for life; spiritually healthy and intellectually thriving |
| Laughs, but usually at others, has little fun | Has regular relationship problems, finds that others often disappoint | Healthy relationships with family and friends, capable of giving and receiving love and affection | High energy, resilient, enjoys challenges, focused |
| Has serious bouts of depression, "down" and tired much of time; has suicidal thoughts | Tends to be cynical/critical of others; tends to have negative/critical friends | Has strong social support, may need to work on improving social skills but usually no major problems | Realistic sense of self and others, sound coping skills, open-minded |
| A "challenge" to be around, socially isolated | Lacks focus much of the time, hard to keep intellectual acuity sharp | Has occasional emotional "dips", but overall good mental/emotional adaptors | Adapts to change easily, sensitive to others and environment |
| Experiences many illnesses, headaches, aches/pains, gets colds/infections easily | Quick to anger, sense of humor and fun evident less often | | Has strong social support and healthy relationships with family and friends |

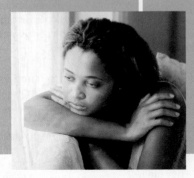
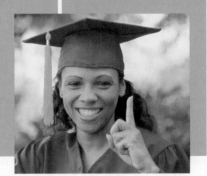

**FIGURE 2.2 Characteristics of Psychologically Healthy and Unhealthy People**
Where do you fall on this continuum?

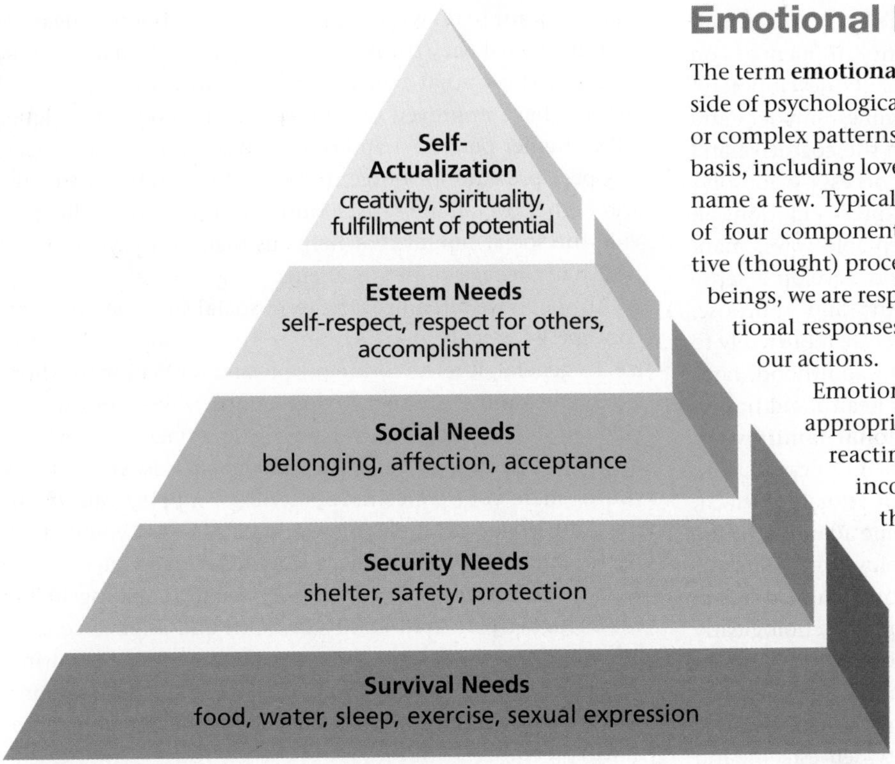

## Emotional Health

The term **emotional health** refers to the feeling, or subjective, side of psychological health. **Emotions** are intensified feelings or complex patterns of feelings that we experience on a regular basis, including love, hate, frustration, anxiety, and joy, just to name a few. Typically, emotions are described as the interplay of four components: physiological arousal, feelings, cognitive (thought) processes, and behavioral reactions. As rational beings, we are responsible for evaluating our individual emotional responses, their causes, and the appropriateness of our actions.

Emotionally healthy people usually respond appropriately to upsetting events. Rather than reacting in an extreme fashion or behaving inconsistently or offensively, they can express their feelings, communicate with others, and show emotions in appropriate ways. In contrast, emotionally unhealthy people are much more likely to let their feelings overpower them. They may be highly volatile and prone to unpredictable emotional responses, which may be followed by inappropriate communication or actions.

Emotional health also affects social and intellectual health. People who feel hostile, withdrawn, or moody may become socially isolated. Because they are not much fun to be around, people may avoid them at the very time they are most in need of emotional support. For students, a more immediate concern is the impact of emotional upset on academic performance. Have you ever tried to study for an exam after a fight with a friend or family member? Emotional turmoil can seriously affect your ability to think, reason, and act rationally.

## Social Health

**Social health** includes your interactions with others on an individual and group basis, your ability to use social resources and support in times of need, and your ability to adapt to a variety of social situations. Socially healthy individuals enjoy a wide range of interactions with family, friends, and acquaintances and are able to have healthy interactions with an intimate partner. Typically, socially healthy individuals can listen, express themselves, form healthy attachments, act in socially acceptable and responsible ways, and find the best fit for themselves in society. Numerous studies have documented the importance of positive relationships with family members, friends, and significant others to overall well-being and longevity.[4]

**Self-Actualization**
creativity, spirituality, fulfillment of potential

**Esteem Needs**
self-respect, respect for others, accomplishment

**Social Needs**
belonging, affection, acceptance

**Security Needs**
shelter, safety, protection

**Survival Needs**
food, water, sleep, exercise, sexual expression

**FIGURE 2.3** Maslow's Hierarchy of Needs

**Source:** From A. H. Maslow, *Motivation and Personality*, 3rd ed., eds. R. D. Frager and J. Fadiman (Upper Saddle River, NJ: Pearson Education, 1987). Reprinted with permission.

 → **VIDEO TUTOR**
Maslow's Hierarchy of Needs

theorist Abraham Maslow developed a *hierarchy of needs* to describe this idea (**FIGURE 2.3**): At the bottom of his hierarchy are basic *survival needs*, such as food, sleep, and water; at the next level are *security needs*, such as shelter and safety; at the third level—*social needs*—is a sense of belonging and affection; at the fourth level are *esteem needs*, self-respect and respect for others; and at the top are needs for *self-actualization* and self-transcendence.

According to Maslow's theory, a person's needs must be met at each of these levels before he or she can be truly healthy. Failure to meet needs at a lower level will interfere with a person's ability to address higher-level needs. For example, someone who is homeless or worried about threats from violence will be unable to focus on fulfilling social, esteem, or actualization needs.[2]

## Mental Health

The term **mental health** is used to describe the "thinking" or "rational" dimension of our health. A mentally healthy person perceives life in realistic ways, can adapt to change, can develop rational strategies to solve problems, and can carry out personal and professional responsibilities. In addition, a mentally healthy person has the intellectual ability to learn and use information effectively and strive for continued growth. This is often referred to as *intellectual health*, a subset of mental health.[3]

**mental health** The thinking part of psychological health; includes your values, attitudes, and beliefs.

**emotional health** The feeling part of psychological health; includes your emotional reactions to life.

**emotions** Intensified feelings or complex patterns of feelings.

**social health** Aspect of psychological health that includes interactions with others, ability to use social supports, and ability to adapt to various situations.

**dysfunctional families** Families in which there is violence; physical, emotional, or sexual abuse; significant parental discord; or other negative family interactions.

**social support** Network of people and services with whom you share ties and from whom you get support.

## The Family

Families have a significant influence on psychological development. Healthy families model and help develop the cognitive and social skills necessary to solve problems, express emotions in socially acceptable ways, manage stress, and develop a sense of self-worth and purpose. Children raised in healthy, nurturing homes are more likely to become well-adjusted, productive adults. In adulthood, family support is one of the best predictors of health and happiness.[5] Children brought up in **dysfunctional families**—in which there is violence; distrust; anger; dietary deprivation; drug abuse; significant parental discord; or sexual, physical, or emotional abuse—may have a harder time adapting to life and may have an increased risk of psychological problems.[6] In dysfunctional families, love, security, and unconditional trust may be so lacking that children become psychologically damaged. Yet not all people raised in dysfunctional families become psychologically unhealthy, and not all people from healthy environments become well adjusted. The difference may lie in their support system, community, self-esteem, and personality.

## Social Supports

Our initial social support may be provided by family members, but as we grow and develop, the support of peers and friends becomes more and more important. We rely on friends to help us figure out who we are and what we want to do with our lives. We often bounce ideas off friends to see if they think we are being logical, smart, or fair. Research shows that college students with adequate social support have improved overall well-being, including higher GPAs, higher perceived ability in math and science courses, less peer pressure for binge drinking, lower rates of suicide, and higher overall life satisfaction.[7] Relationships in life provide the social capital that helps us maintain psychological health in the face of life's challenges.

Although we often hear the term **social support** used, this concept is actually more complex than many people realize. In general, it refers to the people and services with whom we interact and share social connections. These ties can provide *tangible support*, such as babysitting services or money to help pay the bills, or *intangible support*, such as encouraging you to share your concerns. Sometimes, support can just be the knowledge that someone would be there for you in a crisis. Research shows that college students with adequate social support have improved overall well-being, including higher GPAs, higher perceived ability in math and science courses, less stress and depression, less peer pressure for binge drinking, lower rates of suicide, and higher overall life satisfaction.[8] (Look for more information about interpersonal relationships in Chapter 8.)

## Community

The communities we live in can provide social support and have a positive impact on our psychological health through collective actions. For example, neighbors may join together to get rid of trash on the street, participate in a neighborhood watch to keep children and homes safe, help each other with home repairs, or organize community social events. Religious institutions, schools, clinics, and local businesses can also engage in efforts that demonstrate support and caring for community members. Likewise, you are a part of a campus community. That community can support and care for your psychological health by creating a safe environment to explore and develop your mental, intellectual, emotional, social, and spiritual dimensions.

**WHAT DO YOU THINK?**

What are some ways in which people in your community work together toward a common goal?

- What type of groundwork must be established before this type of working together can occur?
- What factors can get in the way of collaboration and cooperation?

## Loneliness

What makes us happiest in life? Some people may point to fabulous fame and fortune. But happiness is most closely connected to having friends and family. Even though our need to connect is innate, some of us always go home alone. You could have people around you throughout the day or even be in a lifelong marriage and still experience a deep, pervasive loneliness. Loneliness is not the same as being alone. Loneliness is a feeling of emptiness or hollowness inside of you, causing people to feel alone and unwanted.

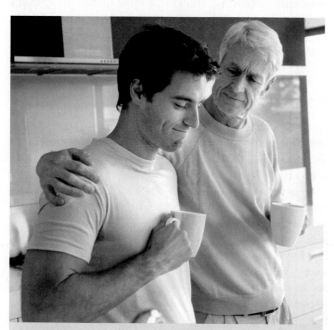

Your family members play an important role in your psychological health. As you were growing up, they modeled behaviors and skills that helped you develop cognitively and socially. Their love and support can give you a sense of self-worth and encourage you to treat others with compassion and care.

There are several possible contributors to increased reports of loneliness in modern society. Most commonly, divorce and death; aging/living longer and losing most of the people who have ever known us; increased use of social media, where we connect with people but may not have as many close social relationships; access to transportation; community structure and walking paths; a more mobile workforce, where people may telecommute or change jobs and locations frequently; and a host of other factors have been discussed as reasons for *social isolation*.[9] A recent study of twins raised apart and together provides preliminary evidence that genetics may play a key role in risk for loneliness. More research is necessary to determine the nature and extent of this relationship.[10]

Loneliness has a wide range of negative effects on both physical and mental health. Some of the health risks of loneliness include depression and suicide; increased stress levels; antisocial behavior; and alcohol and drug abuse.[11]

Finding ways to change feelings of loneliness is key. Recognize the feelings of loneliness and find ways to express these feelings through journaling, writing, or reaching out to a friend or counselor on campus. It is not unusual for other students on campus to experience loneliness. In fact, approximately 59 percent of college students reported feeling lonely in the past year.[12] Becoming engaged in a campus activity or club that you enjoy provides an opportunity to look forward to something and to meet with others that have similar interests.

## Spiritual Health

It is possible to be mentally, emotionally, and socially healthy and still not achieve optimal psychological well-being. For many people, the difficult-to-describe element that gives life purpose is the spiritual dimension.

The term *spirituality* is broader in meaning than religion and is defined as an individual's sense of purpose and meaning in life; it involves a sense of peace and connection to others.[13] Spirituality may be practiced in many ways, including through religion; however, religion does not have to be part of a spiritual person's life. **Spiritual health** refers to the sense of belonging to something greater than the purely physical or personal dimensions of existence. For some, this unifying force is nature; for others, it is a feeling of connection to other people; for still others, the unifying force is a god or other higher power. (**Focus On: Cultivating Your Spiritual Health**, which begins on page 51, explores spiritual health and the role spirituality plays in your overall psychological health in more detail.)

## LO 2 | KEYS TO ENHANCING PSYCHOLOGICAL HEALTH

Discuss the roles of self-efficacy and self-esteem, emotional intelligence, personality, maturity, and happiness in psychological well-being.

- - - - - - - - - - - - - - - - - - - - - - - - - - - - - - - - -

Psychological health is the product of many influences throughout our lives, including family, social supports, and the community in which you live. Your psychological health is also shaped by your sense of self-efficacy and self-esteem, your personality, and your maturity.

## Self-Efficacy and Self-Esteem

During our formative years, successes and failures in school, athletics, friendships, intimate relationships, jobs, and every other aspect of life subtly shape our beliefs about our personal worth and abilities. These beliefs in turn become internal influences on our psychological health.

**Self-efficacy** describes a person's belief about whether he or she can successfully engage in and execute a specific behavior. **Self-esteem** refers to one's realistic sense of self-respect or self-worth. People with high levels of self-efficacy and self-esteem tend to express a positive outlook on life.

Self-esteem results from the relationships we have with our parents and family growing up; with friends as we grow older; with our significant others as we form intimate relationships; and with our teachers, coworkers, and others throughout our lives. While we tend to think of self-esteem as a positive thing, the Health Headlines box on page 30 discusses the possible downside of having too much self-esteem.

**Learned Helplessness versus Learned Optimism** Psychologist Martin Seligman proposed that people who continually experience failure may develop a pattern of response known as **learned helplessness** in which they give up and fail to take action to help themselves. Seligman ascribes this response in part to society's tendency toward *victimology*—blaming one's problems on other people and circumstances.[14] Although viewing ourselves as victims may make us feel better temporarily, it does not address the underlying causes of a problem. Ultimately, it can erode self-efficacy by making us feel that we cannot do anything to improve the situation.

Today, many self-help programs use elements of Seligman's principle of **learned optimism**. The basis for these programs is the idea that we can teach ourselves to be optimistic. By changing our self-talk, examining our reactions, and blocking negative thoughts, we can "unlearn" negative thought processes that have become habitual. Some programs practice positive affirmations with clients, teaching them the habit of acknowledging positive things about themselves. Often we are our own worst critics, and learning to be kinder to ourselves can be difficult.

## Defense Mechanisms

Famed psychoanalyst Sigmund Freud proposed that, in order to deflect negative emotions and stress, we develop defense

**spiritual health** Aspect of psychological health that relates to having a sense of meaning and purpose to one's life, as well as a feeling of connection with others and with nature.

**self-efficacy** Describes a person's belief about whether he or she can successfully engage in and execute a specific behavior.

**self-esteem** One's realistic sense of self-respect or self-worth.

**learned helplessness** Pattern of responding to situations by giving up because of repeated failure in the past.

**learned optimism** Teaching oneself to think positively.

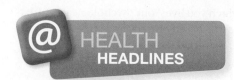

# OVERDOSING ON SELF-ESTEEM?

Fostering self-esteem in children has been seen as key to keeping them away from drugs and violence and to ensuring well-adjusted lives. While it's true people tend to thrive when praised for hard work and accomplishments, society is now seeing a possible downside to handing out trophies just for showing up. There is a fine line between healthy self-esteem and vanity or narcissism, leading some to have an exaggerated self-image, a need for constant compliments, and a sense of feeling entitled to special treatment. In a study conducted on Facebook updates, it was found that extraverts more frequently post about their social activities, those with lower self-esteem tend to relay updates about romantic partners, and

narcissists tend to share content about their achievements, diet, and exercise.

Call it the "soccer trophy effect" if you will, but it appears to have serious downsides. First, preliminary research indicates people who have been protected from failure (perhaps by well-meaning parents and teachers) and have extremely high levels of self-esteem might be more prone to anger, aggression, and other negative behaviors when others don't praise them or meet their needs for instant gratification. Second, learning to lose may teach us valuable lessons. Carol Dweck, a psychology professor at Stanford University, found that after a steady diet of praise, kids collapsed at the first experience of difficulty. Failure can teach us to keep trying—and that

just showing up is not enough to excel in college or the subsequent work world; in real life, there are no participation ribbons.

Psychologists continue to support the idea that self-esteem is important for positive growth and development. More research is needed to examine potential risks of too much self-esteem and the best ways to deal with it once it occurs.

**Sources:** T. Marshall, K. Lefringhausen, and N. Ferenczi, "The Big Five, Self-Esteem, Narcissism as Predictors of the Topics People Write about in Facebook Status Updates," *Personality and Individual Differences* 85 (2015): 35–40; C. Dweck, "Helping Kids Excel," *Scientific American* 23 no. 80 (2015): www.nature.com/scientificamerican/journal/v23/n5s/full/scientificamericangenius0115-80.html; A. Diddaway and E. Rafestesder, "Agenda for Conceptualizing and Researching Praise and Criticism," *Journal of Paediatrics and Child Health* 52, no.1 (2016): 99.

---

mechanisms, strategies we unconsciously use to distort our present reality to help avoid anxiety. While defense mechanisms can be pathological if taken to an extreme, fantasizing about a vacation to cope with work stress or rationalizing why you weren't selected for the lead role in a play can help to relieve stress and disappointment.[15]

## Emotional Intelligence

Intelligence has long been regarded as key to a successful career and healthy social life. It helps us understand the complex interaction of forces in our lives and respond in rational, reasonable ways. In the 1990s, two leading psychologists, Peter Salovey and John Mayer, championed a more comprehensive view of intelligence, known as **emotional intelligence (EI)**.[16] Emotional intelligence is the ability to anticipate, identify, understand, and manage emotions in positive ways (yours and others'); it summarizes how your history and experiences help you deal with other people; and how you communicate, empathize with, and avoid or diffuse potential conflicts.[17]

Essentially, Salovey and Mayer said that just because you are intelligent doesn't mean you "get it" when it comes to daily interactions with others. If you know how to avoid, manage, and deflect negative emotions and

respond to emotionally charged situations in appropriate, rational ways, the end result is more likely to be positive—and to improve well-being.[18] Your *emotional intelligence quotient (EQ)* is an indicator of social and interpersonal skills—your ability to successfully maneuver in sometimes emotionally charged settings. Emotional intelligence typically consists of the following:

- **Self-Awareness.** The ability to recognize your own emotions, moods, and reactions, as well as have an awareness of how others perceive or react to you.
- **Self-Regulation/Self-Management.** The ability to control your emotional impulses, think before responding, and express yourself appropriately.
- **Internal Motivation.** A drive for learning about things, being able to take initiative and follow through, as well as being trustworthy, stable, and consistent.
- **Empathy.** An awareness of what others might be going through, rather than being so engrossed in yourself that you are oblivious to others. Not being judgmental and rigid in thinking and reacting appropriately to others little "mental moments" is part of this element.
- **Social Skills.** Involves identifying social cues, learning to listen and respond appropriately, and knowing how to work with others for the common good and to avoid conflicts with others.

Proponents of EI suggest that developing or increasing your emotional intelligence can help you build stronger relationships, succeed at work, and achieve your goals.[19]

**emotional intelligence (EI)** The ability to anticipate, identify, understand, and manage emotions in positive ways (yours and others'); to communicate effectively with others; and to empathize and avoid/diffuse potential conflicts.

# Personality

Your personality is the unique mix of characteristics that distinguishes you from others. Heredity, environment, culture, and experience influence how each person develops. Personality determines how we react to the challenges of life, interpret our feelings, and resolve conflicts. A leading personality theory called the *Five-Factor Model* distills personality into five traits, often called the "Big Five":[20]

- **Agreeableness.** People who score high are trusting, likable, and demonstrate friendly compliance and love, whereas low scorers are critical and suspicious.
- **Openness to experience.** People who score high demonstrate curiosity, independence, and imagination, whereas low scorers are more conventional and down-to-earth.
- **Neuroticism.** People who score high in neuroticism are anxious and insecure, whereas those who score low show the ability to maintain emotional control.
- **Conscientiousness.** People who score high are dependable and demonstrate self-control, discipline, and a need to achieve, whereas low scorers are disorganized and impulsive.
- **Extroversion.** People who score high adapt well to social situations, demonstrate assertiveness, and draw enjoyment from the company of others, whereas low scorers are more reserved and passive.

Scoring high on agreeableness, openness, conscientiousness, and extroversion, while scoring low on neuroticism, is often related to psychological well-being.

Most recent schools of psychological theory indicate that we have the power to understand our behavior and change it, thus molding our own personalities, even as adults.[21] Although inhospitable social environments make it more difficult, there are opportunities for making changes and improving our long-term psychological well-being.

# Lifespan and Maturity

Although our temperaments are largely determined by genetics, as we age we learn to control the volatile emotions of youth and channel our feelings in more acceptable ways. For example, as children we might have screamed, thrown things, or hit people when upset, but as we mature we learn to control angry outbursts. People who have not completed early developmental tasks may find it impacts their life in later stages. For example, if you did not learn to trust others in childhood, you may have difficulty establishing intimate relationships as an adult.

The college years mark a critical transition period as young adults move away from families and establish themselves as independent adults. This transition is easier for those who have successfully accomplished earlier developmental tasks such as learning how to solve problems, make and evaluate decisions, define and adhere to personal values, and establish both casual and intimate relationships. Graduating from college can also be another transition for many into adulthood and further independence. Anticipating an adjustment period and exploring campus resources for new graduates can help in developing autonomy after graduation.

# Happiness and the Mind–Body Connection

Can negative emotions make us physically ill? Can positive emotions help us stay well? Researchers are exploring the interaction between emotions and health, especially in conditions of uncontrolled, persistent stress. In fact, the National Center for Complementary and Alternative Medicine (NCCAM) and other organizations are investing more and more dollars in large research projects designed to explore the link between mind and body. At the core of the mind–body connection is **psychoneuroimmunology (PNI)**, the study of the interactions of behavioral, neural, and endocrine functions and the functioning of the body's immune system.

One area of study that appears to be particularly promising in enhancing health is **positive psychology**. According to psychologist Martin Seligman, who is seen as its founder, positive psychology is the scientific study of human strengths and virtues.[22] Practitioners of positive psychology believe that science has focused disproportionally on pathology and repair of mental health and paid very little attention to factors that make life worth living. Positive psychology is based on the beliefs that people want to nurture their best qualities, find meaning and fulfillment in their lives,

**psychoneuroimmunology (PNI)** The study of the interactions of behavioral, neural, and endocrine functions and the functioning of the body's immune system.

**positive psychology** The scientific study of human strengths and virtues.

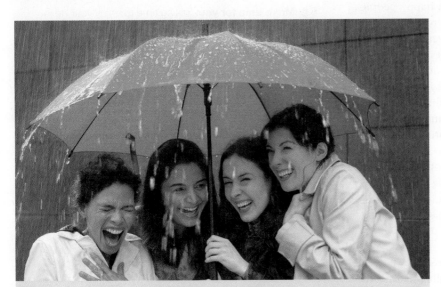

Research suggests that laughter can increase blood flow, boost the immune response, lower blood sugar levels, and facilitate better sleep. Additionally, sharing laughter and fun with others can strengthen social ties and bring joy to your everyday life.

and to enhance the love, work, and play that they experience. Central to the philosophy is the idea of building on an individual's strengths rather than focusing on trying to fix what is broken, as is the case with much of traditional psychotherapy.

People who are described as mentally healthy have certain strengths and virtues in common:

- They have high self-esteem.
- They are realistic.
- They value close relationships with others.
- They approach life with excitement and energy.
- They think things through and examine things from all sides.

Positive psychology interventions have proven effective in enhancing emotional, cognitive, and physical health, reducing depression, lessening disease and disability, and increasing longevity.[23]

Seligman suggests that we can develop well-being by practicing positive psychological actions. He describes five elements of well-being (represented by the acronym PERMA) that help humans flourish:[24]

- **Positive emotion.** How happy and satisfied are you?
- **Engagement.** Can you get completely absorbed in a task?
- **Relationships.** Are there people in life who really care about you?
- **Meaning.** Are you working toward something bigger than yourself?
- **Accomplishment.** How hard will you work for something?

The **Making Changes Today** box provides some suggestions for things you can do to incorporate PERMA principles in your own life.

The study of **happiness**—a collective term for several positive states in which individuals actively embrace the world around them—is part of the study of positive psychology.[25] While no differences have been found between men and women in feelings of happiness, happiness does decrease as we age. There are four characteristics that happy people share: *health* (knowing and partaking in healthy habits); *intimacy* (being able to enjoy the company of friends and family, as well as practice empathy); *resources* (possessing a certain agency over one's conditions in life); and *competence* (the knowledge of and ability to learn new skills).[26] For university students, happiness has been positively related to friendship, altruism, social skills, cooperation, and academic success.[27]

Overall, unhappy people have more health problems. Those who experience more feelings of happiness have fewer mental health issues such as depression, anxiety, and obsessive–compulsive disorders, and fewer behavioral health and physical health (cardiovascular disease, obesity, cancer, etc.) issues.[28] Some of the newest research, however, shows that being happy or unhappy has no direct effect on mortality.[29]

Scientists suggest that people may be biologically predisposed to happiness and well-being. Numerous studies have examined the role of environment and genetics and concluded that

**happiness** A collective term for several positive states in which individuals actively embrace the world around them.

**neurotransmitters** Chemicals that relay messages between nerve cells or from nerve cells to other body cells.

# MAKING **CHANGES** TODAY

## Strategies to Enhance Psychological Health

As we have seen, psychological health involves four dimensions. Attaining self-fulfillment is a lifelong, conscious process that involves enhancing each of these components. Strategies include building self-efficacy and self-esteem, understanding and controlling emotions, maintaining support networks, and employing a positive outlook. Here are some tips and tools for enhancing your psychological health. (See Chapter 3 for more tips for managing stress.)

- ◉ **Develop a support system.** One of the best ways to promote self-esteem is through a support system of peers and others who share your values. Members of your support system can help you feel good about yourself and force you to take an honest look at your actions and choices. Keeping in contact with old friends and family members can provide a foundation of unconditional love that will help you through life's transitions.

- ◎ **Complete required tasks to the best of your ability.** A good way to boost your sense of self-efficacy is to learn new skills and develop a history of success. Most college campuses provide study groups and learning centers that can help you manage time, improve study and writing skills, and prepare for tests.

- ◎ **Form realistic expectations.** If you expect perfect grades, a steady stream of Saturday-night dates, and the perfect job, you may be setting yourself up for failure. Assess your current resources and the direction in which you are heading. Set small, incremental goals that you can likely meet.

- ◎ **Make time for you.** Taking time to enjoy your life is another way to boost your self-esteem and psychological health. View a new activity as something to look forward to and an opportunity to have fun.

- ◎ **Maintain physical health.** Regular exercise fosters a sense of well-being. More and more research supports the role of exercise and good nutrition in improved mental health.

- ◎ **Examine problems and seek help when necessary.** Knowing when to seek help from friends, family, or professionals is an important factor in boosting self-esteem. Sometimes you can handle life's problems alone; at other times, you need assistance.

- ◎ **Get adequate sleep.** Getting enough sleep on a daily basis is a key factor in physical and psychological health. Not only do our bodies need to rest to conserve energy for daily activities, but we also need to restore supplies of many of the **neurotransmitters** that we use up during our waking hours. (For more information on the importance of sleep, see **Chapter 4, Improving Your Sleep** beginning on page 102.)

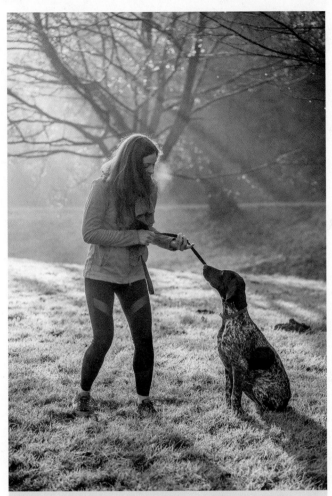
Spending time in the fresh air with your best friend is a simple thing you can do to improve psychological health.

genetic or familial predisposition and excessive, unresolved stress, particularly due to trauma or war or devastating natural or human-caused disaster. Changes in biochemistry due to illness, drug use, or other imbalances may trigger unusual mental disturbances. Car accidents or occupational injuries that cause physical brain trauma are among common threats to brain health. In addition, a mother's exposure to viruses or toxic chemicals while pregnant may play a part, as can having a history of child abuse or neglect.[32] As with physical disease, mental illnesses can range from mild to severe and can exact a heavy toll on quality of life, both for people with the illnesses and for those who interact with them.

Mental disorders are common in the United States and worldwide. The basis for diagnosing mental disorders in the United States is the *Diagnostic and Statistical Manual of Mental Disorders*, Fifth Edition (DSM-5). An estimated 18.5 percent of Americans age 18 and older—just slightly under 1 in 5 adults—suffer from a diagnosable mental disorder in a given year, and nearly half of them have more than one mental illness at the same time. About 4 percent, or approximately 1 in 20, suffer from a serious mental illness requiring close monitoring, residential care in many instances, and medication.[33] Mental disorders are the leading cause of disability worldwide for people age 15–44, costing more than $464 billion annually in the United States alone.[34]

**mental illnesses** Disorders that disrupt thinking, feeling, moods, and behaviors and that impair daily functioning.

each contributes to overall happiness and well-being. Since circumstances interact with genetic predisposition, it may be possible to influence happiness and well-being development.[30]

## LO 3 | WHEN PSYCHOLOGICAL HEALTH DETERIORATES

Describe and differentiate psychological disorders, including mood disorders, anxiety disorders, obsessive–compulsive disorders, posttraumatic stress disorder, personality disorders, and schizophrenia, and explain their causes and treatments.

Sometimes circumstances overwhelm us to such a degree that we need help to get back on track to healthful living. Stress, abusive relationships, anxiety, loneliness, financial upheavals, and other traumatic events can derail our coping resources. Chemical imbalances, drug interactions, trauma, neurological disruptions, and other physical problems may also contribute to mental health problems.

**Mental illnesses** are disorders that disrupt thinking, feeling, moods, and behaviors and cause varying degrees of impaired functioning in daily living. They are believed to be caused by a variety of biochemical, genetic, and environmental factors.[31] Among the most common risk factors are a

# APPROXIMATELY
# 9.3 MILLION
adults seriously CONSIDERED SUICIDE in the past year.

## Mental Health Threats to College Students

Mental health problems are increasingly common among college students, growing in both number and severity.[35] The most recent National College Health Assessment survey found that approximately 1 in 3 undergraduates reported "feeling so depressed it was difficult to function" at least once in the past year, and nearly 9 percent of students reported "seriously considering attempting suicide" in the past year.[36] In all, more than 1 in 4 college students are diagnosed or treated by a professional for a mental health issue each year.[37] Anxiety is the most common (15.8 percent), with depression (13.1 percent) not far behind.[38] Although these data may appear alarming, it is important to note that increases in help-seeking behavior, in addition to actual increases in overall prevalence of disorders,

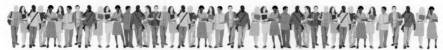

**Felt overwhelmed by all they needed to do: 85.1%**

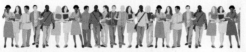

**Felt things were hopeless: 47.8%**

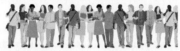

**Felt so depressed that it was difficult to function: 35.3%**

**Seriously considered suicide: 9.6%**

**Intentionally injured themselves: 6.5%**

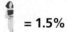 = 1.5%         = 1.45%

**Attempted suicide**

**FIGURE 2.4** Mental Health Concerns of American College Students, Past 12 Months

**Source:** Data from American College Health Association, *American College Health Association—National College Health Assessment II (ACHA-NCHA II): Undergraduate Students, Reference Group Data Report, Fall,* 2015 (Baltimore: American College Health Association, 2016).

---

**chronic mood disorder** Experience of persistent emotional states, such as sadness, despair, hopelessness, or euphoria.

**major depression** Severe depressive disorder with physical effects such as sleep disturbance and exhaustion and mental effects such as the inability to concentrate; also called *clinical depression.*

**attention-deficit (hyperactivity) disorder (ADD/ADHD)** A learning disability usually associated with school-aged children, often involving difficulty concentrating, organizing things, listening to instructions, and remembering details.

**dyslexia** Language-based learning disorder that can pose problems for reading, writing, and spelling.

**dyscalculia** A learning disability involving math.

**dysgraphia** A learning disability involving writing; individuals may have difficulty putting letters, numbers, and words on a page into order.

may contribute to these trends. FIGURE 2.4 shows the mental health concerns reported by American college students.

Although there are many types of mental illnesses, we focus here on those disorders that are most common among college students: mood disorders, anxiety disorders, obsessive–compulsive disorder (OCD), posttraumatic stress disorder (PTSD), personality disorders, and schizophrenia. See the Health Headlines box for information on other brain-based disorders in young adults. (For coverage of addiction, which is classified as a mental disorder, see **Focus On: Recognizing and Avoiding Addiction** beginning on page 299.) For information about other disorders, consult the websites listed at the end of this chapter or ask your instructor for local resources.

## Mood Disorders

**Chronic mood disorders** are disorders that affect how you feel, such as persistent sadness or feelings of euphoria. They include major depression, dysthymic disorder, bipolar disorder, and seasonal affective disorder. In any given year, approximately 10 percent of Americans age 18 or older suffer from a mood disorder.[39]

**Major Depression** Sometimes life throws us a curveball. We experience loss, pain, disappointment, or frustration, and we can be left feeling beaten and bruised. How do we know if these emotions are really signs of **major depression**? Major or clinical depression is not the same as having a bad day or feeling down after a negative experience. It is also not something that can be willed or wished away, nor can a person just "cheer up." Major depression is the most common mood disorder, affecting approximately 8 percent of the U.S. population in a given year.[40] This number, however, does not reflect all those who suffer from depression because many are misdiagnosed or undiagnosed.

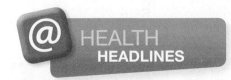
# COLLEGE SUCCESS WITH LEARNING DISABILITIES AND NEURODEVELOPMENTAL DISORDERS

The mental illnesses discussed in this chapter are all based in the brain, but there are other brain-based disorders that are not mental illnesses. Just as people living with mental illness can be successful in college with appropriate counseling, medication, and/or accommodations, people living with learning disabilities (LDs) and neurodevelopmental disorders can also be successful in college when the proper supports are in place.

**Attention-deficit (hyperactivity) disorder (ADD/ADHD)** is a learning disability usually associated with school-age children, but for many people, symptoms persist into adulthood. People with ADD/ADHD are distracted much of the time. Even when they try to concentrate, they find it hard to pay attention. Organizing things, listening to instructions, and remembering details are especially difficult. About 4 percent of the adult population, or slightly over 12 million adults, are living with ADHD. Recent studies indicate that ADHD affects somewhere between 2 and 8 percent of college students. Left untreated, ADHD can disrupt everything from careers to relationships to financial stability. Key areas of disruption might include:

- **Health.** Difficulties around organization and a tendency to be impulsive can lead to health problems. Alcohol and drug abuse, compulsive eating, and forgetting to take important medications are all ways ADHD can impact health.
- **Work and finances.** Difficulty concentrating, completing tasks, listening, and relating to others can lead to trouble at work and at school. Managing finances may also be a concern because a person with ADHD may struggle to pay bills on time, lose paperwork, miss deadlines, or spend impulsively, resulting in debt.
- **Relationships.** If you have ADHD, it might feel like your friends and loved ones regularly prod you to get your things organized, to be tidy, and to get

Disorder and chaos can be headaches for us all, but ADHD sufferers may find them insurmountable obstacles.

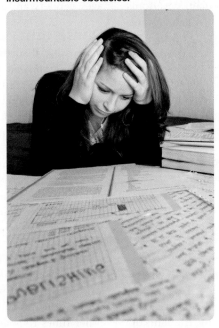

things done. If your romantic partner has ADHD, you might be hurt that your loved one doesn't seem to listen to you, blurts out hurtful things, and leaves you with the bulk of organizing and planning.

**Dyslexia** is a language-based learning disorder that can pose problems for reading, writing, and spelling. Lesser known, but equally challenging, are **dyscalculia** (a learning disability involving math) and **dysgraphia** (a learning disability involving writing). People with dysgraphia may have difficulty putting letters, numbers, and words on a page in order.

**Autism spectrum disorder (ASD)** is not a learning disability, but a neurodevelopmental disorder (an impairment in brain development). People with an ASD will continue to learn and grow intellectually throughout their lives, but struggle to master communication and social behavior skills, which impacts their performance

in school and work. Some adults with an ASD (especially those with high-functioning autism or **Asperger syndrome**) will attend college and go on to succeed in the workforce.

Universities regularly offer a variety of support services to help students with learning disabilities. These may include testing and diagnosis for LDs, including prescribing medication for ADD/ADHD; reading and writing supports; exam accommodations, such as extra time or a quiet location; and classes on study skills and test anxiety. These supports are generally offered at no cost through an office of disability services or health center. Universities are newly considering what supports can be offered to allow more students on the autism spectrum to attend and be successful in college. A small number of campuses have developed programs specifically targeted toward students on the spectrum. Students with ASD will usually need a significant amount of support to be successful in college. In addition to the free services offered to students with LDs, some schools offer additional fee-based assistance including tutoring, help with financial management, and support groups for social interaction and leisure activities.

**Sources:** Centers for Disease Control and Prevention, "Attention-Deficit Hyperactivity Disorder," January 2016, www.cdc.gov/ncbddd/adhd/facts.html; Healthline, "ADHD by the Numbers: Facts, Statistics, and You," September 2014, www.healthline.com/health/adhd/facts-statistics-infographic#1; Helpguide.org, "Adult ADD/ADHD: Signs, Symptoms, Effects, and Treatment," December 2014, www.helpguide.org/articles/add-adhd/adult-adhd-attention-deficit-disorder; National Center for Learning Disabilities, "Types of LD," Accessed February 2014, www.ncld.org/types-learning-disabilities; M. Gormley et al., "First-Year GPA and Academic Service Use Among College Students With and Without ADHD," *Journal of Attention Disorders* (2016), doi:10.1177/1087054715623046; P. Pedrelli et al., "College Students: Mental Health Problems and Treatment Considerations," *Academic Psychiatry* 39 no. 5 (2015): 503–11; A. Fleming et al., "Pilot Randomized Controlled Trial of Dialectical Behavior Therapy Group Skills Training for ADHD Among College Students," *Journal of Attention Disorders* 19, no. 3 (2015): 260–71.

**autism spectrum disorder (ASD)** A neurodevelopmental disorder (an impairment in brain development) where individuals learn and grow intellectually throughout their lives, but struggle to master communication and social behavior skills, impacting school and work performance.

**Asperger syndrome** A form of high functioning autism.

**persistent depressive disorder (PDD)** Type of depression that is milder and harder to recognize than major depression; chronic; and often characterized by fatigue, pessimism, or a short temper. Also called *dysthymic disorder* or *dysthymia*.

**bipolar disorder** Form of mood disorder characterized by alternating mania and depression; also called *manic depressive illness*.

**seasonal affective disorder (SAD)** Type of depression that occurs in the winter months, when sunlight levels are low.

Major depression is characterized by a combination of symptoms that interfere with work, study, sleep, appetite, relationships, and enjoyment of life. Symptoms can last for weeks, months, or years and vary in intensity.[41] Sadness and despair are the main symptoms of depression.[42] Other common signs include:

- Loss of motivation or interest in pleasurable activities
- Preoccupation with failures and inadequacies; concern over what others are thinking
- Difficulty concentrating; indecisiveness; memory lapses
- Loss of sex drive or interest in close interactions with others
- Fatigue, oversleeping, insomnia, and loss of energy
- Feeling agitated, worthless, or hopeless
- Significant weight loss or gain due to appetite changes
- Recurring thoughts that life isn't worth living; thoughts of death or suicide

## Depression in College Students

Mental health problems, particularly depression, have gained increased recognition as major obstacles to healthy adjustment and success in college. Students who have weak communication skills, who find that college isn't what they expected, or who lack motivation often have difficulties. Stressors such as anxiety over relationships, pressure to get good grades and win social acceptance, abuse of alcohol and other drugs, poor diet, and lack of sleep can create a toxic cocktail that can overwhelm even the most resilient students. In a recent survey by the American College Health Association, 13.1 percent of college students reported having been diagnosed with or treated for depression in the past 12 months.[43]

Being far from home without the security of family and friends can exacerbate problems. International students are particularly vulnerable to depression and other mental health concerns. Most campuses have counseling centers

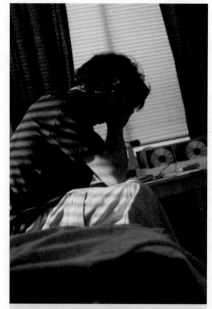

There is more to depression than simply feeling blue. When a person is clinically depressed, he or she finds it difficult to function, sometimes struggling just to get out of bed in the morning or to follow a conversation.

and other services available; however, many students do not use them because of persistent stigma about seeing a counselor. The **Health in a Diverse World** box discusses the differences in depression prevalence across different ages, genders, and ethnicities.

### Persistent Depressive Disorder

**Persistent depressive disorder (PDD)**, formerly called *dysthymic disorder* or *dysthymia*, is a less severe syndrome of chronic mild depression and can be harder to recognize than major depression. Individuals with PDD may appear to function well, but they may lack energy or may fatigue easily; be short-tempered, overly pessimistic, and ornery; or just not feel quite up to par but not have any significant, overt symptoms. People with PDD may cycle into major depression over time. For a diagnosis, symptoms must persist for at least 2 years in adults (1 year in children). This disorder affects approximately 2.5 percent of the adult population in the United States in a given year.[44]

### Bipolar Disorder

People with **bipolar disorder** (also known as *manic-depressive illness*) often have severe mood swings, ranging from extreme highs (mania) to extreme lows (depression). Sometimes these swings are dramatic and rapid; other times they are slow and gradual. When in the manic phase, people may be overactive, talkative, and have tons of energy; in the depressed phase, they may experience some or all of the symptoms of major depression. Bipolar disorder affects approximately 2.6 percent of the adult population in the United States and 11.2 percent of 13- to 18-year-olds in the United States.[45]

Although the cause of bipolar disorder is unknown, biological, genetic, and environmental factors, such as drug abuse and stressful or psychologically traumatic events, seem to be involved in triggering episodes. Once diagnosed, persons with bipolar disorder have several counseling and pharmaceutical options, and most will be able to live a healthy, functional life while being treated.

### Seasonal Affective Disorder

*Seasonal depression*, referred to as **seasonal affective disorder (SAD)**, strikes during the fall and winter months and is associated with reduced exposure to sunlight. People with SAD suffer from extreme fatigue, irritability, apathy, carbohydrate craving and weight gain, increased sleep time, and general sadness. Several factors are implicated in SAD development,

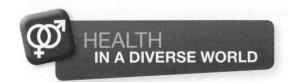

# DEPRESSION ACROSS GENDER, AGE, AND ETHNICITY

Although depression may affect persons of every age, gender, and ethnicity, it does not always manifest itself in the same way across all populations.

## Depression and Gender

Women are almost twice as likely as men to experience depression. Hormonal changes may be one factor. Women also face various stressors related to multiple responsibilities—work, childrearing, single parenthood, household work, and caring for elderly parents—at rates that are higher than those of men. Researchers have observed gender differences in coping strategies (responses to negative events) and suggest that some women's strategies make them more vulnerable to depression. For example, men may try to distract themselves from a depressed mood, whereas women may focus on it. If focusing on negative feelings intensifies these feelings, women who do this may predispose themselves to depression.

Depression in men is often masked by alcohol or drug abuse, or by the socially acceptable habit of working excessively long hours. Typically, depressed men present not as hopeless and helpless, but as irritable, angry, and discouraged—often personifying a "tough guy" image. Men are less likely to admit they are depressed, and doctors are less likely to suspect it, based on what men report during doctor's visits.

Depression can affect men's physical health differently than it can women's health. Although depression is associated with an increased risk of coronary heart disease in both men and women, it is associated with a higher risk of death in men.

## Depression and Age

A recent survey in the United States reported that approximately 11 percent of

**Although mental health problems have increased dramatically among younger adults, they affect people of all ages, with growing numbers of youth affected.**

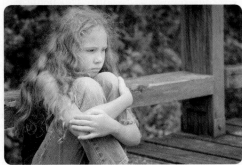

12- to 17-year-olds suffered at least one major depressive episode in the past year. Depressed adolescents may pretend to be sick, refuse to go to school or have a sudden drop in school performance, sleep excessively, engage in self-injury, abuse drugs or alcohol, feel misunderstood, or attempt suicide.

Before adolescence, girls and boys experience depression at about the same rate, but by adolescence and young adulthood, girls experience depression more than boys do. This may be due to biological and hormonal changes; girls' struggles with self-esteem and perceptions of success and approval; and an increase in girls' exposure to traumas, such as childhood sexual abuse, that may contribute to depression.

As adults reach their middle and older years, most are emotionally stable and lead active and satisfying lives. With aging, though, comes higher rates of depression; in fact, depression is considered the most common mental disorder of people age 65 and older. Rates are likely even higher than reported, as the symptoms of depression can be mistaken for dementia and thus be misdiagnosed.

## Depression and Race/Ethnicity

The Centers for Disease Control and Prevention (CDC) reports that rates of depression are higher among African Americans and Latinos than among whites; however, true rates of depression among minority populations are difficult to determine, as members of these groups may have difficulty accessing mental health services because of economic barriers, social and cultural differences, language barriers, and lack of culturally competent providers. African American males specifically may avoid professional help owing to stigma attached to mental illness in the African American community as well as greater distrust of physicians and poor patient–physician communication. Unfortunately, when African Americans do report depression symptoms to a health care provider, they are significantly less likely to receive a depression diagnosis from a health care provider than are non-Hispanic whites, and those who are diagnosed are less likely to be treated for depression.

There is no simple fix for this type of health disparity, but including universal depression screening in all primary care visits would be a good first step to ensure every patient's symptoms were equally considered for a depression diagnosis and treatment.

**Sources:** Mayo Clinic, "Depression in Women: Understanding the Gender Gap," January 2016, www.mayoclinic.org/diseases-conditions/depression/in-depth/depression/art-20047725; HelpGuide.org, "Depression in Men," February 2016, www.helpguide.org/articles/depression/depression-in-men.htm; CDC, "Depression in the U.S. Household Population, 2009–2012," *NCHS Data Brief* 172, December 2014, Available at www.cdc.gov/nchs/data/databriefs/db172.htm; Center for Behavioral Health Statistics and Quality, Behavioral Health Trends in the United States: Results from the 2014 National Survey on Drug Use and Health (HHS Publication No. SMA 15-4927, NSDUH Series H-50), 2015. Retrieved from www.samhsa.gov/data/; Z. Gellis and S. McCracken, "Mental Health in Older Adults: Depressive Disorders in Older Adults," *Council on Social Work Education,* Accessed February 2016, www.cswe.org/File.aspx?id=23509.

including disruption in the body's circadian rhythms and changes in levels of the hormone melatonin and the brain chemical serotonin.[46] Over 500,000 people in the United States suffer from SAD. Nearly three-fourths of those with SAD are women in early adulthood, particularly those living at high latitudes with long winter nights.[47]

The most beneficial treatment for SAD is light therapy, which exposes patients to lamps that simulate sunlight. Other treatments for SAD include diet change (such as eating more complex carbohydrates), increased exercise, stress-management techniques, sleep restriction (limiting the number of hours slept in a 24-hour period), psychotherapy, and prescription medications.

## What Causes Mood Disorders?

Mood disorders are caused by the interaction between multiple factors, including biological differences, hormones, inherited traits, life events, and early childhood trauma.[48] The biology of mood disorders is related to individual levels of brain chemicals called *neurotransmitters*. Several types of depression, including bipolar disorder, appear to have a genetic component. Depression can also be triggered by a serious loss, difficult relationships, financial problems, and pressure to succeed. Early childhood trauma, such as loss of a parent, may cause permanent changes in the brain, making one more prone to depression. Changes in the body's physical health can be accompanied by mental changes, particularly depression. Stroke, heart attack, cancer, Parkinson's disease, chronic pain, type 2 diabetes, certain medications, alcohol, hormonal disorders, and a wide range of other afflictions can cause a person to become depressed, frustrated, or angry. When this happens, recovery is often more difficult, as a person who feels exhausted and defeated may lack the will to fight illness and do what is necessary to optimize recovery.

## Anxiety Disorders

**Anxiety disorders** are characterized by persistent feelings of threat and worry and include generalized anxiety disorder, panic disorders, and phobic disorders. The largest mental health problem in the United States, anxiety disorders affect more than 40 million people in any given year. Anxiety disorders are most prevalent among 13- to 17-year-olds, with a median age of onset of 6 years.[49] Approximately 16 percent of U.S.

undergraduates report being diagnosed with or treated for anxiety in the past year.[50]

## Generalized Anxiety Disorder

One common form of anxiety disorder, **generalized anxiety disorder (GAD)**, is severe enough to interfere significantly with daily life. To be diagnosed with GAD, one must exhibit at least three of the following symptoms for more days than not during a 6-month period: restlessness or feeling keyed up or on edge, being easily fatigued, difficulty concentrating or mind going blank, irritability, muscle tension, and/or sleep disturbances.[51]

## Panic Disorder

Panic disorder is characterized by the occurrence of **panic attacks**, an acute anxiety reaction that brings on an intense physical reaction. Approximately 7.4 percent of college students report being diagnosed or treated for panic attacks in the last year.[52] Panic attacks and disorders are increasing in incidence, particularly among young women.

Although highly treatable, panic attacks may become debilitating and destructive, particularly if they happen often and cause the person to avoid going out in public or interacting with others. A panic attack typically starts abruptly, peaks within 10 minutes, lasts about 30 minutes, and leaves the person tired and drained. Symptoms include increased respiration, chills, hot flashes, shortness of breath, stomach cramps, chest pain, difficulty swallowing, and a sense of doom or impending death.[53]

Although researchers aren't sure what causes panic attacks, heredity, stress, and certain biochemical factors may play a role. Your chances of having a panic attack increase if a close relative has them. Some researchers believe that people who suffer panic attacks are experiencing an overreactive fight-or-flight physical response. (See Chapter 3 for more on the fight-or-flight response.)

## Phobic Disorders

**Phobias**, or phobic disorders, involve a persistent and irrational fear of a specific object, activity, or situation, often out of proportion to the circumstances. Phobias result in a compelling desire to avoid the source of the fear. Between 5 and 12 percent of American adults suffer from specific phobias, such as fear of spiders or snakes or riding in elevators.[54]

Another 7.4 percent of American adults suffer from **social anxiety disorder**, also called *social phobia*.[55] Social phobia is an anxiety disorder characterized by the persistent fear and avoidance of social situations. Essentially, the person dreads these situations for fear of being humiliated, embarrassed, or even looked at. These disorders vary in scope. Some cause difficulty only in specific

Many people are uneasy around spiders, but if your fear of them is debilitating, it may be a phobia.

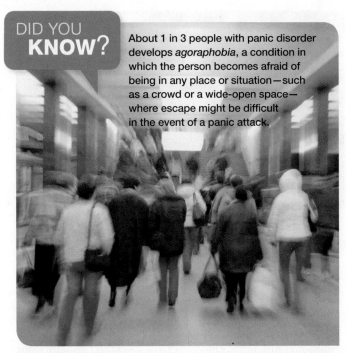
Source: Anxiety and Depression Association of America, "Panic Disorder and Agoraphobia," Accessed February 2016, https://www.adaa.org/understanding-anxiety/panic-disorder-agoraphobia.

situations, such as getting up in front of the class to give a presentation, while in extreme cases, a person avoids all contact with others.[56]

## What Causes Anxiety Disorders?

Because anxiety disorders vary in complexity and degree, scientists have yet to find clear reasons why one person develops them and another doesn't. The following factors are often cited as possible causes:[57]

- **Biology.** Some scientists trace the origin of anxiety to the brain and its functioning. Using sophisticated positron emission tomography (PET) scans, scientists can analyze areas of the brain that react during anxiety-producing events. Families appear to display similar brain and physiological reactivity, so we may inherit tendencies toward anxiety disorders.
- **Environment.** Anxiety can be a learned response. Although genetic tendencies may exist, experiencing a repeated pattern of reaction to certain situations programs the brain to respond in a certain way. For example, if your sibling screamed whenever a large spider crept into view or if other anxiety-raising events occurred frequently, you might be predisposed to react with anxiety to similar events later in life.
- **Social and cultural roles.** Cultural and social roles may also be a factor in risks for anxiety. Because men and women are taught to assume different roles, women may find it more acceptable to scream, tremble, or otherwise express extreme anxiety. Men, in contrast, may have learned to repress anxious feelings rather than act on them.

## Obsessive-Compulsive Disorder

People who feel compelled to perform rituals over and over again; who are fearful of dirt or contamination; who have an unnatural concern about order, symmetry, and exactness; or who have persistent intrusive thoughts, impulses, or images that cause intense anxiety or distress may be suffering from **obsessive–compulsive disorder (OCD).** Approximately 1 percent of Americans age 18 and over have OCD.[58]

Not to be confused with being a perfectionist, a person with OCD often knows the behaviors are irrational, yet is powerless to stop them. According to the DSM-5, OCD diagnosis requires obsessions to consume more than 1 hour per day and interfere with normal social or life activities. Although the exact cause is unknown, genetics, biological abnormalities, learned behaviors, and environmental factors have all been considered. Obsessive–compulsive disorder usually begins in childhood or the teen years; most people are diagnosed before age 20.[59]

Although highly treatable, only one-third of individuals with OCD receive treatment. Treatments vary by disorder type, severity, and other factors. The most effective treatments tend to be a combination of psychotherapy and medications designed to treat symptoms, such as antidepressants or antianxiety medication.[60]

## Posttraumatic Stress Disorder

People who have experienced or witnessed a traumatic event may develop **posttraumatic stress disorder (PTSD).** While only about 4 percent of Americans suffer from PTSD each year, about 7 percent will experience PTSD in their lifetimes, with women experiencing rates twice as high as men.[61] Fourteen percent of U.S. combat veterans who fought in Iraq and Afghanistan have experienced PTSD, and their stories frequent the national news. However, the "worst stressful experiences" reported most frequently by those with PTSD are not war related, but rather the unexpected death, serious illness, or injury of someone close and sexual assault. Others report experiences such as a natural disaster, serious accident, violent assault, or terrorism. PTSD in women appears related to a history of abuse, rape, or assault. Natural disasters, serious accidents, violent assault, and terrorism are all causes of PTSD in both men and women.[62] It is important to understand that PTSD is not rooted in weakness or an inability to cope; traumatic events can actually cause

**social anxiety disorder** Phobia characterized by fear and avoidance of social situations; also called *social phobia*.

**obsessive–compulsive disorder (OCD)** Form of anxiety disorder characterized by recurrent, unwanted thoughts and repetitive behaviors.

**posttraumatic stress disorder (PTSD)** Collection of symptoms that may occur as a delayed response to a traumatic event or series of events.

**SEE IT! VIDEOS**
How can we help veterans who suffer from PTSD? Watch **Battling Post Traumatic Stress**, available on **MasteringHealth.™**

chemical changes in the brain, leading to PTSD.[63] Symptoms of PTSD include:

- Dissociation, or perceived detachment of the mind from the emotional state or even the body
- Intrusive recollections of the traumatic event, such as flashbacks, nightmares, and recurrent thoughts or images
- Acute anxiety or nervousness, in which the person is hyperaroused, may cry easily, or experiences mood swings
- Insomnia and difficulty concentrating
- Intense physiological reactions, such as shaking or nausea, when something reminds the person of the traumatic event

Although these symptoms may be appropriate as initial responses to traumatic events, PTSD may be diagnosed if a person experiences them for at least 1 month following the traumatic event. However, in some cases, symptoms don't appear until months or even years later.

Treatment for PTSD may involve psychotherapy, as well as medications to help with depression, anxiety, and sleep. Group and talk therapy is also often recommended, depending on its nature and severity.

## Personality Disorders

According to the DSM-5, a **personality disorder** is an "enduring pattern of inner experience and behavior that deviates markedly from the expectation of the individual's culture and is pervasive and inflexible."[64] It is estimated that at least 10 percent of adults in the United States have some form of personality disorder as defined by the DSM-5.[65] People who live, work, or are in relationships with individuals suffering from personality disorders often find interactions with them to be challenging and destructive.

One common type of personality disorder is *paranoid personality disorder*, which involves pervasive, unfounded suspicion and mistrust of other people, irrational jealousy, and secretiveness. Persons with this illness have delusions of being persecuted by everyone, from family members and loved ones to the government.

*Narcissistic personality disorders* involve an exaggerated sense of self-importance and self-absorption. Persons with narcissistic personalities are preoccupied with fantasies of how wonderful they are. Typically, they are overly needy and demanding and believe that they are "entitled" to nothing but the best.

Persons with *antisocial personality disorders* display a long-term pattern of manipulation and taking advantage of others, often in a criminal manner. Symptoms include disregard for the safety of others and lack of remorse, arrogance, and anger. Men with antisocial personality disorder far outnumber

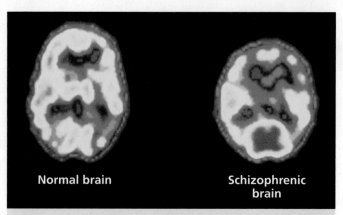

**Normal brain**    **Schizophrenic brain**

These brain images reveal the difference in brain activity in persons with and without schizophrenia. The yellow and red correspond to areas with greatest activity, and blue signifies reduced activity.

women, and it remains one of the hardest to treat of all personality disorders.[66]

*Borderline personality disorder (BPD)* is characterized by severe emotional instability, impulsiveness, mood swings, and poor self-image.[67] High suicide rates, unpredictable mood swings, and erratic and risky behaviors, including gambling, unsafe sex, illicit drug use, daredevil driving, and self-mutilation, are typical.[68] (For more about self-mutilation, see **Student Health Today**.) Although causation is not clear, genetics and environment appear to converge to increase risks. About 1.6 million adults in the United States have BPD in a given year. BPD usually begins during adolescence or early adulthood.[69]

For treating personality disorders, individual and group psychotherapy, skill development, family education, support from peers, and medications can lead to a good long-term prognosis.[70]

## Schizophrenia

**Schizophrenia** is a severe psychological disorder that affects about 1 percent of the U.S. population.[71] Schizophrenia is characterized by alterations of the senses (including auditory and visual hallucinations); the inability to sort and process incoming stimuli and make appropriate responses; an altered sense of self; and radical changes in emotions, movements, and behaviors. Typical symptoms of schizophrenia include fluctuating courses of delusional behavior, hallucinations, incoherent and rambling speech, inability to think logically, erratic movement, odd gesturing, and difficulty with normal activities of daily living.[72] Symptoms usually appear in men in their late teens and 20s and in women in their late 20s and early 30s.[73] Such individuals are often regarded as odd or dangerous, and viewed that way, they have difficulties in social interactions and may withdraw.

For decades, scientists believed that schizophrenia was a form of madness provoked by the environment in which a child lived. They blamed abnormal family interactions or early childhood traumas. In the mid-1980s, magnetic resonance imaging (MRI) and PET scans began allowing scientists to study brain function more closely; based on that knowledge,

**personality disorder** Mental disorder characterized by inflexible patterns of thought and beliefs that lead to socially distressing behavior.

**schizophrenia** Mental illness with biological origins characterized by irrational behavior, severe alterations of the senses, and often an inability to function in society.

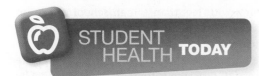

# CUTTING THROUGH THE PAIN

When some people are unable to deal with the pain, pressure, or stress they experience in everyday life, they may resort to self-harm in an effort to cope. **Self-injury**, also termed *self-mutilation, self-harm,* or *nonsuicidal self-injury (NSI)*, is the act of deliberately harming one's body tissue without suicidal attempt and for purposes that are not socially supported.

The most common method of self-harm is cutting (with razors, glass, knives, or other sharp objects). Other methods include burning, bruising, excessive nail biting, breaking bones, pulling out hair, and embedding sharp objects under the skin.

Approximately 4–6 percent of adults in the United States have engaged in NSI at least once in their lifetime. However, the occurrence of NSI is much higher in young adults and adolescents. The prevalence of NSI in college students is estimated to be approximately 6 percent. NSI more commonly occurs in female college students, approximately 7 percent in the past 12 months, versus approximately 4 percent in males. Estimates are higher in the high school population, with the majority of studies reporting between 14 and 18 percent of adolescents and young adults engaging in self-injury at least once in their lifetime. Many people who harm themselves suffer from other mental health conditions and have experienced sexual, physical, or emotional abuse as children or adults. Self-harm is also commonly associated with mental illnesses such as borderline personality disorder, depression, anxiety disorders, substance abuse disorders, posttraumatic stress disorder, and eating disorders.

Signs of self-injury include multiple scars, current cuts and abrasions, and implausible explanations for wounds and ongoing injuries. A self-injurer may attempt to conceal scars and injuries by wearing long sleeves and pants. Other symptoms can include difficulty handling anger, social withdrawal, sensitivity to rejection, or body alienation. If you or someone you know is engaging in self-injury, seek professional help. Treatment is challenging; not only must the self-injurious behavior be stopped, but the sufferer must also learn to recognize and manage the feelings that trigger the behavior.

If you are a recovering self-injurer, some of the following steps may be part of your treatment:

1. Start by being aware of feelings and situations that trigger your urge to hurt yourself.
2. Identify a plan of what you can do instead when you feel the urge.
3. Create a list of alternatives, including:
   - Things that might distract you
   - Things that might soothe and calm you
   - Things that might help you express the pain and deep emotion
   - Things that might help release physical tension and distress
   - Things that might help you feel supported and connected
   - Things that might substitute for the cutting sensation

For more information, visit these resources: S.A.F.E. Alternatives, www.selfinjury.com, and Help Guide, www.helpguide.org/mental/self_injury.htm.

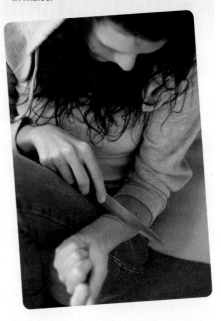

Cutting and scratching behaviors are more common in females, while burning and hitting behaviors are more common in males.

**Sources:** American College Health Association, *ACHA–NCHA II: Reference Group Data Report, Spring 2015* (Baltimore: American College Health Association, 2015); D. Klonsky et al., "The Functions of Nonsuicidal Self-Injury: Converging Evidence for a Two-Factor Structure," *Child Adolescent Psychiatry Mental Health* 9, no. 44 (2015); M. Smith and J. Segal, HelpGuide.org, "Cutting and Self-Harm," updated February 2016, www.helpguide.org/articles/anxiety/cutting-and-self-harm.htm; K. Bresin and M. Schoenleber, "Gender Differences in the Prevalence of Nonsuicidal Self-Injury: A Meta-Analysis," *Clinical Psychology Review* 38 (2015): 55–64.

---

schizophrenia was found to be a biological disease of the brain. The brain damage occurs early in life, possibly as early as the second trimester of fetal development. Fetal exposure to toxic substances, infections, and medications have been studied as a possible risk, and hereditary links are being explored.

Even though theories that blame abnormal family life or childhood trauma for schizophrenia have been discarded in favor of biological theories, a stigma remains attached to the disease. Families of people with schizophrenia frequently experience anger and guilt. They often need information, family counseling, and advice on how to meet the schizophrenic person's needs for shelter, medical care, vocational training, and social interaction.

At present, schizophrenia is treatable but not curable. Treatments usually include some combination of hospitalization,

**self-injury** Intentionally causing injury to one's own body in an attempt to cope with overwhelming negative emotions; also called *self-mutilation, self-harm,* or *nonsuicidal self-injury (NSSI).*

medication, and psychotherapy. Supportive psychotherapy, as opposed to psychoanalysis, can help the patient acquire skills for living in society. With proper medication, public understanding, support of loved ones, and access to therapy, many people with schizophrenia lead normal lives. Without these forms of assistance and treatment, they often have great difficulty.

## LO 4 | UNDERSTANDING SUICIDE

Discuss risk factors and possible warning signs of suicide, as well as actions that can be taken to help a person contemplating suicide.

*"Every 40 seconds a person dies of suicide somewhere in the world . . . another 20 or so more attempt suicide."* These grim statistics and others from the World Health Association's 2014 report highlight the growing international toll of suicide.[74] Each year, over 805,000 deaths are reported internationally. The young, age 15–29, are particularly vulnerable, with suicide being the second leading cause of death in this group internationally.[75] In some of the richest countries, more than 300 percent as many men die of suicide as women. However, in low- and middle-income countries, the male-to-female suicide ratio is only 1.5 men to every woman. Globally, suicides make up 50 percent of all violent deaths for men and over 71 percent for women. The highest rates of suicide are among individuals age 70 years and older.[76]

In the United States, older American suicide rates are comparable to overall international rates. Suicide is the third leading cause of death for 15- to 19-year-olds and the second leading cause of death for 19- to 24-year-olds in the United States.[77] The pressures, disappointments, challenges, and changes of the college years are believed to be partially responsible for the emotional turmoil that can lead a young person to contemplate suicide. According to the 2015 National College Health Assessment, approximately 8 percent of students had seriously considered suicide at some point in their life, and 1 percent had attempted to kill themselves in the past year.[78] However, young adults who do not attend college but who are searching for direction in careers, relationships, and other areas are also at risk; in fact, suicide rates for young adults are higher in the general population than among college students.[79]

### Risk Factors for Suicide

Risk factors include a family history of suicide, previous suicide attempts, excessive drug and alcohol use, prolonged depression, financial difficulties, serious illness in oneself or a loved one, and loss of a loved one through death or rejection. Recent research indicates that lesbian, gay, bisexual, and transgender (LGBT) people are significantly more likely to have thought about or attempted suicide than their heterosexual counterparts, with transgender individuals having the highest rates.[80] Those raised in home and school environments where homophobic teasing is not condoned had significantly lower rates of suicide attempts, whereas those from low-income homes with less than a high school education and with the presence of substance abuse had significantly more suicide attempts.[81]

Whether they are more likely to attempt suicide or are more often successful, nearly four times as many men die by suicide as women.[82] The most commonly used method of suicide among males is firearms; for women, the most common method is poisoning.[83]

### Warning Signs of Suicide

People who commit suicide usually indicate their intentions, although others do not always recognize their warnings.[84] Anyone who expresses a desire to kill him- or herself or who has made an attempt is at risk. Common signs that a person may be contemplating suicide include:[85]

- Recent loss and a seeming inability to let go of grief
- History of depression
- Change in personality, such as sadness, withdrawal, irritability, anxiety, tiredness, indecisiveness, apathy
- Change in behavior, such as inability to concentrate, loss of interest in classes or work, unexplained demonstration

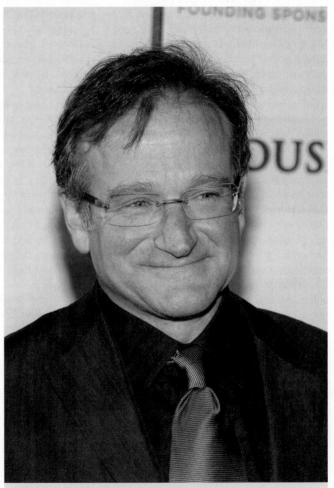

Suicide symptoms are not always obvious. Even "funny, life of the party" people can be struggling inwardly. It was only after his suicide in August 2014 that Robin Williams's struggles with severe depression became widely known.

of happiness following a period of depression, or risk-taking behavior
- Change in sexual interest
- Change in sleep patterns and/or eating habits
- A direct statement (including statements posted on social media) about committing suicide, such as "I might as well end it all"
- An indirect statement (including statements posted on social media), such as "You won't have to worry about me anymore"
- Final preparations such as writing a will, giving away prized possessions, or writing revealing letters or social media posts
- Preoccupation with themes of death
- Marked changes in personal appearance

## Preventing Suicide

Most people who attempt suicide really want to live but see death as the only way out of an intolerable situation. Crisis counselors and suicide hotlines may help temporarily, but the best way to prevent suicide is to get rid of conditions and substances that may precipitate attempts, including alcohol, drugs, loneliness, isolation, and access to guns.

If someone you know threatens suicide or displays warning signs, get involved—ask questions and seek help. Specific actions you can take include:[86]

- **Monitor the warning signals.** Keep an eye on the person or see that someone else is present. Don't leave the person alone.
- **Take threats seriously.** Don't brush them off as "cries for attention." Act now.
- **Let the person know how much you care.** State that you are there to help.
- **Ask directly,** "Are you thinking of hurting or killing yourself?" Don't be judgmental. Let them share their thoughts.
- **Take action.** Remove any firearms or objects that could be used for suicide from the area.
- **Help the person think about alternatives to suicide.** Offer to go for help along with the person. Call your local suicide hotline, and use all available community and campus resources.
- **Tell the person's spouse, partner, parents, siblings, or counselor.** Do not keep your suspicions to yourself. Don't let a suicidal friend talk you into keeping your discussions confidential. If your friend succeeds in a suicide attempt, you may blame yourself.

## LO 5 | SEEKING PROFESSIONAL HELP

Explain the different types of treatment options and professional services available to those experiencing mental health problems.

A physical ailment will readily send most of us to the nearest health professional, but many people view seeking professional help for psychological problems as an admission of personal failure. Although estimates show that while about 20 percent of adults have some kind of mental disorder, only 12–15 percent of adults use mental health counseling services.[87]

> **stigma** Negative perception about a group of people or a certain situation or condition.

Researchers view breakdowns in support systems, high societal expectations, and dysfunctional families as three major reasons why people need more assistance than ever before. Consider seeking help if:

- You feel that you need help or feel out of control.
- You experience wild mood swings or inappropriate emotional responses to normal stimuli.
- Your fears or feelings of guilt frequently distract your attention.
- You begin to withdraw from others.
- You have hallucinations.
- You feel inadequate or worthless or that life is not worth living.
- Your daily life seems to be nothing but a series of repeated crises.
- You are considering suicide.
- You turn to drugs or alcohol to escape your problems.

Low-cost or free counseling sessions or support groups are often available on college campuses to help students deal with all types of issues, including mental illness; recovery from eating disorders, substance abuse, and other addictions; dealing with health conditions such as diabetes or cancer; and addressing other challenges, such as managing stress, overcoming fear of public speaking, becoming more physically fit, or changing eating habits. See the **Money & Health** box on page 44 for tips on how to get good mental health care on a tight budget. You may find certain websites or phone apps useful as well, but be cautious in your selection.

## Mental Illness Stigma

**Stigmas** are negative perceptions about groups of people or about a certain situation or condition. Common stigmas about people with mental illness are that they are dangerous, irresponsible, require constant care, or that they "just need to get over it." In truth, only about 3–5 percent of all violent acts are attributed to people with serious mental illness. It is no more likely for most people with mental health problems to be violent than it is for anyone else, even though the mentally ill are 10 times more likely to become victims of violence. Most

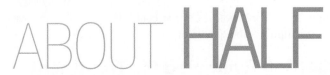

ABOUT HALF
of students with **MENTAL HEALTH PROBLEMS** receive treatment.

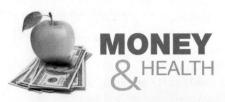

# MONEY & HEALTH | LOW-COST TREATMENT OPTIONS FOR MENTAL HEALTH CONDITIONS

**M**ental health disorders are treatable, yet people don't always seek help. Often the cost of therapy and prescription drugs is a major barrier, since insurance plans may provide only limited coverage of mental health services. If you are on a tight budget and struggle with depression, anxiety, or other mental health issues, it's a good idea to speak with your family physician about low-cost treatment resources in your region and state. Here is a roundup of possible treatment options one can pursue, along with tips on easing the expense.

### Therapy

Cognitive-behavioral therapy (CBT) can cost $100 or more per hour. However, some therapists or clinics offer therapy on a sliding scale, which means the fee fluctuates based on income. Ask about a sliding scale or other payment options when you call or visit for a consultation.

Federally funded health centers can also be a good resource for those with a limited budget. Many of these centers include mental health services, and they also have sliding scales for payment. Finally, some colleges and universities offer low-cost therapy for mental health problems through the health center. You can also call the psychology, psychiatry, or behavioral health department and inquire about sessions with graduate students, who are supervised and can provide services at a lower cost as they gain counseling experience.

### Prescription Drugs

Medication can help reduce symptoms of certain mental health disorders, including anxiety and depression, but for many people drugs can be expensive. Most pharmaceutical companies offer patient-assistance programs for low-income patients. These programs provide prescribed

medication at little to no cost. It's also a good idea to ask your doctor if a generic (non-brand-name) drug might work as well for you as a brand-name drug. The cost difference between generic and brand-name drugs can be substantial. You can also see if your doctor might have medication samples he or she could give you for free.

Note that if you are considering medication, it must be prescribed and monitored by your physician. Do not adjust the dosage or frequency or stop taking it abruptly, even if cost is a factor, without first discussing it with your doctor.

**Sources:** ADAA, "Low Cost Treatment," Accessed February 2016, www.adaa.org/finding-help/treatment/low-cost-treatment; Partnership for Prescription Assistance, Accessed February 2016, "Patient Frequently Asked Questions," www.pparx.org/en/patient_faqs; J. Grohol, "Finding Low-Cost Psychotherapy," *PsychCentral*, Accessed February 2016, http://psychcentral.com/lib/2007/finding-low-cost-psychotherapy.

---

## WHAT DO YOU THINK?

Do you notice a stigma associated with mental illness in your campus? If yes, describe the way(s) stigma appears on campus.

- How often do you hear terms such as "crazy" or "whacko" used to describe people who appear to have a mental health problem? Why are those words harmful?
- What could you do to combat the stigma of mental illness?

hold regular jobs, are productive members of society, and lead normal lives.[88]

The stigma of mental illness often leads to feelings of shame, guilt, loss of self-esteem, and a sense of isolation and hopelessness. Many people who have successfully managed their mental illness report that the stigma they faced was more disabling at times than the illness itself.[89] This stigma may cause people who are struggling with a mental illness to delay seeking treatment or avoid care that could dramatically improve their symptoms and quality of life.

health professional for a thorough examination, which should include three parts:

1. A *physical checkup*, which will rule out thyroid disorders, viral infections, and anemia—all of which can result in depression-like symptoms—and a neurological check of coordination, reflexes, and balance to rule out brain disorders.
2. A *psychiatric history*, which will trace the course of the apparent disorder, genetic or family factors, and any past treatments.
3. A *mental status examination*, which will assess thoughts, speaking processes, and memory, and will include an in-depth interview with tests for other psychiatric symptoms.

Once physical factors have been ruled out, you may decide to consult a professional who specializes in psychological health.

## Getting Evaluated for Treatment

If you are considering treatment for a psychological problem, schedule a complete evaluation first. Consult a credentialed

## Mental Health Professionals

Several types of mental health professionals are available; **TABLE 2.1** provides information on the most common types of

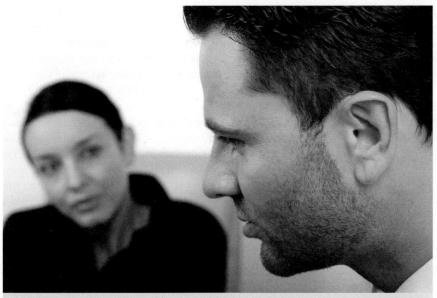

When you begin seeing a mental health professional, you enter into a relationship with that person, and just as with any person, you will connect better with some therapists than others. If one doesn't "feel right," trust your instincts and look for someone else.

practitioners. When choosing a therapist, it is important to verify that he or she has the appropriate training and certification. But the most important factor is whether you feel you can work with him or her. A qualified mental health professional should be willing to answer all your questions during an initial consultation. Questions to ask the therapist or yourself include:

- **Can you interview the therapist before starting treatment?** An initial meeting will help you determine whether this person will be a good fit for you.
- **Do you like the therapist as a person?** Can you talk to him or her comfortably?
- **Is the therapist watching the clock or easily distracted?** You should be the main focus of the session.

## TABLE **2.1** | Mental Health Professionals

| What Are They Called? | What Kind of Training Do They Have? | What Kind of Therapy Do They Do? | Professional Association |
|---|---|---|---|
| Psychiatrist | Medical doctor degree (MD), followed by 4 years of mental health training | Can prescribe medications and may have admitting privileges at a local hospital | American Psychiatric Association www.psych.org |
| Psychologist | Doctoral degree in counseling or clinical psychology (PhD), plus several years of supervised practice to earn license | Various types, such as cognitive-behavioral therapy and specialties including family or sexual counseling | American Psychological Association www.apa.org |
| Clinical/psychiatric social worker | Master's degree in social work (MSW), followed by 2 years of experience in a clinical setting to earn license | May be trained in certain specialties, such as substance abuse counseling or child counseling | National Association of Social Workers www.socialworkers.org |
| Counselor | Master's degree in counseling, psychology, educational psychology, or related human service; generally must complete at least 2 years of supervised practice to obtain a license | Many are trained to provide individual and group therapy; may specialize in one type of counseling, such as family, marital, relationship, children, or substance abuse | American Counseling Association www.counseling.org |
| Psychoanalyst | Postgraduate degree in psychology or psychiatry (PhD or MD), followed by 8–10 years of training in psychoanalysis, which includes undergoing analysis themselves | Based on the theories of Freud and others, focuses on patterns of thinking and behavior and recalling early traumas that block personal growth; treatment lasts 5–10 years, with three to four sessions per week | American Psychoanalytic Association www.apsa.org |
| Licensed marriage and family therapist (LMFT) | Master's or doctoral degree in psychology, social work, or counseling, specializing in family and interpersonal dynamics; generally must complete at least 2 years of supervised practice to obtain a license | Treats individuals or families who want relationship counseling; treatment is often brief and focused on finding solutions to specific relational problems | American Association for Marriage and Family Therapy www.aamft.org |

- **Does the therapist demonstrate professionalism?** Be concerned if your therapist is frequently late or breaks appointments, suggests social interactions outside therapy sessions, talks inappropriately about him- or herself, has questionable billing practices, or resists releasing you from therapy.
- **Will the therapist help you set your own goals and timetables?** A good professional should evaluate your general situation and help you set small goals to work on between sessions.

Note that the use of the title *therapist* or *counselor* is not nationally regulated. Check credentials and make your choice carefully.

## What to Expect in Therapy

Before making an appointment, call for information and briefly explain your needs. Ask about office hours, policies and procedures, fees, and insurance participation. The first trip to a therapist can be unsettling. Most of us have misconceptions about what therapy is and what it can do. The first visit serves as a sizing-up between you and the therapist. If you decide that this professional is not for you, you will at least have learned how to present your problem and what qualities you need in a therapist.

Dress however you feel most comfortable, arrive on time, and expect your visit to last about an hour. The therapist will record your history and details about the problem that has brought you to therapy. Answer honestly and do not be embarrassed to acknowledge your feelings. It is critical to the success of your treatment that you trust the therapist enough to be open and honest.

Do not expect the therapist to tell you what to do or how to behave. The responsibility for improved behavior lies with you. If after your first visit (or even after several visits), you feel you cannot work with this person, say so. You have the right to find a therapist with whom you feel comfortable.

### Treatment Models
Many different types of counseling exist, including psychodynamic therapy, interpersonal therapy, and cognitive-behavioral therapy.

*Psychodynamic therapy* focuses on the psychological roots of emotional suffering. This type of therapy has roots in Freud's theories and involves self-reflection, self-examination, and the use of the relationship between therapist and patient as a window into problematic relationship patterns in the patient's life. Its goal is not only to alleviate the most obvious symptoms, but also to help people lead healthier lives.[90]

*Interpersonal therapy* is a variation of psychodynamic therapy and focuses on social roles and relationships. The patient works with a therapist to evaluate specific problem areas in the patient's life, such as conflicts with family and friends or significant life changes or transition. While past experiences help inform the process, interpersonal therapy focuses mainly on improving relationships in the present.[91]

Treatment for mental disorders can include various cognitive-behavioral therapies. *Cognitive therapy* focuses on the impact of thoughts and ideas on feelings and behavior. It helps a person to look at life rationally and correct habitually pessimistic or faulty thinking patterns. *Behavioral therapy*, as the name implies, focuses on what we do. Behavioral therapy uses the concepts of stimulus, response, and reinforcement to alter behavior patterns. With cognitive-behavioral therapy, you work with a mental health professional in a structured way, attending a limited number of sessions to become aware of inaccurate or negative thinking. Cognitive-behavioral therapy enables you to view challenging situations more clearly and respond to them in a more effective and positive way. This therapy can be a very helpful tool in treating mental anxiety or depression.[92]

## Pharmacological Treatment

Treatment for some conditions combines cognitive-behavioral therapies with psychoactive medication prescribed by the patient's physician or by a psychiatrist. **TABLE 2.2** includes information about the major classes of medications used to treat the most common mental illnesses. Psychoactive drugs require a doctor's prescription and carry approval from the U.S. Food and Drug Administration (FDA). Side effects of psychoactive drugs commonly include dry mouth, headaches, nausea, sexual dysfunction, and weight gain, among others. Additionally, the FDA requires warnings for antidepressant medications, including a black box labeling (black box warnings are the FDA's most stringent a drug can carry) that warns of increased risks of suicidal thinking and behavior during initial treatment in young adults age 18–24.[93]

Potency, dosage, and side effects of drugs can vary greatly. It is vital to talk to your health care provider and completely understand the risks and benefits of any prescribed medication. Likewise, your doctor needs to be notified as soon as possible of any adverse effects you may experience. With some drug therapies, such as antidepressants, you may not feel the therapeutic effects for several weeks, so patience is important. Finally, be sure to follow your doctor's recommendations for beginning or ending a course of any medication.

To avoid the side effects of psychoactive drugs, some patients choose complementary or alternative therapies such as St. John's wort or omega-3 fatty acids for depression and kava or acupuncture for anxiety. While the efficacy of these therapies is not yet conclusive, NCCAM continues to invest in research to explore alternatives to

Many people with mental illnesses live normal lives with help from drugs that keep their illnesses under control.

# TABLE 2.2 | Types of Medications Used to Treat Mental Illness

| **Antidepressants** | **Used to Treat Depression, Panic Disorders, and Anxiety Disorders** | |
|---|---|---|
| Selective serotonin-reuptake inhibitors (SSRIs) | *Examples:* fluoxetine (Prozac), paroxetine (Paxil), escitalopram (Lexapro, Esipram), citalopram (Celexa) | The current standard drug treatment for depression; also frequently prescribed for anxiety disorders |
| Noradrenergic and specific serotonergic antidepressants (NaSSAs) | *Examples:* mirtazapine (Remeron) | Reportedly has fewer sexual dysfunction side effects than do SSRIs |
| Serotonin-norepinephrine reuptake inhibitors (SNRIs) | *Examples:* venlafaxine (Effexor), duloxetine (Cymbalta) | Also sometimes prescribed for ADHD |
| Norepinephrine-dopamine reuptake inhibitors (NDRIs) | *Examples:* bupropion (Wellbutrin) | Also used in smoking cessation; fewer weight gain or sexual dysfunction side effects than SSRIs |
| Tricyclic antidepressants (TCAs) | *Examples:* imipramine (Tofranil), amitriptyline, nortriptyline (Pamelor), and desipramine (Norpramin) | Negative side effects; usually used as a second or third line of treatment when other medications prove ineffective |
| Monoamine oxidase inhibitors (MAOIs) | *Examples:* phenelzine (Nardil), tranylcypromine (Parnate), and isocarboxazid (Marplan) | Dangerous interactions with many other drugs and substances in food; generally no longer prescribed |
| **Anxiolytics (Antianxiety Drugs)** | **Used to Treat Anxiety Disorders, GAD, Panic Disorders, Phobias, OCD, and PTSD** | |
| Benzodiazepines | *Examples:* lorazepam (Ativan), clonazepam (Klonopin), alprazolam (Xanax), diazepam (Valium) | Short-term relief, sometimes taken on an as-needed basis; dangerous interactions with alcohol; possible to develop tolerance or dependence |
| Serotonin 1A agonists | *Examples:* buspirone (BuSpar) | Longer-term relief; must be taken for at least 2 weeks to achieve antianxiety effects |
| **Mood Stabilizers** | **Used to Treat Bipolar Disorder and Schizophrenia** | |
| Lithium | *Examples:* lithium carbonate (Eskalith) | Drug most commonly used to treat bipolar disorder; blood levels must be closely monitored to determine proper dosage and avoid toxic effects |
| Anticonvulsants | *Examples:* valproic acid/divalproex sodium (Depakote) | Used more frequently for acute mania than for long-term maintenance of bipolar disorder |
| **Antipsychotics (Neuroleptics)** | **Used to Treat Schizophrenia, Mania, and Bipolar Disorder** | |
| Atypical antipsychotics | *Examples:* olanzapine, risperidone (Risperdal) | First line of treatment for schizophrenia; fewer adverse effects than earlier antipsychotics |
| First-generation antipsychotics | *Examples:* haloperidol (Haldol), chlorpromazine (Thorazine) | Earliest forms of antipsychotics; unpleasant side effects such as tremor and muscle stiffness |
| **Stimulants** | **Used to Treat ADHD and Narcolepsy** | |
| Methylphenidate | *Examples:* Ritalin, Metadate CD, Concerta | Can lead to tolerance and dependence; frequently abused for both performance enhancement and recreational use |
| Amphetamines | *Examples:* amphetamine (Adderall), dextroamphetamine (Dexedrine, Dextrostat) | Can lead to tolerance and dependence; frequently abused for both performance enhancement and recreational use |

**Sources:** National Institute of Mental Health, "Mental Health Medications," January 2016, www.nimh.nih.gov/health/publications/mental-health-medications/nimh-mental-health-medications.pdf; National Institute of Mental Health, "Attention Deficit Hyperactivity Disorder," Accessed February 2016, www.nimh.nih.gov/health/topics/attention-deficit-hyperactivity-disorder-adhd/index.shtml; Mayo Clinic, "Depression: Monoamine oxidase inhibitors," Accessed February 2016, www.mayoclinic.org/diseases-conditions/depression/in-depth/maois/art-20043992; Mayo Clinic, "Depression: Tricyclic antidepressants and tetracyclic antidepressants," Accessed February 2016, www.mayoclinic.org/diseases-conditions/depression/in-depth/antidepressants/art-20046983.

prescription drugs. While some CAM therapies, such as mindfulness meditation—associated with structural changes in the brain that may reduce symptoms of both anxiety and depression—is unlikely to cause any harm, some therapies, like St. John's wort, can be life-threatening when combined with traditional depression medications. Much research is still needed on both traditional and CAM therapies for mental illness, making it essential to talk to a medical professional when considering any new treatment or change in treatment.

## **ASSESS** YOURSELF

**How is your psychological health?** Want to find out?
Take the **How Psychologically Healthy Are You?** assessment available on

**MasteringHealth.**™

## CHAPTER **REVIEW**

To hear an MP3 Tutor Session, scan here or visit the Study Area in **MasteringHealth**.

### LO **1** What Is Psychological Health?

- Psychological health is a complex phenomenon involving mental, emotional, social, and spiritual dimensions.

### LO **2** Keys to Enhancing Psychological Health

- Many factors influence psychological health, including life experiences, family, the environment, other people, self-esteem, self-efficacy, and personality.
- The mind–body connection is an important link in overall health and well-being. Positive psychology emphasizes well-being as a key factor in determining overall reactions to life's challenges. Psychoneuroimmunology indicates that mental health and physical health are linked.

### LO **3** When Psychological Health Deteriorates

- College is a time when disorders such as depression or anxiety, often related to high stress levels that result from pressures for grades and financial problems, occur.
- Mood disorders include major depression, dysthymic disorder,

bipolar disorder, and seasonal affective disorder.
- Anxiety disorders include generalized anxiety disorder, panic disorders, phobic disorders, obsessive–compulsive disorder, and post-traumatic stress disorder.
- People with OCD often have irrational concern about order, symmetry, or exactness, or have persistent intrusive thoughts.
- PTSD is caused by experiencing or witnessing a traumatic event, such as those that occur in war, natural disasters, or the loss of a loved one.
- Personality disorders include paranoid, narcissistic, antisocial, and borderline personality disorders.
- Schizophrenia is often characterized by visual and auditory hallucinations, an altered sense of self, and radical changes in emotions, among others.

### LO **4** Understanding Suicide

- Suicide is a result of negative psychological reactions to life. People intending to commit suicide often give warning signs of their intentions and can often be helped. Suicide prevention involves eliminating the conditions that may lead to attempts.

### LO **5** Seeking Professional Help

- Mental health professionals include psychiatrists, psychoanalysts, psychologists, social workers, and counselors/therapists. Many therapy

methods exist, including psychodynamic, interpersonal, and cognitive-behavioral therapy.
- Treatment of mental disorders can combine talk therapy and drug therapy using psychoactive drugs, such as antidepressants or anxiolytics.

## POP **QUIZ**

Visit **MasteringHealth** to personalize your study plan with Chapter Review Quizzes and Dynamic Study Modules.

### LO **1** What Is Psychological Health?

1. All of the following traits have been identified as characterizing psychologically healthy people *except*
   a. conscientiousness.
   b. understanding.
   c. openness.
   d. agreeableness.

### LO **2** Keys to Enhancing Psychological Health

2. A person with high self-esteem
   a. possesses feelings of self-respect and self-worth.
   b. believes he or she can successfully engage in a specific behavior.
   c. believes external influences shape one's psychological health.
   d. has a high altruistic capacity.

3. The initial "A" in the PERMA acronym represents which concept?
   a. Activity
   b. Advocacy
   c. Acceptance
   d. Accomplishments

4. Which of the following is *not* part of a good strategy for building self-esteem?
   a. Develop a support system
   b. Concentrate more on mental health than physical health
   c. Make time for you
   d. Form realistic expectations

LO **3** | **When Psychological Health Deteriorates**

5. Which statement below is *false*?
   a. One in five adults in the United States suffers from a diagnosable mental disorder in a given year.
   b. Mental disorders are the leading cause of disability in the United States.
   c. Dysthymia is an example of an anxiety disorder.
   d. Bipolar disorder can also be referred to as manic depressive illness.

6. Every winter, Stan suffers from irritability, apathy, weight gain, and sadness. He most likely has
   a. seasonal depression.
   b. generalized anxiety disorder.
   c. seasonal affective disorder.
   d. chronic mood disorder.

7. Sarah has a compulsion to wash her hands over and over again and she's extremely fearful of dirt. She most likely has
   a. generalized anxiety disorder
   b. panic disorder
   c. obsessive–compulsive disorder
   d. dysthymic disorder

8. This disorder is characterized by a need to perform rituals over and over again; fear of dirt or contamination; or an unnatural concern with order, symmetry, and exactness.
   a. Personality disorder
   b. Obsessive–compulsive disorder
   c. Phobic disorder
   d. Posttraumatic stress disorder

9. How many Americans will experience posttraumatic stress disorder in their lifetime?

   a. 1 percent
   b. 8 percent
   c. 16 percent
   d. 32 percent

10. This type of disorder is characterized by an exaggerated sense of self-importance and self-absorption.
    a. Borderline personality disorder
    b. Narcissistic personality disorder
    c. Antisocial personality disorder
    d. Paranoid personality disorder

11. What percentage of the United States population has schizophrenia?
    a. 1 percent
    b. 5 percent
    c. 10 percent
    d. 20 percent

LO **4** | **Understanding Suicide**

12. For 15- to 24-year-olds in the United States, suicide is the ___ leading cause of death.
    a. first
    b. second
    c. third
    d. fourth

LO **5** | **Seeking Professional Help**

13. A person with a PhD in counseling psychology and training in various types of therapy is a
    a. psychiatrist.
    b. psychologist.
    c. social worker.
    d. psychoanalyst.

*Answers to the Pop Quiz can be found on page A-1. If you answered a question incorrectly, review the section identified by the Learning Outcome. For even more study tools, visit* **MasteringHealth**.

# THINK ABOUT IT!

LO **1** | **What Is Psychological Health?**

1. What is psychological health? What indicates that you are or are not psychologically healthy? Why might the college environment provide a challenge to psychological health?

LO **2** | **Keys to Enhancing Psychological Health**

2. Consider the factors that influence your overall level of psychological health. Which factors can you change? Which ones may be more difficult to change?

3. What connections can you make between physical and psychological health?

LO **3** | **When Psychological Health Deteriorates**

4. What proportion of the student population suffers from some type of mental illness? What types of support networks exist on your campus?

5. What are the symptoms of major depression? How is major depression different from other mood disorders?

6. What are the symptoms of an anxiety disorder? How is feeling anxious different from having an anxiety disorder or having a panic attack?

7. How common is obsessive–compulsive disorder? How is having OCD different from being a perfectionist?

8. What are the causes of posttraumatic stress disorder? Why do some go less reported than others?

9. What are the characteristics of borderline personality disorder? How is it different from other personality disorders?

10. How has our understanding of schizophrenia evolved? What is responsible for this shift in understanding? Why might it be difficult for people with schizophrenia to lead normal lives without support and other treatment?

LO **4** | **Understanding Suicide**

11. What are the warning signs of suicide? Why are some people more vulnerable to suicide than others? What could you do if you heard a classmate say to no one in

particular that he was going to "do the world a favor and end it all"?

LO **5** | **Seeking Professional Help**

12. Describe the various types of mental health professionals and types of therapies. If you felt depressed about breaking off a long-term relationship, which professional and which therapy do you think would be most beneficial to you?

# ACCESS YOUR HEALTH ON THE INTERNET

Visit **MasteringHealth** for links to the websites and RSS feeds.

The following websites explore further topics related to psychological health.

**American Foundation for Suicide Prevention.** Provides resources for suicide prevention and support for family and friends of those who have committed suicide. Includes info on the National Suicide Prevention Hotline, 1-800-273-TALK (8255). **www.afsp.org**

**American Psychological Association Help Center.** Includes information on psychology at work, the mind–body connection, understanding depression, psychological responses to war, and other topics. **www.apa.org/helpcenter/wellness**

**National Alliance on Mental Illness.** Support and advocacy organization of families and friends of people with severe mental illnesses. **www.nami.org**

**National Institute of Mental Health (NIMH).** Provides an overview of mental health information and new research. **www.nimh.nih.gov**

**Helpguide.** Resources for improving mental and emotional health as well as specific information on topics such as self-injury, sleep, depressive disorders, and anxiety disorders. **www.helpguide.org**

**Active Minds.** Campus education and advocacy organization formed to combat the stigma of mental illness, encourage students who need help to seek it early, and prevent tragedies related to untreated mental illness. **www.activeminds.org**

**Jed Foundation.** Works to promote emotional health and prevent suicide among college students. Provides information for parents, students, campus professionals, and friends. **www.jedfoundation.org**

# FOCUS **ON** Cultivating Your Spiritual Health

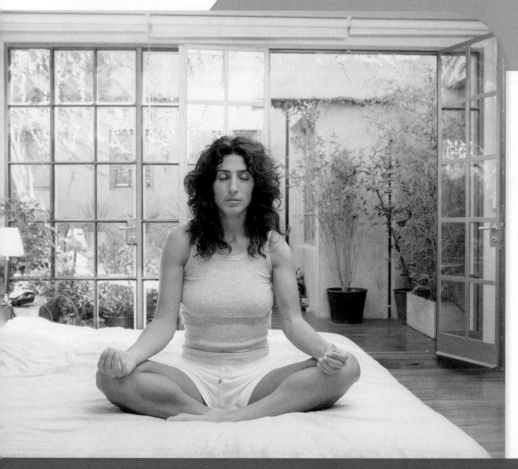

## LEARNING OUTCOMES

LO **1** Define spirituality, describe its three facets, and distinguish between religion and spirituality.

LO **2** Describe the evidence that spiritual health has physical benefits, has psychological benefits, and lowers stress.

LO **3** Describe three ways you can develop your spiritual health.

## WHY SHOULD I CARE?

Spirituality refers to looking for well-being in one's life, particularly regarding relationships, values, and purpose. In practice, spirituality can provide physical and psychological benefits to individuals (such as decreasing blood pressure and reducing stress and anxiety) and can also help communities become stronger and more connected, all important factors for healthy students and a healthy campus. Spiritual practices such as meditation can improve concentration and your brain's ability to process information; it can also reduce stress, anxiety, and depression, all important factors when trying to manage your classes and handle daily demands.

Lia's favorite spot on campus is the secluded Japanese garden on the south side of the library. Whether she's feeling stressed about exams or is mulling over an important decision, a few minutes alone in the garden always seem to help. Sometimes she sits quietly and watches the birds come and go. Sometimes she gets out her camera and photographs particularly brilliant blossoms. Often she simply rests, eyes closed, feeling the sun's warmth on her face, and lets her thoughts turn to gratitude for her health, her loving family,

51

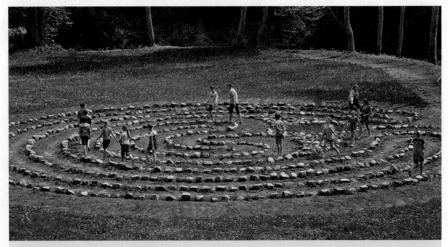

The simple act of walking slowly, mindfully, and with purpose through a maze, or labyrinth, is a way to visualize our path through life as we consider our place in our community and society.

and her opportunity to be in college. However she spends it, her "garden break" leaves Lia feeling refreshed and refocused, with greater confidence in her ability to tackle the challenges of her day.

Lia's desire to find a sense of purpose, meaning, and harmony in her life is shared by a majority of American college students, according to UCLA's Higher Education Research Institute (HERI).[1] Of the 153,015 students at 227 colleges and universities who were surveyed as they entered college in the fall of 2014, nearly 36 percent rated themselves as above average in spirituality.[2]

Spiritual health is one of six key dimensions of health (see **FIGURE 1.4** on page 7 in Chapter 1). This chapter looks at what spiritual health is and why it is beneficial, as well as provides the tools for enhancing your own spiritual health.

## LO 1 | WHAT IS SPIRITUALITY?

**Define spirituality, describe its three facets, and distinguish between religion and spirituality.**

From one day to the next, many of us attempt to satisfy our needs for belonging and self-esteem by acquiring material possessions, hanging with the "right crowd," and being the "best" at everything we do. But new "toys" and keeping up with others don't necessarily bring happiness or improve our sense of self-worth or well-being—nor do they protect us from life's ups and downs. Friends and family can disappoint; relationships can falter; and even the best-laid plans can fail. Buffeted by life, many of us begin to seek more answers—to grow and develop in a way that helps us cope. With

this seeking, our quest for spirituality begins.

But what is spirituality? Let's begin by exploring its root, *spirit*, which in many cultures refers to *breath*, or the force that animates life. When you're "inspired," your energy flows. You're not held back by doubts about the purpose or meaning of your work and life. Indeed, many definitions of spirituality incorporate this sense of transcendence, focused on an internal experience.

Harold G. Koenig, MD, one of the foremost researchers of spirituality and health, defines **spirituality** as "the personal quest for understanding answers to ultimate questions about life, about meaning, and about our relationship with the sacred or transcendent."[3] The sacred or transcendent could be thought of as a higher power or being, or it could refer to the

essential goodness of life, or our relationship with nature or forces we cannot explain.

Spirituality may mean different things to different people; however, there are often several common elements, including:

- Being aware of your impact on people, places, and events
- Actively searching for meaning in your life
- Finding a way to give back, knowing that service to others is a source of true happiness
- Understanding the interconnectedness of humanity, nature, and the universe and respecting all elements
- Nurturing loving relationships with yourself and others
- Living with intention, as if every day matters
- Developing a philosophy of life that guides your daily attitudes and decisions
- Accepting your limitations as well as your strengths

Essentially, spirituality is about actively paying attention to our relationships, our community, and our selves, emphasizing respect and awareness.

**27.5%** of first-year students marked "none" as their **RELIGIOUS PREFERENCE,** nearly doubling the 15.4% who indicated no religious preference in 1971.

**spirituality** An individual's sense of peace, purpose, and connection to others and beliefs about the meaning of life.

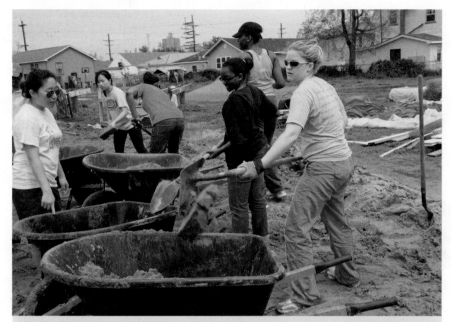

Spiritual and ethical concerns are important to most American college students. One of the ways students express their spirituality is by working to reduce suffering in the world; many contribute their time and skills to volunteer organizations, as these students are doing by working to build homes for Habitat for Humanity.

## Spirituality and Religion

Spirituality and religion are not the same thing. Religion is a set of rituals, beliefs, symbols, and practices intended to enable a feeling of connection to the holy or divine. It is possible to be spiritual and not religious and equally possible to be religious and not spiritual. In fact, while one global survey revealed that nearly 4 out of 5 people worldwide are religiously affiliated, it also showed 16 percent (1.1 billion) are not affiliated, making them the third largest group surveyed.[4] Recent research showed that so-called "millennials," people born roughly between the years 1981 and 1996, are less likely than older Americans to say that religion is very important to them. In contrast, they were just as likely as older Americans to report the importance of spirituality.[5] Many people without religious affiliation still have certain religious or spiritual beliefs.[6] Thus, it's clear that religion does not have to be part of a spiritual person's life. **TABLE 1** identifies some characteristics that can help you distinguish between religion and spirituality.

## Spirituality Integrates Three Facets

Brian Luke Seaward, a professor at the University of Northern Colorado and author of several books on spirituality and mind–body healing, identifies three facets of human existence that together constitute the core of human spirituality: *relationships*, *values*, and *purpose in life* (**FIGURE 1**).[7] Questions arising in these three domains prompt many of us to look for spiritual answers.

## Relationships

Have you ever wondered if someone you were attracted to is really right for you? Or, conversely, wondered if you should break off a long-term relationship? Have you ever wished you had more friends, or that you were a better friend to yourself? For many people, such questions and yearnings are natural triggers for spiritual growth: As we contemplate who we should choose as a life partner or how to mend a quarrel with a friend, we begin to foster our own inner wisdom. At the same time, healthy relationships are a sign of spiritual well-being and problematic relationships can negatively impact many facets of one's life. For example, in 2015, 9 percent of college students who participated in the National College Health Assessment reported that relationship difficulties had negatively impacted their academic performance.[8] When we think well of ourselves, and consequently treat others with respect, honesty, integrity, and love, we are manifesting our spiritual health.

## Values

Our personal **values** are our principles—the set of fundamental rules by which we conduct our lives. It's what we stand for, such as honesty, integrity, and altruism. When we attempt to clarify our values, and then live according to those values, we're moving closer

**values** Principles that influence our thoughts and emotions and guide the choices we make in our lives.

## TABLE 1 | Characteristics Distinguishing Religion and Spirituality

| Religion | Spirituality |
| --- | --- |
| Reverence for a specific higher power | Connections between all things |
| Systematic method of worship | Variety of practices to enhance spiritual growth |
| Institutional and organized | Outside of organized traditions |
| Formal, orthodox | Personalized and individual |
| Behavior-oriented, outward practices | Emotionally oriented, inwardly directed |
| Authoritarian in terms of behaviors | Accountability to self |
| Doctrine separating good from evil | Unifying, not doctrine oriented |

**Source:** R.F. Paloutzian and C.L. Park, *Handbook of the Psychology of Religion and Spirituality,* 2nd ed. (New York: Guilford Press, 2013); National Center for Complementary and Integrative Health (NCCIH), "Prayer and Spirituality in Health: Ancient Practices, Modern Science," *CAM at the NIH* 12, no. 1 (2005): 1–4.

to a spiritually healthy life. Spiritual health is characterized by a personal understanding of one's own values (including how we established our values and why we hold certain values) as well as a respect and curiosity about the values of others in our community.

## Purpose in Life

What things will make you feel happy and "complete"? How do you hope to find "meaning" in your life and your relationships with others? What experiences do you hope to gain? How will family and friends fit into your plans? Is there some "wrong" in the world that you would like to help make "right"? How do these choices reflect what you hold as your purpose in life? At the end of your days, what would you want people to say about how you've lived your life and what your life has meant to others? How will the way you live your life contribute to your community and society? Do you wonder about the meaning your life has? Spiritual growth is fostered by contemplating these questions about our place in the world rather than our individual gains and material possessions. People who are spiritually healthy are able to articulate their search for a global purpose and to make choices that manifest that purpose.

Picture in your mind someone you think has made the world a better place—whether someone close to you, or a global figure such as Gandhi, Martin Luther King, Jr., or Mother Theresa—people whose spiritual quests took on a life-size view of a better world and had a real purpose. Allow yourself to see your life as having its own mission and purpose.

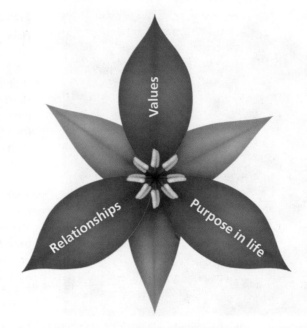

**FIGURE 1** **Three Facets of Spirituality** Most of us are prompted to explore our spirituality because of questions relating to our relationships, values, and purpose in life. At the same time, these three facets together constitute spiritual well-being.

➡ **VIDEO TUTOR**
Facets of Spirituality

## Spiritual Intelligence and Inner Wisdom

Our relationships, values, and sense of purpose together contribute to our overall **spiritual intelligence (SI)**. This term was introduced by physicist and philosopher Danah Zohar, who defined it as "an ability to access higher meanings, values, abiding purposes, and unconscious aspects of the self."[9] Humility, the capacity to consider ideas that fall "outside the box" and tapping in to energies outside the ego all fit in her definition. SI allows us to utilize values (such as gratitude and forgiveness), meanings, and purposes to be more creative and enrich our lives.

Since Zohar introduced the idea of SI, a number of psychologists, clerics, and even some business consultants have taken the liberty of expanding the definition of the term. For example, spiritual intelligence expert Cindy Wigglesworth explains that SI helps us find compassion and wisdom to help guide us through life.[10] SI also helps us maintain our peaceful center. To find out your own spiritual IQ, see the **Assess Yourself** activity in **MasteringHealth**.

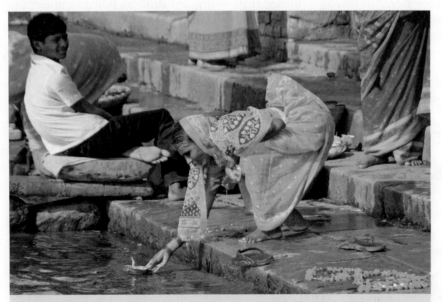

Spirituality and religion are not the same. Many people find that religious practices, for example, attending services or making offerings—such as the small lamp this Hindu woman is placing in the sacred Ganges River—help them to focus on their spirituality. However, religion does not have to be part of a spiritual person's life.

**spiritual intelligence (SI)** The ability to access higher meanings, values, abiding purposes, and unconscious aspects of the self; a characteristic that helps us find a moral and ethical path to guide us through life.

# THE #1

trait millennials look for in a successful career is a "**SENSE OF MEANING**," which seems to be defined as doing things for others, or giving.

## LO 2 | THE **BENEFITS** OF SPIRITUAL HEALTH

Discuss the evidence that spiritual health has physical benefits, has psychological benefits, and lowers stress.

A broad range of large-scale surveys have documented the importance of the mind–body connection to human health and wellness.

### Physical Benefits

The emerging science of mind–body medicine is a research focus of the National Center for Complementary and Integrative Health (NCCIH) and an important objective of the organization's 2011–2015 Strategic Plan. One area under study is the association between spiritual health and general health. The NCCIH cites evidence that spirituality can have a positive influence on physical health and suggests that the connection may be due to improved immune function, cardiovascular function, or a combination of physiological changes.[11] Increasing numbers of studies are examining the effect that certain spiritual practices—such as yoga, deep meditation, and prayer—have on the mind, body, social and emotional health, and behavior, and how these practices may improve health and promote healthy behaviors.[12]

The National Cancer Institute (NCI) contends that when we get sick, spiritual or religious well-being may help restore health and improve quality of life by:[13]

- Decreasing anxiety, depression, anger, discomfort, and feelings of isolation
- Decreasing alcohol and drug abuse
- Decreasing blood pressure and the risk of heart disease
- Increasing the person's ability to cope with the effects of illness and with medical treatments
- Increasing feelings of hope and optimism, freedom from regret, satisfaction with life, and inner peace

Several studies have shown an association between spirituality and/or religion and a person's ability to cope with a variety of physical illnesses, including cancer.[14] However, newer research has questioned the efficacy of many of these studies, citing small sample size and methodological issues.[15]

One recent study of over 33,000 adults found that indicators of "social capital" such as visiting friends or relatives, visiting neighbors, attending church, belonging to clubs, and attending club meetings were associated with improved biomarkers such as cholesterol and blood pressure.[16]

Another recent review of literature found that measures of spirituality were related to biomarkers such as blood pressure, immune factors, cardiac reactivity, and the progression of disease.[17] In addition, spiritual well-being and spiritual growth has been shown to be associated with reports of overall physical health.[18] Recent studies of college students found a relationship between personal spirituality and healthy college behaviors such as physical activity, reduced alcohol use, and reduced nonsuicidal self-harm behaviors.[19]

### Psychological Benefits

Current research also suggests that spiritual health contributes to psychological health. For instance, the NCI and independent studies have found that

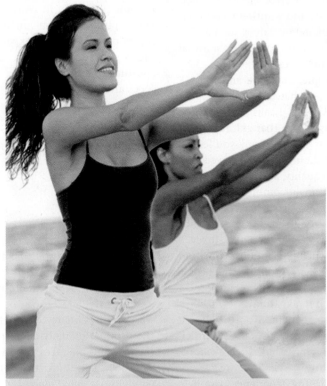

Spirituality is widely acknowledged to have a positive impact on health and wellness, from reductions in overall morbidity and mortality to improved abilities to cope with illness and stress. These students are using the movement techniques of tai chi to improve their spiritual health.

spirituality reduces levels of anxiety and depression.[20] In the case of academic performance, spirituality may provide a protective factor against burnout. In a study of 259 medical students, each completed a survey asking questions intended to measure levels of burnout, spirituality, psychological distress, ability to cope, and general happiness. Results showed students with higher scores of spiritual exercise and well-being to be more satisfied with their lives than students scoring lower.[21]

When people undergo psychological trauma, the meaning of life can be severely challenged. Counselors work with trauma survivors to help them find meaning in their trauma, to change their ways of thinking, and move them toward involvement in meaningful life experiences. Psychologists at the U.S. Department of Veterans Affairs have done extensive clinical work with veterans who are experiencing *posttraumatic stress disorder (PTSD)* as a result of their combat service. An example of the value of spiritual or religious practice may be that, following trauma, powerful emotions such as anger, rage, and wanting to get even may be softened by values such as forgiveness, gratitude, or other spiritual beliefs and practices.[22]

For example, gratitude and forgiveness are values that, when acted upon, can improve our health. Preliminary research has shown that gratitude exercises, such as writing thank-you letters, have a positive impact on perceived well-being, sleep quality, and energy.[23] Gratitude is not an uncommon experience for millennials—76 percent reported "feeling a strong sense of gratitude or thankfulness weekly" in a 2015 survey.[24]

People who have found a **spiritual community**—a group of people meeting together for the purpose of enriching and expanding their spirituality—also benefit from increased social support. For instance, participation in charitable organizations, religious groups, social gatherings, or spiritual learning experiences can help members avoid isolation. A community may include retired members who offer childcare for working parents, support for those with addictions or mental health problems, shelter and food for the homeless, or transportation to medical appointments. Spiritually active members may volunteer or receive help from other volunteers, all of which may enhance feelings of self-worth, security, and belonging. Rooting oneself in a social network in this way can be an important part of spiritual growth.

Additionally, the NCI cites stress reduction as one probable mechanism among spiritually healthy people for improved health and longevity and for better coping with illness.[25] Chapter 3, "Managing Stress and Coping with Life's Challenges," goes into more detail on this topic.

## LO 3 | CULTIVATING YOUR SPIRITUAL HEALTH

Describe three ways you can develop your spiritual health.

Cultivating your spiritual side takes hard work, similar to the work it takes to become physically fit. Ways to develop your spiritual health include tuning in, training your body, expanding your mind, and reaching out. Cultivating spirituality means bringing enhanced focus and mindfulness to all that we do so that we acknowledge, respect, and develop the connections between different aspects of our lives.

## Tune in to Yourself and Your Surroundings

Focusing on your spiritual health has been likened to tuning in on a radio: Inner wisdom is perpetually available to us, but if we fail to tune our "receiver," we won't be able to hear it through all the "static" of daily life. Fortunately, four ancient practices still in use today can help you tune in: *contemplation* (studying), *mindfulness* (observing), *meditation* (quieting), and *prayer* (communing with the divine). These practices have their roots in yoga, traditional Chinese medicine, and Ayurveda.

### Contemplation

In a dictionary, the word *contemplation* means a study of something—whether a candle flame or a theory of quantum mechanics. In the domain of spirituality, **contemplation** refers to concentrating the mind on a spiritual or ethical question or subject, a view of the natural world, or an icon or other image representative of divinity. Most religious and spiritual traditions advocate engaging in the contemplation of gratitude, forgiveness, and unconditional love.

When practicing contemplation, it can be helpful to keep a journal to record any insights that arise, and journaling itself can be a form of contemplation. For example, you might want to make a list of 20 things in your life you are grateful for or write a letter of forgiveness for yourself or a loved one. You might also use your journal to record inspirational quotations that you encounter in your readings. Journaling can fill a larger role in spiritual health and development by providing a sense of overall calmness.

### Mindfulness

A practice of focused, nonjudgmental observation, **mindfulness** is the ability to be fully present in the moment (FIGURE 2). Being "tuned in" could mean being fully present while listening to a mournful song, feeling incredibly happy to have great friends around you, or just enjoying a morning cup of coffee. In any case, mindfulness is an awareness of present-moment reality—a holistic sensation of being totally involved in the moment rather than focused on some worry or being on "autopilot."[26]

The range of opportunities to practice mindfulness is as infinite as the moments of our lives. Living mindfully means allowing ourselves to be

---

**spiritual community** A group of people who meet together for the purpose of enriching and expanding their spirituality.

**contemplation** Practice of concentrating the mind on a spiritual or ethical question or subject, a view of the natural world, or an icon or other image representative of divinity.

**mindfulness** Practice of purposeful, nonjudgmental observation in which we are fully present in the moment.

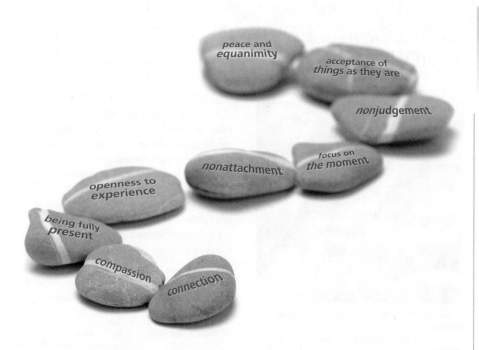

**FIGURE 2** Qualities of Mindfulness

**Source:** M. Greenberg, "Nine Essential Qualities of Mindfulness," *Psychology Today*, February 22, 2012, www.psychologytoday.com/blog/the-mindful-self-express/201202/nine-essential-qualities-mindfulness.

meditation Practice of concentrated focus on a sound, object, visualization, the breath, movement, or attention itself in order to increase awareness of the present moment, reduce stress, promote relaxation, and enhance personal and spiritual growth.

**WHAT DO YOU THINK?**

Why do you think mindfulness practices are gaining more recognition?

- What are benefits of mindfulness?
- In today's fast-paced, multitasking world, do you think it is challenging to practice mindfulness on a regular basis?

present in the current moment—to be wholly aware of what we are feeling in each moment.[27] For instance, the next time you are going to eat an orange, pay attention! What does it feel like to pierce the skin? How does it smell as you peel it? What does the rind really look like?

Pursuing almost any endeavor that requires close concentration can help you develop mindfulness. Even household activities such as cooking or cleaning can foster mindfulness—as long as you pay attention while you do them!

In this era of global environmental concerns, we can also cultivate mindfulness by paying attention to how our choices affect our world. Mindfulness of our environment calls on us to examine our values and behaviors as we share our Earth with all living creatures every moment of each day. It includes having a shared sense of responsibility for improving the world for future generations. See the **Health Headlines** box on page 58 for more information about developing environmental mindfulness.

## Meditation

**Meditation** is a practice of cultivating a still or quiet mind. Although the precise details vary with different schools of meditation, the fundamental task is the same: to quiet the mind's noise (variously referred to as "chatter," "static," or "monkey mind").

Why would you want to cultivate *stillness*? For thousands of years, human beings of different cultures and traditions have found that achieving periods of meditative stillness each day enhances their spiritual health. Today, researchers are beginning to discover why. The NCCIH reports that researchers using brain-scanning techniques found experienced meditators show a significantly increased level of *empathy*—the ability to understand and share another person's experience.[28] Similar research has shown that participants who practiced a specific form of meditation, known as *compassion-meditation*, further increased their levels of compassion toward others.[29] Studies also suggest that meditation improves the brain's ability to process information; reduces stress, anxiety, and depression; reduces insomnia; improves concentration; and decreases blood pressure.[30]

The physiological processes that produce these effects are only partially understood. One theory suggests meditation works by reducing the body's stress response. By practicing deep,

Even the most mundane activities—such as peeling and eating an orange—can have spiritual value if done mindfully.

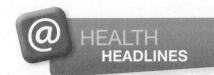
# DEVELOPING ENVIRONMENTAL MINDFULNESS

We know that the earth's oil reserves won't last forever, yet in 2013 many U.S. automakers saw a continued increase in sales of large pickups and sport utility vehicles (SUVs). General Motors reported their sales of pickups increased 15 percent and SUVs 29 percent. Chrysler and Ford Motor Company also reported significant increases in their heavy-duty pickups and large SUVs. We know that beef production releases gobs of greenhouse gases, yet Americans consume nearly 26 billion pounds of beef annually. Why do we make such choices? We want to "go green," so what's in our way? A 2015 Gallup poll suggested that concern for environmental issues is actually decreasing.

If the environmental movement seems to be running out of steam, many activists say that it's due to an overemphasis on our external choices, whereas the real challenge is to change our state of mind. They argue that until we confront the mental habits and identities that fuel our consumption patterns, meaningful change won't happen. In short, they advocate mindfulness. Spiritual growth is driven

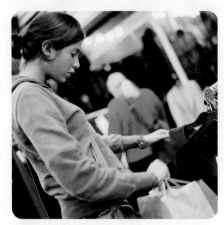

To be mindfully green requires us to ask ourselves some tough questions, such as What is my fair share? and How much do I really need?

by questions about our place in our community and society—this includes thinking about our contributions to the quality of our environment. Perhaps a collective focus on spiritual intelligence can lead to significant environmental improvements. So how do we cultivate environmental mindfulness? Environmentalist and Zen Master Thich Nhat Hanh, in an article for the United

Nations, suggests that we begin to see ourselves as part of Earth, rather than separate from it, saying: "When we breathe with mindfulness, we can experience our interbeing with the Earth's delicate atmosphere, with all the plants, and even with the sun, whose light makes possible the miracle of photosynthesis. With every breath we can experience communion. With every breath we can savor the wonders of life."

**Sources:** J. R. Healey, C. Woodyard, and F. Meier, "Detroit's August Sales Lead the Way, Pickups and SUVs Lead the Way," *USAToday*, September 4, 2013, www.usatoday.com/story/money/cars/2013/09/04/general-motors-gm-ford-chrysler-detroit-sales-august/2760795/; U.S. Department of Agriculture, Economics Research Service, "Statistics and Information," October 31, 2013, www.ers.usda.gov/topics/animal-products/cattle-beef/statistics-information.aspx; Jeffrey M. Jones, "In U.S., Concern About Environmental Threats Eases," *Gallup*, March 25, 2015, Available at www.gallup.com/poll/182105/concern-environmental-threats-eases.aspx?utm_source=Politics&utm_medium=newsfeed&utm_campaign=tiles; Thich Nhat Hanh, "Falling in Love with the Earth," *UN Climate Change Newsroom*, July 14, 2014, http://newsroom.unfccc.int/1758.aspx.

calm contemplation, people who meditate seem to promote activity in the body's systems, leading to a sense of peacefulness and subjective well-being as well as to physical relaxation that may slow breathing, lower blood pressure, improve sleep, and reduce symptoms of digestive problems.[31]

New research has shown actual differences in the brain structures of experienced meditators compared to those with no history of meditation.[32] Other studies have shown meditation to boost gray-matter density in parts of the brain critical to learning and memory and improved psychological and emotional health, compassion, and introspection.[33] At the same time, meditation may decrease gray-matter areas of the brain known to play a key role in anxiety and stress.[34]

So how do you meditate? Detailed instructions are beyond the scope of this text, but most teachers suggest beginning by sitting in a quiet place with low lighting where you won't be interrupted. Many advocate assuming a "full lotus" position, with legs bent fully at the knees, each ankle over the opposite knee. If this is impossible or uncomfortable, you may want to assume a modified lotus position, with your legs simply crossed in front of you. Rest your hands on your knees, palms upward. Beginners usually find it easier to meditate with the eyes closed.

Once you're in position, it's time to start emptying your mind. The various schools of meditation teach different methods to achieve this. Some options include:

- **Mantra meditation.** Focus on a *mantra*, a single word such as *Om*, *Amen*, *Love*, or *God*, and repeat this word silently. When a distracting thought arises, simply set it aside. It may help to imagine the thought as a leaf, and visualize placing it on a gently flowing stream. Do not fault yourself for becoming distracted. Simply notice the thought, release it, and return to your mantra.
- **Breath meditation.** Count each breath: Pay attention to each inhalation, the brief pause that follows, and the exhalation. Together, these equal one breath. When you have counted 10 breaths, return to one. As with mantra meditation, release distractions as they arise, and return to following the breath.

- **Color meditation.** When your eyes are closed, you may perceive a field of color, such as a deep, restful blue. Focus on this color. Treat distractions as in other forms of meditation.
- **Candle meditation.** With your eyes open, focus on the flame of a candle. Allow your eyes to soften as you meditate on this object. Treat distractions as in the other forms of meditation.

After several minutes of meditation, and with practice, you may come to experience a sensation sometimes described as "dropping down," in which you feel yourself release into the meditation. In this state, which can be likened to a wakeful sleep, distracting thoughts are far less likely to arise, and yet you may receive surprising insights.

Initially, try meditating for just 10–20 minutes, once or twice a day. In time, you can increase your sessions to 30 minutes or more. As you meditate for longer periods, you will likely find yourself feeling more rested and less stressed, and you may begin to experience the increased levels of empathy recorded among expert meditators.

## Prayer

In **prayer**, an individual focuses the mind in communication with a transcendent Presence. For many, prayer offers a sense of comfort, a sense that we are not alone. It can be the means of expressing concern for others, for admission of transgressions, for seeking forgiveness, and for renewing hope and purpose. Focusing on the things we are grateful for can move people to look to the future with hope and give them the strength to get through the most challenging times. Research has shown that spiritual practices such as prayer can increase the ability to cope and decrease depressive symptoms among individuals diagnosed with chronic conditions.[35]

## Train Your Body

For thousands of years, in regions throughout the world, spiritual seekers have pursued transcendence through

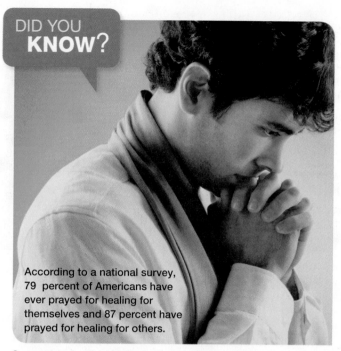

According to a national survey, 79 percent of Americans have ever prayed for healing for themselves and 87 percent have prayed for healing for others.

**Source:** J. Levin, "Prevalence and Religious Predictors of Healing Prayer Use in the USA: Findings from the Baylor Religion Survey," *Journal of Religion and Health*, Published online April 13, 2016, at http://link.springer.com/article/10.1007/s10943-016-0240-9.

physical means. One of the foremost examples is the practice of **yoga**. Although many in the West tend to picture yoga as having to do with a number of physical postures and some controlled breathing, more traditional forms tend to also emphasize chanting, meditation, and other techniques believed to encourage unity with the *Atman*, or spiritual life principle of the universe.

## 31 MILLION

U.S. adults have practiced **YOGA** and 21 million have practiced yoga in the past 12 months. Of these, 18- to 29-year-olds were most likely to practice yoga.

If you are interested in exploring yoga, sign up for a class on campus, at your local YMCA, or at a yoga center. Choose a form that seems right to you: Some, such as *hatha yoga*, focus on developing flexibility, deep breathing, and tranquility, whereas others, such as *ashtanga yoga*, are fast-paced and demanding and thus more focused on developing physical fitness. See Chapter 3 and Chapter 7 for more on various styles of yoga.

The Eastern meditative movement practices of tai chi or qigong can also increase physical activity and mental focus. With roots in Chinese medicine, both have been shown to have beneficial effects on bone health, stress, cardiopulmonary fitness, mood, balance, and quality of life.[36] Recent studies suggest that these practices are associated with improved physical health such as flexibility and balance, as well as cognitive abilities such as learning and

**prayer** Communication with a transcendent Presence.

**yoga** System of physical and mental training involving controlled breathing, physical postures (*asanas*), meditation, chanting, and other practices believed to cultivate unity with the *Atman*, or spiritual life principle of the universe.

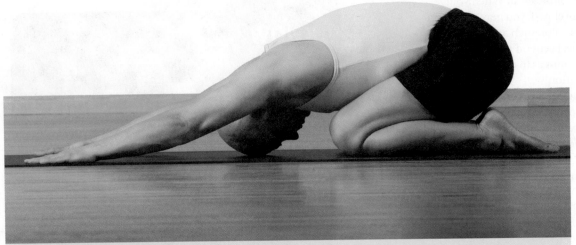

Yoga incorporates a variety of poses (*asanas*), from energetic to restful. This yoga student is performing a restful asana known as *child's pose*.

memory.[37] See Chapter 3 for more on tai chi and qigong.

If you're training your body to improve your spiritual health, you don't necessarily need to take up a formal practice. Jogging, aerobics, dancing, riding your bike, or any other type of regular physical activity can contribute to your spiritual health by energizing your body and sharpening your mental focus. In particular, mindfulness *while* exercising or engaging in physical pursuits can enhance the physical benefits. To shift a purely physical workout toward something more spiritual, start by expressing gratitude for your abilities—for your body, your health, and your wellness; throughout your workout session, be mindful of your breathing.

## Expand Your Mind

For many people, psychological counseling is a first step toward improving their spiritual health. Therapy helps you let go of past hurts, accept your limitations, manage stress and anger, reduce anxiety and depression, and take control of your life—all steps that can lead to spiritual growth. If you've never engaged in therapy, making the first appointment can feel daunting. Your campus health department can usually help by providing a referral. It is important to find

a therapist who is open to the concepts described in this chapter.

Another practical way to expand your mind is to study the sacred texts of the world's major religions and spiritual practices. Libraries and bookstores are filled with volumes that explore the diverse approaches humans take to achieving spiritual fulfillment.

Finally, you can expand your awareness of different spiritual practices by exploring on-campus meditation or service-oriented groups, taking classes in spiritual or religious subjects, attending religious meetings or services, attending public lectures, and checking out the websites of various spiritual and religious organizations. In each case, you can evaluate the messages and ideas you encounter and decide which practices or beliefs hold meaning for you.

## Show Up—Take Action

**Altruism**, the giving of oneself out of genuine concern for others, is a key aspect of a spiritually healthy lifestyle. It's easy to say you care, but it takes real energy, time, and

passion to think beyond the *me*—to tune into and see what others are going through, to advocate for change, and to become a force for "good" and all that is positive in life. It means instead of so much time spent looking in the mirror and perfecting the next selfie pose or taking pictures of our "foodie" exploits, that we look outward more, think more about those who may not know where their next meal is coming from, and those who are less advantaged; to be less narcissistically turned inward and focus on being an advocate for making the world a better place for all living things. The following are just a few

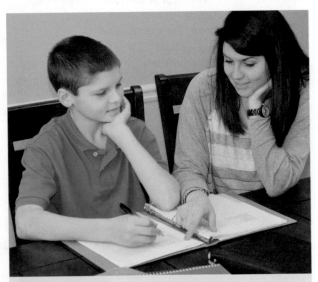

Volunteering can be a fun and fulfilling way to broaden your experience, connect with your community, and focus on your spiritual health.

**altruism** Giving of oneself out of genuine concern for others.

steps we can take to be mindful and increase our spiritual health:

- Advocate for others, write letters to elected leaders, fight for change and against injustice. Don't just talk about it—make a plan and act.
- Contemplate a better world and what you can do to lift others up as you work to be a better you.
- Live generously, compassionately, and with an openness toward others; give more of yourself.
- Listen more, hear more, consciously engage your brain in understanding and working with others.
- Take time to pause, to contemplate, to rise—and give a hand up to others.
- Turn Meaning and things you care most about into action; prioritize and find your purpose.
- Think about the positive things you want to be remembered for; make a list and begin.

Researchers have referred to the benefits of volunteering as a "helper's high," a specific feeling connected with helping others.[38] About 50 percent of people who participated in one study reported feeling more energetic and stronger after helping others; many also said they felt more calm and less depressed, with a greater sense of self-worth.[39]

For more strategies to enhance your spiritual health by reaching out to others, refer to the Making Changes Today box.

## MAKING CHANGES TODAY

### Finding Your Spiritual Side through Service

Recognizing that we are all part of a greater system with responsibilities to and for others is a key part of spiritual growth. Volunteering your time and energy is a great way to connect with others and help make the world a better place while improving your own health. A good way to get started is by identifying your own skills and interests first, then finding opportunities that allow you to build on them.

If you enjoy spending time with children:

- ◉ Organize or participate in an after-school or summertime activity for neighborhood children.
- ◎ Apply to become a Big Brother or Big Sister and mentor a child who may face significant challenges or have poor role models.

If you enjoy spending time with older adults or enjoy spending time in groups with multiple generations:

- ◎ Offer to help elderly neighbors with lawn care or simple household repairs.
- ◎ Volunteer at a local retirement community, reading, playing board games, or talking with residents.

If you value being part of the community by meeting different people, you could:

- ◎ Volunteer with Meals on Wheels, a local soup kitchen, a food bank, or another program that helps people obtain adequate food.
- ◎ Volunteer in a neighborhood challenged by poverty, low literacy levels, or a natural disaster. Or volunteer with an organization such as Habitat for Humanity to build homes or provide other aid to developing communities.

If you feel strongly in environmental awareness and sustainability, you could:

- ◎ Participate in a highway, beach, or neighborhood cleanup; restoration of park trails and waterways; or other environmental preservation projects.
- ◎ Volunteer at the local humane society.
- ◎ Join an organization working on a cause such as global warming or hunger, or start one yourself. Check out these inspiring examples: Students Against Global Apathy (SAGA), Students for the Environment (S4E), the National Student Campaign Against Hunger and Homelessness.

To find out more information on service, the following are some online resources:

Locates service opportunities: **www.volunteermatch.org**
Lists overseas volunteer opportunities: **www.projects-abroad.org**
Oriented toward students: **www.dosomething.org**
Competition for money for service projects: **www.truehero.org**

# STUDY **PLAN**

Customize your study plan—and master your health!—in the Study Area of **MasteringHealth..**

## CHAPTER **REVIEW**

To hear an MP3 Tutor Session, scan here or visit the Study Area in **MasteringHealth**.

### LO **1** | What Is Spirituality?

- Although spirituality is hard to define and can mean something slightly different to everyone, it encompasses an individual's sense of peace, purpose and connection to others, and beliefs about the meaning of life and how to live one's life. It involves a person's values and way of viewing life and how one should behave in the world. It is sometimes guided by a sense of connection to a higher presense.

### LO **2** | The Benefits of Spiritual Health

- Because of the diversity of human spiritual experience and the overlap of spirituality with religious practice, it is often hard to delineate the exact impact of spiritual beliefs and actions. However, in recent years, a number of studies of specific practices such as mindfulness, meditation, and prayer have shown that spiritual health reduces stress, decreases anxiety and depression, increases a person's ability to heal from illness and cope with medical treatment, and can increase feelings of hope and optimism, among other positive benefits.

### LO **3** | Cultivating Your Spiritual Health

- Similar to developing physical fitness, developing spiritual health takes knowledge, guidance, commitment, and consistency. Learning practices such as mindfulness, meditation, contemplation, right-mindedness, prayer, and service, and doing them regularly, will help build a foundation of spiritual health.

## POP **QUIZ**

Visit **MasteringHealth** to personalize your study plan with Chapter Review Quizzes and Dynamic Study Modules.

### LO **1** | What Is Spirituality?

1. Spirituality could be characterized by all of the following except:
   a. Bringing greater awareness to the present moment, such as in the practice of mindfulness.
   b. Focusing on relationships, values, and finding meaningful purpose in life.
   c. Participating in psychotherapy using a short-term, problem-solving model.
   d. Studying teachings from ancient spiritual traditions.

### LO **2** | The Benefits of Spiritual Health

2. Benefits of spiritual health have been shown in all except:

   a. Decrease in blood pressure and risk of heart disease
   b. Increase in muscle mass during regular resistance exercise
   c. Increase in ability to heal from illness
   d. Decrease in drug and alcohol use

### LO **3** | Cultivating Your Spiritual Health

3. The following are purposeful ways to cultivate spiritual health except:
   a. Taking a course on improving relationships that is offered at the university ecuminical ministry center.
   b. Volunteering to help build a Habitat for Humanity home because you want to meet the cute guy or girl in charge of the project.
   c. Taking a hatha yoga class.
   d. Browsing Amazon for books written by spiritual teachers of our time.

*Answers to the Pop Quiz questions can be found on page A-1. If you answered a question incorrectly, review the section identified by the Learning Outcome. For even more study tools, visit **MasteringHealth**.*

# 3 Managing Stress and Coping with Life's Challenges

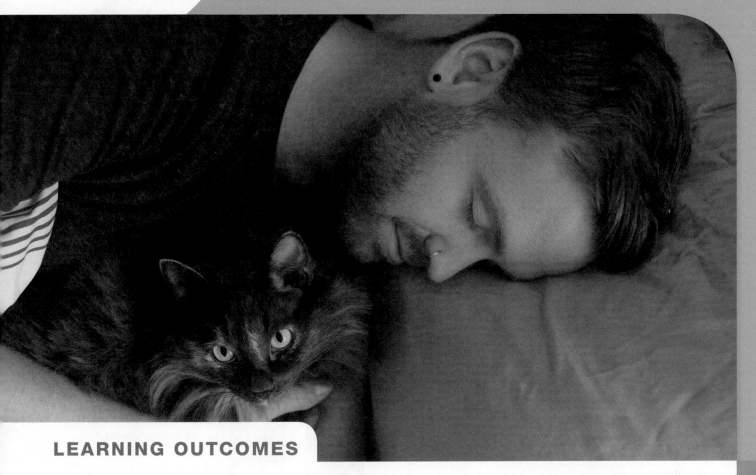

## LEARNING OUTCOMES

**LO 1** Define *stress* and examine its potential impact on health, relationships, and success in college and in life.

**LO 2** Explain key stress theories as well as the emotional, mental, and physiological changes that occur during the stress response.

**LO 3** Examine the physical health risks that may occur with chronic stress.

**LO 4** Examine the intellectual and psychological effects of stress and their impacts on college students.

**LO 5** Discuss sources of stress and examine the unique stressors that affect young adults, particularly college students.

**LO 6** Explain key individual factors that may influence whether or not a person is able to cope with stressors.

**LO 7** Explore stress-management and stress-reduction strategies, ways you can cope more effectively with stress, and ways you can enrich your life experiences to protect against the effects of stress.

Compelling evidence links stress to a wide range of physical and psychological problems.[1] Chronic stress can wreak havoc on your immune system, disrupt several physiological functions, and increase risk for problems with the cardiovascular, immune, gastrointestinal, respiratory, and neurological systems, as well as increase risk for Type 2 diabetes and many other health problems. Not for the faint-hearted, stress can cause issues with sleep, work, relationships, and most aspects of your life. In fact, a new report by the American Psychological Association aptly titled "Stress in America: Paying with our Health provides an overview of stress as a major epidemic of the 21st century."[2] College students and young adults trying to navigate the sometimes murky years where career paths, relationship decisions, family decisions, pressure to fit in, soaring tuition and housing costs, health insurance, and other choices intersect make young adulthood one of the most highly stressed periods in life (FIGURE 3.1).

n today's fast-paced, 24/7-connected world, stress can cause us to feel overwhelmed and zap our energy. Chronic stress inhibits normal functioning for prolonged periods and is a growing public health crisis among people of all ages. According to recent American Psychological Association studies, the health care system is not giving Americans the support they need to cope with stress and build healthy lifestyles. Key findings indicate that:[4]

- Americans consistently report high stress levels (20% report extreme stress), and teenagers are reporting stress levels on par with adults.
- Lower-income populations, Millennials, Gen-Xers, and women are among those likely to report higher levels of stress.
- Fifty-one percent of women say they have lain awake at night due to high stress, compared with 32 percent of men.
- Millennials are more likely to report feeling isolated due to stress in the last month, and are the most likely generation to report stress having a very strong impact on their physical and mental health.
- Only about half of all teens say they feel confident in their ability to handle personal problems.
- The biggest sources of stress for adults ages 18–32 are work, relationships, money, and job stability; when all adults report their sources of stress, money tops the list, followed by work, family, and health.
- Boomers and mature (older) adults report less stress than their younger counterparts and are much more likely to cite personal or family health concerns as a key source of stress.

While key sources of stress are similar for men and women (money, work, family, health), huge gender differences exist in how people experience, report, and cope with stress. Both men and women report above-average levels of stress, but women are more likely to report stress levels that are on the rise and more extreme than men.[5] Women are also more likely to report experiencing negative stress symptoms that affect their eating habits, and prevent them from making lifestyle changes.[6] Additionally, while men recognize and report stress, they are much less likely to take action to reduce it. Being "stressed out" can take a major toll on people at all ages and stages of life.

Is too much stress always a bad thing? Fortunately, the answer is no. How we react to real and perceived threats often is key to whether stressors are enabling or debilitating. Learning to assess our perceptions and to anticipate, avoid, and develop skills to reduce or better manage those stressors is key. The first step in controlling or reducing stress is to understand what stress is and how it affects the body.

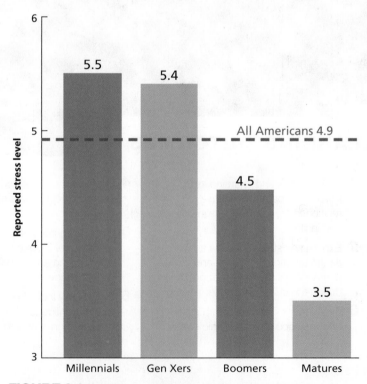

**FIGURE 3.1** **Stress Levels by Age** Stress levels for Gen-Xers and Millennials are above average, particularly compared to older generations.

# 36%

of millenials (ages 18–33) say their stress levels have **INCREASED** in the last year, with 51% of women and 32% of men saying their stress levels keep them awake at night.

## LO 1 | **WHAT** IS STRESS?

Define *stress* and examine its potential impact on health, relationships, and success in college and in life.

Most current definitions of **stress** describe it as the mental and physical response and adaptation by our bodies to real or perceived change and challenges. A **stressor** is any real or perceived physical, social, or psychological event or stimulus that causes our bodies to react or respond. Several factors influence one's response to stressors, including *characteristics of the stressor* (How traumatic is it? Can you control it? Did it catch you by surprise? Has anything in your life experience prepared you for it?); *biological factors* (e.g., your age, gender, health status, or whether you've had enough sleep recently); and *past experiences* (e.g., things that have happened to you, their consequences, and how you felt or responded). Stressors may be *tangible*, such as a failing grade on a test, or *intangible*, such as the angst associated with meeting your significant other's parents for the first time. *Change* can also be a major stressor.

Generally, positive stress is called **eustress**. Eustress presents the opportunity for personal growth and satisfaction and can actually improve health. Getting married, the excitement

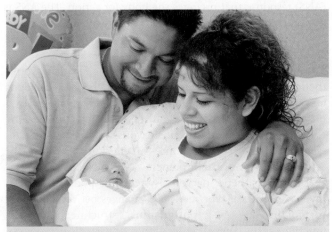

Not all stress is bad for you! Although events that cause prolonged *distress*, such as a natural disaster, can undermine your health, events that cause *eustress*, such as the birth of a child or waiting anxiously to see how you did on a test only to find you got the best grade in the class, can have positive effects on your growth and well-being.

of a first date, or winning a major competition can give rise to the pleasurable rush associated with eustress.

**Distress**, or negative stress, is more likely to occur when you are tired, under the influence of alcohol or other drugs, under pressure to do well, or coping with an illness, financial trouble, or relationship problems. There are several kinds of distress. The most common type, **acute stress**, comes from demands and pressures of the recent past and near future.[7] Usually, acute stress is intense, lasts for a short time, and disappears quickly without permanent damage to your health. The positive reaction to acute stress is that you rise to the occasion and put your most charming self forward: Seeing someone you have a crush on could cause your heart to race and your muscles to tense while you appear cool, calm, and collected on the outside. In contrast, anticipating a class presentation could cause shaking, sweaty hands, nausea, headache, cramping, or diarrhea, along with a galloping heartbeat, stammering, and forgetfulness. **Episodic acute stress** is the state of regularly reacting with wild, acute stress to various situations. Individuals experiencing episodic acute stress may complain about all they have to do and focus on negative events that may or may not occur. These *"awfulizers"* are often reactive and anxious, constantly complaining about their lack of sleep and all they have to do—habits so much a part of them that they seem normal. Others may respond to stress with a "hyperactive, chirpy, happy-happy" persona. Acute stress and episodic acute stress can both cause physical and emotional reactions, but they may or may not result in negative physical or emotional outcomes. In fact, they may serve as a form of self-protection.

In contrast, **chronic stress** can linger indefinitely and wreak silent havoc on your body systems. Caregivers are especially vulnerable to prolonged physiological stress as they watch a loved one struggle with illness. Upon a loved one's eventual death, or the symbolic death of a love relationship gone south, survivors may struggle to balance the need to process emotions with the need to stay caught up in classes, work, and everyday life.

Another type of stress, **traumatic stress**, is often a result of witnessing or experiencing events like major accidents, war, shootings, sexual violence, assault, or natural disasters. Effects of traumatic stress may be felt for years after the event and cause significant disability, potentially leading to posttraumatic stress disorder, or PTSD (see Chapter 2 for a discussion of PTSD).[8]

**stress** A series of mental and physiological responses and adaptations to a real or perceived threat to one's well-being.

**stressor** A physical, social, or psychological event or condition that upsets homeostasis and produces a stress response.

**eustress** Stress that presents opportunities for personal growth; positive stress.

**distress** Stress that can have a detrimental effect on health; negative stress.

**acute stress** The short-term physiological response to an immediate perceived threat.

**episodic acute stress** The state of regularly reacting with wild, acute stress about one thing or another.

**chronic stress** An ongoing state of physiological arousal in response to ongoing or numerous perceived threats.

**traumatic stress** A physiological and mental response that occurs for a prolonged period of time after a major accident, war, assault, natural disaster, or an event in which one may have been seriously hurt, killed, or witness to horrible things.

## LO 2 | THE **STRESS** RESPONSE: WHAT REALLY HAPPENS?

Explain key stress theories as well as the emotional, mental, and physiological changes that occur during the stress response.

Over the years, several theories have evolved explaining what happens (physiologically and psychologically) when a person perceives or experiences a stressor—as well as why some people thrive in stressful situations and others suffer debilitating consequences. One of the most well-developed and respected theories evolved from the idea that the body's efforts to protect itself from threats is part of an evolutionary process. Thousands of years ago, if your ancestors didn't respond to danger by fighting or fleeing, they might have been eaten by a saber-toothed tiger or killed by a marauding enemy clan. Today, when we face real or perceived threats, these same physiological responses kick into gear, but our instinctual reactions to fight, scream, or run must be held in check. While we learn culturally acceptable restraint, our bodies remain charged for battle—sometimes chronically. Over time, this vigilant, simmering stress response can lead to serious health problems.

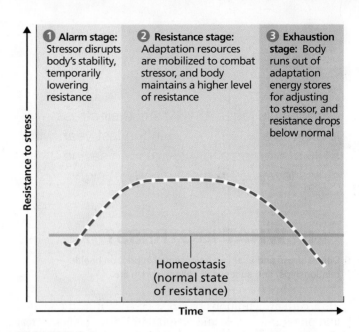

**1 Alarm stage:** Stressor disrupts body's stability, temporarily lowering resistance

**2 Resistance stage:** Adaptation resources are mobilized to combat stressor, and body maintains a higher level of resistance

**3 Exhaustion stage:** Body runs out of adaptation energy stores for adjusting to stressor, and resistance drops below normal

Resistance to stress

Homeostasis (normal state of resistance)

Time

**FIGURE 3.2** General Adaptation Syndrome (GAS) GAS describes the body's method of coping with prolonged stress.

---

**homeostasis** A balanced physiological state in which all the body's systems function smoothly.

**adaptive response** The physiological adjustments the body makes in an attempt to restore homeostasis.

**general adaptation syndrome (GAS)** The pattern followed in the physiological response to stress, consisting of the alarm, resistance, and exhaustion phases.

**fight-or-flight response** Physiological arousal response in which the body prepares to combat or escape a real or perceived threat.

**autonomic nervous system (ANS)** The portion of the central nervous system that regulates body functions that a person does not normally consciously control.

**sympathetic nervous system** Branch of the autonomic nervous system responsible for stress arousal.

**parasympathetic nervous system** Branch of the autonomic nervous system responsible for slowing systems stimulated by the stress response.

**hypothalamus** A structure in the brain that controls the sympathetic nervous system and directs the stress response.

**epinephrine** Also called *adrenaline*, a hormone that stimulates body systems in response to stress.

## Physiology/ Systems Theory: General Adaptation Syndrome

When stress levels are low, the body is often in a state of **homeostasis**, or balance; all body systems are operating smoothly to maintain equilibrium. Stressors trigger a crisis-mode physiological response, after which the body attempts to return to homeostasis by means of an **adaptive response**. First characterized in 1936 by noted endocrinologist and stress researcher Dr. Hans Selye, **general adaptation syndrome (GAS)** (FIGURE 3.2) provides an explanation of the body's internal fight to restore homeostasis when stressed. GAS has three distinct phases: *alarm, resistance,* and *exhaustion.*[9]

### Alarm Phase: The Body in "Protect Mode"

Suppose you are walking home after a night class on a dimly lit campus. You hear someone cough behind you and sense them approaching rapidly. You walk

faster, only to hear the other person's footsteps quicken. Your senses go on high alert, your breathing quickens, your heart races, and you begin to perspire. In desperation you stop, rip off your backpack, and prepare to fling it at your would-be attacker. You turn around, arms flailing, and let out a blood-curdling yell. To your surprise, the would-be attacker screeches back. In relief and a bit of embarrassment, you realize it's just one of your classmates trying to stay close out of her own fear of being alone in the dark! You have just experienced the alarm phase of GAS. Also known as the **fight-or-flight response**, this physiological reaction is one of our most basic, innate survival instincts[10] (FIGURE 3.3).

When the mind perceives a real or imaginary stressor, the cerebral cortex, the region of the brain that interprets the nature of an event, triggers an **autonomic nervous system (ANS)** response that prepares the body for action. The ANS is the portion of the nervous system that regulates body functions normally outside conscious control, such as heart and glandular functions and breathing.

The ANS has two branches: sympathetic and parasympathetic. The **sympathetic nervous system** energizes the body for fight or flight by signaling the release of several key stress hormones, particularly epinephrine, norepeinephrine, and cortisol. The **parasympathetic nervous system** slows systems stimulated by the stress response—in effect, it counteracts the actions of the sympathetic branch.

The sympathetic nervous system's responses to stress involve a series of biochemical exchanges between different parts of the body. The **hypothalamus**, a structure in the brain, functions as the control center of the sympathetic nervous system and determines the overall reaction to stressors. When the hypothalamus perceives that extra energy is needed to fight a stressor, it stimulates the adrenal glands, located near the top of the kidneys, to release the hormone **epinephrine**, also called *adrenaline*. Epinephrine more or less "kicks" the body

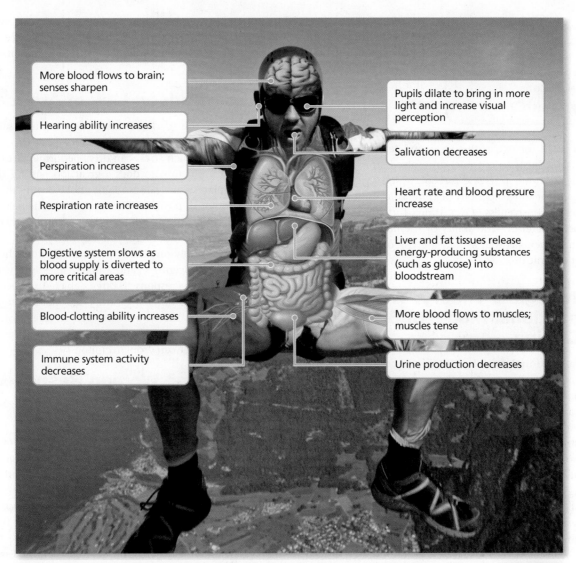

Labels on figure (clockwise from top left):

More blood flows to brain; senses sharpen

Hearing ability increases

Perspiration increases

Respiration rate increases

Digestive system slows as blood supply is diverted to more critical areas

Blood-clotting ability increases

Immune system activity decreases

Pupils dilate to bring in more light and increase visual perception

Salivation decreases

Heart rate and blood pressure increase

Liver and fat tissues release energy-producing substances (such as glucose) into bloodstream

More blood flows to muscles; muscles tense

Urine production decreases

**FIGURE 3.3** **Fight-or-Flight: The Body's Acute Stress Response** Exposure to stress of any kind causes a complex series of involuntary physiological responses.

➤ **VIDEO TUTOR**
Body's Stress Response

into gear, causing more blood to be pumped with each beat of the heart, dilates the airways in the lungs to increase oxygen intake, increases breathing rate, stimulates the liver to release more glucose (which fuels muscular exertion), and dilates the pupils to improve visual sensitivity. In addition to the fight-or-flight response, the alarm phase can trigger a longer-term reaction to stress. The hypothalamus uses chemical messages to trigger the pituitary gland within the brain to release a powerful hormone, *adrenocorticotropic hormone (ACTH)*. ACTH signals the adrenal glands to release **cortisol**, a key hormone that makes stored nutrients more readily available to meet energy demands. Finally, other parts of the brain and body release **endorphins**, which can relieve the pain and anxiety that a stressor may cause.

### Resistance Phase: Mobilizing the Body's Resources
In the resistance phase of GAS, the body tries to return to homeostasis by resisting the alarm responses.

Special hormones such as *oxytocin* (also known as the "cuddle chemical") begin to circulate in an attempt to bring physiological processes back to homeostatis. However, because some perceived stressor still exists, the body does not achieve complete calm or rest. Instead, the body stays activated or "revved up" at a level that causes a higher metabolic rate in some organ tissues.

### Exhaustion Phase: Body Resources Depleted
In the exhaustion phase of GAS, the hormones, chemicals, and systems that trigger and maintain the stress response are depleted by substances such as oxytocin, and the body puts on the stress brakes, beginning to bring systems into balance. You may feel tired or drained as your body returns to normal. In

**cortisol** Hormone released by the adrenal glands that makes stored nutrients more readily available to meet energy demands.

**endorphins** Opioid-like hormones that are manufactured in the human body and con-tribute to natural feelings of well-being.

**allostatic load**, or exhaustive wear and tear on the body. As the body adjusts to chronic, unresolved stress, the adrenal glands continue to release cortisol, which remains in the bloodstream for longer periods of time as a result of slower metabolic responsiveness. Over time, cortisol can reduce **immunocompetence**—the ability of the immune system to respond to attack—as well as increase risk of diabetes, CVD, and other chronic diseases.[11]

## Psychological Theory: The Transactional Model of Stress and Coping

In the **transactional model of stress and coping**, psychologist Richard Lazarus proposed that our reaction to stress is not so much about the nature of a stressor as the interaction between a *person's perception, their coping ability, and the environment*. In other words, your history, experience, and beliefs about a stressor will influence perceptions about whether you should worry or jump into action, remain calm and unreactive, or utilize coping strategies that have worked in the past. According to Lazarus, the transactional model consists of four stages:/ (1) *appraisal*, where you size up whether the stressor is a real threat; (2) *secondary appraisal*, where you assess whether your actions might reduce the threat with the resources you have; (3) *coping*, where you take action to reduce the threat; and (4) *postassessment*, where you examine what happened and decide whether you need to take more action. In this model, your perceptions are key to your stress response. By changing your perceptions, you can reduce the stress effect.

## Minority Stress Perspective

Another theory explaining the role of negative stressors relates to the role that stress plays in the lives of minority populations. According to the **minority stress perspective**, there are unresolved conflicts between minority and dominant group members. As such, minority stress may be explained in large part by disparities and the chronic stress inherent in

situations where stress is chronic, triggers may reverberate in the body, keeping body systems at a heightened arousal state. The prolonged effort to adapt to the stress response leads to

populations where rejection, alienation, and hostility persist. This is especially true in cases where there has been a long history of harassment, maltreatment, discrimination, and victimization.[12]

## Yerkes-Dodson Law of Arousal

According to the **Yerkes-Dodson law of arousal**, when arousal or stress increases, performance goes up—but only to a point. Too much stress can drive performance down. For example, an athlete who does a great job passing the football in regular-season games might choke during the conference championship when NFL scouts are on the field. On the other end, if you are cramming for four exams a mere two days before you have to take them, you may find yourself so wound up, you do horribly on all of the exams. You may be listless, find it hard to concentrate, and watch helplessly as your grade tumbles. This stress response is often depicted as a bell-shaped curve. As your stress increases, the performance curve moves upward; however, once you reach a certain level of stress, performance levels off. If stress persists and increases beyond this point, performance can drop precipitously.[13]

## Do Men and Women Respond Differently to Stress?

Ever since Walter Cannon's landmark studies in the 1930s, it's been thought that humans as well as many species of animals respond similarly to stressful events. However, newer research indicates that men and women may actually respond very differently to stressors. While men may be prone to fighting or fleeing, women may be more likely to *"tend and befriend"* by befriending the enemy or obtaining social support from others to ease stress-related reactions.[14] Many believe that the neurotransmitter oxytocin is key to this response. Essentially, women under stress appear to have higher oxytocin than men under similar circumstances. As such, they are more likely to be empathetic and seek out others when stressed, while men are more likely to withdraw after a stressful day.[15]

Other studies point to the fact that males and females may differ in their stress responses based on the way they perceive stressful events. Perceptions are widely believed to be a result of socialization and the way individuals are raised to play out their issues by repressing or opening up to others.[16]

### LO 3 | **STRESS** AND YOUR HEALTH: THE INCREASING TOLL

**Examine the physical health risks that may occur with chronic stress.**

Researchers have only begun to untangle the complex web of responses that can take a toll on a person's physical, intellectual, and emotional well-being. Stress is often described

---

**allostatic load** Wear and tear on the body caused by prolonged or excessive stress responses.

**immunocompetence** The ability of the immune system to respond to attack.

**transactional model of stress and coping** Theory proposed by psychologist Richard Lazarus, saying that our reaction to stress is about the interaction between perception, coping ability, and environment.

**minority stress perspective** Theory positing that minority stress may be partially explained by disparities and the chronic stress inherent in populations where rejection, alienation, and hostility persist.

**Yerkes-Dodson law of arousal** Theory suggesting that when arousal or stress increases, performance goes up to a point, after which performance declines.

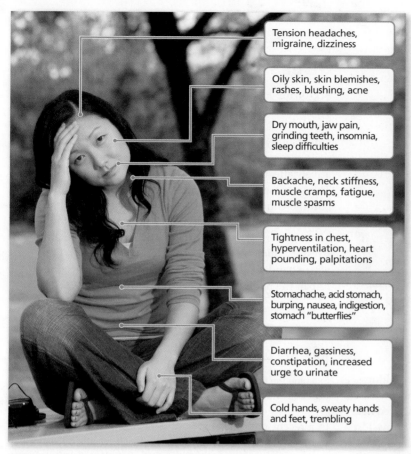

- Tension headaches, migraine, dizziness
- Oily skin, skin blemishes, rashes, blushing, acne
- Dry mouth, jaw pain, grinding teeth, insomnia, sleep difficulties
- Backache, neck stiffness, muscle cramps, fatigue, muscle spasms
- Tightness in chest, hyperventilation, heart pounding, palpitations
- Stomachache, acid stomach, burping, nausea, indigestion, stomach "butterflies"
- Diarrhea, gassiness, constipation, increased urge to urinate
- Cold hands, sweaty hands and feet, trembling

**FIGURE 3.4 Common Physical Symptoms of Stress**
Sometimes you may not even notice how stressed you are until your body starts sending you signals. Do you frequently experience any of these physical symptoms of stress?

as a "disease of prolonged arousal" that leads to a cascade of negative health effects. Some warning symptoms of prolonged stress are shown in **FIGURE 3.4**.

The higher the levels of stress you experience and the longer that stress continues, the greater the likelihood of damage to your physical health.[17] A recent international study indicated a universal tendency toward negative health consequences among those with chronically high stress in their lives.[18] Specifically, the more traumatic life events a person experiences, the greater the risk of a wide range of subsequent illnesses, including cardiovascular diseases, arthritis, gastrointestinal disorders, and others.[19]

## Stress and Cardiovascular Disease

Perhaps the most studied and documented health consequence of unresolved stress is cardiovascular disease. A recent summary of accumulated knowledge indicates that chronic stress plays a significant role in heart rate problems, high blood pressure, and atherosclerosis, as well as increased risk for a wide range of cardiovascular diseases.[20]

Chronic stress has been linked to increased arterial plaque buildup due to elevated cholesterol, hardening of the arteries,

increases in inflammatory responses in the body, alterations in heart rhythm, increased and fluctuating blood pressures, and other CVD risks.[21] In recent decades, research into the relationship between stress and CVD contributors has shown direct links between the incidence and progression of CVD and stressors such as job strain, occupational noise, caregiving, bereavement, and natural disasters.[22] (For more on CVD, see Chapter 16.)

## Stress and Weight Gain

Are you a "*stress eater*" or an "*emotional eater*"? Do you run for the refrigerator when you are under pressure or feeling anxious or down? If you think that when you are extremely stressed, you tend to eat more and gain weight, you probably aren't imagining it. Higher stress levels may increase cortisol levels in the bloodstream, which contributes to increased hunger and seems to activate fat-storing enzymes. Animal and human studies, including those in which subjects suffer from posttraumatic stress, seem to support the theory that cortisol plays a role in laying down extra belly fat and increasing eating behaviors.[23]

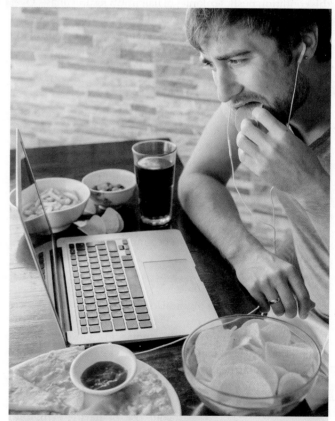

High stress levels may increase cortisol levels in the bloodstream, increasing hunger and encouraging stress eating.

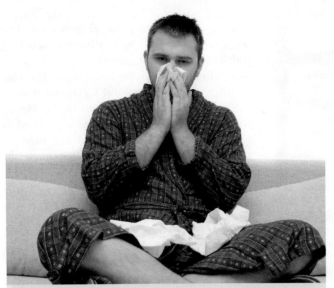
Prolonged stress can compromise the immune system, leaving you vulnerable to infection.

## Stress and Hair Loss

Too much stress can lead to thinning hair, and even baldness, in men and women—ironically, a problem that can increase stress even more! The most common type of stress-induced hair loss is *telogen effluvium*. Often seen in individuals who have lost a loved one or experienced severe weight loss or other trauma, this condition pushes colonies of hair into a resting phase. Over time, hair begins to fall out. A similar stress-related condition known as *alopecia areata* occurs when stress triggers white blood cells to attack and destroy hair follicles, usually in patches.[24]

## Stress and Diabetes

Controlling stress levels is critical for preventing development of type 2 diabetes—and for successful short- and long-term diabetes management.[25] People under a lot of stress often don't get enough sleep, don't eat well, and may drink or take other drugs to help them get through a stressful time. All of these behaviors can alter blood sugar levels and appear to increase the risk of type 2 diabetes.[26] Stress hormones may affect blood glucose levels directly.[27] (For more, see **Focus On: Minimizing Your Risk for Diabetes** beginning on page 446.)

## Stress and Digestive Problems

Digestive disorders are physical conditions for which causes are often unknown. It is widely assumed that an underlying illness, pathogen, injury, or inflammation is already present when stress triggers nausea, vomiting, stomach cramps and gut pain, or diarrhea. Although stress doesn't directly cause these symptoms, it is clearly related and may actually make your risk of having symptoms worse.[28] For example, people with depression or anxiety, or who feel tense, angry, or

**psychoneuroimmunology (PNI)** The study of the interrelationship between mind and body on immune system functioning.

overwhelmed, are more susceptible to dehydration, inflammation, and other digestive problems.[29]

## Stress and Impaired Immunity

A growing area of scientific investigation known as **psychoneuroimmunology (PNI)** analyzes the intricate relationship between the mind's response to stress and the immune system's ability to function effectively. Several recent research reviews suggest that too much stress over a long period can negatively affect various aspects of the cellular immune response. This increases risks for upper respiratory infections and certain chronic conditions, increases adverse fetal development and birth outcomes, and exacerbates problems for children and adults suffering from posttraumatic stress.[30] More prolonged stressors, such as the loss of a loved one, caregiving, living with a handicap, and unemployment, have also been shown to impair the natural immune response over time.[31]

## LO 4 | STRESS AND YOUR MENTAL HEALTH

Examine the intellectual and psychological effects of stress and their impacts on college students.

In a recent national survey of college students, 51 percent of respondents said they felt overwhelmed by all that they had to do within the past 2 weeks, with a similar number reporting they felt exhausted.[32] Nearly 43 percent of students said they had experienced a larger than average amount of stress, and another 11 percent said they had experienced tremendous

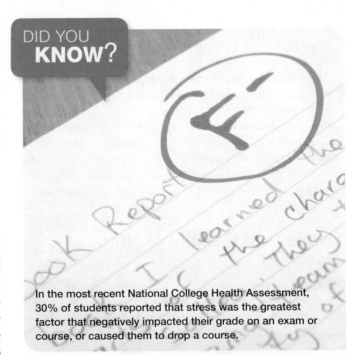
DID YOU **KNOW**?

In the most recent National College Health Assessment, 30% of students reported that stress was the greatest factor that negatively impacted their grade on an exam or course, or caused them to drop a course.

**Source:** Data are from American College Health Association, *American College Health Association-National College Health Assessment II (ACHA-NCHA II): Reference Group Data Report Spring 2015* (Hanover, MD: American College Health Association, 2016)

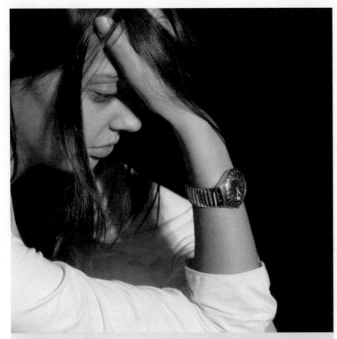

Stress and depression have complicated interconnections based on emotional, physiological, and biochemical processes. Prolonged stress can trigger depression in susceptible people, and prior periods of depression can leave individuals more susceptible to stress.

stress during the past year.[33] Not surprisingly, these same students rated stress as their number one impediment to academic performance, followed closely by anxiety.[34] Stress can play a huge role in whether students stay in school, get good grades, and succeed on their career path. It can also wreak havoc on students' ability to concentrate, understand, and retain information. Having a short fuse or being highly reactive can also cause stress in relationships.

## Stress, Memory, and Concentration

Although the exact ways stress affects grades and job performance are complex, new research provides possible clues. Animal studies suggest *glucocorticoids*—stress hormones released from the adrenal cortex—may affect cognitive functioning and overall mental health. In humans, memory is impaired when acute stress bombards the brain with hormones and neurotransmitters—affecting the way we think, make decisions, and respond in stressful situations.[35] Recent laboratory studies have linked prolonged exposure to cortisol to actual shrinking of the hippocampus, the brain's major memory center.[36] Other research, particularly laboratory studies of mice and other animals, indicates that prolonged exposure to high levels of stress hormones may increase the risk of Alzheimer's disease.[37] More research is needed to determine the validity of these theories.

## Psychological Effects of Stress

Stress may be one of the single greatest contributors to mental disability and emotional dysfunction in industrialized

nations. Recent studies have shown that chronic stress may actually cause structural degeneration and impaired function of the brain, leading to depression, dementia, and Alzheimer's disease as well as an overactive *amygdala* (region of the brain associated with emotional responses) that may increase rates of violence.[38]

## LO 5 | WHAT CAUSES STRESS?

Discuss sources of stress and examine the unique stressors that affect young adults, particularly college students.

On any given day, we all experience eustress and distress from a wide range of sources. The American Psychological Association conducts one of the most comprehensive studies examining sources of stress among various populations annually. The 2014 survey found concerns over money, work, family, and health to be the biggest reported causes of stress for American adults (FIGURE 3.5 on page 72).[39] College students, in particular, face stressors from internal sources, as well as external pressures to succeed in a competitive environment. Awareness of the sources of stress can do much to help you develop a plan to avoid, prevent, or control stressors.

## Adjustment to Change

Any change to your routine can result in stress. Unfortunately, although your first days on campus can be exciting, they can also be among the most stressful you will face in your life. Moving away from home, trying to fit in and make new friends, adjusting to a new schedule, dietary changes, lack of privacy, and learning to live with strangers in housing often lacking the comforts of home can all cause sleeplessness, anxiety, and keep your body in fight-or-flight mode. And while you may have been the shining star in your high school class academically, now your work will be evaluated against a classroom full of former stars.

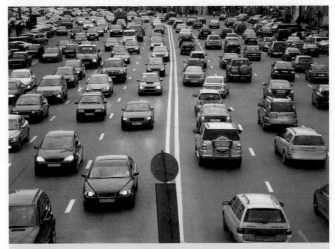

Traffic jams and noise pollution are examples of daily hassles that can add up and jeopardize our health.

## Hassles: Little Things That Bug You

A growing chorus of psychologists propose that the little stressors, frustrations, and petty annoyances, known collectively as *hassles*, can be just as stressful and damaging to your physical and mental health as major life changes[40] Cumulative hassles add up, increasing allostatic load and resulting in wear and tear on body systems. Listening to others monopolize class time, waiting in long lines, hunting for parking, loud music while you are trying to study, and a host of other irritants can push your buttons, triggering fight-or-flight responses. A lifetime of hassles can wreak havoc on the body, triggering mental health issues, high blood pressure, and other chronic health problems.[41] In addition to life and work stressors, electronic devices pose increased stress load for many. See the **Tech & Health** box for more on technostress.

## The Toll of Relationships

It isn't any secret that relationships can trigger some of the biggest fight-or-flight reactions of all. Although romantic relationships are the ones we often think of first, relationships with friends, family, and coworkers can be sources of struggle as easily as support. In addition, job insecurity, jobs with high demands and low control, conflict among coworkers and between workers and management, and unrelenting performance expectations increase the risks of a wide range of health problems.[42] Competition for rewards and systems that favor certain classes of employees or pit workers against one another are among the most stressful job situations.

## Money Worries: Impact on Academics and More

Let's face it, there never seems to be enough money to buy all of the things you want and need. Living in expensive student housing, dressing to look good, socializing, buying food and books, and paying for transportation, insurance, and a cell phone can tax even those whose parents help with the bills. For those without a parental safety net, or whose parents have their own financial troubles, keeping up with expenses can be a major challenge.

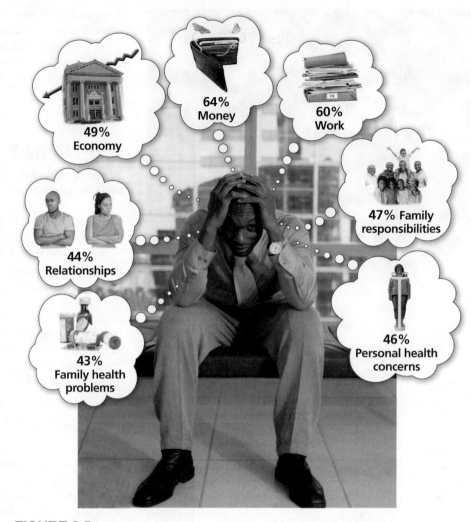

**FIGURE 3.5** **What Do We Say Stresses Us?** Over the past few years, the annual *Stress in America* survey has indicated that large percentages of American adults report experiencing concerns over money, work, and the economy as major sources of stress in their lives.

**Source:** Data from American Psychological Association, *2015 Stress in America: Paying with Your Health. Key Findings,* 2016, www.apa.org.

As college and university tuition soars, increasing numbers of students must hold jobs to stay afloat; others incur massive student loan debt that will be a drag on their lifestyles for years after graduation. According to recent estimates, the 2015 graduating class will be the most indebted class ever, with over 71% of students leaving school with an average of

# 72%

(nearly ¾ of adults) report feeling stressed about money at least some of the time; 26% report feeling stressed about money *all* of the time.

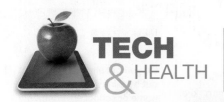

# TECH & HEALTH | TECHNOSTRESS AND TAKING TIME TO UNPLUG

Can you disconnect totally from your smartphone or other device for a day, or would you nervously long to check it? If you are someone who is always connected and finds that even an hour unplugged in class is too much, you may need to reconsider your priorities. *High-frequency cell phone use* is on the rise, and with it comes a variety of problems. According to a new study, college students who can't keep their hands off their mobile devices are reporting higher levels of anxiety, less satisfaction with life, and lower grades than peers who use their devices less often. The average student surveyed spent nearly 5 hours per day using their cell phones for everything from calling and texting (over 77 messages/day), tweeting, checking Facebook, sending e-mails, gaming, and more. Surprised?

Today, the media has a veritable dictionary of words describing the potential negative effects of too much time on social media and other sites. *Technostress* refers to stress created by a dependence on technology and the constant state of connection, which can include a perceived obligation to respond, chat, or tweet. Some have likened this obsessive desire to check in, tweet, text, or "like" to a form of *technologyy addiction*, whereby individuals may check their phones 35-50 times on an average day, even waking in the night to respond. Such obsessive behavior can sap energy, lead to insomnia/sleep

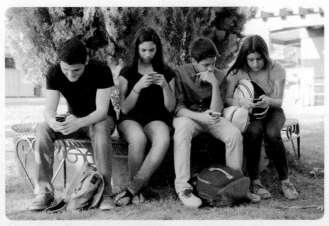

**Technology may keep you in touch, but it can also add to your stress and take you away from real-world interactions.**

disorders, damage relationships and normal in-person relationships, and hurt grades. These negative consequences, known as *iDisorders* are on the rise, along with the surge in smart technology across the globe. If you find yourself in an unhealthy relationship with your smartphone or tablet, it may be time to unplug. Here are some tips that may help:

- **Schedule screen time.** Set time aside to check e-mail, text messages, and Twitter feeds, like once in the morning and once in the evening for no more than a half hour. Resist the urge to check if you're outside your set time frame. NO reading messages in the middle of the night!
- **Unfriend the annoying and offensive.** Lighten your load by focusing only on those who really matter to you and add to your day in a positive way.
- **Connect with your friends in real time.** Socialize with friends in person

rather than spending hours commenting and scrolling through their Facebook pages.

- **Don't overshare.** Refrain from sharing intimate photos or details of your love life.
- **Power devices down.** Turn off all your devices completely (not just silent mode) when you're driving, in class, at work, in bed, having dinner with friends, or on vacation.

**Sources:** S. Deatherage, H. Servaty-Seib, and I. Aksoz, "Stress, Coping and the Internet Use of College Students," Journal of American Health 62, no. 1 (2014): 40-46; Y. Lee et al., "The Dark Side of Smartphone Usage: Psychological Traits, Compulsive Behavior and Technostress," Computers in Human Behavior 31 (2014): 373-81; A. Lepp, J. Barkley, and A. Karpinski, "The Relationship between Cell Phone Use, Academic Performance, Anxiety, and Satisfaction with Life in College Students," Computers in Human Behavior 31 (2014): 343-50; M. Salahan and A. Negahban, "Social Networking on Smartphones: When Mobile Phone Use Becomes Addictive," Computers in Human Behavior 29, no. 6 (2013): 2632-39; L. D. Rosen et al., "Is Facebook Creating 'iDisorders'?: The Link between Clinical Symptoms of Psychiatric Disorders and Technology Use, Attitudes and Anxiety," Computers in Human Behavior 29, no. 3 (2013): 1243-54, Available at http://dx.doi.org/10.1016/j.chb.2012.11.012; NIH Medline Plus, "Avid Cellphone Use by College Kids Tied to Anxiety, Lower Grades," December 2013, www.nlm.nih.gov/;medlineplus/news/fullstory_143389.html; A. Lepp, T. Barkley, and A. Karpinski, "The Relationship between Cell Phone Use, Academic Performance, Anxiety and Satisfaction with Life in College Students," Computers in Human Behavior 31 (2014): 343-50.

$35,000 in loan debt.[43] Worries over finding a job after graduation coupled with student loans underscore the fact that finances are a major source of stress for most students.[44] (For tips on how to head off some financial stressors before they start, see **Focus On: Improving Your Financial Health** on page 90.)

## Frustrations and Conflicts

Whenever there is a disparity between our goals (what we hope to obtain in life) and our behaviors (actions that may or may not lead to these goals), frustration can occur. Conflicts occur when we are forced to decide among competing motives, impulses, desires, and behaviors (e.g., to party or study) or when we are forced to face pressures or demands that are incompatible with our own values and sense of importance (e.g., get good grades or compete in college athletics). College students may face a variety of conflicts among parental values, their own beliefs, and the beliefs of others different from themselves.

## Overload

We've all experienced times in our lives when the demands of work, responsibilities, deadlines, and relationships all seem to be pulling us under. **Overload** occurs when we are overextended and, try as we might, there are not enough hours in the day to do everything. Students suffering from overload may experience depression, sleeplessness, mood swings, frustration, anxiety, or a host of other symptoms. Binge drinking and high consumption of junk food—often coping strategies for stress overload—catch many in a downward spiral as their negative behaviors actually add to their stress load. Unrelenting stress and overload can lead to a state of physical and mental exhaustion known as **burnout**.

**overload** A condition in which a person feels overly pressured by demands.

**burnout** A state of physical and mental exhaustion resulting from unrelenting stress.

**background distressors** Environmental stressors of which people are often unaware.

## Stressful Environments

For many students, living environment causes significant levels of stress. Perhaps you cannot afford safe, healthy housing, a bad roommate constantly makes

life uncomfortable, or loud neighbors keep you up at night. Noise, pressure of people in crowded living situations, and uncertainties over food and housing can keep even the most resilient person on edge.

Natural disasters can cause tremendous stress initially and for years later. Typhoons and hurricanes, earthquakes and tsunamis, killer tornadoes, as well as human disasters such as devastating oil spills, nuclear disasters, terrorist attacks, and the devastation of war have disrupted millions of lives and damaged ecosystems. Even after the initial images of suffering pass and the crisis has subsided, shortages of vital resources such as gasoline, clean water, food, housing, health care, sewage disposal, and other necessities, as well as electricity outages and transportation problems, can wreak havoc in local communities and on campuses and result in epidemics of infectious disease, major injuries, and death. Survivors often suffer from horrific emotional and mental health reactions.

**Background distressors** in the environment, such as noise, air, and water pollution; allergy-aggravating pollen and dust; unsafe food; or environmental tobacco smoke can also be incredibly stressful. As with other challenges, our bodies respond to environmental distressors with GAS. People who cannot escape background distressors may exist in a constant resistance phase.

### WHAT DO YOU THINK?

Do you get stressed out by things in your home or school environment?

■ Which environmental stressors bug you the most?

■ When you encounter these environmental stressors, what actions do you take, if any?

## Bias and Discrimination

Racial and ethnic diversity of students, faculty members, and staff enriches everyone's educational experience on campus. It also challenges us to examine our personal attitudes, beliefs, and biases. Today's campuses include a diverse cultural base of vastly different life experiences, languages, and customs. Bias and discrimination based on race, ethnicity, religious affiliation, age, sexual orientation, or other "differences"—whether in viewpoints, appearance, behaviors, or backgrounds—can take the form of bigotry, insensitivity, harassment, hostility, or simply ignoring a person or group.[45] See **Health in a Diverse World** for more on stress and international students.

**Stress among Minority Populations** Evidence of the health effects of excessive stress in minority groups abounds. For example, African Americans and other minority populations, particularly women and those living in poverty, report higher levels of stress than other populations. They also report less satisfaction with their health care and a perception that they are not receiving the same care as white populations.[46] They suffer higher rates of hypertension, CVD, and most cancers than do whites, and are 33 percent more likely to die from heart disease than other racial and ethnic groups.[47] Although poverty and socioeconomic status are key sources of stress for many, the chronic, physically debilitating stress among African Americans and other marginalized groups

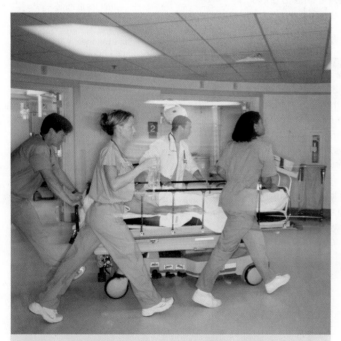

Certain jobs can be especially stressful, particularly those where the stakes are high and coworkers have little control over many outcomes. Individuals such as doctors and nurses face long work hours and a high-stakes work environment that make them especially prone to stress, overload, and burnout.

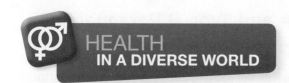

## HEALTH IN A DIVERSE WORLD

# UNIQUE STRESSORS FACING INTERNATIONAL STUDENTS

International students experience unique adjustment issues related to language barriers, cultural barriers, financial issues, and a lack of social support, among other challenges. Academic stress may pose a particular problem for the nearly 974,926 international students who left their native countries to study in the United States in 2014–2015. Accumulating evidence suggests that emotional support from others, on-campus socialization opportunities, and strong host networks are particularly effective ways for students to cope with stressful aculturation issues. Yet, many international students refrain from doing so because of cultural norms, feelings of shame, and the belief that seeking support is a sign of weakness that calls inappropriate attention to both the individual and the respective ethnic group. This reluctance, coupled with language barriers, cultural conflicts, loneliness, and the pressure to succeed, can lead international students

**Language barriers, cultural conflicts, racial prejudices, and a reluctance to seek social support all contribute to a significantly higher rate of stress-related illnesses among international students studying in the United States.**

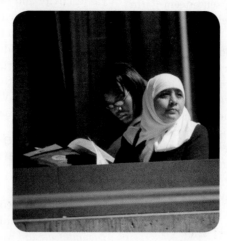

to suffer significantly more stress-related illnesses than their American counterparts.

Many universities are responding to this extra stress by hosting stress-management workshops each term that are geared toward the needs of international students and that encourage them to share stress-management techniques from their home countries. Both American and international students can help each other reduce stress with simple actions: share companionship and communication, and lend a helping hand. To paraphrase a popular Hindu proverb: "Help thy neighbor's boat across and thine own boat will also reach the shore."

**Sources:** Institute of International Education, "Open Doors 2015: Report on International Educational Exchange," January 2016, www.iie.org; K. Cokley et al., "An Examination of the Impact of Minority Status Stress and Imposter Feelings on the Mental Health of Diverse Ethnic Minority College Students," Journal of Multicultural Counseling and Development 41, no. 2 (2013): 82-93; E. Gomez, A. Ursua, and C. R. Glass, "International Student Adjustment to College: Social Networks, Acculturation and Leisure," Journal of Parks and Recreation 32, no. 1 (2014), http://js.sagamorepub.com/jpra/article/view/2972.

---

may also reflect real and perceived effects of institutional racism rather than the stress caused by individual/interpersonal poverty and perceived racism alone. More research is necessary to show direct associations between racism, stress, and hypertension among those who also experience persistent poverty. It is important to realize that all types of "isms" may influence stress-related hypertension and make it more difficult for those affected to engage in healthy lifestyle behaviors.[48]

## LO 6 | **INDIVIDUAL** FACTORS THAT AFFECT YOUR STRESS RESPONSE

Explain key individual factors that may influence whether or not a person is able to cope with stressors.

Although stress can come from the environment and external sources, it can also be a result of internal or individual factors: the "baggage" that we carry with us from a lifetime of real and perceived experiences. Low self-esteem, negative appraisal, lack of self-compassion, fears and anxiety, narciscistic tendencies, and other learned behaviors and coping mechanisms can increase stress levels. Fortunately, there are also many things

you can do to help innoculate yourself against potential stress threats. Developing positive self-esteem and self-efficacy, recognizing that past experiences can help you get through stressful situations, having a strong support network, developing coping skills, and buffering your reactions to stressors through exercise, diet, and sleep are among the many things that will help you keep excess stress in check.

### Appraisal

A lot of times, our **appraisal** of life's demands, not the demands themselves, result in experiences of stress. Appraisal is defined as the interpretation and evaluation of information provided to the brain by the senses. As new information becomes available, appraisal helps us recognize stressors, evaluate them based on past experiences and emotions, and decide whether we can cope. When you feel that the stressors of life are overwhelming and you lack control, you are more likely to feel strain and distress.

### Self-Esteem

Recall that *self-esteem* refers to your sense of self-worth: how you judge yourself in

> **appraisal** The interpretation and evaluation of information provided to the brain by the senses.

**suicidal ideation** A desire to die and thoughts about suicide.

**psychological hardiness** A personality trait characterized by control, commitment, and the embrace of challenge.

**psychological resilience** The capacity to maintain or regain psychological well-being in the face of adversity, trauma, tragedy, threats, or significant sources of stress.

comparison to others. Research with adolescents and young adults indicates that high stress and low self-esteem significantly predict depression and **suicidal ideation**, a desire to die and thoughts about suicide. Fortunately, research has shown that you can improve your ability to cope with stress by increasing self-esteem.[49] (In Chapter 2 we discussed several ways to develop and maintain self-esteem.)

While a healthy dose of self-esteem has long been regarded as necessary for mental health, questions over its potential dark side have arisen. Is there a point where a person can have too much self-esteem, or be so focused on proving their worth to others that it becomes a detriment to mental health and social interactions?[50] Critics of the self-esteem movement point to the fact that today's college students have the highest level of narcissism ever recorded and that the quest to have thousands of Facebook "friends" or huge Twitter followings can be huge stressors.[51] Environments where individuals are always compared to others as indicators of self-worth may contribute to elitism, bullying in a quest for power, prejudice between groups, and a host of other negative self-esteem behaviors. Those caught between their own self-esteem perceptions and the worry that they may not measure up may, in fact, experience high levels of debilitating stress.

## Self-Efficacy

*Self-efficacy*, or confidence in one's skills and ability to cope with life's challenges, appears to be a key buffer in preventing negative stress effects. Research has shown that people with high levels of confidence in their skills and ability to cope with life's challenges tend to feel more in control of stressful situations and, as such, report fewer stress effects.[52] Self-efficacy is considered one of the most important personality traits to influence psychological and physiological stress responses.[53] Developing self-efficacy is also vital to coping with and overcoming academic pressures and worries.[54] High test anxiety has been shown to account for up to 15 percent of the variance in student performance on exams.[55] By learning to handle test anxiety, research suggests that your confidence may increase and test scores improve, leading to better performance overall.[56] Tips on how to deal with test-taking anxiety and build your testing self-efficacy can be found in the Making Changes Today box. (For more on self-efficacy, see Chapters 1 and 2.)

## Type A and Type B Personalities

It's no surprise that personality can have an impact on whether you are happy and socially well-adjusted or sad and socially isolated. But personality may also be a critical factor in stress levels, as well as in your risk for CVD, cancer, and other chronic and infectious diseases.

In 1974, physicians Meyer Friedman and Ray Rosenman published a book indicating that Type A individuals had a greatly increased risk of heart disease due to increased physiological reactivity and prolonged activation of the stress response, including increased heart rate and blood pressure.[57] *Type A* personalities have historically been defined as hard-driving, competitive, time-driven perfectionists. In contrast, *Type B* personalities are described as being relaxed, noncompetitive, and more tolerant of others. Today, most researchers recognize that none of us are wholly Type A or Type B; we may exhibit either type in selected situations, sometimes with varying outcomes.

### Thriving Type As: Hardiness, Psychological Resilience, and Grit

In the 1970s, psychologist Susan Kobasa noted that many people who were super stressed didn't have the negative health consequences one might expect. She aptly described the theory of **psychological hardiness** indicating that hardy individuals were unique in their *control*, *commitment*, and *willingness to embrace challenges* in life, rather than succumb to them.[58] Fast forward nearly four decades and Kobasa's work has been expanded and refined to suggest that not only are certain individuals hardy, but some seem to thrive on their supercharged lifestyles, at least in the short term. These individuals are described as being **psychologically resilient**—a dynamic process in which people exposed to sustained adversity or traumatic challenges adapt positively.[59] They pick themselves up when knocked down and recover quickly from illness, adversity, changes, or challenges. These high-achieving *thrivers* often demonstrate (1) a positive and proactive personality; (2) experience and learning history that contributes to self-efficacy; (3) a sense of control, flexibility, and adaptability—an ability to "go with the flow"; (4) balance and perspective in their reactions; and (5) a perceived safety net of social support.[60] Newer researchers have focused their attention on yet another factor contributing to thriving and resilience despite stress: **grit**, a combination of passion and perseverance for a singularly important goal that high achievers demonstrate in all walks of life.[61] Studies of youth have shown that stress management and mindfulness training may help people develop resilience and grit, particularly if they have strong social support, healthy family environments, and community supports during the stress management programming.[62]

How daunting that pile of books and homework is depends on your appraisal of it.

### Type As and a Toxic Core

In contrast to those who thrive, some Type As exhibit a "toxic core," that is, they demonstrate a disproportionate amount of anger, distrust, and a cynical, glass-half-empty approach to life—a set of characteristics referred to as **hostility**. These individuals have an increased risk for heart disease and a host of other health issues.[63] In addition, those who have high-stress work environments, are exposed to traumatic events, suffer from depression, or who have personalities that lead to conflict with others have an increased risk for type 2 diabetes.[64]

## Type C and Type D Personalities

In addition to CVD, personality types have often been linked to increased risk for a variety of other illnesses. A type commonly discussed is the *Type C* personality: a suppressor who is stoic, denies their feelings or the existance of problems in their world, conforms to the wills of others, and appears calm and in control, even as their world swirls around them. This personality appears to be more susceptible to illnesses such as asthma, multiple sclerosis, autoimmune disorders, and

cancer; however, more research is necessary to support this relationship.[65]

A more recently identified personality type is *Type D* (distressed), characterized by a tendency toward excessive negative worry and anxiety, lack of patience with others, and a quick temper. Type D individuals tend to be direct and decisive, with an abundance of self-confidence. They are often in leadership and management positions, are risk-takers and problem-solvers, are relied on for leadership, and enjoy being in charge. Several recent studies have indicated that Type D people may be up to eight times more likely to die of a heart attack or sudden death.[66]

> **grit** A combination of passion and perseverance for a singularly important goal.
>
> **hostility** The cognitive, affective, and behavioral tendencies toward anger, distrust, and cynicism.
>
> **shift and persist** A strategy of reframing appraisals of current stressors and focusing on a meaningful future that protects a person from the negative effects of too much stress.

## Shift and Persist

Some young people who face extreme poverty, abuse, and unspeakable living conditions as they grow up seem to thrive, despite bleak conditions. Why? An emerging body of sociological research proposes that in the midst of extreme, persistent adversity, young people—often with the help of positive role models in their lives—are able to reframe appraisals of current stressors more positively (*shifting*), while *persisting* in focusing on the future. This outlook enables people to endure the present by adapting, holding on to meaningful things in their lives, and staying optimistic. These "**shift and persist**" strategies are among the most recently identified factors that protect against the negative effects of stress in our lives.[67]

## LO 7 | MANAGING STRESS IN COLLEGE

Explore stress-management and stress-reduction strategies, ways you can cope more effectively with stress, and ways you can enrich your life experiences to protect against the effects of stress.

College students thrive under a certain amount of stress; however, excessive stress can leave them overwhelmed and unable to cope. Recent studies of college students indicate that the emotional health self-rating of first-year college students compared to their peers is at an all-time low, with increasing numbers frequently feeling overwhelmed.[68] Students spend more time studying and less time socializing with friends, and nearly 10 percent report that they are frequently depressed. In contrast, sophomores and juniors reported fewer problems with these issues, and seniors reported the fewest problems. This may indicate students' progressive emotional growth through experience, maturity, increased awareness of support services, and more social connections.[69]

Although you can't eliminate all life stressors, you can train yourself to recognize the events that cause stress and to

# 43%

of those with no emotional support report **SIGNIFICANT INCREASES** in overall stress levels in last year compared to 26% with no emotional support reporting stress increases.

anticipate your reactions to them. **Coping** is the act of managing events or conditions to lessen the physical or psychological effects of excess stress (see the **Student Health Today** box for more on how people try to cope with stress).[70] One of the most effective ways to combat stressors is to build coping strategies and skills, known collectively as *stress-management techniques*.

> **coping** Managing events or conditions to lessen the physical or psychological effects of excess stress.
>
> **stress inoculation** Stress-management technique in which a person consciously anticipates and prepares for potential stressors.

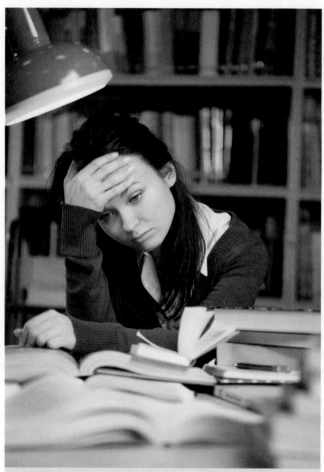

College students face a unique set of stressors as they search for meaning in their lives, try to live up to expectations, and struggle to find a career path that may influence the rest of their lives. Social and academic demands often collide, leading to increased challenges.

## Practicing Mental Work to Reduce Stress

Stress management isn't something that just happens. It calls for getting a handle on what is going on in your life, taking a careful look at yourself, and coming up with a personal plan of action. Because your perceptions are often part of the problem, assessing your self-talk, beliefs, and actions are good first steps. Why are you so stressed? How much of it is due to perception rather than reality? What's a realistic plan of action for you? Think about your situation and map out a strategy for change. The tools in this section will help you.

**Journaling to Reduce Stress** Assessing what is really going on in your life is an important first step to solving problems and reducing your stress. Journaling can help you examine your stressors, factors that contribute to them, and help you visualize what options might reduce your stress. Here's how:

- Start tracking. Write down your worries and the things that are "bugging" you at the moment. Do you have friends or family that drain your emotional reserves, keep you stirred up, bring you down, or push your buttons? Are competitive, high-stress classmates putting you on edge? Are your schedule and time management, your finances, your living conditions, your classes, your relationships, or other issues in your life causing you distress? Journaling can help you get to the heart of your daily challenges, and give you ideas about where to start making changes. Think about when your stress is greatest, who is around you, and how you respond.
- Examine the causes of your stress. Which are tangible? Intangible?
- List your options and the potential consequences of each.
- Outline an action plan, and then *act*. Remember that even little things can sometimes make a big difference and that you shouldn't expect immediate results.
- After you act, evaluate. How did you do? How do you feel about your actions? How can you change to achieve better outcomes?

One useful way of coping with your stressors is to consciously anticipate and prepare for specific ones, a technique known as **stress inoculation**. For example, if speaking in front of a class scares you, practice in front of friends or a video camera to prevent freezing up on the day of the presentation. If a friend is constantly dragging you down or upsetting you, try to change the subject gently or be less available. If interactions don't enhance your life, think about why you are having them.

# 42%

of adults say they are not doing enough to manage their **STRESS**; 1 in 5 (20%) never engage in activity to relieve or manage stress.

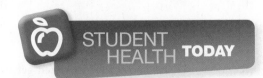

# HOW WE COPE WITH STRESS

People choose a wide range of behaviors to deal with the stress in their lives. Younger populations, particularly Millennials, are most likely to choose "sedentary" or "vegging out" stress-management techniques—more so than any other generation. Not only do they suffer from the most stress; their strategies to reduce stress may increase their risk of obesity and related health issues that can result in major problems down the road.

**Differences in Stress-Management Strategies by Age (What They Report Doing)**

| Actions | Millennials | Gen-Xers | Boomers | Matures |
|---|---|---|---|---|
| Listening to music | 57% | 42% | 39% | 29% |
| Watching TV 2+ hrs/day | 44% | 37% | 42% | 35% |
| Going online | 46% | 33% | 37% | 31% |
| Eating too much/unhealthy food | 35% | 35% | 29% | 21% |

**Source:** American Psychological Association, "Stress In America: Paying with our Health," February 2015, Available at https://www.apa.org/news/press/releases/stress/2014/stress-report.pdf.

## Practicing Self-Compassion in Self-Talk/Self-Thought

Have you ever noticed how we are often more kind to people that we don't know than we are to ourselves and the people we are closest to? We say things to our loved ones that we would never say to others and we beat ourselves up over little things—like the size of our hips, a bulge or two in the middle, a nose that is too big, and other bodily imperfections. All this negative self-talk can increase our stress and zap the joy out of our lives.

While several types of negative self-talk exist, the most common are *pessimism*, or focusing on the negative; *perfectionism*, or expecting superhuman standards; *"should-ing,"* or reprimanding yourself for things that you should have done; *blaming* yourself or others for circumstances and events; and *dichotomous thinking*, in which everything is either black or white (good or bad). To combat negative self-talk, we must first become aware of it, then stop it, and finally replace the negative thoughts with positive ones—a process called **cognitive restructuring**. Once you realize that some of your thoughts may be negative, irrational, or overreactive, interrupt this self-talk by saying, "Stop" (under your breath or aloud), and make a conscious effort to think positively.

Psychologist Kristin Neff says that we need to treat ourselves with the same kindness, caring, and compassion we show to good friends or people we want to impress. **Self-compassion** means that rather than harshly judging and bashing yourself for various inadequacies or shortcomings, you are understanding and kind in the face of real or perceived personal shortcomings. It involves self-kindness, common humanity, and mindfulness.[71] Increasing studies point to the benefits of this mindfulness-oriented, compassionate self as a key to stress management and control.[72] See the Making Changes Today box for other suggestions of ways to rethink your thinking habits.

## Developing a Support Network

If you are stressed-out and considering a plan for stress management, remember the importance of social networks and social bonds. Friendships are important for inoculating yourself against harmful stressors. A recent study of adult women indicates that social support from friends can inoculate you against negative stress symptoms within hours of that friend support.[73] Studies of college students have demonstrated the importance of social support in *buffering* individuals from the

---

## MAKING CHANGES TODAY

### Rethink Your Thinking Habits

- **Reframe a distressing event from a positive perspective.** For example, if you feel frustrated that you aren't the best in every class, change your perspective. Focus on your strengths!

- **Tolerate mistakes.** Rather than getting upset by mishaps, evaluate what happened and learn from it. Take yourself less seriously. Cut yourself some slack via self-compassion and changing self-talk.

- **Break the worry habit.** If you are preoccupied with what-ifs and worst-case scenarios, the following suggestions can help slow the worry drain:

  - If you must worry, create a 20-minute "worry period" when you can journal or talk about it each day. After that, block the worry if it pops up again.
  - Try to focus on what is going right, rather than what *might* go wrong.
  - Learn to accept what you cannot change. Each of us must learn to live with some uncertainty.
  - Seek help. Anxiety is increasing at all levels of society. If you are feeling overwhelmed by life, talk with someone you trust or make an appointment with a counselor.

---

**cognitive restructuring** The modification of thoughts, ideas, and beliefs that contribute to stress.

**self-compassion** Treating yourself with as much understanding and care as you would a loved one.

effects of stress. Social support in the form of social media appears to be particularly effective in reducing stress and improving life satisfaction among international students.[74] Social support has also been shown to be a significant buffer against negative outcomes for those suffering from PTSD and other chronic stress situations.[75]

Family members and friends can be a steady base of support when the pressures of life seem overwhelming. Additionally, most colleges and universities offer counseling services at no cost for short-term crises. Clergy, instructors, and residence hall supervisors may also be excellent resources.

In order to have a healthy social support network, you have to invest time and energy. Cultivate and nurture the relationships that matter: those built on trust, mutual acceptance and understanding, honesty, and genuine caring. If you want others to be there for you to help you cope with life's stressors, you need to be there for them. Spend more time in face-to-face interactions.

## Cultivating Your Spiritual Side

One of the most important factors in reducing stress in your life is taking the time and making the commitment to cultivate your spiritual side: finding your purpose in life and living your days more fully. Spiritual health and spiritual practices can be vital components of your support system, often linking you to a community of like-minded individuals and giving you perspective on the things that truly matter in your life. (For information on spirituality and how it can affect your overall health, see **Focus On: Cultivating Your Spiritual Health**, beginning on page 51.)

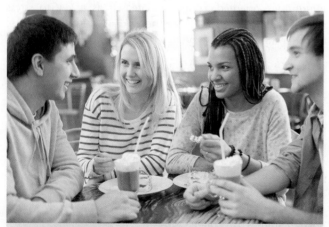

Spending time socializing face-to-face can be an important part of building a support network and reducing your stress level.

## Managing Emotional Responses

Have you ever gotten all worked up about something only to find that your perceptions were totally wrong? We often get upset not by realities, but by our faulty perceptions. Social networking sites and e-mails are often perfect places for reading meaning into things that are said and perceiving issues that don't exist. Interactions where body language, voice intonation, and opportunities for clarification are present are much better for interpreting true meanings than are cryptic texts or e-mails.

Stress management requires examining your emotional responses. With any emotional response to a stressor, you are responsible for the emotion and the resulting behaviors. Learning to tell the difference between normal emotions and emotions based on irrational beliefs or expressed and interpreted in an over-the-top manner can help you stop the emotion or express it in a healthy and appropriate way.

**Fight the Anger Urge** Major sources of anger include (1) perceived *threats* to self or others we care about; (2) *reactions to injustice*, such as unfair actions, policies, or behaviors; (3) *fear*, which leads to negative responses (for more on this topic, see the **Health Headlines** box); (4) *faulty emotional reasoning*, or misinterpretation of normal events; (5) *low frustration tolerance*, often fueled by stress, drugs, lack of sleep, and other factors; (6) *unreasonable expectations* about ourselves and others; and (7) *people rating*, or applying derogatory ratings to others.

There are three main approaches to dealing with anger: *expressing it*, *suppressing it*, or *calming it*. You may be surprised to find out that expressing anger is probably the healthiest thing to do in the long run, if you express anger in an assertive rather than in an aggressive way. There are several strategies you can use to keep aggressive reactions at bay:[76]

- **Identify your anger style.** Do you express anger passively or actively? Do you hold anger in, or do you explode?
- **Learn to recognize patterns in your anger responses and how to de-escalate them.** For 1 week, keep track of everything that angers you or keeps you stewing. What thoughts or feelings lead up to your boiling point? Explore ways to interrupt patterns of anger, such as counting to 10, getting a drink of water, or taking some deep breaths.
- **Find the right words to de-escalate conflict.** When conflict arises, be respectful and state your needs or feelings rather than shooting zingers at the other person. Avoid "you always" or "you never" and instead say, "I feel_____ when you_____" or "I would really appreciate it if you could_____." If you find yourself continually revved up for battle, consider taking a class or workshop on assertiveness training or anger management.
- **Plan ahead.** Explore options to minimize your exposure to anger-provoking situations, such as traffic jams.
- **Vent to your friends.** Find a few close friends you trust and who can be honest with you. Allow them to listen and

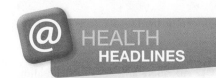
# AN EPIDEMIC OF FEAR IN AMERICA
## Stressing Ourselves Out Needlessly, Or Real Threat?

If someone were to ask you what you were most afraid of—what your greatest fear was right now—what would you respond? It may not surprise you, but when a sample of Americans was asked to rate their top 10 fears in 2015, these things were rated highly by significant percentages of respondents:

- Corruption of government officials (58.0%)
- Cyber-terrorism (44.8%)
- Corporate tracking of personal information (44.6%)
- Terrorist attacks (44.4%)
- Government tracking of personal information (41.4%)
- Bio-warfare (40.9%)
- Identity theft (39.6%)
- Economic collapse (39.2%)
- Running out of money in the future (37.4%)
- Credit card fraud (36.9%)

Consider the following "self-checks" whenever your fears seem to be hindering your behaviors:

1. Are my fears rational or irrational? Where is the evidence that because a shooting took place in Florida, that I will be shot at a concert or football game in my community? What is the threat to me here and now based on statistics? What safety nets are in place to protect me?

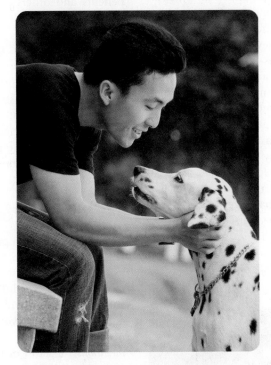

**Four-legged friends can be great stress relievers as they allow you to focus on something besides yourself and can add laughter to your life.**

2. Can I do anything about it? Are there things I can do to protect myself?
3. Where is the evidence that government officials are corrupt? Is it real or just part of the growing viciousness of political campaigns and ways that people discredit others in the media to gain advantage. Am I being manipulated by myths/misperceptions about

situations to win votes? Even if part of the corruption in politics is true, are there things I can do to change the situation?

4. Have I educated myself about the facts? Is the Zika Virus present in my area right now? Because a restaurant had a foodborne outbreak, should I avoid similar restaurants? What can I do to ensure my safety? What can I do to find out more about a situation and actions I can take?
5. Have I thought about what is triggering my fears? Is there anyone I can talk to about it? Are there any support groups or speakers in my area where I can go to discuss issues, vent and express my concerns?
6. Have my fears prevented me from doing something I really like to do or from going places I would love to go? If so, answering items 1-5 above might help me get a grip on my fears and better understand that my beliefs are unrealistic and causing me to alter my lifestyle in negative and unnecessary ways. If you find out that your fears are real, take action to stay safe, seek support from others.

**Source:** S. Ledbetter, "America's Top Fears, 2015," *The Chapman University Survey of American Fears, 2015,* October 13, 2015, https://blogs.chapman.edu/wilkinson/2015/10/13/americas-top-fears-2015/.

---

give their perspective, but don't wear down your supporters with continual rants.

- **Develop realistic expectations of yourself and others.** Are your expectations of yourself and others realistic? Try talking about your feelings with those involved at a time when you are calm.
- **Turn complaints into requests.** When frustrated or angry with someone, try reworking the problem into a request. Instead of screaming and pounding on the wall because your neighbors are blaring music at 2:00 A.M., talk with them. Think about the words you will use, and try to reach an agreement that works for everyone.
- **Leave past anger in the past.** Learn to resolve issues and not bring them up over and over. Let it go. If you can't, seek the counsel of a professional to learn how.

**Learn to Laugh, Be Joyful, and Cry** Have you ever noticed that you feel better after a belly laugh or a good cry? Adages such as "Laughter is the best medicine" and "Smile and the world smiles with you" didn't come from nowhere. Humans have long recognized that actions such as smiling, laughing, singing, and dancing can elevate our moods, relieve stress, and improve our relationships. Learning to take yourself less seriously is a good starting place. Crying can have similar positive physiological effects in relieving tension. Several preliminary studies indicate that laughter and joy may increase endorphin levels, increase oxygen levels in the blood, decrease stress levels, relieve pain, help in recovery from cardiovascular disease, improve relationships, and even reduce risks of chronic disease; however, the evidence for *long-term* effects must be validated through larger, more rigorous studies.[77]

## Taking Physical Action

Are you often feeling sluggish, hard to get out of bed, or ready to nap? Or, are you feeling wired, restless, and ready to explode? Either could be the result of too much stress.

**Get Enough Exercise** Remember that the human stress response is intended to end in physical activity. Exercise "burns off" existing stress hormones by directing them toward their intended metabolic function.[78] Exercise can also help combat stress by raising levels of endorphins—mood-elevating, painkilling hormones—in the bloodstream, increasing energy, reducing hostility, and improving mental alertness. Still, according to a recent meta-analysis of stress and exercise research, those who would benefit most—particularly sedentary, overweight individuals—are more likely to eat when they are stressed and less likely to exercise. Motivating people unready to exercise for health and stress relief is a major challenge; however, the health benefits to be achieved

**sympathomimetics** Food substances that can produce stresslike physiological responses.

**procrastinate** To intentionally put off doing something.

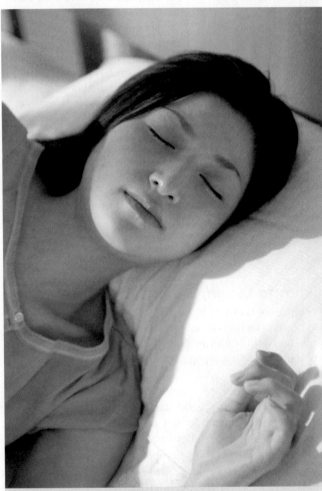

Taking care of your physical health—through quality sleep, sufficient exercise, and healthful nutrition—is a crucial component of stress management.

are significant.[79] (For more on the beneficial effects of exercise, see Chapter 7.)

**Get Enough Sleep** Adequate amounts of sleep allow you to refresh your vital energy, cope with multiple stressors more effectively, and be productive when you need to be. In fact, sleep is one of the biggest stress busters of them all. (These benefits and others are discussed in much more depth in Chapter 4.)

**Eat Healthfully** Although we receive countless messages to "eat this and not that," if we want to remain healthy and reduce stress, the actual mechanisms verifying that diet plays a significant role in stress management remain unclear. It is known that undereating, overeating, and eating the wrong kinds of foods can create distress in the body. In particular, avoid **sympathomimetics**, substances in foods that produce (or mimic) stresslike responses, such as caffeine. (For more information about the benefits of sound nutrition, see Chapter 5.)

## Managing Your Time

Ever put off writing a paper until the night before it was due? We all **procrastinate**, or voluntarily delay some task despite expecting to be worse off for the delay. Procrastination can result in academic difficulties, financial problems, relationship problems, and a multitude of stress-related ailments.

How can you avoid the temptation to procrastinate? According to recent research, setting clear "*implementation intentions*," a series of goals to accomplish toward a specific end, is key.[80] Having a plan that includes specific deadlines (and rewards for meeting deadlines) can help you stay on task. Another strategy is to get started early and set a personal end date that is well ahead of the deadline.

Keep a journal for 2 days to become aware of how you spend your time. Write down your activities every day—everything from going to class to doing your laundry to texting your friends—and the amount of time you spend doing each. What can you do to make better use of your time? Use the following time-management tips in your stress-management program:

- **Do one thing at a time.** Don't multitask. Instead of watching TV, doing laundry, and writing your term paper all at once, pick one and stay focused.
- **Clean off your desk.** Sort your desk, tossing unnecessary paper and mail and filing important papers in labeled folders. (For more on organizing to destress, see the Student Health Today box.)
- **Prioritize your tasks.** Make a daily "to-do" list and stick to it. Categorize the things you must do today, the things that must eventually get done, and the things that it would be nice to do. Consider the "nice to do" items only if you finish the others (or if they include something fun).
- **Find a clean, comfortable place to work, and avoid interruptions.** Schedule uninterrupted time for work. Don't answer the phone; close your door and post a "Do Not Disturb" sign; or go to a quiet room in the library or student union.

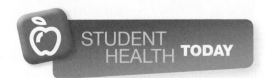
# *FENG SHUI* FOR STRESS RELIEF

Today, many space designers are trying to create peaceful "me caves" for reducing the stress of harried lives. One strategy, known as *feng shui* (translation "wind and water"), is part of an ancient Chinese art designed to restore balance of *chi* and create peace and harmony with help from the built environment. Here are several tips for reducing stress in your bedroom area:

- **Declutter.** Get rid of any extra "things" in your space. Pick up and put things away each day.
- **Paint.** Use peaceful and welcoming colors. Coordinate linens and tapestry colors to enhance warmth.
- **Relocate.** Your bed should never be in line with the door; nightstands should be balanced on either side of the bed, and mirrors should *never* reflect the bed.

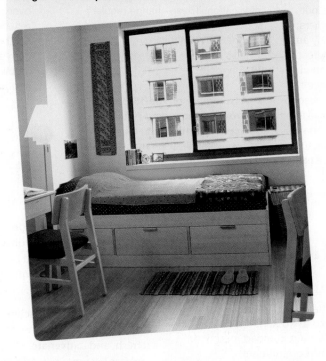

Keeping your room clear of clutter and well organized using feng shui techniques can reduce stress.

- **Shut out the world.** Use shades that allow you to darken or dim the room.
- **Beautify.** Include things that make you feel peaceful.
- **Invest.** Get a set of soft sheets, a duvet cover, and a blanket. Plump and soften pillows.
- **Refresh.** Open windows to remove stale odors. If needed, use relaxing fragrances such as lavender.
- **Block.** If you can't get rid of a desk covered in work, use a curtain to keep things out of sight. Put your phone away, and *relax*.

**Source:** Feng Shui DeStress, "Using Feng Shui to Reduce Stress," Accessed February 2016, www.destress.com/relax/lifestyle/using-feng-shui-to-reduce-stress.htm.

- **Reward yourself for work completed.** When you finish a task, do something nice for yourself. Rest breaks give you time to recharge.
- **Work when you're at your best.** If you're a morning person, study and write papers in the morning, and take breaks when you start to slow down.
- **Break overwhelming tasks into small pieces, and allocate a certain amount of time to each.** If you are floundering in a task, move on and come back to it when you're refreshed.
- **Remember that time is precious.** Many people learn to value their time only when they face a terminal illness. Try to value each day. If you have trouble saying no to people and projects that steal your time, see the Making Changes Today box on page 84 for some suggestions.

## Consider Downshifting: Living Simply

Today's lifestyles are hectic, and stress often comes from trying to keep up. Many people are questioning whether "having it all" is worth it, and are working to simplify their lives. This trend has been labeled **downshifting**, or *voluntary simplicity*.

The Tiny Home movement is one example, as are giving up high-stress jobs for ones you enjoy, house decluttering, and making other life changes.

Deciding what is most important in life, cutting down on "things," and considering your environmental footprint are part of downshifting. When you contemplate any form of downshift (or start your career this way), it's important to move slowly and consider the following:

- Are you spending your money on things you *want* or things you *need*? What can you do without? What things are necessities? (See **Focus On: Improving Your Financial Health** for more on assessing your finances.)
- Choose your career based on what you love; consider the importance of salary versus really liking what you do. Can you be happy taking a lower-paying job if it is less stressful?
- Don't let money and possessions dictate who you are or rule your life. Save, be prudent, but don't be excessive in everything you do. Build a reserve for emergencies.

**downshifting** Taking a step back and simplifying a lifestyle that is hectic, packed with pressure and stress, and focused on trying to keep up; also known as *voluntary simplicity*.

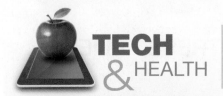

# APPS FOR THE RELAXATION RESPONSE

Looking for a way to relax that you can carry with you? Check out the yearly reviews of apps put out by consumer groups and others, making sure to note whether they are affiliated or have conflicts of interest with manufacturers. Pay close attention to the costs, amount of space used on your device, whether subscriptions are necessary after the initial free period, which devices are supported, privacy issues, and consumer ratings. Note that these are not scientific reviews of effectiveness; rather, they are designed to provide you with basic information. These change regularly and a simple Google search will get you there. Two noteworthy summary reviews of stress and anxiety apps for 2015 are:

1. **A Summary of The 15 Best Anxiety iPhone and Android Apps of 2015** can be found at www.healthine.com/health/anxiety/top-iphone-android-apps.

2. **A second review put out by *Tech Times* in 2015** provides an overview of 12 mobile apps that reduce stress and anxiety. This can be found at www.techtimes.com/articles/57571/20150605/12-mobile-apps-that-help-relieve-stress-and-anxiety.htm

---

## MAKING CHANGES TODAY

### Learn to Say No and Mean It!

Is your calendar so full you barely have time to breathe? When you are asked to do something you don't really want to do or are overextended, practice the following tips to avoid overcommitment:

- ◉ **Be sympathetic, but firm.** Explain that although you think it's a great cause or idea, you can't participate right now. Don't waver if they persist or pressure you.

- ◎ **Don't say you want to think about it and will get back to them.** This only leads to more forceful requests later.

- ◎ **Don't give in to guilt.** Stick to your guns. Remember you don't owe anyone your time.

- ◎ **Even if something sounds good, avoid spontaneous "yes" responses.** Make a rule that you will take at least a day to think about committing your time.

- ◎ **Schedule time for yourself first.** If you don't have time for the things you love to do, stop and prioritize your activities. Don't let your time be sucked up by things that you really don't want to do.

## Relaxation Techniques for Stress Management

Relaxation techniques to reduce stress have been practiced for centuries and offer opportunities for calming your nervous energy and coping with life's challenges. Some common techniques include yoga, qigong, tai chi, deep breathing, meditation, visualization, progressive muscle relaxation, massage therapy, biofeedback, and hypnosis. Newer forms of relaxation may be found in the latest technology; see the **Tech & Health** box for more information.

**Yoga** Yoga is an ancient practice that combines meditation, stretching, and breathing exercises designed to relax, refresh, and rejuvenate. It began about 5,000 years ago in India and has become increasingly popular among Americans. Over 80 million Americans (34% of the population) say that, over the next year, they are very likely or somewhat likely to practice yoga.[81] Today, people are flocking to yoga as a form of stress release as well as for balance and flexibility and for overall health and fitness.

*Classical yoga* is the ancestor of nearly all modern forms of yoga. Breathing, poses, and verbal mantras are often part of classical yoga. Of the many branches of classical yoga, *Hatha yoga* is the most well known; it is body focused, involving the practice of breath control and *asanas*—held postures and choreographed movements that enhance strength and flexibility. Recent research shows increased evidence of the benefits of Hatha yoga in reducing inflammation, boosting mood, increasing relaxation, and reducing stress among those who practice regularly.[82] Although studies have shown yoga to have similar benefits in treating insomnia and PTSD, reducing anxiety, lowering heart rate and blood pressure, improving fitness and flexibility, reducing pain, and other benefits, much of this research could benefit from more rigorous investigation.[83] (See **Focus On: Cultivating Your Spiritual Health**, starting on page 51, for additional information on yoga.)

**Qigong and Tai Chi** Qigong (pronounced "chee-kong"), one of the fastest-growing, most widely accepted forms of mind–body health exercise, is used by some of the country's largest health care organizations, particularly for people suffering from chronic pain or stress. An ancient Chinese practice, Qigong involves awareness and control of vital body energy known as *qi* (or *chi*, pronounced "chee"). A complex system of internal pathways called *meridians* are believed to carry *qi* throughout your body. If *qi* becomes stagnant or blocked, you'll feel sluggish or powerless. Qigong incorporates a series of flowing movements, breath techniques, mental visualization exercises, and vocalizations of healing sounds that are designed to restore balance and integrate and refresh the mind and body.

Another popular form of mind–body exercise is *tai chi* (pronounced "ty-chee"), often described as "meditation in motion." Originally developed in China over 2,000 years ago, this graceful form of exercise began as a form of self-defense. Tai chi is noncompetitive, self-paced, and involves a defined series of postures or movements done in a slow, graceful manner. Each movement or posture flows into the next without pause. Tai chi has been widely practiced in China for centuries and is now becoming increasingly popular around the world, both as a basic exercise program and as a key component of stress reduction and balance and flexibility programs. Research demonstrating the effectiveness of these benefits is only in its infancy.

**Diaphragmatic or Deep Breathing** Typically, we breathe using only our upper chest and thoracic region. Simply stated, diaphragmatic breathing is deep breathing that maximally fills the lungs by involving the movement of the diaphragm and lower abdomen. This technique is commonly used in yoga exercises and in other meditative practices. Try the diaphragmatic breathing exercise in **FIGURE 3.6** right now and see whether you feel more relaxed!

**Meditation** There are many different forms of **meditation**. Most involve sitting quietly for 15–20 minutes, focusing your thoughts, blocking the "noise" in your life, controlling breathing, and ultimately, relaxing. Practiced by Eastern religions for centuries, meditation is believed to be an important form of introspection and personal renewal. When used as an aid in destressing, it is believed to calm the physiological responses of stress and has been reported to reduce risks of illness. According to a recent review of key *randomized controlled trials (RCTs)* by the American Heart Association, one form of meditation, *transcendental meditation (TM)*, appeared to be most effective in lowering blood pressure, overall mortality, and

**meditation** A relaxation technique that involves deep breathing and concentration.

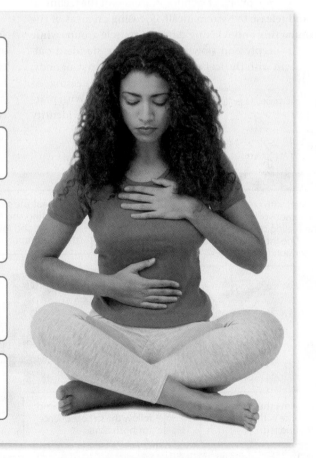

① Assume a natural, comfortable position either sitting up straight with your head, neck, and shoulders relaxed, or lying on your back with your knees bent and your head supported. Close your eyes and loosen binding clothes.

② In order to feel your abdomen moving as you breathe, place one hand on your upper chest and the other just below your rib cage.

③ Breathe in slowly and deeply through your nose. Feel your stomach expanding into your hand. The hand on your chest should move as little as possible.

④ Exhale slowly through your mouth. Feel the fall of your stomach away from your hand. Again, the hand on your chest should move as little as possible.

⑤ Concentrate on the act of breathing. Shut out external noise. Focus on inhaling and exhaling, the route the air is following, and the rise and fall of your stomach.

**FIGURE 3.6 Diaphragmatic Breathing** This exercise will help you learn to breathe deeply as a way to relieve stress. Practice this for 5–10 minutes several times a day, and soon diaphragmatic breathing will become natural for you.

CVD events. Other forms of meditation appeared to have little or no effect on these health risks.[84] More rigorous, controlled research must be done to better understand the potential benefits of meditation. (Meditation and other aspects of spiritual health are discussed in detail in **Focus On: Cultivating Your Spiritual Health**, beginning on page 51.) Meditation can be performed alone or in a group. Many colleges and universities offer classes on how to meditate. Check with your campus wellness center.

**Visualization** Often our thoughts and imagination provoke distress by conjuring up worst-case scenarios. Our imagination, however, can also be tapped to reduce stress. In **visualization**, you use your imagination to create calming mental scenes. The choice of mental images is unlimited, but natural settings such as ocean beaches, deep forests, and mountain lakes often conjure up soothing sights, sounds, and smells. These sensory experiences can replace stressful stimuli with peaceful or pleasurable thoughts. Think of a place that is "quieting" for you. Try to imagine yourself there, sitting quietly. Breathe deeply and allow yourself to be in that space/moment.

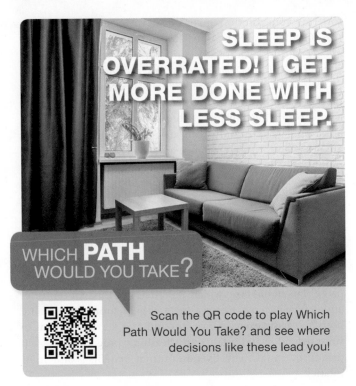

WHICH **PATH** WOULD YOU TAKE?

Scan the QR code to play Which Path Would You Take? and see where decisions like these lead you!

**Progressive Muscle Relaxation** Progressive muscle relaxation involves teaching awareness of the feeling of tension and release by systematically focusing on areas of the body; contracting and relaxing different muscle groups while breathing in deeply and slowly exhaling. The standard pattern is to begin with the feet and work your way up your body, contracting and releasing as you go (**FIGURE 3.7**). With practice, you can quickly identify

**visualization** The creation of mental images to promote relaxation.

tension in your body and consciously release that tension to calm yourself.

**Massage Therapy** Massage not only feels great, it is also an excellent way to relax. Techniques vary from deep-tissue massage to the gentler acupressure, use of hot rocks on tense muscle groups, and a wide range of other techniques. Although a variety of studies have been carried out to assess the health effects of massage, much of this research is poorly

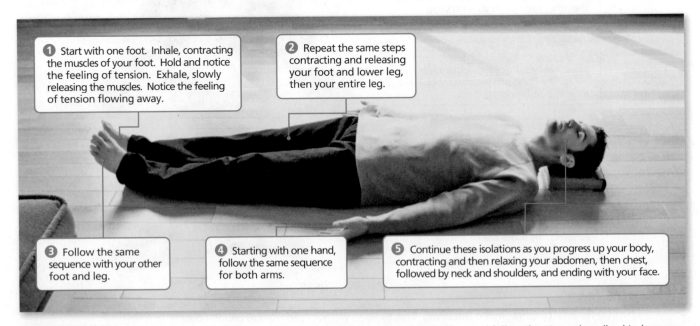

**1** Start with one foot. Inhale, contracting the muscles of your foot. Hold and notice the feeling of tension. Exhale, slowly releasing the muscles. Notice the feeling of tension flowing away.

**2** Repeat the same steps contracting and releasing your foot and lower leg, then your entire leg.

**3** Follow the same sequence with your other foot and leg.

**4** Starting with one hand, follow the same sequence for both arms.

**5** Continue these isolations as you progress up your body, contracting and then relaxing your abdomen, then chest, followed by neck and shoulders, and ending with your face.

**FIGURE 3.7 Progressive Muscle Relaxation** Sit or lie down in a comfortable position and follow the steps described to increase your awareness of tension in your body and your ability to release it.

controlled, lacks sufficient sample size, and results are preliminary or conflicting. However, there is a growing body of evidence indicating that massage may ease back pain, as well as potentially increase quality of life for cancer patients, as well as those with HIV/AIDS and depression.[85] Though promising, this research is in its infancy.

**Biofeedback** Biofeedback is a technique in which a person learns to use the mind to consciously control bodily functions, such as heart rate, body temperature, and breathing rate. Using devices from those as simple as stress dots that change color with body temperature variation to sophisticated electrical sensors, individuals learn to listen to their bodies and make necessary adjustments, such as relaxing certain muscles, changing breathing, or concentrating to slow heart rate and relax. Eventually, individuals develop the ability to recognize and lower stress responses without machines and can practice it anywhere.

**biofeedback** A technique using a machine to self-monitor physical responses to stress.

**Hypnosis** A trancelike state that allows people to become unusually responsive to suggestion.

**Hypnosis** Hypnosis requires a person to focus on one thought, object, or voice, thereby freeing the right hemisphere of the brain to become more active. The person then becomes unusually responsive to suggestion. Whether self- or other-induced, hypnosis can reduce certain types of stress.

# STUDY **PLAN**

Customize your study plan—and master your health!—in the Study Area of **MasteringHealth**.

## **ASSESS** YOURSELF

**Is stress negatively affecting your life?** Want to find out? Take the **How Stressed Are You?** assessment available on

## MasteringHealth.™

## CHAPTER **REVIEW**

To hear an MP3 Tutor Session, scan here or visit the Study Area in **MasteringHealth**.

### LO **1** | **What Is Stress?**

■ Stress is an inevitable part of our lives. *Eustress* refers to stress associated with positive events; *distress* refers to stress associated with negative events. Both forms can have a negative physiological impact on your health.

### LO **2** | **Body Responses to Stress**

■ Several theories attempt to explain what happens when a person experiences real or perceived stress. The alarm, resistance, and exhaustion phases of general adaptation syndrome (GAS) involve physiological responses to both real and imagined stressors and cause complex hormonal reactions. The transactional theory, minority stress theory, and Yerkes-Dodson law of arousal help explain other factors that influence how stress is perceived, how people cope at varying levels of stress, and how health disparities can influence stress levels.

### LO **3** | **Physical Effects of Stress**

■ Undue stress for extended periods of time can compromise the immune system and result in serious health consequences. Stress has been linked to numerous health problems, including cardiovascular disease, weight gain, hair loss, diabetes, digestive problems, and increased susceptibility to infectious diseases. *Psychoneuroimmunology* is the science that analyzes the relationship between the mind's reaction to stress and the function of the immune system.

### LO **4** | **Stress and Your Mental Health**

■ Stress can have negative impacts on your intellectual and psychological health, including impaired memory, poor concentration, depression, anxiety, and other disorders.

## LO 5 | What Causes Stress?

- Psychosocial and physical sources of stress include change, hassles, relationships, academic and financial pressure, frustrations and conflict, overload, bias/discrimination, and environmental stressors.

## LO 6 | Individual Factors That Affect Your Stress Response

- Some sources of stress are internal and are related to appraisal, self-esteem, self-efficacy, personality types, hardiness and resilience, grit, shift and persist, and other factors.

## LO 7 | Managing Stress in College

- College and the transition to independent adulthood can be especially stressful. Managing stress begins with learning coping skills. Managing emotional responses, taking mental or physical action, developing a support network, practicing self-compassion, cultivating spirituality, downshifting, learning time management, managing finances, or learning relaxation techniques—all will help you better cope with stress in the long run.

# POP QUIZ

Visit **MasteringHealth** to personalize your study plan with Chapter Review Quizzes and Dynamic Study Modules.

## LO 1 | What Is Stress?

1. Even though Andre experienced stress when he graduated from college and moved to a new city, he viewed these changes as an opportunity for growth. What is Andre's stress called?
   a. Strain
   b. Distress
   c. Eustress
   d. Adaptive response

## LO 2 | Body Responses to Stress

2. In which stage of general adaptation syndrome does the fight-or-flight response occur?
   a. Exhaustion stage
   b. Alarm stage
   c. Resistance stage
   d. Response stage

3. The branch of the autonomic nervous system that is responsible for energizing the body for either fight or flight and for triggering many other stress responses is the
   a. central nervous system.
   b. parasympathetic nervous system.
   c. sympathetic nervous system.
   d. endocrine system.

## LO 3 | Physical Effects of Stress

4. The area of scientific investigation that analyzes the relationship between the mind's response to stress and the immune system's ability to function effectively is called
   a. psychoneuroimmunology.
   b. immunocompetence.
   c. psychoimmunology.
   d. psychology.

## LO 4 | Stress and Your Mental Health

5. When Jesse encounters a stressful situation, he adapts well and tends to bounce back easily, even though the same situation may derail others. What protective factor is Jesse exhibiting to deal with stress?
   a. Cognitive restructuring
   b. Type A personality
   c. High self-esteem
   d. Psychological resilience

## LO 5 | What Causes Stress?

6. Losing your keys is an example of what psychosocial source of stress?
   a. Pressure
   b. Inconsistent behaviors
   c. Hassles
   d. Conflict

7. A state of physical and mental exhaustion caused by excessive stress is called
   a. conflict.
   b. overload.
   c. hassles.
   d. burnout.

## LO 6 | Individual Factors That Affect Your Stress Response

8. Which of the following statements is *correct* regarding factors that affect your stress response?
   a. Type A individuals are characterized by anger and toxic core behaviors that inevitably lead to negative health outcomes.
   b. Individuals who thrive under challenges typically demonstrate qualities of hardiness and resilience
   c. People with grit are those who are bull-headed and rigid and who typically experience negative health outcomes.
   d. People with high self-efficacy typically have little control over what happens to them; people with high self-esteem are typically much more in control of their environment than those with high self-efficacy.

## LO 7 | Managing Stress in College

9. Which of the following is the best strategy to avoid test-taking anxiety on an exam?
   a. Do the majority of your studying the night before the exam so it is fresh in your mind.
   b. Plan ahead and study over a period of time for the exam with a limited, yet thorough, review the night before.
   c. Drink a caffeinated beverage right before the exam because sympathomimetics are known to reduce stress.
   d. Go through the exam as quickly as possible so you don't dwell on potential mistakes.

10. Which of the following describes the stress management strategy that focuses on improving your self-talk?
    a. Adaptation
    b. Conflict resolution
    c. Self-compassion
    d. Meditation

*Answers to the Pop Quiz questions can be found on page A-1. If you answered a question incorrectly, review the section identified by the Learning Outcome. For even more study tools, visit **MasteringHealth**.*

# THINK ABOUT IT!

## LO 1 | What Is Stress?

1. Define *stress*. What are some examples of scenarios where you might feel distress? Eustress?

## LO 2 | Body Responses to Stress

2. Describe the alarm, resistance, and exhaustion phases of general adaptation syndrome and the body's physiological response to stress. Does stress lead to more irritability or emotionality, or does irritability or emotionality lead to stress? Provide examples from your own life or from friends or family.

## LO 3 | Physical Effects of Stress

3. What are some of the health risks that result from chronic stress? How does the study of psychoneuroimmunology link stress and illness? What are your biggest stressors right now and do you think you are experiencing any physical or mental effects?

## LO 4 | Stress and Your Mental Health

4. Why might stress and the occurrence of mental disorders be correlated? Can you think of examples from recent headlines where acute or chronic stress has led to increases in violence or other social problems?

## LO 5 | What Causes Stress?

5. Why are the college years often high stress for many? How do you think stress may differ between people your age who go to college and those that do not? What factors increase stress risks for both groups?

## LO 6 | Individual Factors That Affect Your Stress Response

6. What are the characteristics of people who thrive by being resilient and demonstrating grit? How do you think you measure up in terms of these characteristics?

## LO 7 | Managing Stress in College

7. What are three important actions you can take right now to help manage your stressors?

8. How does anger affect the body? Discuss the steps you can take to manage your own anger and help your friends control theirs.

9. How much of a procrastinator are you? What sorts of situations make you the most likely to procrastinate? What could you do to reduce the likelihood of procrastinating in these situations?

# ACCESS YOUR HEALTH ON THE INTERNET

Visit **MasteringHealth** for links to the websites and RSS feeds.

The following websites explore further topics and issues related to stress.

**American College Counseling Association.** The website of the professional organization for college counselors offers useful links and articles. www.collegecounseling.org

**American College Health Association.** This site provides yearly information and data from the National College Health Assessment survey, which covers stress, anxiety, and other health issues for students. www.acha.org

**American Psychological Association.** Here you can find current information and research on stress and stress-related conditions as well as an annual survey. www.apa.org

**Higher Education Research Institute.** This organization provides annual surveys of first-year and senior college students that cover academic, financial, and health-related issues and problems. www.heri.ucla.edu

**National Institute of Mental Health.** A resource for information on all aspects of mental health, including the effects of stress. www.nimh.nih.gov

# FOCUS ON Improving Your Financial Health

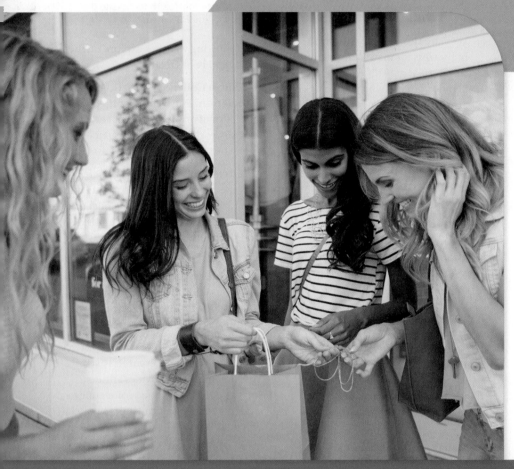

## WHY SHOULD I CARE?

In addition to enabling you to buy the food, clothing, health care, books, technology, and other goods and services you need such as health insurance, financial health allows you to choose a safe place to live, pursue your education, keep stressors in control, and have leisure time to exercise, maintain your friendships, travel, and volunteer. A key characteristic of financial health is a good credit history, which will help you get a car loan, mortgage, or other funding to pursue your dreams.

They say money can't buy happiness or love—but can it buy health? Individuals of a greater **socioeconomic status (SES)** tend to live healthier and longer lives than those living in poverty.[1] This phenomenon is known as the **health–income gradient (FIGURE 1)**. Based on this gradient, a lower-income individual has more to gain, healthwise, with a smaller increase in income.

**socioeconomic status (SES)** An individual or family's social and economic position in relation to others with regard to education, income, and occupation.

**health–income gradient** The relationship between the health of individuals or communities and income, where health outcomes increase as income increases.

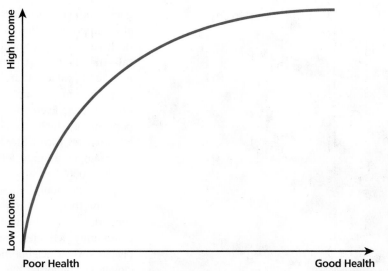

**FIGURE 1** The Health–Income Gradient The health–income gradient shows a steeper curve in the lower income levels and flattens out toward higher income levels. Individuals at the lower end of the gradient typically have poorer health outcomes.

**VIDEO TUTOR**
Financial Health

**Source:** Based on W. Evans, B. Wolfe, and N. Adler, "The Income–Health Gradient," *Institute for Research on Poverty: Focus* 30, no. 1 (2013), Available at www.irp.wisc.edu/publications/focus/pdfs/foc301b.pdf.

The gradient between poverty and health can be demonstrated worldwide, whether it's based on individual income, community wealth, or a country's gross national product.[2] People living in wealthy, developed countries have much longer life expectancies than do those in poor countries (**FIGURE 2**). This is in part because smoking, alcohol abuse, a poor-quality diet, and exposure to environmental pollutants and occupational risks, as well as lack of access to health care are more common among low-income populations. These factors and others found in low income populations increase the risk for heart disease, stroke, cancer, and diabetes.

That said, a higher income doesn't *guarantee* better health. For example, the United States has the highest household wealth and highest disposable income per capita in the world, yet lags behind many nations in life expectancy and infant mortality. An assortment of factors, from social connectedness to work–life balance, contribute to a population's health.[3] While good health is never a sure thing, money makes attaining it much easier. This chapter addresses some of the factors that influence health and wealth and what you can do now to increase your financial health.

## LO 1 | THE LINK BETWEEN HEALTH AND WEALTH

List and explain factors that influence the relationship between health and wealth.

The relationship between health and wealth is based on a complex interplay of factors, including the *determinants of health* introduced in Chapter 1. For example, research has linked higher rates of smoking, a behavior associated with a wide range of negative health effects, with lower socioeconomic status.[4] (See Chapter 12 for more on the impacts of smoking.) Many factors contribute to higher smoking rates in poorer populations worldwide, including lower cost of cigarettes; fewer bans on smoking in public places; fewer limits on tobacco advertising; illiteracy, which contributes to reduced awareness of tobacco's health effects; reduced social support for quitting; and reduced availability of smoking-cessation programs and drug therapies.[5] In addition, low-income individuals may turn to smoking to reduce stress, or may have become addicted at an early age after witnessing family members smoking.

Let's take a closer look at additional risks low-income individuals face and factors that influence the link between health and socioeconomic status.

## Money and Stress

Have you ever been embarrassed that you couldn't afford a concert ticket when everyone else is going? Or have you been jealous of your roommate's new smartphone when you're stuck with an older model? On the whole, we have a tendency to compare ourselves

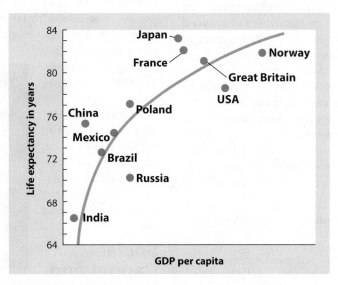

**FIGURE 2** Life Expectancy at Birth and GDP per Capita, 2013 (or latest year)

**Source:** Based on FIGURE 3.2, *OECD Health Statistics 2015*, http://dx.doi.org/10.1787/health-data-en.

to others. Because we value money as an indicator of status and success, those with long-term financial insecurity may experience increased feelings of inferiority, low self-esteem, and self-doubt. These feelings are in part due to **relative deprivation**—the inability of lower-income groups to sustain the same lifestyle as higher-income groups in the same community.

For low-income individuals, experiencing constant feelings of inferiority, anxiety, and insecurity in a money-driven society can lead to chronic stress. In addition, lacking money for basic needs can cause acute stress. Financial stress is associated with negative health outcomes such as mental health issues, cardiovascular disease, immune system issues, gastrointestinal problems, and increased risk for infectious diseases.[6]

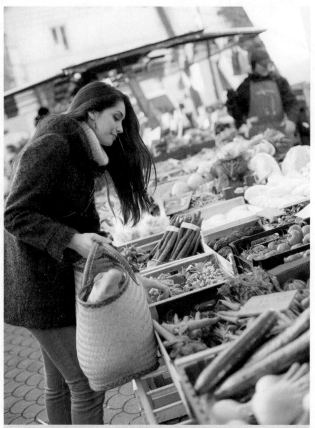

Living in an area with more farmers' markets and grocery stores than fast-food chains and liquor stores provides ample access to healthy foods.

## Money and Access to Resources

People of lower SES often live in areas where they lack access to social services and support, such as nearby medical facilities, educational opportunities, safe housing, or clean water. Researchers have found higher obesity rates in areas with a greater density of fast-food restaurants and lower obesity rates in areas with better access to healthy foods in supermarkets.[7] Areas where people lack access to affordable, nutritious foods that make up a full and healthy diet are known as **food deserts**.[8] The difference between living in a fast food–dense neighborhood and a place that promotes good health—a safe, walkable neighborhood with weekend local

organic farmers' markets, for instance—usually comes down to money.

Access to health care and health insurance is strongly linked to levels of chronic disease, disease management, and life expectancy. One 2016 study found the prevalence of obesity to be 20 percent lower in communities with "robust" access to primary care providers.[9] Moreover, the American Cancer Society reports that "uninsured patients are far more likely to receive cancer diagnoses at a later stage, when treatment is usually more extensive, more expensive, and less successful.[10]

## Social Capital and Health

Clearly, health depends on access to material

goods and services. But research also supports a link between health and access to **social capital**—the shared bonds, behaviors, and values that enable people to support and to trust one another. Even for low-SES populations, high social capital correlates with better health. For example, a study following nearly 5,000 low SES mothers in U.S. cities found those with someone they could rely on for support, who participated in community activities, and who perceived their neighborhood as closely knit reported higher levels of health, and retained those higher levels through up to 9 years of follow-up.[11] On the other hand, living in a high-income area with ample access to material resources frequently fails to correlate with good health when area residents experience low levels of social capital.

## Poverty, Early Care, and Education

Disadvantages early in life can have a lasting impact on health. For example, pregnant women of low SES may face increased risks for nutrient deficiencies, high stress, smoking, and drug or alcohol abuse—all of which can harm the fetus. They may also have reduced access to preconception and prenatal

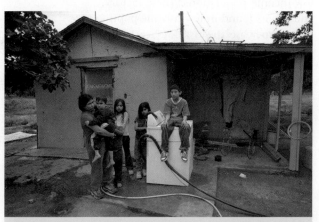

Experiencing poverty in childhood makes people susceptible to a variety of health problems, including obesity, infections, asthma, type 2 diabetes, violence, and mental health issues.

**relative deprivation** The inability of lower-income groups to sustain the same lifestyle as higher-income groups in the same community, often resulting in feelings of anxiety and inferiority.

**food desert** Neighborhood or region where people lack access to affordable, nutritious food.

**social capital** The shared bonds, behaviors, and values that enable people to support and to trust one another.

care, including regular medical check-ups, diet planning, alcohol and drug counseling, and smoking-cessation programs. Access to these services promotes the growth and development of a healthy child. (More about preconception care and prenatal care in Chapter 10.)

Compared to children in moderate and high-income households, children living in poverty experience reduced physical health, greater developmental delay, lower school achievement, and more behavioral and emotional problems.[12] Low-SES parents may be unable to provide appropriate cognitive stimulation to their developing child, or the stress of poverty, menial labor, poor health, or substance abuse may foster negative parenting skills. Early childhood education can help, but quality education may be lacking in low-SES populations. See the **Money & Health** box on page 99 for more on poverty and poor health.

## LO 2 | FINANCIAL STRUGGLES IN COLLEGE

Describe common financial struggles college students face and the impact these may have on their health and well-being.

Many first feel the burden of financial struggles in college. The 2008 recession resulted in widespread layoffs and huge reductions in the value of families' savings and investments, followed by several years of sluggish economic growth from which many have yet to recover. As a result, parents have had to limit the financial support they can offer their children in college just when increased demands on state governments have reduced budgets for higher education and increased tuition and fees. Adjusted to 2015 dollars, the average cost of tuition and fees at public 4-year colleges and universities in 2006–2007—just prior to the recession—was $6,800. It is now nearly $9,500, an increase of more than 38 percent.[13] Other costs, such as course materials, housing, food, and travel expenses, can more than double this figure: In 2015–2016, the average full-time undergraduate budget for a student living on-campus at a 4-year in-state public institution was $24,061.[14]

It's not surprising that a recent survey of students at over 1,500 U.S. colleges and universities found that more than 60 percent worried often or very often about meeting regular expenses, and over 55 percent also worried frequently about paying for school.[15] Over one-third of undergraduate students queried in a different survey said finances have been "traumatic or very difficult to handle" in the past year, and nearly 7 percent said that concerns about their finances had negatively affected their grades.[16]

## Making College More Affordable

In a recent survey of incoming first-year students, over 92 percent of lower-SES students and 62 percent of higher-SES students said their financial aid package was a somewhat or very important factor in their college choice, and 74 percent of students crossed colleges off their list because of cost.[17] Over 60 percent of students said that the ability to obtain a good job upon graduation was a very important consideration in their choice of school.[18] More than half of lower SES students borrow at least $3,000 to pay for their first year of school, and nearly 36 percent borrow at least $15,000.[19] On average, about 22 percent of college costs are paid for with borrowed funds.[20]

During his 8 years in office, President Barack Obama took several actions to rein in college costs, such as increasing the size of federal Pell grants by nearly $1,000 and expanding eligibility to receive them.[21] The Obama Administration also established an education tax credit to help offset college costs for families, and instituted income-based repayment, which caps student loan repayments at 10 percent of income.[22] Most ambitiously, the administration called for the first 2 years of community college to be free to responsible students.[23] Although several countries in Europe and South America have free tuition at all public colleges and universities, this proposal has been hotly debated in the United States, including in the 2016 election cycle. Its fate as of this writing is uncertain.

Families are also taking steps to make college more affordable, including having students work while earning their degree, reduce spending, or take on another roommate (**FIGURE 3**).[24] While these solutions can help, there are some drawbacks. For example, having a job in college looks good on a resumé and helps reduce borrowing, but the difficulty of balancing work and school can cause students to spend less time on

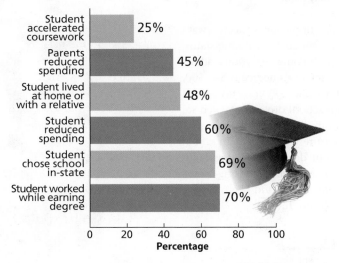

**FIGURE 3** How Families Cut Costs to Make College More Affordable

**Source:** Data are from Sallie Mae, "How America Pays for College 2015," 2016, www.salliemae.com.

Do you think the federal government should provide financial aid to colleges based on how long it takes students to graduate, or the average salary of graduates, or how well they serve low- and middle-income students?

- Should such funding be reduced if colleges don't perform well?
- What constitutes a valuable education?

coursework or drop out altogether. And while many students tightly restrict their discretionary spending, expenditures for books, supplies, and transportation are largely beyond their control. In the United States, only 58 percent of first-time college students at public universities and 65 percent at private colleges complete their degree within 6 years.[25] One common reason students drop out is growing debt.

## LO 3 | ACTIONS TO IMPROVE YOUR FINANCIAL HEALTH

**Explain how to successfully manage finances through budgeting, understanding debt and credit, and avoiding identity theft.**

College is one of the most effective ways to improve your socioeconomic status. The median income for young adults holding a bachelor's degree is $48,500, compared to $30,000 for those with only a high school diploma.[26] Even so, learning to manage your finances now will help ensure you can stay in school and earn your degree, as well as manage postcollege debt, housing costs, advanced education, and begin to save and invest in your future.

### SEE IT! VIDEOS
Imagine living debt-free. Watch **This Frugal Family Has Mastering Living Cheaply,** available on **MasteringHealth.™**

## Prioritizing Health Insurance

Purchasing health insurance may be low on your financial priority list. What's the point in spending money on health care you don't need? While college-age students generally suffer low rates of chronic diseases, individuals aged 15 to 24 are at significant risk of infections and injuries. In 2015, 16 percent of college students were treated for a sinus infection, 10 percent for strep throat, and 6 percent for a fracture or sprain.[27] If you're injured, having insurance could be the difference between quick recovery and financial ruin. Say you were to break your ankle—the costs for medical and surgical care without health insurance range from a minimum of $40,000 to as much as $140,000 for patients who develop complications.[28] Planning for potentially devastating outcomes from an unexpected injury or illness is one key to financial health.

## Making a Budget

Learning skills to effectively manage your money will help you become financially secure. Creating a **budget** during tough economic times may strike you as downright depressing. But how often do you worry vaguely about money? If you feel a little tense every time you open your wallet, then determining how much you can afford to spend may actually be a stress reducer. Here are a few tips for getting started.

### Set Goals
Budgeting should be goal oriented. For students, goal number one is to avoid debt as much as possible. If you have more resources, your goal may be to graduate with no debt at all, or to save for occasional indulgences like a vacation. At other points in life, you may budget to save for buying a car, supporting a family, or retiring. Whenever your life circumstances change, draw up a new budget to match current income level, expenses, and priorities.

### Track Expenses
Start your budget by listing the things you must buy and services you must use. Tuition and fees, rent, mortgage, utilities, phone service, a monthly bus pass, gas, insurance premiums, and routine

**budget** An estimate of spending and income over a set period of time.

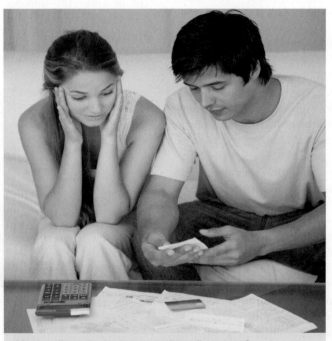

Many college students worry about finances. Smart spending, such as investing in health insurance, can buffer against unexpectedly large costs and the debt that goes along with them.

visits (such as dental and vision) not covered by insurance are just a few examples of *fixed expenses*, meaning their cost does not change much in the short term. Student loan payments may be deferred, depending on the type of loan, if you are in school at least half time. But other debts such as credit card balances can't be deferred and need to be listed as monthly expenses.

Next, figure out how much you spend on food, clothing, entertainment, and personal products or services. Some of these items are **discretionary spending**, things you like but don't necessarily need. Of course, food is essential, but be careful how you classify it. Unless you eat only at a school dining hall that has a fixed fee, chances are you are spending much more on restaurants and store-bought food than you strictly need to.

## Track Income

Income is the money you have to spend. It generally includes wages from work or interest payments from investments. It may also include financial aid payments, allowances or stipends, and other gifts. Some students will also be withdrawing money from college savings accounts to pay for living expenses and tuition.

When you earn more than you spend, you have a **budget surplus**. If expenses are greater than income, you have a **budget deficit**. As mentioned before, the goal with budgeting should be to create a surplus and build savings. College is a unique time when many people run budget deficits while earning a degree, trusting that future wage gains from their education make the debt feasible. Sometimes this leads people to feel that, because they are already going into debt, they might as well borrow as much as they can to make life easier or more fun in the short term. Avoid this thought process. Every dollar of debt you take on matters. With compound interest and loan terms, a "few extra" thousand dollars can take many extra years to pay off.

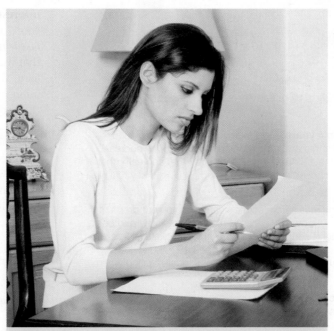

A budget helps you put limits on spending and save for your goals. No matter the income level, a budget is important.

## Making the Math Work

Both income and expenses may be concentrated at the beginning of each academic term when scholarship and loan money arrive and tuition is due. Students receiving lump-sum payments may overspend early on and find themselves unexpectedly broke before finals. Accurate budgets can smooth out spending and help you avoid that problem.

Let's say you create a budget that shows there should be $100 surplus at the end of each month, but that theoretical surplus never appears. The problem could be that you're failing to track all of your discretionary spending. Forgetting to include the purchase of a daily cup of coffee, an occasional movie, and other minor expenditures can quickly add up to that missing $100 per month of savings.

To track spending accurately, watch your expenses for several weeks at a time. Write everything down and keep receipts. Use the **Assess Yourself** budget worksheet on **MasteringHealth** or try a personal finance app or program that tracks spending and income. Many universities also offer free spreadsheets for student budgeting. Check your own school's website for options.

Budget cutting is hard, but taking control of your money builds self-efficacy, and should leave you with more money in the future. Once the adjustment period is over, you might find that your "new financial normal" feels empowering. The Making Changes Today box on page 96 gives some examples of little things you can do to help trim spending.

## Understanding Consumer Credit

It would be nearly impossible for you to function in the modern world if you had to pay for every expense in cash. Just as a majority of college students need loans to obtain their bachelor's degree, consumer credit—typically in the form of a credit card—is actually required for some purchases, like many rental cars and hotel reservations. Used wisely, consumer credit can support your financial health. But overuse of credit—and falling into debt—is a primary stressor. In general, student debt is associated with poorer psychological functioning, anxiety, physical disorders, and poor self-reported health; moreover, credit card debt of $1,000 or more is linked to an increased risk for substance abuse.[29]

## Principles of Debt and Credit

**Debt** is the condition of owing money for something that was purchased. **Credit** is the ability to purchase things in advance of paying for them; put another way, credit is a loan. The original amount borrowed is referred to as the loan **principal**. Loans also include

**discretionary spending** Goods and services that are not life essentials.

**budget deficit** Spending more money than your income.

**budget surplus** Money left over for savings after expenses have been paid.

**debt** Money owed for goods and services that have been purchased.

**credit** The ability to buy goods and services in advance of paying for them.

**principal** Either the original loan amount or the amount left outstanding on a loan, excluding interest.

# MAKING **CHANGES** TODAY

## Creative Ways to Cut Costs

Changes in behavior can add up to big savings. Consider some of the following:

- ⦿ **Commit to graduating in 4 years.** Meet with your advisor s to plan a way to complete all classes that are mandatory for your major as soon as possible. Every semester that you're still in school is another semester that you're not working in your chosen career. Graduating on time is key to limiting your debt.

- ◎ **Cook for yourself.** Making meals from scratch can save you hundreds of dollars each month. Pack your own lunches. At dinner, cook large portions of rice and beans, pasta, lentil soup, and other healthful meals, and freeze the leftovers for fast meals. Invest in a crockpot: spend 15 minutes loading it up before class, set it on low, and you'll have several meals waiting when you get home.

- ◎ **Save on personal services.** Maybe your university has a school of dentistry or dental hygiene where you can get routine dental care free of charge from students, or an optometry school that offers free vision exams. Perhaps a cosmetology school nearby offers free haircuts, or a nearby theater, ballet, or symphony is looking for ushers who get to attend the program for free. Opportunities like these can save you hundreds of dollars.

- ◎ **Consider alternatives to spending.** Before making a purchase, stop. Ask yourself if you could share it, rent it, swap for it, or get it used. If you decide you have to buy retail, comparison-shop, both online and in person. When you've chosen the retailer with the best price, ask for a student discount.

- ◎ **Leave your credit and bank cards at home.** Withdraw a set amount of cash each week for daily expenses and live on it. Reserve your credit cards for infrequent, big-ticket buying.

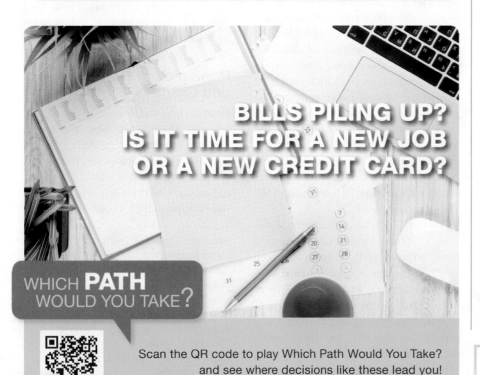

**BILLS PILING UP? IS IT TIME FOR A NEW JOB OR A NEW CREDIT CARD?**

WHICH **PATH** WOULD YOU TAKE?

Scan the QR code to play Which Path Would You Take? and see where decisions like these lead you!

---

**interest** harges, sometimes described as "rent" for using someone else's money. *Fixed interest rate loans* have payments that will not fluctuate for the life of the loan. *Variable interest rate loans* have interest rates that fluctuate over time.

Credit cards are *unsecured loans*, meaning the only thing guaranteeing their repayment is your promise. This differs from *secured loans* such as home mortgages, where the loan giver is allowed to seize an asset (for home mortgages, the house itself) if payments are not made on time.

## Credit Card Interest and Fees

Credit card interest can be variable or fixed, and the rates charged can vary widely. In 2015, the **annual percentage rate (APR)**, the interest rate you pay over a 1-year period, averaged about 12 percent; however, the APR on credit cards issued to students can be much higher.[30] Without existing credit, it is hard for companies to judge how much of a risk it is to lend to you. To compensate, companies typically charge students higher interest rates.

Many credit cards do not charge interest if you pay the balance off in full by the date the payment is due. For example, if you purchased a bus ticket in mid-December, but paid your bill in full before the due date of January 7, you would pay no interest—even though the credit card company had lent you the funds for 3 weeks. Knowing what day of the month your payment is due can allow you to avoid interest charges.

Credit card companies also charge fees. *Cash advance fees* are charged when you withdraw money from a credit card at an ATM. *Annual fees* are charged once every 12 months. *Late fees*, discussed in more detail shortly, are charged when you fail to pay at least your minimum monthly amount due on time.

## Using Your Credit Card Wisely

What counts as your official "first credit card" is one created in your name only,

---

**interest** A fee paid by the borrower of a loan.
**annual percentage rate (APR)** The yearly cost of a credit card account, including interest and certain fees, expressed as a percentage.

# $15,762

is the average amount of U.S. **CREDIT CARD DEBT.**

with no cosigner who is guaranteeing that charges will be covered. This card will probably have a high APR and a low **credit limit**, allowing you to build credit history without going far into debt. Keep just a single credit card account. Most people get into trouble when they run up balances on multiple cards.

Getting your first credit card is an important—but potentially dangerous—rite of passage. On the positive side, it can allow you to rent a car or book a hotel or flight, things that are almost impossible to do without a credit card. Likewise, many high-end cards provide purchase protection programs, so if your new phone falls into the bathtub, your card may actually compensate for the loss.

Credit cards can sometimes make shopping *too* easy: You wouldn't buy that new jacket because you don't have $200 to spare, but you can put it on your credit card and pay it off over several months. Unfortunately, you'll also pay a high percentage in interest, significantly increasing the total cost of the jacket. In 2013, although the median credit card debt owed by college students was just $136, the average debt was $499, suggesting that many college students are carrying well above $500 debt in what are essentially high-interest loans.[31]

There are over 400 million open credit card accounts in the United States today, which averages to more than one card for every man, woman, and child.[32] More than 7 percent of these credit card accounts are currently more than 90 days delinquent.[33] Why is this harmful? Every time you fail to make at least the minimum credit card payment on or before the due date, the credit card company is allowed to charge you a penalty—up to $25 for an occasional slip, and up to $35 for a repeat offense. If you miss two consecutive payments, the credit card company is allowed to increase your interest rate. Once spending is out of control, these penalties and increased, compounding interest can make your debt balloon fast. This, in turn, will reduce your **credit score**, that is, the number financial institutions assign to indicate your ability to repay a loan. To learn more about your credit report and score, see the **Student Health Today** box on page 98.

## Know Your Consumer Credit Rights

If you apply for a credit card and your application is rejected, investigate. The rejection may indicate identity theft, discussed shortly, or a credit report mistake. After rejection, you can always apply for a credit card somewhere else. A "no" at one company doesn't automatically mean "no" elsewhere.

For many years, credit card companies were criticized for enticing college students to get multiple cards. Interest rates and fees were high, and penalties for missed payments extreme. In 2009, the Credit Card Accountability Responsibility and Disclosure (CARD) Act was enacted. It included several new rules to prevent predatory practices, such as "plain language" disclosure of fees and rates. It also requires all applicants under the age of 21 to provide proof of adequate income to repay amounts borrowed. This rule can only be waived if the application is co-signed by someone over age 21 with the financial means to cover potential debts. The CARD Act also stipulates that credit limits on cards with a co-signature cannot be raised without written permission of the cosigner.[34]

The Consumer Financial Protection Bureau (CFPB) is a federal agency established in 2010 whose goals include educating consumers about personal finances and enforcing federal consumer financial laws. The CFPB website (www.consumerfinance.gov) is the place to look for recent developments in credit card rules and other financial information.

## Protecting against Fraud and Identity Theft

**Identity theft** occurs when someone steals personal information (name, address, Social Security number, credit card, or bank account numbers) and uses it without permission. Identity crimes have always existed, but they exploded when online banking and shopping became widespread. In 2014, 12.7 million Americans experienced identity theft, costing them about $16 billion.[35]

## Responding to Credit or Debit Card Theft

If your credit or debit card is lost or stolen, call your bank immediately. Do the

---

**credit limit** The maximum amount a person can charge on a credit card account.

**credit score** Numerical measure of an individual's creditworthiness.

**identity theft** Stealing personal information and using it without permission.

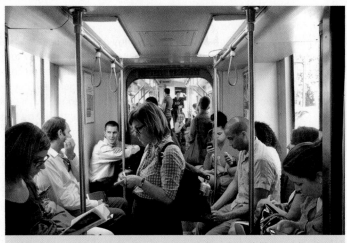

Wireless technology increases people's vulnerability to identity theft.

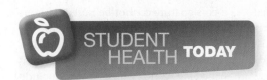

# PROTECTING YOUR CREDIT REPORT

If you've ever borrowed money, then you have a credit report. Knowing its contents—especially your credit score, what it means, and how to improve or protect it—is critical to your present and future financial health.

A credit score is a three-digit number used by lenders to determine whether or not you're creditworthy—whether they trust your ability to pay back funds they allow you to borrow. It's often referred to as a FICO score because the most commonly used score in the United States is from the Fair Isaac Corporation (FICO). The number can range from 300 to 850. The higher the score, the better; however, because different lenders use the score in different ways, it's not possible to say what constitutes a good score for any particular lender.

Your credit report includes vital information factored into your credit score. The most important factor is your payment history—a record of all of your loans and credit accounts, with details about any late or missed payments, the number of accounts that show no late payments, and any foreclosure, wage attachment, bankruptcy, or other legal action related to paying your debts.

Another important factor in your score is the length of your credit history—the length of time you've borrowed from any particular lender. Sticking with one credit card for 5 years makes you a safer bet than opening and closing three or four different credit card accounts in 5 years. Other factors include the total amount you already owe, and the mix of credit sources you use.

Negative information on your report, such as late or missed payments, can remain on your report for up to 7 years. Thus, overextending yourself can have long-term implications for your ability to borrow many years from now, at a time when you might have an urgent need for funds.

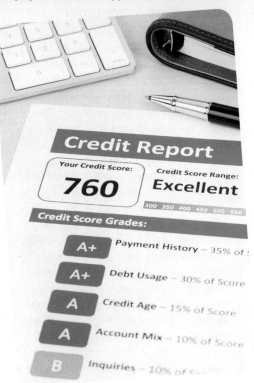

Your credit score is an indication of your financial reliability—to banks, apartment rental agencies, car dealerships, wireless services, and other companies with which you wish to transact business. Some employers also check applicants' credit scores.

**Credit Report**

Your Credit Score: **760**

Credit Score Range: **Excellent**

300 350 400 450 500 550

Credit Score Grades:

- **A+** Payment History — 35% of
- **A+** Debt Usage — 30% of Score
- **A** Credit Age — 15% of Score
- **A** Account Mix — 10% of Score
- **B** Inquiries — 10% of

All potential lenders and other agencies with a legitimate business need have a right to obtain a copy of your credit report. In addition to financial institutions, other businesses with a legal right to obtain your credit report include:

- **Employers.** Potential employers are allowed under federal law to obtain a copy of your credit report to help them make hiring decisions. They need your permission to do so, but if you don't give permission, they'll be less likely to hire you.
- **Rental agencies.** Property owners can obtain a copy of your credit report to evaluate your potential to pay rent in full and on time. Depending on what the report indicates, they can deny you the rental, require a co-signer on the lease, or require a higher deposit.

- **Insurance companies.** On average, people with good credit make fewer insurance claims than people with poor credit; thus, insurance companies are legally allowed to obtain your credit report, and to adjust the rate they charge accordingly.

For all of these reasons, protecting your credit is critical. The most fundamental step is to always pay your bills on time. Stick with one credit card, keep the balance low, and don't apply for any form of credit you don't need. If an emergency arises—for example, if you become too ill to work or a parent who supports you loses his or her job, contact your creditors immediately. They may be able to restructure your loans or refer you to a credit agency that can help.

Review your credit report regularly. You're entitled to a free copy once every 12 months from each of the three credit reporting agencies that lenders use (Equifax, Experian, and TransUnion). To obtain your free copy, visit www.annualcreditreport.com; it's the only site authorized by the federal government to help consumers obtain their free credit report. Your free report will not include your three-digit credit score; however, you can obtain your credit score for a small fee.

If you obtain a copy of your credit report and you find any inaccuracies, contact the reporting agency that issued it, as well as the bank, credit card company, or other creditor that supplied the erroneous information. For more information on disputing errors in credit reports, visit the Federal Trade Commission's web page on Disputing Errors on Credit Reports at www.ftc.gov.

**Sources:** SallieMae Bank, "Fair Isaac Corporation's Frequently Asked Questions About the FICO Score," Accessed March 2016, https://www.salliemae.com/landing/fico/; Fair Isaac Corporation, "The 5 FICO Score Ingredients," Accessed March 2016, www.scoreinfo.org/overview-of-fico-scores/5-fico-score-ingredients/; Federal Trade Commission, "Employment Background Checks," November 2014, https://www.consumer.ftc.gov/articles/0157-employment-background-checks.

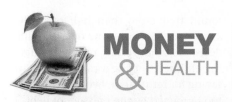

# MONEY & HEALTH | THE POOR AND POOR HEALTH

The evidence is pretty clear that financial health can increase stress, which can also wreak havoc on people's health. But persistent poverty can have devastating consequences for individuals and their loved ones that go well beyond just stress. Consider the following effects of poverty on health:

- Marginalizes people, putting them into groups that routinely live in poor, unsafe neighborhoods, which makes it less likely they will have health insurance and increases risks that they will access health care with late-stage disease instead of more treatable disease.
- Results in unsafe, unsanitary, and overcrowded housing or homelessness.
- Vaccinations and prevention of infectious diseases are less likely to be up-to-date, even nonexistent.
- Makes it less likely that you will eat healthy foods, more likely that you will not eat enough fruits and vegetables, and more likely that you will be obese.
- Makes it less likely that you will be engaged in physical activity or live in an area where low-cost fitness facilities and walking areas are available.
- Makes it more likely that you will have to work two jobs to survive, that you will not have health insurance benefits, and that you will live paycheck to paycheck with few benefits.
- Individuals are more likely to have lower education levels and lower paying jobs.
- Individuals are more likely to smoke cigarettes; suffer from depression; suffer from asthma; have higher rates of obesity and high blood pressure; and have increased risk of heart attack and chronic disease.
- Children are at higher risk for a wide range of negative health effects.

This is not a comprehensive list of all of the potential negative health consequences of a life of poverty and food insecurity. Can you think of other health effects for those without sufficient means?

**Source:** D. Simon, "Poverty Fact Sheet: Poor and in Poor Health," Institute for Research and and Poverty, July 2016, https://morgridge.wisc.edu/documents/Poor_and_In_Poor_Health.pdf; D. Kurzleben, et al., "Americans in Poverty at Greater Risk for Chronic Health Problems," *U.S. News and World Report*, October 30, 2012, http://www.usnews.com/news/articles/2012/10/30/americans-in-poverty-at-greater-risk-for-chronic-health-problems.

---

same if you see unfamiliar charges on your statement. You will not be held responsible for charges once you report the loss, theft, or fraudulent activity. However, if you allow time to elapse before reporting, you may be liable for charges. For example, reporting debit card fraud 2 to 60 days after a crime leaves you liable for up to $500 of losses, and if you discover the problem after 60 days, you will be unable to recover *any* lost money.[36] Watch those bank cards and balances carefully!

## Protecting Personal Information and Avoiding Scams

Sometimes accounts are compromised through data breaches at credit card and banking facilities. The companies in question should notify you of the problem and, if necessary, close the compromised accounts and transfer your balances to new accounts.

While you don't have control over identity breaches, there are other types of fraud you can help prevent. Here are some tips:

- **Steer clear of phishers.** Phishing is an e-mail scam where someone impersonates a bank, credit card company, or other entity in an attempt to trick you into divulging account numbers or passwords. Most financial institutions will not contact you via e-mail asking for personal information. Never supply personal information without verifying the request is genuine. Look up contact information independently to verify the requester.
- **Be wary of Wi-Fi.** Scammers can access your data when you use public Wi-Fi hotspots. Whenever you're in public, your Wi-Fi should be turned off unless you're using it.
- **Update software regularly.** When security vulnerabilities are discovered, programmers "bug patch" them quickly to resolve threats. But you remain open to attack if you don't update to newer versions.
- **Lock your devices.** If you don't put a password on your devices, they become a goldmine of names, numbers, and other information for identity thieves when stolen.
- **Use irregular passwords, and change them frequently.** Create passwords that include letters, numbers, and symbols, and are more like phrases than single words. Don't use the same password for multiple sites.
- **Watch your numbers.** Do not divulge your Social Security number or credit card number to any source you do not completely trust. Don't throw away old credit card statements or any communications containing sensitive information unless it has been rendered unreadable.
- **Keep personal information off social media accounts.** Sharing birth dates and other life details on social media sites makes you vulnerable to fraud.

# 44%
## of IDENTITY FRAUD
involves Internet transactions.

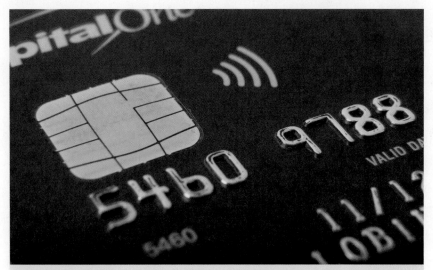

Smart debit or credit cards contain a microchip and are much more secure from fraud than are cards that only have a magnetic strip.

## Get a Smart Card

Traditional credit and debit cards have magnetic strip technology that is fairly easy to steal from. New smart cards contain microchips that make it harder to hijack account information. Merchants and banks in the United States have increasingly adopted smart cards.

## Clean Up Identity Theft Messes

If you discover identity theft, place a fraud alert on your credit reports and ask for report copies to review for problems. Close any accounts that were misused or set up fraudulently. Fill out dispute forms so related debts won't be held against you. Visit the Federal Trade Commission website at www.ftc.gov to learn more about complaint forms and how to correct credit reports. You should also file a police report to document the crime.

## Taking Steps to Improve Your Financial Health

Taking steps to improve and protect your financial health now will pay dividends for decades. A 2015 survey found that more than half of adults aged 18 to 35 are putting off major life decisions, from getting married to having children, buying a car or home, or saving for retirement, because they feel too burdened by the pressure of debt— much of it from student loans. And the trouble doesn't suddenly disappear thereafter: 43 percent of adults over age 35 still defer major purchases because of concerns about their level of debt.[37]

What can you do? First, as suggested earlier, finish your degree on time. Then, once you've landed a steady job in your field, visit a financial planner for planning to pay off your debt while still saving for your future. For information on credit counseling and other options, visit the "Dealing with Debt" page at www.usa.gov/debt.

If debt is causing you severe anxiety, depression, or hopelessness, seek psychological counseling, either through your workplace or community services. In addition, draw on your social capital. Talking to others can help you realize that debt is nothing to be ashamed of, and that many people have concerns just like yours. Social support can also help you stay positive as you seek, find, and share resources and solutions, and celebrate your progress along the way. Curtail all unnecessary spending and come up with a payment plan. Try not to borrow money to pay off loans for borrowed money.

# STUDY **PLAN**

Customize your study plan—and master your health!—in the Study Area of **MasteringHealth**.

## ASSESS YOURSELF

**Want to improve your budgeting skills?** Complete the **Budgeting for College Students** worksheet available on

MasteringHealth.™

## CHAPTER **REVIEW**

To hear an MP3 Tutor Session, scan here or visit the Study Area in **MasteringHealth**.

### LO 1 | The Link between Health and Wealth

- Wealthier populations tend to enjoy better health than lower-income populations, in part because relative deprivation and other stressors associated with poverty increase the risk for poor health. Poorer communities also have higher rates of tobacco use, reduced access to nutritious foods and quality health care, and higher rates of social and environmental problems affecting fetal, infant, and childhood health.

### LO 2 | Financial Struggles in College

- The cost of higher education has increased dramatically over the past decade. Students are borrowing, working part time, living at home, and finding other ways to decrease their expenses to make college more affordable.

### LO 3 | Actions to Improve Your Financial Health

- You can improve your financial health by prioritizing health insurance and creating a budget. Track your income and expenses—especially your discretionary expenditures—closely to avoid shortfalls.

- Strictly limit credit card purchases and pay off your balance monthly to avoid high interest charges. If you must carry a balance, pay more than the minimum, and pay on time to avoid late fees and increased interest rates.

- You can reduce your risk for identity theft by monitoring your personal information. If you suspect fradulent activity on one of your accounts, contact the financial institution immediately to limit losses or liability for unauthorized charges.

## POP **QUIZ**

Visit **MasteringHealth** to personalize your study plan with Chapter Review Quizzes and Dynamic Study Modules.

### LO 1 | The Link between Health and Wealth

1. Which of the following statements helps to explain the association between low socioeconomic status (SES) and poor health in the United States?
   a. The lower a county's income, the greater the prevalence of underweight, which contributes to poor health.
   b. Greater government spending on social services in low-SES counties fosters dependency.
   c. For low-SES individuals, experiencing constant feelings of inferiority, anxiety, and insecurity can progress to chronic stress, which is a risk factor for poor health.
   d. All of the above statements are true.

### LO 2 | Financial Struggles in College

2. A majority of college students
   a. worry about meeting regular expenses and about paying for school.
   b. admitted to their top-choice college decide not to attend because they are not offered aid.
   c. who are enrolled in college for the first time fail to earn their degree within 6 to 8 years.
   d. report that they make college more affordable by living at home or with a relative.

### LO 3 | Actions to Improve Your Financial Health

3. The interest rate you pay over a year-long period is your
   a. credit limit.
   b. annual percentage rate.
   c. annual fee.
   d. grace period.

*Answers to the Pop Quiz questions can be found on page A-1. If you answered a question incorrectly, review the section identified by the Learning Outcome. For even more study tools, visit **MasteringHealth**.*

# 4 Improving Your Sleep

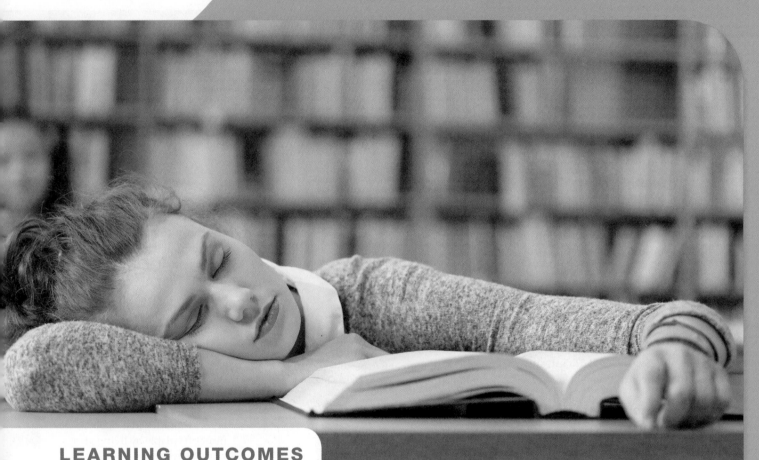

## LEARNING OUTCOMES

LO **1** Describe the problem of sleep deprivation in the United States, including the unique challenges of sleep deprivation on campus.

LO **2** Explain why we need sleep and what happens if we don't get enough, including potential physical, emotional, social, and safety threats to health.

LO **3** Explain the processes of sleep, including the two-stage model, circadian rhythm, and sleep–wake cycle, and how they work, as well as their importance for restful sleep.

LO **4** Describe some common sleep disorders, including risk factors and what can be done to prevent or treat them.

LO **5** Explore ways to improve your sleep through cognitive-behavioral therapy for insomnia, changing daily habits, modifying your environment, avoiding sleep disruptors, using sleep aids responsibly, and other sound sleep hygiene strategies.

Sleeping for fewer than 7 hours per night may be one of our greatest public health threats—associated with an increased risk for obesity, diabetes, high blood pressure, coronary heart disease, cancer, stroke, gastrointestinal issues, frequent mental distress, and all-cause mortality. It can also have a major effect on cognitive performance, which can increase the likelihood of motor vehicle and other transportation accidents, industrial accidents, medical errors, loss of work productivity, memory loss, and our relationships with others. College students, in particular, report high levels of sleeplessness and stress. But there are things you can do now to ensure healthy and restorative sleep each night.[1]

## LO 1 | SLEEPLESS IN AMERICA

Describe the problem of sleep deprivation in the United States, including the unique challenges of sleep deprivation on campus.

Nearly every night, we leave our waking world and slide into a series of sleep stages, punctuated by changes in heart rate, respiration rate, blood pressure, and other bodily processes. We all need sleep—the stages and changes that allow the body to repair, restore, and refresh itself. However, over 83 million people in the United States don't get the sleep they need, with as many as 70 million individuals suffering from an actual sleep disorder.[2]

Inadequate sleep isn't just an American problem; in fact, people in the United States and Japan have the dubious distinction of being the most sleep-deprived countries in the world, consistently racking up fewer hours of sleep each night than people in the United Kingdom, Germany, Canada, and Mexico. Overall, poor sleep affects quality of life, productivity, physical and mental health, and social interactions of 45 percent of the world's population, and those numbers are increasing.[3] FIGURE 4.1 compares average nightly sleep times across a number of countries.

Just how serious is **sleep deprivation**, a condition that occurs when sleep is insufficient for a given age? How many suffer from **somnolence**—drowsiness, sluggishness, and a lack of mental alertness that can affect daily performance in the United States?[4] Although recent surveys of nearly 450,000 U.S. adults' self-reported sleep habits indicate that just over 65 percent had slept the recommended 7 hours in the last 24 hours, the other 35 percent—over 83 million people—did not. Over 38 percent of Americans reported unintentionally falling asleep during the day at least once in the last month.[5]

While falling asleep in class or studying for an exam can have serious implications, one of the greatest potential risks for drowsiness occurs when a tired individual gets behind the wheel of a motor vehicle. Over 5 percent of all drivers reported falling asleep at the wheel, and 1 in 25 report actually falling asleep at the wheel in the last month![6] Drowsy driving was responsible for nearly 83,000 crashes, 37,000 injuries, and 850 deaths in the United States in 2014—not to mention 45,000 property-only crashes each year.[7]

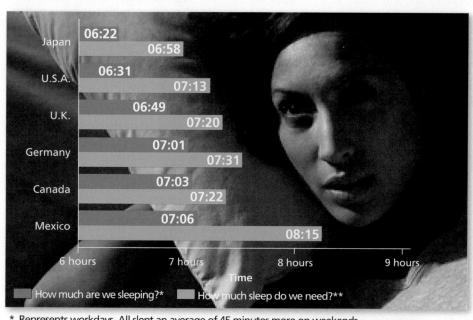

* Represents workdays. All slept an average of 45 minutes more on weekends.
** Represents the number of hours needed for respondents to function at their best the next day (self-reported).

**FIGURE 4.1** International Sleep Statistics

**Source:** Data from National Sleep Foundation, *2013 International Sleep Poll: Summary of Findings* (Arlington, VA: National Sleep Foundation, 2014), Available at http://sleepfoundation.org/sites/default/files/RPT495a.pdf.

**sleep deprivation** A condition that occurs when sleep is insufficient.

**somnolence** Drowsiness, sluggishness, and lack of mental alertness that can affect your daily performance and lead to life-threatening sleepiness while driving.

## Sleepless on Campus: Tired and Dragged-Out Students?

College students seem to be particularly vulnerable to sleep problems. In a recent survey from the American College Health Association (ACHA), only 11.8 percent of students reported getting enough sleep to feel well rested in the morning 6 or more days a week.[8] Nearly 61 percent of students aged 18 to 29 say they often stay awake late and get up early.[9] Not surprisingly, over 68 percent of students said that, in the last 7 days, they felt sleepy during the day on 3–6 or more days per week. They also indicated that sleep is more than a little problem (24.9 percent), a big problem (11.9 percent), or a very big problem (4.7 percent) in the last week.[10] Sleep deficiencies have been linked to a host of student issues, including poor academic performance, weight gain, increased alcohol abuse, accidents, daytime drowsiness, relationship issues, depression, and other problems.[11] Despite large numbers of students reporting sleep problems, less than 5 percent have sought treatment for insomnia, and just over 2 percent have sought treatment for other sleep problems.[12] Clearly there is room for greater awareness about possible resources and easier access to sleep resources on America's campuses.

Approximately 20 percent of the U.S. population suffers from a condition known as **excessive daytime sleepiness** or **excessive sleepiness**—a major compulsion to sleep, along with persistent sluggishness and fatigue, that can cause individuals to nod off at inopportune times and interfere with most aspects of life.[13] Adults aged 18 to 25 and those over age 65 are

## TABLE 4.1 | Adults Reporting Selected Sleep Behaviors in 12 States

| Age (Years) | Unintentionally Fell Asleep During the Day at Least Once in the Past Month | Nodded Off or Fell Asleep While Driving in the Past Month |
|---|---|---|
| 18 to <25 | 43.7% | 4.5% |
| 25 to <35 | 36.1% | 7.2% |
| 35 to <45 | 34.0% | 5.7% |
| 45 to <55% | 35.3% | 3.9% |
| 55 to <65 | 36.5% | 3.1% |
| >65 | 44.6% | 2.0% |

**Source:** Centers for Disease Control and Prevention, "Insufficient Sleep is a Public Health Problem," September 3, 2015, www.cdc.gov/features/dssleep/.

the most likely to nod off during the day. (See **TABLE 4.1**.)[14] In clinical terms, **primary idiopathic hypersomnia** refers to excessive daytime sleepiness without narcolepsy or the associated features of other sleep disorders.[15]

## Why So Sleep Deprived?

Several factors can lead to sleep deprivation:

- **Shift work.** Changing shifts or shifts that are outside the normal 9-to-5 work schedule can disrupt biological clocks and lead to sleeplessness, insomnia, and a host of other problems.[16] Chronic insomnia and disruptions in biological clocks can result in high levels of on-the-job errors; in fact, sleepy workers are 70 percent more likely to be involved in accidents than those getting enough sleep.[17] Some train crashes, cruise ship crashes, and other serious accidents appear to be sleep-related. Drowsy workers are also more likely to be depressed, miss work, and have motor vehicle accidents when commuting.[18]
- **Long-haul driving.** Sleep deprivation is common among truckers, particularly those who drive commercially over 60 hours per week and drive alone.[19]
- **Drugs and medications.** As noted on warning labels, prescription,

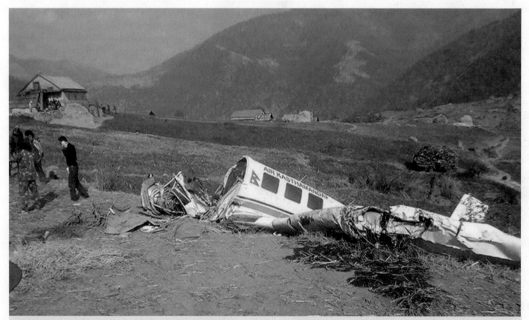
Many of the major transportation and industrial accidents occur among shift workers or those who suffer from chronic sleep deprivation.

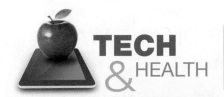

## TECH & HEALTH

## WIRED AND TIRED
### *Technology's Toll on Our Sleep*

Why are younger Americans so tired? According to some sources, the average 18- to 34-year-old college student has up to seven tech devices (including TVs) and may be using a smartphone from 1 to 4 hours each day! In fact, according to a recent poll, technology invades the bedrooms of millions, with over 96 percent of young adults reporting using electronic devices before bed and during the night. Is it any wonder that sleep may suffer?

Sleep experts indicate that increased exposure to interactive technology and "multiscreening" with several devices at a time may increase alertness compared to just watching television. Researchers in a recent study assessing biological changes associated with using blue-light devices such as tablets or smartphones showed significant decreases in *melatonin*, a hormone that helps people fall asleep. While sleepless nights are an initial threat, long-term melatonin drops may increase risk of diabetes, certain types of cancer, and migraines, among others.

Here are a few ways to avoid the melatonin-draining effects of blue light on your sleep and health:

- Stick to small screens, and keep them far away from your eyes.
- Dim your screen and home lights as dusk settles in.
- Purchase amber-tinted glasses that block blue light.
- Allow yourself only an hour or two of screen time after dark.

**Sources:** Marketing Charts, "College Students Own an Average of 7 Tech Devices," June 2013, www.marketingcharts.com/wp/topics/demographics/college-students-own-anaverage-of-7-tech-devices-30430; A. M. Chang et al., "Evening Use of Light-Emitting eReaders Negatively Affects Sleep, Circadian Timing, and Next-Morning Alertness," *Proceedings of the National Academy of Sciences* (2014): 201418490; S. L. Chellappa et al., "Acute Exposure to Evening Blue-Enriched Light Impacts on Human Sleep," *Journal of Sleep Research* 22, no. 5 (2013): 573–80; G. Gaggiaoni et al., "Neuroimaging, Cognition, Light and Circadian Rhythms," *Frontiers in Systems Neuroscience* 8 (2014): 126.

# 17–23

The age of males at **HIGHEST RISK** for drowsy-driving accidents. These accidents are typically single-car accidents that run off the road with little evidence of braking between the hours of midnight and 6:00 AM.

over-the-counter, and illicit drugs can lead to excessive sleepiness.

- **Sleep habits.** Burning the candle at both ends, exercising before bed, and hours of time on smartphones or tablets can lead to excess sleepiness. See the **Tech & Health** box for more on adverse effects of too much screen time.
- **Gender.** Women have twice the sleep difficulties of men, believed due to be caused by hormonal factors, pregnancy, pain syndromes, and psychological issues such as anxiety and depression.[20] See the **Health in a Diverse World** box on page 106 for more on gender and sleep.
- **Sleep disorders.** Numerous studies point to sleep disorders such as sleep apnea as major risks for excessive daytime sleepiness and subsequent automobile accidents.[21]

## LO 2 | THE **IMPORTANCE** OF SLEEP

Explain why we need sleep and what happens if we don't get enough, including potential physical, emotional, social, and safety threats to health.

When there just aren't enough hours in the day, sleep can get short-changed. Because Americans are managing to function with less sleep, you might conclude that sufficient sleep isn't all that necessary. In fact, evidence for the importance of adequate sleep to overall health and daily functioning grows daily. Sleep serves to maintain your physical health, affect your ability to function effectively, and enhance your psychological health by serving at least two biological purposes:

- **It conserves body energy.** When you sleep, your core body temperature and the rate at which you burn calories drop. This leaves you with more energy to perform activities throughout your waking hours.
- **It restores you both physically and mentally.** Certain reparative chemicals are released while you sleep. There is also some evidence, discussed shortly, that during sleep the brain is cleared of daily minutiae, learning is synthesized, and memories are consolidated.

### Sleep and Health

Sleep has beneficial effects on most body systems. That's why, when you consistently don't get a good night's rest, your body doesn't function as well, and you become more vulnerable to

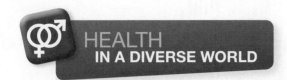
# MIRROR, MIRROR ON THE WALL
*Who's Sleepiest of Them All?*

Judging by the scope and number of cosmetics designed to get rid of dark circles under the eyes, baggy eyelids, and other "sleep-deprived afflictions," women have far more products to help them when they look tired and dragged out than their male counterparts. But are women really more tired and sleepy than men—enough to justify the thousands of sleepy-eyed look "cures" on the market?

At all ages and stages of life, women are much less likely to get enough sleep than men, and the sleep deficit differences accelerate with each decade of life, increasing dramatically at menopause and beyond. Typically, women have more problems falling asleep and staying asleep, waking up more frequently, and finding it hard to get back to sleep once awakened. Possible reasons include:

1. **Hormonal changes.** In general, estrogen and progesterone fluctuate throughout a woman's life with the menstrual cycle. With increasing age, hormone levels decrease; these changes may have an impact on sleep regulation and circadian rhythms. The side effects of menopause, such as hot flashes and night sweats, may also cause sleeplessness and increase insomnia.

2. **Pregnancy.** During pregnancy, discomfort from weight gain, swelling of feet and legs, baby movement, cramping, and increased frequency of urination may cause repeated trips to the bathroom in the night due to pressure on the bladder. Sleep apnea and restless legs syndrome increase during pregnancy. After birth, feeding schedules, baby wakefulness and fussing, and worry over the newborn may influence sleep patterns.

3. **Menopause.** With menopause, the increased potential for weight gain, sleep apnea, insomnia, arthritis, and other chronic ailments can make it difficult for women to get to sleep and stay asleep. More women (58 percent) suffer from nighttime pain than their male counterparts (48%). One in 4 women report that pain in the night keeps them awake three nights per week or more.

4. **Depression, anxiety, worry, and stress.** Women tend to report and experience more stress, anxiety, worry, obsessive–compulsive behaviors, and emotional volatility both at home and at work. These can all wreak havoc on sleep.

While several factors converge to make women more sleep deprived than men throughout the life cycle, men aren't immune. Possible reasons for this include:

1. **Sleep apnea.** Men are at greater risk for development of sleep apnea, with African American and Hispanic men at highest risk. Men often seek help after their partner complains of loud snoring, stoppage of breathing, and other symptoms that cause concern.

2. **Men are less likely to seek help.** Anxiety-prone, worry-prone, depressed, emotionally volatile, and feeling out of control? If you are a male, you are less likely to seek help than your female counterpart. If you fail to report these concerns to a physician or counselor, you won't receive treatment and will remain sleepless and feeling down and exhausted.

3. **Chronic ailments that come with age.** Men often experience more pain from ailments and conditions that disrupt sleep patterns as they age. Older men are particularly susceptible to enlarged prostates that cause them to have to urinate often or heart medications that increase urine production.

**Sources:** National Sleep Foundation, "Women & Sleep," Accessed March 2016, https://sleepfoundation.org/sleep-topics/women-and-sleep; C. Nugent and L. Black, "Sleep Duration, Quality of Sleep, and Use of Sleep Medication, by Sex and Family Type, 2013–2014," *NCHS Data Brief* 230 (2016), Available at www.cdc.gov/nchs/data/databriefs/db230.pdf.

a wide variety of health problems.[22] Researchers are only just beginning to explore the physical benefits of sleep, summarized briefly here.

■ **Sleep helps maintain your immune system.** The common cold, strep throat, flu, mononucleosis, cold sores, and a variety of other ailments are more common when your immune system is depressed. If you aren't getting enough sleep, immune response is weakened. In fact, poor sleep quality and shorter sleep duration increase susceptibility to diseases like the common cold.[23] Other studies have shown that sleep disruption, particularly when circadian rhythms are disturbed repeatedly, disrupts overall immune function.[24] In contrast, adolescents getting more than 9 hours of sleep per night showed improvements in markers of immune functioning.[25]

■ **Sleep helps reduce your risk for cardiovascular disease.** Several recent studies suggest a link between short sleep duration and chronic inflammation, coronary artery disease, risk of stroke, hypertension, and other cardiovascular risks. In addition, people with untreated sleep apnea and nighttime oxygen deprivation have a significant risk of CVD issues.[26] Several studies indicate that high blood pressure is more common in people who get fewer than 7 hours of sleep a night.[27] Newer research points to a strong association between short-duration sleep and increased risk of developing and/or dying from cardiovascular disease.[28]

■ **Sleep contributes to a healthy metabolism.** Chemical reactions in your body's cells break down food and synthesize compounds that the body needs. The sum of all these reactions is called *metabolism*. Several recent studies

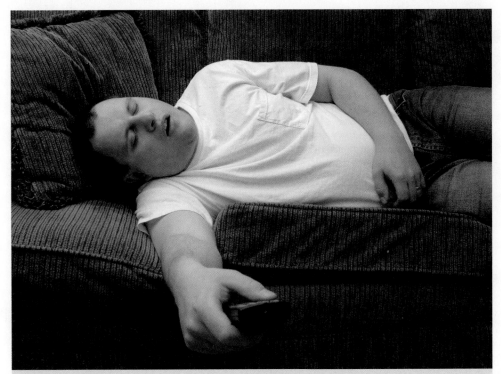
Being overweight can increase your risk of certain sleep disorders.

SEE IT! VIDEOS

What kind of sleep keeps your memory sharp? Watch **How Sleep Affects Your Memory**, available on MasteringHealth.™

suggest that sleep contributes to healthy metabolism and possibly a healthy body weight. In fact, those who sleep less than 5 hours per night have a 40 percent higher risk of becoming obese than those sleeping 7 to 8 hours per night.[29] Sleeping less is associated with eating more—particularly high-fat, high-protein foods—and exercising less.[30]

- **Short sleep increases risk of type 2 diabetes.** There is evidence that sleep deficiencies, particularly sleep disorders such as sleep apnea, can increase the risk of *type 2 diabetes*, a disorder of glucose metabolism.[31]
- **Sleep may be a factor in male reproductive health.** Although issues with sexual interest and sexual performance are common problems for tired people, new research suggests sleep deprivation may affect males more than they realize. Young males who suffered from chronic sleep deficits were shown to have reduced semen quality, reduced sperm motility, and smaller testicular size than men with higher sleep levels.[32] More research is necessary to determine the mechanisms contributing to these problems.
- **Sleep contributes to neurological/mental functioning.** Restricting sleep can cause a wide range of neurological problems, including lapses of attention, slowed or poor memory, reduced cognitive ability, difficulty concentrating, and a tendency for your thinking to get "stuck in a rut."[33] Studies of college students consistently show pulling an "all-nighter" to be a bad idea if you want to perform well on exams or be productive. Sleep before and after a task improves performance and is important to memory consolidation and retention.[34] Several studies have shown

that chronic lack of sleep can affect memory, particularly for simple tasks, and may increase risk of dementia.[35]

- **Sleep improves motor tasks.** Sleep also has a restorative effect on motor function, or the ability to perform tasks such as shooting a basket, playing a musical instrument, or driving a car. Motor function is affected by sleep throughout the lifespan among otherwise healthy individuals.[36] Some researchers contend that a night without sleep impairs your motor skills and reaction time as much as driving drunk.[37]

- **Sleep plays a role in stress management and mental health.** The relationship between sleep and stress is highly complex: Stress can cause or contribute to sleep problems, and sleep problems can cause or increase your level of stress. The same is true of clinical psychiatric conditions such as depression and anxiety disorders: Reduced or poor-quality sleep can trigger these disorders, but it's also a common symptom resulting from them. Individuals who suffer from chronic insomnia have over twice the risk of developing depression.[38]

SEE IT! VIDEOS

How you can avoid nodding off behind the wheel? Watch **Dozing and Driving**, available on MasteringHealth.™

## LO 3 | THE **PROCESSES** OF SLEEP

Explain the processes of sleep, including the two-stage model, circadian rhythm, and sleep–wake cycle, and how they work, as well as their importance for restful sleep.

If you've ever taken a flight that crossed two or more time zones, you've probably experienced *jet lag*, a feeling that your body's "internal clock" is out of sync with the hours of daylight and darkness at your destination. Jet lag happens because the new day/night pattern disrupts the 24-hour biological clock by which you are accustomed to going to sleep, waking

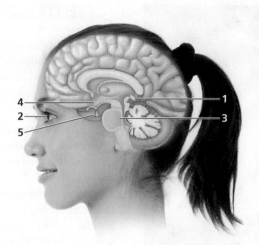

**1. Pineal Body**
Responsible for releasing the drowsiness-inducing hormone called melatonin as light dims and the sun goes down. During the day, the pineal gland is inactive and you remain awake.
**2. Retina**
Light travels through the retina and triggers the regulation of melatonin, slowing its production in daylight and encouraging it in darkness, helping to regulate the sleep cycle.
**3. Pons**
The *pons*, one of the smallest areas of the brain, is a major message transmitter, and is responsible for much of what happens in our sleep/wake cycle. Unless disrupted, the pons helps you enter REM sleep and keeps you down and out, with muscles essentially immobilized.
**4. Hypothalamus**
With parts that function as your body's clock, regulating your circadian rhythm, the hypothalamus stimulates the pineal gland to secrete melatonin.
**5. Pituitary gland**
After being stimulated by the hypothalamus, the pituitary gland releases human growth hormone, signaling the body to repair worn tissues.

**FIGURE 4.2** Parts of the Brain Involved in Sleep

---

**circadian rhythm** The 24-hour cycle by which you are accustomed to going to sleep, waking up, and performing habitual behaviors.

**melatonin** A hormone that affects sleep cycles, increasing drowsiness.

**REM sleep** A period of sleep characterized by brain-wave activity similar to that seen in wakefulness in which rapid eye movement and dreaming occur.

**non-REM (NREM) sleep** A period of restful sleep dominated by slow brain waves; during non-REM sleep, rapid eye movement is rare.

up, and performing habitual behaviors. This cycle, known as your **circadian rhythm**, is regulated by a master clock that coordinates the activity of nerve cells, protein, and genes. The *hypothalamus* and a tiny gland in your brain called the *pineal gland*—responsible for the drowsiness-inducing hormone called **melatonin**—are key to these cyclical rhythms.[39] See **FIGURE 4.2** for more on brain structures involved in sleep.

## Stages and Cycles of Sleep

Humans should spend roughly one-third of every day asleep. Sleep researchers generally distinguish between two primary sleep stages. During **REM sleep**, rapid eye movement and dreams occur, and brain-wave activity appears similar to that

when you are awake. **Non-REM (NREM) sleep**, in contrast, is the period of restful sleep with slowed brain activity that does *not* include rapid eye movement. During the night, you alternate between periods of NREM and REM sleep, repeating one full cycle about once every 90 minutes.[40] Overall, you spend about 75 percent of each night in NREM sleep and 25 percent in REM sleep (**FIGURE 4.3**).

**Non-REM Sleep Is Restorative** During non-REM sleep, the body rests. Both your body temperature and your energy use drop; sensation is dulled; and your brain waves, heart rate, and breathing slow. In contrast, digestive processes speed up, and your body stores nutrients. In NREM sleep—also called *slow-wave sleep*—you do not typically dream. Four distinct stages of NREM sleep have been distinguished by their characteristic brain-wave patterns as shown on an electroencephalogram (EEG), a test detecting electrical activity in the brain.

*Stage 1* is the lightest stage of sleep, lasts only a few minutes, and involves the transition between waking and sleep.

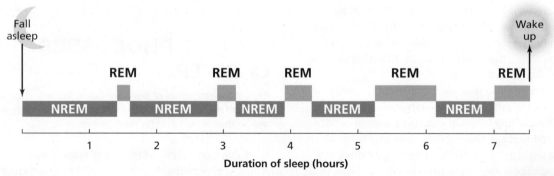

**FIGURE 4.3** **The Nightly Sleep Cycle** As the number of hours you sleep increases, your brain spends more and more time in REM sleep. Thus, sleeping for too few hours could mean you're depriving yourself primarily of essential REM sleep.

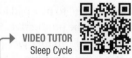

VIDEO TUTOR
Sleep Cycle

Your brain begins to produce *theta waves* (slow brain waves), and you may experience sensations of falling with quick, jerky muscle reactions. During *stage 2*, your eyes close, body movement slows, and you disengage from your environment. During *stages 3 and 4*, a sleeper's brain generates slow, large-amplitude *delta waves*. Blood pressure drops, your heart rate and respiration slow considerably, and you enter deep sleep. The hypothalamus stimulates the pituitary gland to release human growth hormone, signaling the body to repair worn tissues. Speech and movement are rare during the final stage (but sometimes people sleepwalk, cook, clean, or drive during this stage!).

**REM Sleep Energizes** Dreaming takes place primarily during REM sleep. On an EEG, a REM sleeper's brain-wave activity is almost indistinguishable from that of someone who is wide awake, and the brain's energy use is higher than that of a person who is performing a difficult math problem![41] The *pons*, one of the smallest areas of the brain, is a major message transmitter, and is responsible for much of what happens in our sleep–wake cycle. Unless disrupted, the pons helps you enter REM sleep and keeps you down and out, with muscles essentially immobilized. You may dream that you're rock climbing, but your body is incapable of movement. Almost the only exceptions are your respiratory muscles, which allow you to breathe, and the tiny muscles of your eyes, which move your eyes rapidly as if you were following the scenario of your dream. This *rapid eye movement* gives REM sleep its name.

Research indicates that deep phases of slow-wave sleep consolidate and organize the day's information, while REM sleep stabilizes consolidated memory.[42] Without adequate slow-wave sleep and REM sleep, your short-term memory may suffer.

## Your Sleep Needs

Recently, a major U.S. consensus statement was published, providing guidelines for how much sleep a healthy adult should get each night. Their key recommendations are:[43]

- Adults should sleep 7 or more hours each night to promote optimal health.
- Getting fewer than 7 hours of sleep per night on a regular basis increases risks of adverse health outcomes.
- Regularly getting more than 9 hours of sleep may be appropriate for young adults, people trying to recover from sleep debt, and those recovering from illness. For others, it's not clear whether getting that much sleep is associated with health risks.

Keep in mind that sleep needs vary from person to person; your gender, health, and lifestyle will also affect how much rest your body demands. For example, women need more sleep than men, overall.[44]

It is worth noting that sleep patterns change over the lifespan. Newborns need 16 to 18 hours of sleep daily, and teens and younger adults need 8 to 9 hours per night, slightly more than the adult average. Older adults may experience sleep difficulties that result in fewer hours of rest per night, owing to health conditions, pain, and the need to use the bathroom more frequently.[45]

Of concern for young adults are the results of a recent study of healthy undergraduate males indicating that short sleep cycles resulted in significant prolonged elevations in heart rate and diastolic pressure recovery after exposure to stressful stimuli as compared to those with longer sleep cycles.[46] Many scientists believe that diabetes, obesity, and other metabolic disorders may be linked with biological clock activity.[47] In general, those who get adequate sleep live longer and enjoy more quality days than those who don't.[48]

**Sleep Debt** In addition to your body's physiological need, consider your current **sleep debt**. That's the total number of hours of missed sleep you're carrying around with you, either because you got up before you were fully rested or because your sleep was interrupted. Let's say that last week you managed just 4 to 5 hours of sleep a night Monday through Thursday while cramming for a Friday exam. Even if you get 7 to 8 hours a night Friday through Sunday, your unresolved sleep debt of 8 to 12 hours will leave you tired and groggy when you start the week again. Research has consistently shown that accruing several days of sleep deprivation can not only make you sleepy, it can also affect your performance over a wide range of activities, lead to inflammation, and negatively affect the immune system. Those with chronic sleep debt may have up to four times the

> **sleep debt** The difference between the number of hours of sleep an individual needed in a given time period and the number of hours he or she actually slept.

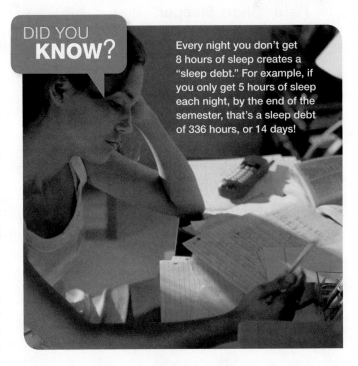

**DID YOU KNOW?**

Every night you don't get 8 hours of sleep creates a "sleep debt." For example, if you only get 5 hours of sleep each night, by the end of the semester, that's a sleep debt of 336 hours, or 14 days!

**sleep inertia** A state characterized by cognitive impairment, grogginess, and disorientation that is experienced upon rising from short sleep or an overly long nap.

**sleep disorders (somnipathy or dyssomnia)** Any medical disorders that have a negative effect on sleep patterns.

**sleep study** A clinical assessment of sleep in which the patient is monitored while spending the night in a sleep disorders center.

risk of catching the common cold or other illnesses.[49]

So, can you make up for lost sleep by sleeping in on the weekend? Some research shows that you *can* catch up if you go about it sensibly. Trying to catch up may make you feel more wide awake, as well as reduce lines and baggy eyelids. It also may reduce stress-related cortisol levels that shoot up while you are sleep deprived. On the other side of the coin, that catch-up sleep is not likely to make much difference in your performance levels, won't restore your functioning, and is likely to disrupt your circadian rhythm. It's best to work on your sleep hygiene to help ensure you get a healthy amount of sleep throughout the week.[50]

**Napping: A Good Idea?** Speaking of catching up, do naps count? Although naps can't entirely cancel out a significant sleep debt, they can improve your mood, alertness, and possibly performance, if your sleep debt is more an occasional deficit than a chronic problem. Regular naps may also improve immune functioning and help ward off infections, as well as improve performance and reduce sleepiness.[51] It's best to nap in the early to mid-afternoon, when the pineal gland in your brain releases a small amount of melatonin and your body experiences a natural dip in its circadian rhythm. Never nap in the late afternoon, as it could interfere with your ability to fall asleep that night. Keep your naps short because a nap of more than 30 minutes can leave you in a state of **sleep inertia**, characterized by cognitive impairment, nausea, light-headedness, grogginess, and a disoriented feeling.

**The Rare "Short Sleeper"** Although many people who don't get enough sleep suffer the consequences, a small group of people—perhaps fewer than 1 percent—seem to thrive on less than 6 hours of sleep per night. Recent research points to a possible gene—the *DEC2 gene*—that affects circadian rhythms and changing normal day/night cycles. Individuals with this gene sleep less and seem to have few adverse affects. They do not accrue the negative consequences of typical sleep-debt individuals and, as such, are considered to be unique in the sleep literature.[52]

## LO 4 | **SLEEP** DISORDERS

Describe some common sleep disorders, including risk factors and what can be done to prevent or treat them.

**Sleep disorders**, also known as **somnipathy** or **dyssomnia**, are any medical disorders with a negative effect on sleep patterns. While millions of people don't get enough sleep on any given night, as many as 70 million suffer from an actual sleep-related disorder.[53] Over 61 percent of college students aged 18

to 29 report staying awake late and getting up early—a recipe for sleep deprivation.[54] Although more than 4 percent of college students report being treated for insomnia, the vast majority go it alone when trying to get enough sleep.[55] Nearly 2.5 percent of students report having sleep disorders other than insomnia.[56] Nearly 29 percent of students say that they have had sleep difficulties in the last year that were traumatic or difficult to handle.[57] If you're following the advice in this chapter and still aren't sleeping well, it's time to visit your health care provider. To aid in diagnosis, you will probably be asked to keep a sleep diary like the one in **FIGURE 4.4**. You may also be referred to a sleep disorders center for an overnight clinical **sleep study**. While you are asleep in the sleep center, sensors and electrodes record data that will be reviewed by a sleep specialist who will work with your doctor to diagnose and treat your sleep problem.

The American Academy of Sleep Medicine identifies more than 80 sleep disorders. The most common disorders in adults are *insomnia*, *sleep apnea*, *restless legs syndrome*, and *narcolepsy*.

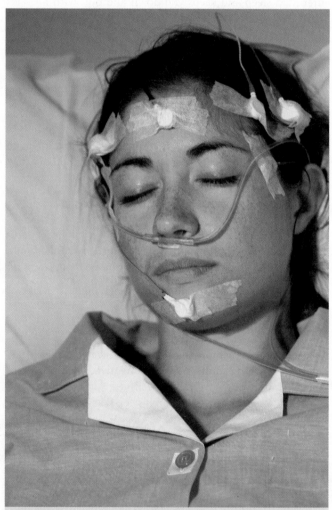

There are more than 80 different clinical sleep disorders affecting 50 to 70 million Americans. One of the most common disorders is sleep apnea, which typically requires a sleep study for a definitive diagnosis.

|  | Day 1 | Day 2 | Day 3 |
|---|---|---|---|
| **Fill out in morning** | | | |
| Bedtime | 11 pm | 11:30 pm | |
| Wake time | 7:30 am | 8:30 am | |
| Time to fall asleep | 45 min | 30 min | |
| Awakenings (how many and how long?) | 2 times / 1 hour | 1 time / 45 min | |
| Total sleep time | 6.75 hrs | 7.75 hrs | |
| Feeling at waking (refreshed, groggy, etc.) | Still tired | Energized | |
| **Fill out at bedtime** | | | |
| Exercise (what, when, how long?) | Jog at 2 pm / 30 min | Soccer practice at 4 pm; 2 hrs | |
| Naps (when, where, how long?) | 4 pm, my bed / 30 min | 2 pm, library / 1 hour | |
| Caffeine (what, when, how much?) | 2 cups coffee at 8 am | 1 latte at 10 am; 1 soda at 4 pm | |
| Alcohol (what, when, how much?) | 1 beer at 8 pm | None | |
| Evening snacks (what, when, how much?) | Bag of popcorn at 10 pm | Chips and soda at 4 pm | |
| Medications (what, when, how much?) | None | None | |
| Feelings (happiness, anxiety, major cause, etc.) | Stressed about paper | Worried about sister | |
| Activities 1 hour before bed (what and how long?) | Wrote paper | Watched TV | |

**FIGURE 4.4 Sample Sleep Diary** Using a sleep diary such as this one can help you and your health care provider discover behavioral factors that might be contributing to your sleep problem.

# Insomnia

**Insomnia**—difficulty in falling asleep, frequent arousals during sleep, or early-morning awakening—is the most common sleep complaint. Young adults aged 18 to 29 experience the most insomnia, with 68 percent reporting symptoms.[58] Somewhat fewer adults (59 percent) aged 30 to 64 experience regular symptoms, and only 44 percent of those over age 65 have regular symptoms.[59] Adults with children in the household tend to report more insomnia symptoms than those without children.[60] Approximately 10 to 15 percent of Americans have chronic insomnia that lasts longer than a month.[61]

Symptoms of insomnia include difficulty falling asleep, waking up frequently during the night, difficulty returning to sleep, waking up too early in the morning, unrefreshing sleep, daytime sleepiness, and irritability. Sometimes, insomnia is related to stress and worry. In other cases, it may be related to disrupted circadian rhythms, which may occur with travel across time zones, shift work, and other major schedule changes. Insomnia can also occur as a side effect from taking certain medications. Left untreated, long-term insomnia may be associated with depression, drug and alcohol use, and heart disease.[62]

**Mind-Based Treatments for Insomnia** Sometimes, hormonal changes or issues with the gastrointestinal tract or bladder may be an underlying cause of insomnia. Excess stress can also be a key factor, and strategies designed to treat or control the underlying contributors can be helpful in reducing insomnia. CBTi—a type of cognitive-behavioral therapy specific to insomnia, discussed in greater detail later in the chapter—can be very effective.

**insomnia** A disorder characterized by difficulty in falling asleep quickly, frequent arousals during sleep, or early-morning awakening.

Relaxation strategies, including yoga and meditation, can be helpful in preparing the body to sleep. Exercise, done early in the day, can also help reduce stress and promote deeper sleep. Talk to a health professional if insomnia is unresolved in spite of your best efforts to make changes.

## Sleep Apnea

**Sleep apnea** is a disorder in which breathing is briefly and repeatedly interrupted during sleep.[63] *Apnea* refers to a breathing pause that lasts at least 10 seconds. Sleep apnea affects more than 18 million Americans, or 1 in every 15 people; it affects all age groups and both sexes.[64]

**Types of Sleep Apnea** There are two major types of sleep apnea: central and obstructive. *Central sleep apnea* occurs when the brain fails to tell the respiratory muscles to initiate breathing. Consumption of alcohol, certain illegal drugs, and certain medications can contribute to central sleep apnea.

*Obstructive sleep apnea (OSA)* is more common and occurs when air cannot move in and out of a person's nose or mouth, even though the body tries to breathe. Typically, OSA occurs when a person's throat muscles and tongue relax during sleep and block the airways, causing snorting, snoring, and gagging. These sounds occur because falling oxygen saturation levels in the blood stimulate the body's autonomic nervous system to trigger inhalation, often via a sudden gasp of breath. This response may wake the person, preventing deep sleep and causing the person to wake in the morning feeling like he or she hasn't slept.

People who are overweight often have sagging internal throat tissue, which puts them at higher risk for sleep apnea. In

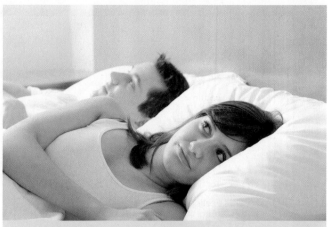

Sleeping with people who have restless legs syndrome can lead to major sleep disruptions for the partner, causing two individuals to be sleep deprived.

addition to overweight, other risk factors include smoking and alcohol use, being age 40 or older, and ethnicity—sleep apnea occurs at higher rates in African Americans, Pacific Islanders, and Hispanics.[65] Anatomical risk factors for OSA can include a small upper airway (or large tongue, tonsils, or uvula), a recessed chin, small jaw or a large overbite, and a large neck size. Because OSA runs in some families, genetics may also play a role.[66] OSA is associated with higher risk for chronic high blood pressure, irregular heartbeats, heart attack, and stroke. Apnea-associated sleeplessness may also increase the risk of type 2 diabetes, immune system deficiencies, and a host of other problems.[67]

**Treatment for Sleep Apnea** The most effective method for preventing and treating sleep apnea is to lose weight, along with avoiding some of the factors that appear to increase risk. The most commonly prescribed therapy for OSA is *continuous positive airway pressure (CPAP)*, which consists of an airflow device, long tube, and mask (see **FIGURE 4.5**). People with sleep apnea wear this mask during sleep, and air is forced into the nose to keep the airway open. The FDA recently approved an implantable *upper airway stimulator (UAS)* called Inspire for use among people who cannot tolerate CPAP devices. Implanted under the skin in the upper chest, Inspire is a small pulsing device that stimulates airway muscle action and improved breathing and can be programmed remotely by a doctor. It is turned on before bed each night and turned off in the morning.[68]

Other methods for treating OSA include dental appliances, which reposition the lower jaw and tongue, and surgery to remove tissue in the upper airway. In general, these approaches are most helpful for mild disease or heavy snoring.

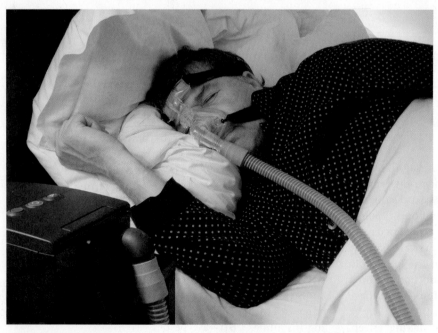

**FIGURE 4.5 Continuous Positive Airway Pressure (CPAP) Device**
People with sleep apnea can get a better night's sleep by wearing a CPAP device. A gentle stream of air flows continuously into the nose through a tube connected to a mask. This steady stream of air helps keep the sleeper's airway open.

## Restless Legs Syndrome

**Restless legs syndrome (RLS)** is a neurological disorder characterized by unpleasant sensations in the legs when at rest combined with an uncontrollable urge to move in an effort to relieve these feelings. These sensations range in severity from mildly uncomfortable to painful. Some researchers estimate that RLS affects over 10 percent of the U.S. population, with increasing diagnosis in all age groups.[69] RLS sensations are often described as burning, creeping, or tugging, or like insects crawling inside the legs. In general, the symptoms are more pronounced at night. Lying down or trying to relax activates the symptoms, and moving the legs relieves the discomfort, so people with RLS often have difficulty falling and staying asleep.

In most cases, the cause of RLS is unknown. A family history of the condition is seen in approximately 50 percent of cases, suggesting some genetic link. In other cases, RLS appears to be related to other conditions, including Parkinson's disease, kidney failure, diabetes, peripheral neuropathy, and anemia. Pregnancy or hormonal changes can worsen symptoms.[70]

If there is an underlying condition, treatment of that condition may provide relief. Other treatment options include prescribed medications, decreasing tobacco and alcohol use, and applying heat to the legs. For some people, relaxation techniques or stretching exercises can alleviate symptoms.

## Narcolepsy

**Narcolepsy** is a neurological disorder caused by the brain's inability to properly regulate sleep–wake cycles. The result is excessive, intrusive sleepiness and daytime sleep attacks. Narcolepsy occurs in about 1 of every 3,000 people.[71] Narcolepsy is not rare, but it is an underrecognized and underdiagnosed condition.

Narcolepsy is characterized by overwhelming and uncontrollable sleepiness during the day. Narcoleptics are prone to falling asleep at inappropriate times and places—in class, at work, while driving or eating, or even mid-conversation. These sleep attacks can last from a few seconds to several minutes. Other symptoms include *cataplexy* (the sudden loss of voluntary muscle tone, often triggered by emotional stimuli), hallucinations during sleep onset or upon awakening, and brief episodes of paralysis during sleep–wake transitions.

In most cases narcolepsy appears to be caused by a deficiency of chemicals in the brain that regulate sleep. Genetics may also play a role.[72] Other possible factors include having another sleep disorder, using certain medications, or having a mental disorder or substance abuse disorder.

Narcolepsy is commonly treated with medications that improve alertness, and antidepressants may be prescribed to treat cataplexy, hallucinations, and sleep paralysis. Behavioral therapy can also help narcoleptics cope with their condition. Some lifestyle changes, such as scheduling brief naps during the day or eating smaller meals on a regular schedule, may be helpful.

## Other Parasomnias

**Parasomnias** include all of the abnormal things that disrupt sleep outside the major problems such as sleep apnea. Among the most common parasomnias are *circadian rhythm disorder*, where there are abnormalities in the sleep–wake cycle due to jet lag and adjustments to shift work; *sleep phase disorder*, in which a person either wakes up or goes to sleep too early; *sleep-related eating disorder*, in which people may be found munching away in the kitchen with no memory of eating an entire cake or bucket of ice cream; *sleep-walking*, in which individuals may wander around the house, or even go for a drive and not remember it; *night terrors*, in which a person wakes up frightened and screaming, often without knowing why (probably because they often occur in non-REM sleep cycles); *sexsomnia*, in which a person may have sex while asleep and have no recollection of the event; *bedwetting* or *enuresis*, in which a person wets the bed without knowing it; and *snoring*, in which inhaled air passes over loose tissue in the back of the throat or nasal passages and causes a rattling sound. Snoring, by itself, is not a problem unless the loose tissue interferes with breathing. In many cases, medications (such as some prescription sleep aids) and other drugs contribute to some of these parasomnias. Trauma, underlying illnesses, or other neurological conditions may also be factors. For others, the causes are unknown. With many sleep disorders, the family or person living or sleeping with the sufferer is often the sleep-deprived person—and isn't tabulated in our overall sleep deficiency statistics!

> **restless legs syndrome (RLS)** A neurological disorder characterized by an overwhelming urge to move the legs when they are at rest.
>
> **narcolepsy** A neurological disorder that causes people to fall asleep involuntarily during the day.
>
> **parasomnias** All of the abnormal things that disrupt sleep, not including some of the major problems such as sleep apnea.
>
> **sleep hygiene** The wide range of practices that can help you manage and create a systematic approach leading to normal, quality nighttime sleep and full daytime alertness.

## LO 5 | GETTING A GOOD NIGHT'S SLEEP

Explore ways to improve your sleep through cognitive-behavioral therapy for insomnia, changing daily habits, modifying your environment, avoiding sleep disruptors, using sleep aids responsibly, and other sound sleep hygiene strategies.

- - - - - - - - - - - - - - - - - - - - - -

Many of us struggle with getting a good night's sleep on a regular basis. For problem sleepers, the good news is that there are many things you can do to improve sleep quality and duration. **Sleep hygiene** refers to the wide range of practices that can help you create and maintain normal, quality nighttime sleep and full daytime alertness.[73] The following sections provide proven strategies for improving your daily sleep patterns and getting the most out of your time spent sleeping.

## Create a Sleep-Promoting Environment

Where you sleep has much to do with how well you sleep. As such, making your bedroom into a calming, wind-down retreat is essential to setting the stage for restful and restorative sleep. Consider the Making Changes Today box and other strategies for improving your sleep.

1. **Chill.** Literally. Turn down the thermostat. The best sleep occurs in a cool bedroom—according to experts, one that is around 65 degrees. Normally, as you get sleepy, your body temperature starts to drop and conserve energy through most of the sleeping hours, gradually increasing your temperature just before dawn. As light hits your room, body temperature goes up, along with your energy levels as part of normal circadian rhythms. In a room that is too hot, or if you are sleeping with too many clothes, blankets, or next to a person who exudes heat, the higher temperature may actually interfere with your natural body rhythms, making it harder to enter or remain in deep sleep, with resultant insomnia and other problems.[74] Everyone has an ideal sleep temperature based on percent body fat and other metabolic differences; finding out what seems to work best for you in different temperature and humidity situations is key to the environmental regulation of sleep. If you or your partner run hot and cold in ideal sleep temperatures, finding a good compromise temperature can help maintain sleep.

2. **Create a Sleep "Cave."** As bedtime approaches, keep your bedroom quiet, calm, and dark, with sensory stimuli at a minimum. Avoid exposure to bright light, particularly *blue light*, by turning off electronic devices or wearing an eye mask. Blue light is a key factor in our secretion of melatonin, a sleep hormone. If you get a lot of blue-light exposure from that big glowing cell phone or computer in your room, melatonin production will drop and you may find it hard to fall asleep or stay asleep.

3. **Associate bed with sleep.** Make your bed a place for comfort and relaxation—a place for you to get the sleep you need to be productive and healthy; it shouldn't serve as your office. Invest in a good mattress. Buy sheets that are smooth and relaxing and pillows that are right for you. Wash bedding weekly or biweekly and keep your bedroom clean and smelling fresh. Get rid of clutter and keep things organized. Free yourself from intrusions by turning off the ringer on your phone, and charge your cell phone or tablet in a place that is out of reach—so you aren't tempted to look at it during sleep time. If you must have a TV in your bedroom, set it to go off after an hour and put the remote far from you bed so you aren't tempted to turn it back onxs!

4. **Only go to bed when you are tired.** If you get in bed and can't sleep within 20 to 30 minutes, get up, keep the lights dim, and listen to relaxing music or meditate. Don't get into heavy studying on your computer or try to memorize complex details for an exam; this will keep you awake.

5. **Establish bedtime and waking rituals.** Go to bed and get up at the same time each day. Establishing a bedtime ritual signals to your body that it's time for sleep. Listen to a quiet song, practice meditation and deep breathing exercises, take a warm shower, or read something that lets you quietly wind down. Upon awakening, make your bed and air out your room. Cool sheets and bedding and a lavender-scented room have been shown to be calming and help you sleep better.[75]

## Adjust Your Daytime Habits

While we often focus on what happens in the bedroom as the key to sleep, what we do during the day can also have a significant impact on sleep quality and duration.

### Get Adequate Daytime Light Exposure

According to Kelly Brown, MD, at the Vanderbilt Sleep Disorders Center, light is the best tool for controlling your internal clock. Light travels through the retina and regulates melatonin, slowing its production in daylight and encouraging it in darkness, helping to regulate the sleep cycle.[76] If you want to stay awake in the daytime and sleep at night, get as much exposure to natural light outdoors during the day as you can. Open your blinds. Look for lights and bulbs that are recommended for therapy with seasonal ailments and for helping with daytime alertness. These special lights increase your exposure to light and can help protect against other problems on dark winter days, in areas where daylight is in short supply, and if *seasonal affective disorder* is a problem.

### Exercise in the Morning or Afternoon
Have you ever noticed that after a day out hiking or a long swim or bike ride that you are tired when you get into bed? In fact, exercise may just be the great elixir when it comes to sleep.[77] You just need to make sure you exercise 3-4 hours before you go to bed. Why? Because exercise revs up your metabolism, makes you more alert, and depletes energy stores, while raising body temperature. It takes hours to bring physiological changes down. Get in a workout in the morning or afternoon and you will be awake for studying or writing that term paper. However, set a cutoff time for relaxing and cooling off the body for optimum sleep. Take time out for yourself. If you must walk the dog or want to go for a walk

before bed or in the evening, keep it to a slow stroll, focusing on the things around you. Block negative thoughts and worries. Don't allow your mind to wander to problems you face, or to get worked up over assignments due or upcoming tests. Focus on you and the moment and the sights and sounds around you.

**Watch Your Diet, Particularly in the Hours before Bed** Avoid eating heavy meals within 2 to 3 hours of bedtime. Foods containing *tryptophan*, an amino acid (found in nut butters, bananas, tuna, eggs, chicken, turkey, yogurt and milk, and pork, as well as in high-carbohydrate foods such as bread and pastries) may encourages sleepiness, particularly if you eat foods containing it on an empty stomach. However, foods high in protein and containing *tyramine* (such as sausage, eggplant, bacon, raspberries, chocolate, avocado, nuts, soy, and red wine) and greasy or spicy foods may keep you awake.[78]

## Avoid Common Sleep Disruptors

Several factors play major roles in whether or not you can fall asleep and stay asleep. Some of the biggest sleep disruptors are common and you'll recognize them right away. Other, lesser-known disruptors may be among the factors that hit you when you least expect them, leaving you staring at the ceiling when you should be sawing logs. See the **Student Health Today** box on page 116 on medicines that disrupt sleep. Avoid some of these behaviors and sleep on.

1. **Go easy on the caffeine.** Long recognized for its ability to increase vigilance and alertness and decrease sleepiness when you need to stay awake to finish that last-minute term paper, consuming too much caffeine (particularly in the late afternoon or evening) can be bad news for your sleep.

   A recent study indicated that effects of caffeine can last 5.5 to 7.7 hours or more—depending on how "stiff" your coffee or energy drink really is. An ever-increasing body of research points to risks of cardiac irregularities, psychological problems, and neurological side effects, including headaches and migraines, from high-caffeine drinks, particularly energy drinks.[79] Excess consumption of caffeine can severely disrupt circadian cycles, leading to the inability to fall asleep and stay asleep.

2. **Avoid nicotine, alcohol, and liquids before bed.** Like caffeine, these will also increase the likelihood of sleep disturbances. Although alcohol may make you sleepy initially, it disturbs other stages of sleep, keeping you from the restorative, deeper levels of sleep you need.[80] Alcohol has been shown to be a key sleep disruptor, particularly after binge drinking.[81] Heavy consumption of any liquids late in the day (even those without caffeine) can lead to **nocturia**, or overactive bladder, meaning you have to get up several times during the night (pregnant women often suffer from this, particularly in the first trimester).

3. **Turn off screens.** Watching TV, playing computer games, hanging out on Facebook or other social media sites, working on your latest paper on your blue-screen laptop or tablet into the wee hours of the morning—all of these things can keep the mind alert and expose you to blue light, wreaking havoc on a good night's sleep.

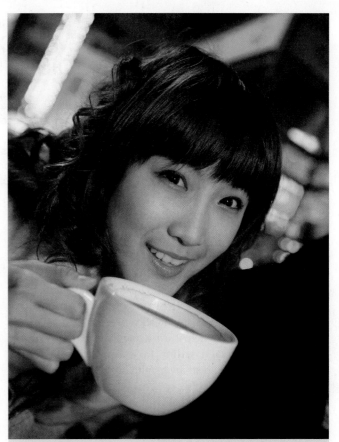

After-dinner coffee? Not unless it's decaf. Caffeine promotes alertness by blocking the neurotransmitter adenosine in your brain—a useful thing when you are studying, but a potential problem when you are trying to sleep.

4. **Tune out on conflict.** Avoid late-night phone calls, texts, or e-mails that can end up in arguments, disappointments, and other emotional stressors. If something does jazz you up before bed, journal about it briefly, then promise yourself that you'll make time the next day to explore your feelings more deeply.

## Mental Strategies to Improve Your Sleep

A major new "study of studies" indicates that **cognitive-behavioral therapy for insomnia (CBTi)** is one of the best first-line defenses for people who can't get to sleep, or who wake up during the night and can't get back to sleep.[82] Essentially CBT is a form of therapy that helps people better understand the thoughts and feelings that influence their behaviors. CBTi focuses on changing the habits that disrupt sleep. For example, a person who has trouble falling asleep because a trip to bed means wide-eyed rehashing of all the real and imaginary threats they have faced during the day would be asked to focus

> **nocturia** Frequent urination at night caused by an overactive bladder.
>
> **cognitive-behavioral therapy for chronic insomnia (CBTi)** A form of therapy that helps people better understand the thoughts and feelings that influence their behaviors and focus on changing habits that disrupt sleep.

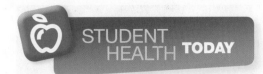

# MEDICATIONS AS SLEEP DISRUPTORS

Just as caffeine, alcohol, nicotine, and other substances can wreak havoc with sleep, so can other medications—even those you may not even think of as sleep disruptors. Some of the most common ones that can negatively affect sleep cycles include:

- **Statins and fibrates** such as Crestor, Lipitor, and Zocor used to decrease cholesterol
- **Antidepressants**, particularly the SSRIs (selective serotonin reuptake inhibitors) such as Proszac, Lexapro, and Celexa
- **Corticosteroids**, such as Cortizone and Prednisone

- **Alpha and beta blockers**, used for hypertension, benign prostatic hyperplasia (BPH), and Raynaud's disease
- **Glucosamine/chondroitin dietary supplements** used to relieve joint inflammation and pain

---

on strategies and develop skills to keep from ruminating on things when they should be falling asleep. Strategies such as thought blocking, thought refocusing, learning to meditate, listening to relaxing music, biofeedback, deep breathing, and other actions can all help turn an anxiety-prone bedroom experience into a calm setting for sleep. Today, increasing numbers of sleep therapists are helping to coach people on better sleep hygiene.

## Sleep Aids: What Works and What Doesn't?

In spite of reports of risks associated with prescription and over-the-counter sleeping pills and other aids, Americans spent an estimated $41 billion on them in 2015—and that number is expected to increase to over $52 billion by 2020![83] The problem is, according to a recent review, the benefits of these sleep remedies may be less than expected. And the risks, such as sleepy driving, may be greater than reported.[84]

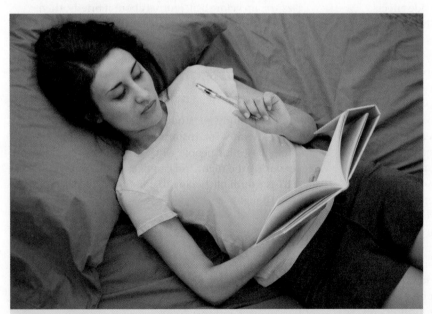

If a worry keeps you awake, jot it down in a journal. You'll be better prepared to handle it in the morning after a good night's sleep.

**Prescription Pills for Sleep** Nearly 9 million people—or 4 percent of U.S. adults—use prescription sleeping pills for sleep problems. The majority of users are older white women aged 50 to 59; however, people of all ages and stages of life are popping pills designed to put them to sleep, keep them asleep, or keep them awake when they should be sleeping.[85] Concerns over the limited effectiveness of many sleep drugs and their potential risks have raised questions over when and if people should use them. A recent study of one of the newer prescription sleep meds marketed widely on television ads showed that people using the drug every night for 3 months fell asleep only 6 minutes faster—and slept only 16 minutes longer—than those on a placebo. People on the sleep meds actually felt more tired the next day than those using a placebo. Similar results were noted with other well-known sleep aids. While benefits were minimal, risks were elevated for daytime drowsiness, headache, dizziness, falls, fractures, auto accidents, constipation, dry mouth, and other issues.[86] (See the **Student Health Today** box on melatonin's effectiveness.)

**White Noise Machines or White Noise Apps** Tools that provide soothing nature sounds and block out disrupting noise are being used by increasing numbers of people. These machines are portable and apps are increasingly available on smartphones. However, these machines and apps vary in cost and may not be the ticket to sleep for you. The advantage of phone apps is that there are many available on iOS and Android devices and you can take them with you anywhere.

**Sleep Trackers** Consumers now have many choices for tracking their sleep besides just looking in the mirror or feeling tired. These range from *mobile phone apps* that can sync with your computer to assess movement patterns (tossing and turning), *wearable devices* (fitness bands, watches, or devices that can be attached to shoes or clothing),

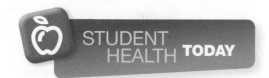
# MELATONIN
*One Popular OTC Sleep Medication*

Although choices for over-the-counter drugs for sleep are abundant, *Melatonin* is America's OTC sleep aid of choice—used by over 34 million Americans, and accounting for nearly $380 million in sales in 2014. What is it? Melatonin is a natural hormone produced by the body's pineal gland. Most pills you buy OTC are synthetic versions of the natural hormone and claim to work in much the same way. During the day, or when there is bright light, the pineal gland is inactive and you remain awake. However, as lights dim

and the sun goes down, the pineal gland turns on, producing melatonin, which enters the bloodstream just as your prime-time TV shows are ending—and you start feeling drowsy and ready to sleep. As you drift off, elevated melatonin levels keep you there for a good night's sleep for some people.

While melatonin can work for those who have real disruptions in their sleep due to shift work or jet lag, it doesn't appear to significantly increase sleep among others. Side effects can include grogginess, headache, and interference with the

effectiveness of some blood pressure, diabetes, and other medications. Since it is considered to be a supplement, it is not regulated by the FDA and labs that produce it are not regulated. If you are considering it, talk with your doctor and do your homework about dosage, possible drug interactions, and the reputation of the maker.

**Sources:** National Sleep Foundation, "Melatonin and Sleep," Accessed March 2016, http://sleepfoundation.org/sleep-topics/melatonin-and-sleep/page/0/2; Consumer Reports, "Does Melatonin Really Help You Sleep?" January 5, 2016, www.consumerreports.org/vitamins-supplements/does-melatonin-really-help-you-sleep/.

---

*embedded devices* (integrated into mattresses, furniture, or other fixtures in the bedroom), and *conventional desktop/website resources*. Many help you get a better sense of the quality and quantity of your sleep, and some actually provide educational messages about sleep and increase your awareness of the sleep disruptors that affect you. The downside is that many are costly. Some questions you might ask are: Do I really need this? What is the value-added element in this product for me? Is there a simpler device that I can purchase to find out similar information? Whatever you decide, be sure to check online reviews by unbiased consumer groups for notes on reliability,

function, and ease of use. Also consider privacy concerns to determine who might access your data.

**New Blue-Light Glasses and Protective Screens** Recent newcomers in the sleep technology area are blue-light glasses designed to protect you from the risks of the blue-light wavelengths believed to affect sleep and vision. Check reviews on these glasses before investing. Not only do they vary significantly in price, some also work better than others in their blue light–blocking capacity. The impact of these on actual sleep has not been fully investigated. Stay tuned.

---

# STUDY **PLAN**

Customize your study plan—and master your health!—in the Study Area of **MasteringHealth**.

## ASSESS YOURSELF

**Are you getting enough sleep?** Want to find out?
Take the **Are You Sleeping Well?** assessment available on
**MasteringHealth.™**

---

# CHAPTER **REVIEW**

To head an MP3 Tutor Session, scan here or visit the Study Area in **MasteringHealth**.

### LO **1** | Sleepless in America

■ Sleep deprivation, or insufficient sleep, is a major problem in America,

affecting 50 to 70 million adults overall and nearly 61 percent of students, resulting in major problems with excessive daytime sleepiness and increased risks of drowsy-driving accidents.

### LO **2** | The Importance of Sleep

■ Sleep serves as a mental and physical restorer, helps conserve energy, reduces

risks of CVD and other chronic ailments, enhances immune functioning, aides in healthy metabolism and neurological functioning, improves motor tasks, and helps manage stress.

### LO **3** | The Processes of Sleep

■ Sleep is regulated by two biological processes that work together to keep your sleep patterns within a healthy range: your circadian rhythm regulates internal processes and alertness, and the sleep–wake cycle regulates sleep substances in the brain and works to keep the body's sleep levels in a state of balance.

- The biological clock, also referred to as the circadian rhythm or circadian clock, regulates alertness, body temperature, brain-wave activity, hormone production, glucose and insulin levels, and several other elements. Several factors, including melatonin, are important to regulating the sleep cycle.
- REM and NREM sleep occur throughout the night; NREM sleep is slow-wave, restful sleep, while REM sleep mimics wakened states.
- How much sleep you need varies by age throughout the lifespan and physical condition.

## LO 4 | Sleep Disorders

- Sleep disorders, also known as somnipathy or dyssomnia, are any medical disorders that have a negative effect on sleep patterns. Although there are many sleep disorders, insomnia, sleep apnea, restless leg syndrome, and narcolepsy are among the most prevalent, with varying symptoms, causes, prevention, and treatement options.

## LO 5 | Getting a Good Night's Sleep

- Practicing good sleep hygeine, including creating a sleep-promoting environment, modifying your daytime habits, avoiding common sleep disruptors, practicing mental strategies designed to help you sleep, and being responsible in use of sleep aids are all important to a good night's sleep.

## POP QUIZ

Visit **MasteringHealth** to personalize your study plan with Chapter Review Quizzes and Dynamic Study Modules.

### LO 1 | Sleepless in America

1. Which of the following statements is *not* correct?
   a. Between 50 and 70 million Americans are sleep deprived
   b. Only 20 percent of Americans report that they got more than 7 hours of sleep in the last 24 hours.
   c. America and Japan are among the most sleep-deprived countries of the world.
   d. The highest risk for drowsy-driving accidents is among males aged 17 to 23.

### LO 2 | The Importance of Sleep

2. The age groups most likely to fall asleep unintentionally during the day are:
   a. 18–25 and 65+
   b. 55–65 and 65+
   c. 18–25 and 55-65
   d. Under 18

### LO 3 | The Processes of Sleep

3. Which of the following occurs when your body's circadian rhythm becomes out of sync with daylight hours?
   a. Jet lag
   b. REM sleep
   c. NREM sleep
   d. Somnolence

### LO 4 | Sleep Disorders

4. Which sleep disorder involves difficulty falling asleep, waking up during the night, and/or difficulty falling back asleep?
   a. Obstructive sleep apnea
   b. Narcolepsy
   c. Restless legs syndrome
   d. Insomnia

### LO 5 | Getting a Good Night's Sleep

5. Which of the following is *not* recommended if you want to get a good night's sleep?
   a. Getting adequate exposure to light, particularly sunlight during the day.
   b. Exercising each day
   c. Paying careful attention to your sleep environment, including clean scents and cool temperatures
   d. Consuming lots of fluids and foods that make you feel sleepy/full just prior to sleeping.

*Answers to the Pop Quiz questions can be found on page A-1. If you answered a question incorrectly, review the section identified by the Learning Outcome. For even more study tools, visit **MasteringHealth**.*

## THINK ABOUT IT!

### LO 1 | Sleepless in America

1. Why do you think America has the dubious distinction of being one of the most sleep-deprived nations in the world? Although college students have high rates of sleeplessness, few seek help. Why do you think this is the case?

### LO 2 | The Importance of Sleep

2. Why is sleep so important to you right now? In the future?

### LO 3 | The Processes of Sleep

3. What factors inferfere or disrupt the normal sleep cycles and cause sleep processes to be challenged?

### LO 4 | Sleep Disorders

4. If you were diagnosed with a sleep disorder, what behavior changes might you make to help you with a specific problem?

5. What actions can you take to help get a good night's sleep? From what you have learned in this chapter, what are five things you might tell your sleep-deprived mother or father to do to promote improved sleep?

# ACCESS YOUR HEALTH ON THE INTERNET

Visit **MasteringHealth** for links to the websites and RSS feeds.

The following websites explore further topics related to sleep.

**National Sleep Foundation.** Information source for national and international sleep statistics, conducts National Sleep in America survey each year, and provides general sleep information for consumers. Covers a variety of sleep topics by experts in the field. https://sleepfoundation.org

**CDC Sleep and Sleep Disorders.** Provides national data/information about sleep, vetted by experts in the field. www.cdc.gov/sleep/index.html

**National Center on Sleep Disorders Research.** Information and research on major sleep disorders. https://www.nhlbi.nih.gov/about/org/ncsdr/

**Annual reviews of sleep apps.** Includes overviews and costs. Updated each year with details of the newest apps and consumer ratings. www.healthline.com/health/healthy-sleep/top-insomnia-iphone-android-apps

# 5 Nutrition: Eating for a Healthier You

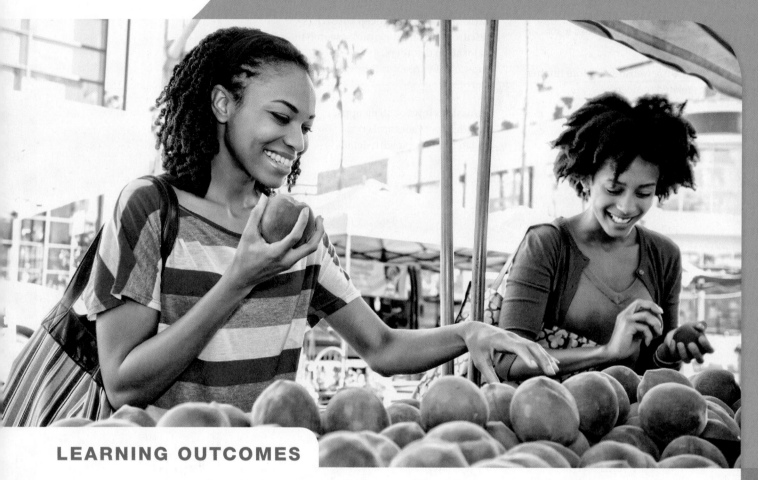

## LEARNING OUTCOMES

LO **1** List the six classes of nutrients, and explain the primary functions of each.

LO **2** Explain how the Dietary Guidelines for Americans and the MyPlate food guidance system can help you follow a healthful eating pattern.

LO **3** Discuss strategies for healthful eating, including how to read food labels, the role of vegetarian diets and dietary supplements, and how to choose healthful foods on and off campus.

LO **4** Explain food safety concerns facing Americans and people in other regions of the world.

## WHY
### SHOULD I CARE?

A poor-quality diet is a major risk factor for three of the top five causes of death: heart disease, cancer, and stroke. The food and beverage choices you make now can have both immediate and long-term effects on your health.

When was the last time you ate because you felt truly hungry? True **hunger** occurs when our brains initiate a physiological response that prompts us to seek food for the energy and **nutrients** that our bodies require to maintain proper functioning. Often, people in wealthy nations don't eat in response to hunger—instead, we eat because of **appetite**, a learned psychological desire to consume food. The sight and smell of food, food advertising, cultural factors, our social interactions, emotions, finances, and even the time of day can influence the choices we make to satisfy our appetites. Given all these influences, how can we make more healthful choices more often?

**Nutrition** is the science that investigates the relationship between physiological function and the essential elements of the foods we eat. With an understanding of nutrition, you will be able to make more informed choices about your diet. What you eat, how much you eat, and the amount of exercise you engage in are key determinants of your health. This chapter focuses on fundamental principles of nutrition—or how you can eat for a healthier you.

## LO 1 | ESSENTIAL NUTRIENTS FOR HEALTH

List the six classes of nutrients, and explain the primary functions of each.

Foods and beverages provide the chemicals needed to maintain the body's tissues and perform its functions. *Essential nutrients* are those the body cannot synthesize (or cannot synthesize in adequate amounts); we must obtain them from our diet. Of the six groups of essential nutrients, the four we need in the largest amounts—water, proteins, carbohydrates, and fats—are called *macronutrients*. The other two groups—vitamins and minerals—are needed in smaller amounts, so they are called *micronutrients*.

Before the body can use food, the digestive system must break it down into smaller molecules that can cross from the small intestine into the bloodstream. The **digestive process** is the sequence of functions by which the body breaks down foods chemically and mechanically, absorbs their nutrients, and excretes waste. (See **FIGURE 5.1** on page 122.)

### Recommended Intakes for Nutrients

In the next sections, we discuss each nutrient group and identify how much of each you need. These recommended amounts are known as the **Dietary Reference Intakes (DRIs)** and are published by the Food and Nutrition Board of the Institute of Medicine. The DRIs establish the amount of each nutrient needed to prevent deficiencies or reduce the risk of chronic disease, as well as identify maximum safe intake levels for healthy people. The DRIs are umbrella guidelines and include the following categories:

- **Recommended Dietary Allowances (RDAs)** are daily nutrient intake levels meeting the nutritional needs of 97–98 percent of healthy individuals.
- **Adequate Intakes (AIs)** are daily intake levels assumed to be adequate for most healthy people. AIs are used when there isn't enough research to support establishing an RDA.
- **Tolerable Upper Intake Levels (ULs)** are the highest amounts of a nutrient that an individual can consume daily without risking adverse health effects.
- **Acceptable Macronutrient Distribution Ranges (AMDRs)** are ranges of protein, carbohydrate, and fat intake that provide adequate nutrition and are associated with a reduced risk for chronic disease.

Whereas the RDAs, AIs, and ULs are expressed as amounts—usually grams, milligrams (mg), or micrograms (µg)—AMDRs are expressed as percentages. The AMDR for protein, for example, is 10–35 percent, meaning that no less than 10 percent and no more than 35 percent of the calories you consume should come from proteins. But that raises a new question: What are calories?

### Calories

A *kilocalorie* is a unit of measure used to quantify the amount of energy in food. On nutrition labels and in consumer publications, the term is shortened to **calorie**. *Energy* is defined as the

**HEAR IT! PODCAST**

Want a study podcast for this chapter? Download the podcast **Nutrition: Eating for Optimum Health**, available on **MasteringHealth.™**

**hunger** The physiological impulse to seek food.

**nutrients** The constituents of food that sustain humans physiologically: water, proteins, carbohydrates, fats, vitamins, and minerals.

**appetite** The learned desire to eat; normally accompanies hunger but is more psychological than physiological.

**nutrition** The science that investigates the relationship between physiological function and the essential elements of foods eaten.

**digestive process** The process by which the body breaks down foods into smaller components and either absorbs or excretes them.

**Dietary Reference Intakes (DRIs)** Set of recommended intakes for each nutrient published by the Institute of Medicine.

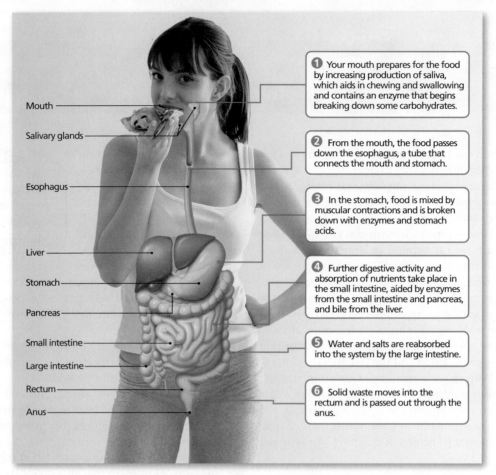

Mouth

Salivary glands

Esophagus

Liver

Stomach

Pancreas

Small intestine

Large intestine

Rectum

Anus

**1** Your mouth prepares for the food by increasing production of saliva, which aids in chewing and swallowing and contains an enzyme that begins breaking down some carbohydrates.

**2** From the mouth, the food passes down the esophagus, a tube that connects the mouth and stomach.

**3** In the stomach, food is mixed by muscular contractions and is broken down with enzymes and stomach acids.

**4** Further digestive activity and absorption of nutrients take place in the small intestine, aided by enzymes from the small intestine and pancreas, and bile from the liver.

**5** Water and salts are reabsorbed into the system by the large intestine.

**6** Solid waste moves into the rectum and is passed out through the anus.

**FIGURE 5.1** **The Digestive Process** The entire digestive process takes approximately 24 hours.

capacity to do work. We derive energy from the energy-containing nutrients in the foods we eat. These energy-containing nutrients—proteins, carbohydrates, and fats—provide calories. Vitamins, minerals, and water do not. **TABLE 5.1** shows the average caloric needs for individuals of various ages.

## Water: A Crucial Nutrient

The human body consists of 50–70 percent water by weight. This water is contained within cells, as well as in the blood and tissue fluids in which cells are bathed. It is essential for the chemical reactions upon which life depends; aids in fluid, electrolyte, and acid–base balance; helps regulate body temperature; and, as the primary component of blood and lymph, carries oxygen, nutrients, and hormones and other substances to body cells and removes metabolic wastes. For all these reasons, humans can survive for several weeks without food, but only for several days without water.

Individual needs for water vary according to dietary factors, age, size, overall health, environmental temperature and humidity levels, and exercise. The DRI for women is approximately 9 cups of water and other beverages each day and for men is about 13 cups.[1] However, critics have questioned whether we

**calorie** A unit of measure that indicates the amount of energy obtained from a particular food.

really need to consume this much additional water as the average healthy person gets considerable water in the foods they eat.[2] In fact, fruits and vegetables are 80–95 percent water, meats are more than 50 percent water, and even dry bread and cheese are about 35 percent water!

According to Robert A. Huggins, PhD, at the University of Connecticut, fluid needs change depending on circumstances and should vary with the individual, based on elements like environmental conditions, biological sex, how often and how hard a person exercises, age, health status, general diet, and level of heat acclimatization, rather than having a set recommendation for everyone. He suggests that the best way to gauge whether you're getting enough water is to pay attention to your thirst and watch the color of your urine before you flush. It should look like lemonade. If it is starting to look darker, like an amber ale, it's time to drink more water.[3] Other groups echo newer recommendations about daily water intake being individualized, particularly if you are exercising heavily.[4]

Contrary to popular opinion, caffeinated drinks, including coffee, tea, and soda, also count toward total fluid intake. Consumed in moderation, caffeinated beverages have not been found to dehydrate people whose bodies are used to caffeine.[5]

## TABLE 5.1 | Estimated Daily Calorie Needs

| | Calorie Range | |
|---|---|---|
| | Sedentary[a] | Active[b] |
| **Children** | | |
| 2–3 years old | 1,000 | → | 1,400 |
| **Females** | | |
| 4–13 years old | 1,200–1,600 | → | 1,400–2,200 |
| 14–18 | 1,800 | → | 2,400 |
| 19–25 | 2,000 | → | 2,400 |
| 26–50 | 1,800 | → | 2,200–2,400 |
| 51+ | 1,600 | → | 2,000–2,200 |
| **Males** | | |
| 4–12 years old | 1,200–1,800 | → | 1,600–2,400 |
| 13–18 | 2,000–2,400 | → | 2,600–3,200 |
| 19–20 | 2,600 | → | 3,000 |
| 21–40 | 2,400 | → | 2,800–3,000 |
| 41–60 | 2,200 | → | 2,800 |
| 61+ | 2,000 | → | 2,400–2,600 |

[a]A lifestyle that includes only the light physical activity associated with typical day-to-day life.

[b]A lifestyle that includes physical activity equivalent to walking more than 3 miles per day at 3–4 miles per hour, in addition to the light physical activity associated with typical day-to-day life.

**Source:** U.S. Department of Agriculture and U.S. Department of Health and Human Services, *2015–2020 Dietary Guidelines for Americans*, 8th ed., Appendix 2, Table A2-1. (Washington, DC: U.S. Government Printing Office).

There are situations in which a person needs additional fluids in order to avoid **dehydration**, a state of abnormal depletion of body fluids. Dehydration can develop within a single day, especially when you engage in strenuous physical activity in a hot climate. When you sweat profusely, you need extra water to keep your body's core temperature within a normal range. Dehydration is also a risk when you have a fever or an illness involving vomiting or diarrhea, and in people with kidney disease, diabetes, or cystic fibrosis. Older adults and the very young are also at increased risk for dehydration.

Excessive water intake can also pose a serious health risk if it prompts *hyponatremia*, a condition characterized by low blood levels of the mineral sodium. Sodium is essential for the transmission of nerve impulses; sodium in the fluid outside of cells balances potassium in the fluid inside of cells to keep cells properly hydrated. When the level of sodium in the bloodstream and tissue spaces is excessively diluted, water flows into cells, which swell. This can cause a potentially fatal swelling of the brain and other tissues.

**DO IT! NUTRITOOLS**

Complete the **Know Your Protein Sources** activity, available on MasteringHealth.™

If you are an athlete and wonder about water consumption, visit the American College of Sports Medicine's website (www.acsm.org) to download its brochure, "Selecting and Effectively Using Hydration for Fitness."[6]

# Proteins

Next to water, **proteins** are the most abundant compounds in the human body. In fact, proteins are major components of all living cells. They are called the "body builders" because of their role in developing and repairing bone, muscle, skin, and blood cells. They are the key elements of antibodies that protect us from disease, enzymes that control chemical activities in the body, and many hormones that regulate body functions. Proteins also supply an alternative source of energy to cells when fats and carbohydrates are not available. Specifically, every gram of protein you eat provides 4 calories. (There are about 28 grams in an ounce by weight.) Adequate protein in the diet is vital to many body functions and ultimately to survival.

Your body breaks down proteins into their nitrogen-containing building blocks, known as **amino acids**. Nine of the 20 different amino acids needed by the body are termed **essential amino acids**, which means the body must obtain them from the diet; the other 11 amino acids are considered nonessential because the body can make them. Dietary proteins that supply all the essential amino acids are called **complete proteins**. Typically, protein from animal products is complete, and soy is a complete plant protein. Other proteins from plant sources are **incomplete proteins** that lack one or more of the essential amino acids. However, it is easy to combine plant foods to produce a complete protein meal (**FIGURE 5.2** on page 124). Plant foods rich in incomplete proteins include *legumes* (beans, lentils, peas, and peanuts); *grains* (e.g., wheat, corn, rice, and oats); and *nuts and seeds*. Certain vegetables, such as leafy green vegetables and broccoli, also contribute valuable plant proteins. Consuming a variety of foods from these categories will provide all the essential amino acids.

Although protein deficiency poses a threat to the global population (see the **Health in a Diverse World** box on page 124), few Americans suffer from protein deficiencies. In fact, the average American age 20 and over consumes 83 grams of protein daily, much of it from high-fat animal flesh and dairy products.[7] The AMDR for protein is 10–35 percent of calories. The RDA is 0.8 gram (g) per kilogram (kg) of body weight.[8] To calculate your protein needs, divide your body weight in pounds by 2.2 to get your weight in kilograms, then multiply by 0.8. The result is your recommended protein intake per day. For example, a woman who weighs 130 pounds should consume about 47 grams of protein each day. A 6-ounce steak provides 53 grams of protein—more than she needs!

**dehydration** Abnormal depletion of body fluids.

**proteins** Large molecules made up of chains of amino acids; essential constituents of all body cells.

**amino acids** The nitrogen-containing building blocks of protein.

**essential amino acids** The nine nitrogen-containing building blocks of human proteins that must be obtained from foods.

**complete proteins** Proteins that contain all nine of the essential amino acids.

**incomplete proteins** Proteins that lack one or more of the essential amino acids.

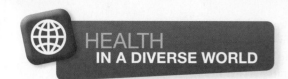
# MALNUTRITION AND FOOD INSECURITY *Hunger Globally and Here at Home*

Worldwide, nearly 800 million people—about 1 in 9—do not have enough to eat. **Severe acute malnutrition (SAM)** causes tissue wasting and stunted growth in at least 17 million children, impairs brain development, diminishes work capacity, and perpetuates poverty within communities. Inadequate protein intake is especially dangerous, weakening the immune system and increasing the risk of death from common infections. In developing nations, the major cause of chronic hunger is unequal distribution of food because of poverty. Wars, climate events, epidemics of disease, lack of infrastructure, and overpopulation are also contributing factors.

Many Americans also experience hunger. The Economic Research Service of the USDA estimates that, in 2014, 14 percent of American households (over 17 million households) were **food insecure**. This means that, during the year, the household members did not have reliable access to an adequate supply of nourishing food. At highest risk for food

**Poverty, hunger, and obesity can coexist within the same family or even within the same individual.**

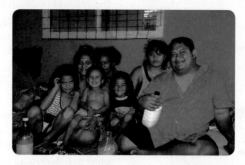

insecurity are households with incomes below 185 percent of the federal poverty threshold. In 2015, for example, the federal poverty threshold for a family of four was $24,250; thus, a family of four earning below $44,863 was at high risk for food insecurity.

Both worldwide and in the United States, the prevalence of obesity is increasing, including among the poor, and even among those experiencing hunger. What could explain this paradox? One of the most common theories is that

low-income people choose cheap, shelf-stable foods that are high in calories but low in protein. Foods low in protein are less satiating; thus, the person must consume more calories in order to feel full. Another link between poverty and obesity may be stress; that is, the chronic stress of having insufficient resources causes oversecretion of the stress hormone cortisol, which slows metabolism. Comfort foods high in sugar may be particularly appealing during times of stress because sugar consumption decreases cortisol levels, and thus is calming.

**Source:** Food and Agriculture Organization of the United Nations, "The State of Food Insecurity in the World," 2015, www.fao.org/3/a-i4646e.pdf; Economic Research Service, "Household Food Security in the United States in 2014," September 2015, www.ers.usda.gov/publications/err-economic-research-report/err194.aspx; U.S. Department of Health and Human Services, "2015 Poverty Guidelines," September 3, 2015, https://aspe.hhs.gov/2015-poverty-guidelines; J. Haushofer and E. Fehr, "On the Psychology of Poverty," *Science* 344, no. 6186 (2014): 862–67. M. S. Tryon et al., "Excessive Sugar Consumption May Be a Difficult Habit to Break: A View from the Brain and Body," *Journal of Clinical Endocrinology and Metabolism* 100, no. 6 (2015): 2239–47.

**severe acute malnutrition** Lack of nutritious food that causes tissue wasting and stunted growth, impairs brain development, diminishes work capacity, and perpetuates poverty within communities.

People who have a higher RDA for protein include pregnant women and patients fighting a serious infection, recovering from surgery or blood loss, or recovering from burns. In these instances, proteins that are lost to cellular repair and development need to be replaced. Athletes also have a higher need for protein, requiring from 1.2 to 2.0 g per kg of body weight to build and repair muscle fibers.[9] In addition, a sedentary person may find it easier to stay in energy balance when consuming a diet with a higher percentage of protein and a

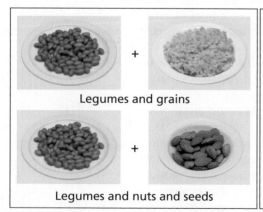

Legumes and grains

Legumes and nuts and seeds

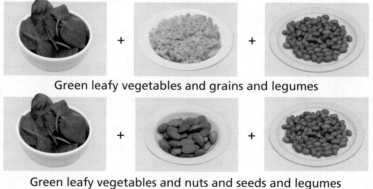

Green leafy vegetables and grains and legumes

Green leafy vegetables and nuts and seeds and legumes

**FIGURE 5.2 Foods Providing Complementary Amino Acids** Complementary combinations of plant-based foods can provide all essential amino acids. In some cases, you might need to combine three sources of protein to supply all nine; however, the foods do not necessarily have to be eaten in the same meal. Here, two of the limited amino acids in leafy green vegetables are supplied by either grains or nuts and seeds, and the third is found in legumes.

lower percentage of carbohydrate. Why? Proteins make a person feel full for a longer period of time because protein takes longer to digest than carbohydrates. Protein also releases certain satiety hormones that contribute to feeling full longer.

## Carbohydrates

**Carbohydrates** supply us with the energy we need to sustain normal daily activity. In comparison to proteins or fats, carbohydrates are broken down more quickly and efficiently, yielding a fuel called *glucose*. All body cells can burn glucose for fuel; moreover, glucose is the only fuel that red blood cells can use and is the primary fuel for the brain. Carbohydrates are the best fuel for moderate to intense exercise because they can be readily broken down to glucose even when we're breathing hard and our muscle cells are getting less oxygen.

Like proteins, carbohydrates provide 4 calories per gram. The RDA for adults is 130 grams of carbohydrate per day.[10] There are two major types: simple and complex.

### Simple Carbohydrates

**Simple carbohydrates** or *simple sugars* are found naturally in fruits, many vegetables, and dairy. The most common form of simple carbohydrates is *glucose*. Fruits and berries contain *fructose* (commonly called *fruit sugar*). Glucose and fructose are **monosaccharides**. Combinations of two monosaccharides yield **disaccharides**. Perhaps the best-known example is *sucrose* (granulated table sugar). *Lactose* (milk sugar), found in milk and milk products, and *maltose* (malt sugar) are other common disaccharides. Eventually, the human body converts all types of simple sugars to glucose to provide energy to cells.

Sugar is also added to a wide range of processed foods and beverages. A classic example is soda: there are more than 10 teaspoons per can! Moreover, such diverse items as breakfast cereals, yogurts, and even some peanut butters can be high in added sugars. Research is increasingly linking high consumption of added sugars not only to obesity but also to chronic diseases, including heart disease and cancer.[11] Read food labels carefully before purchasing. If *sugar* or one of its aliases (including *high-fructose corn syrup*) appears near the top of the ingredients list, then that product is high in added sugars and is probably not your best nutritional bet.

### Complex Carbohydrates: Starches and Glycogen

**Complex carbohydrates** are found in grains, cereals, legumes, and other vegetables. Also called *polysaccharides*, they are formed by long chains of glucose. *Starches, glycogen,* and *fiber* are the main types of complex carbohydrates.

**Starches** make up the majority of the complex carbohydrate group and come from cereals, breads, pasta, rice, corn, oats, barley, potatoes, legumes, starchy vegetables, and related foods. The body breaks down starches into glucose, which can be easily absorbed by cells and used as energy or stored in the muscles and the liver as **glycogen**. When the body requires a sudden burst of energy, the liver converts glycogen into glucose and releases it into the bloodstream.

### Complex Carbohydrates: Fiber

**Fiber**, sometimes referred to as "bulk" or "roughage," is the indigestible portion of plant foods that helps move foods through the digestive system, delays absorption of cholesterol and other nutrients, and softens stools by absorbing water. Dietary fiber is found only in plant foods, such as fruits, vegetables, nuts and seeds, and grains.

Fiber is either *soluble* or *insoluble*. Soluble fibers, such as pectins, gums, and mucilages, dissolve in water, form gel-like substances, and can be digested easily by bacteria in the colon. Major food sources of soluble fiber include citrus fruits, berries, oat bran, dried beans, and some other vegetables. Insoluble fibers, such as lignins and cellulose, typically do not dissolve in water and cannot be fermented by bacteria in the colon. They are found in most fruits and vegetables and in **whole grains**, such as brown rice, wheat, bran, and whole-grain breads and cereals (see **FIGURE 5.3**). The AMDR for

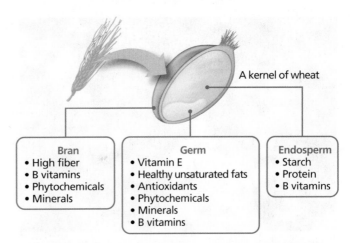

**FIGURE 5.3 Anatomy of a Whole Grain** Whole grains are more nutritious than refined grains because they contain the bran, germ, and endosperm of the seed—sources of fiber, vitamins, minerals, and beneficial phytochemicals (chemical compounds that occur naturally in plants).

*Bran*
- High fiber
- B vitamins
- Phytochemicals
- Minerals

*Germ*
- Vitamin E
- Healthy unsaturated fats
- Antioxidants
- Phytochemicals
- Minerals
- B vitamins

*Endosperm*
- Starch
- Protein
- B vitamins

A kernel of wheat

**Source:** Adapted from Joan Salge Blake, Kathy D. Munoz, and Stella Volpe, *Nutrition: From Science to You,* 3rd ed. © 2015, page 132. Printed and electronically reproduced by permission of Pearson Education, Inc., Upper Saddle River, New Jersey.

**DO IT! NUTRITOOLS**
Complete the **Know Your Carbohydrate Sources** activity, available on **MasteringHealth.™**

---

**food insecure** Lack of access to an adequate supply of nourishing food.

**carbohydrates** Basic nutrients that supply the body with glucose, the energy molecule most readily used by cells.

**simple carbohydrates** A carbohydrate made up of only one or two sugar molecules; also called *simple sugars.*

**monosaccharides** One-molecule sugars; include fructose and glucose.

**disaccharides** Sugars combining two monosaccharides; include lactose, maltose, and sucrose.

**complex carbohydrates** Polysaccharides composed of long chains of glucose.

**starches** Polysaccharides that are the storage forms of glucose in plants.

**glycogen** The polysaccharide form in which glucose is stored in the liver and, to a lesser extent, in muscles.

**fiber** The indigestible portion of plant foods that helps move food through the digestive system and softens stools by absorbing water.

**whole grains** Grains that retain the bran, germ, and endosperm, with only the husk removed.

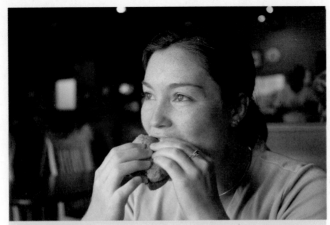

A recent study following more than 367,000 participants over 14 years found that the higher the consumption of whole grains, the lower the risk for death from cardiovascular disease, diabetes, and cancer. The risk of death was reduced by an average of 17%. Unfortunately, nearly 100% of Americans fail to meet their recommended intakes for whole grains.

Sources: T. Huang et al., "Consumption of Whole Grains and Cereal Fiber and Total and Cause-Specific Mortality: Prospective Analysis of 367,442 Individuals," *BMC Medicine* 13, no. 1 (2015): 59; Scientific Report of the 2015 Dietary Guidelines Advisory Committee, "Advisory Report to the Secretary of Health and Human Services and the Secretary of Agriculture," 2015, Available at: http://health.gov/dietaryguidelines/2015-scientific-report/.

carbohydrates is 45–65 percent of total calories, and health experts recommend that the majority of this intake be fiber-rich carbohydrates.

Fiber is associated with a reduced risk for obesity, heart disease, constipation, and possibly even type 2 diabetes and colon and rectal cancers. The DRI for dietary fiber is 25 grams per day for women and 38 grams per day for men.[12] What's the best way to increase your intake? Eat fewer refined carbohydrates in favor of more fiber-rich carbohydrates, including whole-grain breads and cereals, fresh fruits, legumes and other vegetables, nuts, and seeds. As with most nutritional advice, however, too much of a good thing can pose problems. A sudden increase in dietary fiber may cause flatulence (intestinal gas), cramping, or bloating. Consume plenty of water or other (sugar-free!) liquids to reduce such side effects. Find out more about the benefits of fiber in the Making Changes Today box.

## Fats

Cholesterol and triglycerides (commonly called fats) are two forms of a large group of biological compounds known as *lipids*, which are not soluble in water.

### Cholesterol

Cholesterol is commonly referred to as a fat, but it's technically a *sterol*, an oily substance found in both plant and animal cells. Plant sterols are present in small amounts

**cholesterol** A type of lipid classified as a sterol and found in animal-based foods; it is also synthesized by the body.

**high-density lipoproteins (HDLs)** Compounds that facilitate the transport of cholesterol in the blood to the liver for metabolism and elimination from the body.

## MAKING **CHANGES** TODAY

### Bulk Up Your Fiber Intake!

You can increase your fiber intake by improving your skills at finding and choosing foods that are high in fiber. Try the following:

- Whenever possible, select whole-grain breads, especially those made without added sugars. Choose breads with 3 or more grams of fiber per serving. Look for the word *whole* on the label. Many breads are called "wheat bread," and colored brown by adding molasses. This doesn't mean they are whole-wheat breads.

- Eat whole, unpeeled fruits and vegetables rather than drinking their juices. The fiber in the whole fruit tends to slow the release of glucose into your bloodstream and helps you feel full longer.

- Substitute whole-grain pastas, bagels, and pizza crust for the refined, white flour versions.

- Add whole-grain bread crumbs, brown rice, or ground seeds to meatloaf and burgers to increase fiber intake.

- Enhance your fiber intake with quinoa, an edible seed that is also a complete protein.

- Toast grains to bring out their nutty flavor and make foods more appealing.

- Sprinkle ground flaxseed on cereals, yogurt, and salads, or add to casseroles, burgers, and baked goods. Flaxseeds have a mild flavor and are also high in beneficial fatty acids.

in plant oils, whole grains, corn, and soy, whereas cholesterol is obtained from animal-based foods such as meats, cheese, and egg yolks. In the body, cholesterol is an essential component of the cell membrane and of many important functional chemicals, including certain hormones. Although we can't live without cholesterol, we don't have to consume it in our diet because the liver synthesizes it from other food substances. Thus, it's not an essential nutrient.

Many people believe that all cholesterol circulating in the bloodstream is "bad" and increases the risk for cardiovascular disease (which can lead to a heart attack or stroke). This isn't strictly true. Cholesterol is transported in the bloodstream in compounds called *lipoproteins* that contain, as their name suggests, a variety of lipids as well as protein. There are three main types, two of which are clinically important:

- **High-density lipoproteins (HDLs)** are about 50 percent protein. The rest of the compound is made up of lipids, including cholesterol. HDLs are "high density" because their high protein content makes these compounds more dense than other lipoproteins, which have less protein.

HDLs are produced in the liver and circulate in the bloodstream, picking up cholesterol and transporting it back to the liver for recycling or excretion. Cholesterol removed from the bloodstream cannot collect in, and damage, the blood vessel lining. Thus, a high level of HDLs reduces an individual's risk for the blood-vessel damage (called atherosclerosis) that leads to cardiovascular disease.

■ **Low-density lipoproteins (LDLs)** are about 22 percent protein, 50 percent cholesterol, and 28 percent other lipids. LDLs transport cholesterol to the body cells that require it. LDLs not taken up by cells are degraded by the liver, which releases their cholesterol load into the bloodstream. There, this cholesterol can accumulate in the lining of blood vessels, eventually leading to atherosclerosis and cardiovascular disease.

For this reason, a high level of HDL-cholesterol in the blood is desirable, as is a low level of LDL-cholesterol. However, for most people, cholesterol intake is not correlated with the levels of cholesterol circulating in the bloodstream. Surprisingly, fiber intake is! A diet high in fiber reduces blood cholesterol, mainly because fiber increases the body's excretion of bile, a cholesterol-containing compound synthesized by the liver. As bile is lost in feces, the liver must remove cholesterol from the bloodstream to make more. (See Chapter 16 for information about recent research on cholesterol, inflammation, and other risks for cardiovascular disease.)

### Triglycerides
The term *dietary fats* technically refers to **triglycerides**. At 9 calories per gram, they are our most significant source of fuel for low-to-moderate levels of activity, and during rest and sleep. They also play a vital role in insulating body organs against cold and shock, as well as maintaining healthy skin and hair. When we consume too many calories from any source, the liver converts the excess into triglycerides, which are stored in fat cells throughout the body. Dietary fats are also broken down into components that contribute to cell structures and many important body chemicals. Finally, you need to consume dietary fat in order for your body to absorb the fat-soluble vitamins A, D, E, and K.

Triglycerides are compounds made up of a molecule called glycerol attached to three *fatty acids*, chains of oxygen, carbon, and hydrogen atoms. Fatty acid chains that cannot hold any more hydrogen in their chemical structure are called **saturated fats**. They generally come from animal sources, such as meat, dairy, and poultry products, and are solid at room temperature. Saturated fats have long been associated with an increased risk for heart disease and stroke, largely because they appear to decrease the removal of LDL-cholesterol from the blood. New research has begun to question the strength of this association;[13] however, the *2015–2020 Dietary Guidelines for Americans* still suggest limiting your intake of saturated fat to less than 10% of your daily calories.

**Unsaturated fats** have regions where carbon atoms are double-bonded together instead of to hydrogen. Thus, they are not "saturated" with hydrogen. They generally come from plants, are liquid at room temperature, and include most vegetable oils. *Monounsaturated fatty acids* (*MUFAs*) have one double-carbon bond in their chain, and *polyunsaturated fatty acids* (*PUFAs*) have more than one double bond. Although most animal and plant-based foods provide a combination of fats, in general, peanut, canola, and olive oils are higher in monounsaturated fats, and corn, sunflower, and safflower oils are higher in polyunsaturated fats. All unsaturated fats are considered more healthful than saturated fats. Replacing saturated fats with unsaturated fats, especially PUFAs, is associated with reduced blood levels of LDL-cholesterol.[14] For a breakdown of the types of fats in common vegetable oils, see **FIGURE 5.4**.

**DO IT! NUTRITOOLS**

Complete the **Know Your Fat Sources** activity, available on **MasteringHealth.™**

**low-density lipoproteins (LDLs)** Compounds that facilitate the transport cholesterol in the blood to body cells.

**triglycerides** The most common lipids in our food supply and in the body; made up of glycerol and three fatty acid chains; commonly referred to as *fats*.

**saturated fats** Fats that are unable to hold any more hydrogen in their chemical structure; derived mostly from animal sources; solid at room temperature.

**unsaturated fats** Fats that have regions not saturated with hydrogen; derived mostly from plants; liquid at room temperature.

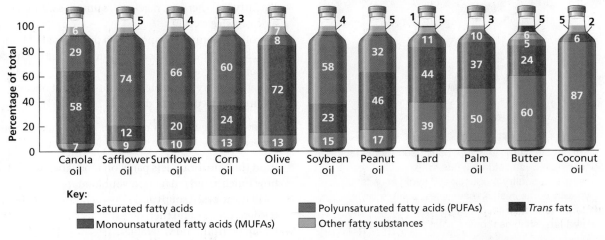

**Key:**
- ■ Saturated fatty acids
- ■ Monounsaturated fatty acids (MUFAs)
- ■ Polyunsaturated fatty acids (PUFAs)
- □ Other fatty substances
- ■ *Trans* fats

**FIGURE 5.4** Percentages of Saturated, Polyunsaturated, Monounsaturated, and *Trans* Fats in Common Vegetable Oils

Two specific types of polyunsaturated fatty acids essential to a healthful diet are *omega-3 fatty acids* (found in many types of fatty fish; dark green, leafy vegetables; walnuts; and flaxseeds) and *omega-6 fatty acids* (found in corn, soybean, peanut, sunflower, and cottonseed oils). Both are classified as *essential fatty acids*—that is, those we must receive from our diets—because the body cannot synthesize them, yet requires them for functioning. The most important fats within these groups are *linoleic acid*, an omega-6 fatty acid, and *alpha-linolenic acid*, an omega-3 fatty acid. The body needs these to make hormone-like compounds that control immune function, pain perception, and inflammation, to name a few key benefits. You may also have heard of EPA (eicosapentaenoic) and DHA (docosahexaenoic acid). These are derivatives of alpha-linolenic acid that are found abundantly in oily fish such as salmon and tuna and are associated with a reduced risk for heart disease.[15]

**trans fats (trans fatty acids)** Fatty acids typically produced from the hydrogenation of polyunsaturated oils.

### Avoiding *Trans* Fatty Acids
For decades, Americans shunned butter, lard, and other foods high in saturated fats, and used margarine and solid shortenings instead. What they didn't know is that these fats, called **trans fatty acids**, increase the risk for cardiovascular disease even more than saturated fats. Research shows that consuming *trans* fats decreases levels of HDL-cholesterol and increases levels of LDL-cholesterol. For every 2 percent increase in intake of *trans* fats, the risk for cardiovascular disease increases 23 percent.[16]

Although a small amount of *trans* fatty acids do occur naturally in some animal products, the great majority are in processed foods made with partially hydrogenated oils (PHOs).[17] PHOs are produced when food manufacturers add hydrogen to a plant oil, solidifying it, helping it resist rancidity, and giving the food in which it is used a longer shelf-life. The hydrogenation process straightens out the fatty acid chain so that it is more like a saturated fatty acid, and it has similar harmful effects, lowering HDLs and raising LDLs. *Trans* fats have been used in margarines, many commercial baked goods, and restaurant deep-fried foods.

In 2015, the U.S. Food and Drug Administration (FDA) ruled that PHOs are no longer "generally recognized as safe" for consumption. Food companies have until July 2018 to remove PHOs from their products.[18] In the meantime, *trans* fats are being removed from most foods. The FDA allows foods with less than 1 gram of *trans* fat per serving to be labeled as *trans*-fat free. However, if you see the words *partially hydrogenated oils, fractionated oils, shortening, lard,* or *hydrogenation* on a food label, then *trans* fats are present, even if the amount listed on the label is zero.

### Fat Intake Recommendations
The AMDR for fats is 20–35 percent of total calories. Saturated fat should make up less than 10 percent of your total calories, and you should keep *trans*-fat intake to an absolute minimum.[19] Instead of trying to eat a low-fat diet, replace the saturated and *trans* fats you eat with healthful unsaturated fats from plants and fish. Many studies have shown that balanced higher-fat diets such as the Mediterranean diet, which is rich in plant oils and fish, produce significant improvements in body weight and cardiovascular risk factors.[20]

Follow these guidelines to add more healthful fats to your diet:

- Eat fatty fish (herring, mackerel, salmon, sardines, or tuna) at least twice weekly.
- Use olive, peanut, soy, and canola oils instead of butter or lard. See **Health Headlines** for more information on coconut oil.
- Add green leafy vegetables, walnuts, walnut oil, and ground flaxseed to your diet.

Follow these guidelines to reduce your intake of saturated and *trans* fats:

- Read the Nutrition Facts panel on food labels to find out how much saturated fat is in your food.
- Chill meat-based soups and stews, scrape off any fat that hardens on top, and then reheat to serve.
- Fill up on fruits and vegetables.
- Hold the creams and sauces.

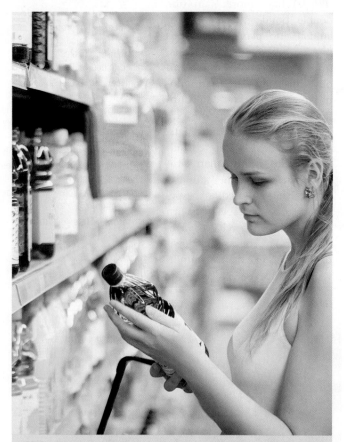

All fats are not the same, and your body needs some fat to function. Try to reduce saturated fats, which are in meat, full-fat dairy, and poultry products, and avoid trans fats, which typically come in stick margarines, commercially baked goods, and deep-fried foods. Replace these with unsaturated fats, such as those in plant oils, fatty fish, and nuts and seeds.

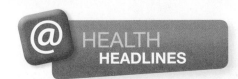
# COCONUT OIL
## Friend or Foe?

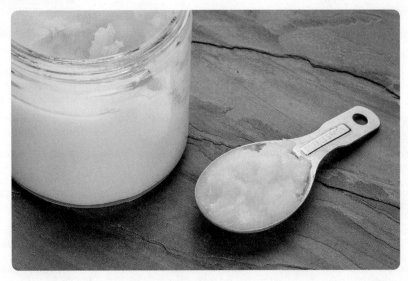

If you're a label reader, you've probably noticed coconut oil on the ingredients list of milk, spreads, and yogurt. Or maybe you've seen jars filled with this semi-solid milky-white fat on the grocery store shelves. Once thought of as unhealthy, coconut oil consumption is now being touted for several beneficial effects, including a reduced risk for cardiovascular disease. Let's see what the science says.

Whereas most plant oils are about 7–17 percent saturated fat, 87 percent of the fatty acids in coconut oil are saturated. Coconut oil also doesn't contain any essential fatty acids. It's known to raise levels of LDL-cholesterol as well. Still, it also raises levels of HDL-cholesterol, and is rich in vitamin E and a variety of phytochemicals.

The original study that sparked interest in coconut oil was observational. It found that Polynesian people, who have a low prevalence of cardiovascular disease, ingest mostly fat from coconuts. This association between consumption of coconut oil and reduced rates of cardiovascular disease does not, of course, prove cause and effect. More recently, however, some clinical studies have demonstrated mechanisms—such as reductions in blood pressure and metabolic stress—by which coconut oil does appear to exert a cardio-protective effect.

Health professionals are therefore divided over whether to recommend replacing heart-healthy polyunsaturated vegetable oils with coconut oil. There is a larger body of research in humans that monounsaturated and polyunsaturated fatty acids lower LDL-cholesterol levels and reduce the risk of cardiovascular disease, but only a few studies support coconut oil as beneficial for heart health. At this point, the American Heart Association advises against adding coconut oil to your diet.

**Source:** F. Hamam, "Specialty Lipids in Health and Disease," *Food and Nutrition Sciences* 4 (2013): 63–70; A. S. Babu et al., "Virgin Coconut Oil And Its Potential Cardioprotective Effects," *Postgraduate Medicine* 126, no. 7 (2014): 76–83; Y. Kamisah et al., "Cardioprotective Effect of Virgin Coconut Oil in Heated Palm Oil Diet-Induced Hypertensive Rats," *Pharmaceutical Biology* 53, no. 9 (2015): 1243–49; American Heart Association, "Fats and Oils: AHA Recommendations," Accessed April 2015, Available at www.heart.org.

- Avoid all products with *trans* fatty acids. Use *trans*-fat-free margarines, vegetable spreads, bean spreads, nut butters, low-fat cream cheese, etc.
- Choose lean meats, fish, or skinless poultry. Broil or bake whenever possible. Drain off fat after cooking.
- Choose fewer cold cuts, bacon, sausages, hot dogs, and organ meats.
- Select nonfat and low-fat dairy products.

## Vitamins

**Vitamins** are organic compounds that promote growth and are essential to life and health. Every minute of every day, vitamins help maintain nerves, skin, blood, and bones, heal wounds, fight metabolic stress, enable vision, and convert food energy to body energy—and they do all this without adding any calories to your diet.

Vitamins are classified as either *fat soluble*, which means they are absorbed through the intestinal tract with the help of fats, or *water soluble*, which means they are absorbed through the intestinal tract directly into the bloodstream. Vitamins A, D, E, and K are fat soluble; B-complex vitamins and vitamin C are water soluble. Fat-soluble vitamins can be stored in the body's fat tissues, and toxic levels can accumulate if people regularly consume more than the UL. Excesses of water-soluble vitamins are generally excreted in the urine and rarely cause toxicity problems. In a recent survey of college students, 42 percent reported taking a multivitamin/multimineral supplement.[21] See **TABLE 5.2** on page 130 for functions, recommended intake amounts, and food sources of specific vitamins.

**Vitamin D** Vitamin D, the "sunshine vitamin," is formed from a compound in the skin when exposed to the sun's ultraviolet rays. In most people, an adequate amount of vitamin D can be synthesized with 5–30 minutes of sun on the face, neck, hands, arms, and legs twice a week, without sunscreen.[22] However, the sun is not high enough in the sky during late fall to early spring in northern climates to allow for vitamin D synthesis. For

**vitamins** Essential organic compounds that promote metabolism, growth, and reproduction.

# TABLE 5.2 | A Guide to Vitamins

| Vitamin Name | Primary Functions | Recommended Intake | Reliable Food Sources |
|---|---|---|---|
| Thiamin | Carbohydrate and protein metabolism | Men: 1.2 mg/day<br>Women: 1.1 mg/day | Pork, fortified cereals, enriched rice and pasta, peas, tuna, legumes |
| Riboflavin | Carbohydrate and fat metabolism | Men: 1.3 mg/day<br>Women: 1.1 mg/day | Beef liver, shrimp, dairy foods, fortified cereals, enriched breads and grains |
| Niacin | Carbohydrate and fat metabolism | Men: 16 mg/day<br>Women: 14 mg/day | Meat/fish/poultry, fortified cereals, enriched breads and grains, canned tomato products |
| Vitamin $B_6$ | Carbohydrate and amino acid metabolism | Men and women aged 19–50: 1.3 mg/day | Garbanzo beans, meat/fish/poultry, fortified cereals, white potatoes |
| Folate | Amino acid metabolism and DNA synthesis | Men: 400 µg/day<br>Women: 400 µg/day | Fortified cereals, enriched breads and grains, spinach, legumes, liver |
| Vitamin $B_{12}$ | Formation of blood cells and nervous system | Men: 2.4 µg/day<br>Women: 2.4 µg/day | Shellfish, all cuts of meat/fish/poultry, dairy foods, fortified cereals |
| Pantothenic acid | Fat metabolism | Men: 5 mg/day<br>Women: 5 mg/day | Meat/fish/poultry, shiitake mushrooms, fortified cereals, egg yolks |
| Biotin | Carbohydrate, fat, and protein metabolism | Men: 30 µg/day<br>Women: 30 µg/day | Nuts, egg yolks |
| Vitamin C | Collagen synthesis, iron absorption, and promotes healing | Men: 90 mg/day<br>Women: 75 mg/day<br>Smokers: 35 mg more per day than RDA | Sweet peppers, citrus fruits and juices, broccoli, strawberries, kiwi |
| Vitamin A | Immune function, maintains epithelial cells, healthy bones and vision | Men: 900 µg<br>Women: 700 µg | Beef and chicken liver, egg yolks, milk<br>Carotenoids found in spinach, carrots, mango, apricots, cantaloupe, pumpkin, yams |
| Vitamin D | Promotes calcium absorption and healthy bones | Adults aged 19–70: 15 µg/day (600 IU/day) | Canned salmon and mackerel, milk, fortified cereals |
| Vitamin E | Protects cell membranes and acts as a powerful antioxidant | Men: 15 mg/day<br>Women: 15 mg/day | Sunflower seeds, almonds, vegetable oils, fortified cereals |
| Vitamin K | Blood coagulation and bone metabolism | Men: 120 µg/day<br>Women: 90 µg/day | Kale, spinach, turnip greens, Brussels sprouts |

**Note:** Values are for all adults aged 19 and older, except as noted. Values increase among women who are pregnant or lactating. Data from Food and Nutrition Board, Institute of Medicine, National Academies, "Dietary Reference Intakes (DRIs): Estimated Average Requirements," Accessed February 2016, Available at https://iom.nationalacademies.org/~/media/Files/Activity%20Files/Nutrition/DRIs/5_Summary%20Table%20Tables%201-4.pdf.

people who cannot rely on the sun to meet their daily vitamin D needs, consuming vitamin D–fortified milk, yogurt, soy milk, cereals, and fatty fish, such as salmon, can also supply this vitamin.

Vitamin D promotes the body's absorption of calcium, the primary mineral component of bone. It also assists in the processes of bone growth, repair, and remodeling. For these reasons, a deficiency of vitamin D can promote loss of bone density and strength, a condition called *osteoporosis*. The risk of fractures (broken bones) is greatly increased in people with osteoporosis. Two other bone disorders—*rickets* in children, and its adult version, *osteomalacia*, both of which cause softening and distortion of the bones—can also be prevented with adequate intake of vitamin D.[23] An adequate level of vitamin

D may also reduce the risk for cardiovascular disease, diabetes, and some forms of cancer.

More is not always better, however.[24] As just noted, vitamin D is stored in the body's fat tissues, and an excessive intake can be toxic.

## Folate

One of the B vitamins, folate is needed for the production of compounds necessary for DNA synthesis in body cells. It is particularly important for proper cell division during embryonic development; folate deficiencies during the first few weeks of pregnancy, typically before a woman even realizes she is pregnant, can prompt a neural tube defect such as spina bifida, in which the primitive tube that eventually forms the brain and spinal cord fails to close properly. The FDA requires that all bread, cereal, rice, and pasta products sold in the United States be fortified with folic acid, the synthetic form of folate, to reduce the incidence of neural tube defects.

## Minerals

**Minerals** are inorganic, indestructible elements that build body tissues and assist body processes. They are readily absorbed and excreted. *Major minerals* are those that the body needs in fairly large amounts: sodium, calcium, phosphorus, magnesium, potassium, sulfur, and chloride. *Trace minerals* include iron, zinc, manganese, copper, fluoride, selenium, chromium, and iodine. Although only very small amounts of trace minerals are needed, they are just as important as the major minerals. (See **TABLE 5.3**.)

Even if you never use table salt, you still may be getting excess sodium in your diet.

**Sodium** Sodium is necessary for the regulation of blood volume and blood pressure, fluid balance, transmission of nerve impulses, heart activity, and certain metabolic functions. It enhances flavors, acts as a preservative, and tenderizes meats, so it's often present in high quantities in the foods we eat. A common misconception is that table salt and sodium are the same thing: Table salt is a compound containing both sodium and chloride. It accounts for only 15 percent of our sodium intake. The majority of sodium in our diet comes from processed foods that are infused with sodium to enhance flavor and for preservation. Pickles, fast foods, salty snacks, processed cheeses, canned and dehydrated soups, frozen dinners, many breads and bakery products, and smoked meats and sausages often contain several hundred milligrams of sodium per serving.

The AI for sodium is just 1,500 milligrams, which is about 0.65 of a teaspoon.[25] The *2015–2020 Dietary Guidelines for Americans* suggest keeping your sodium intake below 2,300 mg/day. Unfortunately, 89 percent of Americans exceed this limit.[26]

Why is high sodium intake a concern? Salt-sensitive individuals respond to a high-sodium diet with an increase in blood pressure (hypertension), which contributes to heart disease and stroke. Although the cause of the majority of cases of hypertension is unknown, lowering sodium intake reduces the risk. See the Making Changes Today box on page 132 for tips on how to reduce your sodium intake.

**Calcium** Calcium is the primary mineral component of bones and teeth. It is also essential for muscle contraction, nerve

**minerals** Inorganic, indestructible elements that aid physiological processes and build body structures.

## TABLE 5.3 | A Guide to Minerals

| Mineral Name | Primary Functions | Recommended Intake | Reliable Food Sources |
|---|---|---|---|
| Sodium | Fluid and acid–base balance; nerve impulses and muscle contraction | Adults: 1.5 g/day (1,500 mg/day) | Table salt, pickles, most canned soups, snack foods, luncheon meats, canned tomato products |
| Potassium | Fluid balance; nerve impulses and muscle contraction | Adults: 4.7 g/day (4,700 mg/day) | Most fresh fruits and vegetables: potato, banana, tomato juice, orange juice, melon |
| Phosphorus | ATP, fluid balance and bone formation | Adults: 700 mg/day | Milk/cheese/yogurt, soy milk and tofu, legumes, nuts, poultry |
| Selenium | Regulates thyroid hormones and reduces oxidative stress | Adults: 55 µg/day | Seafood, milk, whole grains, and eggs |
| Calcium | Part of bone; muscle contraction, acid–base balance, and nerve transmission | Adults: 1,000 mg/day | Milk/yogurt/cheese, sardines, collard greens and spinach, calcium-fortified juices |
| Magnesium | Part of bone; muscle contraction | Men: 400 mg/day Women: 310 mg/day | Spinach, kale, collard greens, whole grains, seeds, nuts, legumes |
| Iodine | Synthesis of thyroid hormones | Adults: 150 µg/day | Iodized salt, saltwater seafood |
| Iron | Part of hemoglobin and myoglobin | Men: 8 mg/day Women: 18 mg/day | Meat/fish/poultry, fortified cereals, legumes |
| Zinc | Immune system function; growth and sexual maturation | Men: 11 mg/day Women: 8 mg/day | Meat/fish/poultry, fortified cereals, legumes |

**Note:** Values are for all adults aged 19 and older. Data from Food and Nutrition Board, Institute of Medicine, National Academies, "Dietary Reference Intakes (DRIs): Estimated Average Requirements," Accessed February 2016, Available at https://iom.nationalacademies.org/~/media/Files/Activity%20Files/Nutrition/DRIs/5_Summary%20Table%20Tables%201-4.pdf.

impulse transmission, blood clotting, and acid–base balance. The issue of calcium consumption has gained national attention with the rising incidence of osteoporosis among older adults. Calcium is an underconsumed "nutrient of public health concern"; that is, most Americans do not consume the recommended 1,000–1,300 milligrams of calcium per day.[27]

Milk is one of the richest sources of dietary calcium. Calcium-fortified soymilk is an excellent vegetarian alternative. Many green leafy vegetables are good sources of calcium, but some contain oxalic acid, which makes their calcium harder to absorb. Spinach, chard, and beet greens are not particularly good sources, whereas broccoli, cauliflower, kale, collard greens, and many peas and beans are rich in absorbable calcium.

It is generally best to consume calcium-rich foods and fluids throughout the day, with foods containing protein, vitamin D, and vitamin C for optimal absorption. Many dairy products are both excellent sources of calcium and fortified with vitamin D, which assists in calcium absorption. Avoid taking calcium supplements unless advised by your health care provider.[28] Supplements have not been associated with a reduced risk for fractures, and are associated with a variety of gastrointestinal side effects, including constipation, as well as an increased risk for kidney stone formation and cardiovascular disease.[29]

Do you consume carbonated soft drinks? Be aware that the added phosphoric acid (phosphate) in these drinks can cause you to excrete extra calcium, which may result in calcium loss from your bones. One study of 2,500 men and women found that in women who consumed at least three cans of cola per week, even diet cola, bone density of the hip was 4–5 percent lower than in women who drank fewer than one cola per month. Colas did not seem to have the same effect on men.[30] There may also be a "milk displacement" effect, meaning that people who drank soda were not drinking milk, thereby decreasing their calcium intake.

**anemia** Condition that results from the body's inability to produce adequate hemoglobin.

**functional foods** Foods believed to have specific health benefits beyond their basic nutrients.

**antioxidants** Substances believed to protect against oxidative stress and resultant cell damage.

**Iron** Worldwide, iron deficiency is the most common nutrient deficiency, affecting more than 2 billion people, nearly 30 percent of the world's population.[31] In the United States, iron deficiency is less prevalent; however, because iron is a key component of red blood cells, deficiency can develop with blood loss and in menstruating women who fail to maintain a balanced diet. Women aged 19–50 need about 18 milligrams of iron per day, and men aged 19–50 need about 8 milligrams.[32]

Iron deficiency can lead to *iron-deficiency anemia*. **Anemia** results from the body's loss of, or insufficient production of, healthy red blood cells. Iron is the oxygen-carrying component of a protein called hemoglobin in blood cells. When iron-deficiency anemia occurs, blood cells pick up less oxygen from the lungs, and transport less oxygen to body tissues, including the brain. As a result, the iron-deficient person feels confused, tired, and weak. Iron is also important for energy metabolism, DNA synthesis, and other body functions.

Iron toxicity is typically due to consuming iron supplements. Symptoms of toxicity include nausea, vomiting, diarrhea, rapid heartbeat, weak pulse, dizziness, shock, and confusion. Excess iron intake has also been associated with an increased risk for neurological disorders, including dementia, as well as cardiovascular disease and cancer.[33]

## Beneficial Non-Nutrient Components of Foods

Increasingly, nutrition research is focusing on components of foods that are not nutrients themselves, but interact with nutrients to promote human health.[34] Foods that may confer health benefits beyond the nutrients they contribute to the diet—whole foods, fortified foods, enriched foods, or enhanced foods—are called **functional foods**. When functional foods are included as part of a varied diet, they have the potential to positively impact health.[35]

Some of the most popular functional foods today are those containing **antioxidants**. These substances appear to protect against oxidative stress, a complex process in which *free radicals*

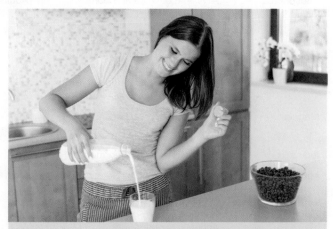

Milk is a great source of calcium and other nutrients. If you don't like milk or can't drink it, make sure to get enough calcium—at least 1,000 milligrams a day—through other sources.

(atoms with unpaired electrons) destabilize other atoms and molecules, prompting a chain reaction that can damage cell membranes, cell proteins, or genetic material in the cells. Free radical formation occurs as a result of normal cell metabolism. Antioxidants combat it by donating their electrons to stabilize free radicals; activating enzymes that convert free radicals to less-damaging substances; or reducing or repairing the damage they cause. Free radical damage is associated with many chronic diseases, including cardiovascular disease, cancer, age-related vision loss, and other diseases of aging.

Some antioxidants are nutrients. These include vitamins C and E, as well as the minerals copper, iron, manganese, selenium, and zinc. Other potent antioxidants are **phytochemicals**, compounds that occur naturally in plants and are thought to protect them against ultraviolet radiation, pests, and other threats. Common examples include the following:

*Carotenoids* are pigments found in red, orange, and dark green fruits and vegetables. Beta-carotene, the most researched carotenoid, is a precursor of vitamin A, meaning that vitamin A can be produced in the body from beta-carotene. Along with beta-carotene, other carotenoids, such as lutein, lycopene, and zeaxanthin, are associated in numerous studies with a reduced risk for chronic disease.[36]

*Polyphenols*, which include a group known as flavonoids, are the largest class of phytochemicals. They are found in an array of fruits and vegetables as well as soy products, tea, and chocolate. Like carotenoids, they are thought to have potent antioxidant properties.[37]

Although research supporting the health benefits of antioxidant nutrients and phytochemicals is not conclusive, studies do show that individuals deficient in antioxidant vitamins and minerals have an increased risk for age-related diseases, and that antioxidants consumed in whole foods, mostly fruits and vegetables, may reduce these individuals' risks.[38] In contrast, antioxidants consumed as supplements do not necessarily confer such a benefit, and some studies suggest they may be harmful, acting as "pro-oxidants" and increasing the risk of certain cancers and overall mortality in some populations, such as smokers.[39]

Foods rich in nutrients and phytochemicals are increasingly being referred to as "superfoods." Do they live up to their name? See the **Health Headlines** box on page 134.

> Blueberries are a great source of antioxidants.

The U.S. Department of Health and Human Services and the U.S. Department of Agriculture (USDA) publish two tools for consumers to make healthy eating easy: the Dietary Guidelines for Americans and the MyPlate food guidance system.

> **phytochemicals** Naturally occurring non-nutrient plant chemicals believed to have beneficial properties.

# LO 2 | NUTRITIONAL GUIDELINES

Explain how the Dietary Guidelines for Americans and the MyPlate food guidance system can help you follow a healthful eating pattern.

Americans consume about 900 more calories per day than they did fifty years ago (see **FIGURE 5.5**).[40] When this trend combines with our increasingly sedentary lifestyle, it is not surprising that we have seen a dramatic rise in obesity.

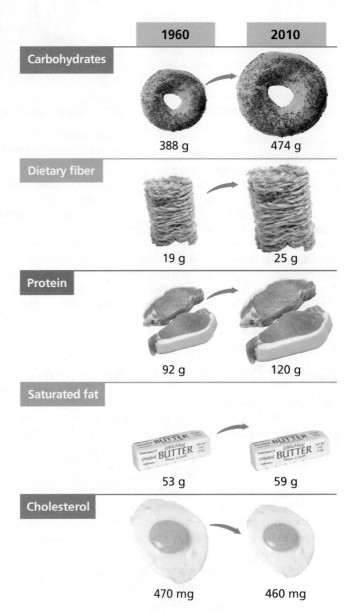

| | 1960 | 2010 |
|---|---|---|
| Carbohydrates | 388 g | 474 g |
| Dietary fiber | 19 g | 25 g |
| Protein | 92 g | 120 g |
| Saturated fat | 53 g | 59 g |
| Cholesterol | 470 mg | 460 mg |

**FIGURE 5.5 Trends in Per Capita Nutrient Consumption** Since 1960, Americans have increased their caloric intake from 3,100 to 4,000 and their daily consumption of carbohydrates, protein, and saturated fat.

**Source:** Data are from the USDA Center for Nutrition Policy and Promotion, February 1, 2015, www.ers.usda.gov/data-products/food-availability-(per-capita)-data-system/.aspx#26715.

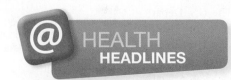
# HEALTH CLAIMS OF SUPERFOODS

Functional foods contain both nutrients and other active compounds that may improve overall health, reduce the risk for certain diseases, or delay aging. These foods are increasingly being referred to as "superfoods." But do they live up to their name? Let's look at a few.

Salmon is a rich source of the omega-3 fatty acids EPA and DHA, which combat inflammation, improve HDL/LDL blood profiles, and reduce the risk for cardiovascular disease. These essential fatty acids may also promote a healthy nervous system, reducing the risk for mood disorders and age-related dementia.

Yogurt makes it onto most superfood lists because it contains living, beneficial bacteria called probiotics. You will see their genus name—for example, *Lactobacillus* or *Bifidobacterium*—in the list of ingredients on the product's label. Probiotics colonize the large intestine, where they help complete digestion and produce certain vitamins, and may reduce the risk of diarrhea and other bowel disorders,

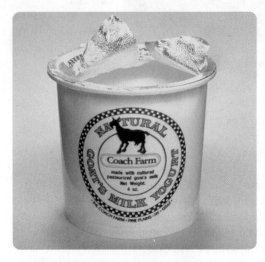

**Yogurt and kefir (a fermented milk drink) are dairy products containing beneficial bacteria called *probiotics*.**

boost immunity, and help regulate body weight.

Cocoa is particularly rich in phytochemicals called flavonols that have been shown in many studies to reduce the risk for cardiovascular disease, diabetes, and even arthritis. Dark chocolate has a higher level of flavonols than milk chocolate.

Given such claims, it's easy to get carried away by the idea that superfoods, like superheros, have superpowers. But eating a square of dark chocolate won't rescue you from the ill effects of a fast-food burger and fries. What matters is your whole diet. Focus on including superfoods as components of a varied diet rich in fresh fruits, legumes and other vegetables, whole grains, lean sources of protein, and nuts and seeds. These are the "everyday heroes" of a super-healthful diet.

**Source:** Academy of Nutrition and Dietetics, "Position of the Academy of Nutrition and Dietetics: Functional Foods," *Journal of the Academy of Nutrition and Dietetics* 113 (2013): 1096–1103; S. C. Dyall, "Long-Chain Omega-3 Fatty Acids and the Brain: A Review of the Independent and Shared Effects of EPA, DPA, and DHA," *Frontiers in Aging Neuroscience* 7 (2015): 52; A. P. S. Hungin et al., "Systematic Review: Probiotics in the Management of Lower Gastrointestinal Symptoms in Clinical Practice–An Evidence-Based International Guide," *Alimentary Pharmacology and Therapeutics* 38, no. 8 (2013): 864–86; N. Khan et al., "Cocoa Polyphenols and Inflammatory Markers of Cardiovascular Disease," *Nutrients* 6, no. 2 (2014): 844–880.

## Dietary Guidelines for Americans

The Dietary Guidelines for Americans (DGAs) are recommendations for eating a healthy, nutritionally adequate diet. They are revised every 5 years. The most recent, the *2015–2020 Dietary Guidelines for Americans*, include the following five key guidelines.[41]

1. **Follow a healthy eating pattern across the lifespan.** An eating pattern is the totality of what you habitually eat and drink. Following a healthful eating pattern requires you to recognize that every food and beverage choice you make throughout the day can positively influence your health, providing you nutrients and fiber at an appropriate calorie level to help you achieve and maintain a healthy body weight, and reduce your risk for chronic disease. The DGAs identify the following components of a healthful eating pattern:

   - A variety of vegetables of different types and colors, from leafy green to red, orange, and yellow, plus legumes (beans, peas, and lentils)
   - Fruits, especially whole fruits

   - Grains, at least half of which are whole grains
   - Fat-free or low-fat dairy choices, including milk, cheese, yogurt, and/or fortified soy milk
   - A variety of lean-protein foods, including seafood, lean meats and poultry, eggs, legumes, soy products, and nuts and seeds
   - Oils

   A healthful eating pattern should be accompanied by regular physical activity. The DGAs advise at least 150 minutes of physical activity each week, along with muscle-strengthening exercise on 2 or more days each week. For more information on improving your physical fitness, see Chapter 7.

2. **Focus on variety, nutrient density, and amount.** To meet your nutrient needs, yet stay within your budget of calories, choose the most nutrient-dense versions of foods

**SEE IT! VIDEOS**

Cut back on sugar while satisfying your sweet tooth! Watch **Ditching Sugar**, available on **MasteringHealth.™**

within all food groups. Nutrient-dense foods provide a relatively high level of nutrients and fiber for a relatively low number of calories. For example, a slice of whole-grain toast with peanut butter provides healthful unsaturated fats, protein, and fiber-rich carbohydrates, as well as vitamins and minerals, for about 300 calories, whereas another breakfast choice, a plain waffle with butter and maple syrup, provides little more than refined carbohydrates, saturated fats, and added sugars, for about 400 calories. The toast with peanut butter is also more satiating, so you won't be as likely to feel hungry as quickly.

3. **Limit calories from added sugars and saturated fats, and reduce sodium intake.** Specifically, the DGAs advise you to:

   ■ Consume less than 10 percent of calories per day from added sugars. This means avoiding sugary drinks such as soft drinks, energy drinks, flavored milks, and specialty coffees, and making candy, cookies, ice cream, and other desserts occasional treats.

   ■ Consume less than 10 percent of calories per day from saturated fats. Limiting your intake of animal-based foods such as fatty meats, cheese, and ice cream will help you meet this goal.

   ■ Consume less than 2,300 mg per day of sodium. Review the Making Changes Today box on page 132 for tips on how.

   ■ If alcohol is consumed, it should be consumed in moderation—up to one drink per day for adult women and two drinks per day for adult men. For more information, see Chapter 11.

4. **Shift to healthier food and beverage choices.** Choose nutrient-dense foods and beverages across and within all food groups in place of less healthy choices. For example, more than three-fourths of Americans consume a diet that is low in vegetables, fruits, dairy, and healthful fish and plant oils. The DGAs recommend you shift your intake of these foods upward, by replacing snack foods like chips and cheese curls with raw veggies; meat-based entrées with fish and legumes; sugary drinks with milk or soy milk; and desserts high in added sugars, like cookies and brownies, with whole fruits.

5. **Support healthy eating patterns for all.** The DGAs affirm that everyone has a role in helping to create and support healthy eating patterns wherever we are, from home to campus to work to within our communities. Citing the social-ecological model of health, the DGAs point out that each of your choices—while shopping, eating out, standing in line at your campus dining hall, or cooking for friends—can promote the availability of healthy foods aligned with the Dietary Guidelines. You can also encourage others to join you in physical activity.

## MyPlate Food Guidance System

To help consumers understand and implement the Dietary Guidelines, the USDA has developed an easy-to-follow graphic and Web-based guidance system called MyPlate, which can

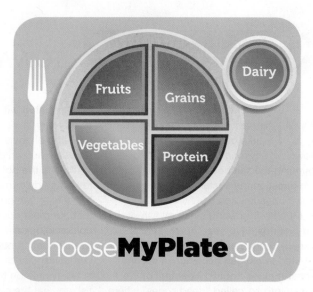

**FIGURE 5.6 The MyPlate System** The USDA MyPlate food guidance system takes a new approach to dietary and exercise recommendations. Each colored section of the plate represents a food group, and an interactive tool at *www.choosemyplate.gov* helps you analyze and track your foods and physical activity and provides helpful tips to personalize your plans.

**Source:** U.S. Department of Agriculture, 2013, www.choosemyplate.gov.

be found at www.choosemyplate.gov and is illustrated in **FIGURE 5.6.** The MyPlate food guidance system takes into consideration the dietary and caloric needs for a wide variety of individuals, such as pregnant or breastfeeding women, those trying to lose weight, and adults with different activity levels. The interactive website can create personalized dietary and exercise recommendations based on the individual information you enter.

MyPlate's key messages, which support the Dietary Guidelines, include the following:

■ **Eat nutrient-dense foods.** While eating the recommended number of servings from MyPlate, make the most nutrient-dense choices within a given food group. Again, these are foods and beverages that have a high nutritional value for their caloric content.

■ **Eat seafood twice a week.** Replace red meat or poultry with grilled, broiled, or baked seafood twice a week. In addition to salmon, tuna, and other fatty fin fish, clams, mussels, oysters, and calamari are all high in omega-3 fatty acids. See Student Health Today on page 136 for information on making environmentally responsible seafood choices.

# 6 OR MORE

teaspoons of **SUGAR** are present in most national brands of fruit yogurt per serving!

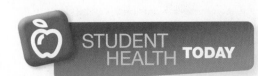
# TOWARD SUSTAINABLE SEAFOOD

MyPlate recommends consuming fish twice a week to boost your intake of omega-3 fatty acids. However, environmental concerns surrounding the seafood industry today call into question the sustainability and safety of fish consumption.

Much of the world's natural fishing grounds have been overfished, and climate change and pollution have contributed to oxygen depletion in ocean water, making about 10 percent of the ocean into so-called "dead zones" where fish and shellfish can no longer live. To counteract the loss of wild fish populations, increasing numbers of fish are being farmed, a technology that poses its own health and environmental risks. In the United States, the Environmental Protection Agency (EPA) regulates effluents from fish farms; nevertheless, the contamination of river, lake, and ocean waters with runoff from fish farms containing feed, waste, and other pollutants continues. In addition, some seafood is contaminated with industrial toxins such as mercury, a neurotoxin, and polychlorinated biphenyls (PCBs) and dioxins, probable human carcinogens.

What's the bottom line? A recent review study comparing the risks and benefits of fish consumption concluded that, for most adults, the overwhelming epidemiological evidence supports regular fish consumption to reduce the risk for cardiovascular disease. Thus, the best strategy may be to find out where the fish you eat are caught and the methods by which they are caught. Check out the EPA's website on safe fish consumption at www.epa.gov/choose-fish-and-shell-fish-wisely. Several environmental groups also offer guides to inform consumers of safe and sustainable seafood choices. Visit the website of the Monterey Bay Aquarium in California at www.seafood-watch.org and download their free seafood-watch app. Another great resource is the FishPhone service offered by the Blue Ocean Institute. Simply send a text message to 30644 with the word FISH and the type of fish you want to know about, and it will send you information about any health or environmental concerns. Purchasing seafood from responsible sources will support fisheries and fish farms that are healthier for you and the environment.

**Source:** S. E. Moffitt et al., "Response of Seafloor Ecosystems to Abrupt Global Climate Change," *Proceedings of the National Academy of Sciences,* 112, no. 15 (2015): 4684–89; U.S. Environmental Protection Agency, "EPA Study Reveals Widespread Contamination of Fish in U.S. Lakes and Reservoirs," February 23, 2016, http://yosemite.epa.gov; A. Gil and F. Gil, "Fish, a Mediterranean Source of n-3 PUFA: Benefits Do Not Justify Limiting Consumption," *British Journal of Nutrition* 113, Supplement 2 (2015): S58–67.

- **Avoid *empty calories*.** MyPlate refers to calories from added sugars and saturated fats as empty calories. Here are some examples of empty-calorie foods:[42]
  - **Sausages, hot dogs, bacon, and ribs.** Adding a sausage link to your breakfast adds 96 empty calories.
  - **Cheese.** Switching from whole-milk mozzarella cheese to nonfat mozzarella cheese saves you 76 empty calories per ounce.
  - **Refined grains, including crackers, bagels, and white rice.** Switching to whole-grain versions can save you 25 or more empty calories per serving.
  - **Cakes, cookies, pastries, and ice cream.** Approximately 75 percent of the calories in a slice of chocolate cake or a serving of ice cream are empty calories.
  - **Wine, beer, and all alcoholic beverages.** A whopping 155 empty calories are consumed with each 12 fluid ounces of beer.
- **Engage in physical activity.** Any activity that gets your heart pumping counts, including walking on campus, playing basketball, and dancing. MyPlate offers personalized recommendations for weekly physical activity. (For more on physical fitness, see Chapter 7.)

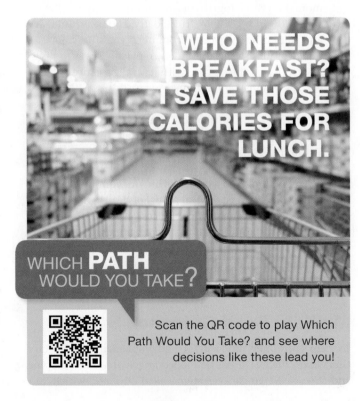

WHO NEEDS BREAKFAST? I SAVE THOSE CALORIES FOR LUNCH.

WHICH **PATH** WOULD YOU TAKE?

Scan the QR code to play Which Path Would You Take? and see where decisions like these lead you!

## LO 3 | **HOW** CAN I EAT MORE HEALTHFULLY?

Discuss strategies for healthful eating, including how to read food labels, the role of vegetarian diets and dietary supplements, and how to choose healthful foods on and off campus.

Whether you follow a vegetarian diet, eat only organic foods, take dietary supplements, or choose to eat locally grown foods, there are ways to improve the nutrient density of your meals. Let's begin with how to read a food label.

## Read Food Labels

How do you know what nutrients the packaged foods you eat are contributing to your diet? To help consumers evaluate the nutritional values of packaged foods, the FDA and the USDA developed the Nutrition Facts label that is typically displayed on the side or back of packaged foods. One of the most helpful items on the label is the **% Daily Values (%DVs)** list, which tells you how much of an average adult's allowance for a particular substance (protein, fiber, calcium, etc.) is provided by a serving of the food. The %DV is calculated based on a 2,000-calorie per day diet, so your values may be different from those listed on a label. The label also includes information on the serving size and calories. In 2016, the FDA published a new label that is more helpful for consumers. It identifies the calories per serving in much larger type, and uses a serving size that better reflects the amount of the food that people typically eat. **FIGURE 5.7** walks you through the former and new Nutrition Facts labels. For the latest information on the new label, go to www.fda.gov and search "Nutrition Facts label."

Food labels contain other information as well, such as the name and manufacturer of the product, an ingredients list, and sometimes claims about the product's contents or effects. The FDA allows three types of claims on the packages of foods and dietary supplements:[43]

- **Health claims** describe a relationship between a food product and health promotion, but no food label is allowed to claim that a food can treat or cure a disease. FDA-approved health claims are supported by current scientific evidence and meet the standard for *significant scientific agreement* (*SSA*) among experts. If there is agreement that a food may reduce your risk of a disease and experts are confident their opinion won't change with more scientific study, the health claim is approved.

> **% Daily Values (%DVs)** Percentages on food and supplement labels identifying how much of each listed nutrient or other substance a serving of food contributes to a 2,000 calorie/day diet.

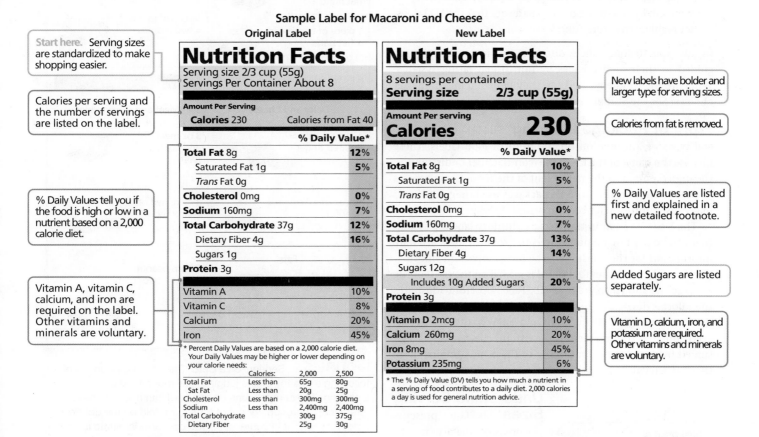

**Sample Label for Macaroni and Cheese**

**FIGURE 5.7** Reading a Food Label

**Source:** U.S. Food and Drug Administration, "How to Understand and Use the Nutrition Facts Panel," April 2015, www.fda.gov/Food/IngredientsPackagingLabeling/LabelingNutrition/ucm274593.htm; U.S. Food and Drug Administration, "Changes to the Nutrition Facts Label," August 2016, http://www.fda.gov/Food/GuidanceRegulation/GuidanceDocumentsRegulatoryInformation/LabelingNutrition/ucm385663.htm.

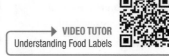

▸ **VIDEO TUTOR**
Understanding Food Labels

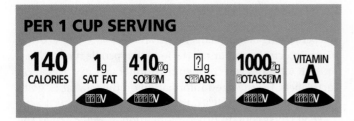

**PER 1 CUP SERVING**

| 140 CALORIES | 1g SAT FAT | 410🅐g SO🅐🅐M | 🅐g S🅐🅐ARS | 1000🅐g 🅐OTASSI🅐M | VITAMIN A |

**FIGURE 5.8** **Facts Up Front** Information is placed on the front of the package for a quick and accurate nutritional profile of a serving of the food.

For example, an approved health claim on a package of whole-grain bread may state, "In a low-fat diet, whole-grain foods like this bread may reduce the risk of heart disease."

- Nutrient content claims indicate a specific nutrient is present at a certain level. For example, a product label might say "High in fiber" or "Low in fat" or "This product contains 100 calories per serving." Nutrient content claims can use the following words: *more, less, fewer, good source of, free, light, lean, extra lean, high, low, reduced*. The claims are strictly regulated and reflect the nutrient data on the Nutrition Facts label.

- Structure and function claims describe the effect that a component in the food product has on the body. For example, the label of a carton of milk is allowed to state, "Calcium builds strong bones." Be aware that the FDA does not regulate structure-function claims.

In addition to food labels, shoppers are increasingly being guided in their food choices by nutritional rating systems. What are these systems, and can they help you make smarter choices? See the **Student Health Today** box for answers.

**Front of Package Labeling** The FDA requires several types of information on the front of food labels. These include the name of the food, the manufacturer or distributor, the ingredients, and the net weight of the food. Other aspects of the labeling on the front of packages are unregulated and may cause confusion for consumers.

The *Facts Up Front* initiative is a voluntary labeling system that can be used by manufacturers to provide quick, accurate information for the consumer. The most important information from the Nutrition Facts label is placed on the front of the package. As shown in **FIGURE 5.8**, Facts Up Front illustrates the kilocalories, saturated fat, sodium, and added sugars per serving. It also lists the amount and %DV of other "encouraged" micronutrients, such as potassium, that are underconsumed by Americans, if a serving of the food contains more than 10 percent.

**Understand Serving Sizes** MyPlate presents personalized dietary recommendations based on servings of particular nutrients. But how much is one serving? Is it different from a portion? Although these two terms are often used interchangeably, they actually mean very different things. A *serving* is the recommended amount you should consume, and it's found on the Nutrition Facts label. A *portion* is the amount you choose to eat at any one time. The saying "your eyes are bigger than your stomach" is rooted in truth—most of us select portions that are much bigger than recommended servings. If a food label says that a serving size of 1 cup is 250 calories, but you eat a portion of 1.5 cups, you've consumed 375 calories. See **FIGURE 5.9** for a handy pocket guide with tips on recognizing serving sizes.

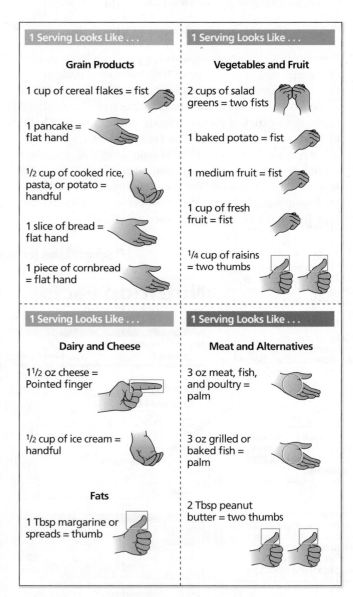

**1 Serving Looks Like . . .**

**Grain Products**

1 cup of cereal flakes = fist

1 pancake = flat hand

½ cup of cooked rice, pasta, or potato = handful

1 slice of bread = flat hand

1 piece of cornbread = flat hand

**1 Serving Looks Like . . .**

**Vegetables and Fruit**

2 cups of salad greens = two fists

1 baked potato = fist

1 medium fruit = fist

1 cup of fresh fruit = fist

¼ cup of raisins = two thumbs

**1 Serving Looks Like . . .**

**Dairy and Cheese**

1½ oz cheese = Pointed finger

½ cup of ice cream = handful

**Fats**

1 Tbsp margarine or spreads = thumb

**1 Serving Looks Like . . .**

**Meat and Alternatives**

3 oz meat, fish, and poultry = palm

3 oz grilled or baked fish = palm

2 Tbsp peanut butter = two thumbs

**FIGURE 5.9** **Serving-Size Card** One of the challenges of following a healthy diet is judging how much food constitutes a serving. The comparisons on this card can help. For easy reference, photocopy or cut out the card, fold on the dotted lines, and keep it in your wallet. You can even laminate it for long-term use.

**Sources:** National Heart, Lung and Blood Institute, "Serving Size Card," Accessed April 2015, http://hp2010.nhlbihin.net/portion/servingcard7.pdf; National Dairy Council, "Serving Size Comparison Chart," Accessed April 2015, www.healthyeating.org/Portals/0/Documents/Schools/Parent%20Ed/Portion_Sizes_Serving_Chart.pdf.

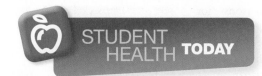
# NUTRITION RATING SYSTEMS

Next time you're at the grocery store, take a close look at the tags on the store shelves. Do you see anything different—stars, perhaps, or numbers inside blue hexagons? If so, you're looking at a nutrition rating system designed to help you quickly locate healthful foods. Four of the most popular systems in American markets are the following:

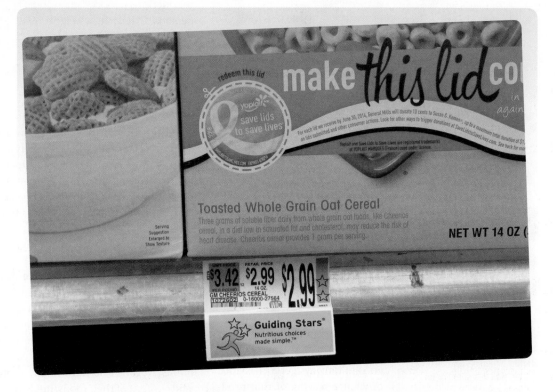

- **Guiding Stars.** This system rates the nutritional quality of foods using zero to three stars, with three indicating the highest nutritional quality. A fresh tomato, for example, gets three stars. What the system lacks in subtlety it makes up for in simplicity—even consumers who haven't been introduced to it can quickly understand the basic message behind it: The product with the most stars "wins."

- **NuVal.** The NuVal System uses a scale of 1 to 100. The higher the number, the higher the nutritional quality. In rating each food, the system considers more than 30 dietary components—not just nutrients, but fiber and phytochemicals, too. In this system, a tomato gets a top score of 100 points. The 100-point rating scale allows consumers to make more subtle distinctions between very similar foods; for example, two brands of whole-grain bread get scores of 48 versus 29: the bread with the higher score is lower in calories and sodium and higher in fiber.

- **American Heart Association Heart Check.** The AHA Heart Check identifies foods that promote heart health. To receive a Heart Check rating, the food must meet specific criteria for levels of saturated fat, sodium, and other nutrients. For example, to receive a Heart Check rating, a serving of food cannot contain more than 20 milligrams of cholesterol, and cannot contain any partially hydrogenated oils (PHOs). Each serving must also contain 10 percent or more of the Daily Value for dietary fiber or at least one of the following nutrients: protein, vitamin A, vitamin C, iron, or calcium.

- **Aggregate Nutrient Density Index (ANDI).** This index ranks foods based on the number of micronutrients per calorie and takes into account as many known beneficial phytochemicals as possible. It does not, however, consider macronutrient density, such as the amount of high-quality protein or essential fatty acids in the food. A top score is 1,000. How does this system rate our tomato? It gets just 164 points! In contrast, kale gets a top score of 1,000. Here's why: A medium-sized tomato and two-thirds of a cup of kale have about the same number of calories, yet the kale has more vitamin C, calcium, and beta-carotene.

Do these ranking systems prompt shoppers to choose more healthful foods? Research suggests they might. A recent study following shoppers in 150 supermarkets for two years found that the systems may be most effective in discouraging unhealthful choices: sales of less nutritious foods fell by as much as 31 percent, resulting in an average purchase of more nutritious foods overall. Moreover, an evaluation of the AHA Heart Check system found that people purchasing the AHA-approved foods have a higher diet quality and a lower risk of cardiovascular disease and diabetes.

**Source:** J. Cawley et al., "The Impact of a Supermarket Nutrition Rating System on Purchases of Nutritious and Less Nutritious Foods," *Public Health Nutrition* 18, no. 1 (2015): 8–14; A. H. Lichtenstein et al., "Food-Intake Patterns Assessed by Using Front-of-Pack Labeling Program Criteria Associated with Better Diet Quality and Lower Cardiometabolic Risk," *American Journal of Clinical Nutrition* 99, no. 3 (2014): 454–62.

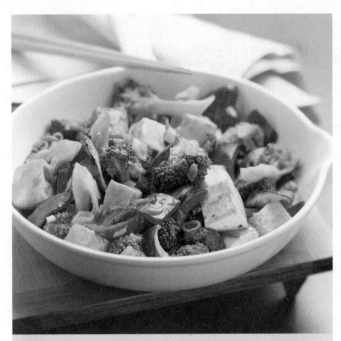

A vegetarian diet can be a very healthy way to eat. Make sure you get complementary essential amino acids throughout the day. Meals like this tofu and vegetable stir-fry can be further enhanced by adding a whole grain, such as brown rice.

**vegetarian** A person who follows a diet that excludes some or all animal products.

**dietary supplements** Products taken by mouth and containing dietary ingredients such as vitamins and minerals that are intended to supplement existing diets.

Even when we read the label, we don't always get a clear idea of what a serving of that product really is. Consider a bottle of chocolate milk: The food label may list one serving size as 8 fluid ounces and 150 calories. However, note the size of the entire bottle. If it holds 16 ounces, drinking the whole thing serves up 300 calories.

## Vegetarianism: A Healthy Diet?

The word **vegetarian** means different things to different people. Strict vegetarians, or *vegans*, avoid all foods of animal origin, including dairy products and eggs. Their diet is based on vegetables, grains, fruits, nuts, seeds, and legumes. Far more common are *lacto-vegetarians*, who eat dairy products but avoid flesh foods and eggs. *Ovo-vegetarians* add eggs to a vegan diet, and *lacto-ovo-vegetarians* eat both dairy products and eggs. *Pesco-vegetarians* eat fish, dairy products, and eggs, and *semivegetarians* eat chicken, fish, dairy products, and eggs. Some people in the semivegetarian category prefer to call themselves "non–red meat eaters."

According to a poll conducted by the Vegetarian Resource Group, 3.4 percent of U.S. adults, approximately 8 million adults, are vegetarians or vegans.[44] Among young adults (ages 18–34), 6 percent are vegetarian.[45]

Common reasons for pursuing a vegetarian lifestyle include concern for animal welfare, the environmental costs of meat production, food safety, personal health, weight loss, and weight maintenance. Generally, people who follow a balanced vegetarian diet weigh less and have better cholesterol levels, fewer problems with irregular bowel movements (constipation and diarrhea), and a lower risk of heart disease than do nonvegetarians. A recent analysis of 29 studies involving a total of more than 20,000 participants found that people who follow a vegetarian diet have an average blood pressure several points lower than that of nonvegetarians.[46] Some studies suggest that vegetarianism may also reduce the risk of some cancers, particularly colon cancer.[47]

With proper meal planning, vegetarianism provides a healthful alternative to a meat-based diet. Eating a variety of healthful foods throughout the day helps to ensure proper nutrient intake. Vegan diets are of greater concern than diets that include dairy products and eggs. Vegans may be deficient in vitamins $B_2$ (riboflavin), $B_{12}$, and D, as well as calcium, iron, zinc, and other minerals; however, many foods are fortified with these nutrients, or vegans can obtain them from supplements. Vegans also have to pay more attention to the amino acid content of their foods, but eating a variety of types of plant foods throughout the day will provide adequate amounts of protein. Pregnant women, older adults, sick people, and families with young children who are vegans need to take special care to ensure that their diets are adequate. In all cases, seek advice from a health care professional if you have questions.

## Supplements: Research on the Daily Dose

**Dietary supplements** are products containing one or more dietary ingredients taken by mouth and intended to supplement existing diets. Ingredients range from vitamins, minerals, and herbs to enzymes, amino acids, fatty acids, and organ tissues. They can come in tablet, capsule, liquid, powder, and other forms. A majority of Americans—68 percent—take at least one dietary supplement.[48] Among supplements users, 98 percent take vitamin/mineral supplements.[49]

It is important to note that dietary supplements are not regulated like foods or drugs. The FDA does not evaluate the safety and efficacy of supplements prior to their marketing, and it can take action to remove a supplement from the market only after the product has been proved harmful. Currently, the United States has no formal guidelines for supplement marketing and safety, and

WHAT DO **YOU** THINK?

Why are so many people becoming vegetarians?

- How easy is it to be a vegetarian on your campus?
- What concerns about vegetarianism do you have, if any?

supplement manufacturers are responsible for self-monitoring the safety and effectiveness of their products.

Do you really need to take dietary supplements? The Office of Dietary Supplements, part of the National Institutes of Health, states that some supplements may help ensure that you get adequate amounts of essential nutrients, but warns that supplements cannot take the place of a varied, healthful diet. They are also not intended to prevent or treat disease, and recently the U.S. Preventive Services Task Force concluded that there is insufficient evidence to recommend that healthy people take multivitamin/mineral supplements to prevent cardiovascular disease or cancer.[50] Those who may benefit from using multivitamin/mineral supplements include pregnant and breastfeeding women, older adults, vegans, people on a very low-calorie weight-loss diet, individuals dependent on alcohol, and patients with malabsorption problems or other significant health problems. On the other hand, many dietary supplements are unproven. The benefit of fish consumption in reducing the risk for cardiovascular disease is well established, for example, but studies have yielded conflicting results about fish-oil supplements.[51]

As noted earlier in this chapter, taking high-dose supplements of the fat-soluble vitamins, especially vitamin A, can be harmful or even fatal. You should also be aware that supplements can interact with certain medications, including aspirin, diuretics, and steroids, resulting in potential problems. Moreover, supplements often do not contain the ingredients listed on the label; in 2015, the New York State Office of the Attorney General required several national supplements retailers to cease selling a variety of herbal supplements found to entirely lack the ingredients indicated on the label and to be contaminated with plant products not identified on the label. Only 4 percent of the supplements tested from Walmart stores, for example, had DNA matching the plants identified on the ingredients list.[52]

If you do decide to take dietary supplements, choose brands that contain the U.S. Pharmacopeia or Consumer Lab seal. This ensures that the supplement is free of toxic ingredients and contains the ingredients stated on the label. Store your supplements in a dark, dry place (not the bathroom or other damp spots), make sure they are out of reach of small children, and check the expiration date.

## Eating Well in College

Many college students find it hard to fit a well-balanced meal into the day, but breakfast and lunch are important if you are to keep energy levels up and get the most out of your classes. Eating a complete breakfast that includes fiber-rich carbohydrates, protein, and healthy unsaturated fat (such as a banana, peanut butter, and whole-grain bread sandwich or a bowl of oatmeal topped with dried fruit and nuts) is key. If you are

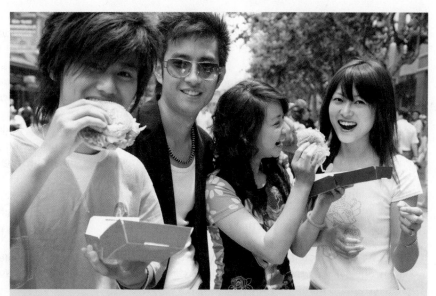

Meals like this one may be convenient, but they are high in saturated fat, sodium, and calories. Even when you are short on time and money, it is possible—and worthwhile—to make healthier choices. If you are ordering fast food, ask for lean meat, poultry, fish, or a vegetarian option prepared by grilling, baking, or roasting, not frying.

short on time, bring a container of plain yogurt and a handful of almonds to your morning class.

If your campus is like many others, your lunchtime options include a variety of fast-food restaurants. Generally speaking, you can eat more healthfully and for less money if you bring food from home or eat at your campus dining hall. If you must eat fast food, follow the tips below to get more nutritional bang for your buck:

- Ask for nutritional analyses of menu items. The FDA requires that most restaurants provide calorie and other nutritional information on menus or menu boards. Read, compare, and make the most nutrient-dense choices accordingly.
- Order salads, but be careful about what you add to them. Taco salads and Cobb salads are often high in fat, calories, and sodium. Ask for low-fat dressing on the side, and use it sparingly. Stay away from high-fat add-ons, such as bacon bits, croutons, and crispy noodles.
- If you crave french fries, try baked "fries," which are typically low in saturated fat.

**SEE IT! VIDEOS**

How accurate are restaurant calorie counts? Watch **Menu Calorie Counts**, available on **MasteringHealth.**™

ONLY 5.4%

of college students eat the recommended five or more servings of **FRUITS AND VEGETABLES** a day.

- Avoid large portion sizes. At one national chain, a large burger, fries, and cola add up to 1,320 calories, whereas a small burger, fries, and water total 470 calories—a difference of 850 calories!
- At Asian restaurants, avoid meats and vegetables swimming in sauces high in sugar and sodium. Also find out the sodium content of ramen, miso soup, and other dishes and ask if lower-sodium versions are available.
- At Mexican restaurants, order chicken or bean burritos or enchiladas, instead of beef, and ask that they be prepared with less cheese. Or order veggie fajitas with beans and rice for a meal high in plant protein and low in saturated fat.
- Out for pizza? You guessed it: order a veggie pizza with a whole-grain crust and request that it be prepared with less cheese or low-fat cheese.
- Wherever you dine, refrain from ordering extra sauce, bacon, cheese, and other toppings that add calories, saturated fat, and sodium.
- Limit sodas, shakes, and other beverages high in added sugars.
- If you typically order a burger, sandwich, or wrap with beef, swap for a chicken, turkey, fish, or vegetarian version.

In the dining hall, try these ideas:

- Choose lean meats, grilled chicken, fish, or vegetable dishes. Avoid fried chicken, fatty cuts of red meat, or meat dishes smothered in cream sauce.
- Hit the salad bar and load up on leafy greens, beans, tuna, or tofu. Choose items such as avocado or nuts for "good" fat. Go easy on the dressing, or substitute vinaigrette or low-fat dressings.
- Choose pasta dishes with vegetables (primavera) or with marinara (tomato) sauce rather than alfredo (cream) sauce or macaroni and cheese.
- Look for beans or lentils over brown rice with a variety of vegetables. Add a sprinkle of nuts or seeds for extra protein.
- Build yourself a veggie taco or burrito using black or red beans, vegetables, and a tablespoon of shredded cheese.
- When choosing items from a made-to-order food station, ask the preparer to hold the butter or oil, mayonnaise, sour cream, or cheese- or cream-based sauces.
- Avoid going back for seconds and consuming large portions.
- If there is something you'd like but don't see in your dining hall, speak to your food service manager and provide suggestions.
- Pass on foods high in added sugars and saturated fats, such as sugary cereals, ice cream, and other sweet treats. Choose fruit over plain yogurt to satisfy your sweet tooth.

Between classes, avoid vending machines. Reach into your backpack for an apple, banana, some dried fruit and nuts, a single serving of unsweetened applesauce, or whole-grain crackers spread with peanut butter. Energy bars can be a nutritious option if you choose right. Check the Nutrition Facts label for bars that are below 200 calories and provide at least 3 grams of dietary fiber. Cereal bars usually provide less protein than energy bars; however, some are low in added sugars and high in fiber.

Maintaining a nutritious diet within the confines of a typical college student's budget can be challenging. The **Money & Health** box identifies ways to include fruits and vegetables in your diet without breaking the bank.

## LO 4 | FOOD SAFETY: A GROWING CONCERN

**Explain food safety concerns facing Americans and people in other regions of the world.**

Eating unhealthy food is one thing. Eating food that has been contaminated with a pathogen, toxin, or other harmful substance is quite another. As outbreaks of foodborne illness (commonly called food poisoning) make the news, the food industry has come under fire. The Food Safety Modernization Act, passed into law in 2011, included new requirements for food processors to take actions to prevent contamination of foods. The act gave the FDA greater authority to inspect food-manufacturing facilities and to recall contaminated foods.[53]

## Choosing Organic or Locally Grown Foods

Concerns about the health effects of chemicals used to grow and produce food have led many people to turn to foods and beverages that are **organic**—produced without the use of toxic and persistent pesticides or fertilizers, antibiotics, hormones, irradiation, or genetic modification. Any food sold in the United States as organic has to meet criteria set by the USDA under the National Organic Rule and can carry a USDA seal verifying products as "certified organic." Under this rule, a product that is certified may carry one of the following terms:

- "100 percent Organic" (100% compliance with organic criteria)
- "Organic" (must contain at least 95% organic materials)
- "Made with Organic Ingredients" (must contain at least 70% organic ingredients)
- "Some Organic Ingredients" (contains less than 70% organic ingredients—usually listed individually).

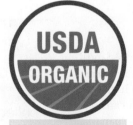

USDA label for organic foods.

**organic** Grown without use of toxic and persistent pesticides, chemicals, or hormones.

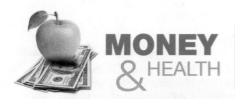

In contrast, the term *natural* on food labels is not currently regulated. However, the FDA is currently investigating concerns related to the use of the term and may shortly develop regulations on its use.[54]

The market for organic foods has been increasing faster than food sales in general for many years. Whereas only a small subset of the population once bought organic, 84 percent of all U.S. families now buy organic foods at least occasionally, and sales of organic foods represent nearly 5 percent of total food sales.[55] In 2015, annual organic food sales were estimated to be over $39 billion.[56]

Is organic food more nutritious? That depends on what aspect of the food is being studied and how the research is conducted. Two recent review studies, both of which examined decades of research into the nutrient quality of organic versus traditionally grown foods, reached opposite conclusions: One found organic foods more nutritious, and the other did not.[57]

Both of the studies just mentioned confirmed higher pesticide residues on conventionally grown produce. Pesticide exposure is a health risk because various types have been associated with significant adverse effects, from hormonal disorders to an increased risk for cancer.[58] The U.S. Environmental Protection Agency regulates pesticide use, and while ensuring Americans that only low levels of pesticide residue remain on conventionally grown foods, advises consumers to scrub

produce under running water and, if possible, peel it.[59]

The word **locavore** has been coined to describe people who eat mostly food grown or produced locally, usually within close proximity to their homes. Because these foods are transported only a few miles from farm to market, they are assumed to use fewer resources and cause the emission of a lower level of greenhouse gases, as well as to be fresher and to stay fresh longer after they're sold. Consumers should not assume, however, that these foods are organic, or that they are less likely to be contaminated with microorganisms. Pesticide residues and harmful bacteria can be found in foods shipped to markets from distant countries, as well as in foods purchased from local farms.[60]

## Foodborne Illnesses

Are you concerned that the chicken you are buying doesn't look pleasingly pink or your "fresh" fish smells a little *too* fishy? You may have good reason to be worried. The Centers for Disease Control and Prevention (CDC) estimates that foodborne

**SEE IT! VIDEOS**

Is organic produce better for you? Watch **Organic Produce**, available on **MasteringHealth.**™

**locavore** A person who primarily eats food grown or produced locally.

# TABLE 5.4 | Five Most Common Foodborne Illnesses

| Microbe | Illnesses per year | Description |
|---|---|---|
| Norovirus | 5.4 million | Transmitted through contact with the vomit or stool of infected people, norovirus is the most common cause of foodborne illness in the United States annually. Symptoms include nausea, vomiting, and diarrhea. Most cases are self-limiting, but about 800 Americans die of infection each year. There is no treatment, but washing hands and all kitchen surfaces can help prevent transmission. |
| *Salmonella* | 1 million | Commonly found in the intestines of birds, reptiles, and mammals, it can spread to humans through foods of animal origin. Infection by *Salmonella* usually consists of fever, diarrhea, and abdominal cramps. Salmonellosis can be life-threatening if the bacteria invade the bloodstream, as is more likely in people with poor health or weakened immune systems. |
| *Clostridium perfringens* | 966,000 | Bacterial species found in the intestinal tracts of humans and animals, as well as in the environment. Infection causes abdominal cramping and diarrhea. |
| *Campylobacter* | 845,000 | Most raw poultry has *Campylobacter* in it, and this bacterial infection most frequently results from eating undercooked chicken, raw eggs, or foods contaminated with juices from raw chicken. Shellfish and unpasteurized milk are also sources. Infection causes fever, diarrhea, and abdominal cramps. |
| *Staphylococcus aureus* | 241,000 | *Staph* lives on human skin, in infected cuts, and in the nose and throat. Infection causes severe nausea, vomiting, and diarrhea that lasts 1–3 days. |

Source: Data are from Centers for Disease Control and Prevention, CDC Estimates of Foodborne Illness in the United States, "CDC 2011 Estimates: Findings," Updated January 8, 2014, from www.cdc.gov/foodborneburden/2011-foodborne-estimates.html.

illnesses sicken 1 in 6 Americans (over 48 million people) and cause some 128,000 hospitalizations and 3,000 deaths in the United States annually.[61] Although the incidence of infection with certain microbes has declined, the incidence of infection with other microbes has risen or stayed essentially unchanged; thus, the CDC reports that foodborne infections are an ongoing public health concern requiring improved prevention.[62]

Several common types of microorganisms cause most foodborne infections and illnesses. **TABLE 5.4** lists the five most common culprits. Norovirus, by far the most common, shows up routinely on college campuses. A less common foodborne illness that is especially harmful during pregnancy and older adulthood is listeriosis, caused by the bacterium *Listeria monocytogenes*. About 1,600 cases occur annually, causing about 260 deaths.[63] About 14% of infections occur in pregnant women, and 58% occur in older adults.[64] Potential food sources include ready-to-eat foods such as hot dogs, luncheon meats, cold cuts and other deli meats, fermented or dry sausage, soft cheeses, and unpasteurized milk.[65] Illness from *Listeria* causes fever, chills, headache, abdominal pain, and diarrhea; a pregnant woman may experience miscarriage or stillbirth, and infection in older adults may be fatal.[66]

Foodborne illnesses can also be caused when a bacterium in the food secretes a toxin. These toxins resist heating and freezing, and therefore can produce illness even if the microbes that produced them have been destroyed. For example, the Staphylococcus bacterium produces an intestinal toxin that can cause

a self-limiting illness characterized by nausea, vomiting, and diarrhea. In contrast, *Clostridium botulinum*, another bacterium, produces the botulism toxin, which is the most deadly nerve toxin known. Botulism is rare, and most cases occur in home-canned vegetables; however, store-bought foods from

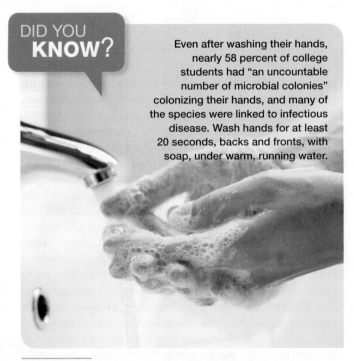

**DID YOU KNOW?**

Even after washing their hands, nearly 58 percent of college students had "an uncountable number of microbial colonies" colonizing their hands, and many of the species were linked to infectious disease. Wash hands for at least 20 seconds, backs and fronts, with soap, under warm, running water.

Source: Data are from K. J. Prater et al., "Poor Hand Hygiene by College Students Linked to More Occurrences of Infectious Diseases, Medical Visits, and Absence from Classes," *American Journal of Infection Control* 44, no. 1 (2016): 66–70.

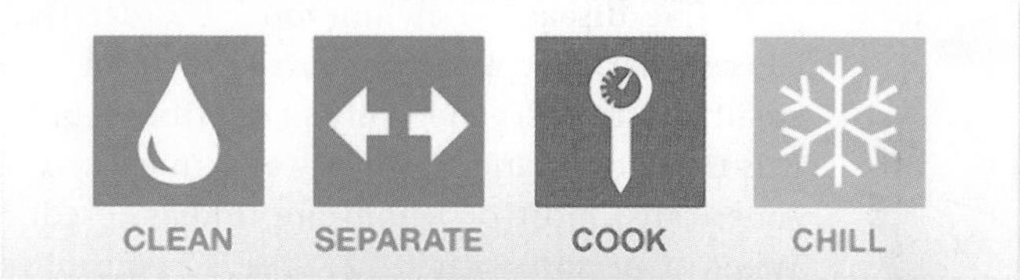

CLEAN    SEPARATE    COOK    CHILL

**FIGURE 5.10 The Four Core Practices** This logo reminds consumers how to prevent foodborne illness.

Source: Foodsafety.gov, "Check Your Steps," Accessed March 2016, www.foodsafety.gov/keep/basics/.

cans that are dented, pierced, leaking, or bulging may also harbor the botulism toxin.[67]

Signs of foodborne illnesses vary tremendously and usually include one or several symptoms: diarrhea, nausea, cramping, and vomiting. Depending on the amount and virulence of the pathogen, symptoms may appear as early as 30 minutes after eating contaminated food or as long as several days or weeks later. Most of the time, symptoms occur 5–8 hours after eating and last only a few hours to a day or two. For certain populations, such as the very young, older adults, or people with severe illnesses such as cancer, diabetes, kidney disease, or AIDS, foodborne diseases can be serious or even fatal.

Several factors contribute to foodborne illnesses, including inadequate oversight of both foreign and domestic suppliers by uncoordinated and underfunded federal agencies. Moreover, federal agencies can be slow to identify and respond to outbreaks.[68] The task, however, is enormous: Food can become contaminated in the field by contaminated irrigation water or runoff from nearby animal feedlots, or during harvesting if farm laborers have not washed their hands properly after using the toilet. Food-processing equipment, facilities, or workers may contaminate food, or it can become contaminated if not kept clean and cool during transport or on store shelves. The bacterium *Escherichia coli*, species of which produce a dangerous toxin, is present in unprocessed cow manure, which is commonly used as a fertilizer on both organic and conventional farms. Although its level drops significantly within 60 days, it can survive on fields for up to 120 days and can even be resuscitated after heavy rains.[69] No regulations prohibit farmers from using animal manure to fertilize crops. In addition, *E coli* quickly reproduces in summer months as cattle await slaughter in crowded, overheated pens. This increases the chances of meat coming to market already contaminated.

## Avoiding Risks in the Home

Although 75 percent of cases of foodborne illness are due to foods consumed in restaurants, delis, or banquet facilities, about 9 percent result from unsafe handling of food at home.[70] Four basic steps reduce the likelihood of contaminating your food (see **FIGURE 5.10**). Among the most basic precautions are to wash your hands and to wash all produce before eating it. Also, avoid cross-contamination in the kitchen by using separate cutting boards and utensils for meats, produce, and

breads. Temperature control is also important—refrigerators must be set at 40°F or lower. Cook meats to the recommended temperature to kill contaminants before eating. Keep hot foods hot and cold foods cold to avoid unchecked bacterial growth. Eat leftovers within 3 days, and if you're unsure how long something has been sitting in the fridge, don't take chances. When in doubt, throw it out. See the Making Changes Today box for more tips about reducing risk of foodborne illness.

**food allergy** Immune hypersensitivity response to normally harmless proteins in foods, prompting the production of antibodies, which triggers symptoms.

## MAKING **CHANGES** TODAY

### Reduce Your Risk for Foodborne Illness

- When shopping, put perishable foods in your cart last. Check for cleanliness throughout the store, especially at the salad bar and at the meat and fish counters. Never buy dented cans of food; report them to the store manager. Check the "sell by" or "use by" date on foods.

- Once you get home, put dairy products, eggs, meat, fish, and poultry in the refrigerator immediately. If you don't plan to eat meats within 2 days, freeze them. You can keep an unopened package of hot dogs or luncheon meats for about 2 weeks. Once the package is opened, you should use hotdogs within 1 week and luncheon meats within 5 days.

- When refrigerating or freezing raw meats, make sure their juices can't spill onto other foods.

- Never thaw frozen foods at room temperature. Put them in the refrigerator to thaw or thaw in the microwave, following manufacturer's instructions.

- Wash your hands with soap and warm water before preparing food. Wash fruits and vegetables before peeling, slicing, cooking, or eating them—but not meat, poultry, fish, or eggs! Wash cutting boards, countertops, and other utensils and surfaces with detergent and hot water after food preparation.

- Don't cross-contaminate. Dedicate one cutting board for meats, another for breads, and another for produce. Wash each after use in hot, soapy water. After a plate has held raw meat, wash it. Do not use it to carry cooked meat—or any other food—to the table.

- Use a meat thermometer to ensure that meats are completely cooked. To find out proper cooking temperatures for different types of meat, visit http://food-safety.gov/keep/charts/mintemp.html.

- Refrigeration slows the secretion of bacterial toxins into foods. Never leave leftovers out for more than 2 hours. On hot days, don't leave foods out for longer than 1 hour.

# Food Irradiation

Food irradiation is a process that exposes foods to low doses of radiation, or ionizing energy, to break down the DNA of

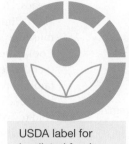

USDA label for irradiated foods.

harmful bacteria, destroying them or keeping them from reproducing. Essentially, the rays pass through the food without leaving any radioactive residue.[71]

Irradiation lengthens food products' shelf-life and prevents the spread of deadly microorganisms, particularly in high-risk foods such as ground beef and pork. Thus, the minimal costs of irradiation result in lower overall costs to consumers and reduce the need for toxic chemicals to preserve foods. Use of food irradiation is limited because of consumer concerns about safety and because irradiation facilities are expensive to build. Still, food irradiation is now common in over 40 countries. Foods that have been irradiated are marked with the "radura" logo.

## Food Sensitivities, Allergies, and Intolerances

Although many people today *think* they have a food allergy, it is estimated that only 5 percent of children and 4 percent of adults actually do.[72] A **food allergy**, or hypersensitivity, is an abnormal response to a component—usually a protein—in food that is triggered by the immune system. Symptoms of an allergic reaction vary in severity and may include a tingling sensation in the mouth; swelling of the lips, tongue, and throat; difficulty breathing; skin hives; vomiting; abdominal cramps; and diarrhea. A severe reaction called *anaphylaxis* can cause widespread inflammation, difficulty breathing, and cardiovascular problems such as a sudden drop in blood pressure that can be life-threatening.[73] Anaphylaxis may occur within seconds to hours after eating the foods to which one is allergic.

The Food Allergen Labeling and Consumer Protection Act (FALCPA) requires food manufacturers to label foods clearly to indicate the presence of (or possible contamination by) any of the eight major food allergens: milk, eggs, peanuts, wheat, soy, tree nuts (walnuts, pecans, cashews, pistachios, etc.), fish, and shellfish. Although over 160 foods have been identified as allergy triggers, these eight foods account for 90 percent of all food allergies in the United States.[74]

Peanuts are an excellent source of plant proteins and beneficial unsaturated fats, but they are among the eight most common food allergens.

**Celiac disease** is an immune disorder that causes malabsorption of nutrients from the small intestine in genetically susceptible people. It is thought to affect as many as 1 in every 141 Americans, most of whom are undiagnosed.[75] When a person with celiac disease consumes gluten—a protein found in wheat, rye, and barley—the person's immune system responds with inflammation. This degrades the lining of the small intestine and reduces nutrient absorption. Pain, abdominal cramping, diarrhea, constipation, nausea, vomiting, and other symptoms are common. Untreated, celiac disease can lead to long-term health problems, such as nutritional deficiencies, tissue wasting, osteoporosis, seizures, liver disease, and cancer of the small intestine. Blood tests and intestinal biopsies are used to diagnose celiac disease. Individuals who have been diagnosed are encouraged to consult a dietitian for help designing a gluten-free diet.

The mechanisms behind another disorder related to gluten are less clearly understood. Called *nonceliac gluten sensitivity*, it is diagnosed when an individual who has tested negative for celiac disease experiences any of a wide variety of symptoms, from abdominal bloating to diarrhea to joint pain, upon consumption of gluten—yet symptoms improve or resolve on a gluten-free diet.[76] See the **Health Headlines** box for more on gluten-free diets.

**Food intolerance** can cause you to have symptoms of digestive upset, but the upset is not the result of an immune system response. Probably the best example of a food intolerance is *lactose intolerance*, an inability to adequately digest the disaccharide lactose, which is in dairy products. The problem is common, although the number of Americans with the condition is unknown.[77] Lactase is an enzyme produced by the small intestine that helps break the bonds in the lactose molecule. If you don't have enough lactase, undigested lactose remains in the small intestine, drawing water by osmosis. This dilates the small intestine and speeds the transit of the food mass, resulting in diarrhea. When the undigested lactose reaches the large intestine, it is fermented by gut bacteria. Gas is formed, and the person experiences bloating and abdominal pain.

If you suspect that you have a food allergy, celiac disease, or a food intolerance, see your doctor. Because these diseases can have some common symptoms, as well as share symptoms with other gastrointestinal disorders, clinical diagnosis is essential.

## Genetically Modified Food Crops

Cultivation of genetically modified crops is expanding rapidly around the world. Genetic modification involves the insertion or deletion of genes into the DNA of an organism.

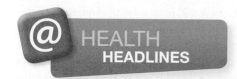
# GLUTEN-FREE DIETS

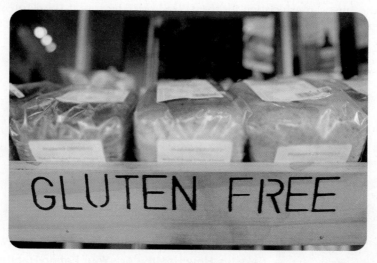

Gluten-free diets have become a fad. In a 5-year period ending in 2014, the sale of gluten-free products grew by more than 34 percent. According to a 2015 national poll, 1 in 5 Americans purchases gluten-free foods and 1 in 6 actively avoids foods with gluten. This is far more people than the number who have been clinically diagnosed with celiac disease or nonceliac gluten sensitivity (NCGS). Is this wise?

A gluten-free diet entirely excludes gluten, which is found in breads, cereals, and other grain products made with wheat, barley, and rye, as well as in many processed foods. The diet is highly restrictive, but for people with celiac disease, it is essential to survival.

In contrast, for people who do not have celiac or NCGS, a gluten-free diet does not provide any nutritional benefits over a varied diet containing gluten. In fact, many whole-grain foods that contain gluten provide more dietary fiber, vitamins, and minerals than gluten-free versions. These versions are often made with refined, unenriched sorghum and rice flours, which are low in essential nutrients and fiber and high in calories—not to mention expensive. In fact, people who follow a gluten-free diet may have inadequate intakes of several micronutrients, including iron, calcium, and the B vitamins riboflavin, thiamin, folate, and niacin.

If you have been diagnosed with celiac disease or NCGS, consult a dietitian for advice on avoiding gluten while still following a healthy eating pattern. Many nutritious foods are naturally free of gluten, including beans, peas, lentils, all other vegetables, fruits, nuts, seeds, all animal-based foods, and even several grains such as oats, cornmeal, brown rice, and quinoa. When buying foods on a gluten-free diet, fresh, unprocessed foods are the best choice. When buying packaged foods, look for the words "certified gluten-free." The FDA requires that, to use a gluten-free label, the product must contain less than 20 parts per million of gluten. For all other packaged foods, carefully study the ingredients list before buying, as many unfamiliar food ingredients contain gluten.

**Source:** Packaged Facts, *Gluten-free Foods and Beverages in the US*, 5th ed. (Rockville, MD: Packaged Foods, 2015), Available from www.packagedfacts.com/Gluten-Free-Foods-8108350/; R. Riffkin, "One in Five Americans Include Gluten-Free Foods in Diet," *Gallop, Inc.*, July 23, 2015, www.gallup.com/poll/184307/one-five-americans-include-gluten-free-foods-diet.aspx; S. J. Shepherd and P. R. Gibson, "Nutritional Inadequacies of the Gluten-free Diet in Both Recently-Diagnosed and Long-Term Patients with Celiac Disease," *Journal of Human Nutrition and Dietetics* 26, no. 4 (2013): 349–58.

In the case of **genetically modified (GM) foods**, usually this genetic cutting and pasting is done to enhance production, for example, by increasing a crop's tolerance to common herbicides (weed killers), making disease- or insect-resistant plants, or improving yield. In fact, GM crops grow faster and have average yields 22 percent higher than traditional crops, and thus are credited with contributing to the global decline in hunger prevalence since their widespread adoption in the 1990s.[78] In addition, GM foods are sometimes created to boost the level of specific nutrients. For example, currently under development is a GM variety of rice high in vitamin A and iron. Another use under development is the production and delivery of vaccines through GM foods.

The long-term safety of GM foods—for humans, other species, and the environment—is still in question. Although the genetic engineering of insect-resistant crops has reduced the use of insecticides, it has simultaneously increased the use of herbicides, leading to the evolution of so-called "superweeds," while also killing off beneficial weeds such as milkweed.[79] As a result, butterfly populations that depend on these weeds, particularly the monarch butterfly, have been decimated.[80] However, climate change and other factors have also contributed to the threat to monarchs. In addition, unintentional transfer of potentially allergy-provoking proteins has occurred, and although rigorous, validated tests of crops are performed to screen for known allergens, there is a potential for the transfer of new, unknown allergens.[81] Loss of crop diversity is another potential threat, as GM varieties of certain plants have been found several miles from

> **genetically modified (GM) foods** Foods derived from organisms whose DNA has been altered using genetic engineering techniques.

their origin. Moreover, monocultures—genetically identical crops—are far more vulnerable to climate events and plant diseases than diverse crops; thus, populations that depend on monocultures for food are at increased risk for food shortages.

Despite these concerns, the American Association for the Advancement of Science reports that foods containing GM ingredients are no more a risk than are the same foods composed of crops modified over time with conventional plant breeding techniques, and the World Health Organization states that no adverse effects on human health have been shown from consumption of GM foods in countries that have approved their use.[82] The debate surrounding GM foods is not likely to end soon.

# STUDY **PLAN**

Customize your study plan—and master your health!—in the Study Area of **MasteringHealth.**

## **ASSESS** YOURSELF

**Do you eat healthfully?** Want to find out?
Take the **How Healthy Are Your Eating Habits?** assessment available on
**MasteringHealth.**™

## CHAPTER **REVIEW**

To hear an MP3 Tutor Session, scan here or visit the Study Area in **MasteringHealth.**

### LO 1 | Essential Nutrients for Health

■ Nutrition is the science of the relationship between physiological function and the essential elements of the foods we eat. The Dietary Reference Intakes (DRIs) are recommended nutrient intakes for healthy people.

■ The essential nutrients include water, proteins, carbohydrates, fats, vitamins, and minerals. Water makes up 50–60 percent of our body weight and is necessary for nearly all life processes. Proteins are major components of our cells and tissues and are key elements of antibodies, enzymes, and hormones. Carbohydrates are our most readily available source of energy. Fiber is a non-digestible carbohydrate that enhances bowel function and reduces the risk for obesity, heart disease, and constipation. Fats provide energy while we are at rest

and for long-term activity. They also play important roles in maintaining body temperature, cushioning and protecting organs, and promoting healthy cell function. Unsaturated fats, including the essential fatty acids, are critical to health. Vitamins are organic compounds, and minerals are inorganic elements. We need these micronutrients in small amounts to maintain healthy body structure and function. Antioxidant nutrients and phytochemicals help protect the body from oxidative stress.

### LO 2 | Nutritional Guidelines

■ The *2015–2020 Dietary Guidelines for Americans* and the MyPlate graphic and website are tools developed by the U.S. Department of Health and Human Services and the U.S. Department of Agriculture to help Americans maintain a healthy diet and reduce their risk for obesity and chronic disease. The Guidelines emphasize following a healthy eating pattern across the lifespan; focusing on variety, nutrient density,

and amount; limiting calories from added sugars and saturated fats; reducing sodium; shifting to healthier choices; and supporting healthy eating patterns for all.

### LO 3 | How Can I Eat More Healthfully?

■ The Nutrition Facts label on packaged foods identifies the serving size, number of calories per serving, and amounts of various nutrients, as well as the %DV, which is the percentage of recommended daily values those amounts represent.

■ With a little menu planning, vegetarianism can be a healthful lifestyle choice, providing plenty of nutrients, plus fiber and phytochemicals, typically with less saturated fat and fewer calories.

■ Although some people may benefit from taking vitamin and mineral supplements, a healthy diet is the best way to give your body the nutrients it needs.

■ College students face unique challenges in eating healthfully. Learning to make better choices, to eat healthfully on a budget, and to eat nutritionally in the dorm are all possible when you use the information in this chapter.

## LO 4 | Food Safety: A Growing Concern

- Organic foods are grown and produced without the use of toxic and persistent synthetic pesticides, fertilizers, antibiotics, hormones, or genetic modification. The USDA offers certification of organic farms and regulates claims regarding organic ingredients used on food labels.

- Foodborne illnesses sicken over 48 million Americans each year. They can be traced to contamination of food at any point from fields to the consumer's kitchen. Viruses, bacteria, and bacterial toxins are the most common culprits. To keep food safe at home, follow four steps: clean, separate, cook, and chill.

- A food allergy is an immune hypersensitivity response to a component, usually a protein, in a food. Celiac disease is characterized by erosion of the lining of the small intestine because of an immune response to gluten, a protein in wheat, rye, and barley. Food intolerances such as lactose intolerance are caused by an inability to adequately digest a component of a food.

- Genetically modified (GM) crops grow faster on average and have higher yields, factors that have helped reduce global hunger. Nevertheless, health and environmental concerns—including generation of superweeds, potential loss of crop diversity, and negative effects on other species—remain.

## POP QUIZ

Visit **MasteringHealth** to personalize your study plan with Chapter Review Quizzes and Dynamic Study Modules.

### LO 1 | Essential Nutrients for Health

1. Which of the following nutrients is most critical for the growth, repair, and maintenance of body tissues?

   a. Carbohydrates
   b. Proteins
   c. Essential fatty acids
   d. Vitamins

2. Which of the following substances helps move food through the intestinal tract?

   a. Folate
   b. Fiber
   c. Glycogen
   d. Starch

3. What substance provides energy, promotes healthy skin and hair, insulates body organs, helps maintain body temperature, and contributes to healthy cell function?

   a. Fats
   b. Fibers
   c. Proteins
   d. Carbohydrates

4. Which of the following fats is the most healthful?

   a. *Trans* fat
   b. Saturated fat
   c. Unsaturated fat
   d. Partially hydrogenated oils

5. Which vitamin helps maintain bone health?

   a. $B_{12}$
   b. D
   c. $B_6$
   d. Niacin

### LO 2 | Nutritional Guidelines

1. Which of the following foods or beverages is the most *nutrient-dense*?

   a. Low-fat milk
   b. Cheddar cheese
   c. Chocolate milk
   d. Fruit-flavored yogurt

2. The *2015–2020 Dietary Guidelines for Americans* recommend that you

   a. stop smoking and walk daily.
   b. consume one alcoholic beverage a day.
   c. follow an eating pattern low in total fat and cholesterol.
   d. limit your intake of added sugars, saturated fats, and sodium.

### LO 3 | How Can I Eat More Healthfully?

1. The %DV on a Nutrition Facts label tells you

   a. the Dietary Reference Intake for the particular food component.
   b. how much of your daily need for a particular food component is met by the food in the package.
   c. how much of an average adult's allowance for a particular food component is provided by one serving of the food.
   d. the relative level (high, low, etc.) of a specific component (fiber, sodium, etc.) in a food.

2. Carrie eats dairy products and eggs, but she does not eat fish, poultry, or meat. Carrie is considered a(n)

   a. vegan.
   b. lacto-ovo-vegetarian.
   c. ovo-vegetarian.
   d. pesco-vegetarian.

### LO 4 | Food Safety: A Growing Concern

1. Lucas's doctor diagnoses him with celiac disease. Which of the following foods must Lucas avoid?

   a. Shellfish
   b. Milk
   c. Peanut butter
   d. Whole-wheat bread

*Answers to the Pop Quiz can be found on page A-1. If you answered a question incorrectly, review the section tagged by the Learning Outcome. For even more study tools, visit* **MasteringHealth**.

## THINK ABOUT IT!

### LO 1 | Essential Nutrients for Health

1. Which factors influence a person's dietary patterns and behaviors? What factors have been the greatest influences on your eating behaviors?

2. What are the six types of nutrients that you need to obtain from your diet? What are their most important functions? For each of the six nutrients, list one particularly healthful food or beverage high in that nutrient.

## LO 2 | Nutritional Guidelines

3. State the first key guideline from the *2015–2020 Dietary Guidelines for Americans*. Explain the role of nutrient density in following this guideline.

4. Identify the major food groups in the MyPlate plan. From which groups do you eat too few servings? What can you do to increase your intake of these foods?

## LO 3 | How Can I Eat More Healthfully?

5. Distinguish among varieties of vegetarianism. Which types are most likely to lead to nutrient deficiencies, and which are the nutrients of concern? How can a strict vegetarian consume enough of these nutrients?

6. What are the major problems you face when trying to eat right? List five actions that you and your classmates could take immediately to improve your eating.

## LO 4 | Food Safety: A Growing Concern

7. Imagine you're preparing a barbecue of grilled chicken and salad for friends. What four steps should you take to reduce your risk for foodborne illnesses?

8. How does a food intolerance differ from a food allergy?

# ACCESS YOUR HEALTH ON THE INTERNET

Visit **MasteringHealth** for links to the websites and RSS feeds.

The following websites explore further topics and issues related to nutrition.

**Academy of Nutrition and Dietetics.** The academy provides information on a full range of nutrition topics; the site also links to scientific publications and information on scholarships and public meetings. **www.eatright.org**

**U S. Food and Drug Administration (FDA).** The FDA provides information about food labeling, food safety, supplements, and many other topics. It also provides links to other sources of nutrition information. **www.fda.gov**

**Food and Nutrition Information Center.** This site offers a wide variety of information related to food and nutrition. **http://fnic.nal.usda.gov**

**National Institutes of Health, Office of Dietary Supplements.** This is the site of the International Bibliographic Database of Information on Dietary Supplements (IBDIDS), updated quarterly. **http://dietary-supplements. info.nih.gov**

**U S. Department of Agriculture, USDA: Choose MyPlate.** Use this site to design a personalized diet and physical activity plan based on the MyPlate program, and find sample menus, recipes, and tips for healthy eating. **www.choosemyplate.gov**

**U S. Department of Health and Human Services: Food Safety.** This is the federal government's official gateway to food safety information, including recalls and alerts, news, and more. **www.foodsafety.gov**

# 6 Reaching and Maintaining a Healthy Weight

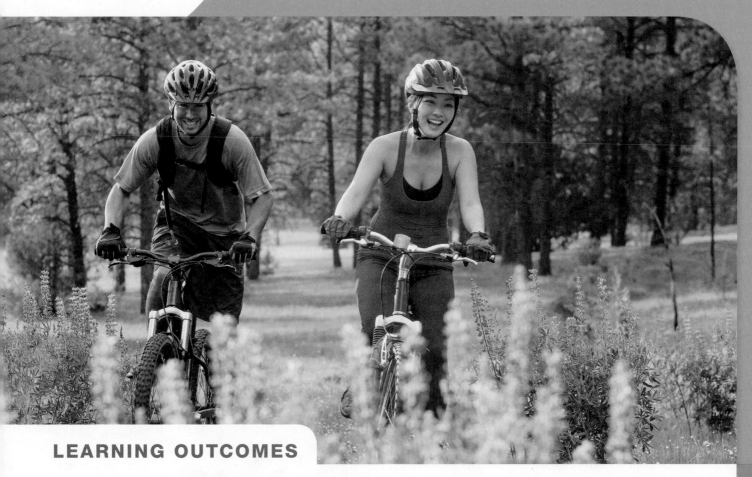

## LEARNING OUTCOMES

**LO 1** Describe the current epidemic of overweight/obesity in the United States and globally and the health risks associated with excess weight.

**LO 2** Describe factors that put people at risk for overweight and obesity, distinguishing between controllable and uncontrollable factors.

**LO 3** Learn reliable options for determining a healthy weight and body fat percentage.

**LO 4** Explain the effectiveness and potential pros/cons of various weight control strategies, including exercise, diet, lifestyle modification, supplements/diet drugs, surgery, and other options.

The United States is currently among the fattest developed nations on Earth. Young and old, rich and poor, rural and urban, educated and uneducated, Americans share one thing in common—they are fatter than virtually all previous generations.[2] The word **obesogenic** refers to environmental conditions that promote obesity, such as the availability and marketing of unhealthy foods, social and cultural norms that lead to high calorie consumption, and lack of physical activity—an apt descriptor of our society.

## LO 1 | OVERWEIGHT AND OBESITY: A GROWING CHALLENGE

Describe the current epidemic of overweight/obesity in the United States and globally and the health risks associated with excess weight.

Categorized by *class* (reflecting both severity and increasing risks based on percent body fat), **obesity** refers to a body weight that is more than 20 percent above recommended levels for health, or a **body mass index (BMI)**—a description of body weight relative to height that we cover in more depth later—over 30. *Class 1 obesity* refers to those with a BMI ≥30 but less than 35. *Class 2 obesity* includes those with a BMI of ≥35 but less than 40, and *Class 3 obesity* includes those with a BMI ≥40, often referred to as *morbidly obese*.[3] Less extreme, but still damaging, is *overweight*, which is body weight more than 10 percent above healthy levels or a BMI between 25 and 29.

**obesogenic** Refers to environmental conditions that promote obesity, such as the availability of unhealthy foods, social and cultural norms that lead to high calorie consumption, and lack of physical activity.

**obesity** Having a body weight more than 20 percent above healthy recommended levels; in an adult, a BMI of 30 or more.

**body mass index (BMI)** A number calculated from a person's weight and height that is used to assess risk for possible present or future health problems.

## Overweight and Obesity in the United States

**FIGURE 6.1** illustrates just how high levels of obesity have risen in the United States, as a percentage of the population, since the 1960s. Indeed, the prevalence of obesity has steadily increased in recent decades, with disproportionate risks among some populations.[4] Children aged 2 to 5 have shown slight decreases overall in prevalence in recent years; however rates remain high with over 17

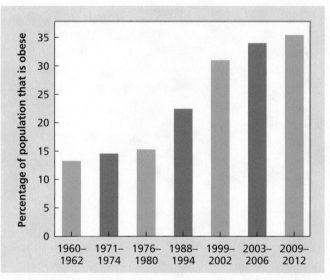

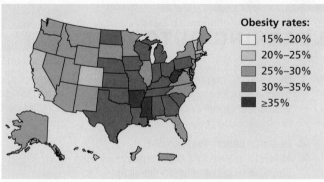

Obesity rates:
- 15%–20%
- 20%–25%
- 25%–30%
- 30%–35%
- ≥35%

**FIGURE 6.1** Obesity in the United States

**Sources:** Centers for Disease Control and Prevention, "Health, United States, 2014, Table 64, Healthy weight, overweight, and obesity among adults aged 20 and over, by selected characteristics: United States, selected years 1960–1962 through 2009–2012," 2014, www.cdc.gov/nchs/data/hus/2014/064.pdf; Centers for Disease Control and Prevention, "Prevalence of Self-Reported Obesity Among U.S. Adults by State and Territory, BRFSS, 2014," September 2015, www.cdc.gov/obesity/data/prevalence-maps.html.

percent of children and adolescents being obese and 5.8 percent extremely obese.[5] Children and adolescents living in low-income, low-education, and higher-unemployment homes are at significantly greater risk of developing obesity, while those from higher-income homes with more educated parents have decreasing risk.[6]

Unfortunately, in spite of massive efforts aimed at prevention of obesity, new research indicates that the epidemic of obesity is worsening. According to the latest statistics, nearly 37 percent of U.S adults are now obese and another 33 percent are overweight, meaning we've reached the highest obesity levels in history in the United States. Rates of obesity are particularly high among women, rising to over 40 percent in the last decade. Men are not far behind with rates of obesity slightly over 35%.[7] More than 5% of men and 10% of women are now morbidly obese..[8]

Research points to higher obesity rates and risks among some ethnic groups in the United States. Hispanic men (80 percent) and non-Hispanic white men (73 percent) are more likely to be overweight/obese than are non-Hispanic black men (69 percent).[9] Non-Hispanic black women (82 percent) and Hispanic women (76) percent) are more likely to be overweight or obese than are non-Hispanic white women (61 percent).[10] In sharp contrast, between 51 and 68 percent of Asian populations are at a healthy weight.[11]

**WHAT DO YOU THINK?**

Can you think of factors in your particular environment that are contributing to your own risks for obesity? Risks of your family and friends?

- What actions could you take to combat them?
- What could be done on your campus to help make weight control easier for students?

## An Obesogenic World

The United States is not alone in the obesity epidemic. In fact, obesity has more than doubled globally since 1980, with over 1.9 billion overweight and 600 million obese adults.[12] While obesity was once predominantly a problem in high-income countries, today increasing numbers of low- and middle-income countries have overweight/obesity problems.[13] The global epidemic of high rates of overweight and obesity in multiple regions of the world has come to be known as **globesity**. See the **Health in a Diverse World** box on page 154 for more on this epidemic.

## Health Risks of Excess Weight

Although smoking is still the leading cause of preventable death in the United States, obesity is rapidly gaining ground. Cardiovascular diseases, such as diseases of the heart, stroke and hypertension, certain cancers, diabetes, digestive problems, gallstones, sleep apnea, depression, osteoarthritis, and other ailments lead the list of life-threatening, weight-related problems. **FIGURE 6.2** on page 155 summarizes these and other potential health consequences of obesity.

Consider the following facts about specific risks for obese individuals compared to their nonobese counterparts:[14]

- They have a 104 percent increase in risk of heart failure.
- BMI greater than 30 reduces their life expectancy by 2 to 4 years.
- BMI greater than 40 costs 8 to 10 years of life expectancy—similar to a long-term smoker.
- Nearly 55 percent of obese children are still obese in adolescence; 80 percent of obese adolescents will be obese adults—with 70 percent of those continuing to be obese after age 30.[15]

Diabetes, strongly associated with overweight and obesity, is another major concern. Over 29 million Americans have diabetes, and another 86 million adults have prediabetes.[16] **Focus On: Minimizing Your Risk for Diabetes** on page 446 discusses the devastating effects of obesity on diabetes-related risks and the benefits of prevention. (See the **Money & Health** box on page 156 for information on the costs of obesity.)

CVD and chronic, killer diseases are not the only risks associated with overweight and obesity. The costs of social isolation, bullying in school, stigmatization, discrimination, and diminished quality of life can also be devastating. Obese individuals suffer more major disability and difficulty with activities of daily living (ADLs) than do their nonobese counterparts. They are also more likely to experience falls and injury, with the exception of morbidly obese individuals—who may fall less—perhaps because they are less active, and seem to be less prone to injury when they fall.[17]

## LO 2 | FACTORS CONTRIBUTING TO OVERWEIGHT AND OBESITY

Describe factors that put people at risk for overweight and obesity, distinguishing between controllable and uncontrollable factors.

The reasons for our soaring rates of overweight and obesity are complex, and not all of them are within easy individual control. Although diet and exercise are two major contributors, other factors, including genetics and physiology, are also important. Newer thinking regarding reducing obesity risk involves a more ecological approach that seeks to change obesogenic environmental and contextual factors. Learned behaviors in the home; influences at school and in social environments; media influences; and the environments where we live, work, and play are important to our weight profiles.[18]

## Physiological, Genetic, and Hormonal Factors

Are some people born to be fat? Obese people may be more likely than thin people to satisfy their appetite and eat for reasons other than nutrition. In fact, obesity appears to involve

**globesity** Global rates of obesity.

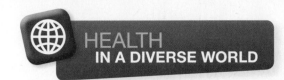
# THE EMERGING CRISIS OF GLOBESITY

According to a newly published report by the International Commission on Ending Childhood Obesity, the obesity epidemic may in fact have the potential to cancel out many of the health benefits that have contributed to longer life expectancy around the world.

Just how bad is the problem? Since 1980, worldwide obesity has more than doubled, with nearly 2 billion (39 percent) of adults 18 years and older being overweight and millions more being obese or severely obese. Unfortunately, in spite of efforts to combat the burgeoning waistlines of the world, things are getting worse, with increases in both rich and poor countries, among young and old alike, among the educated and uneducated, and among nearly all racial/ethnic groups. Consider these global statistics:

- Overweight and obesity are responsible for more deaths globally than underweight.
- One in 10 men and 1 in 7 women in the world today are obese; at current

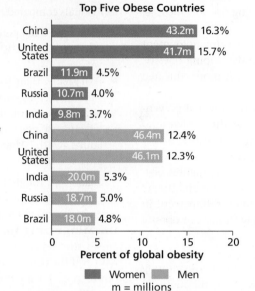

**Top Five Obese Countries**

This figure shows some of the world's most obese countries. What factors do you think influence average weights in these nations? If we continue at our current rate, what do you think this figure will look like in another decade?

rates, by 2025, 18 percent of men and 21 percent of women are projected to be obese.

- In the last 40 years, we have gone from a world where underweight was nearly twice as common as overweight, to one where obesity prevalence is more common than underweight.
- Among high-income countries, Japanese adults have the lowest BMIs, whereas the U.S. and China have the highest BMIs overall and the most obese people.
- In India and Bangledesh, one-fifth of men and one-fourth of women are underweight.

And, among youth, the picture is bleak.

- In 2014, an estimated 41 million children under the age of 5 years were affected by overweight or obesity.
- In Africa, the number of overweight or obese children has grown by almost 100 percent since 1990, to 10.3 million up from 5.4 million. In 2014, of children under 5 years of age who were overweight, 48 percent lived in Asia and 25 percent in Africa.

**Sources:** NCD Risk Factor Collaboration, "Trends in adult body-mass index in 200 countries from 1975 to 2014: a pooled analysis of 1698 population-based measurement studies with 19.2 million participants," *The Lancet* 387, no. 10026 (2016): 1377–96; R. Dobbs et al., "How the world could better fight obesity," *Mckinsey Global Institute,* November 2014, www.mckinsey.com/industries/healthcare-systems-and-services/our-insights/how-the-world-could-better-fight-obesity; WHO, "Obesity and Overweight: Fact Sheet," January 2015, www.who.int/mediacentre/factsheets/fs311/en/#.

**satiety** The feeling of fullness or satisfaction at the end of a meal.

In spite of decades of research, the exact role of genes in one's predisposition toward obesity remains in question. Countless observational studies back up the theory that fat parents tend to have fat children. Whether that is due to learned eating and exercise behaviors, environmental cues, genes, or a combination is unclear. Early support for a genetic basis for obesity came from twin research where adopted individuals tended to be similar in weight to their biological parents and identical twins were twice as likely to weigh the same as were fraternal twins, even if they were raised separately. These studies suggest that genes may contribute significantly (as much as 50 to 90 percent) to adiposity—severe or morbid overweight.[20]

### FTO, Ghrelin, and Leptin: Genes and Hormones at Work?
New research suggests that there is a genetic basis for our appetite and that some people inherit

complex genetic, hormonal, physiological, and environmental interactions.[19]

a lower sensitivity to **satiety**, or feeling full.[21] As such, some people may be more prone to grazing and food cravings than others. One in particular, the *fat mass and obesity-associated (FTO) gene,* may be among the most important.[22] Much research has centered on the role of genes such as FTO on regulating *ghrelin*—a hormone shown to play a key role in determining appetite and food intake control (particularly in controlling satiety), gastrointestinal motility, gastric acid secretion, endocrine and exocrine pancreatic secretions, glucose and lipid metabolism, and cardiovascular and immunological processes.[23]

Another hormone that has gained increased attention and research is *leptin,* an appetite regulator produced by fat cells in mammals. As fat tissue increases, levels of leptin in the blood increase, and when levels of leptin in the blood rise, appetite drops. Scientists believe leptin serves as a form of "adipostat" that signals you are getting full, slows food intake, and promotes energy. When leptin levels are low, researchers believe that people will be more prone to overeating and weight gain.

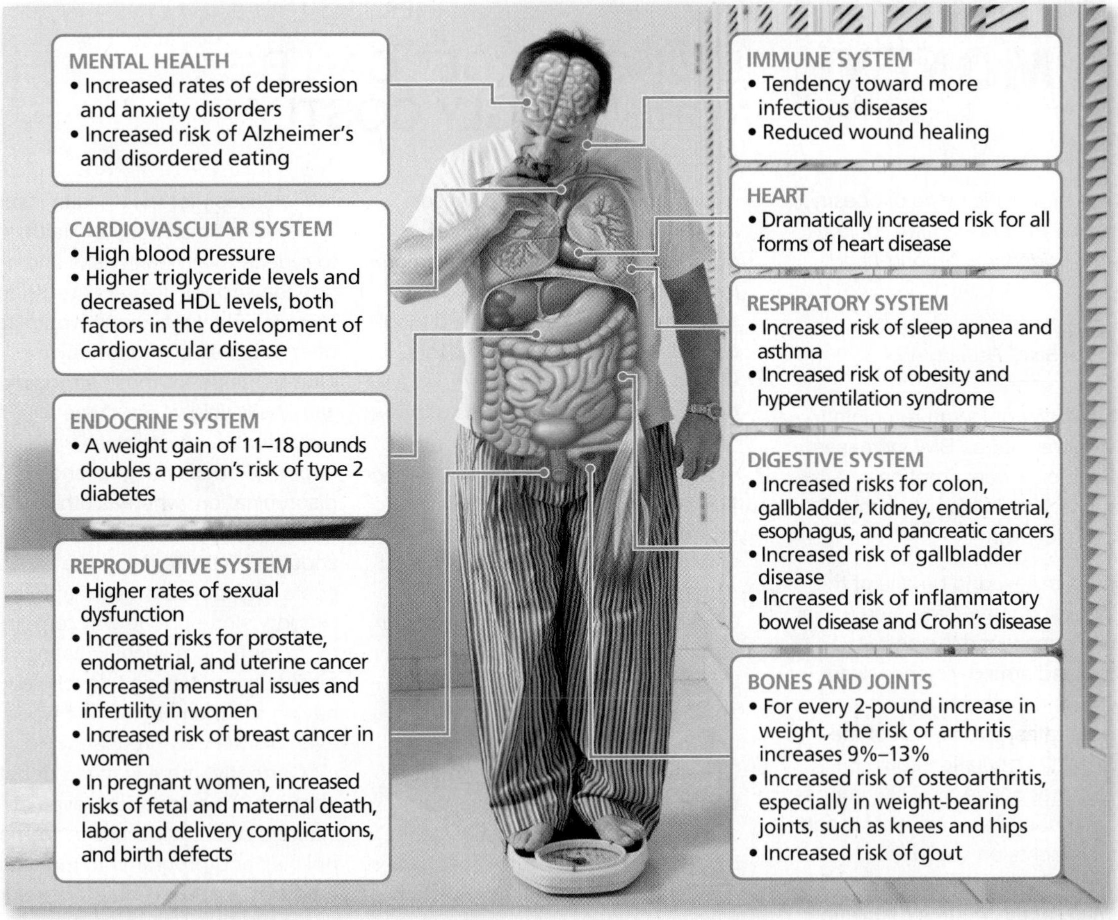

**FIGURE 6.2** Potential Negative Health Effects of Overweight and Obesity

**MENTAL HEALTH**
- Increased rates of depression and anxiety disorders
- Increased risk of Alzheimer's and disordered eating

**CARDIOVASCULAR SYSTEM**
- High blood pressure
- Higher triglyceride levels and decreased HDL levels, both factors in the development of cardiovascular disease

**ENDOCRINE SYSTEM**
- A weight gain of 11–18 pounds doubles a person's risk of type 2 diabetes

**REPRODUCTIVE SYSTEM**
- Higher rates of sexual dysfunction
- Increased risks for prostate, endometrial, and uterine cancer
- Increased menstrual issues and infertility in women
- Increased risk of breast cancer in women
- In pregnant women, increased risks of fetal and maternal death, labor and delivery complications, and birth defects

**IMMUNE SYSTEM**
- Tendency toward more infectious diseases
- Reduced wound healing

**HEART**
- Dramatically increased risk for all forms of heart disease

**RESPIRATORY SYSTEM**
- Increased risk of sleep apnea and asthma
- Increased risk of obesity and hyperventilation syndrome

**DIGESTIVE SYSTEM**
- Increased risks for colon, gallbladder, kidney, endometrial, esophagus, and pancreatic cancers
- Increased risk of gallbladder disease
- Increased risk of inflammatory bowel disease and Crohn's disease

**BONES AND JOINTS**
- For every 2-pound increase in weight, the risk of arthritis increases 9%–13%
- Increased risk of osteoarthritis, especially in weight-bearing joints, such as knees and hips
- Increased risk of gout

> VIDEO TUTOR
> Obesity Health Effects

For unknown reasons, obese people seem to have excess ghrelin production and faulty leptin receptors, although the exact reasons why these hormones function improperly is not clear. It may be that environmental and psychological cues are stronger than biological signals in some individuals.[24] Specifically, people with certain genetic variations may tend to graze for food more often, eat more meals, and consume more calories every day, as well as display patterns of seeking out high-fat food groups. Also, different genes may influence weight gain at certain periods of life, particularly during adolescence and young adulthood.[25] Rather than acting individually, the effects of the genes may be in clusters, influencing the regulation of food intake through action in the central nervous system, as well as influencing fat cell synthesis and functioning.

So, if your genes play a key role in obesity tendencies, are you doomed to a lifelong battle with your weight? Probably not. A healthy lifestyle may be able to override "obesity" genes. Results of a recent study of 5,079 adult twin pairs indicates that physical activity suppresses genetic variability in BMI, indicating that exercise may override genetic influences on risk of obesity.[26]

### Are You Thrifty or a Spendthrift?: Impact on Weight Loss
Another potential genetic basis for obesity was identified as a result of observational studies of certain Native American and African tribes. Labeled the *thrifty gene theory*, researchers noted higher body fat and obesity levels in some of these tribes than in the general population.[27] Because their ancestors struggled through centuries of famine, members of the tribes appear to have survived by adapting metabolically to periods of famine with slowed metabolism. Over time, ancestors may have passed on a genetic, hormonal, physiological/biological, or metabolic predisposition toward fat storage that makes losing fat more difficult.

New research appears to support the theory that the ease with which one person loses weight and another hangs on to it may be influenced by individual biology. In a carefully controlled lab study, 12 obese men and women were asked to fast for one day and remain as inpatients for 6 weeks, consuming

## OVER 60%
of college students are at **HEALTHY WEIGHT**. Nearly 23% are overweight, over 16% are obese, and just over 4% are underweight.

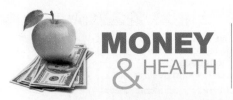

## MONEY & HEALTH | "LIVING LARGE" CAN BE INCREASINGLY COSTLY

*The startling economic costs of obesity, often borne by the non-obese, could become the epidemic's second-hand smoke.*

—Sharon Begley, "As America's Waistline Expands, Costs Soar," Reuters, April 30, 2012

A large body of literature points to evidence that as BMI increases, health care consumption and associated costs also increase. Consider the following:

- Obesity is believed to be one of the three largest human-generated social burdens in the world, along with smoking and armed violence, war, and terrorism.
- At current rates, almost half of the world's adult population could be overweight or obese by 2030, imposing tremendous personal, social, and economic costs on society.
- More than 2.1 billion people, almost 30 percent of the world's population, are overweight or obese—more than 2.5 times the number of people who are undernourished.
- Obesity is responsible for nearly 5 percent of all the deaths each year globally. Its economic impact hits international gross domestic product hard, costing nearly $2.0 trillion— right up there with smoking ($2.1 trillion), armed violence ($2.1 trillion), war and terrorism ($2.1 trillion), and alcoholism ($1.4 trillion).
- Obese populations have a 36 percent higher annual health care cost than healthy-weight populations. Lifetime medical costs for major diseases increase by over 50 percent for obese individuals—twice that amount for severely obese. Longer hospital stays, recovery, and increased medications are all part of these costs.
- Obese populations incur 37 percent higher prescription drug costs than healthy-weight populations.
- Obese individuals miss nearly 2 days of work more than their healthy-weight counterparts, accounting for between 6.5 to 12.6 percent of total absenteeism costs each year.
- Obese individuals are more likely to suffer from "presenteeism" where they are less likely to be productive and have less stamina than their healthy-weight counterparts.
- Obesity may mean increased transportation costs for more fuel consumption and larger vehicles/seats, bigger ambulances, and other issues.
- A recent study of 150,000 Swedish brothers indicated that *being obese is as costly as not having an undergraduate degree*; an "obesity penalty" is equivalent to earning over 16 percent less than their normal-weight counterparts.

Many insurance companies are charging more for people who are overweight and refuse to participate in available "wellness" programs. In fact, the U.S. Patient Protection and Affordable Care Act has a provision that allows employers to charge obese workers significantly higher premiums (between 30 and 50 percent more in some cases!) for their health insurance if they don't make a good-faith effort to reduce their health risks and must provide support for services to help them lose weight. Some workplaces offer counseling and free gym memberships for those struggling with their weight. Are these fair? Many argue that such penalties unfairly reflect a form of obesity stigma and size discrimination, whereas others argue that those within a normal weight range shouldn't have to subsidize excess costs. Still others argue that this is a slippery slope on the way to paying more for factors such as eating high-fat foods and having high cholesterol, having too many beers in a week, or even unintended pregnancy.

Currently, there is much debate about these extra costs, even as many insurers and businesses implement policies and programs to motivate employees and members of insurance groups to take action, "or else."

**Sources:** A. Dee et al., "The Direct and Indirect Costs of Both Overweight and Obesity: A Systematic Review," *BMC Research Notes* 7, no. 1 (2014): 242; T. Andreyeva et al., "State-Level Estimates of Obesity-Attributable Costs of Absenteeism," *Journal of Occupational and Environmental Medicine* 56, no. 11 (2014): 1120–7; P. Lunderg et al., "Body Size, Skills and Income: Evidence from 150,000 Teenage Siblings," *Demography* 51, no. 5 (2014): 1573–96; C. Roberts et al., "Patchy Progress on Obesity Prevention: Emerging Examples, Entrenched Barriers and New Thinking," *The Lancet* 385, no. 9985 (2015): 2400–9; McKinsey & Company, "How the World Could Better Fight Obesity," November 2014, www.mckinsey.com/insights/economic_studies/how_the_world_could_better_fight_obesity.

50 percent of their normal calories each day. Those who lost the least during the time period were those whose metabolism slowed down significantly in response to caloric restriction.[28] These individuals have what researchers refer to as *thrifty metabolism*. In contrast, those with tendency toward a *spendthrift metabolism* had metabolisms that kept chugging along when caloric intake decreased, losing significantly more weight than the thrifty group. Researchers are unsure whether these responses to dieting have a genetic basis or develop over time in individuals. Regardless, it appears that some obese individuals may have a harder time losing weight than others and that fasting and other extreme low-calorie diets may actually slow your metabolism, offsetting potential weight loss.

### Metabolic Rates

Several other aspects of your metabolism also help determine whether you gain, maintain, or lose weight. Each of us has an innate energy-burning capacity called **basal metabolic rate (BMR)**—the minimum rate at which the body uses energy to maintain basic vital functions. A BMR for the average, healthy adult is usually between 1,200 and 1,800 calories per day. Technically, to measure BMR, a

**basal metabolic rate (BMR)** The rate of energy expenditure by a body at complete rest in a neutral environment.

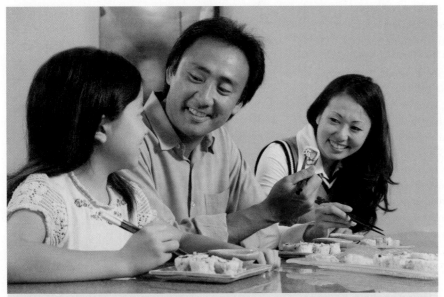

Many factors help determine weight and body type, including heredity and genetic makeup, hormones, environment, and learned eating patterns, which are often connected to family habits.

occurs during physical activity. For most of us, these calories come from light daily activities, such as walking, climbing stairs, and mowing the lawn.

Your BMR and RMR fluctuate through life, and are highest during infancy, puberty, and pregnancy. Generally, the younger you are, the higher your BMR, partly because cells undergo rapid subdivision during periods of growth, consuming lots of energy. After age 30, a person's BMR slows down 1 to 2 percent a year; older people commonly find an extra helping of ice cream harder to burn off. Slower BMR, coupled with less activity, age-related muscle loss, and shifting priorities from fitness to family and career obligations contribute to the weight gain of many middle-aged people.

Anyone who has ever lost weight only to reach a point at which, try as they might, they can't lose another ounce may be a victim of **adaptive thermogenesis,** whereby the body slows metabolic activity and energy expenditure as a form of defensive protection against possible starvation. With increased weight loss may come increased hunger sensations, slowed energy expenditure, and a tendency to regain weight or make further weight loss more difficult.[29]

person would be awake, but all major stimuli (including stressors to the sympathetic nervous system and digestion) would be at rest. Usually, the best time to measure BMR is after 8 hours of sleep and after a 12-hour fast.

A more practical way of assessing your energy expenditure levels is the **resting metabolic rate (RMR).** Slightly higher than the BMR, the RMR includes the BMR plus any additional energy expended through daily sedentary activities such as food digestion, sitting, studying, or standing. The **exercise metabolic rate (EMR)** accounts for the remaining percentage of all daily calorie expenditures and refers to the energy expenditure that

**Yo-yo diets** refer to when people cycle between periods of weight loss and gain. Typically, after weight loss, BMR is lower due to the fact that the body has less muscle mass and weight and requires less energy for basic functioning. When dieters resume eating after their weight loss, due to the related BMR decrease, calories burn more slowly, and they regain weight. Repeated cycles of dieting and regaining weight may actually increase the likelihood of getting heavier over time. Increased age and overall loss of muscle mass through inactivity also tend to result in lowered BMR.

On the other side of the BMR equation is **set point theory,** which suggests that our bodies fight to maintain weight around a narrow range or set point. If we go on a drastic starvation diet or fast, BMR slows to conserve energy. Set point theory, which suggests that our own bodies may sabotage our weight loss efforts by holding on to calories, explains why people tend to stay near a certain weight threshold and why moving to a different level of weight loss is difficult. The good news is that set points can be changed; however, these changes may take time to be permanent.

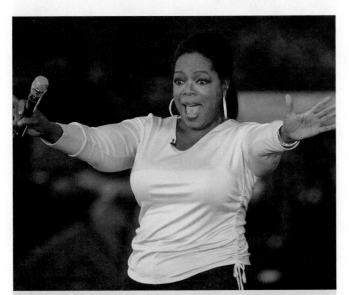

Oprah Winfrey, part owner and spokesperson for Weight Watchers, has been candid about her struggles with yo-yo dieting. Such a pattern disrupts the body's metabolism and makes future weight loss more difficult and permanent changes even harder to maintain.

## Fat Cells and Predisposition to Fatness

Some obese people may have excessive numbers of fat cells.

**resting metabolic rate (RMR)** The energy expenditure of the body under BMR conditions plus other daily sedentary activities.

**exercise metabolic rate (EMR)** The energy expenditure that occurs during exercise.

**adaptive thermogenesis** Theoretical mechanism by which the brain regulates metabolic activity according to caloric intake.

**yo-yo diets** Cycles in which people diet and regain weight.

**set point theory** Theory that a form of internal thermostat controls our weight and fights to maintain this weight around a narrowly set range.

**hyperplasia** A condition characterized by an excessive number of fat cells.

**hypertrophy** The act of swelling or increasing in size, as with cells.

Where an average-weight adult has approximately 25 to 35 billion fat cells and a moderately obese adult 60 to 100 billion, an extremely obese adult has as many as 200 billion.[30] This condition, often referred to as **hyperplasia**, usually appears in early childhood and perhaps, due to the mother's dietary habits, even prior to birth. The most critical periods for the development of hyperplasia are the last 2 to 3 months of fetal development, the first year of life, and the period between ages 9 and 13. Central to this theory is the belief that the number of fat cells in a body does not increase appreciably during adulthood. However, the ability of each of these cells to swell (**hypertrophy**) and shrink does carry over into adulthood. People with large numbers of fat cells may be able to lose weight by decreasing the size of each cell in adulthood, but with the next calorie binge, cells swell and sabotage weight-loss efforts. Weight gain may be tied to both the number of fat cells in the body and the capacity of individual cells to enlarge (**FIGURE 6.3**).

## Environmental Factors

Environmental factors have come to play a large role in weight maintenance. Automobiles, remote controls, desk jobs, and sedentary habits contribute to decreased physical activity and energy expenditure. Coupled with our culture of eating more, it's a recipe for weight gain.

**Greater Access to High-Calorie Foods** More foods that are high in calories and low in nutrients exist today compared to the past. Even though the new *Dietary Guidelines for Americans* (see Chapter 5) point to a need for more fruits and

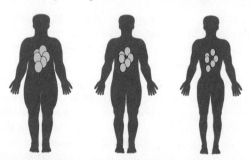

| | Before body weight reduction | Initial weight reduction | Second weight reduction |
|---|---|---|---|
| Body weight | 328 lb | 227 lb | 165 lb |
| Fat cell size | 0.9 µg/cell | 0.6 µg/cell | 0.2 µg/cell |
| Fat cell number | 75 billion | 75 billion | 75 billion |

**FIGURE 6.3** **One Person at Various Stages of Weight Loss** Note that, according to the hyperplasia theory, the number of fat cells remains constant, but their size decreases when weight is lost.

## OVER 34%

of children and adolescents in the United States get a significant portion of their nutrition from high-fat, high-carbohydrate, **PROCESSED FAST FOOD** each day.

vegetables in the diet, decreases in animal fats, and increases in healthy fats and other recommendations, Americans continue to fall short of these guidelines. Why do so many ignore sound dietary advice and go for the high-calorie options? There are many environmental factors that can prompt us to take the high-calorie path:

- Because of constant advertising, we are bombarded with messages to eat, eat, eat, and taste often trumps nutrition.
- Super-sized portions are now the norm (see the **Student Health Today** box), leading to increased calorie and fat intake.

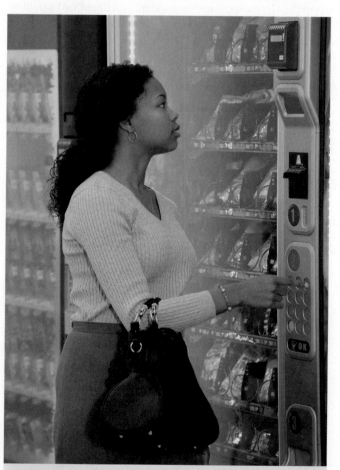

The easy availability of high-calorie foods, such as those found in most vending machines, is one of the environmental factors contributing to the obesity problem in the United States today.

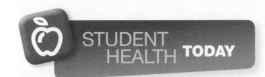

# BE WISE ABOUT SIZE
## *Flip Your Restaurant Priorities*

How many times have you ordered something at a restaurant and sat wide-eyed as the heaping dish is placed in front of you? For many, that "wow" response is synonymous with good restaurant ratings. A quick check on Trip Advisor or Yelp will clearly show "bigger is better" for many, with large portions being synonymous with good food value. But is that really the case?

Many researchers believe that the main reason Americans are gaining weight is that people no longer recognize a normal serving size. The National Heart, Lung, and Blood Institute has developed a pair of "Portion Distortion" quizzes that show how today's portions compare with those of 20 years ago. Test your knowledge of portion size online at www.nhlbi.nih.gov/health/educational/wecan/eat-right/portion-distortion.htm.

Of course, you can still get good value and be wise by flipping your perspective and following these simple strategies when you sit down for your next meal out

■ Check out the menu before you get to the restaurant. If you have to have a big portion, cut it in half and take a portion home for the next day. That way, you'll get two meals for the same price and it will really be a good value! Alternately, split an entrée with a friend and order a side salad for each of you. Decide before the food is put in front of you that you will cut the portion in half and not touch serving #2!

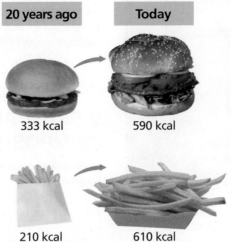

| 20 years ago | Today |
|---|---|
| 333 kcal | 590 kcal |
| 210 kcal | 610 kcal |

**Today's bloated portions.**

**Source:** Data are from National Heart, Lung, and Blood Institute, "Portion Distortion," Accessed April 1, 2015, www.nhlbi.nih.gov/health/educational/wecan/eat-right/portion-distortion.htm.

■ Be wise about size. More isn't better quality. Much of what you see as size is you being duped. Remember that many restaurants use less expensive filler foods (potatoes, rice, salad, bread) and cheaper cuts of meat and protein to make servings look larger and fill you up faster. That way you may not realize that your piece of chicken or other protein is small or tough, or that in that "all-you-can-eat" area, you're full to the brim way before the main course is served.

■ Think about taste and quality first, not portion size. Prioritize fresh, protein-rich foods, particularly those with unique tastes and seasonings. Think about combining two to three different appetizers or tapas into a meal, choosing things that are healthy. Happy-hour menus can allow you to combine some smaller plates and save money, while eating foods you wouldn't find on your meal plan or cook yourself!

■ Take your time. Go slow, and taste your food. Chew more, talk more, set your fork down more often between bites, and don't wash your food down with a beverage. Savor the flavor.

■ Order condiments and dressings on the side and don't use the entire container! Lightly dip your food in dressings or gravies rather than pouring on extra calories.

■ Avoid buffets and all-you-can-eat establishments. If you go to them, use small plates and fill them with salads, vegetables, and other high-protein, low-calorie, low-fat options.

■ Pay careful attention to newly required menu labeling for fast-food restaurants. These can be helpful in making sure you choose the best alternative for healthy dining. Focus on the entrée and avoid the biggie fries or super-size drinks.

**Source:** Data are from National Heart, Lung, and Blood Institute, "Portion Distortion: Eat Right," April 1, 2015, www.nhlbi.nih.gov/health/educational/wecan/eat-right/portion-distortion.htm.

---

■ Recent popularity of high-fat foods such as bacon and red meat adds significantly to totally calories consumed.
■ Widespread availability of high-calorie coffee and sugary drinks lure people in for a form of break/reward between meals, which really add up in calories over time.
■ Misleading food labels confuse consumers about serving sizes.

Although we still consume about 500 calories per day more today than we did in 1970, daily consumption of some healthy foods appears to have increased, with some noteworthy declines in others. In 2013, each American had access to an average of 57 more pounds of commercially grown vegetables than they did in 1970; 9 more pounds of caloric sweeteners; a full 23 more pounds of fruit; 36 more pounds of poultry; 3 more pounds of seafood; 38 more pounds of products made with grains; and 22 more pounds of cheeses.[31] On the flipside, each American, on average, had 34 fewer pounds of red meat available to consume, 8 fewer gallons of coffee, about 4 dozen fewer eggs, and another dozen fewer gallons of milk.[32] If we are consuming healthier foods in some groups, why aren't we seeing major changes in obesity rates? One possibility is that we are exercising less than ever, thereby offsetting potential weight loss.

## Lack of Physical Activity
Although heredity, metabolism, and environment all have an impact on weight management, the way we live our lives is also responsible. In general, Americans are eating more and moving less than ever before—and becoming overfat as a result.

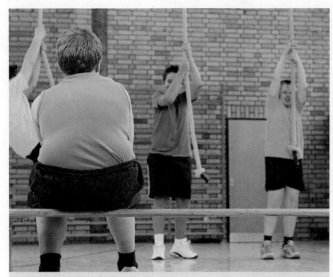
Stigmatization of people who are obese can contribute to depression and loss of self-esteem.

According to data from the 2015 *National Health Interview Survey*, just over 41 percent of adults age 18 and over in the United States met the guidelines for aerobic activity through involvement in leisure-time activity.[33] Only 20.8 percent met the minimum guidelines for both aerobic exercise and muscle strengthening.[34]

**WHAT DO YOU THINK?**

- Why do you think the United States has become one of the "fattest" nations on Earth, even though we have policies and educational programs in place to fight our epidemic of obesity/overweight? What should we do differently (policies/programs, etc.) to motivate people to lose weight and keep it off?

## Psychosocial and Socioeconomic Factors

The relationship of weight problems to emotional insecurities, needs, and wants remains difficult to assess. What we do know is eating tends to be a focal point of people's lives and is in part a social ritual associated with companionship, celebration, and enjoyment. *Comfort food* is also used to help you feel good when other things in life are not going well. Our friends and loved ones are often key influences in our eating behaviors. In fact, according to recent research, young adults who are overweight and obese tend to befriend and date overweight and obese people in much the same way that smokers or exercisers tend to hang out with other smokers or exercisers. People may gain or lose weight based on support for loss or social undermining of weight loss attempts ("Let's go out for ice cream!").[35]

Socioeconomic status can have a significant effect on risk for obesity. When times are tough, people tend to eat more inexpensive, high-calorie processed foods. People living in poverty may have less access to fresh, nutrient-dense foods and have less time to cook nutritious meals due to shift work, longer commutes, or multiple jobs. Counselors, fitness center memberships, and other supports for weight loss are often too expensive or unavailable. Additionally, unsafe neighborhoods and poor infrastructure, such as lack of sidewalks or parks, can make it difficult for less-affluent people to exercise.[36]

## LO 3 | ASSESSING BODY WEIGHT AND BODY COMPOSITION

Learn reliable options for determining a healthy weight and body fat percentage.

Everyone has his or her own ideal weight, based on individual variables such as body structure, height, and fat distribution. Traditionally, experts used measurement techniques such as height-weight charts to determine whether an individual was an ideal weight, overweight, or obese. These charts can be misleading because they don't take body composition—a person's ratio of fat to lean muscle—or fat distribution into account. More accurate measures of evaluating healthy weight and disease risk focus on a person's percentage of body fat and how that fat is distributed in his or her body.

It's important to remember that body fat isn't all bad. In fact, some fat is essential for healthy body functioning. Fat regulates body temperature, cushions and insulates organs and tissues, and is the body's main source of stored energy. Body fat is composed of two types: essential fat and storage fat. *Essential fat* is the fat necessary for maintenance of life and reproductive functions. *Storage fat*, the nonessential fat that many of us try to shed, makes up the remainder of our fat reserves.

Being **underweight**, or having extremely low body fat, can cause a host of problems, including hair loss, visual disturbances, skin problems, a tendency to fracture bones easily, digestive system disturbances, heart irregularities, gastrointestinal problems, difficulties in maintaining body temperature, and loss of menstrual period in women.

### Body Mass Index

As mentioned earlier, BMI is a description of body weight relative to height—numbers that are highly correlated with your total body fat. Find your BMI in inches and pounds in **FIGURE 6.4**, or calculate your BMI now by dividing your weight in kilograms by height in meters squared. The mathematical formula is

$$\text{BMI} = \text{weight (kg)/height squared (m}^2)$$

A BMI calculator is also available from the National Heart, Lung, and Blood Institute at www.nhlbi.nih.gov/guidelines/obesity/BMI/bmicalc.htm, along with their standard classification system.

**underweight** Having a body weight more than 10 percent below healthy recommended levels; in an adult, having a BMI below 18.5.

|  | 100 |  | 120 |  | 140 |  | 160 |  | 180 |  | 200 |  | 220 |  | 240 |  | 260 |
|---|---|---|---|---|---|---|---|---|---|---|---|---|---|---|---|---|---|
| 4'6" | 24 | 27 | 29 | 31 | 34 | 36 | 39 | 41 | 43 | 46 | 48 | 51 | 53 | 55 | 58 | 60 | 63 |
| 4'8" | 22 | 25 | 27 | 29 | 31 | 34 | 36 | 38 | 40 | 43 | 45 | 47 | 49 | 52 | 54 | 56 | 58 |
| 4'10" | 21 | 23 | 25 | 27 | 29 | 31 | 33 | 36 | 38 | 40 | 42 | 44 | 46 | 48 | 50 | 52 | 54 |
| 5'0" | 20 | 22 | 23 | 25 | 27 | 29 | 31 | 33 | 35 | 37 | 39 | 41 | 43 | 45 | 47 | 49 | 51 |
| 5'2" | 18 | 20 | 22 | 24 | 26 | 27 | 29 | 31 | 33 | 35 | 37 | 38 | 40 | 42 | 44 | 46 | 48 |
| 5'4" | 17 | 19 | 21 | 22 | 24 | 26 | 28 | 29 | 31 | 33 | 34 | 36 | 38 | 40 | 41 | 43 | 45 |
| 5'6" | 16 | 18 | 19 | 21 | 23 | 24 | 26 | 27 | 29 | 31 | 32 | 34 | 36 | 37 | 39 | 40 | 42 |
| 5'8" | 15 | 17 | 18 | 20 | 21 | 23 | 24 | 26 | 27 | 29 | 30 | 32 | 33 | 35 | 37 | 38 | 40 |
| 5'10" | 14 | 16 | 17 | 19 | 20 | 22 | 23 | 24 | 26 | 27 | 29 | 30 | 32 | 33 | 34 | 36 | 37 |
| 6'0" | 14 | 15 | 16 | 18 | 19 | 20 | 22 | 23 | 24 | 26 | 27 | 29 | 30 | 31 | 33 | 34 | 35 |
| 6'2" | 13 | 14 | 15 | 17 | 18 | 19 | 21 | 22 | 23 | 24 | 26 | 27 | 28 | 30 | 31 | 32 | 33 |
| 6'4" | 12 | 13 | 15 | 16 | 17 | 18 | 20 | 21 | 22 | 23 | 24 | 26 | 27 | 28 | 29 | 30 | 32 |
| 6'6" | 12 | 13 | 14 | 15 | 16 | 17 | 19 | 20 | 21 | 22 | 23 | 24 | 25 | 27 | 28 | 29 | 30 |
| 6'8" | 11 | 12 | 13 | 14 | 15 | 17 | 18 | 19 | 20 | 21 | 22 | 23 | 24 | 25 | 26 | 28 | 29 |
| 6'10" | 11 | 12 | 13 | 14 | 15 | 16 | 17 | 18 | 19 | 20 | 21 | 22 | 23 | 24 | 25 | 26 | 27 |
| 7'0" | 10 | 11 | 12 | 13 | 14 | 15 | 16 | 17 | 18 | 19 | 20 | 21 | 22 | 23 | 24 | 25 | 26 |

Height (feet and inches) — Weight (pounds)

**Key:**
- Underweight
- Normal weight
- Overweight
- Obese

**FIGURE 6.4 Body Mass Index (BMI)** Locate your height, read across to find your weight, and then read up to determine your BMI. Note that BMI values have been rounded off to the nearest whole number.

Desirable BMI levels may vary with age and by sex; however, most BMI tables for adults do not account for such variables and as such should viewed as a general guide. **Healthy weight** is defined as having a BMI of 18.5 to 24.9, the range of lowest statistical health risk.[37] A BMI of 25 to 29.9 indicates **overweight** and potentially significant health risks.[38] A BMI of 30 to 39.9 is classified as **obese**.[39] A BMI of 40+ is often labeled extremely or **morbidly obese**, and some sources add a new class known as **super obese** for those with a BMI of 50 or higher—one increasing in numbers.[40] Nearly 5 percent of obese men and almost 10 percent of obese women are morbidly obese (see **TABLE 6.1** on page 162).[41]

## Limitations of BMI
Like other assessments of fatness, the BMI has its limitations. Water, muscle, and bone mass are not included in BMI calculations, and BMI levels don't account for the fact that muscle weighs more than fat. BMI levels can be inaccurate for people who are under 5 feet tall, are highly muscled, or who are older and have little muscle mass. Although a combination of measures might be most reliable in assessing fat levels, BMI continues to be a quick, inexpensive, and useful tool for developing basic health recommendations.[42]

## Youth and BMI
Although BMI levels in youth are calculated in the same way as BMI levels in adults, they are interpreted and discussed differently. Today, over 30 percent of youth in America are obese, three times higher than rates in the 1980s.[43] Although the labels *obese* and *morbidly obese* have been used for years for adults, there is growing concern that such labels increase bias and *obesity stigma* against youth. According to a recent study, when subjected to bias and discrimination, the person who is the recipient of stigma is actually more likely to eat more, rather than curtailing eating behavior.[44] BMI ranges above a normal weight for children and teens are often labeled differently, as "at risk of overweight" and "overweight," to avoid the sense of shame such words may cause. In addition, BMI ranges for children and teens take into account normal differences in body fat between boys and girls and the differences in body fat that occur at various ages.

# 69%
of U.S. adults are OVERWEIGHT INCLUDING OBESITY. Nearly 37% of adults overall—36.3% of those aged 20 and over, 32.3% of those 20–39, 40.4% of those 40–59 and 37% of those 60 plus—are obese.

**healthy weight** Those with BMIs of 18.5 to 24.9, the range of lowest statistical health risk.

**overweight** Having a body weight more than 10 percent above healthy recommended levels; in an adult, having a BMI of 25 to 29.9.

**morbidly obese** Having a body weight 100 percent or more above healthy recommended levels; in an adult, having a BMI of 40 or more.

**super obese** Having a body weight higher than morbid obesity; in an adult, having a BMI of 50 or more.

| | BMI (kg/m²) | Obesity Class | Disease Risk* Relative to Normal Weight and Waist Circumference | |
|---|---|---|---|---|
| | | | Men 102 cm (40 in) or less Women 88 cm (35 in) or less | Men > 102 cm (40 in) Women > 88 cm (35 in) |
| Underweight | < 18.5 | | — | — |
| Normal | 18.5–24.9 | | — | — |
| Overweight | 25.0–29.9 | | Increased | High |
| Obesity | 30.0–34.9 | I | High | Very high |
| | 35.0–39.9 | II | Very high | Very high |
| Extreme/Morbid Obesity | 40.0+ | III | Extremely high | Extremely high |

\* Disease risk for type 2 diabetes, hypertension, and CVD.
+ Increased waist circumference also can be a marker for increased risk, even in persons of normal weight.

**Source:** National Heart, Lung and Blood Institute, "Classification of Overweight and Obesity by BMI, Waist Circumference, and Associated Disease Risks," Accessed April 2016, https://www.nhlbi.nih.gov/health/educational/lose_wt/BMI/bmi_dis.htm.

Specific guidelines for calculating youth BMI are available at the Centers for Disease Control and Prevention website at www.cdc.gov.

## Waist Circumference and Ratio Measurements

Knowing where your fat is carried may be more important than knowing how much you carry. Men and postmenopausal women tend to store fat in the upper regions of the body, particularly in the abdominal area. Premenopausal women usually store fat in the lower regions of their bodies, particularly the hips, buttocks, and thighs. Waist circumference measurements, including *waist circumference* only, the *waist circumference-to-hip ratio*, and the *waist circumference-to-height ratio*, have all been used to measure abdominal fat as an indicator of obesity and health risk. Where you carry the weight may be of particular importance in determining whether you develop diabetes, cardiovascular disease, hypertension, or stroke.[45]

A waistline greater than 40 inches (102 centimeters) in men and 35 inches (88 centimeters) in women may be particularly

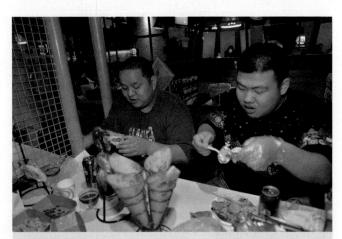

Abdominal obesity puts individuals at increased risk of CVD, stroke, and diabetes, particularly among men.

indicative of greater health risk.[46] If a person is less than 5 feet tall or has a BMI of 35 or above, waist circumference standards used for the general population might not apply.

The waist circumference-to-hip ratio measures regional fat distribution. The higher your waist-to-hip ratio is, the greater chance of having increased health risks.[47] Newer research has pointed to waist-to-hip ratio being more effective than waist circumference alone or BMI use when measuring body fat in children and adolescents.[48] A waist circumference-to-height ratio is a simple screening tool that says that your waist should be approximately one-half of your height; if you are 70 inches tall, your waist shouldn't be more than 35 inches.

## Measures of Body Fat

There are numerous ways to assess whether your body fat levels are too high. One low-tech way is simply to look in the mirror or consider how your clothes fit now compared with how they fit last year. For those who wish to take a more precise measurement of their percentage of body fat, more accurate techniques are available, several of which are described and depicted in **FIGURE 6.5**. These methods usually involve the help of a skilled professional and typically must be done in a lab or clinical setting. Before undergoing any procedure, make sure you understand the expense, potential for accuracy, risks, and training of the tester. Also, consider why you are seeking this assessment and what you plan to do with the results.

## LO 4 | MANAGING YOUR WEIGHT: INDIVIDUAL ROLES

Explain the effectiveness and potential pros/cons of various weight control strategies, including exercise, diet, lifestyle modification, supplements/diet drugs, surgery, and other options.

At some point in our lives, almost all of us will decide to lose weight. Many will have mixed success and others will

**Underwater (hydrostatic) weighing:**
Measures the amount of water a person displaces when completely submerged. Fat tissue is less dense than muscle or bone, so body fat can be computed within a 2%–3% margin of error by comparing weight underwater and out of water.

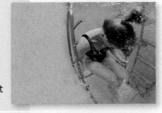

**Skinfolds:**
Involves "pinching" a person's fold of skin (with its underlying layer of fat) at various locations of the body. The fold is measured using a specially designed caliper. When performed by a skilled technician, it can estimate body fat with an error of 3%–4%.

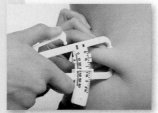

**Bioelectrical impedance analysis (BIA):**
Involves sending a very low level of electrical current through a person's body. As lean body mass is made up of mostly water, the rate at which the electricity is conducted gives an indication of a person's lean body mass and body fat. Under the best circumstances, BIA can estimate body fat with an error of 3%–4%.

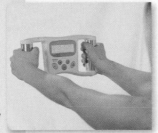

**Dual-energy X-ray absorptiometry (DXA):**
The technology is based on using very-low-level X ray to differentiate between bone tissue, soft (or lean) tissue, and fat (or adipose) tissue. The margin of error for predicting body fat is 2%–4%.

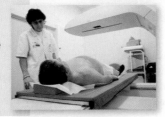

**Bod Pod:**
Uses air displacement to measure body composition. This machine is a large, egg-shaped chamber made from fiberglass. The person being measured sits in the machine wearing a swimsuit. The door is closed and the machine measures how much air is displaced. That value is used to calculate body fat, with a 2%–3% margin of error.

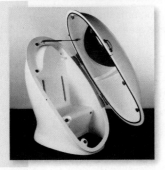

**FIGURE 6.5** Overview of Various Body Composition Assessment Methods

**Source:** Adapted from J. Thompson and M. Manore, *Nutrition: An Applied Approach,* 4th ed., © 2015. Printed and electronically reproduced by permission of Pearson Education, Inc., Upper Saddle River, New Jersey.

fail. Failure is often related to thinking about losing weight in terms of short-term "dieting" rather than adjusting long-term behaviors. Drugs and intensive counseling can contribute to positive weight loss, but even then, many people regain weight after treatment. Maintaining a healthful body takes constant attention and nurturing. The **Student Health Today** box on page 164 looks at characteristics of successful weight losers.

# Understanding Calories and Energy Balance

A *calorie* is a unit of measure that indicates the amount of energy gained from food or expended through activity. Each time you consume 3,500 calories more than your body needs to maintain weight, you gain a pound of storage fat. Conversely, each time your body expends an extra 3,500 calories, you lose a pound of fat. If you consume 140 calories (the amount in one can of regular soda) more than you need every single day and make no other changes in diet or activity, you would gain 1 pound in 25 days (3,500 calories ÷ 140 calories per day = 25 days). Conversely, if you walk for 30 minutes each day at a pace of 15 minutes per mile (172 calories burned) in addition to your regular activities, you would lose 1 pound in 20 days (3,500 calories ÷ 172 calories per day = 20.3 days). **FIGURE 6.6** illustrates the concept of energy balance.

# Diet and Eating Behaviors

Successful weight loss requires shifting energy balance. The first part of the equation is to reduce calorie intake through modifying eating habits and daily diet.

**Improving Your Eating Habits** Before you can change an unhealthy eating habit, you must first determine what causes or triggers it. Keeping a detailed daily log of eating triggers—when, what, where, and how much you eat—for at least a week can give clues about what causes you to want food. Typically, dietary triggers center on patterns and problems in everyday living rather than real hunger pangs. Many people eat compulsively when stressed; however, for other people, the same circumstances diminish their appetite, causing them to

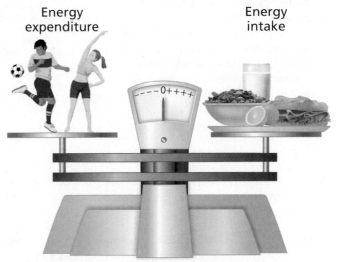

**Energy expenditure = Energy intake**

**FIGURE 6.6** **The Concept of Energy Balance** If you consume more calories than you burn, you gain weight. If you burn more than you consume, you lose weight. If both are equal, your weight will not change.

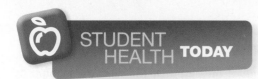
# WHO WINS AT LOSING?
## *Characteristics of Successful Losers*

Millions of Americans start their New Year with the most popular resolution: to lose weight and keep it off. Even so, the majority who lose some weight ultimately regain it. But what about those few losers who manage to keep it off?

In general, the literature indicates success rates between 2 and 15 percent, using a variety of weight and BMI parameters, as well as timelines for defining success. Based on recent studies, characteristics of those likely to be successful include:

- Those who have strong initial weight loss in the first month are most likely to be successful at one year; hence, having supports for change and incentives to keep going are critical to early and sustained success.
- Those who attend group sessions for support in those first months are more likely to be successful.
- High self-esteem and self-efficacy (success breeds success) are important.
- A strong locus of control—being motivated by internal rather than external factors.
- Having awareness of their current risks and reasonable knowledge of healthy nutrition.
- Knowing how to access and utilize community resources is important.
- People who journal and track calories, nutrients, and/or portion sizes, as well as monitor weight regularly. Using electronic tracking/monitoring devices shows great promise in motivating change.

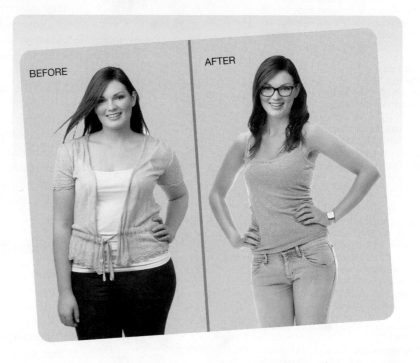

BEFORE    AFTER

- Making a commitment to follow a healthy, realistic eating and exercise pattern.
- Staying positive, practicing self-compassion, and avoiding becoming discouraged by setbacks.
- Using weight loss programs that include exercise have greater chances of success.

**Sources:** CDC, "Keeping it Off," May 15, 2015, www.cdc.gov/healthyweight/losing_weight/keepingitoff.html; C. Pellegrini et al., "Smartphone Applications to Support Weight Loss: A Current Perspective," *Journal of Medical Internet Research* 1 (2015): 13–22; S. Guendelman, M. Rittermann Weintraub, and M. Kaufer-Horwitz, "Weight Loss Success Among Overweight and Obese Women of Mexican-Origin Living in Mexico and the United States: A Comparison of Two National Surveys," *Journal of Immigrant and Minority Health*

(2016): 1–9; M. Ortner Hadziabdic et al., "Factors Predictive of Drop-out and Weight Loss Success in Weight Management for Obese Patients," *Journal of Human Nutrition and Dietetics* 28, no. 2 (2015): 24–32; J. Dombrowski et al., "Long Term Maintenance of Weight Loss with Non-surgical Interventions in Obese Adults: Systematic Review and Meta-Analyses of Randomized Controlled Trials," *British Medical Journal* 348 (2014): g2646; Look AHEAD Research Group, "Eight Year Weight Losses with an Intensive Lifestyle Intervention: The Look Ahead Study," *Obesity* 22, no 1 (2014): 5–13; J. Moreno and C. Johnston, "Success Habits of Weight Losers," *American Journal of Lifestyle Medicine* 6, no. 2 (2012): 113–5; S. Ramage et al., "Healthy Strategies for Successful Weight Loss and Weight Maintenance: A Systematic Review," *Applied Physiology, Nutrition, and Metabolism* 39, no. 1 (2013): 1–20; R. Goode et al., "Socio-Demographic, Anthropometric, and Psychosocial Predictors of Attrition Across Behavioral Weight-Loss Trials," *Eating Behaviors* 20 (2016): 27–33.

---

lose weight. See the Making Changes Today box on page 166 for tips on healthy snacking, and see FIGURE 6.7 for ways to adjust your eating triggers.

### Choosing a Diet Plan
Once you have determined your triggers, begin to devise a plan for improved eating by doing the following:

- Seeking assistance from reputable sources such as MyPlate (www.choosemyplate.gov), a registered dietitian (RD), some physicians, health educators, or exercise physiologists with nutritional training.

- Being wary of nutritionists or nutritional life coaches, since there is no formal credential for those titles.

- Avoiding weight-loss programs that promise quick, "miracle" results or that are run by "trainees," often people with short courses on nutrition and exercise that are designed to sell products or services.

**SEE IT! VIDEOS**

What makes one diet plan work better than another? Watch **Low-Carb Diet Trumps Low Fat in Weight-Loss Study**, available on **MasteringHealth.™**

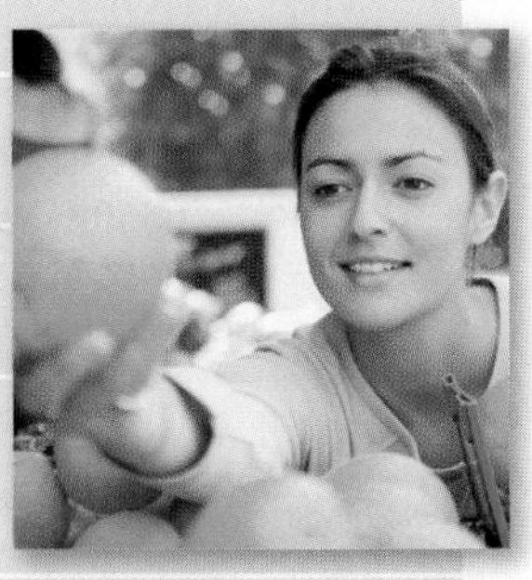

| If your trigger is . . . | then → try this strategy . . . |
|---|---|
| A stressful situation | Acknowledge and address feelings of anxiety or stress, and develop stress management techniques to practice daily. |
| Feeling angry or upset | Analyze your emotions and look for a noneating activity to deal with them, such as taking a quick walk or calling a friend. |
| A certain time of day | Change your eating schedule to avoid skipping or delaying meals and overeating later; make a plan of what you'll eat ahead of time to avoid impulse or emotional eating. |
| Pressure from friends and family | Have a response ready to help you refuse food you do not want, or look for healthy alternatives you can eat instead when in social settings. |
| Being in an environment where food is available | Avoid the environment that causes you to want to eat: Sit far away from the food at meetings, take a different route to class to avoid passing the vending machines, shop from a list and only when you aren't hungry, arrange nonfood outings with your friends. |
| Feeling bored and tired | Identify the times when you feel low energy and fill them with activities other than eating, such as exercise breaks; cultivate a new interest or hobby that keeps your mind and hands busy. |
| The sight and smell of food | Stop buying high-calorie foods that tempt you to snack, or store them in an inconvenient place, out of sight; avoid walking past or sitting or standing near the table of tempting treats at a meeting, party, or other gathering. |
| Eating mindlessly or inattentively | Turn off all distractions, including phones, computers, television, and radio, and eat more slowly, savoring your food and putting your fork down between bites so you can become aware of when your hunger is satisfied. |
| Spending time alone in the car | Get a book on tape to listen to, or tape your class notes and use the time for studying. Keep your mind off food. Don't bring money into the gas station where snacks are tempting. |
| Alcohol use | Drink plenty of water and stay hydrated. Seek out healthy snack choices. After a night out, brush your teeth immediately upon getting home and stay out of the kitchen. |
| Feeling deprived | Allow yourself to eat "indulgences" in moderation, so you won't crave them; focus on balancing your calorie input to calorie output. |
| Eating out of habit | Establish a new routine to circumvent the old, such as taking a new route to class so you don't feel compelled to stop at your favorite fast-food restaurant on the way. |
| Watching television | Look for something else to occupy your hands and body while your mind is engaged with the screen: Ride an exercise bike, do stretching exercises, doodle on a pad of paper, or learn to knit. |

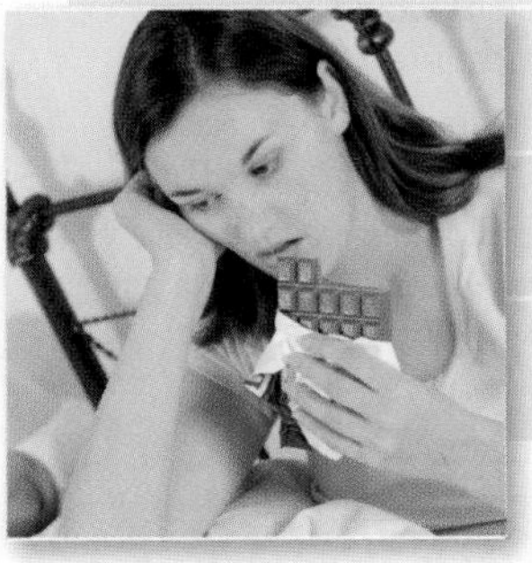

FIGURE 6.7 **Avoid Trigger-Happy Eating** Learn what triggers your "eat" response—and what stops it—by keeping a daily log.

■ Assessing the nutrient value of any prescribed diet, verifying dietary guidelines are consistent with reliable nutrition research, and analyzing the suitability of the diet to your tastes, budget, and lifestyle.

Any diet that requires radical behavior changes or sets up artificial dietary programs through prepackaged products is likely to fail. The most successful plans allow you to make food choices in real-world settings and do not ask you to sacrifice everything you enjoy. See **TABLE 6.2** on page 167 for an analysis of some popular diets marketed today. For information on other plans, check out the regularly updated list of reviews on the website of the Academy of Nutrition and Dietetics (formerly the American Dietetic Association) at www.eatright.org.

## Including Exercise

Any increase in the intensity, frequency, and duration of daily exercise can lead to an increase in muscle mass, which can have a significant impact on total calorie expenditure because lean (muscle) tissue is more metabolically active than fat tissue. Exact estimates vary, but experts currently think that 2 to 50 more calories per day are burned per pound of muscle than each pound of fat tissue. Thus, the base level of calories needed

## MAKING CHANGES TODAY

### Tips for Sensible Snacking

- ⦿ **Keep healthy munchies around.** Buy 100 percent whole-wheat breads, and if you need something to spice it up, use low-fat or soy cheese, low-fat cream cheese, peanut butter, hummus, or other high-protein healthy favorites. Some baked or popped crackers are low in fat and calories and high in fiber.

- ◎ **Keep "crunchies" on hand.** Apples, pears, green or red pepper sticks, popcorn, snap peas, and celery all are good choices. Wash the fruits and vegetables and cut them up to carry with you; eat them when a snack attack comes on.

- ◎ **Choose natural beverages.** Drink plain water, 100 percent juice in small quantities, or other low-sugar choices to satisfy your thirst. Hot tea, coffee (black), or soup broths are also good choices.

- ◎ **Eat nuts instead of candy.** Although relatively high in calories, nuts are also loaded with healthy fats and are healthy when consumed in moderation.

- ◎ **If you must have a piece of chocolate, keep it small and dark.** Dark chocolate has more antioxidants.

- ◎ **Avoid high-calorie energy bars.** Eat these only if you are exercising hard and don't have an opportunity to eat a regular meal. Select ones with a good mixture of fiber and protein and that are low in fat, sugar, and calories.

## DID YOU KNOW?

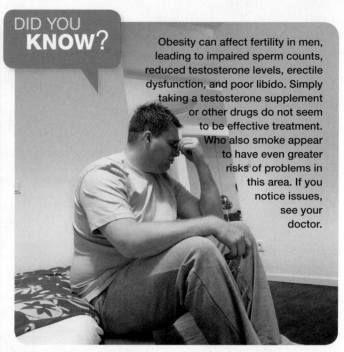

Obesity can affect fertility in men, leading to impaired sperm counts, reduced testosterone levels, erectile dysfunction, and poor libido. Simply taking a testosterone supplement or other drugs do not seem to be effective treatment. Who also smoke appear to have even greater risks of problems in this area. If you notice issues, see your doctor.

**Source:** V. Stokes et al., "How Does Obesity Affect Fertility in Men– and What Are the Treatment Options?," *Clinical Endocrinology* 82, no. 5 (2015): 633–38.

to maintain a healthy weight varies greatly from person to person.

The number of calories spent through physical activity depends on three factors:

1. The number and proportion of muscles used
2. The amount of weight moved
3. The length of time the activity takes

An activity involving both the arms and legs burns more calories than one involving only the legs. An activity performed by a heavy person burns more calories than the same activity performed by a lighter person. And, an activity performed for 40 minutes requires twice as much energy as the same activity performed for only 20 minutes. See the **Student Health Today** box on page 169 for more on diet and exercise.

## Keeping Weight Control in Perspective

Weight loss is a struggle for many people, and many factors influence success or failure. To reach and maintain a healthy weight, develop a program of exercise and healthy eating behaviors that you can maintain. Remember, you didn't gain your weight in a week or two, and it is both unrealistic and potentially dangerous to take drastic weight loss measures. Instead, try to lose a healthy 1 to 2 pounds during the first week, and stay with this slow and easy regimen. Adding exercise and cutting back on calories to expend about 500 calories more than you consume each day will help you lose weight at a rate of 1 pound per week. You may find tracking your intake and activity easier with one of the apps described in the **Tech & Health** box on page 170. See the **Making Changes Today** box on page 171 for strategies to help your weight management program succeed.

### WHAT DO YOU THINK?

**If you wanted to lose weight, what strategies would you most likely choose?**

- ▪ Which strategies, if any, have worked for you before?
- ▪ What factors might serve to help or hinder your weight-loss efforts?

## Considering Drastic Weight Loss Measures?

When nothing seems to work, people become frustrated and pursue high-risk, unproven methods of weight loss or seek medical interventions. Dramatic weight loss may be recommended in cases of extreme health risk. Even in such situations, drastic dietary, pharmacological, or surgical measures should be considered carefully and discussed with several knowledgeable, licensed health professionals working in accredited facilities.

## TABLE 6.2 | Popular Diet Programs

| Diet Name | Basic Principles | Good for Diabetes and Heart Health? | Weight Loss Effectiveness | Pros, Cons, and Other Things to Consider |
|---|---|---|---|---|
| DASH (Dietary Approaches to Stop Hypertension) | A balanced plan developed to fight high blood pressure. Eat fruits, veggies, whole grains, lean protein, and low-fat dairy. Avoid sweets, fats, red meat, and sodium. | Yes | Not specifically designed for weight loss. | A balanced, safe, and healthy diet, rated the number one best diet overall by *U.S. News & World Report* in 2016. Although not designed for weight reduction per se, it is regarded as very effective in improving cholesterol levels and other biomarkers long term. |
| TLC (Therapeutic Lifestyle Change) | Developed by NIH. Focus on CVD risk reduction with fruits and veggies, lean protein, low fat, etc. Balanced and effective. | Yes | Weight loss likely; cholesterol key. | Safe, balanced, and healthy diet, tied for number two diet with the MIND diet by *U.S. News & World Report* in 2016. Particularly good for heart health and cholesterol reduction. |
| Mediterranean | A plan that emphasizes fruits, vegetables, fish, whole grains, beans, nuts, legumes, olive oil, and herbs and spices. Poultry, eggs, cheese, yogurt, and red wine can be enjoyed in moderation, whereas sweets and red meat are saved for special occasions. | Yes | Effective | Widely considered to be one of the more healthy, safe, and balanced diets. Weight loss may not be as dramatic but long-term health benefits have been demonstrated. Tied for fourth best overall and third for best healthy eating diet by *U.S. News & World Report* in 2016. Relatively easy to follow. |
| Weight Watchers | New "Beyond the Scale" program, which emphasizes three components: eating healthier, fitness that fits your life, and "developing skills and supportive connections to help you stay on track." Involves tracking food, nutritional values, and exercise. Total points allowed depend on activity level and personal weight goals. In-person group meetings or online membership are options. | Yes (depending on individual choices) | Effective | Consistently rated by experts as one of the top, most effective weight loss programs. Flexible programs that don't deny foods, but rather teach about healthy choices. Works for both short- and long-term weight loss. Support groups are available, but can do online in privacy of home with coaches. Planning for indulgences helps maintain control. Check your campus or community for meeting times and watch for specials. While not as expensive as some plans, there are membership fees. Rated number one weight loss diet by *U.S. News & World Report* in 2016. |
| MIND Diet | Combines best elements of DASH and Mediterranean diets into a healthy dietary regimen. | Yes | Effective | Number two best overall diet rating by *U.S. News and World Report* in 2016. Noteworthy for potential to boost brain power and reduced risk of cognitive decline. |
| Jenny Craig | Prepackaged meals do the work of restricting calorie intake. Members get personalized meal and exercise plans, plus weekly counseling sessions. | Yes | Effective short term; long-term results dependent on adopting healthful eating later | Support and premade meals make weight loss easier; however, it may be difficult to maintain long term. Cons include cost, which will run hundreds of dollars per month for food alone, plus membership fees. Lactose- and gluten-intolerant individuals cannot join due to available foods. |
| Biggest Loser | Four servings a day of fruits and vegetables, three of protein foods, two of whole grains, and no more than 200 calories of "extras" like desserts. Exercise, food journals, portion control, and calculating personal calorie allowances are all stressed. | Yes | Effective | This diet is effective at weight loss. Ranked number one by *U.S. News and World Report* in 2016 for those with prediabetes or diabetes. Helps reduce blood glucose levels and reduces other biomarkers such as cholesterol, triglycerides, etc. |

*continued*

TABLE **6.2** | Popular Diet Programs (*continued*)

| Diet Name | Basic Principles | Good for Diabetes and Heart Health? | Weight Loss Effectiveness | Pros, Cons, and Other Things to Consider |
|---|---|---|---|---|
| **Nutrisystem** | Low-calorie, prepackaged meals are ordered online and delivered to your home. | Not for heart health per se, but may help reduce diabetes risks | Effective short term; long-term results dependent on adopting healthful eating later | Nutrisystem is quite safe and easier to follow than many other diets, and has few nutritional deficiencies if followed as directed, according to experts. It is also expensive (similar to Jenny Craig) due to the cost of ordering food and may not help you learn to eat healthfully after diet is done. |
| **Medifast** | Dieters eat six meals a day, five of them 100-calorie Medifast products. After goal weight loss, people wean from Medifast food and gradually add back in starchy veggies, whole grains, fruits, and low-fat dairy products. | Likely yes | Effective in short term; long-term results unproven | Medifast scored above average in short-term weight loss but gets lower marks for keeping weight off. Because of the extremely low-calorie intakes on the program, it is hard to stay on the program for long; doesn't teach healthy eating as part of plan. |
| **Low-carb diets (Atkins, South Beach, and other variations)** | Carbs—sugars and "simple starches" such as potatoes, white bread, and rice—are avoided, and some minimize all carb-based foods. Emphasis on proteins and fat from meat and eggs are embraced. | Not likely with so much fat eaten | Effective in short term; mixed long-term results | Low-carb diets in most forms are often extremely effective at short-term weight loss, but many experts worry that fat intake is up to three times higher than standard daily recommendations and some even omit fruits, vegetables, and healthy grains. |
| **Paleo** | Based on the theory that digestive systems have not evolved to deal with many modern foods such as dairy, legumes, grains, and sugar; this plan emphasizes meats, fish, poultry, fruits, and vegetables. | Unknown (too few studies) | Unknown (too few studies) | Gets low marks by health and nutrition experts due to avoidance of grains, legumes, and dairy, and is higher in fat than the government recommends. Missing essential nutrients; costly to maintain. It can be hard to follow long term and has had only few very small studies done to document effectiveness. |
| **Fast Diet (also known as the 5:2 diet or Intermittent Fasting Diet)** | Based on the theory that by drastically reducing calories on two days (500 cal/day) each week and eating normally the other five, you will lose weight. | Not likely, as it doesn't follow guidelines for carbohydrates; should talk with registered dietician or health care provider | Effective, but weight loss is relatively slow unless calorie intake is monitored on nonfast days and exercise is part of regimen | Exceeds dietary guidelines for fat and protein and falls short on carbohydrate recommendation. Does encourage fruits and veggies, but feast-and-famine regimen is hard to sustain. |

**Sources:** Opinions on diet pros and cons are based on *U.S. News & World Report*, "Best Diets Overall," 2016, http://health.usnews.com/best-diet/best-overall-diets?int=9c2508; dietary reviews are available online from registered dieticians at the Academy of Nutrition and Dietetics, 2015; B. Johnson et al., "Comparisons of Weight Loss Among Diet Programs in Overweight and Obese Adults: A Meta-Analysis," *Journal of the American Medical Association* 312, no. 9 (2014): 923–33.

## Very-Low-Calorie Diets

In severe cases of obesity that are not responsive to traditional dietary strategies, medically supervised, powdered formulas with daily values of 400 to 700 calories plus vitamin and mineral supplements may be given to patients. Many of these diets emphasize high protein and very low carbohydrates. Such **very-low-calorie diets (VLCDs)** should never be undertaken without strict medical supervision. They do not teach healthy eating, and persons who manage to lose weight on VLCDs or prolonged fasts may experience significant weight regain. Problems associated with any form of severe caloric restriction include blood sugar imbalance, cold

**very-low-calorie diets (VLCDs)** Diets with a daily caloric value of 400 to 700 calories.

**SEE IT!** VIDEOS

A new strategy to keep off the weight? Watch **Experiment Shows Portion Control is the Key to Healthy Eating**, available on MasteringHealth.™

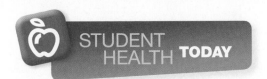
# WHICH IS BEST FOR WEIGHT LOSS?
*Diet, Exercise, or Both?*

Although the debate has raged for decades, recent research supports the idea that calories consumed ultimately are more important than exercise in a weight loss regimen. It turns out that if the experts are right, you really can't outrun a bad diet!

According to the above researchers, by most indicators, diet trumps exercise when it comes to weight loss and maintenance. If you want to lose weight in the short term, portion control and healthy eating habits are both key to success. Eat fewer calories and you will lose weight. Of course, there continue to be critics of the "diet is the key" philosophy. Numerous studies have shown that the combination of diet and exercise is the best way to lose weight. Other studies have found that exercise plus calorie restriction achieves the same weight loss as calorie restriction alone, and very few people exercise enough to affect weight in the long term. Many that increase physical activity increase their caloric intake, and when they do, calories win out.

Does that mean you can just starve yourself, lose weight, and ignore exercise? Of course not. There are numerous benefits of exercise that are important to overall health and well-being. Diet and exercise, when working together in perfect harmony, continue to be the most powerful long-term strategy for weight control. Combined, they also are important in reducing blood lipids, blood pressure, and reducing risks of cardiovascular disease and type 2 diabetes.

**Sources:** A. Myers et al., "Associations among Sedentary and Active Behaviours, Body Fat and Appetite Dysregulation: Investigating the Myth of Physical Inactivity and Obesity," *British Journal of Sports Medicine* (2016): doi:10.1136/bjsports-2015-095640; P. Kelly et al., "Critique of the 'Physical Activity Myth' Paper: Discussion of Flawed Logic and Inappropriate Use of Evidence," *British Journal of Sports Medicine* (2015): doi10:1136/bjsports-2015-095120; B. Johnson et al., "Comparison of Weight Loss Among Named Diet Programs in Overweight Obese Adults: A Meta-Analysis," *Journal of the American Medical Association* 312, no. 9 (2014): 923–33; A. Luke and R. S. Cooper, "Physical Activity Does Not Influence Obesity Risk: Time to Clarify the Public Health Message," *International Journal of Epidemiology* 42, no. 6 (2013): 1831–6; Academy of Medical Royal Colleges, "Exercise—The Miracle Cure," February 2015, www.aomrc.org.uk/general-news/exercise-the-miracle-cure.html; A. Malhotra, T. Noakes, and S. Phinney, "It is Time to Bust the Myth of Physical Inactivity and Obesity: You Cannot Outrun a Bad Diet," *British Journal of Sports Medicine* 49, no. 15 (2015): 967–8.

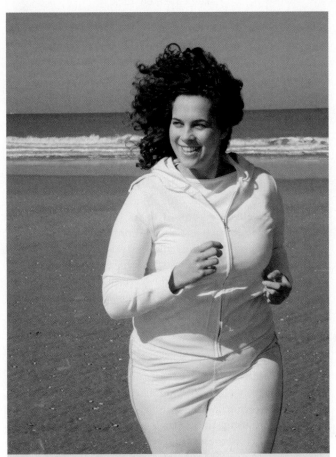

Participating in daily physical activity is key to managing your weight, as well as overall fitness and health.

intolerance, constipation, decreased BMR, dehydration, diarrhea, emotional problems, fatigue, headaches, heart irregularities, kidney infections and failure, loss of lean body tissue, and *ketosis*, a condition that happens when glucose levels decline drastically (as in extremely low carb diets) and begins to burn fat which can lead to a build up of acidic chemicals known as *ketones*. Over time on VLCDs or starvation diets, these ketones can increase and you may not feel hungry or thirsty and weight loss may occur. As ketones increase and ketosis progresses, *ketoacidosis* or acidic blood levels are likely. This is a potentially dangerous complication of VLCD diets or starvation diets. weakness, and the potential for coma and death.

Early symptoms may include excessive thirst, excessive urination, and high blood sugar, progressing to extreme fatigue, nausea, vomiting, abdominal pain, "fruity breath," fainting, possible coma, and death. Extreme diets that allow very few carbohydrates and/or calories are often the culprits. People with untreated diabetes can experience diabetic ketoacidosis as well as individuals with anorexia or bulimia are also at high risk.

## Weight Loss Supplements and Over-the-Counter Drugs
Thousands of over-the-counter supplements and drugs that claim to make weight loss fast and easy are available for purchase. It's important to note that U.S. Food and Drug Administration (FDA) approval is not required for over-the-counter "diet aids" or supplements. The lack of regular and continuous monitoring of supplements in the United States leaves consumers vulnerable to fraud and potentially toxic "remedies." Most dietary supplements contain

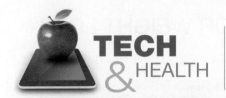

# TECH & HEALTH

## TRACKING YOUR DIET OR WEIGHT LOSS? *There's an App for That*

Studies consistently report that people who keep detailed food and exercise journals lose more weight and keep it off longer than those who do not. Want to track what you ate today in terms of total calories and amount of nutrients? There's an app for that. Want to track your walking, running, swimming, lifting, and sleeping activities? There are apps for that, too.

The best programs combine food and physical activity logs, so if you splurge on dessert, you can figure out how many miles you'll need to jog to burn it off. These apps often feature calculators for determining daily calorie intake goals as well as barcode scanners that allow you to quickly add packaged foods to your log. Here are just a few of the latest free apps for iPhone and Android users:

- **My Fitness Pal Calorie Counter and Diet Tracker.** Easy-to-use app for those interested in tracking details of diet, calories, and exercise. Includes easy data entry, barcode scanning via phone to analyze food purchases, and meal logs to help you assess progress and set goals.
- **Fooducate.** Uses a combination of food lists, barcode scanners via phone to help you determine what is in the food you eat—helping you make healthy food choices while watching calories and daily intake.
- **Instant Heart Rate.** Want to know what your heart rate is as you begin and maintain a diet and exercise

regimen? Want to do it without wearing or strapping on all kinds of devices during the day? This app allows you to use your smartphone as a heart rate monitor. Just put your finger on the camera lens to get your pulse. Allows you to track resting heart rate, track progress, and set goals aimed at an optimum heart rate.
- **Fitocracy.** "Fitocrats" play against each other on this app to help motivate diet and exercise "wannabes." In the game, users begin at the first level, and, depending on how frequently, how long, and how hard they work out, they earn points, eventually moving to the next level. They also offer support and advice to each other to keep them on track.

---

stimulants, such as caffeine, or diuretics, and their effectiveness in promoting weight loss has been largely untested and unproved by any scientific studies. In many cases, the only thing that users lose is money. Virtually all persons who used supplements and diet pills in review studies regained their weight once they stopped taking them.[49]

Supplements containing *Hoodia gordonii*, an African cactus-like plant, have become popular in recent years, and there are many off-market brands produced, including some that contain more unproven ingredients such as bitter orange and other stimulants. Hoodie has not yet received FDA approval.

Products containing *ephedra* can cause rapid heart rate, tremors, seizures, insomnia, headaches, and raised blood pressure, all without significant effects on long-term weight control. *St. John's wort* and other alternative medicines reported to enhance serotonin, suppress appetite, and reduce the side effects of depression have not been shown to be effective in weight loss, either.

Historically, FDA-approved diet pills have been available only by prescription and are closely monitored. These lines were blurred in 2007 when the FDA approved the first over-the-counter weight loss pill—a half-strength version of the prescription drug *orlistat* (brand name *Xenical*), marketed as Alli. This drug inhibits the action of lipase, an enzyme that helps the body to digest fats, causing about 30 percent of fats consumed to pass through the digestive system undigested, leading to reduced overall caloric intake. Known side effects of orlistat include gas with watery fecal discharge; oily stools and

spotting; frequent, often unexpected, bowel movements; and possible deficiencies of fat-soluble vitamins.

**Prescription Weight Loss Drugs** Several FDA-approved weight loss drugs are now available after nearly 13 years of inactivity. *Belviq* and *Qsymia* were among the first available and were met with much controversy and carry several warnings and restrictions. Qsymia is an appetite suppressant and antiseizure drug that reduces the desire for food. Belviq affects serotonin levels, helping patients feel full. Newer drugs, such as *Contrave* combine antidepressants with other approved drugs and carry warnings specific to both. Other weight loss drugs that have been on the market for some time, such as *Meridia*, continue to be marketed. Before taking any weight loss supplements and herbal remedies or prescription drugs, you should always discuss risks, benefits, and options with your doctor and carefully read FDA warnings.

When used as part of a long-term, comprehensive weight-loss program, weight-loss drugs can potentially help those who are severely obese lose weight and keep it off; however, they are not without adverse side effects. Check with your doctor before using these drugs and investigate side effects before considering these options.

**Surgery** When all else fails, particularly for people who are severely overweight and have weight-related diseases, a person may be a candidate for weight-loss surgery. Generally,

## MAKING **CHANGES** TODAY

### Keys to Successful Weight Management

**MAKE A PLAN**

- ◉ Establish short- and long-term plans. What are the diet and exercise changes you can make this week? Once you do 1 week, plot a course for 2 weeks, and so on.

- ◎ Look for balance. Remember it's calories taken in and burned over time that make the difference.

**CHANGE YOUR HABITS**

- ◉ Be adventurous. Expand your usual foods to enjoy a wider variety.

- ◎ Eat small portions, less often and savor the flavor.

- ◎ Notice whether you are hungry before starting a meal. Eat slowly, noting when you start to feel full, and *stop* before you are full.

- ◎ Eat breakfast, especially low-fat foods with whole grains and protein. This will prevent you from being too hungry and overeating at lunch.

- ◎ Keep healthful snacks on hand for when you get hungry.

**INCORPORATE EXERCISE**

- ◉ Be active and slowly increase your time, speed, distance, or resistance levels.

- ◎ Vary your physical activity. Find activities that you really love and try things you haven't tried before.

- ◎ Find an exercise partner to help you stay motivated.

these surgeries fall into one of two major categories: *restrictive surgeries*, such as gastric banding or lap banding, that limit food intake, and *malabsorption surgeries*, such as gastric bypass, which decrease the absorption of food into the body (see **FIGURE 6.8**).

To select the best option, a physician will consider the operation's benefits and risks and the patient's age, BMI, eating behaviors, obesity-related health conditions, mental history, dietary history, and previous operations. Like drugs prescribed for weight loss, surgery for obesity also carries risks for consumers.[50] Recently, several groups have begun listing obesity as a *disease*, prompting considerable controversy in the media. Some health advocates have proposed that obesity be classified as a disability, which could potentially affect a physician's decision on recommending surgery.

In gastric banding and other restrictive surgeries, the surgeon uses an inflatable band to partition off part of the stomach. The band is wrapped around that part of the stomach and is pulled tight, like a belt, leaving only a small opening between the two parts of the stomach. The upper part of the stomach is smaller, so the person feels full more quickly, and food digestion slows so that the person also feels full longer. Although the bands are designed to stay in place, they can be removed surgically. They can also be inflated to different levels to adjust the amount of restriction.

*Sleeve gastrectomy* is another form of restrictive weight loss that is often done laparoscopically. In this surgery, about 75 percent of the stomach is removed, leaving only a tube (about the size of a banana) or sleeve that is connected directly to the intestines. Usually, this procedure is done on extremely obese or ill patients who need an interim, less invasive procedure before more invasive gastric bypass. However, this procedure isn't reversible and potential risks may be higher.

*Gastric bypass* is one of the most common types of weight loss surgery and it combines restrictive and malabsorption elements. It can be done laparoscopically or via full open surgery.

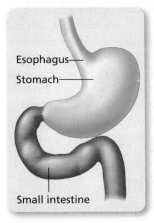

**a** Normal anatomy

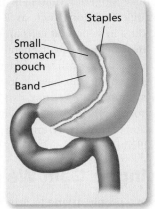

**b** Sleeve gastrectory

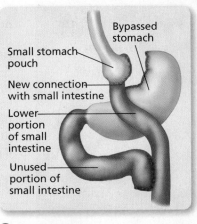

**c** Gastric bypass

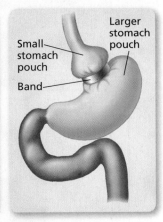

**d** Gastric banding

**FIGURE 6.8** Weight-Loss Surgery Alters the Normal Anatomy of the Stomach

**Source:** Adapted from J. Thompson and M. Manore, *Nutrition: An Applied Approach*, 4th ed., ©2015. Printed and electronically reproduced by permission of Pearson Education, Inc. Upper Saddle River, New Jersey.

In this surgery, a major section (as much as 70 percent) of the stomach is sutured off, restricting the amount of food you can eat and absorb. The remaining pouch is hooked up directly to the small intestine. Results are fast and dramatic, with health issues related to obesity, such as diabetes, high blood pressure, arthritis, sleep apnea, and other problems, diminishing or being reduced drastically in a short time.

While weight loss tends to be maintained and health problems decline after gastric bypass surgery, there are many risks, including nutritional deficiencies, blood clots in the legs, a leak in a staple line in the stomach, pneumonia, infection, and, although rare, even death. Another risk is rapid gastric emptying, commonly referred to as "dumping," in which undigested foods rush through the small intestine, causing cramping and problems with uncontrollable diarrhea.[51] Because the stomach pouch that remains after surgery is only the size of a lime, the person can drink only a few tablespoons of liquid and consume only a very small amount of food at a time. For this reason, other possible side effects include nausea, vitamin and mineral deficiencies, and dehydration. Additional risks

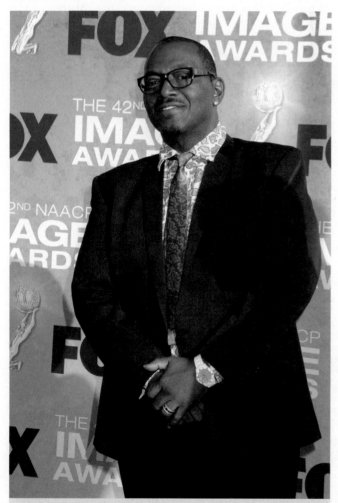

Former *American Idol* judge and record producer Randy Jackson underwent gastric bypass surgery to shed well over 100 pounds and reduce the risks of serious chronic diseases such as type 2 diabetes.

include the potential for excess bleeding, ulcers, hernia, and the typical risks from anesthesia.

A technique gaining in popularity because it is even more effective than gastric bypass for rapid weight loss is the *biliopancreatic diversion* or *duodenal switch procedure*, which combines elements of restrictive and malabsorption surgeries. The patient receives a partial gastrectomy to reduce the size of the stomach (less than gastric bypass's reduction) while bypassing less of the small intestine. The pyloric valve remains intact, which helps prevent dumping syndrome, ulcers, blockages, and other problems that can occur with other techniques. This surgery is one of the most difficult and highest risk surgeries for patients, with the risk of death and other complications higher than those of other options.[52]

Considerable research has demonstrated exciting, unexpected results from gastric surgeries: Even prior to weight loss, patients have shown complete remission of type 2 diabetes in the majority of cases, with drastic reductions in blood glucose levels in others. Add postsurgical exercise to the formula and both weight loss and relief of type 2 diabetes occur.[53] While extremely promising, newer research indicates that about one-third of those who have gastric surgery with remission of diabetic symptoms will relapse and begin to show diabetic symptoms within 5 years after surgery. For those at high risk from these diseases, the choice of undergoing surgery may ultimately be similar to the risk of maintaining their current weight.

*Bariatric arterial embolization* (BAE) is a new nonsurgical alternative to gastric bypass in which a catheter is inserted through the wrist or groin and targets blood vessels in the stomach where the "hunger hormone" ghrelin is produced. Tiny, microscopic beads designed to block ghrelin production are injected in the vessels, causing the patient to be less hungry. With lifestyle and dietary modifications as well as exercise, results of limited early trials appear promising. Thus, other options for weight loss via surgical or nonsurgical treatments are not a panacea for weight loss. All have risks, with diet and exercise as part of a sound weight control program being the best option for most.

Unlike surgeries that help make weight loss easier, or nonsurgical options such as BAE, *liposuction* is a surgical procedure in which fat cells are actually removed from specific areas of the body. Generally, liposuction is considered cosmetic surgery rather than true weight loss surgery, even though people who have it lose weight and contour their bodies. Liposuction is not risk-free. If you are considering this procedure, check the credentials of the surgeon, the certification of the facility, and the proximity to emergency care if problems arise.

## Trying to Gain Weight

For some people, trying to gain weight is a challenge. If you have trouble, the first priority is to determine why you cannot gain weight. Perhaps you're an athlete and you burn more calories than you eat. Perhaps you're stressed out and skip meals to increase study time. Among older adults, senses of taste and smell may decline, making food less pleasurable to eat.

Visual problems and other disabilities may make meals more difficult to prepare, and dental problems may make eating more difficult. People who engage in extreme energy-burning sports and exercise routines may be at risk for caloric and nutritional deficiencies, which can lead not only to weight loss, but also to immune system problems and organ dysfunction; weakness, which leads to falls and fractures; slower recovery from diseases; and a host of other problems. Underweight individuals need to examine diet and exercise behaviors and take steps to achieve and maintain a healthy weight.

# STUDY PLAN

## CHAPTER REVIEW

### LO 1 Overweight and Obesity: A Growing Challenge

- Overweight, obesity, and weight-related health problems have reached epidemic levels globally, termed *globesity*, and threatens the health of many countries. Societal costs from obesity include increased health care costs and lowered worker productivity. Individual health risks from overweight and obesity include increased chance of developing cardiovascular diseases, arthritis, stroke, diabetes, gastrointestinal problems, and low back pain, among others. Overweight individuals are also at risk of struggling with depression, low self-esteem, and high levels of stress.

### LO 2 Factors Contributing to Overweight and Obesity

- It is important to consider environmental, cultural, and socioeconomic factors when working to prevent obesity. In addition to genetics, metabolism, hormonal influences, excess fat cells, and physical risks, key environmental influences, such as poverty, socioeconomic status, education level, and lack of access to nutritious food, and lifestyle factors, including sedentary lifestyle and high calorie consumption, all make weight loss challenging.

### LO 3 Assessing Body Weight and Body Composition

- Percentage of body fat is a fairly reliable indicator for levels of overweight and obesity. There are many different methods of assessing body fat. Body mass index (BMI) is one of the most commonly accepted measures of weight based on height. *Overweight* is most commonly defined as a BMI of 25 to 29.9 and *obesity* as a BMI of 30 or greater. Waist circumference, or the amount of fat in the belly region, is believed to be related to the risk for several chronic diseases, particularly type 2 diabetes.

### LO 4 Managing Your Weight: Individual Roles

- Increased physical activity, a balanced, healthy diet that controls caloric intake, and other strategies are recommended for controlling your weight. When these options fail and risks increase, doctor-recommended prescription medications, weight loss surgery, and other strategies are used to maintain or lose weight. However, sensible eating behavior and aerobic and muscle-strengthening exercises offer the best options for weight loss and maintenance.

## POP QUIZ

### LO 1 Overweight and Obesity: A Growing Challenge

1. All of the following statements are true *except*:
   a. Hispanic and non-Hispanic white men are more likely to be overweight/obese than non-Hispanic black or Asian men.
   b. Children and adolescents living in higher-income homes where parents are more educated have a greatly increased risk of obesity over those living

in low-income homes where parents are less educated and/or unemployed.

c. Non-Hispanic black and Hispanic women are more likely to be overweight or obese than non-Hispanic white women.

d. The United States has the distinction of being one of the fattest developed nations on Earth.

LO 2 **Factors Contributing to Overweight and Obesity**

2. The rate at which your body consumes food energy to sustain basic functions is your
   a. basal metabolic rate.
   b. resting metabolic rate.
   c. body mass index.
   d. set point.

3. All of the following statements are true *except*:
   a. A slowing basal metabolic rate may contribute to weight gain after age 30.
   b. Hormones are increasingly implicated in hunger impulses and eating behavior.
   c. The more muscles you have, the fewer calories you will burn.
   d. Yo-yo dieting can make weight loss more difficult.

4. The theory that suggests there may be a genetic predisposition toward fat storage that makes losing fat more difficult for certain individuals is called
   a. thrifty gene theory.
   b. stingy gene theory.
   c. hoarder theory.
   d. spendthrift theory.

LO 3 **Assessing Body Weight and Body Composition**

5. The proportion of your total weight that is made up of fat is called
   a. body composition.
   b. lean mass.
   c. percentage of body fat.
   d. BMI.

6. All of the following statements about BMI are true *except*:
   a. BMI is based on height and weight measurements.
   b. BMI is accurate for everyone, including athletes with high amounts of muscle mass.
   c. Very low and very high BMI scores are associated with greater risk of mortality.
   d. BMI stands for "body mass index."

7. Which of the following body circumferences is most strongly associated with risk of heart disease and diabetes?
   a. Hip circumference
   b. Chest circumference
   c. Waist circumference
   d. Thigh circumference

LO 4 **Managing Your Weight: Individual Roles**

8. One pound of additional body fat is created through consuming how many extra calories?
   a. 1,500 calories
   b. 3,500 calories
   c. 5,000 calories
   d. 7,000 calories

9. Successful weight maintainers are most likely to do which of the following?
   a. Eat two large meals a day before 1:00 P.M.
   b. Skip meals
   c. Drink diet sodas
   d. Eat high-volume but low-calorie foods

10. Successful, healthy weight loss is characterized by
    a. a lifelong pattern of healthful eating and exercise.
    b. cutting out all fats and carbohydrates and eating a lean, high-protein diet.
    c. never eating foods that are considered bad for you and rigidly adhering to a plan.
    d. a pattern of repeatedly losing and regaining weight.

*Answers to the Pop Quiz can be found page A-1. If you answered a question incorrectly, review the section tagged by the Learning Outcome. For even more study tools, visit* **MasteringHealth**.

# THINK ABOUT IT!

LO 1 **Overweight and Obesity: A Growing Challenge**

1. Why do you think that obesity rates are rising in both developed and less-developed regions of the world? What strategies can we take collectively and individually to reduce risks of obesity nationally? Internationally?

LO 2 **Factors Contributing to Overweight and Obesity**

2. List the risk factors for your being overweight or obese right now. Which seem most likely to determine whether you will be obese in middle age? What factors do you think might help your weight loss? Which might sabotage your weight loss?

LO 3 **Assessing Body Weight and Body Composition**

3. Which measurement would you choose to assess your fat levels? Why? What would be the "normal" BMI for you right now?

LO 4 **Managing Your Weight: Individual Roles**

4. Are you satisfied with your body weight? If so, what do you do to maintain a healthy weight? If not, what are some lifestyle changes you could make to improve your weight and overall health?

# ACCESS YOUR HEALTH ON THE INTERNET

Visit **MasteringHealth** for links to the websites and RSS feeds.

The following websites explore further topics and issues related to obesity.

**Academy of Nutrition and Dietetics.** This site includes recommended dietary guidelines and other current information about weight control. **www.eatright.org**

**Weight Control Information Network.** This is an excellent resource for diet and weight control information. **http://win.niddk.nih.gov/index.htm**

**The Rudd Center for Food Policy and Obesity.** This website provides excellent information on the latest in obesity research, public policy, and ways we can stop the obesity epidemic at the community level. **www.uconnruddcenter.org**

**The Obesity Society.** Key site for information/education about our national obesity epidemic, including statistics, research, consumer issues, and fact sheets. **www.obesity.org**

# FOCUS ON Enhancing Your Body Image

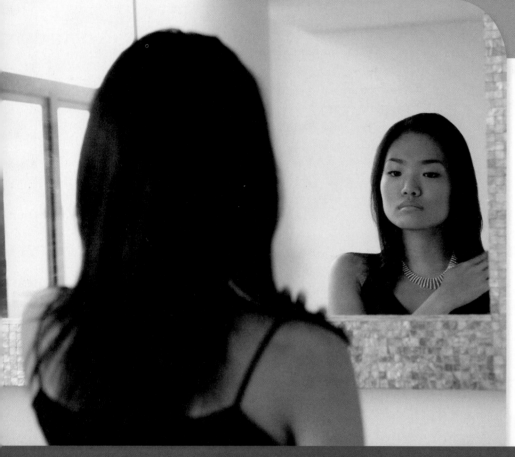

## LEARNING OUTCOMES

LO **1** Define body image, list the factors that influence it, and identify the difference between being dissatisfied with your appearance and having body dysmorphic disorder.

LO **2** Describe the signs and symptoms of disordered eating, as well as the physical effects and treatment options for anorexia nervosa, bulimia nervosa, orthorexia nervosa, and binge-eating disorder.

LO **3** List the criteria, symptoms, and treatment options for exercise disorders such as muscle dysmorphia and female athlete triad.

## WHY SHOULD I CARE?

All-too-common dissatisfaction with one's appearance and shape can foster unhealthy attitudes and thought patterns, as well as disordered eating and compulsive exercise behaviors.

**W**hen you look in the mirror, do you like what you see? If you feel dissatisfied, frustrated, or even angry, you're not alone. In a recent national poll, 67% of women and 53% of men reported worrying about their appearance regularly—women, more than every other issue in their lives, and men, more than every issue but finances.[1] For both women (69%) and men (52%), the body part of greatest concern is the abdomen.[2] Concerns about weight and shape are central to many people's body dissatisfaction. As body mass increases, dissatisfaction increases, particularly during transitional periods in life. Females, in particular, seem to experience peak levels of body dissatisfaction when transitioning from high school to young adulthood.[3] Sadly, dissatisfaction with your body can result in behaviors that disrupt your relationships, undermine your goals, affect your mental health, and lead to life-threatening illness. Developing and maintaining a healthy body image can enhance your interactions with others, reduce stress, give you an increased sense of personal empowerment, and bring confidence and joy to your life.

LO **1** | **WHAT** IS BODY IMAGE?

Define body image, list the factors that influence it, and identify the difference between being dissatisfied with your appearance and having body dysmorphic disorder.

**Body image** refers to what you believe or emotionally feel about your body's shape, weight, and general appearance. More than what you see in the mirror, it includes the following:[4]

- How you see yourself in your mind
- What you believe about your own appearance (including beliefs about how others view you)
- How you feel about your body, including your height, weight, and shape
- How you sense and control your body as you move

A *negative body image* is defined as either a distorted perception of your shape or feelings of discomfort, shame, or anxiety about your body. It may involve being certain that only other people are attractive and that your body's shape is a sign of personal failure. Negative body image is associated with many negative health outcomes including emotional distress, unhealthy eating patterns, anxiety, depression, eating disorders, sexual risk-taking, and social withdrawal.

In contrast, a *positive body image* is a true perception of your appearance: You see yourself as you really are. You are comfortable and confident in your skin. You understand that everyone is different, and you celebrate your uniqueness— including perceived "flaws," which have nothing to do with your value as a person.

**SEE IT! VIDEOS**

The dangers of chasing an "ideal" body image. Watch **Young Boys Exercising to Extremes**, available on MasteringHealth.™

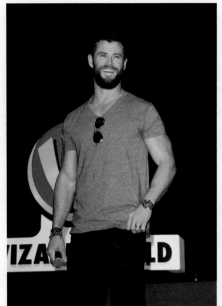
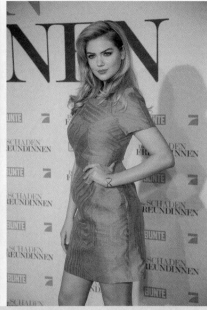

Although the exact nature of the "in" look may change from generation to generation, unrealistic images of both male and female celebrities are nothing new. *People* magazine's 2014's Sexiest Man and Woman Alive, Chris Hemsworth and Kate Upton, both exhibit physical features difficult for the average person to achieve, no matter how hard they might work.

Is your body image negative, positive, or somewhere in between? Researchers have developed a body image continuum that may help you decide (see **FIGURE 1** on page 178). Notice that the continuum identifies behaviors associated with particular states, from total dissociation to body acceptance.

## Many Factors Influence Body Image

You're not born with a body image, but you do begin to develop one at an early age. One recent study found that by age 7 one in four kids has engaged in dieting behavior and that one-half of girls and one-third of boys as young as 7 think their ideal weight is thinner than their current size.[5] Let's look at the factors that play a role in body image development.

### The Media and Popular Culture

Media images tend to set the standard for what we find attractive, leading some people to go to dangerous extremes to have bigger biceps or fit into smaller jeans. Changing our bodies to better achieve what the current society identifies as "attractive" has long been part of American culture. During the early twentieth century, while men idolized the strong, hearty outdoorsman President Teddy Roosevelt, women pulled their corsets ever tighter to achieve unrealistically tiny waists. In the 1920s and 1930s, men emulated the burly cops and robbers in gangster films, while women dieted and bound their breasts to achieve the boyish "flapper" look. By the 1960s, tough guys were the male ideal, where rail-thin supermodels were the standard of female beauty. Today's societal obsession around celebrity appearance—even when we know many images are "Photoshopped" (i.e., altered) or the person has had cosmetic surgery—hasn't evolved very much.

Today's college students grew up with the added pressure of social media, which has increased concerns about appearance.[6] In fact, people who spend more time on Facebook report more body dissatisfaction, more drive for thinness, and paying more attention to their physical appearance.[7] These feelings may be due to constantly comparing one's appearance to others' and

**body image** How you see yourself in your mind, what you believe about your appearance, and how you feel about your body.

| Body hate/ disassociation | Distorted body image | Body preoccupied/ obsessed | Body acceptance | Body is not an issue |
|---|---|---|---|---|
| I often feel separated and distant from my body—as if it belonged to someone else. | I spend a significant amount of time exercising and dieting to change my body. | I weigh and measure myself a lot. | I pay attention to my body and my appearance because it is important to me, but it only occupies a small part of my day. | I feel fine about my body. |
| I hate my body, and I often isolate myself from others. | My body shape and size keeps me from dating or finding someone who will treat me the way I want to be treated. | I spend a significant amount of time viewing myself in the mirror. | I would like to change some things about my body, but I spend most of my time highlighting my positive features. | I don't worry about changing my body shape or weight. |
| I don't see anything positive or even neutral about my body shape and size. | I have considered changing (or have changed) my body shape and size through surgical means. | I compare my body to others. | My self-esteem is based on my personality traits, achievements, and relationships—not just my body image. | I never weigh or measure myself. |
| I don't believe others when they tell me I look okay. | I wish I could change the way I look in the mirror. | I have days when I feel fat. | | My feelings about my body are not influenced by society's concept of an ideal body shape. |
| I hate the way I look in the mirror. | | I accept society's ideal body shape and size as the best body shape and size. | | I know that the significant others in my life will always love me for who I am, not for how I look. |
| | | I'd be more attractive if I were thinner, more muscular, etc. | | |

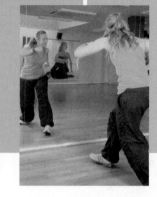

**FIGURE 1 Body Image Continuum** This continuum shows a range of attitudes and behaviors toward body image, from full acceptance to disassociation.

Source: Adapted from Smiley/King/Avery, "Eating Issues and Body Image Continuum," Campus Health Service 1996. Copyright © 1997 Arizona Board of Regents for University of Arizona.

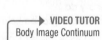

▶ VIDEO TUTOR
Body Image Continuum

that the pictures posted often show idealized curated images, not real ones. While many social media sites actively warn against posts promoting or glorifying self-harm, messages promoting unhealthy body images are common. Such messages are often disguised as a type of encouragement—images of unrealistically thin bodies coupled with catch phrases telling people to get "thin" or be "fit."[8] See **Student Health Today** for more on "thinspiration."

With more than two-thirds of American adults 20 years and older overweight or obese, a significant disconnect exists between the media's idealized images and the typical American body.[9] The images of "beauty" we are bombarded with are unrealistic for all but a small fragment of the population. These messages can damage our body image, as no amount of dieting or exercise can shift a person to the size or shape of a Photoshopped body.

## Family, Community, and Cultural Groups

People we interact with regularly strongly influence the way we see ourselves. Parents are especially influential in body image development. For instance, it's common and natural for fathers of adolescent girls to experience feelings of discomfort related to their daughters' changing bodies. If they are able to navigate these feelings and validate the acceptability of their daughters' appearance throughout puberty, they'll help their daughters maintain a positive body image.[10] Even subtle judgments about their changing bodies may prompt girls to question how males

view their bodies in general. In addition, mothers who model body acceptance or body ownership may be more likely to foster a positive body image in their daughters, whereas mothers who are frustrated with or ashamed of their own bodies may foster negative attitudes in their children.[11]

Interactions with other relatives, peers, teachers, coworkers, and other community members can also influence body image development. Being overweight is now the most commonly reported reason children are bullied at school,[12] and peer harassment (teasing and bullying) is widely acknowledged to contribute to a negative body image. Associations within one's cultural group are also an influence on body image. For example, studies have found that white females experience the highest rates of

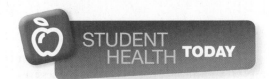
# THINSPIRATION AND INSPIRATION

The pro-anorexia movement has a host of websites, chatrooms, blogs, and discussion boards mostly created and hosted by girls and women struggling with eating disorders. One study found that 13% of young females have visited a pro–eating disorder website and the sites were Googled 13 million times last year. Along with dangerous and incorrect information about restrictive eating, metabolism, bingeing, and laxative abuse, many include "thinspiration"—pictures and quotes intended to inspire visitors to thinness—as well as tips and tricks to hide and maintain disordered eating.

Despite the support and understanding that participating women get from each other, they also encourage each other to remain sick. Ambivalent messages about thinness and weight loss coincide with tips on "how to become anorexic." Some people meet on the website and then compete with each other to see who can lose the most weight. This is not the type of inspiration girls and women need!

We can be inspired, however, by some changes in the modeling industry. The French government recently passed a law that models must have a BMI of 18 or over to prevent the use of "excessively thin" models. The bill also requires that Photoshopped images—in particular those that make a model's silhouette "narrower or wider"—be labeled as "retouched."

In the United States there has also been a recent surge of more normal-sized models gracing magazine pages. Retailer Modcloth had its employees, of all shapes and sizes, model the site's new swimsuits; Calvin Klein recently featured a size-10 model in its "Perfect Body" campaign; and in 2016, for the first time ever, the cover of the *Sports Illustrated* swimsuit issue featured a plus-sized model, Ashley Graham. The tag "real-sized" (instead of plus-sized) is now commonly used for popular models like Tocarra Jones and Robyn Lawley. This acceptance of a variety of beauty is the kind of inspiration we need!

**Sources:** National Eating Disorder Information Centre; MPA Website, Accessed May 2015, www.myproana.com/index.php/blogs/; M. Persad, "Average-Size Models Could Be Better For Business, Study Says" May 14, 2015, http://www.huffingtonpost.com/2015/05/14/average-size-models-study-advertising_n_7275376.html; Vogue News, "France Passes Model Health Law," December 21, 2015, http://www.vogue.co.uk/news/2015/12/21/french-model-law-bmi-medical-certificate-for-models-in-france; S. Jett et al., "Impact of Exposure to Pro-Eating Disorder Websites on Eating Behavior in College Women," *European Eating Disorders Review* 18 (2010): 410–6.

## WHAT DO YOU THINK?

**What different cultural ideals of beauty do different race/ethnic groups hold?**

- Why do you think this is? How do you think body-image pressure is different for males and females?
- How do you think they are the same?

body dissatisfaction, but the body dissatisfaction levels of minority women increase the more they are acculturated within and exposed to mainstream media.[13]

## Physiological and Psychological Factors

Neurological research suggests that people diagnosed with a body image disorder show differences in the brain's ability to regulate mood-linked chemicals called *neurotransmitters*.[14] Poor regulation of neurotransmitters is also involved in depression, anxiety disorders, and obsessive–compulsive disorder. One study linked distortions in body image to a malfunction in the brain's visual processing region.[15] Another theory suggests genetic differences in the level of the neurotransmitter serotonin in the brain of those with a body image disorder.[16] These findings suggest that some people are more biologically susceptible to developing a body image disorder. They also indicate that there is a small number of people that could

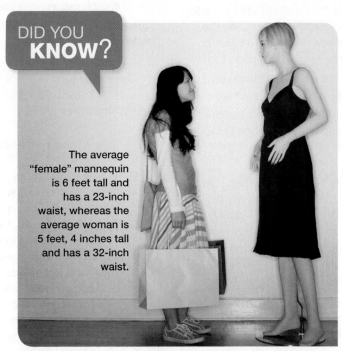

## DID YOU KNOW?

The average "female" mannequin is 6 feet tall and has a 23-inch waist, whereas the average woman is 5 feet, 4 inches tall and has a 32-inch waist.

**Sources:** R. Duyff, *American Dietetic Association Complete Food and Nutrition Guide*, 4th ed. (Hoboken, NJ: John Wiley & Sons, 2012), 50; C. Fryar, Q. Gu, and C. Ogden, "Anthropometric Reference Data for Children and Adults: United States, 2007–2010," National Center for Health Statistics, *Vital and Health Statistics*, Series 11, no. 252 (2012), www.cdc.gov/nchs/data/series/sr_11/sr11_252.pdf.

# 30%

of college males and 45% of college females **REPORT DIETING** in the past 30 days to lose weight.

benefit from medication, such as SSRIs, to improve their body image.[17]

## Building a Positive Body Image

To develop a more positive body image, you can start by challenging some commonly held myths and attitudes in contemporary society.[18]

- **Myth 1: How you look is more important than who you are.**
  Fact: Your appearance does not determine who you are or what you are capable of.

- **Myth 2: Anyone can look like the celebrities if they work hard enough.**
  Fact: While exercise and healthy eating can improve anyone's health status, not everyone has the genes to be muscular, tall, or curvy. We can exercise and eat our way to health, but not to a particular shape.

- **Myth 3: Extreme dieting is an effective weight-loss strategy.**
  Fact: Extreme dieting is dangerous and quick weight loss is rarely sustainable. (See Chapter 6 for more on weight loss techniques.)

- **Myth 4: Things will go better for me after I achieve the perfect body.**
  Fact: A certain shape or weight is not the key to a happy, wonderful life. Investing in healthy relationships and working toward life goals can bring lasting happiness.

For ways to build a more positive body image, check out the Making Changes Today box.

---

**body dysmorphic disorder (BDD)** Psychological disorder characterized by an obsession with one's appearance and a distorted view of one's body or with a minor or imagined flaw in appearance.

## Body Dysmorphic Disorder

Although most Americans report being dissatisfied with some aspect of their appearance, very few have a true body image disorder. The difference lies in the degree of dissatisfaction and the actions taken to chase satisfaction. Approximately 2 percent of people in the United States suffer from **body dysmorphic disorder (BDD)**.[19] Persons with BDD are obsessively concerned with their appearance and have a distorted view of their own body to the extent that it impairs their social or occupational functioning. Although the cause of the disorder isn't known, an anxiety disorder or obsessive–compulsive disorder is often also present. (See Chapter 2 for more discussion of anxiety disorders.) Contributing factors may include genetic susceptibility, childhood teasing, physical or sexual abuse, low self-esteem, and rigid sociocultural expectations of attractiveness.[20] Males and females show similar prevalence, although they usually focus on different perceived defects.[21]

---

## MAKING CHANGES TODAY

### Ten Steps to a Positive Body Image

One way to turn negative thoughts positive is to think about how to look more healthfully and happily at yourself and your body. The more you try, the better you will feel about who you are and the body you naturally have.

◉ **Step 1.** Appreciate all of the amazing things your body does for you—running, dancing, breathing, laughing, dreaming.

◎ **Step 2.** Make a list of things you like about yourself—things that aren't related to how much you weigh or how you look. Add to it as you notice new things.

◎ **Step 3.** Remind yourself that true beauty is not skin deep. When you feel good about yourself and who you are, you carry yourself with a sense of confidence, self-acceptance, and openness that makes you beautiful.

◎ **Step 4.** Look at yourself as a whole person. When you see yourself in a mirror or in your mind, choose not to focus on specific body parts.

◎ **Step 5.** Surround yourself with positive people. It is easier to feel good about yourself when you are around those who are supportive and who recognize the importance of liking yourself as you naturally are.

◎ **Step 6.** Shut down those voices in your head that tell you your body is not "right" or that you are a "bad" person.

◎ **Step 7.** Wear comfortable clothes that make you feel good about your body. Work with your body, not against it.

◎ **Step 8.** Become a critical viewer of social and media messages. Pay attention to images, slogans, and attitudes that make you feel bad about your appearance.

◎ **Step 9.** Show appreciation for your body. Take a bubble bath, make time for a nap, or find a peaceful place outside to relax.

◎ **Step 10.** Use the time and energy you might have spent worrying about food, calories, and your weight to do something to help others. Reaching out to other people can help you feel better about yourself and make a positive change in our world.

**Source:** "10 Steps to Positive Body Image," from National Eating Disorders Association website, Accessed February 13, 2016. National Eating Disorders Association. Reprinted with permission. For more information, visit www.NationalEatingDisorders.org or call NEDA's helpline at 1-800-931-2237.

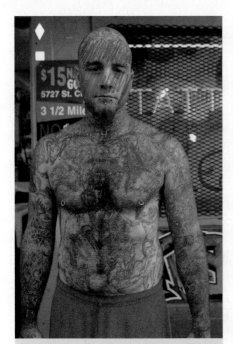

It's nearly impossible to spot people who are highly dissatisfied with their bodies. People who cover their bodies with tattoos may have a strong sense of self-esteem. On the other hand, extreme tattooing can be an outward sign of a severe body image disturbance known as body dysmorphic disorder.

People with BDD may try to fix their perceived flaws through abuse of steroids, excessive bodybuilding, cosmetic surgeries, extreme tattooing, or other appearance-altering behaviors. It is estimated that 10 percent of people seeking dermatology or cosmetic treatments have BDD.[22] Not only do such actions fail to address the underlying problem, but they also are actually considered diagnostic signs of BDD. Psychiatric treatment, including psychotherapy and/or antidepressant medications, can help.

## LO 2 | DISORDERED EATING AND EATING DISORDERS

Describe the signs and symptoms of disordered eating, as well as the physical effects and treatment options for anorexia nervosa, bulimia nervosa, orthorexia nervosa, and binge-eating disorder.

People with a negative body image can fixate on a wide range of self-perceived "flaws." The so-called flaw that distresses the majority of people with negative body image is feeling overweight. Some people channel weight-related anxiety into self-defeating thoughts and harmful behaviors. The far left of the eating issues continuum (**FIGURE 2** on page 182) identifies a pattern of thoughts and behaviors associated with **disordered eating**, including chronic dieting, rigid eating patterns, abusing diet pills and laxatives, self-induced vomiting, and body hatred, among others.

Far more people follow disordered eating patterns than actually have an eating disorder. In fact, research suggests that up to 50% of Americans have problematic or disordered relationships with food.[23] Persons with disordered eating patterns take dieting to the extreme; they may obsessively count calories, fear gaining small amounts of weight, lie about the amount of food eaten, abstain from certain types of food, or obsess about their weight. Although not severe enough to qualify as a mental illness, disordered eating creates an unhealthy relationship with food and weight.

To avoid disordered eating patterns, you can avoid dieting rules that are highly restrictive, fast only for medical reasons, stop fat talk, separate food from mood, and focus on eating mindfully (see **Focus On: Cultivating Your Spiritual Health** on page 51 for more on mindfulness).

A small number of people who exhibit disordered eating patterns progress to a clinical **eating disorder**. The eating disorders defined by the American Psychiatric Association (APA) in the *Diagnostic and Statistical Manual of Mental Disorders, Fifth Edition (DSM-5)* are *anorexia nervosa*, *bulimia nervosa*, *binge-eating disorder*, and a cluster of less-distinct conditions collectively referred to as *other specified feeding or eating disorder (OSFED)*.[24]

Twenty million women and 10 million men in the United States will suffer from some sort of eating disorder over their lifetimes.[25] Although anorexia nervosa and bulimia nervosa primarily affect people in their teens and 20s, increasing numbers of children as young as age 7 have been diagnosed, as have women as old as age 80.[26] In 2015, 2.6 percent of college students reported having been diagnosed with anorexia or bulimia.[27] While anyone can have an eating disorder, they are more common among ballet dancers and athletes, particularly athletes in sports with an aesthetic component (e.g., figure skating or gymnastics), lean sports (cross-country running), or sports tied to a weight class (e.g., tae kwon do or wrestling).[28]

Eating disorders are on the rise among men, who make up nearly 25 percent of all anorexia and bulimia patients.[29] Many men suffering from eating disorders fail to seek treatment because these illnesses are traditionally thought of as a woman's problem.

What factors put individuals at risk? Many people with eating disorders feel controlled in other aspects of their lives and try to gain a sense of power through food. Many are clinically depressed, suffer from obsessive–compulsive disorder, or have other psychiatric problems. In addition, individuals with low self-esteem, negative body image, and a high tendency for perfectionism are at risk.[30] **FIGURE 3** on page 183 shows how individual and social factors can interact to increase the risk of an eating disorder.

## Anorexia Nervosa

**Anorexia nervosa** is a persistent, chronic eating disorder characterized by deliberate food restriction and severe, life-threatening weight loss. It has the highest death rate (20%) of any psychological illness.[31] It involves self-starvation motivated by an intense fear of gaining weight and an extremely distorted body image. Initially, most people with anorexia nervosa lose weight by reducing total food intake, particularly of high-calorie foods. Eventually, they progress to restricting their intake of almost all foods. The little they do eat, they may purge through vomiting or using laxatives. Although

**disordered eating** A pattern of atypical eating behaviors that is used to achieve or maintain a lower body weight.

**eating disorder** A psychiatric disorder characterized by severe disturbances in body image and eating behaviors.

**anorexia nervosa** Eating disorder characterized by deliberate food restriction, self-starvation, or extreme exercising to achieve weight loss, as well as an extremely distorted body image.

| Eating disordered | Disruptive eating patterns | Food preoccupied/ obsessed | Concerned in a healthy way | Food is not an issue |
|---|---|---|---|---|
| I worry about what I will eat or when I will exercise all the time. | My food and exercise concerns are starting to interfere with my school and social life. | I think about food a lot. | I pay attention to what I eat in order to maintain a healthy body. | I am not concerned about what or how much I eat. |
| I follow a very rigid eating plan and know precisely how many calories, fat grams, or carbohydrates I eat every day. | I use food to comfort myself. | I'm obsessed with reading books and magazines about dieting, fitness, and weight control. | Food and exercise are important parts of my life, but they only occupy a small part of my time. | I feel no guilt or shame no matter what I eat or how much I eat. |
| I feel incredible guilt, shame, and anxiety when I break my diet. | I have tried diet pills, laxatives, vomiting, or extra time exercising in order to lose or maintain my weight. | I sometimes miss school, work, and social events because of my diet or exercise schedule. | I enjoy eating, and I balance my pleasure with my concern for a healthy body. | Exercise is not really important to me. I choose foods based on cost, taste, and convenience, with little regard to health. |
| I regularly stuff myself and then exercise, vomit, or use laxatives to get rid of the food. | I have fasted or avoided eating for long periods of time in order to lose or maintain my weight. | I divide food into "good" and "bad" categories. | I usually eat three balanced meals daily, plus snacks, to fuel my body with adequate energy. | My eating is very sporadic and irregular. |
| My friends and family tell me I am too thin, but I feel fat. | If I cannot exercise to burn off calories, I panic. | I feel guilty when I eat "bad" foods or when I eat more than what I feel I should be eating. | I am moderate and flexible in my goals for eating well and being physically active. | I don't worry about meals; I just eat whatever I can, whenever I can. |
| I am out of control when I eat. | I feel strong when I can restrict how much I eat. | I am afraid of getting fat. | Sometimes I eat more (or less) than I really need, but most of the time I listen to my body. | I enjoy stuffing myself with lots of tasty food at restaurants, holiday meals, and social events. |
| I am afraid to eat in front of others. | I feel out of control when I eat more than I wanted to. | I wish I could change how much I want to eat and what I am hungry for. | | |
| I prefer to eat alone. | | | | |

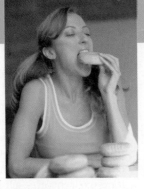

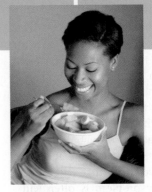

**FIGURE 2** **Eating Issues Continuum** This continuum shows progression from eating disorders to healthy eating, with healthy attention to food as the goal.

**Source:** Adapted from Smiley/King/Avery, "Eating Issues and Body Image Continuum," Campus Health Service 1996. Copyright © 1997 Arizona Board of Regents for University of Arizona.

they lose weight, people with anorexia nervosa never feel thin enough. An estimated 0.3 percent of females suffer from anorexia nervosa in their lifetime.[32] The DSM-5 criteria for anorexia nervosa are as follows:[33]

- Refusal to maintain body weight at or above a minimally normal weight for age and height
- Intense fear of gaining weight or becoming fat, even though considered underweight by all medical criteria

- Disturbance in the way in which one's body weight or shape is experienced, undue influence of body weight or shape on self-evaluation, or denial of the seriousness of the current low body weight

FIGURE 4 on page 183 illustrates physical symptoms and negative health consequences associated with anorexia nervosa.

Causes of anorexia nervosa are complex and variable. Many people with anorexia have other coexisting psychiatric problems, including low self-esteem, depression, an anxiety disorder such as obsessive–compulsive disorder, and substance abuse. Some people have a history of being physically or sexually abused, and others have troubled interpersonal relationships. Cultural norms that value appearance and glorify thinness as beauty are factors, as are weight-based shame, peer comparisons, and weight bias.[34] Physical factors are thought to include an imbalance of neurotransmitters and genetic susceptibility.[35]

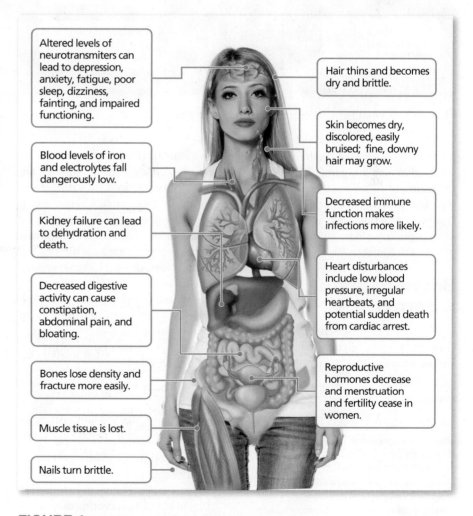

## Figure 3 diagram (top left)

**Sociocultural factors**
- Family and personal relationships
- History of being teased
- History of abuse
- Cultural norms
- Media influences
- Economic status

**Psychological factors**
- Low self-esteem
- Feelings of inadequacy or lack of control
- Unhealthy body image
- Perfectionism
- Lack of coping skills

**Biological factors**
- Inherited personality traits
- Genes that affect hunger, satiety, and body weight
- Depression or anxiety
- Brain chemistry

**FIGURE 3** Factors That Contribute to Eating Disorders

other medications; fasting; or excessive exercise
- Binge eating and inappropriate compensatory behavior occurs on average at least once a week for 3 months
- Body shape and weight unduly influence self-evaluation

**FIGURE 5** on page 184 illustrates the physical symptoms and negative health consequences associated with bulimia nervosa.

A combination of genetic and environmental factors is thought to cause bulimia nervosa.[38] A family history of obesity, an underlying anxiety disorder, and an imbalance in neurotransmitters are all possible contributing factors. In support of the role of neurotransmitters,

**bulimia nervosa** Eating disorder characterized by binge eating followed by inappropriate purging measures or compensatory behavior, such as vomiting or excessive exercise, to prevent weight gain.

# Bulimia Nervosa

Individuals with **bulimia nervosa** binge on huge amounts of food—often with a feeling of being out of control—and then engage in some kind of purging or compensatory behavior, such as vomiting, taking laxatives, or exercising excessively, to lose the calories they have just consumed. People with bulimia are obsessed with their bodies, weight gain, and appearance, but unlike those with anorexia, their problem is often hidden from the public eye because their weight may fall within a normal range or they may be overweight. Up to 3 percent of adolescents and young women are bulimic; rates among men are about 10 percent of the rate among women.[36] The DSM-5 diagnostic criteria for bulimia nervosa are as follows:[37]

- Recurrent episodes of binge eating (defined as eating, in a discrete period of time, an amount of food that is larger than most people would eat during a similar period of time and under similar circumstances, and experiencing a sense of lack of control over eating during the episode)
- Recurrent inappropriate compensatory behavior to prevent weight gain, such as self-induced vomiting; misusing laxatives, diuretics, or

## Figure 4 labels

- Altered levels of neurotransmiters can lead to depression, anxiety, fatigue, poor sleep, dizziness, fainting, and impaired functioning.
- Blood levels of iron and electrolytes fall dangerously low.
- Kidney failure can lead to dehydration and death.
- Decreased digestive activity can cause constipation, abdominal pain, and bloating.
- Bones lose density and fracture more easily.
- Muscle tissue is lost.
- Nails turn brittle.
- Hair thins and becomes dry and brittle.
- Skin becomes dry, discolored, easily bruised; fine, downy hair may grow.
- Decreased immune function makes infections more likely.
- Heart disturbances include low blood pressure, irregular heartbeats, and potential sudden death from cardiac arrest.
- Reproductive hormones decrease and menstruation and fertility cease in women.

**FIGURE 4** What Anorexia Nervosa Can Do to the Body

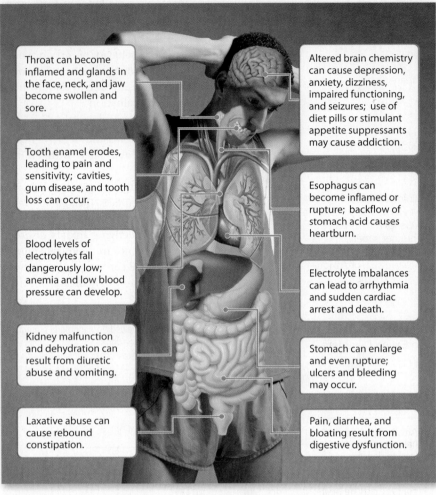

Throat can become inflamed and glands in the face, neck, and jaw become swollen and sore.

Tooth enamel erodes, leading to pain and sensitivity; cavities, gum disease, and tooth loss can occur.

Blood levels of electrolytes fall dangerously low; anemia and low blood pressure can develop.

Kidney malfunction and dehydration can result from diuretic abuse and vomiting.

Laxative abuse can cause rebound constipation.

Altered brain chemistry can cause depression, anxiety, dizziness, impaired functioning, and seizures; use of diet pills or stimulant appetite suppressants may cause addiction.

Esophagus can become inflamed or rupture; backflow of stomach acid causes heartburn.

Electrolyte imbalances can lead to arrhythmia and sudden cardiac arrest and death.

Stomach can enlarge and even rupture; ulcers and bleeding may occur.

Pain, diarrhea, and bloating result from digestive dysfunction.

**FIGURE 5** What Bulimia Nervosa Can Do to the Body

a study showed that brain circuitry involved in regulating impulsive behavior seems to be less active in women with bulimia than in healthy women.[39] However, it is unknown whether such differences exist before bulimia develops or arise as a consequence of the disorder.

## Binge-Eating Disorder

Individuals with **binge-eating disorder** gorge themselves, but do not take excessive measures to lose the weight gained

> **binge-eating disorder** A type of eating disorder characterized by gorging on food once a week or more, but not typically followed by a purge.
>
> **other specified feeding or eating disorder (OSFED)** Eating disorders that are a true psychiatric illness but that do not fit the strict diagnostic criteria for anorexia nervosa, bulimia nervosa, or binge-eating disorder.
>
> **orthorexia nervosa** An eating disorder characterized by fixation on food quality and purity.

(as in bulimia). Thus, they are often clinically obese. Binge-eating episodes are typically characterized by eating large amounts of food rapidly, even when not feeling hungry, and feeling guilty or depressed after overeating.[40] Binge eaters often report eating to avoid dealing with problems, often feeling powerless, shameful, and socially isolated.

A national survey reported a lifetime prevalence of binge-eating disorder in the study participants of 1.4 percent.[41] The DSM-5 criteria for binge-eating disorder are as follows:[42]

- Recurrent episodes of binge eating (defined as eating, in a discrete period of time, an amount of food that is larger than most people would eat during a similar period of time and under similar circumstances, and experiencing a sense of lack of control over eating during the episode)

- Binge-eating episodes are associated with three (or more) of the following: (1) eating much more rapidly than normal; (2) eating until feeling uncomfortably full; (3) eating large amounts of food when not feeling physical hunger; (4) eating alone because of embarrassment over how much one is eating; (5) feeling disgusted with oneself, depressed, or guilty after overeating
- Experiencing marked distress regarding binge eating
- The binge eating occurs, on average, at least once a week for 3 months
- The binge eating is not associated with the recurrent use of inappropriate compensatory behavior (e.g., purging) and does not occur exclusively during the course of bulimia nervosa or anorexia nervosa

## Other Specified Feeding or Eating Disorders

The APA recognizes that some patterns of disordered eating qualify as a legitimate psychiatric illness but don't fit into the strict diagnostic criteria for anorexia, bulimia, or binge-eating disorder. Called **other specified feeding or eating disorders (OSFED)**, this group of disorders includes five specific subtypes: *night eating syndrome, purging disorder, binge-eating disorder of low frequency/limited duration, bulimia nervosa of low frequency/duration,* and *atypical anorexia nervosa.* Atypical anorexia nervosa is defined in this category as displaying anorexic features without low weight.[43] All of these subtypes can cause remarkable distress or impairment but don't exhibit the full criteria of another feeding or eating disorder; some people may cross over between types of eating disorders over time. About one-third of people who seek treatment for eating disorders have OSFED.[44]

## Orthorexia Nervosa

Literally meaning "fixation on righteous eating," **orthorexia nervosa** is an unhealthy obsession with what would otherwise be healthy eating. What typically begins as a simple attempt to eat more healthfully can become a fixation with food quality and purity. Those with orthorexia nervosa become consumed with what and how much to eat and how to deal with eating mistakes. While not categorized as an eating disorder by the DSM-5, eventually, food choices become so restrictive that health suffers.

## Treatment for Eating Disorders

Because eating disorders are caused by a combination of factors, there are no simple solutions. Without treatment, approximately 20 percent of people with a serious eating disorder will die as a result; the highest fatality risk of any psychiatric disorder. With treatment, long-term full recovery rates range from 44 to 76 percent for anorexia nervosa and from 50 to 70 percent for bulimia nervosa.[45]

Treatment often focuses first on reducing the threat to life. Once the patient is stabilized, long-term therapy focuses on the psychological, social, environmental, and physiological factors that have led to the problem. Through therapy, the patient works on adopting new eating behaviors, building self-confidence, and finding healthy ways to deal with life's problems. Support groups can help the family and the individual learn positive actions and interactions. Treatment of an underlying anxiety disorder or depression may also be a focus.

## Helping Someone with Eating Issues

Although every situation is different, there are several things you can do if you suspect someone you know is struggling with disordered eating or an eating disorder:[46]

- **Know the facts** about weight, nutrition, exercise, disordered eating, and eating disorders. Accurate information can help you reason against excuses used to maintain a disordered eating pattern.
- **Be honest** and talk openly about your concerns.
- **Be caring, but be firm** because caring about your friend does not mean allowing him or her to

**WHAT DO YOU THINK?**

Is attention to the national obesity epidemic likely to worsen problems with eating disorders? Why or why not?

- What do you think can be done to increase awareness of eating disorders in the United States?
- What resources are available on your campus for people with food and exercise issues?

manipulate you. Your friend must be responsible for his or her actions and the consequences of those actions. Avoid making threats that you cannot or will not uphold. Don't badger or get angry. Stay calm and be reassuring.

- **Compliment** your friend's personality, successes, and accomplishments.
- **Be a good role model** for healthy eating, exercise, and self-acceptance.
- **Tell someone**, and don't wait until your friend's life is in danger. Addressing disordered eating patterns in their beginning stages offers your friend the best chance for working through these issues and becoming healthy again.

There are many resources for people who are considering seeking help or finding out if they are at risk for developing an eating disorder. The National Eating Disorders Association has a general online screening tool allowing individuals to assess their own patterns to determine if they should seek professional help (*www.nationaleatingdisorders.org/online-eating-disorder-screening*). They also have additional information and a helpline (1-800-931-2237) for guidance, treatment referrals, and support.[47]

## LO 3 | CAN TOO MUCH EXERCISE BE UNHEALTHY?

List the criteria, symptoms, and treatment options for exercise disorders such as muscle dysmorphia and female athlete triad.

Although exercise is generally beneficial, in excess it can be a problem. In addition to being a common compensatory behavior used by people with anorexia or bulimia, exercise can become a compulsion or contribute to more complex disorders such as muscle dysmorphia or the female athlete triad.

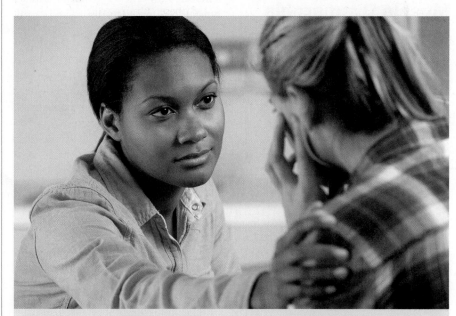

When talking to a friend about an eating disorder or disordered eating patterns, avoid blaming, preaching, or offering unsolicited advice. Instead, be a good listener, let the person know that you care, and offer your support.

## Compulsive Exercise

In a recent study, researchers showed that participants used excessive exercise or **compulsive exercise** as a way to regulate their emotions.[48] Also called *anorexia athletica*, compulsive exercise is characterized not by a *desire* to exercise but a *compulsion*; that is, the person struggles with guilt and anxiety if he or she doesn't work out. Compulsive exercisers, like people with eating disorders, often define their self-worth externally. They overexercise in order to feel more in control of their lives, to relieve guilt, or sometimes to purge calories—similar to a person with bulimia nervosa purging after a food binge. Disordered eating or an eating disorder is often part of the picture also.

Compulsive exercise can contribute to a variety of injuries, such as sprains, strains, or stress fractures. It can also put significant stress on the heart, especially if combined with disordered eating. Signs that exercise has crossed over to compulsion include feeling anxious or depressed when exercise isn't possible, missing other commitments to exercise, and exercising despite injury. Psychologically, people who engage in compulsive exercise are often plagued by anxiety and/or depression. Their social life and academic success can suffer as they fixate more and more on exercise.

## Muscle Dysmorphia

**Muscle dysmorphia** is a form of body image disturbance and exercise disorder

**SEE IT! VIDEOS**

Can you go too far with extreme exercise? Watch **Young Boys Exercising to Extremes**, available on MasteringHealth.™

compulsive exercise  Disorder characterized by a compulsion to engage in excessive amounts of exercise and feelings of guilt and anxiety if the level of exercise is perceived as inadequate.

muscle dysmorphia  Body image disorder in which men believe that their bodies are insufficiently lean or muscular.

amenorrhea  The absence of menstruation.

female athlete triad  A syndrome of three interrelated health problems seen in some female athletes: disordered eating, amenorrhea, and poor bone density.

in which a person (most commonly a male) believes his body is insufficiently lean or muscular.[49] Men who have muscle dysmorphia believe, despite looking normal or even unusually brawny, that they look "puny." Because of their adherence to a meticulous diet and time-consuming workout schedule, and their shame over their perceived appearance flaws, important social or occupational activities may fall by the wayside. Other behaviors characteristic of muscle dysmorphia include comparing oneself unfavorably to others, checking one's appearance in the mirror, and camouflaging one's appearance. Men with muscle dysmorphia are also likely to abuse anabolic steroids and dietary supplements.[50] Who will suffer? Those with low self-esteem are at greatest risk.[51] As society, via sports and media, glorifies certain types of bodies, we will likely see more. To help a friend, be supportive, do not equate worth to size or musculature, and do not mock people about size or shape.[52]

## The Female Athlete Triad

In an effort to reach their athletic potential, some women may put themselves at risk for developing a syndrome called the **female athlete triad**. *Triad* means "three," and the three interrelated problems are low energy (calorie) intake, typically prompted by disordered eating behaviors; menstrual dysfunction, such as **amenorrhea**; and poor bone density (**FIGURE 6**).[53]

This cycle begins when a chronic pattern of low energy intake and intensive exercise alters normal body functions. For example, when an athlete restricts her eating, she can deplete her body stores of essential nutrients. At the same time, her body begins to burn its stores of fat tissue for energy. Since adequate body fat is essential to maintaining healthy levels of the female reproductive hormone *estrogen*, when an athlete isn't getting enough food, estrogen levels decline. The body, using all calories to keep the athlete alive, then shuts down nonessential body functions, such as menstruation, causing amenorrhea and increasing risk for future infertility. In addition, fat-soluble vitamins, calcium, and estrogen, all essential for dense, healthy bones, are not stored, so their depletion weakens the athlete's bones, leaving her at high risk for fracture and early osteoporosis.

The female athlete triad is particularly prevalent in women who participate in highly competitive individual sports or activities that emphasize leanness and require body-contouring clothing. Cross-country runners, gymnasts, figure skaters, weight-class athletes like rowers, and ballet dancers are among those at highest risk for the female athlete triad.

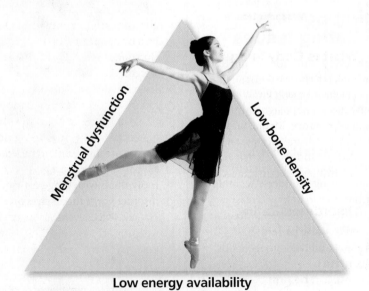

**FIGURE 6** The Female Athlete Triad

Menstrual dysfunction

Low bone density

**Low energy availability**

Warning signs of the female athlete triad include dry skin; light-headedness/fainting; lanugo (fine, downy hair covering the body); multiple injuries; and muscle cramps, weakness, and fatigue.[54] Behaviors associated with the female athlete triad include preoccupation with food and weight, compulsive exercise, use and abuse of weight-loss products or laxatives, increased anxiety, and depression. Treatment can be challenging, and requires a multidisciplinary approach involving the athlete's coach and trainer, a sports medicine team, and a psychologist, as well as family members and friends.

## Health at Every Size

Too many college students and their friends and loved ones struggle with disordered eating, eating disorders, and unhealthy exercise patterns. They fail to well nourish and strengthen their bodies for the days and years to come. At the same time, most Americans who are overweight put on their extra pounds through high calorie intake and low energy expenditure. One model that takes all of these issues into account is the Health At Every Size (HAES) philosophy.[55] HAES posits that well-being and healthy eating and exercise habits are more important than any number on a scale, so all of us, no matter our size, should accept our size—not waiting for a different weight to begin self-acceptance. Then, we can adopt a healthy lifestyle full of movement, nutritious foods, and mindful eating while embracing size diversity. We need to recognize that humans come in a variety of shapes and sizes—all of which need to work toward our healthiest selves, all of which are deserving of love and respect.

---

# STUDY **PLAN**

Customize your study plan—and master your health!—in the Study Area of **MasteringHealth**.

## **ASSESS** YOURSELF

**Could you be suffering from an eating or exercise disorder?**
Take the **Are Your Efforts to Be Thin Sensible—Or Spinning Out of Control?** assessment available on

## MasteringHealth.™

---

## CHAPTER **REVIEW**

To head an MP3 Tutor Session, scan here or visit the Study Area in **MasteringHealth**.

### LO **1** | **What Is Body Image?**

- Body image refers to what you believe or emotionally feel about your body's shape, weight, and general appearance. Media, family, community, cultural groups, and psychological and physiological factors all influence body image.

### LO **2** | **Disordered Eating and Eating Disorders**

- Most Americans report some dissatisfaction with their appearance. Based on the degree of that dissatisfaction, they may develop a disordered realtionship with food.

- Disordered eating is the following of strict food rules, but not to the degree of an eating disorder.
- Anorexia nervosa is a persistent, chronic eating disorder characterized by deliberate food restriction and severe, life-threatening weight loss.
- Individuals with bulimia nervosa rapidly consume large amounts of food and purge either with vomiting or laxative abuse or by using non-purging techniques such as excessive exercise and/or fasting.
- Individuals with binge-eating disorder gorge themselves but do not take excessive measures to lose weight.
- Orthorexia nervosa is an unhealthy obsession with a rigid diet focused on food quality and purity.
- Eating disorders are caused by a combination of many factors, and there are no simple solutions. Without treatment, approximately 20 percent of people with a serious eating disorder will die from it. Long-term treatment focuses on the psychological, social, environmental, and physiological factors that have led to the problem.

### LO **3** | **Can Too Much Exercise Be Unhealthy?**

- Compulsive exercise is used as a way to regulate emotions. Also called *anorexia athletica*, compulsive exercise is characterized by a compulsion to exercise, resulting in guilt and anxiety if the person doesn't work out.
- Muscle dysmorphia, typically found in men, is characterized by a distorted belief that their body is

insufficiently muscular or lean. As a result, they spend an inordinate amount of time working out.

- The female athlete triad occurs when female athletes restrict their food intake and train intensively, altering their normal body functions. Three interrelated problems occur: low energy intake, amennorrhea, and poor bone density. Treatment requires a multidisciplinary approach involving the coach, psychologist, and family members.
- Health At Every Size is a model that encourages all people to accept their size while working toward an active, healthy life.

# POP QUIZ

Visit **MasteringHealth** to personalize your study plan with Chapter Review Quizzes and Dynamic Study Modules.

## LO 1 | What Is Body Image?

1. All of the statements about body image are true *except* which?

a. The American obsession with having bigger biceps or being able to wear skinnier jeans began in the late 1990s.

b. Concerns about weight seem to be central to many people's dissatifaction with their body.

c. People who have been diagnosed with a body image disorder show differences in the brain's ability to regulate neurotransmitters.

d. Positive body image is possessing a true perception of your appearance.

## LO 2 | Disordered Eating and Eating Disorders

2. Orthorexia nervosa is

a. an excessive focus on eating foods high in calcium and vitamin D.

b. characterized by a fixation on the quality and purity of food.

c. an obsession with bone health.

d. a condition that results from bingeing and purging.

## LO 3 | Can Too Much Exercise Be Unhealthy?

3. Muscle dysmorphia

a. is a muscular disease that results from an autoimmune disorder.

b. occurs only in women.

c. results in menstrual dysfunction.

d. occurs most often in men.

*Answers to the Pop Quiz questions can be found on page A-1. If you answered a question incorrectly, review the section identified by the Learning Outcome. For even more study tools, visit **MasteringHealth**.*

# 7

# Improving Your Personal Fitness

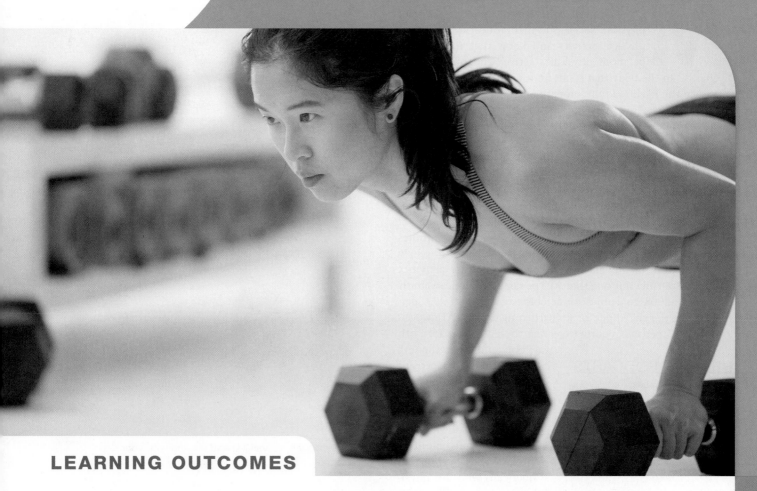

## LEARNING OUTCOMES

LO **1** Describe how physical activity can improve physical and psychological health and how inactivity contributes to the increased risk of poor health outcomes.

LO **2** Distinguish between the physical activity required for health, physical fitness, and performance.

LO **3** Identify lifestyle obstacles to physical activity, describe ways to surmount them, and make a commitment to getting physically fit.

LO **4** Use the FITT (frequency, intensity, time, and type) principles for the health-related components of physical fitness.

LO **5** Devise a plan to implement your safe and effective fitness program.

LO **6** Describe optimal food and fluid consumption recommendations for exercise and recovery.

LO **7** Explain how to prevent and treat common exercise injuries.

Most Americans are aware of the wide range of physical, social, and mental health benefits of physical activity and know that they should be more physically active. The physiological changes in the body that result from regular physical activity reduce the likelihood of coronary artery disease, high blood pressure, type 2 diabetes, obesity, and other chronic diseases. Furthermore, engaging in physical activity regularly helps to control stress, increases self-esteem, and contributes to that "feel-good" feeling.[1]

Despite knowledge of the importance of physical activity for health and wellness, most people are not sufficiently active to obtain these optimal health benefits. It is recommended that adults participate in at least 150 minutes of moderate-intensity aerobic activity per week, 75 minutes of vigorous-intensity aerobic activity per week, or a weekly combination of moderate- and vigorous-intensity activity.[2] Recent statistics indicate that 50.2 percent of American adults met the 2008 guidelines for aerobic exercise, and 29.6 percent met the guidelines for strengthening exercise.[3] However, only 20.2 percent reported meeting the guidelines for both aerobic and strengthening exercise, and 26.3 percent reported no leisure activities.[4] These statistics are based on activity reported during one's "down" time in the previous month.[5] The growing percentage of Americans who live physically inactive lives has been linked to the current high incidences of obesity, type 2 diabetes, and other chronic and mental health diseases.[6] So, why don't people get enough activity? The reasons vary, but competing demands (school, work, social activities, screen time, etc.) and lack of time, motivation, or access are common reasons for not getting enough activity.[7] Safety concerns of the physical environment, lack of resources that support activity in the environment, and an inadequate support network also prevent people from being physically active.[8]

In general, college students are more physically active than older adults, but a recent survey indicated that 56.9 percent of college women and 49.3 percent

**HEAR IT! PODCASTS**

Want a study podcast for this chapter? Download **Personal Fitness: Improving Health through Exercise**, available on **MasteringHealth.**™

**physical activity** Refers to all body movements produced by skeletal muscles, resulting in substantial increases in energy expenditure.

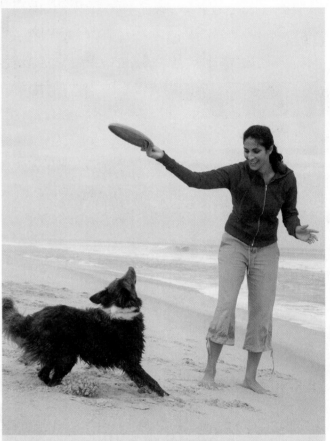

Activities such as walking and playing with your dog count toward your recommended daily physical activity.

of college men do get the recommended 3 to 5 days of moderate to vigorous physical activity per week.[9] Extracurricular activities, screen time, studying, and social activities can be physical activity barriers for college students.

## LO 1 | PHYSICAL ACTIVITY FOR HEALTH

Describe how physical activity can improve physical and psychological health and how inactivity contributes to the increased risk of poor health outcomes.

**Physical activity** refers to all body movements produced by skeletal muscles that result in substantial increases in energy

## WHAT DO **YOU** THINK?

**Why do you think most college students aren't more physically active?**

■ Why do you think women are less likely than men to obtain sufficient levels of physical activity?

■ Do you think your college or university years are a good time to become more physically active? Why or why not?

expenditure. Physical activities can vary by intensity: light, moderate, or vigorous. For example, walking on a flat surface at a casual pace requires little effort (light), whereas walking uphill is more intense and harder to do (moderate). Jogging and running are examples of vigorous-intensity physical activities. There are three general categories of physical activity defined by the purpose for which they are done: leisure-time physical activity (e.g., exercise, walking the dog), occupational physical activity (e.g., restaurant server, summer camp counselor), and lifestyle physical activity (e.g., walking to class, housework).

**Exercise** is defined as planned, repetitive, and structured bodily movement undertaken to maintain or better any number of physical fitness components—for example, cardiorespiratory fitness, body composition, muscular strength or endurance, or flexibility. Although all exercise is physical activity, not all physical activity would be considered exercise. For example, walking from your car to class is physical

# 150 MINUTES

of moderate physical activity a week—along with strength exercises 2 days a week—provides substantial **HEALTH BENEFITS**. More is even better!

activity, whereas going for a brisk 30-minute walk to maintain a healthy body weight is considered exercise.

Adding more physical activity to your day, such as walking or cycling to school, can benefit your health.[10] We know that physical activity is good for health, and we also know that physical inactivity contributes to increased risk of negative health outcomes. Physical inactivity is defined as not meeting the minimum activity recommendations for health (see **TABLE 7.1**).[11] It is not just a problem in the United States, but it is a worldwide health concern. A recent analysis of sitting time across 54 countries indicated that sitting more the 3 hours per day was responsible for over 400,000 deaths, which is 3.8% of all causes of mortality.[12]

> **exercise** Planned, structured, and repetitive bodily movement done to improve or maintain one or more components of physical fitness.

## TABLE **7.1** | 2008 Physical Activity Guidelines for Americans

|  | Key Guidelines for Health* | For Additional Fitness or Weight Loss Benefits* | Additional Exercises |
|---|---|---|---|
| **Adults** | 150 min/week moderate-intensity physical activity<br><br>OR<br><br>75 min/week of vigorous-intensity physical activity<br><br>OR<br><br>Equivalent combination of moderate- and vigorous-intensity physical activity (e.g., 100 min moderate intensity + 25 min vigorous intensity) | 300 min/week moderate-intensity physical activity<br><br>OR<br><br>150 min/week of vigorous-intensity physical activity<br><br>OR<br><br>Equivalent combination of moderate- and vigorous-intensity physical activity (e.g., 200 min moderate intensity + 50 min vigorous intensity)<br><br>OR<br><br>More than the previously described amounts | Muscle-strengthening activities for all the major muscle groups at least 2 days/week |
| **Older adults** | If unable to follow above guidelines, then as much physical activity as their condition allows. Physician's clearance is recommended for older adults with health problems. | If unable to follow above guidelines, then as much physical activity as their condition allows | In addition to muscle-strengthening activities, those with limited mobility should add exercises to improve balance and reduce risk of falling. |
| **Children and youth** | 60 min or more of moderate- or vigorous-intensity physical activity daily; should include at least 3 days/week of vigorous activity | At least 60 min of moderate- or vigorous-intensity physical activity on every day of the week | Include muscle-strengthening activities at least 3 days/week. Include bone-strengthening activities at least 3 days/week. |

*Avoid inactivity (some activity is better than none), accumulate physical activity in sessions of 10 minutes or more at one time, and spread activity throughout the week.
**Source:** Office of Disease Prevention and Health Promotion, U.S. Department of Health and Human Services, *2008 Physical Activity Guidelines for Americans: Be Active, Healthy, and Happy!* (Washington, DC: U.S. Department of Health and Human Services, 2008), ODPHP Publication No. U0036, www.health.gov.

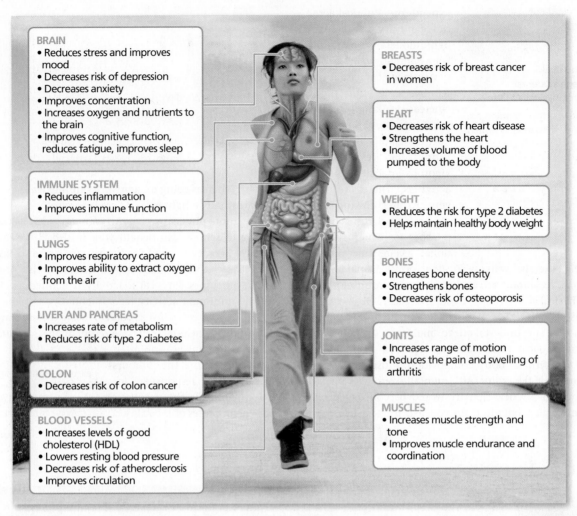

**FIGURE 7.1** Selected Health Benefits of Regular Exercise

➔ VIDEO TUTOR
Health Benefits of Regular
Exercise

Based on this statistic, the researchers determined that a decrease in sitting time of just 30 minutes per day could reduce 0.6% of the deaths attributed to excess sitting time.[13] When considering major chronic diseases, it is estimated that physical inactivity is responsible for 30 percent of the cases of ischemic heart disease, 27 percent of cases of type 2 diabetes, and 21–25 percent of cases of breast and colon cancer worldwide.[14]

**Sedentary** time is generally considered time spent while sitting or reclining in an activity that does not increase energy expenditure more than 1.5 times the resting level (1.5 **METS**, or metabolic equivalents).[15] Sedentary time, however, should not be confused with inactivity. Common sedentary activities include screen time, reading, and driving. Keep in mind that someone who gets regular activity can also participate in high levels of sedentary behaviors. Those individuals who exercise but still report a lot of sedentary time have been referred to as "active couch potatoes."[16]

Although regular exercise and high levels of physical activity can protect against disease and premature death, sedentary time has an independent effect on disease and mortality.[17] Research shows that risk for cardiovascular disease, cancers, and type 2 diabetes is increased with high amounts of sitting time.[18] So, moving is important! You can get activity through your lifestyle choices, your job, or leisure-time activity and exercise.

Regular participation in physical activity improves more than 50 different physiological, metabolic, and psychological aspects of human life. **FIGURE 7.1** summarizes some of these major health-related benefits, and **TABLE 7.2** highlights popular fitness equipment.

## Reduced Risk of Cardiovascular Diseases

Aerobic activity is good for your cardiovascular system (the heart, lungs, and blood vessels) and it reduces the risk for heart-related diseases and premature death. High blood pressure (hypertension), unhealthy cholesterol profiles (dyslipidemia), coronary heart disease, and stroke are among the

**sedentary** Activity that expends no more than 1.5 times the resting energy level while seated or reclined.

**MET** A metabolic equivalent or resting level of energy expenditure (3.5 ml·kg⁻¹·min⁻¹)

# TABLE 7.2 | Popular Fitness Equipment

| 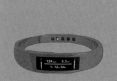 Heart Rate Monitor |  Pedometer | 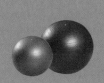 Stability Ball |  Balance Board |  Resistance Band | Medicine Ball |
|---|---|---|---|---|---|

A device that measures heart rate and other vitals during training.

- Provides instant and continuous feedback about the intensity of your workout
- Some versions include a chest strap; strap must fit well; can be uncomfortable (most women tuck the strap under the bottom strap of their sport bras).

Cost: $50–500

A battery-operated device, usually worn on your belt or wrist, that measures the number of steps taken. Some models also monitor calories, distance, and speed.

- Great motivation and feedback regarding the recommended 10,000 steps per day.
- Must be calibrated for your height, weight, and stride length.

Cost: $25–100

Ball made of burst-resistant vinyl that can be used for strengthening core muscles or to improve flexibility.

- Balls must be inflated correctly to be most effective.

Cost: $25–100

A board with a rounded bottom that can be used to improve balance, core muscle strength, and flexibility.

- Great for improving agility, coordination, reaction skills, and ankle strength.
- Can be difficult initially for new users. Caution new users with weak ankles, as there is a risk of straining ligaments and tendons.

Cost: $40–80

Rubber or elastic material, sometimes with handles, that can be used to build muscular strength and endurance. Can also be used in yoga or Pilates to provide assistance in flexibility training.

- Improves muscular strength and endurance, balance, coordination, and flexibility.
- Lightweight, durable, and portable.
- Breaks down over time; need to inspect regularly to avoid injury if it breaks during use.

Cost: $5–35

A heavy ball, about 14 inches in diameter, used in rehabilitation and strength training. Weight varies from 2 to 25 lb. Some made with handles.

- Can be used effectively to increase explosive power.
- Also used to develop core body strength.
- If used incorrectly, there is potential for lower back injuries.

Cost: $10–150

| 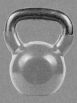 Kettlebell | 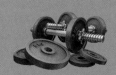 Free Weights | 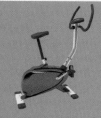 Elliptical Trainer |  Stationary Bike | 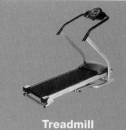 Treadmill |
|---|---|---|---|---|

A heavy ball with a handle used for full-body muscular strength and endurance exercises. Weight varies from 5 to 100 lb.

- Can be used effectively to increase muscular fitness, core strength, and explosive power.
- Movements can be complex, and if used incorrectly, there is potential for lower back and/or wrist injuries.

Cost: $10–150

Rubber, plastic, or metal dumbbells or barbells, often with adjustable weight; can be used with a weight bench.

- Traditional method for building muscular strength and endurance.
- A full set allows you to increase resistance as you train, allowing for greater improvements in muscular strength.
- Potential for injury if form is incorrect; must concentrate on body alignment and ensuring sufficient core body strength.

Cost: $1–300

A stationary exercise machine that stimulates walking or running without impact on the bones and joints. Some machines include arm movements.

- Nonimpact; less wear and tear on the joints and risk of shin splints.
- Readout and programs vary.

Cost: $300–4,000

A lower-body exercise machine designed to simulate bike riding.

- Generally easy to use; does not require balance.
- Comes with varied resistance programs.
- Recumbent styles offer less strain on back and knees and are useful for individuals struggling with back pain.

Cost: $200–3,000

Exercise machine for walking or running on a moving platform while remaining in one place.

- Generally easy to use; comes with an emergency shutoff.
- Different models have varied readouts and programmability.
- Less impact on joints than running on most pavements.

Cost: $500–4,000

cardiovascular conditions prevented or improved by physical activity. Additionally, regularly getting enough physical activity eases the performance of everyday tasks.

Regular aerobic activity makes the cardiovascular and respiratory systems more efficient by strengthening the heart muscle. One change you typically notice a few weeks after the adoption of a regular aerobic activity program is a decrease in your resting heart rate. As your heart becomes stronger, it can pump more blood with each beat (increased stroke volume). Basically, the heart can beat fewer times per minute and still get the same amount of blood throughout the body. The number of capillaries (small blood vessels that allow gas exchange between blood and surrounding tissues) increases with regular aerobic activity in the trained skeletal muscles. This change enables more blood and oxygen to get to the working muscles. Aerobic activity also improves the respiratory system by increasing the amount of oxygen that is inhaled with each breath and distributed to body tissues. In sum, regular exercise encourages changes that ultimately contribute to an increased level of aerobic fitness.[19]

Regular physical activity of moderate intensity can reduce hypertension, or chronic high blood pressure, a cardiovascular disease itself and a significant risk factor for other coronary heart diseases and stroke (see Chapter 16).[20] Regular aerobic activity also improves the blood lipid profile. It typically increases high-density lipoproteins (HDLs, or "good" cholesterol), which are associated with lower risk for coronary artery disease because of their role in removing plaque built up in the arteries.[21] Triglycerides (a blood fat) typically decrease with aerobic activity. Low-density lipoproteins (LDLs, or "bad" cholesterol) and total cholesterol are often improved with exercise due to weight loss and the improvements in HDL and triglycerides.[22]

## Reduced Risk of Metabolic Syndrome and Type 2 Diabetes

Regular physical activity reduces the risk of metabolic syndrome, a combination of heart disease and diabetes risk factors that produces a synergistic increase in risk.[23] Specifically, metabolic syndrome includes high blood pressure, abdominal obesity, low levels of HDLs, high levels of triglycerides, and impaired glucose tolerance.[24] Regular participation in moderate- to vigorous-intensity physical activities reduces risk for each factor individually and collectively.[25]

Research indicates that a healthy dietary intake combined with sufficient physical activity could prevent many of the current cases of type 2 diabetes, as well as help manage blood glucose levels in those who have already been diagnosed with type 2 diabetes.[26] Meeting the recommendation of 150 minutes of moderate- to vigorous-intensity aerobic activity per week has been shown to improve glucose tolerance and insulin sensitivity to manage diabetes.[27] The importance of resistance exercise in diabetes prevention and management should also be noted. Resistance exercise performed 2 to 3 days per week improves muscular fitness and is associated with improved management of insulin response and improved glucose control.[28] Physical activity intervention for the prevention and management of type 2 diabetes should be comprehensive,

including regular aerobic and resistance exercise. (For more on diabetes prevention and management, see **Focus On: Minimizing Your Risk for Diabetes** on page 446.)

## Reduced Cancer Risk

After decades of research, most cancer epidemiologists believe that 25 to 37 percent of cancers can be avoided by healthier lifestyle and environmental choices.[29] The American Cancer Society reports that approximately one-third of cancers could be prevented with regular physical activity and healthy diet choices.[30] Regular physical aerobic activity appears to lower the risk for some specific cancers, particularly colon, rectal, and breast cancer.[31] Recent research assessing the impact of sedentary time on cancer indicates that the risk for several types of cancer is associated with high levels of sedentary time.[32] Research on exercise and breast cancer survivors has shown that aerobic and resistance exercise can improve health and quality-of-life outcomes.[33] However, one study reported that breast cancer survivors were not optimistic about exercise decreasing treatment effects.[34]

## Improved Bone Mass and Reduced Risk of Osteoporosis

A common affliction for older people is *osteoporosis*, a disease characterized by low bone mass and deterioration of bone tissue, which increases fracture risk. It is estimated that behavioral risk factors contribute 20 to 40 percent to the development of osteoporosis.[35] The National Osteoporosis Foundation issued a 2016 position stand on peak bone mass and lifestyle factors, stressing the importance of physical activity and calcium intake in youth and adolescence for the development of bone density and mass.[36] Regular weight-bearing and strength-building physical activities are recommended to maintain bone health and prevent osteoporotic fractures for girls and women.[37] Although men and women are both negatively affected by osteoporosis, it is more common in women. Due to this difference, much of the research focuses on women, but there is support for weight-bearing and strength-building exercise improving bone health in men and women.[38] However, it appears that the full bone-related benefits of physical activity can only be achieved with sufficient hormone levels (estrogen in women, testosterone in men) and adequate calcium, vitamin D, and total caloric intakes.[39]

## Improved Weight Management

For many people, the desire to lose weight or maintain a healthy weight is the main reason for physical activity. On the most basic level, physical activity requires your body to generate energy through calorie expenditure; if calories expended exceed calories consumed over a span of time, the net result will be weight loss. Some activities are more intense or vigorous than others and result in more calories used. FIGURE 7.2 on page 196 shows the caloric cost of various activities when done for 30 minutes.

There has been some discussion over the best weight loss methods. Should diet or exercise be the emphasis? While diet

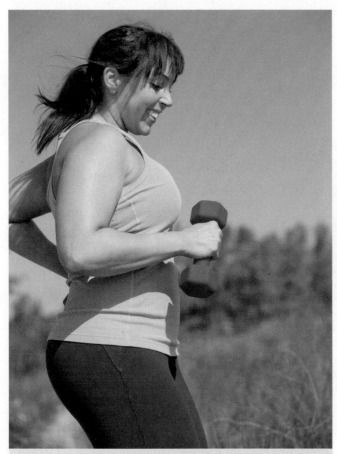

If you want to lose weight, you need to move more and often!

and caloric intake may ultimately hold the key to weight loss (see Chapter 6), exercise certainly has its place in maintaining overall health and fitness. Research supports the comprehensive lifestyle changes that include both exercise and diet changes for weight loss.[40] Dietary recommendations for weight loss can vary depending on comorbid conditions. For example, an individual at increased risk for diabetes or with diabetes will need to consider the glycemic index of food more carefully than one with lesser concerns over blood sugar levels. When it comes to trimming excess pounds, the amount of exercise recommended for weight loss is greater than the amount recommended for general health benefits (exercise recommendations are discussed later in the chapter). Generally, exercise for weight loss is an accumulation of 300 minutes of aerobic exercise per week versus 150 minutes for general health maintenance.[41]

One interesting recent finding supported the idea of frequent weighing in as being an integral part of successful weight loss plans. Participants who weighed themselves daily or on most days lost more weight than participants who weighed themselves infrequently.[42] Participants who weighed themselves more frequently were more likely to make health behavior dietary and physical activity choices that support weight loss and maintenance, and as a result lost more weight than those who didn't weigh themselves regularly.[43]

Ultimately, when you're trying to lose weight and keep it off, it is important to make changes that can be maintained long term, to manage your weight after initial weight loss.

Activity seems to be a key component of the weight maintenance phase.[44] The National Weight Control Registry (NWCR) is comprised of individuals who have lost at least 30 pounds and have maintained the loss for at least a year.[45] Ninety percent of individuals on the registry report an average of 60 minutes of daily exercise.[46] A decrease in physical activity among individuals on the NWCR has been associated with weight regain. More specifically, data from one study showed that 44 percent of NWCR participants who had regained weight after shedding pounds reported decreases in physical activity.[47] All of this is to say that weight loss should not be considered a one-time event. If you have some success getting down to your target weight, keep up with the routine that got you there to maintain a healthy weight.

In addition to the calories expended during activity, physical activity has a direct positive effect on metabolic rate, keeping it elevated for several hours following vigorous physical activities.[48] This increase in metabolic rate can lead to an increased number of calories expended, which helps to prevent weight gain and improve weight loss. If you are currently at a healthy body weight, regular physical activity can prevent significant weight gain.

## Improved Immunity

Research shows that regular moderate-intensity physical activity reduces individual susceptibility to disease through improving the body's ability to fight infections.[49] Regular exercise has also been shown to reduce body inflammation that is associated with higher risk of chronic conditions such as cardiovascular disease or cancer.[50] Just how regular physical activity positively influences immunity is not well understood. We know that moderate-intensity physical activity temporarily increases the number of white blood cells, which are responsible for fighting infection.[51] Often, the relationship of physical activity to immunity, or more specifically to disease susceptibility, is described as a J-shaped curve.[52] Susceptibility to disease decreases with moderate activity, but then increases as you move to extreme levels of physical activity or exercise (e.g., marathons or triathlons) or if you continue to exercise without adequate recovery time and/or dietary intake.[53]

## Improved Mental Health and Stress Management

Mental health is an area of growing concern for many college students. Recent data show that the factors with the biggest impact on academic performance reported by college students include stress, anxiety, sleep difficulties, and depression.[54] Fortunately, acute (each session) and regular exercise (a training program) can help. A comprehensive study assessing the effects of an exercise intervention on several mental health issues supported the role of exercise in improving sleep quality and reducing fatigue in

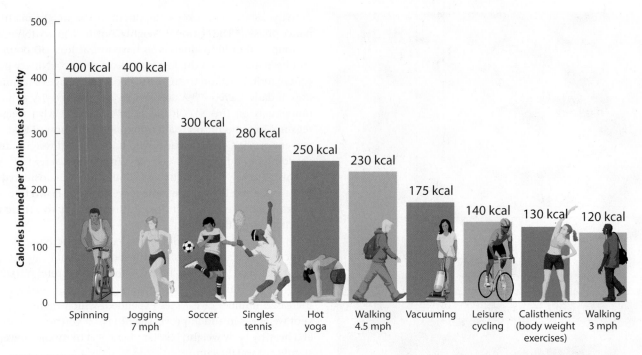

**FIGURE 7.2 Calories Burned by Different Activities** The harder your physical activity, the more energy you expend. Estimated calories burned for various moderate and vigorous activities are listed for 30 minutes of activity. Note that the number of calories burned depends on body weight (generally, the higher your body weight, the greater the number of calories you'll burn).

college students.[55] These effects were seen both immediately postintervention and at follow-up 1 and 3 months later.[56] Physical activity is also associated with improvement in depression.[57] It is important to note that improvements are seen in those who are experiencing some depression symptoms as well as those who are diagnosed with major depressive disorders.[58] Most evidence is for the role of moderate- to vigorous-intensity aerobic activity in the management of depression, with the same physical activity recommendations for general health benefits being effective in managing symptoms.[59] Stress management is also a benefit of regular physical activity. Not only can regular physical activity provide a break from stressors such as work and everyday worries, but aerobic activity has also been shown to improve the way the body handles stress by its effect on neurotransmitters associated with mood enhancement. Physical activity might also help the body recover from the stress response more quickly as fitness increases.[60]

People who engage in regular physical activity are likely to notice the psychological benefits, such as feeling better about oneself and an overall sense of well-being.[61] Although these mental health benefits are difficult to quantify, they are frequently mentioned as reasons for continuing to be physically active. Learning new skills, developing increased ability and capacity in recreational activities, and sticking with a physical activity plan also improve self-esteem.[62] In addition, regular physical activity can improve a person's physical appearance, further increasing self-esteem.[63]

There is increasing evidence that regular physical activity positively impacts cognitive function across the lifespan. Research has associated regular activity and fitness levels with academic performance in school.[64] Results from a large longitudinal study of middle school students showed that

significant increases in fitness were associated with greater improvements in academic ranking compared to those with no change in overall fitness.[65] Although much of the research on academic performance has a focus on youth, there are studies that support the role of exercise improving aspects of cognitive function in college students.[66] Study-related fatigue and performance on laboratory tasks to assess executive cognitive

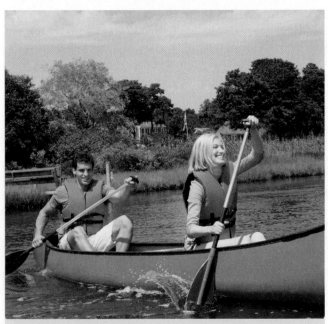

Although physical activity actually stimulates the stress response, a physically fit body adapts efficiently to the eustress of it, and as a result is better able to tolerate and effectively manage stress of all kinds.

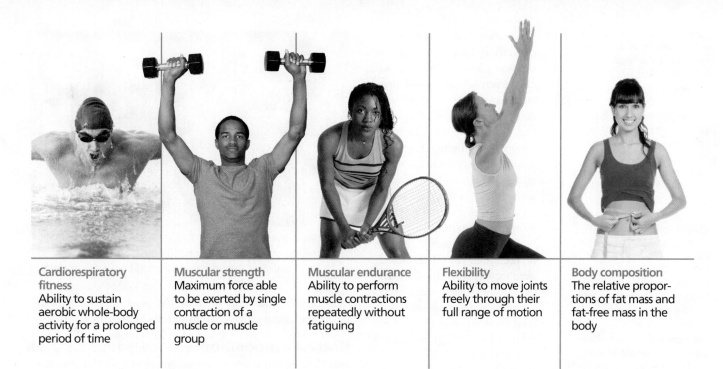

| Cardiorespiratory fitness | Muscular strength | Muscular endurance | Flexibility | Body composition |
|---|---|---|---|---|
| Ability to sustain aerobic whole-body activity for a prolonged period of time | Maximum force able to be exerted by single contraction of a muscle or muscle group | Ability to perform muscle contractions repeatedly without fatiguing | Ability to move joints freely through their full range of motion | The relative proportions of fat mass and fat-free mass in the body |

**FIGURE 7.3** Health-Related Components of Physical Fitness

functions improved with regular aerobic exercise, and these effects were seen both immediately postintervention and during follow-ups 1 and 3 months later.[67] Results from another study supported a positive relationship between aerobic exercise participation and grade point average, also suggesting that resistance exercise might also have a positive association.[68] First-year medical students who reported using the recreation center frequently in the 3 weeks before an exam had higher scores on exams than those using it less frequently.[69] The most frequent use was associated with the highest exam scores.[70]

Recent research indicates that the relationship between physical activity and executive cognitive function is reciprocal. In other words, both physical activity and executive cognitive function may impact each other.[71] Those with poor executive function experienced greater reductions in physical activity over time compared to those with higher function. Promoting physical activity as we age is important to prevent the decline in cognitive function, which in turn can help maintain regular activity.[72] Regular aerobic activity, even when initiated as an adult, has also been associated with reduced risk for and improvement of dementia and Alzheimer's disease in adults.[73]

## Longer Lifespan

Experts have long debated the relationship between physical activity and longevity. Several studies indicate significant decreases in long-term health risk and increases in years lived, particularly among those who have several risk factors and who use physical activity as a means of risk reduction.[74] The largest benefits from physical activity occur in sedentary individuals who add a little physical activity to their lives, with additional benefits as physical activity levels increase.[75] Additionally, data from a national sample show that a sedentary lifestyle as associated with a reduced ability to perform activities of daily

living.[76] The more sedentary time adults report, the greater reduction in the ability to perform activities of daily living. It is not just structured exercise that is important, but moving as much as possible and sitting as little as possible.

## LO 2 | PHYSICAL ACTIVITY FOR FITNESS AND PERFORMANCE

Distinguish between the physical activity required for health, physical fitness, and performance.

**Physical fitness** refers to a set of attributes that are either health or skill related.

## Health-Related Components of Physical Fitness

The health-related attributes—cardiorespiratory fitness, muscular strength and endurance, flexibility, and body composition—allow you to perform moderate- to vigorous-intensity physical activities on a regular basis without getting too tired and with energy left over to handle physical or mental emergencies. **FIGURE 7.3** identifies the major health-related components of physical fitness.

### Cardiorespiratory Fitness
Cardiorespiratory fitness is the ability of the heart, lungs, and blood vessels to supply the body with oxygen efficiently.

> **physical fitness** A balance of health-related attributes that allows you to perform moderate to vigorous physical activities on a regular basis and complete daily physical tasks without undue fatigue.
>
> **cardiorespiratory fitness** The ability of the heart, lungs, and blood vessels to supply oxygen to skeletal muscles during sustained physical activity.

**aerobic exercise** Prolonged exercise that requires oxygen to make energy for activity.

**aerobic capacity (power)** The functional status of the cardiorespiratory system; refers specifically to the volume of oxygen the muscles consume during exercise.

**muscular strength** The amount of force that a muscle is capable of exerting in one contraction.

**muscular endurance** A muscle's ability to exert force repeatedly without fatiguing or the ability to sustain a muscular contraction for a length of time.

**flexibility** The range of motion, or the amount of movement possible, at a particular joint or series of joints.

**body composition** The relative proportions of fat and fat-free (muscle, bone, water, organs) tissues in the body.

The primary category of physical activity known to improve cardiorespiratory fitness is **aerobic exercise**. The word *aerobic* means "with oxygen" and describes any type of exercise that requires oxygen to make energy for prolonged activity. Aerobic activities, such as swimming, cycling, and jogging, are among the best exercises for improving or maintaining cardiorespiratory fitness.

Cardiorespiratory fitness is measured by determining **aerobic capacity** (power), the volume of oxygen the muscles consume during exercise. Maximal aerobic power (commonly written as $VO_{2max}$) is defined as the volume of oxygen that the muscles consume per minute during maximal exercise. The most common measure of maximal aerobic capacity is a walk or run test on a treadmill. For greatest accuracy, this is done in a lab with specialized equipment and technicians to measure the precise amount of oxygen entering and exiting the body during the exercise session. To get a more general sense of cardiorespiratory fitness, submaximal tests performed in the classroom or field can predict maximal aerobic capacity.

**Muscular Strength** Muscular strength refers to the amount of force a muscle or group of muscles can generate in one contraction. The most common way to assess the strength of a particular muscle or muscle group is to measure the maximum amount of weight you can move one time (and no more) or your one repetition maximum (1 RM).

**Muscular Endurance** Muscular endurance is the ability of a muscle or group of muscles to exert force repeatedly without fatigue or the ability to sustain a muscular contraction. The more repetitions you can perform successfully (e.g., push-ups) or the longer you can hold a certain position (e.g., flexed arm hang), the greater your muscular endurance.

**Flexibility** Flexibility refers to the range of motion, or the amount of movement possible, at a particular joint or series of joints: the greater the range of motion, the greater the

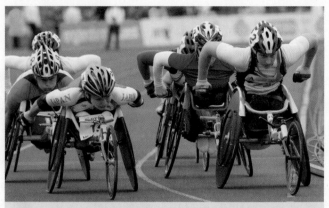

It is important for all people, including those with disabilities, to develop optimal levels of physical fitness and participate in physical activities they enjoy—including competitive sports.

flexibility. Various tests measure the flexibility of the body's joints, including range-of-motion tests for specific joints.

**Body Composition** **Body composition** is the fifth and final health-related component of physical fitness. Body composition describes the relative proportions and distribution of fat and fat-free (muscle, bone, water, organs) tissues in the body. (For more details on body composition, including its measurement, see Chapter 6.)

## Skill-Related Components of Physical Fitness

In addition to the five health-related components of physical fitness, physical fitness for athletes involves attributes that improve their ability to perform athletic tasks. These attributes, called the *skill-related components* of physical fitness, also help recreational athletes and general exercisers increase fitness levels and their ability to perform daily tasks. The skill-related components of physical fitness (also called sport skills) are *agility, balance, coordination, power, speed,* and *reaction time.* Note that some of the skill-related fitness components can impact health. For example, consider the importance of balance and coordination for older adults who are at increased risk for falls.

## LO 3 | COMMITTING TO PHYSICAL FITNESS

Identify lifestyle obstacles to physical activity, describe ways to surmount them, and make a commitment to getting physically fit.

To succeed at incorporating physical fitness into your life, you need to design a fitness program that takes obstacles into account and that is founded on the activities you enjoy most.

## What if I Have Been Inactive for a While?

If you have been physically inactive for the past few months or longer, first make sure that your physician clears you for

# 20.2%
of American adults meet guidelines for both cardiorespiratory and muscular FITNESS.

exercise. Consider consulting a personal trainer or fitness instructor to help you get started. In this phase of a fitness program, known as the *initial conditioning stage*, you may begin at levels lower than those recommended for physical fitness. For example, you might start your cardiorespiratory program by simply moving more each day and reducing your sedentary time. Take the stairs instead of the elevator, walk farther from your car to the store, and plan for organized movement each day, such as a 10- to 15-minute walk. In addition, you can start your muscle fitness program with simple body weight exercises, emphasizing proper technique and body alignment before adding any resistance.

## Overcoming Common Obstacles to Physical Activity

People have real and perceived barriers that prevent regular physical activity, ranging from personal ("I do not have time") to environmental ("I do not have a safe place to be active") to social ("I do not have a workout partner"). Some people may be reluctant to exercise if they are overweight, feel embarrassed to work out with their more "fit" friends, or feel they lack the knowledge and skills required.

Think about your obstacles to physical activity and write them down. Consider anything that gets in your way of exercising, however minor. Some of the barriers reported by college students include lack of motivation, self-discipline, or enjoyment coupled with the enjoyment of sedentary activities, such as screen time and the use of technology.[77] "Partying" and social networks that do not support physical activity are also reported as barriers.[78] Commute time to school, studying, school demands, and equipment cost also get in the way of college students getting enough physical activity.[79] Once you honestly evaluate why you are not as physically active as you want to be, review **TABLE 7.3** for suggestions on overcoming your hurdles. Once you determine your biggest obstacles, develop and write out specific plans to address them (more on setting attainable fitness goals later in this chapter).

## TABLE 7.3 | Overcoming Obstacles to Physical Activity

| Obstacle | Possible Solution |
|---|---|
| Lack of time | ■ Look at your schedule. Where can you find 30-minute time slots? Perhaps you need to focus on shorter times (10 minutes or more) throughout the day.<br>■ Multitask. Read while riding an exercise bike or listen to lectures or podcasts while walking.<br>■ Be physically active during your lunch and study breaks as well as between classes. Skip rope or throw a Frisbee with a friend.<br>■ Select activities that require less time, such as brisk walking or jogging.<br>■ Ride your bike to class, or park (or get off the bus) farther from your destination. |
| Social influence | ■ Invite family and friends to be active with you.<br>■ Join an exercise class to meet new people.<br>■ Explain the importance of exercise and your commitment to physical activity to people who may not support your efforts.<br>■ Find a role model to support your efforts.<br>■ Plan for physically active dates—walking, dancing, or bowling. |
| Lack of motivation, willpower, or energy | ■ Schedule your workout time just as you would any other important commitment. Prioritize you.<br>■ Enlist the help of an exercise partner to make you accountable for working out.<br>■ Give yourself an incentive or reward for meeting short-term goals and longer-term goals.<br>■ Schedule your workouts when you feel most energetic. If you are too tired to walk a mile, do what you can do. Every little bit helps—and every small step is a positive achievement•Remind yourself that exercise gives you more energy.<br>■ Get things ready; for example, if you choose to walk in the morning, set out your clothes and shoes the night before. |
| Lack of resources | ■ Select an activity that requires minimal equipment, such as walking, jogging, jumping rope, lifting small free weights, or using resistance bands.<br>■ Identify inexpensive resources on campus or in the community.<br>■ Whenever possible, walk, bike, or select active transportation rather than riding.<br>■ Take advantage of no-cost opportunities, such as playing catch or Frisbee. Get into a pickup game of basketball, volleyball, or soccer in the park or green space on campus. |
| Environmental barriers | ■ Develop a plan for inclement or extreme weather, such as an indoor option or home exercise if driving is hazardous.<br>■ Have a workout partner or use a gym if safety is a concern.<br>■ Increase lifestyle activity and decrease sedentary time. |

**Source:** Adapted from National Center for Chronic Disease Prevention and Health Promotion, "How Can I Overcome Barriers to Physical Activity?," Updated May 2011, www.cdc.gov.

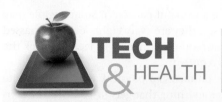
## GADGETS TO TRACK YOUR FITNESS *Which One Is Right for You?*

Activity trackers and apps are all the rage. Everyone seems to have one, but are they accurate and do they encourage behavior change? Research shows that some features such as heart rate and step counting can be very accurate, while measures like caloric expenditure and sleep variables are less accurate. The impact on behavior change will likely depend on the individual. With all of the options, how do you choose one?

**Cost.** There are many free and low-cost apps that can be downloaded or that come preloaded on your cell phone. There are also monitors that cost a couple hundred dollars. Be sure to find an option that works for your budget.

**What do you want to track?** If your goal is to monitor steps and exercise time, your phone may be an ideal option, especially if cost is a concern. However, for continuous monitoring, your phone might not be a good choice. For estimates of energy expenditure, sleep, heart rate, and sedentary time, you will have to spend a little money. Fortunately, there are several affordable monitors.

**Behavior change features.** Regardless of cost, all fitness trackers and apps have some behavior change elements. Keeping track of your activity is self-monitoring, which is helpful in maintaining a new behavior. Look for monitors that have features that fit with strategies that motivate you. Setting goals, connecting with friends or social media, and reminders to exercise are

all behavior change features to consider. Trackers that have websites to download your information are great for tracking progress to meet long-term goals. Good tracker websites provide up-to-date scientific information about fitness and exercise as a resource. Wrist monitors wear like a watch, which makes it easy to remember on a daily basis. Some even look more like jewelry than a fitness gadget for those who do not want to compromise style for function. Whatever you do, be sure to search for reviews and compare devices before you make a purchase.

**Source:** K. R. Evenson et al., "Systematic Review of the Validity and Reliability of Consumer-Wearable Activity Trackers," *International Journal of Behavioral Nutrition and Physical Activity* 12, no. 1 (2015): 1–22.

## Incorporating Physical Activity in Your Life

When designing your fitness program, there are several factors to consider. First, choose activities that are appropriate for you, are convenient, and that you genuinely enjoy. For example, choose jogging because you like to run and there are beautiful trails nearby versus swimming when you do not really like the water and the pool is difficult to get to. Likewise, choose activities that are suitable for your current fitness level. If you are overweight or have not exercised in months, start slowly, plan fun activities, and progress to more challenging physical activities as your physical fitness improves. You may choose to simply walk more in an attempt to achieve the recommended goal of 10,000 steps per day; keep track with a pedometer, fitness app, or physical activity tracker. (See the **Tech & Health** box for more on choosing the right activity tracker for your needs and lifestyle.) Try to make physical activity a part of your routine by incorporating it into something you already have to do—such as getting to class or work. See the **Health Headlines** box for more on using your transportation for fitness.

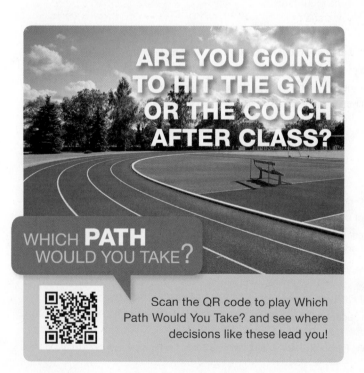

ARE YOU GOING TO HIT THE GYM OR THE COUCH AFTER CLASS?

WHICH **PATH** WOULD YOU TAKE?

Scan the QR code to play Which Path Would You Take? and see where decisions like these lead you!

## LO 4 | **CREATING** YOUR OWN FITNESS PROGRAM

Use the FITT (frequency, intensity, time, and type) principles for the health-related components of physical fitness.

The first step in creating a personal physical fitness program is identifying your goals. Do you want to be better at sports or feel better about your body? Is your goal to manage stress or reduce your risk of chronic diseases? Perhaps your most vital goal will be to establish a realistic schedule of diverse physical activities that you can maintain and enjoy throughout your life. Your physical fitness goals and objectives

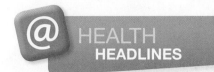
# TRANSPORT YOURSELF!

Once again, many people are embracing a movement toward more active transportation. *Active transportation* means using your own power to get from place to place—whether walking, riding a bike, skateboarding, or roller skating. A bicycle is an excellent and cost-effective way to get to and around campus. Check to see whether your city has a bike share program at http://bikeshare.com. Here are just a few of the many reasons to make active transportation a bigger part of your life:

- You will be adding more exercise into your daily routine. People who use active forms of transportation to complete errands are more likely to meet physical activity guidelines.
- Walking or biking can save you money. It is significantly less expensive to own a bike than a car when you consider gas and maintenance. It is estimated that it is costs 30 times more to maintain a car than a bike! Also consider that you will save the cost of a parking permit and any parking tickets.
- Walking or biking may save you time! Short commutes of 3 to 5 files are usually as fast or faster via bicycle rather than via car.
- You will enjoy being outdoors. Research is emerging on the physical and mental health benefits of nature and being outdoors. So much of what we do is inside, with recirculated air and artificial lighting, that our bodies are deficient in fresh air and sunlight.

**Hop on that bike and join the green revolution! Active transportation is an excellent want to protect the environment and add physical activity to your day, especially on nonexercise days.**

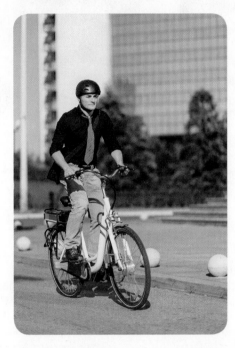

- You will make a significant contribution to reducing air pollution. Choosing to walk or bike instead of driving only 2 days a week can reduce greenhouse gas emissions by an average of 4,000 pounds a year.
- You will help reduce traffic. More active commuters means fewer cars on the roads and less traffic congestion.
- You will contribute to global environmental health. Reducing vehicle trips will help reduce overall greenhouse gas emissions and the need to source more fossil fuel. Swapping walking or cycling for the car when taking short trips is estimated to save over 10 billion gallons of fuel per year.

Safety is paramount, so make sure you consider the following recommendations:

- Always wear a bike helmet! Even for short trips, you should wear a helmet that fits well and has not been damaged.
- Obey traffic rules. Cycle with the flow of traffic, obey traffic lights and signs, and use bike lanes when available.
- Be seen. Avoid dark clothing, wear reflective clothing, have reflectors and head and tail lights for your bike. Be aware of your surroundings. Remember that drivers often do not look for pedestrians and cyclists.
- Use caution when carrying items. Use a backpack or rack for carrying books, class materials, and groceries.

**Sources:** Rails-to-Trails Conservancy, "Investing in Trails: Cost-Effective Improvements—for Everyone," 2013, www.railstotrails.org/resourcehandler. ashx?id=3629; M. Woodruff, "13 Reasons You Should Start Biking to Work," *Business Insider,* October 2012, www.businessinsider. com/13-reasons-you-should-bike-to-work-2012-10#ixzz3fFS2Ovre; U.S. Environmental Protection Agency, "Climate Change: What You Can Do: On the Road," Updated April 2014, www.epa.gov/climatechange/wycd/road.html; B. McKenzie, "Modes Less Traveled—Bicycling and Walking to Work in the United States: 2008–2012," U.S. Department of Commerce, May 2014, www.census.gov/prod/2014pubs/acs-25.pdf.

should be both achievable for you and in line with what you truly want.

## Set SMART Goals

Goal setting done correctly can provide direction and help you develop a plan that works. Ideally, goals should be difficult so you will work hard. However, they must also be attainable so you will not set yourself up for failure and get discouraged. To set successful goals, try using the *SMART* system. SMART goals are specific, measurable, action-oriented, realistic, and time-oriented.

A vague goal would be "Improve fitness by exercising more." A SMART goal would be as follows:

- *Specific*—"I'll participate in a resistance training program that targets all of the major muscle groups 3 to 5 days per week."
- *Measurable*—"I'll improve my fitness from the average classification to the above average classification by increasing the amount of weight I lift by 20 percent."
- *Action-oriented*—"I'll meet with a personal trainer to learn how to safely do resistance exercises and to plan a workout for the gym and home. The trainer will assess my fitness level to make sure the goal is realistic."

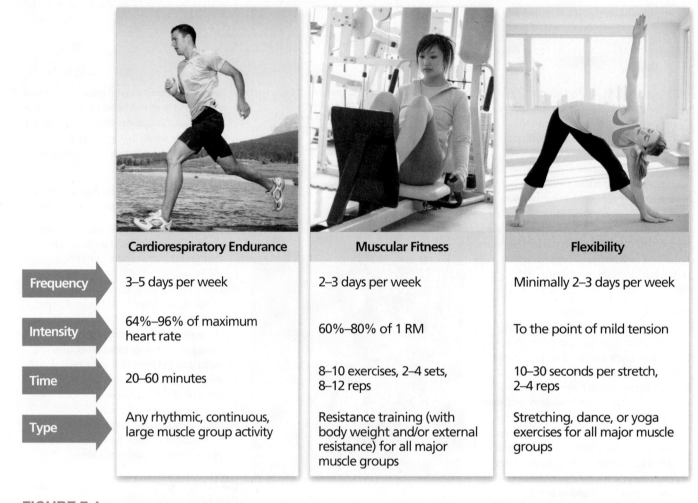

| | Cardiorespiratory Endurance | Muscular Fitness | Flexibility |
|---|---|---|---|
| **Frequency** | 3–5 days per week | 2–3 days per week | Minimally 2–3 days per week |
| **Intensity** | 64%–96% of maximum heart rate | 60%–80% of 1 RM | To the point of mild tension |
| **Time** | 20–60 minutes | 8–10 exercises, 2–4 sets, 8–12 reps | 10–30 seconds per stretch, 2–4 reps |
| **Type** | Any rhythmic, continuous, large muscle group activity | Resistance training (with body weight and/or external resistance) for all major muscle groups | Stretching, dance, or yoga exercises for all major muscle groups |

**FIGURE 7.4** The FITT Principle Applied to Cardiorespiratory Fitness, Muscular Strength and Endurance, and Flexibility

- *Realistic*—"I'll increase the weight I can lift by 20 percent."
- *Time-oriented*—"I'll try my new weight program for 8 weeks, then reassess."

Setting both short- and long-term goals is important. The short-term goals can help to maintain motivation and help to determine whether the long-term goal should be adjusted. If you are a novice exerciser, you might need help with setting realistic goals. Getting a fitness assessment or consulting with a trainer can help you set realistic goals.

## Use the FITT Principle

To improve your health-related physical fitness (or performance-related physical fitness), use the **FITT** (frequency, intensity, time, and type)[80] principle to define your exercise program. The FITT prescription (**FIGURE 7.4**) uses the following criteria:

- **Frequency** refers to the number of times per week you need to engage in particular exercises to achieve the desired level of physical fitness in a particular component.
- **Intensity** refers to how hard your workout must be to achieve the desired level of physical fitness.
- **Time**, or *duration*, refers to how many minutes or repetitions of an exercise are required at a specified intensity during any one session to attain the desired level of physical fitness for each component.
- **Type** refers to what kind of exercises should be performed to improve the specific component of physical fitness.

## The FITT Principle for Cardiorespiratory Fitness

The most effective aerobic exercises for building cardiorespiratory fitness are total body activities involving the large muscle groups. The FITT prescription for cardiorespiratory fitness includes 3 to 5 days per week of vigorous, rhythmic,

**FITT** Acronym for frequency, intensity, time, and type; the terms that describe the essential components of a program or plan to improve a health-related component of physical fitness.

**frequency** As part of the FITT prescription, refers to how many days per week a person should exercise.

**intensity** As part of the FITT prescription, refers to how hard or how much effort is needed when a person exercises.

**time** As part of the FITT prescription, refers to the duration of an exercise session.

**type** As part of the FITT prescription, refers to what kind of exercises a person needs to do.

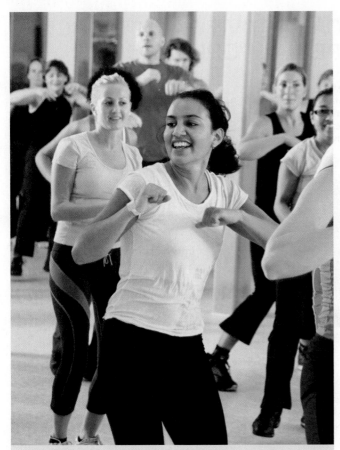

One great way to motivate yourself is to sign up for an exercise class. The structure, schedule, social interaction, and challenge of learning a new skill can be the motivation you need to get moving!

continuous activity at 64 to 96 percent of your estimated maximal heart rate for 20 to 60 minutes.[81]

**Frequency** The frequency of your program is related to your intensity. If you choose to do moderate-intensity exercises, you should aim for a frequency of at least 5 days (frequency drops to at least 3 days per week with vigorous-intensity activities). Newcomers to exercise can still improve by doing less intense exercise (light to moderate level), but doing it more days during the week. In this case, follow the recommendations from the Centers for Disease Control and Prevention (CDC) for moderate physical activity (refer to **TABLE 7.1** on page 191).

**Intensity** The most common methods used to determine the intensity of cardiorespiratory endurance exercises are target heart rate, rating of perceived exertion, and the talk test. The exercise intensity required to improve cardiorespiratory endurance is a heart rate between 64 and 96 percent of your maximum heart rate (moderate to vigorous intensity). Before calculating your **target heart rate**, you must first estimate your maximal heart rate with the formula [207 – 0.7 (age)]. The example below is based on a 20-year-old. Substitute your age to determine your target heart rate training range, then multiply by 0.64 and 0.94 to determine the lower and upper limits

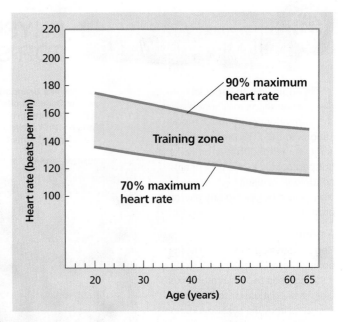

**FIGURE 7.5** **Target Heart Rate Ranges** These ranges are based on calculating the maximum heart rate as [206.9 – 0.67 (age)] and the training zone as 64 to 96 percent of maximum heart rate. Individuals with low fitness levels should start below or at the low end of these ranges.

of your target range. **FIGURE 7.5** shows a range of target heart rates for various ages.

1.  207 – 0.7 (20) = target heart rate for a 20-year-old
2.  207 – 14 = 193 (maximal heart rate)
3.  193(0.64) = 123.52 (lower target limit)
4.  193.5 (0.94) = 185.28 (upper target limit)
5.  Target range = 124–186 beats per minute

To determine how close you are to your target heart rate, take your pulse. Lightly place your index and middle fingers (not your thumb) over the carotid artery in your neck or on the radial artery on the inside of your wrist (**FIGURE 7.6**). Count your pulse while exercising, if

> **target heart rate** The heart rate range of aerobic exercise that leads to improved cardiorespiratory fitness (i.e., 64 to 96% of maximal heart rate).

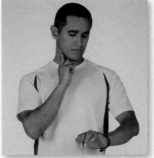
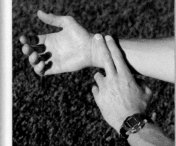

**a** Carotid pulse     **b** Radial pulse

**FIGURE 7.6** **Taking a Pulse** Palpation of the carotid (neck) or radial (wrist) artery is a simple way of determining heart rate. You can also use an activity tracker or cell phone to take your heart rate.

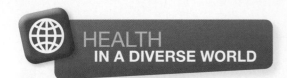
# PHYSICAL ACTIVITY AND EXERCISE FOR SPECIAL POPULATIONS

People with the special considerations mentioned below might need to make modifications to the FITT prescription. It is recommended that all individuals, but particularly those with health conditions, consult with a physician before beginning any exercise program.

## Asthma

Regular physical activity provides benefits for individuals with asthma. It strengthens the respiratory muscles, making it easier to breathe; improves immune system functioning; and helps maintain weight.

Before engaging in exercise, ensure that your asthma is under control. Ask about adjusting your medications (e.g., your doctor may recommend you use your inhaler 15 minutes prior to exercise). Keep your inhaler nearby. Warm up and cool down properly; it is particularly important that you allow your lungs and breathing rate to adjust slowly. Protect yourself from your asthma triggers when exercising (e.g., pollution or cold environments). If you have symptoms while exercising, stop and use your inhaler; if an asthma attack persists, call 9-1-1.

## Obesity

Obese individuals may have limitations such as heat intolerance, shortness of breath during physical activity, lack of flexibility, frequent musculoskeletal injuries, and difficulty with balance. Programs should emphasize physical activities that can be sustained for longer periods of time such as walking, swimming, or bicycling. Use caution when performing these activities in hot or humid environments.

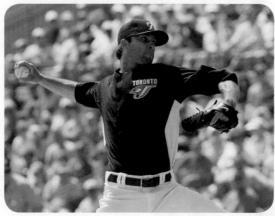

**Athletes like Brandon Morrow, a Major League Baseball pitcher and a type 1 diabetic, are living proof that chronic conditions needn't prevent you from achieving your physical activity goals.**

Although it is recommended to start slow (5 to 10 minutes of activity) and at a lower intensity (55 to 65% of maximal heart rate), the ultimate goal for weight loss and prevention of regain is to perform at least 30 to 60 minutes of exercise per day—150 to 300 minutes per week. Regardless of the amount of weight lost, evidence suggests that individuals who are obese improve their health with cardiorespiratory and resistance training activities.

## Coronary Heart Disease

Although regular physical activity reduces risk of coronary heart disease, vigorous-intensity activity acutely increases risk of sudden cardiac death and myocardial infarction (heart attack). Individuals with coronary heart disease must consult their physicians and might need to participate in a supervised exercise program for individuals with heart disease.

## Hypertension

Using the FITT prescription, individuals who are hypertensive should engage in physical activity on most, if not all, days of the week, at a moderate intensity (12 to 13 on the Borg RPE scale), for 30 minutes or more.

## Diabetes

Physical activity benefits individuals with diabetes in many ways. It controls blood glucose (for individuals with type 2) by improving transport into the cells, controls body weight, and reduces risk for heart disease.

Before people with type 1 diabetes engage in physical activity, they must learn how to manage their resting blood glucose levels. Individuals should have an exercise partner; eat 1 to 3 hours prior to the activity; eat complex carbohydrates after the activity; avoid late-evening exercise; and monitor their blood glucose before, during, and after activity.

One of the most important factors for individuals with type 2 diabetes is the time or length of their physical activity. Because a critical objective of the management of type 2 diabetes is to reduce body fat (obesity), the recommendations for time are longer—at least 30 minutes, working up to 60 minutes per session or 300 minutes per week. Multiple 10-minute sessions can be used to accumulate these totals. For sessions of this length, it is prudent to reduce the intensity of the activity to a target heart rate range of 40 to 60 percent of maximal heart rate.

**Source:** P. Williamson, *Exercise for Special Populations* (Philadelphia: Lippincott Williams & Wilkins, 2011); American College of Sports Medicine, *ASM's Guidelines for Exercise Testing and Prescription,* 9th ed. (Baltimore: Lippincott Williams & Wilkins, 2014).

possible, or start counting your pulse immediately after you stop exercising, as your heart rate decreases rapidly when you stop. Using a watch or a clock, take your pulse for 10 seconds (the first pulse is "0" if you are starting a stopwatch, but 1 if you are using a watch that is already running) and multiply this number by 6 to get the number of beats per minute. You can also use your cell phone or activity tracker if you have one.

**perceived exertion** The subjective perception of effort during exercise that can be used to monitor exercise intensity

Another way to determine the intensity of cardiorespiratory exercise is to use Borg's rating of perceived exertion (RPE) scale. **Perceived exertion** refers to how hard you feel you are working, which you might base on your heart rate, breathing rate, sweat, and level of fatigue. This scale uses a rating from 6 (no exertion at all) to 20 (maximal exertion). An RPE of 12 to 16 is generally recommended for training the cardiorespiratory system.

The easiest method of measuring cardiorespiratory exercise intensity is the "talk test." A "moderate" level of exercise (heart rate at 64 to 76 percent of maximum) is a conversational level of exercise. At this level you are able to talk with a partner while exercising. If you can talk, but only in short fragments and not sentences, you may be at a "vigorous" level of exercise (heart rate at 76 to 96 percent of maximum). If you are breathing so hard that speaking at all is difficult, the intensity of your exercise may be too high. Conversely, if you are able to sing or laugh heartily while exercising, the intensity of your exercise is light and may be insufficient for maintaining or improving cardiorespiratory fitness.

**Time** For cardiorespiratory fitness benefits, the American College of Sports Medicine (ACSM) recommends that vigorous activities be performed for at least 20 minutes at a time, and moderate activities for at least 30 minutes.[82] See also the **Health in a Diverse World** box for recommendations for individuals with chronic diseases or conditions that require alterations to the FITT prescription.

Free time for exercise can vary from day to day, so you can also set a time goal for the entire week as long as you keep your sessions to at least 10 minutes (150 minutes per week for moderate intensity and 75 minutes per week for vigorous intensity). See the **Student Health Today** box on page 206 for information on a few exercise programs that can really give you a lot of bang for your buck.

**Type** Any sort of rhythmic, continuous, and physical activity that can be done for 20 or more minutes will improve cardiorespiratory fitness. Examples include walking briskly, cycling, jogging, fitness classes, and swimming.

## The FITT Principle for Muscular Strength and Endurance

The FITT prescription for muscular strength and endurance includes 2 to 3 days per week of exercises that train the major muscle groups, using enough sets, repetitions, and resistance to maintain or improve muscular strength and endurance.[83]

**Frequency** For frequency, training the major muscle groups 2 to 3 days a week is recommended. It is believed that overloading the muscles, a normal part of resistance training described below, causes microscopic tears in muscle fibers, and the rebuilding process that increases the muscle's size and capacity takes about 24 to 48 hours. Thus, resistance training exercise programs should include at least 1 day of rest between workouts before the same muscles are overloaded again. But don't wait too long between workouts: One of the important principles of strength training is the idea of *reversibility*. Reversibility means that if you stop exercising, the body responds by deconditioning. Within 2 weeks, muscles begin to revert to their untrained state.[84] The saying "use it or lose it" applies!

**Intensity** To determine the intensity of exercise needed to improve muscular strength and endurance, you need to know

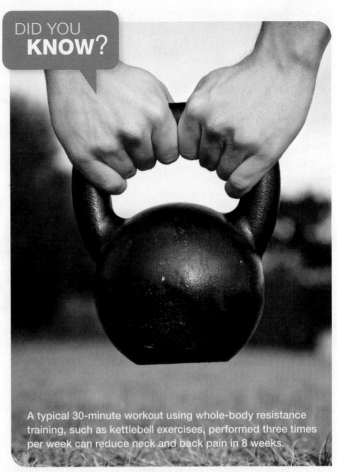

A typical 30-minute workout using whole-body resistance training, such as kettlebell exercises, performed three times per week can reduce neck and back pain in 8 weeks.

**Source:** K. Jay et al., "Kettlebell Training for Musculoskeletal and Cardiovascular Health: A Randomized Controlled Trial," *Scandinavian Journal of Work, Environment, and Health* 37, no. 3 (2011): 196–203.

the maximum amount of weight you can lift (or move) in one contraction. This value is called your **one repetition maximum (1 RM)**. Once your 1 RM is determined, it is used as the basis for intensity recommendations for improving muscular strength and endurance. Muscular strength is improved when resistance loads are greater than 60 percent of your 1 RM, whereas muscular endurance is improved using loads less than 50 percent of your 1 RM.

Everyone begins a resistance training program at an initial level of strength. To become stronger, you must *overload* your muscles; that is, you must regularly create a degree of tension in your muscles that is greater than what they are accustomed to. Overloading them forces your muscles to adapt by getting larger, stronger, and capable of producing more tension. If you "underload" your muscles, you will not increase strength. If you create too great an overload, you may experience muscle injury, muscle fatigue, and potentially a loss in strength.

**Time** The time recommended for muscular strength and endurance exercises is measured not in minutes of exercise, but rather in repetitions and sets.

**one repetition maximum (1 RM)** The amount of weight or resistance that can be lifted or moved only once.

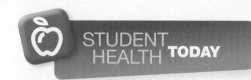
# IS HIGH-INTENSITY INTERVAL TRAINING RIGHT FOR YOU?

CrossFit and high-intensity interval training (HIIT) are two methods of training that are increasing in popularity. CrossFit is a strength and conditioning program that utilizes a broad range of high-intensity functional movements and activities. CrossFit is typically performed in a CrossFit gym or "Box" within a group or class. It is an intense specialized training program, so there are special requirements and certifications to become a CrossFit trainer or coach.

HIIT is a type of training that combines alternating high-intensity bouts and active rest bouts within your exercise session. For example, after the warm-up phase, you might do 2 minutes of a near-maximal-paced run, and then jog for 2 minutes to rest. This type of training can provide a very efficient workout. The volume of exercise is generally less than a continuous bout at a constant pace, but similar fitness gains can be seen with the lower volume of exercise as with

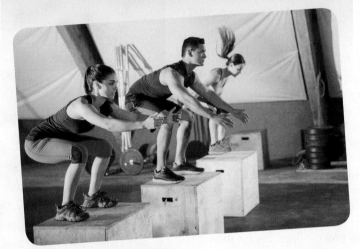

CrossFit and high-intensity interval training (HIIT) are two methods of training that are increasing in popularity. If you're healthy enough—and up for the challenge—they might be right for you.

the traditional exercise bout. The intervals can be varied depending on your fitness level and goals.

How do you know whether either type of training is right for you? If you are a beginner, have risk factors for cardiovascular disease or musculoskeletal disorders, are obese, or have been sedentary, make sure you get clearance from your health care provider. After getting checked out, find a fitness professional who can

help you get started. Both types of training can be modified to accommodate varying levels of fitness.

If you like a challenge, a variety of exercises, and the motivation of the gym, CrossFit might be right for you. HIIT might be a good option if time is a barrier or you are trying to improve your performance. Because both are high-intensity activities, it is important to allow your body time to rest and recover to reduce the risk of injury. Using different activities on consecutive days and not doing more than 3 consecutive days of exercise are recommendations for CrossFit. HIIT should be alternated with other activities throughout the week. If you are up for the challenge, give one of these nontraditional training programs a try.

**Sources:** CrossFit, "What is Crossfit?" Accessed April 2016, www.crossfit.com; L. Kravitz, "High-Intensity Interval Training," ACSM, 2014, www .acsm.org/docs/brochures/high-intensity-interval-training.pdf.

- **Repetitions and sets.** To increase muscular strength, you need higher intensity and fewer repetitions and sets: Use a resistance of at least 60 percent of your 1 RM, performing 8 to 12 repetitions per set, with two to four sets performed overall. If improving muscular endurance is your goal, use less resistance and more repetitions: Perform one to two sets of 15 to 25 repetitions using a resistance that is less than 50 percent of your 1 RM.
- **Rest periods.** Resting between exercises is crucial to reduce fatigue and help with performance and safety in subsequent sets. A rest period of 2 to 3 minutes is recommended when using the guidelines for general health benefits. However, the rest period when working to develop strength or endurance will vary. Note that the rest period refers specifically to the muscle group being exercised. For example, you can alternate a set of push-ups with curl-ups, as the muscle groups worked in one set can rest while you are working the other muscle groups.

**Type** To improve muscular strength or endurance, it is recommended that resistance training use either the body's weight or devices that provide a fixed or variable resistance (see **TABLE 7.4**). When selecting strength-training exercises, there are three important principles to bear in mind: specificity, exercise selection, and exercise order. According to the *specificity principle*, the effects of resistance exercise training are specific to the muscles exercised; thus, to improve total body strength, include exercises for all the major muscle groups.

The second important concept is *exercise selection*. It is important to select exercises that will meet your goals. Selecting 8 to 10 exercises targeting all major muscle groups is generally recommended and will ensure that exercises are balanced for opposing muscle groups.

Finally, for optimal training effects, pay attention to *exercise order*. When training all major muscle groups in a single workout, complete large muscle group exercises (e.g., the bench press or leg press) before small muscle group exercises, multiple-joint exercises before single-joint exercises (e.g., biceps

TABLE **7.4** | Methods of Providing Muscular Resistance

| Body Weight Resistance (Calisthenics) | Fixed Resistance | Variable Resistance |
|---|---|---|
| 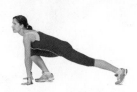 | 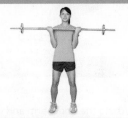 | 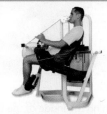 |
| ■ Uses your own body weight to develop muscular strength and endurance<br><br>■ Improves overall muscular fitness and, in particular, core body strength and overall muscle tone | ■ Provides a constant resistance through-out the full range of movement<br><br>■ Requires balance and coordination; promotes development of core body strength | ■ Resistance altered so that the muscle's effort is consistent throughout the full range of motion<br><br>■ Provides more controlled motion and isolates certain muscle groups |
| **Examples:** Push-ups, pull-ups, curl-ups, dips, leg raises, chair sits, etc. | **Examples:** Free weights, such as barbells, dumbbells, medicine balls, and kettlebells | **Examples:** Weight machines |

curls, triceps extension), and high-intensity exercises before lower-intensity exercises.

## The FITT Principle for Flexibility

Although often overshadowed by cardiorespiratory and muscular fitness training, flexibility is important. Stretching is important in helping maintain range of motion, improve aspects of performance, and manage lower-back problems.[85] Improved flexibility also means less tension and pressure on joints, resulting in less joint pain and joint deterioration.[86] This means that remaining flexible can help prevent the decreased physical function that often occurs with aging.[87]

**Frequency** The FITT principle calls for a minimum of 2 to 3 days per week for flexibility training.

**Intensity** Intensity recommendations for flexibility are that you perform or hold stretching positions at an individually determined "point of mild tension." You should be able to feel tension or mild discomfort in the muscle(s) you are stretching, but the stretch should not hurt.[88]

**Time** The time recommended to improve flexibility is based on time per stretch. Once you are in a stretching position, you should hold at the "point of tension" for 10 to 30 seconds for each stretch and repeat two to four times in close succession.[89]

**Type** The most effective exercises for increasing flexibility involve stretching the major muscle groups of your body when the body is already warm, such as after your cardiorespiratory workout. The safest exercises for improving flexibility involve **static stretching**. The primary strategy is to decrease the resistance to stretch (tension) within a tight muscle targeted for increased range of motion.[90] To do this, you repeatedly stretch the muscle and its tendons of attachment to elongate them. With each repetition of a static stretch, your range of motion improves temporarily due to the slightly lessened sensitivity of tension receptors in the stretched muscles; when done regularly, range of motion increases. Data from a recent review support the role of the post-stretching dynamic to maximize benefits of stretching, but did not find consistent evidence for the reduced risk of injury.[91] **FIGURE 7.7** on page 208 illustrates some basic stretching exercises to increase flexibility.

## LO 5 | IMPLEMENTING YOUR FITNESS PROGRAM

Devise a plan to implement your safe and effective fitness program.

As your physical fitness improves, you need to adjust the frequency, intensity, time, and type of your exercise to maintain or continue to improve your level of physical fitness. Below are a few suggestions to get started and stay on track. (If you're looking for a little more direction, the **Money & Health** box on page 209 offers suggestions on choosing a personal trainer or fitness coach.)

**static stretching** Stretching techniques that slowly and gradually lengthen a muscle or group of muscles and their tendons.

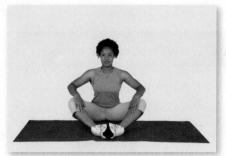 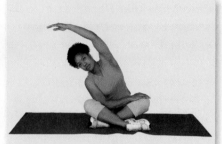 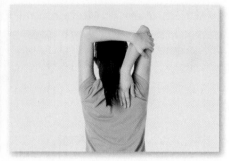

(a) Stretching the inside of the thighs

(b) Stretching the upper arm and the side of the trunk

(c) Stretching the triceps

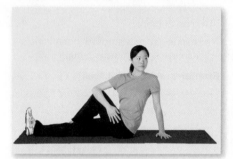 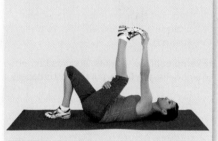 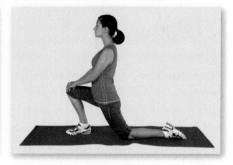

(d) Stretching the trunk and the hip

(e) Stretching the hip, back of the thigh, and the calf

(f) Stretching the front of the thigh and the hip flexor

**FIGURE 7.7 Stretching Exercises to Improve Flexibility** Use these stretches as part of your cool-down. Hold each stretch for 10 to 30 seconds, and repeat two to four times for each limb.

## Develop a Progressive Plan

Experts recommend beginning an exercise regimen by picking an exercise that you enjoy. Keep in mind that you might have to try a few activities to find an exercise or activity that is fun for you, so do not get discouraged if you do not enjoy your first trip to the gym. Once you find exercises and activities that you like, gradually increase the frequency or time of your workouts. For example, in week 1, you might exercise 3 days for 20 minutes per day, and then move to 4 days in week 3 or 4. Then, consider increasing your duration to 30 minutes per session over the next couple of weeks. Gradual increases in intensity are typically made once the duration and frequency goals are met.

Finding a variety of exercises can reduce the risk of overuse injuries. Choosing different exercises for your workouts will also provide for a more complete training program by targeting more muscle groups. Reevaluate your physical fitness goals and action plan monthly to ensure that they are still working for you. A mistake many people make when they decide to become more physically active (or to make any other behavior change) is putting a lot of effort into getting started,

but failing to develop a long-term plan for action and maintenance phases. The Making Changes Today box on page 211 offers more tips on starting and sticking with an exercise plan.

## Design Your Exercise Session

A comprehensive workout should include a warm-up, cardiorespiratory and/or resistance training, and then a cool-down to finish the session.

**Warm-Up** The warm-up prepares the body physically and mentally for cardiorespiratory and/or resistance training. A warm-up should involve large body movements, generally using light cardiorespiratory activities, followed by range-of-motion exercises of the muscle groups to be used during the exercise session. Usually 5 to 15 minutes long, a warm-up is shorter when you are ready to go and longer when you are struggling to get moving or your muscles are cold or tight. The warm-up provides a transition from rest to physical activity by slowly increasing heart rate,

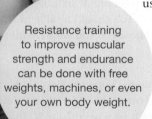

Resistance training to improve muscular strength and endurance can be done with free weights, machines, or even your own body weight.

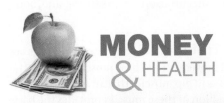

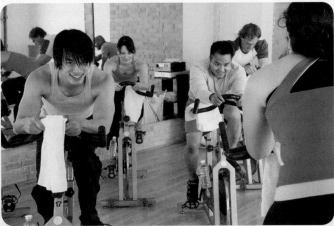

## MONEY & HEALTH | ALL CERTIFICATIONS ARE NOT CREATED EQUAL

Using a personal trainer or fitness trainer is a great way to get on track with a new exercise program. So, how do you select the best fit for you and your goals?

First, make sure your trainer is certified and carries personal liability insurance, but be careful! There are a lot of certifications available, and not all are reputable. You can use the Internet to review the organizations that award certifications. Consider the following characteristics when reviewing certifications:

■ **Quality of certification.** Avoid using a trainer with a certification that is very easily obtainable. The reputable certifications have workshops, test review materials, online study materials, and minimal standards to qualify (e.g., a high school diploma). The National Commission for Certifying Agencies, an accrediting agency for health professions (www.credentialingexcellence.org/p/cm/ld/fid=121), lists accredited fitness certifications.

Before you sign on the dotted line, check out the classes, equipment, and personnel a fitness center offers.

■ **Continuing education credits.** Review the continuing education requirements to maintain the certification. Workshops, professional conferences, tests in scientific journals, and online courses should be options for maintaining the certification. It's a good sign when other certifying bodies use an organization's conferences and classes for continuing education.

■ **Readily available information.** You should be able to readily find information about the certification or organization that provides the certification.

In addition to certification, also consider characteristics of the trainer and get recommendations from those you trust.

■ The trainer's area of specialty should fit with your goals (e.g., weight loss, improved athletic performance).
■ The trainer should teach you about fitness, and not just give you a workout plan. And, the trainer should explain things to you at a level you understand.

Consider the trainer's education level.
■ You should not feel judged by the trainer.
■ The trainer's style should match your needs. For example, if you need a lot of encouragement and reinforcement, select a trainer who will provide those things.

**Sources:** ACE, "How to Choose the Right Personal Trainer," 2015, www.acefitness.org/acefit/healthy_living_fit_facts_content.aspx?itemid=19; ACSM, "Using a Personal Trainer," www.acsm.org/docs/default-source/brochures/using-a-personal-trainer.pdf?sfvrsn=4.

blood pressure, breathing rate, and body temperature. These gradual changes improve joint lubrication, increase muscle and tendon elasticity, and enhance blood flow throughout the body, facilitating performance during the next stage of the workout. Static or **dynamic stretching** can be included in the warm-up phase. Any stretching should be performed after light cardiovascular activity. When stretching, make sure you target the muscles that are dominant in your workout.

### Cardiorespiratory and/or Resistance Training

The next stage of your workout may involve cardiorespiratory training, resistance training, or a little of both. If completing aerobic and resistance exercise in the same session, it is often recommended to perform your aerobic exercise first. This order will provide additional warm-up for the resistance

session, and your muscles will not be fatigued for the aerobic workout.

### Cool-Down and Stretching

A cool-down is an essential component of a fitness program; it involves another 10 to 15 minutes of activity time. Start your cool-down with 5 to 10 minutes of moderate- to low-intensity activity, and follow it with approximately 5 to 10 minutes of stretching. Because of the body's increased temperature, the cool-down is an excellent time to stretch to improve flexibility. The purpose and importance of the cool-down is to gradually reduce your heart rate, blood pressure, and body temperature to pre-exercise levels. In addition, the cool-down reduces the risk of blood pooling in the extremities and facilitates quicker recovery between exercise sessions.

**dynamic stretching** Gradual transitions in movement and body position that progressively increase the range of motion through repeating the movements.

## Explore Activities That Develop Multiple Components of Fitness

Some forms of activity have the potential to improve several components of physical fitness and thus improve your everyday functioning ("functional" exercises). For example, core strength training improves posture and can prevent back pain. In addition, yoga, tai chi, and Pilates improve flexibility, muscular fitness and endurance, balance, coordination, and agility. They also develop the mind–body connection through concentration on breathing and body position.

**Core Strength Training** The body's core muscles are the foundation for all movement.[92] These muscles include the deep back, abdominal, and hip muscles that attach to the spine and pelvis. The contraction of these muscles provides the basis of support for movements of the upper and lower body and powerful movements of the extremities. A weak core generally results in poor posture, low back pain, and muscle injuries. A strong core provides a more stable center of gravity and, as a result, a more stable platform for movement, thus reducing the chance of injury.

You can develop core muscular fitness by doing various exercises, including calisthenics, yoga, or Pilates. Holding yourself in a front or reverse plank (an upward-facing version of a push-up position) or doing abdominal curl-ups are examples of exercises that increase core strength. Increased core strength does not happen from one single exercise, but rather from a structured regime of postures and exercises.[93] The use of instability devices (stability ball, wobble boards, etc.) and exercises to train the core have become popular.[94]

**Yoga** Yoga, based on ancient Indian practices, blends the mental and physical aspects of exercise—a union of mind and body that participants often find relaxing and satisfying. The practice of yoga focuses attention on controlled breathing as well as physical exercise and incorporates a complex array of static stretching and strengthening exercises expressed as postures (*asanas*). Done regularly, yoga improves flexibility, vitality, posture, agility, balance, coordination, and core muscular fitness and endurance. Many people report an improved sense of general well-being, too.

**Tai Chi** Tai chi is an ancient Chinese form of exercise that combines stretching, balance, muscular endurance, coordination, and meditation. It increases range of motion and flexibility while reducing muscular tension. It involves continuously performing a series of positions called *forms*. Tai chi is often described as "meditation in motion" because it promotes serenity through gentle movements that connect the mind and body.

**Pilates** Pilates was developed by Joseph Pilates in 1926 as an exercise style that combines stretching with movement against resistance, frequently aided by devices such as tension springs or heavy rubber bands. It differs from yoga and tai chi in that it includes a component specifically designed to increase strength. Some movements are carried out on specially designed equipment, whereas others can be performed on mats. It teaches body awareness, good posture, and easy, graceful body movements while improving flexibility, coordination, core strength, muscle tone, and economy of motion.

Some people set themselves up to succeed in terms of their fitness goals by participating in group activities or exercise classes. For some guidance on how best to choose the right fitness class for you, see the Making Changes Today box.

## LO **6** | **TAKING** IN PROPER NUTRITION FOR EXERCISE

Describe optimal food and fluid consumption recommendations for exercise and recovery.

It's important to evaluate your eating habits in light of your exercise habits. Whether you're a seasoned fitness buff or a beginner, the importance of proper nutrition for exercise can't be overstated.

## Foods for Exercise and Recovery

To make the most of your workouts, follow the recommendations from the MyPlate plan and make sure that you eat sufficient carbohydrates, the body's main source of fuel. Your body stores carbohydrates as glycogen primarily in the muscles and liver and then uses this stored glycogen for energy when you are physically active. Fats are also an important source of energy, packing more than double the energy per gram compared to carbohydrates. Protein plays a role in muscle repair and growth, but is not normally a source of energy.

When you eat is almost as important as what you eat. Eating a large meal before exercising can cause upset stomach, cramping, and diarrhea because your muscles have to compete with your digestive system for energy. After a large meal, wait 3 to 4 hours before you begin exercising. Smaller meals (snacks) can be eaten about an hour before activity. Not eating at all before a workout can cause low blood sugar levels that in turn cause weakness and slower reaction times.

After your workout, help your muscles recover by eating a snack or meal that contains plenty of carbohydrates and a little protein, too. Today, there is a burgeoning market for dietary supplements that claim to deliver the nutrients needed for muscle recovery, as well as additional "performance-enhancing" ingredients; one thing to keep in mind, especially if you consider these products, is that there are few standards and virtually no Food and Drug Administration (FDA) approval needed for many to grace store shelves. (See **TABLE 7.5** on page 212 for some of the most popular performance-enhancing drugs and supplements, their purported benefits, and associated risks.)

## Fluids for Exercise and Recovery

In addition to eating well, staying hydrated is also crucial. How much fluid do you need? Keep in mind that the goal of fluid replacement is to prevent excessive dehydration (greater than 2% loss of body weight). The ACSM and the National Athletic Trainers' Association recommend consuming 5 to 7 milliliters per kilogram of body weight (approximately 0.7 to 1.07 ounces per 10 pounds body weight) 4 hours prior to exercise.[95] A good way to monitor how much fluid you need to replace

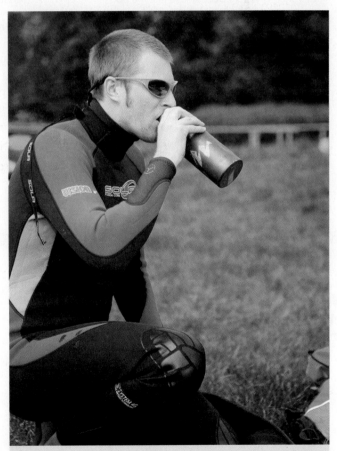

The American College of Sports Medicine and the National Athletic Trainers' Association recommend consuming 14 to 22 ounces of fluid several hours prior to exercise and about 6 to 12 ounces per 15 to 20 minutes during—assuming you are sweating.

# TABLE 7.5 | Performance-Enhancing Dietary Supplements and Drugs—Their Uses and Effects

| Supplement/Drug | Primary Uses | Side Effects |
|---|---|---|
| *Creatine* Naturally occurring compound that helps supply energy to muscle | ■ Improve postworkout recovery<br>■ Increase muscle mass<br>■ Increase strength<br>■ Increase power | ■ Weight gain, nausea, muscle cramps<br>■ Large doses can impair kidney function |
| *Ephedra and ephedrine* Stimulant that constricts blood vessels and increases blood pressure and heart rate*Illegal; banned by FDA in 2008; banned by sports organizations | ■ Lose Weight<br>■ Increase performance | ■ Nausea, vomiting<br>■ Anxiety and mood changes<br>■ Hyperactivity<br>■ Rarely seizures, heart attack, stroke, psychotic episodes |
| *Anabolic steroids* Synthetic versions of the hormone testosterone *Nonmedical use is illegal; banned by major sports organizations | ■ Improve strength, power, and speed<br>■ Increase muscle mass | ■ In adolescents, stops bone growth; therefore reduced adult height<br>■ Masculinization of females; feminization of males<br>■ Mood swings<br>■ Severe acne, particularly on the back<br>■ Sexual dysfunction<br>■ Aggressive behavior<br>■ Potential heart and liver damage |
| *Steroid precursors* Substances that the body converts into anabolic steroids, for example, androstenedione (andro), dehydroepiandrosterone (DHEA)*Nonmedical use is illegal; banned by major sports organizations | ■ Converted in the body to anabolic steroids to increase muscle mass | ■ In addition to side effects noted with anabolic steroids:body hair growth, increased risk of pancreatic cancer |
| *Human growth hormone* Naturally occurring hormone secreted by the pituitary gland that is essential for body growth*Nonmedical use is illegal; banned by major sports organizations | ■ Antiaging agent<br>■ Improve performance<br>■ Increase muscle mass | ■ Structural changes to the face<br>■ Increased risk of high blood pressure<br>■ Potential for congestive heart failure |

**Sources:** Mayo Clinic Staff, "Performance-Enhancing Drugs and Your Teen Athlete," MayoClinic.com, August 2013, www.mayoclinic.com/health/performance-enhancing-drugs/SM00045; Office of Diversion Control, Drug and Chemical Evaluation Section, "Drugs and Chemicals of Concern: Human Growth Hormone," August 2013, www.deadiversion.usdoj.gov/drug_chem_info/hgh.pdf; Office of Dietary Supplements, National Institutes of Health, "Ephedra and Ephedrine Alkaloids for Weight Loss and Athletic Performance," reviewed July 2004, http://ods.od.nih.gov/factsheets/EphedraandEphedrine.

**SEE IT! VIDEOS**

Will that fancy sports drink help you exercise better? Watch **Sports Drinks Science: Is It Hype?** available on **MasteringHealth.™**

is to weigh yourself before and after your workout. The difference in weight is how much you should drink. So, for example, if you lost 2 pounds during a training session, you should drink 32 ounces of fluid.[96]

For exercise sessions lasting less than 1 hour, plain water is sufficient for rehydration. If your exercise session exceeds 1 hour—and you sweat profusely—consider a sports drink containing electrolytes. The electrolytes in these products are minerals and ions such as sodium and potassium that are needed for proper functioning of your nervous and muscular systems. Replacing electrolytes is particularly important for endurance athletes. In endurance events lasting more than 4 hours, an athlete's overconsumption of plain water can dilute the sodium concentration in the blood with potentially fatal results, an effect called **hyponatremia**, or water intoxication.

Although water is the best choice in most cases, there are situations in which you might need to choose something different. Some people are likely to consume more when their drink is flavored because the taste is more appealing than water, a point that may be significant in ensuring proper hydration. Recently, research has considered low-fat chocolate milk as a recovery drink.[97] Chocolate milk is a liquid that not only hydrates, but also is a source of sodium, potassium, carbohydrates, and protein. Consuming carbohydrates and protein immediately after exercise will help replenish muscle and liver glycogen stores and stimulate muscle protein synthesis for better recovery from exercise. The protein in milk, whey protein, is ideal because it contains all of the essential amino acids and is rapidly absorbed by the body.

**hyponatremia or water intoxication** Overconsumption of water, which leads to a dilution of sodium concentration in the blood, with potentially fatal results.

## LO 7 | PREVENTING AND TREATING FITNESS-RELATED INJURIES

Explain how to prevent and treat common exercise injuries.

Two basic types of injuries stem from fitness-related activities: traumatic injuries and overuse injuries. **Traumatic injuries** occur suddenly and usually by accident. Typical traumatic injuries are broken bones, torn ligaments and muscles, contusions, and lacerations. If a traumatic injury causes a noticeable loss of function and immediate pain or pain that does not go away after 30 minutes, consult a physician.

**Overuse injuries** result from the cumulative effects of day-after-day stresses. These injuries occur most often in repetitive activities such as swimming, running, bicycling, and step aerobics. The forces that occur normally during physical activity are not enough to cause a ligament sprain or muscle strain as in a traumatic injury, but when these forces are applied daily for weeks or months, they can result in an overuse injury. Factors such as overweight or obesity, running mechanics, and poor choice of shoe can also contribute to overuse injury.

The three most common overuse injuries are *runner's knee*, *shin splints*, and *plantar fasciitis*. Runner's knee is a general term describing a series of problems involving the muscles, tendons, and ligaments around the knee. Shin splints is a general term used for any pain that occurs below the knee and above the ankle in the shin. Plantar fasciitis is an inflammation of the plantar fascia, a broad band of dense, inelastic tissue in the foot. Wearing the appropriate athletic shoes, including warm-up and cool-down phases, maintaining a healthy body weight, and having proper mechanics for your activity can help reduce your risk.[98] However, if you do develop one of these conditions, rest, variation of routine, and stretching are the first lines of treatment for any of these overuse injuries. If pain continues, visit a physician. Orthotics, physical therapy, or steroid shots are possible treatment options.

## Preventing Injuries

To reduce your risk of overuse or traumatic injuries, use common sense and the proper gear and equipment. Vary your physical activities throughout the week, setting appropriate and realistic short- and long-term goals. Listen to your body when working out. Warning signs include muscle stiffness and soreness, bone and joint pain, and whole-body fatigue that simply does not go away.

**Appropriate Footwear** Proper footwear, replaced in a timely manner, can decrease the likelihood of foot, knee, hip, or back injuries. Running, jumping, and other high-impact activities have a significant impact on your joints. Consider the impact for a runner who has poor mechanics or an overweight individual who participates in weight-bearing activities. The force not absorbed by the running shoe is transmitted upward into the foot, leg, thigh, and back. Our bodies can absorb forces such as these but may be injured by the cumulative effect of

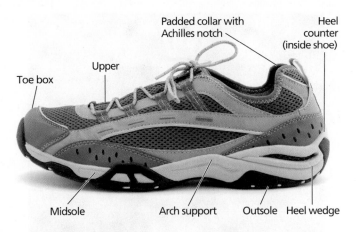

**FIGURE 7.8 Anatomy of a Running Shoe** A good running shoe should fit comfortably; allow room for your toes to move; have a firm, but flexible midsole; and have a firm grip on your heel to prevent slipping.

repetitive impact (such as running 40 miles per week). Thus, the shoes' ability to absorb shock is critical— not just for those who run, but for anyone engaged in weight-bearing activities.

In addition to absorbing shock, an athletic shoe should provide a good fit for maximal comfort and performance (see **FIGURE 7.8**). To get the best fit, shop at a sports or fitness specialty store where there is a large selection and the salespeople are trained in properly fitting athletic shoes. Try on shoes later in the day when your feet are largest, and check to make sure there is a little extra room in the toe and that the width is appropriate. Because different activities place different stresses on your feet and joints, you should choose shoes specifically designed for your sport or activity. Shoes of any type should be replaced once they lose their cushioning. A common rule of thumb is that running shoes ought to be replaced after 300 to 500 miles of use, which is typically between 3 and 9 months, depending on your activity level.

**Appropriate Protective Equipment** It is essential to use well-fitted, appropriate protective equipment for your physical activities. For example, using the correct racquet with the proper tension helps prevent the general inflammatory condition known as tennis elbow. As another example, eye injuries can occur in virtually all physical activities, although some activities (such as baseball, basketball, and racquet sports) are more risky than others.[99] As many as 90 percent of eye injuries could be prevented by wearing appropriate eye protection, such as goggles with polycarbonate lenses.[100]

Wearing a helmet while bicycle riding is an important safety precaution. An estimated 66 to

**WHAT DO YOU THINK?**

**How do your physical activities put you at risk of injury?**

- What changes can you make to your approach to training, your training program, equipment, or footwear to reduce these risks?

**traumatic injuries** Injuries that are accidental and occur suddenly.

**overuse injuries** Injuries that result from the cumulative effects of day-after-day stresses placed on tendons, muscles, and joints.

Padded collar with Achilles notch
Heel counter (inside shoe)
Upper
Toe box
Midsole
Arch support
Outsole   Heel wedge

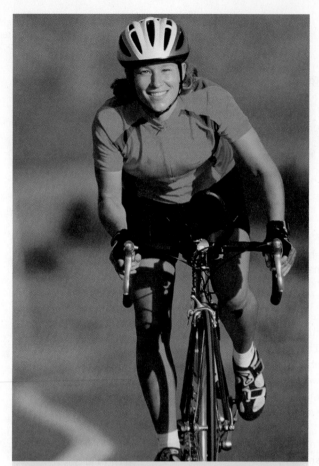

Reducing risk for exercise injuries requires common sense and preventative measures, including wearing protective gear (helmets, knee pads, elbow pads, eyewear).

88 percent of head injuries among cyclists can be prevented by wearing a helmet.[101] In a recent study of college students, 43.8 percent of students who rode a bike in the past 12 months reported never wearing a helmet, and 23.6 percent said they wore one only sometimes or rarely.[102] The direct medical costs from cyclists' failure to wear helmets is an estimated $81 million a year.[103] Cyclists aren't the only ones who should be wearing helmets. People who skateboard, ski, in-line skate, snowboard, play contact sports, or use kick-scooters should also wear helmets. Look for helmets that meet the standards established by the American National Standards Institute or the Snell Memorial Foundation.

## Exercising in the Heat

Exercising in hot or humid weather increases your risk of a heat-related illness. In these conditions, your body's rate of heat production can exceed its ability to cool itself. The three different heat stress illnesses, progressive in their level of severity, are heat cramps, heat exhaustion, and heatstroke.

**heat cramps** Involuntary and forcible muscle contractions that occur during or following exercise in hot and/or humid weather.

**heat exhaustion** A heat stress illness caused by significant dehydration resulting from exercise in hot and/or humid conditions.

**heatstroke** A deadly heat stress illness resulting from dehydration and overexertion in hot and/or humid conditions.

**hypothermia** Potentially fatal condition caused by abnormally low body core temperature.

**Heat cramps** (heat-related involuntary and forcible muscle contractions that cannot be relaxed), the least serious problem, can usually be prevented by adequate fluid replacement and a dietary intake that includes the electrolytes lost during sweating.

**Heat exhaustion** is actually a mild form of shock, in which the blood pools in the arms and legs away from the brain and major organs of the body. It is caused by excessive water loss because of intense or prolonged exercise or work in a hot and/or humid environment. Symptoms of heat exhaustion include nausea, headache, fatigue, dizziness and faintness, and, paradoxically, goose bumps and chills. When you are suffering from heat exhaustion, your skin will be cool and moist.

**Heatstroke**, often called *sunstroke*, is a life-threatening emergency condition with a high morbidity and mortality rate.[104] Heatstroke occurs during vigorous exercise when the body's heat production significantly exceeds its cooling capacities. Core body temperature can rise from normal (98.6°F) to 105 to 110°F within minutes after the body's cooling mechanism shuts down. A rapid increase in core body temperature can cause brain damage, permanent disability, and death. Common signs of heatstroke are dry, hot, and usually red skin; very high body temperature; and rapid heart rate. If you experience any of the symptoms mentioned here, stop exercising immediately. Move to the shade or a cool spot to rest and drink plenty of cool fluids for heat cramps and exhaustion. If heatstroke is suspected, seek medical attention immediately.

You can prevent heat stress by following certain precautions. First, acclimatize yourself to hot or humid weather. The process of heat acclimatization, which increases your body's cooling efficiency, requires about 10 to 14 days of gradually increased physical activity in the hot environment. Second, reduce your risk of dehydration by replacing fluids before, during, and after exercise. Third, wear clothing appropriate for the activity and the environment—for example, light-colored nylon shorts and a mesh tank top. Finally, use common sense. For example, on a day when the temperature is 85°F and the humidity is around 80 percent, postpone lunchtime physical activity until the evening when it is cooler or exercise indoors where the conditions are controlled.

## Exercising in the Cold

When you exercise in cool weather, especially in windy and damp conditions, your body's rate of heat loss is frequently greater than its rate of heat production. These conditions may lead to **hypothermia**—a condition in which the body's core temperature drops below 95°F.[105] Temperatures need not be frigid for hypothermia to occur; it can also result from prolonged, vigorous exercise in 40 to 50°F temperatures, particularly if there is rain, snow, or a strong wind.

As body core temperature drops from the normal 98.6°F to about 93.2°F, shivering begins. Shivering—the involuntary contraction of nearly every muscle in the body—increases body temperature by using the heat given off by muscle activity. You may also experience cold hands and feet, poor judgment, apathy, and amnesia. Shivering ceases in most hypothermia victims as body core temperatures drop to between 87 and 90°F, a sign that the body has lost its ability to generate heat. Death usually occurs at body core temperatures between 75 and 80°F.[106]

To prevent hypothermia, analyze weather conditions before engaging in outdoor physical activity. Remember that wind and humidity are as significant as temperature. Have a friend join you for safety when exercising outdoors in cold weather, and wear layers of appropriate clothing to prevent excessive heat loss and frostbite (polypropylene or woolen undergarments, a windproof outer garment, and a wool hat and gloves). Keep your head, hands, and feet warm. Finally, do not allow yourself to become dehydrated.[107]

## Treating Injuries

First-aid treatment for virtually all fitness training–related injuries involves RICE: rest, ice, compression, and elevation.

- *Rest* is required to avoid further irritation of the injured body part.

Applying ice to an injury such as a sprain can help relieve pain and reduce swelling. To prevent frostbite, never apply ice directly to the skin.

- *Ice* is applied to relieve pain and constrict the blood vessels to reduce internal or external bleeding or the inflammatory response. To prevent frostbite, wrap the ice or cold pack in a layer of wet toweling or elastic bandage before applying it to your skin. A new injury should be iced for approximately 20 minutes every hour for the first 24 to 72 hours.
- *Compression* of the injured body part can be accomplished with a 4- or 6-inch-wide elastic bandage; this applies indirect pressure to damaged blood vessels to help stop bleeding and reduce inflammation. Be careful, though, that the compression wrap does not interfere with normal blood flow. Throbbing or pain indicates that the compression wrap should be loosened.
- *Elevation* of an injured extremity above the level of your heart also helps control internal or external bleeding and reduce the inflammatory response by making the blood flow upward to reach the injured area.

**RICE** Acronym for the standard first-aid treatment for virtually all traumatic and overuse injuries: rest, ice, compression, and elevation.

# STUDY PLAN

Customize your study plan—and master your health!—in the Study Area of **MasteringHealth.**

## ASSESS YOURSELF

**Want to measure your muscular strength, flexibility, and cardiovascular endurance?** Take the **How Physically Fit Are You?** assessment available on

## MasteringHealth.™

# CHAPTER REVIEW

To hear an MP3 Tutor Session, scan here or visit the Study Area in **MasteringHealth.**

## LO 1 Physical Activity for Health

- Benefits of regular physical activity include reduced risk of cardiovascular diseases, metabolic syndrome and type 2 diabetes, and cancer, as well as improved blood lipoproteins, bone mass, weight control, immunity to disease, mental health, stress management, and lifespan. Sedentary activity and the time spent sitting also increase the risk of poor health outcomes. The risk for type 2 diabetes, cardiovascular disease, some cancers, and premature death is independently increased by high amounts of sitting time.

## LO 2 Physical Activity for Fitness and Performance

- Physical fitness involves achieving minimal levels in the health-related components of fitness: cardiorespiratory, muscular strength, muscular endurance, flexibility, and body composition. Skill-related components of fitness—such as agility, balance, reaction time, speed, coordination, and power—are essential for elite and recreational athletes to increase their performance in and enjoyment of sport.

## LO 3 Committing to Physical Fitness

- Commit to your new lifestyle of physical activity and increased fitness levels by incorporating fitness activities into your life. If you are new to exercise, start slowly, keep your fitness program simple, and consider consulting your physician and/or a fitness instructor for recommendations. Overcome your barriers or obstacles to exercise by identifying them and then planning specific strategies to address them. Choose activities that are fun and convenient to increase your likelihood of sticking with them.

## LO 4 | Creating Your Own Fitness Program

- The FITT principle can be used to develop a progressive program of physical fitness. For general health benefits, every adult should participate in moderate-intensity activities for 30 minutes at least 5 days a week. To improve cardiorespiratory fitness, you should engage in vigorous, continuous, and rhythmic activities 3 to 5 days per week at an exercise intensity of 64 to 96 percent of your maximum heart rate for 20 to 30 minutes.

- Three key principles for developing muscular strength and endurance are overload, specificity of training, and reversibility. Muscular strength is improved by engaging in resistance training exercises two to three times per week, using an intensity of greater than 60 percent of 1 RM, and completing two to four sets of 8 to 12 repetitions. Muscular endurance is improved by engaging in resistance training exercises two to three times per week, using an intensity of less than 50 percent of 1 RM, and completing one to two sets of 15 to 25 repetitions.

- Flexibility is improved by engaging in two to four repetitions of static stretching exercises at least 2 to 3 days a week, where each stretch is held for 10 to 30 seconds.

## LO 5 | Implementing Your Fitness Program

- Planning to improve your physical fitness involves setting goals and designing a program to achieve these goals. A comprehensive workout should include a warm-up with some light stretching, strength-development exercises, aerobic activities, and a cool-down period with a heavier emphasis on stretching exercises. Core strength training is important for mobility, stability, and preventing back injury. The popular exercise forms of yoga, tai chi, and Pilates all develop core strength as well as flexibility, strength, and endurance.

## LO 6 | Taking in Proper Nutrition for Exercise

- Fueling properly for exercise involves eating a balance of healthy foods 3 to 4 hours before exercise. In exercise sessions lasting an hour or more, performance can benefit from some additional calories ingested during the exercise session. Hydrating properly for exercise is important for performance and injury prevention. Chocolate milk is a source of carbohydrates and protein for postexercise recovery.

## LO 7 | Preventing and Treating Common Fitness-Related Injuries

- Physical activity–related injuries are generally caused by overuse or trauma. The most common overuse injuries are plantar fasciitis, shin splints, and runner's knee. Proper footwear and protective equipment help to prevent injuries. Exercising in the heat or cold requires taking special precautions. Minor exercise injuries should be treated with RICE (rest, ice, compression, and elevation).

## POP QUIZ

Visit **MasteringHealth** to personalize your study plan with Chapter Review Quizzes and Dynamic Study Modules.

### LO 1 | Physical Activity for Health

1. What is physical fitness?
   a. The ability to respond to routine physical demands
   b. Having enough physical reserves to cope with a sudden challenge
   c. A balance of cardiorespiratory, muscle, and flexibility fitness
   d. All of the above

2. Which of the following is *not* a health benefit associated with regular exercise?
   a. Reduced risk for some cancers
   b. Reduced risk for cardiovascular diseases
   c. Elimination of chronic diseases
   d. Improved mental health

### LO 2 | Physical Activity for Fitness and Performance

3. The maximum volume of oxygen consumed by the muscles during exercise defines
   a. target heart rate.
   b. muscular strength.
   c. aerobic capacity.
   d. muscular endurance.

4. Flexibility is the range of motion around
   a. specific bones.
   b. a joint or series of joints.
   c. the tendons.
   d. the muscles.

### LO 3 | Committing to Physical Fitness

5. Miguel is thinking about becoming more active. Which of the following is *not* a good piece of advice to offer him?
   a. Incorporate physical activity into your daily life.
   b. Make multiple changes to diet and exercise routines simultaneously.
   c. Identify the habits and environmental elements that keep him from being active.
   d. Set SMART goals.

### LO 4 | Creating Your Own Fitness Program

6. Janice has been lifting 95 pounds while doing three sets of six leg curls. To become stronger, she began lifting 105 pounds while doing leg curls. What principle of strength development does this represent?
   a. Reversibility
   b. Overload
   c. Flexibility
   d. Specificity of training

7. The "talk test" measures
   a. exercise intensity.
   b. exercise time.
   c. exercise frequency.
   d. exercise type.

## LO 5 | Implementing Your Fitness Program

8. At the start of an exercise session, you should always
   a. stretch before doing any activity.
   b. do 50 crunches to activate your core muscles.
   c. warm up with light cardiorespiratory activities.
   d. eat a meal to ensure that you are fueled for the activity.

## LO 6 | Taking in Proper Nutrition for Exercise

9. Chocolate milk is good for
   a. preworkout energy boost.
   b. postworkout recovery.
   c. slimming down.
   d. staying hydrated during exercise.

## LO 7 | Preventing and Treating Common Fitness-Related Injuries

10. Overuse injuries can be prevented by
    a. monitoring the quantity and quality of your workouts.
    b. engaging in only one type of aerobic training.
    c. working out daily.
    d. working out with a friend.

*Answers to the Pop Quiz can be found on page A-1. If you answered a question incorrectly, review the section identified by the Learning Outcome. For even more study tools, visit* **MasteringHealth**.

# THINK ABOUT IT!

## LO 1 | Physical Activity for Health

1. How do you define *physical fitness*? Identify at least four physiological and psychological benefits of physical activity. How would you promote these benefits to nonexercisers?

## LO 2 | Physical Activity for Fitness and Performance

2. How are muscle strength and muscle endurance different? What are some ways you might work to increase muscle strength and muscle endurance?

## LO 3 | Committing to Physical Fitness

3. What do you do to motivate yourself to engage in physical activity on a regular basis? What and who helps you to be physically active?

## LO 4 | Creating Your Own Fitness Program

4. Describe the FITT prescription for cardiorespiratory fitness, muscular strength and endurance, and flexibility training.

## LO 5 | Implementing Your Fitness Program

5. Why is core strength important? What are some ways to increase your core strength every day?

## LO 6 | Taking in Proper Nutrition for Exercise

6. Why is when you eat as important as what you eat? How might your exercise preparation and routine differ in hot and cold climates?

## LO 7 | Preventing and Treating Common Fitness-Related Injuries

7. What precautions do you need to take when exercising outdoors in the heat and in the cold?

# ACCESS YOUR HEALTH ON THE INTERNET

Visit **MasteringHealth** for links to the websites and RSS feeds.

The following websites explore further topics and issues related to personal fitness.

**American College of Sports Medicine.** This site is the link to the American College of Sports Medicine and all its resources. **www.acsm.org**

**American Council on Exercise.** Information is found here on exercise and disease prevention. **www.acefitness.org**

**Centers for Disease Control and Prevention, National Center for Chronic Disease Prevention and Health Promotion, Division of Nutrition, Physical Activity, and Obesity.** This site is a great resource for current information on exercise and health. **www.cdc.gov/nccdphp/dnpao**

**National Strength and Conditioning Association.** This site is a resource for personal trainers and others interested in conditioning and fitness. **www.nsca.com**

# 8 Connecting and Communicating in the Modern World

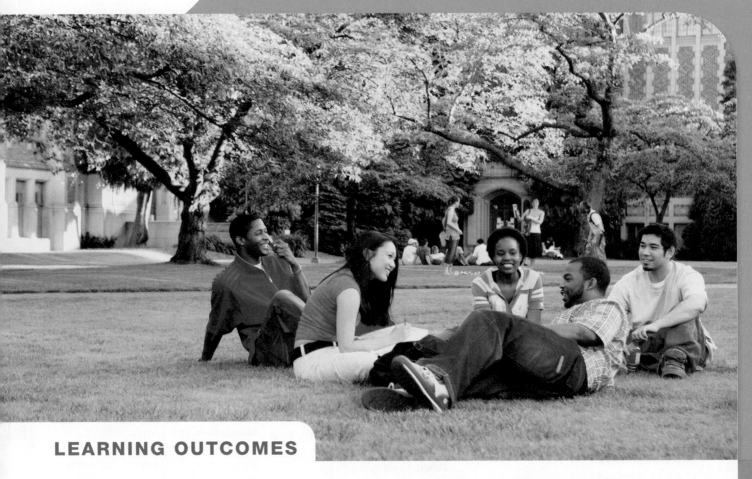

## LEARNING OUTCOMES

LO **1** Describe the types of social support available and the impact of social networks on health status.

LO **2** Discuss the purpose and common forms of intimate relationships.

LO **3** Discuss ways to improve communication skills and interpersonal interactions, particularly in the digital environment.

LO **4** Identify the characteristics of successful relationships, including how to overcome common conflicts, and discuss how to cope when relationships end.

LO **5** Compare and contrast the types of committed relationships and lifestyle choices.

Humans are social beings—we have a basic need to belong and to feel loved, accepted, and wanted. We can't thrive without relating to and interacting with others. Strong connections to others reduce depression, build our immune systems, improve sleep, and strengthen our resolve.[2] In fact, people with positive, fulfilling relationships with spouses, family members, friends, and coworkers are 30 percent more likely to survive over time than people with poor relationships.[3] However, having a healthy social life is not a given, even for people who regularly interact with many others. Contrary to what many people think, loneliness does not result from being physically alone; it is caused by feeling disconnected from others.[4] In this chapter, we examine the vital role relationships play in our lives and the communication skills necessary to create and maintain them.

**HEAR IT! PODCASTS**

Want a study podcast for this chapter? Download the podcast **Healthy Relationships and Sexuality: Making Commitments**, available on **MasteringHealth.**™

## LO 1 | THE **VALUE** OF RELATIONSHIPS

Describe the types of social support available and the impact of social networks on health status.

Historically, research examining the benefits of intimate relationships has focused on marriage; however, recent studies report that all types of close relationships are good for our health.[5] The benefits range from a decreased likelihood of catching a cold, to a faster recovery from stressful tasks, to a longer lifespan. On the flip side, those with poor social connections—lonely people—have decreased immune function, higher blood pressure, and higher rates of depression, pain, and fatigue.[6] Having weak ties to a community or a small number of friends can be as harmful to your overall health as alcohol abuse or smoking roughly a pack of cigarettes per day.[7] One recent study analyzing data from more than 14,000 people over decades revealed that the effects of social isolation are long lasting, raising future risk for increased blood pressure, body mass index, waist circumference, and inflammation (a risk factor for heart disease and cancer).[8]

Why do relationships make us healthier? First, they impact our choices. For example, we eat healthier when our friends eat healthy foods.[9] Second, friends often provide us with **social support**—the type of help we receive from our contact with others. Social support is delivered in four forms: emotional, instrumental, informational, and belonging.[10] For a college student who breaks her leg playing basketball, social support might be:

- **Emotional support.** Displays of caring, love, trust, and empathy; for example, when close friends and family members provide a listening ear about frustrations and pain.
- **Instrumental support.** Concrete help and service; for example, a roommate carrying her backpack to class as she learns to use her crutches and keeping the apartment tidy so she doesn't trip.
- **Informational support.** Advice, suggestions, and information, for example, when an aunt shows her some tricks to better navigate on crutches.
- **Belonging support.** Sharing activities or a sense of belonging, for example, when her teammates still encourage her to come to practice while she recovers.

Another theory suggests that having friends can change your perspective of how challenging a task is. In one clever study, a group of students were taken to the foot of a steep hill and fitted with a heavy backpack. They were then told to estimate how steep the hill was. Students standing with friends estimated the hill to be less steep than students who stood alone. The hill appeared even less steep the longer the friends had known each other. Evidence suggests that with support, challenges look easier to us—thus reducing our stress.[11]

> **social support** Help we receive from people in our social network in the form of emotional, instrumental, informational, and appraisal support.

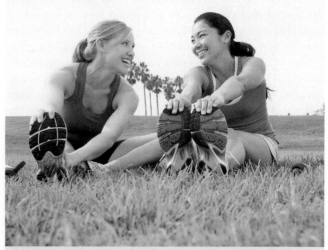

Healthy relationships can come in all shapes and sizes, but they do have some characteristics in common, including communication, caring, respect, and support.

**social network** People you know who can provide social support when needed.

**social capital** Collective value of all the people in your social network and the likelihood of those people providing social support when you need it.

**relational connectedness** Mutually rewarding face-to-face contacts.

**collective connectedness** Feeling that you are part of a community or group.

**intimate connectedness** A relationship that makes you feel who you are is affirmed.

**intimate relationships** Relationships with family members, friends, and romantic partners, characterized by behavioral interdependence, need fulfillment, emotional attachment, and emotional availability.

That the length of the friendship impacted the students' estimate of the difficulty of the climb comes as no surprise. Research shows that it is the quality of our friendships, not the quantity, that matters when it come to health. There's a lot of wisdom in that quip often attributed to Al Capone, "I'd rather have 4 quarters than 100 pennies." He was right; a few close friends are worth far more to our health than 100 acquaintances—or a thousand Facebook friends. The good news is that the average number of confidants reported by Americans is on the rise, averaging a little over two per person; sadly, 9 percent of Americans report they have no one they can turn to for discussing important matters.[12]

Besides our closest relationships, we all have a constellation of neighbors, relatives, classmates, coworkers, and friends of friends that make up our **social network**. The collective value of all the people in your social network—and the likelihood of those people providing social support when you need it—determines your **social capital**. The more social capital we have, the happier and healthier we are.[13]

To build social capital, we can both strengthen our existing ties and widen our existing network. John Cacioppo, a leading researcher on loneliness, describes these actions as building relational connectedness and collective connectedness.[14]

**Relational connectedness** comes from mutually rewarding face-to-face contact. We deepen our relational connectedness each time we interact positively with people in our social network, strengthening our ties and increasing the likelihood of someone coming to our aid when asked.

**Collective connectedness**, on the other hand, comes from the feeling that you are part of a group beyond yourself. It manifests itself in feelings like trust and having a sense of community, as well as in actions like voting and volunteering. The groups you belong to deepen your collective connectedness and can expand your social network. People find collective connectedness in many ways: cheering for the same sports team, volunteering together, or worshipping at the same temple. The important thing is feeling that you are a part of something, even when you might not have intimate ties to the group.

Collective connectedness appears to be on the rise. Seventy-four percent of Americans now belong to a sports league, worship community, charitable organization, or another type of local group. Additionally, 12 percent more Americans report knowing their neighbors by name than just a few years ago. Some believe this increase is due to economic changes, encouraging Americans to turn to neighbors and community groups for social support during harder times.[15] No matter the reason, feeling connected to your community is connected to improved health.

## LO 2 | INTIMATE RELATIONS: WHEN CONNECTING GETS PERSONAL

Discuss the purpose and common forms of intimate relationships.

We all need people in our lives who affirm who we are and provide **intimate connectedness**.[16] These **intimate relationships** often include four characteristics: *behavioral interdependence, need fulfillment, emotional attachment,* and *emotional availability.* Each of these characteristics may be related to interactions with family, close friends, and romantic partners.

*Behavioral interdependence* refers to the mutual impact that people have on each other as their lives intertwine. What one person does influences what the other person wants to do and can do. Behavioral interdependence usually becomes stronger over time, to the point that each person would feel a great void if the other were gone.

Intimate relationships are also a means of *need fulfillment.* Through relationships with others, we fulfill our needs for:

- **Intimacy**—someone with whom we can share our feelings freely.
- **Social integration**—someone with whom we can share worries and concerns.
- **Nurturance**—someone we can take care of and who will take care of us.
- **Assistance**—someone to help us in times of need.
- **Affirmation**—someone who will reassure us of our own worth.

In mutually rewarding intimate relationships, partners and friends meet each other's needs. They disclose feelings, share

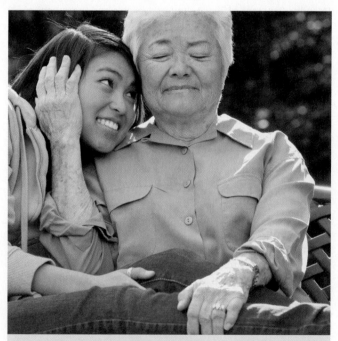

The emotional bonds that characterize intimate relationships often span the generations and help individuals gain insight into and understanding of each other's worlds.

confidences, and provide support and reassurance. Each person comes away feeling better for the interaction and validated by the other person.

In addition to behavioral interdependence and need fulfillment, intimate relationships involve strong bonds of *emotional attachment*, or feelings of love. When we hear the word *intimate*, we often think of a sexual relationship. Although sex can play an important role in emotional attachment to a romantic partner, relationships can be intimate without being sexual; for example, two people can be emotionally intimate (share feelings) or spiritually intimate (share spiritual beliefs and practices) without being sexually intimate.

*Emotional availability*, the ability to give emotionally to and receive emotionally from others without fear of being hurt or rejected, is the fourth characteristic of intimate relationships. At times, it is healthy to limit our emotional availability. For example, after a painful breakup, we may decide not to jump into another relationship immediately, or we may decide to talk about it only with close friends. Holding back can offer time for introspection, healing, and for considering lessons learned. Some people who have experienced intense trauma find it difficult to ever be fully available emotionally, which can limit their ability to experience intimate relationships.[17]

## Caring for Yourself

You have probably heard the old saying that you must love yourself before you can love someone else. What does this mean, exactly? Learning how you function emotionally and how to nurture yourself through all life's situations is a lifelong task. You should certainly not postpone intimate connections with others until you achieve this state. However, a certain level of individual maturity will help you maintain relationships.

Two personal qualities that are especially important to any good relationship are *accountability* and *self-nurturance*. **Accountability** means that you recognize responsibility for your own choices and actions. You don't hold others responsible for positive or negative experiences. **Self-nurturance** means developing individual potential through a balanced and realistic appreciation of self-worth and ability. To make good choices in life, a person must balance many physical and emotional needs—sleeping, eating, exercising, working, relaxing, and socializing. When the balance is disrupted, self-nurturing people are patient with themselves as they put things back on course. Learning to live in a balanced and healthy way is a lifelong process. Individuals who are on a path of accountability and self-nurturance have a much better chance of achieving this balance and maintaining satisfying relationships with others.

Important factors that affect your ability to nurture yourself and maintain healthy relationships with others include the way you define yourself (*self-concept*) and the way you evaluate yourself (*self-esteem*). Your self-concept is like a mental mirror that reflects how you view your physical features, emotional states, talents, likes and dislikes, values, and roles. A person might define herself as an activist, a mother, an honor student,

an athlete, or a musician. As we discuss in other chapters, how you feel about yourself or evaluate yourself constitutes your self-esteem.

Your perception and acceptance of yourself influences your relationship choices. If you feel unattractive, insecure, or inferior to others, you may choose not to interact with other people or to avoid social events. You may even unconsciously seek out individuals who confirm your negative view of yourself by treating you poorly. Conversely, if you are secure about your unique characteristics and talents, that positive self-concept will make it easier to form relationships with people who support and nurture you and to interact with a variety of people in a healthy, balanced way.

## Family Relationships

A family is a recognizable group of people with roles, tasks, boundaries, and personalities whose central focus is to protect, care for, love, and socialize with one another. Because the family is a dynamic institution that changes as society changes, the definition of *family* changes over time. Historically, most families have been made up of people related by blood, marriage or long-term committed relationships, or adoption. Today, however, many groups of people are recognized and function as family units. Although there is no "best" family type, we do know that a healthy family's key roles and tasks include nurturance and support. Healthy families foster a sense of security and feelings of belonging that are central to growth and development.

During the childhood years, families provide our most significant relationships. It is from our **family of origin**, the people present in our household during our first years of life, that we initially learn about feelings, problem solving, love, intimacy, and gender roles. We learn to negotiate relationships and have opportunities to communicate effectively, develop attitudes and values, and explore spiritual belief systems. It is not uncommon when we establish relationships outside the family to rely on these initial experiences and on skills modeled by our family of origin.

## Friendships

Friendships are often the first relationships we form outside our immediate families. Establishing and maintaining strong friendships may be a good predictor of your success in establishing romantic relationships, as both require shared interests and values, mutual acceptance, trust, understanding, respect, and self-confidence.

Developing meaningful friendships is more than merely "friending" someone on Facebook. Getting to know someone well requires time, effort, and commitment. But the effort is worth it—a good friend can be a trustworthy companion, someone who respects your strengths and

**accountability** Accepting responsibility for personal decisions, choices, and actions.

**self-nurturance** Developing individual potential through a balanced and realistic appreciation of self-worth and ability.

**family of origin** People present in the household during a child's first years of life—usually parents and siblings.

**consummate love** A relationship that combines intimacy, compassion, and commitment.

accepts your weaknesses, someone who can share your joys and your sorrows, and someone you can count on for support.

## Romantic Relationships

At some point, most people choose to enter an intimate romantic and sexual relationship with another person. Beyond the characteristics of friendship, romantic relationships typically include the following characteristics related to passion and caring:

- **Fascination.** Lovers tend to pay attention to the other person even when they should be involved in other activities. They are preoccupied with the other and want to think about, talk to, and be with the other.
- **Exclusivity.** Lovers have a special relationship that usually precludes having the same kind of relationship with a third party. The love relationship often takes priority over all others.
- **Sexual desire.** Lovers desire physical intimacy and want to touch, hold, and engage in sexual activities with the other.
- **Giving the utmost.** Lovers care enough to give the utmost when the other is in need, sometimes to the point of extreme sacrifice.
- **Being a champion or advocate.** Lovers actively champion each other's interests and attempt to ensure that the other succeeds.

**Theories of Love** There is no single definition of *love*, and the word may mean different things to different people, depending on cultural values, age, gender, and situation. Although we may not know how to put our feelings into words, we know it when the "lightning bolt" of love strikes.

Several theories related to how and why love develops have been proposed. In his classic triangular theory of love, psychologist Robert Sternberg proposed the following three key components to loving relationships (**FIGURE 8.1**):[18]

- **Intimacy.** The emotional component, which involves closeness, sharing, and mutual support.
- **Passion.** The motivational component, which includes lust, attraction, and sexual arousal.
- **Commitment.** The cognitive component, which includes the decision to be open to love in the short term and commitment to the relationship in the long term. See the **Student Health Today** box for a discussion of hooking up.

According to Sternberg, the quality of a love relationship is related to the level of intimacy, passion, and commitment each person brings to the relationship over time. He suggests that relationships including two or more of those components are more likely to endure than those that include only one. He uses the term **consummate love** to describe a combination of intimacy, passion, and commitment—an ideal and deep form of love that is, unfortunately, all too rare.[19]

Quite different from Sternberg's approach are theories of love and attraction based on brain circuitry and chemistry. Anthropologist Helen Fisher, among others, hypothesizes that attraction and falling in love follow a fairly predictable pattern based on (1) *imprinting*, in which our evolutionary patterns, genetic predispositions, and past experiences trigger a romantic reaction; (2) *attraction*, in which neurochemicals produce feelings of euphoria and elation; (3) *attachment*, in which endorphins (natural opiates) cause lovers to feel peaceful, secure, and calm; and (4) *production of a cuddle chemical*; that is, the brain secretes the hormone oxytocin, which stimulates sensations during lovemaking and elicits feelings of satisfaction and attachment.[20]

According to Fisher's theory, lovers who claim to be swept away by passion may not be far from the truth. A love-smitten

**WHAT DO YOU THINK?**

What factors do you consider most important in a potential partner?

- Are any absolute musts?
- Does what you believe to be important in a relationship differ from what your parents might feel is important?

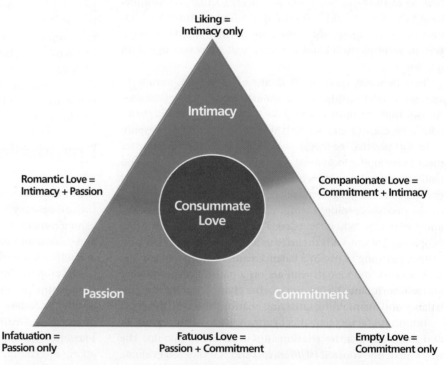

**FIGURE 8.1 Sternberg's Triangular Theory of Love** According to Sternberg's model, three elements—intimacy, passion, and commitment—existing alone or in combination, form different types of love. The most complete, ideal type of love in the model is consummate love, which combines balanced amounts of all three elements.

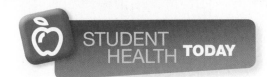
# HOOKING UP
## *The New Norm or Nothing New?*

"Hooking up" is a vague term often used to describe sexual encounters, from kissing to intercourse, without the expectation of commitment. While the media often report about the new "hookup culture" on campus, research tells a different story. Longitudinal data tells us that young adults' sexual behavior hasn't changed much in the past few decades. College students are not having more sex or a greater number of partners than their counterparts 20 or 30 years ago. Today's college students are, however, more likely to describe their sex partner as a "friend" than in the past, but today's college students are still twice as likely to have sex with a romantic partner than with a hookup.

While hookup behavior may not be as pervasive as some think, college students should understand the risks involved:

1. **Recognize the role of emotions in sex.** Sternberg's Triangle of Love would place hooking up in the "infatuation" category, passion with no commitment or intimacy, far from Sternberg's picture of "ideal." Additionally, according to Fisher, attraction and sex create a chemical reaction in the brain that fosters an emotional response, even if we say, "It's just about the sex."

2. **Recognize the role of alcohol in hooking up.** In a recent study of college hookups, students reported that they were more likely to hook up if they had been drinking alcohol. Among participants who consumed alcohol prior to their last hookup, 31 percent of females and 28 percent of males indicated that they would likely not have hooked up with their partners had alcohol not been involved.

3. **Recognize the risk of unintended pregnancy and STIs.** In one study, only 70 percent of students reported condom use during their last hookup. Reduced inhibitions due to alcohol plus a lack of communication with a new partner increase the risk of unprotected sex and thus the risk for unintended pregnancy and STIs.

**Sources:** M. A. Monto and A. G. Carey, "A New Standard of Sexual Behavior?: Are Claims Associated with the 'Hookup Culture' Supported by General Social Survey Data?," *Journal of Sex Research* 56, no. 6 (2014): 605–15; R. L. Fielder, J. L.??? Walsh, K. B. Carey, and M. P. Carey, "Sexual Hookups and Adverse Health Outcomes: A Longitudinal Study of First-Year College Women," *Journal of Sex Research* 51, no. 2 (2014): 131–44; J. M. Bearak, "Casual Contraception in Casual Sex: Life-Cycle Change in Undergraduates' Sexual Behavior in Hookups," *Social Forces* 93, no. 2 (2014): 483–513.

---

person's endocrine system secretes chemical substances such as dopamine and norepinephrine.[21] Attraction may in fact be a "natural high"; however, this passion "buzz" lessens over time as the body builds up a tolerance. Fisher speculates that some people become attraction junkies, seeking out the intoxication of new love much as a drug user seeks a chemical high.

**Choosing a Romantic Partner** *Attraction theory* suggests that more than just chemical and psychological processes influence who a person falls in love with. This theory suggests proximity, similarities, reciprocity, and physical attraction also play strong roles.[22] *Proximity* is being in the same place at the same time. When you are out and about in the community, it is more likely that an interaction will occur than if you stay at home. And if you meet a person while at work, at the dog park, or at a religious event, it is likely that you may share interests. While physical proximity is important, with the growth of Internet dating sites, it has become easier to meet people outside your geographic proximity.

You also choose a partner based on *similarities* (in attitudes, values, intellect, interests, education, and socioeconomic status); the old adage that "opposites attract" usually isn't true, at least not in the long run. If your potential partner expresses interest, you may react with mutual regard—*reciprocity*. The more you express interest, the safer it is for someone else to reciprocate, continuing the cycle and strengthening the connection.

A final factor that plays a significant role in selecting a partner is *physical attraction*. Attraction is a complex notion, influenced by social, biological, and cultural factors.[23] People seem to seek out "similarly attractive" partners, meaning more attractive people seek out more attractive partners and vice versa; however, as relationships evolve, status and personality become more important and the importance of personal appearance diminishes.[24]

## LO 3 | BUILDING COMMUNICATION SKILLS

Discuss ways to improve communication skills and interpersonal interactions, particularly in the digital environment.

From the moment of birth, we struggle to be understood. We flail our arms, cry, scream, smile, frown, and make sounds and gestures to attract attention or to communicate our wants or needs. By adulthood, each of us has developed a unique way of communicating through gestures, words, expressions, and body language. No two people communicate exactly the same way or have the same need for connecting with others, yet we all need to connect.

Different cultures have different ways of expressing feelings and using body language. Members of some cultures gesture broadly; others maintain a closed body posture. Some are offended by direct eye contact; others welcome a steady gaze. Men and women also tend to have different styles of communication, largely dictated by culture and socialization (see the **Health in a Diverse World** box on page 224).

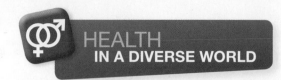

# HE SAYS/SHE SAYS

There are some gender-specific communication patterns and behaviors that are obvious to the casual observer (see graphic). However, according to Dr. Cynthia Burggraf Torppa at Ohio State University, the bigger difference is the way in which men and women interpret or process the same message.

She indicates that women are more sensitive to interpersonal meanings "between the lines," and men are more sensitive to subtle messages about status or social hierarchy. Recognizing these differences and how they make us unique is a good first step in avoiding unnecessary frustrations and miscommunications.

**Sources:** C. Burggraf Torppa, Family and Consumer Sciences, Ohio State University Extension, "Gender Issues: Communication Differences in Interpersonal Relationships," 2010, http://ohioline.osu.edu/flm02/pdf/fs04.pdf; J. Wood, *Gendered Lives: Communication, Gender, and Culture*, 11th ed. (Boston, MA: Wadsworth Publishing, 2014).

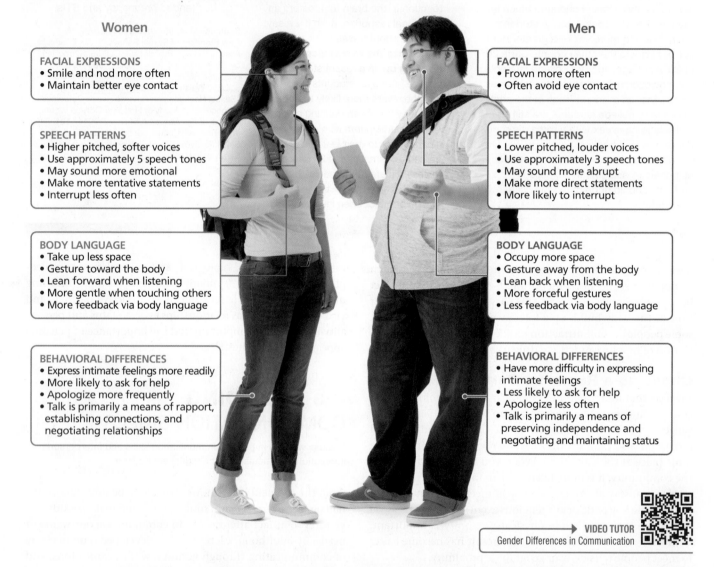

### Women

**FACIAL EXPRESSIONS**
• Smile and nod more often
• Maintain better eye contact

**SPEECH PATTERNS**
• Higher pitched, softer voices
• Use approximately 5 speech tones
• May sound more emotional
• Make more tentative statements
• Interrupt less often

**BODY LANGUAGE**
• Take up less space
• Gesture toward the body
• Lean forward when listening
• More gentle when touching others
• More feedback via body language

**BEHAVIORAL DIFFERENCES**
• Express intimate feelings more readily
• More likely to ask for help
• Apologize more frequently
• Talk is primarily a means of rapport, establishing connections, and negotiating relationships

### Men

**FACIAL EXPRESSIONS**
• Frown more often
• Often avoid eye contact

**SPEECH PATTERNS**
• Lower pitched, louder voices
• Use approximately 3 speech tones
• May sound more abrupt
• Make more direct statements
• More likely to interrupt

**BODY LANGUAGE**
• Occupy more space
• Gesture away from the body
• Lean back when listening
• More forceful gestures
• Less feedback via body language

**BEHAVIORAL DIFFERENCES**
• Have more difficulty in expressing intimate feelings
• Less likely to ask for help
• Apologize less often
• Talk is primarily a means of preserving independence and negotiating and maintaining status

**VIDEO TUTOR**
Gender Differences in Communication

Although people differ in the ways they communicate, this doesn't mean that one gender, culture, or group is better at communication than another. We have to be willing to accept differences and work to keep lines of communication open and fluid. Remaining interested, actively engaging, and being open and willing to exchange ideas and thoughts are all things we can typically learn with practice. By understanding how to deliver and interpret information, we can enhance our relationships.

## Learning Appropriate Self-Disclosure

Sharing personal information with others is called **self-disclosure**. If you are willing to share personal information with others, they will likely share personal information with you. Likewise, if you want to learn

**self-disclosure** Sharing feelings or personal information with others.

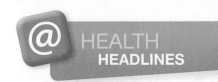

## LIFE IS AN OPEN (FACE)BOOK

Headlines like "Lamar Odom Found Unconscious at Brothel" and "Kylie Jenner Shocked To See Tyga's Nude Photos" confirm that celebrities have no expectation of privacy in a world where nearly everyone has a camera phone and an Internet connection. But headlines such as "Gay Students Accidentally Outed to Parents via Facebook" remind us that we cannot expect complete privacy either. We are just one photo tag away from a family member or potential employer seeing us in less than flattering circumstances or knowing information we'd prefer kept quiet.

"Social media screening," the practice of searching out all possible information on a prospective employee, is done by about a third of employers. Increasingly, job applicants are being asked to share their Facebook pages to see if they are a good fit for a job! Mostly they want to see if job candidates present themselves professionally, are a good fit for company

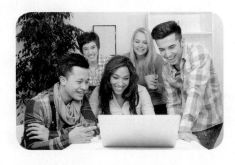

culture, have good communication skills, or are lying about their qualifications. Employers also report looking for inappropriate photos or evidence of drug or alcohol abuse.

If you are concerned about your privacy, make sure your publicly available information is what you want prospective employers, family, and other people to see. Tighten your privacy settings and untag yourself in photos you don't want people to see. Due to cached sites and reposts, you can't erase everything, so you may need to prepare an explanation

for past posts, photos, and other information. As our "private" lives get more public all the time, we may have to accept that what we do in private always has the potential to become public knowledge.

**Sources:** Z. Seemayer and P. Ng, "Lamar Odom Found Unconscious in Nevada Brothel, Transported to Las Vegas Hospital," *Enerntainment Tonight Online*, February 27, 2015, www.etonline.com/news/173939_lamar_odom_reportedly_found_unconscious_nevada_brothel/; S. Shankar, " Kylie Jenner-Tyga Update: Kylie 'Shocked' To See Tyga's Nude Photos, Demands To Know Who He Sent It To," *International Business Times*, July 8, 2015, www.ibtimes.com/kylie-jenner-tyga-update-kylie-shocked-see-tygas-nude-photos-demands-know-who-he-sent-1999206; HuffPost Live, "Blogger Bobbie Duncan Recalls Getting Outed Accidentally On Facebook," *Huffington Post*, January 08, 2014, www.huffingtonpost.com/2014/01/08/outed-on-facebook_n_4563522.html; J. Smith, How Social Media Can Help (or Hurt) You in Your Job Search," *Forbes*, January 10, 2013, www.forbes.com/sites/jacquelynsmith/2013/01/10/how-to-use-social-media-to-make-sales-2/.

more about someone, you have to be willing to share some of your personal background and interests with that person. Self-disclosure is not only storytelling or sharing secrets; it is also sharing emotions about what you are currently experiencing in life and providing any information about the past that is relevant to the other person's understanding of your current reactions.

Self-disclosure can be a double-edged sword because there is risk in divulging personal insights and feelings. If you sense that sharing feelings and personal thoughts will result in a closer relationship, you will likely take such a risk. But if you believe that the disclosure may result in rejection or alienation, you may not open up so easily. If the confidentiality of previously shared information has been violated, you may hesitate to be as open in the future. However, the risk in not disclosing yourself to others is a lack of intimacy in relationships.[25]

If self-disclosure is a key element in creating healthy communication, but fear is a barrier to that process, what can be done? The following suggestions can help:

- **Get to know yourself.** Remember that your *self* includes your feelings, beliefs, thoughts, and concerns. The more you know about yourself, the more likely you will be able to share yourself with others.
- **Become more accepting of yourself.** No one is perfect or has to be.
- **Choose a safe context for self-disclosure.** When and where you make such disclosures and to whom may greatly

influence the response you receive. Choose a setting where you feel safe to let yourself be heard.

- **Be willing to talk about sex.** The U.S. culture puts many taboos on discussions of sex, so it's no wonder we find it hard to disclose our sexual past to those with whom we are sexually intimate. However, the threats of unintended pregnancy and sexually transmitted infections make it important for partners to discuss sexual history.
- **Be thoughtful about self-disclosure via social media.** Self-disclosure can be an effective method of building intimacy with another person, but not with large groups. Sharing too much information or information that is too personal on Facebook or Twitter may cause you to feel vulnerable or embarrassed later. See the Health Headlines box for more about social media and privacy.

## Becoming a Better Listener

Listening is a vital part of interpersonal communication. Good listening skills enhance our relationships, improve our grasp of information, and allow us to more effectively interpret what others say. We listen best when (1) we believe that the message is somehow important and relevant to us; (2) the speaker holds our attention through humor, dramatic effect, or other techniques; and (3) we are in the mood to listen (free of distractions

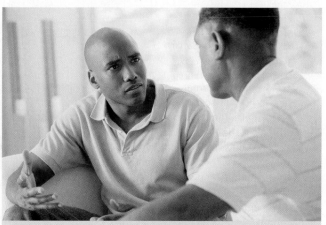

One way to communicate better is to pay attention to your body language. Much of our message is conveyed by nonverbal cues.

and worries). See the Making Changes Today box for suggestions on improving your listening skills.

## The Three Basic Listening Modes
There are three main ways in which we listen:

- *Competitive listening* happens when we are more interested in explaining our own point of view than in understanding someone else's.[26]
- *Passive listening* occurs when we are listening but not providing either verbal or nonverbal feedback to the speaker. The speaker may feel unsure if the message is being received.[27]
- *Active listening* is when we not only hear the words, but also are trying to understand what is really being said. The listener confirms understanding by restating or paraphrasing the speaker's message before responding. By actively listening, we show genuine interest in what the other person is thinking and feeling.[28]

## Using Nonverbal Communication

Understanding what someone is saying usually involves more than listening and speaking. Often, what is not said may speak louder than any words could. Rolling the eyes, looking at the floor or ceiling rather than maintaining eye contact, body movements, and hand gestures—all these nonverbal clues influence the way we interpret messages.

**nonverbal communication**
Unwritten and unspoken messages, both intentional and unintentional.

Nonverbal communication includes all unwritten and unspoken messages, both intentional and unintentional, including touch, gestures, interpersonal space, body language, tone of voice, and facial expressions.[29] Ideally, our nonverbal communication matches and supports our verbal communication, but this is not always the case. Research shows that when verbal and nonverbal communication doesn't match, we are more likely to believe the nonverbal cues.[30] This is one reason it is important to be aware of the nonverbal cues we use regularly and to understand how others might interpret them.

While facial expressions like smiling are believed to have near universal meaning, other facial expressions and most body language is culturally specific.[31] A gesture of agreement or approval in one culture can be offensive in another. To communicate as effectively as possible, it is important to recognize and use appropriate nonverbal cues that support and help clarify your verbal messages. Awareness and practice of your verbal and nonverbal communication will help you better understand others.

## Connecting Digitally: Too Much of a Good Thing?

You may have noticed a few pages ago that, in the definition of *relational connectedness*, Dr. Cacioppo specifically describes the contact as "face-to-face." Does Facetime count? Is oxytocin—the hormone that make us feel happy when we interact with friends in person—released when we receive a Snap? Or when we comment on a friend's Facebook post?

While preliminary research shows some similarities, we don't really know yet. We do know that digital communication is different from face-to-face communication in many ways. Digital communication often lacks the nonverbal cues that make face-to-face communication so rich. With no accompanying tone of voice, eye roll, or smile, interpreting text-based communication can be challenging.

On the flip side, digital communication allows us to have a more diverse social network and easily keep in touch over long distances.[32] According to some reports, Americans spend more time on *social networking sites (SNSs)* that any other online activity.[33] These connections seem to strengthen our social

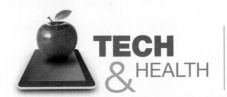
# LOVE IN THE TIME OF TWITTER

Technology has revolutionized our access to information and the ways we communicate. Couples can meet on Tinder, keep in constant contact via texting, and inform the world of their relationship highs and lows via Facebook and Twitter. With all these tools available, it can be easy to share TMI (too much information). Kim Stolz, author of *Unfriending My Ex: Confessions of a Social Media Addict*, suggests the ways we interact with each other have fundamentally changed because of social media. At its best, social media can bring people closer together; at its worst, it can be used intentionally or unintentionally to embarrass or hurt. Consider the following suggestions to safeguard yourself:

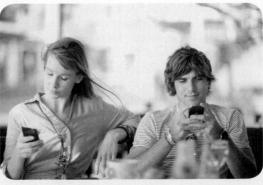

### When meeting:

- If you join a dating site, be honest about yourself; state your own interests and characteristics fairly, including things that you think might be less attractive than stereotypes and cultural norms dictate.
- If you meet someone online and want to meet in person, put safety first! Plan something brief, preferably during daylight hours. Meet in a public place, like a coffee shop. Do not meet with anyone who wants to keep the time and location a secret. Tell a friend or family member the details of when and where you are meeting and any information you have on the person you are meeting.

### While dating:

- Discuss limits with your partner on the type of information you each want shared online. Agree to share only within those limits.
- Recognize that constant electronic updates throughout the day can leave little to share when you are together. Save some information for face-to-face talks!
- Sober up before you click "Submit." Things that seem funny under the influence may not seem funny the next morning.
- Remember that the Internet is forever. Once a picture or a post is sent, it can never be completely erased.

Never post anything that would embarrass someone if it was seen by a family member or potential employer.

- Respect your partner's privacy. Logging onto his or her e-mail or Facebook account to look at private messages is a breach of trust.
- Know that the GPS in a phone can be used to track your location, and cell phone spyware can be installed that allows e-mail and texts to be read from another device. If you think you may be a victim of "cyberstalking" by a current or former partner, get a new phone or ask the phone company to reinstall the phone's operating system to wipe out the software.

### If breaking up:

- Do not break up with someone via text/e-mail/tweet/Facebook/chat. People deserve the respect of a more personal breakup.
- Upon breaking up, be sure to change any passwords you may have confided in your partner. The temptation to use those for ill may be too strong to resist.

**Sources:** K. Stolz, *Unfriending My Ex: Confessions of a Social Media Addict* (New York: Scribner, 2015).

networks, as frequent Facebook users report 9 percent more close core ties than other Internet users.[34] Frequent Facebook users also report higher levels of perceived social support, specifically in emotional and instrumental support.[35] The boost is significant too—it is about half the total support you would expect from being married.[36] See the **Tech & Health** box for more on social media and relationships.

While some worry that SNS users are becoming more socially isolated and have weaker social ties, according to Pew Research, SNS users actually have larger social networks, both online and in real life.[37] The more frequently someone uses SNSs, the larger that person's network tends to be and the more close ties he or she has. So, in some ways, Facebook can "support intimacy, rather than undermine it."[38]

However, while SNSs can be a source of connection and social support, they also have a downside. Studies show that when people spend more time on Facebook, they report higher levels of depression.[39] Researchers first thought the depression was related to envy of the activities and lifestyles of their friends, but newer research shows that "social comparison" (paying attention to how one does things compared with how others do things) is what mediates the depressive symptoms—no matter if the comparison is upward, downward, or neutral,

# 27%

of 18- to 24-year-olds have used **ONLINE DATING**—triple the rates of just 2 years ago.

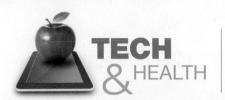

## TECH & HEALTH | SOCIAL MEDIA MEANNESS

t's not your imagination; people are more rude online than in person.

- Three in five people report someone is rude to them on social media more than once a month.
- Three in four people report that there is more rudeness in the virtual world than in the real world.

Why does technology seem to bring out the worst in people? Psychologists often call anonymity and invisibility the culprits for this lack of restraint. When people feel anonymous, they are more willing to say things they normally wouldn't. And even when we aren't anonymous, impulse control is reduced because we can respond or vent immediately.

Perhaps another reason is that we can't see the person when commenting. At the University of Haifa in Israel, a group of researchers

tested this hypothesis, asking 71 pairs of unacquainted college students to use Instant Messenger to debate an issue. Pairs chatted under different conditions, some shared personal info, some could see the person's body, and some were asked to look directly into the other person's eyes onscreen. More than any other condition, whether or not participants had to make eye contact with each other predicted how poorly they treated each other. In the absence of eye contact, subjects were 200 percent more likely to be impolite. The lead researcher, Noam Lapidot-Lefler, suggests that "seeing a partner's eyes helps you understand the other person's feelings, the signals that the person is trying to send you"—something that often gets lost in the anonymity of the online environment.

What can you do when people are rude or are trolling you?

- Try not to respond emotionally. Don't type anything you wouldn't say to the person's face.
- When you are angry, press "Pause," not "Send." Take a while to think about your response.
- Watch your words. Reread your response and think about how your words may be interpreted without the benefit of tone of voice or other nonverbal cues.
- End the conversation. If you want to respond without continuing the rudeness, you can thank the person for giving you their thoughts, ask to meet to talk about it in person, or "agree to disagree."

**Sources:** D. Archer, "Rude Technology," *Psychology Today*, September 27, 2014, www.psychologytoday.com/blog/reading-between-the-headlines/201409/rude-technology; M. W. Moyer, "Eye Contact Quells Online Hostility," *Scientific American*, August 2, 2012, www.scientificamerican.com/article/rudeness-on-the-internet/.

or if the user is male or female.[40] Thus, it may be wise to limit the time spent on social media. When using social media, remember, people often show the most flattering image of themselves possible; it is not always an accurate representation of their lives. And regardless, the number of likes or followers you have is not a reflection of your worth as a person.

Another concern about SNS use is the lack of nonverbal communication in text-based digital communication, which can lead to confusion and misunderstanding.[41] Some experts are concerned that, over time, reduced exposure to nonverbal communication may reduce people's ability to read facial expressions—impacting their in-person communication skills.[42] See the **Tech & Health** box for more on the impact of facial expressions on how we communicate.

Today, there are more questions than answers about technology's impact on society in general, and on communication specifically. The bottom line is that real hugs and kisses cannot be replaced by typing XOXO, and the lack of accompanying nonverbal communication with most digital communication can create confusion and conflict due to a lack of clarity. While technology allows us to be more connected than during any other time in history, we must be sure to use digital communication as a complement to other ways of communicating—not a replacement.

**conflict** Emotional state that arises when opinions differ or the behavior of one person interferes with the behavior of another.

**conflict resolution** Concerted effort by all parties to constructively resolve differences or points of contention.

## Managing Conflict through Communication

A **conflict** is an emotional state that arises when the behavior of one person interferes with that of another. Conflict is inevitable whenever people live or work together. Not all conflict is bad; in fact, airing feelings and coming to resolution over differences can sometimes strengthen a relationship. **Conflict resolution** and successful conflict management form a systematic approach to resolving differences fairly and constructively, rather than allowing them to fester. The goal of conflict resolution is to solve differences peacefully and creatively.

Here are some strategies for conflict resolution:

1. **Identify the problem or issue.** Talk with each other to clarify exactly what the conflict is. Try to understand both sides. In this first stage, you must say what you want and listen to what the other person wants. Focus on using "I" messages and avoid "you" messages. Be an active listener: Repeat what the other person has said and ask questions for clarification.
2. **Generate several possible solutions.** Base your search for solutions on the goals and interests identified in the first step. Come up with several different alternatives, and avoid evaluating any of them until you have finished brainstorming.

| In an unhealthy relationship . . . | In a healthy relationship . . . |
|---|---|
| You care for and focus on another person only and neglect yourself or you focus only on yourself and neglect the other person. | You both love and take care of yourselves before and while in a relationship. |
| One of you feels pressure to change to meet the other person's standards and is afraid to disagree or voice ideas. | You respect each other's individuality, embrace your differences, and allow each other to "be yourselves." |
| One of you has to justify what you do, where you go, and whom you see. | You both do things with friends and family and have activities independent of each other. |
| One of you makes all the decisions and controls everything without listening to the other's input. | You discuss things with each other, allow for differences of opinion, and compromise equally. |
| One of you feels unheard and is unable to communicate what you want. | You express and listen to each other's feelings, needs, and desires. |
| You lie to each other and find yourself making excuses for the other person. | You both trust and are honest with yourselves and with each other. |
| You don't have any personal space and have to share everything with the other person. | You respect each other's need for privacy. |
| Your partner keeps his or her sexual history a secret or hides a sexually transmitted infection from you, or you do not disclose your history to your partner. | You share sexual histories and information about sexual health with each other. |
| One of you is scared of asking the other to use protection or has refused the other's requests for safer sex. | You both practice safer sex methods. |
| One of you has forced or coerced the other to have sex. | You both respect sexual boundaries and are able to say no to sex. |
| One of you yells and hits, shoves, or throws things at the other in an argument. | You resolve conflicts in a rational, peaceful, and mutually agreed upon way. |
| You feel stifled, trapped, and stagnant. You are unable to escape the pressures of the relationship. | You both have room for positive growth, and you both learn more about each other as you develop and mature. |

**FIGURE 8.2** Healthy versus Unhealthy Relationships

Source: Advocates for Youth, Washington, DC, 2006, www.advocatesforyouth.org. Copyright © 2000. Used with permission.

3. **Evaluate the alternative solutions.** Narrow solutions to one or two that seem to work for both parties. Be honest with each other about a solution that feels unsatisfactory, but also be open to compromise.
4. **Decide on the best solution.** Choose a solution that is acceptable to both parties. You both need to be committed to the decision for it to be effective.
5. **Implement the solution.** Discuss how the decision will be carried out. Establish who is responsible to do what and when. The solution stands a better chance of working if you agree on how it will be implemented.
6. **Follow up.** Evaluate whether the solution is working. Check in with the other person to see how he or she feels about it. Are you satisfied with the way the solution is working out? If something is not working

as planned, or if circumstances have changed, discuss revising the plan. Remember that both parties must agree to any changes to the plan, as they did with the original idea.

## LO 4 | RELATIONSHIPS: FOR BETTER AND WORSE

Identify the characteristics of successful relationships, including how to overcome common conflicts, and discuss how to cope when relationships end.

Success in intimate relationships is often defined by whether a couple stays together and remains close over time. Perhaps this isn't the best measure though, as we can still benefit from

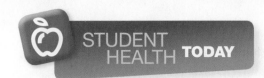
We know technology like dating sites can help couples meet, and texting can help people get to know each other better, but what about after a relationship begins? Does technology help or hurt? Two University of Nevada–Las Vegas researchers attempted to find out by interviewing 410 college students about the good and bad of technology in relationships.

**The Good:** Not surprisingly, text messaging was highly praised for its ability to keep couples in constant contact. People also reported using the Internet to search for information to improve their relationship, on topics from relationship building to sexual positions. Couples appreciated that they could make their relationship public, both by setting a status to "in a relationship," as well as posting pictures that their friends could see.

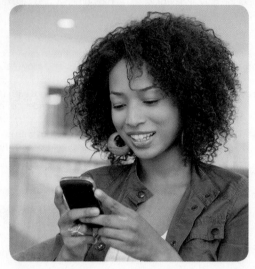

Using technology as a way to manage conflict was also a common theme. People reported it was easier to use text messaging to apologize, to test the waters after a fight, and to argue slowly and more clearly.

**The Bad:** Texting sometimes seemed impersonal and detached, especially sexting. The presence of phones made people feel they did not always have the full attention of their partner. Trust was also an issue. People were concerned with who else their partner might be in contact with—that a phone is "another outlet for infidelity." Finally, the lack of nonverbal cues made it harder to interpret messages, creating opportunities for misunderstanding and for information to be taken out of context.

**Source:** K. Herlein and K. Ancheta, "Advantages and Disadvantages of Technology in Relationships: Findings from an Open-Ended Survey," *Qualitative Report* 19, no. 22 (2014): 1–11, Available at www.nova.edu/ssss/QR/QR19/hertlein22.pdf.

---

relationships that come to an end or lose closeness. Either way, learning to communicate, respecting each other, and sharing a genuine fondness are crucial to relationship success. Many social scientists agree that the happiest committed relationships are ones flexible enough to allow partners to grow throughout their lives.

## Characteristics of Healthy and Unhealthy Relationships

Satisfying and stable relationships are based on good communication, intimacy, friendship, and other factors. A key ingredient is *trust*, the degree to which each partner feels he or she can rely on the integrity of the other. Without trust, intimacy will not develop, and the relationship will likely fail. Trust includes three fundamental elements:

- **Predictability**—the ability to predict your partner's behavior based on past actions.
- **Dependability**—the ability to rely on your partner to emotionally support you in all situations, particularly those in which you feel threatened or hurt.
- **Faith**—belief in your partner having positive intentions and behavior.

What does a healthy relationship look and feel like? Healthy and unhealthy relationships are contrasted in **FIGURE 8.2.** Answering some basic questions can also help you determine if a relationship is working.

- Do you love and care for yourself to the same extent that you did before the relationship? Can you be yourself in the relationship?
- Is there genuine caring and goodwill? Do you share interests, values, and opinions? Is there mutual respect for differences?
- Is there mutual encouragement? Do you support each other unconditionally?
- Do you trust each other? Are you honest with each other? Can you comfortably express your feelings, opinions, and needs?
- Is there room in your relationship for growth as you both evolve and mature?

Relationships are nurtured by consistent communication, actions, and self-reflection. Poor communication can weaken bonds and create mistrust. We all need to reflect periodically on how we typically relate to others through our words and actions. Have we been honest, direct, and fair in our conversations? Have we listened to others' thoughts, wants, and needs? Have we behaved in ways consistent with our words, values, and beliefs?

**WHAT DO YOU THINK?**

What has been your experience with rudeness in digital communication?

- Have you ever ended a friendship because of rude online behavior?
- What kind of actions would lead you to "unfriend" someone on Facebook?
- What are some examples of bad behavior you have seen online?

Breakdowns in relationships often begin with a change in communication, however subtle. Either partner may stop listening and cease to be emotionally present for the other. In turn, the other feels ignored, unappreciated, or unwanted. Unresolved conflicts increase, and unresolved anger can cause problems in sexual relations, which can further increase communication difficulties. New communication technologies add a whole new dimension (see the **Student Health Today** box for more on the pros and cons).

College students, particularly those who are socially isolated and far from family and hometown friends, may be particularly vulnerable to staying in unhealthy relationships. They may become emotionally dependent on a partner. Mutual obligations, such as shared rental, financial, or transportation arrangements, and sometimes childcare, can complicate a decision to end an unhealthy relationship. It's also easy to mistake sexual advances for physical attraction or love. Without a strong social network to validate feelings or share concerns, a student can feel stuck in an unhealthy relationship.

Honesty and verbal affection are usually positive aspects of a relationship. In a troubled relationship, however, they can be used to cover up irresponsible or hurtful behavior. Saying "at least I was honest" is not an acceptable substitute for acting in a trustworthy way, and claiming "but I really do love you" is not a license for being inconsiderate or hurtful.

## Confronting Couples Issues

Couples seeking a long-term relationship must confront a number of issues that can either enhance or diminish their chances of success. These issues can involve jealousy, sharing power and responsibility, and communication about unmet expectations.

**Jealousy** **Jealousy** is a negative reaction evoked by a real or imagined relationship involving one's partner and another person. Contrary to what many people believe, jealousy is not a sign of intense devotion. Instead, jealousy often indicates underlying problems, such as insecurity or possessiveness—significant barriers to a healthy relationship. Often, jealousy is rooted in past experiences of deception or loss. Other causes of jealousy typically include:

- **Overdependence on the relationship.** People who have few social ties and rely exclusively on their partners tend to be overly fearful of losing them.
- **Severity of the threat.** People may feel uneasy if someone with good looks or a great personality appears to be interested in their partner.
- **High value on sexual exclusivity.** People who believe that sexual exclusivity is

a crucial indicator of love are more likely to become jealous.

- **Low self-esteem.** People who think poorly of themselves are more likely to fear that someone else will gain their partner's affection.
- **Fear of losing control.** Some people need to feel in control of every situation. Feeling that they may be losing control over a partner can cause jealousy.

In both men and women, jealousy is also related to believing it would be difficult to find another relationship if the current one ends. Although a certain amount of jealousy can be expected in any loving relationship, it doesn't have to threaten the relationship as long as partners communicate openly about it.[43]

**Sharing Power and Responsibility** **Power** can be defined as the ability to make and implement decisions. Historically, men have been the primary wage earners and, consequently, had decision-making power. Women exerted much influence, but ultimately, they needed a man's income for survival. As increasing numbers of women have entered the workforce and generated their own financial resources, the power dynamics between women and men have shifted considerably. The increase in the divorce rate in the past century was partly due to working women gaining the ability to support themselves rather than stay in difficult or abusive relationships solely for financial reasons.

While gender roles and tasks were more rigid in the past, modern society has very few gender-specific roles. Both women and men work, care for children, drive, run businesses, manage family finances, and perform equally well in the tasks of daily living. Rather than taking on traditional female and male roles, many couples find it makes more sense to divide tasks on the basis of schedule, convenience, and preference. However, while many women work as many hours outside the home as men, the division of labor at home is rarely equal. The Bureau of Labor Statistics estimates that on a typical day, 49 percent of women do household chores like laundry, where the same is true of only 20 percent of men; over two-thirds of women prepare food or clean up afterward, while less than half

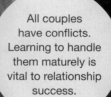

All couples have conflicts. Learning to handle them maturely is vital to relationship success.

**jealousy** Aversive reaction evoked by a real or imagined relationship involving a person's partner and a third person.

**power** Ability to make and implement decisions.

> **WHAT DO YOU THINK?**
>
> **Have you ever felt jealousy in a relationship?**
>
> - Can you identify what actions or events caused you to feel this way?
> - Did you have actual facts to support your feelings, or was your response based on suspicions?

of men share those tasks.[44] Over time, if couples can't communicate how they feel about sharing power and responsibility and arrive at an equitable solution, the relationship is likely to suffer.

**Unmet Expectations** We all have expectations of ourselves and our partners—how we will spend our time and our money, how we will express love and intimacy, and how we will grow together as a couple. Expectations are an extension of our values, beliefs, hopes, and dreams for the future. When communicated and agreed upon, these expectations help relationships thrive. If we are unable to communicate our expectations, we set ourselves up for disappointment and hurt. Partners in healthy relationships can communicate wants and needs and have honest discussions when things aren't going as expected.

## When and Why Relationships End

Relationships end for many reasons, including illness, financial concerns, career problems, and personality conflicts. Many people enter a relationship with certain expectations about how they and their partner will behave. Failure to communicate these beliefs can lead to resentment or disappointment. Differences in sexual needs may also contribute to the demise of a relationship. Under stress, communication and cooperation between partners can break down. Conflict, negative interactions, and a general lack of respect between partners can erode even the most loving relationship.

What behaviors signal trouble? Based on 35 years of research and couples therapy, therapist John Gottman has identified four behavior patterns in couples that predict future divorce with 85 percent or better accuracy:[45]

- **Criticism.** Phrasing complaints in terms of a partner's defect; for example, "You never talk about anyone but yourself. You are self-centered."
- **Defensiveness.** Righteous indignation as a form of self-protection; for example, "It's not my fault we missed the flight; you always make us late."
- **Stonewalling.** Withdrawing emotionally from a given interaction; for example, the listener seems to ignore the speaker as he or she speaks, giving no indication that the speaker was heard.
- **Contempt.** Talking down to a person; for example, "How could you be so stupid?"

Of these, contempt is the biggest predictor of divorce. While these behaviors do not guarantee that an individual couple will divorce, they are "red flags" for relationships at high risk for failure.

## Coping with Failed Relationships

No relationship comes with a guarantee. Losing love is as much a part of life as falling in love. That being said, uncoupling can be very painful. Whenever we risk getting close to another person, we also risk getting hurt if things don't work out. Consider the following tips for coping with a failed relationship:[46]

- **Acknowledge that you've gone through a rough spot.** You may feel grief, loneliness, rejection, anger, guilt, relief, sadness, or all of these. Seek out trusted friends and, if needed, professional help.
- **Let go of negative thought patterns and habits.** Engage in activities that make you happy. Take a walk, read, listen to music, go to the movies or a concert, spend time with fun friends, volunteer with a community organization, or write in a journal. Seek out joy!
- **Make a promise to yourself: no new relationships until you have moved past the last one.** You need time to resolve your experience rather than escape from it. It can be difficult to be trusting and intimate in a new relationship if you are still working on getting over a past relationship. Heal first, before looking for love again.

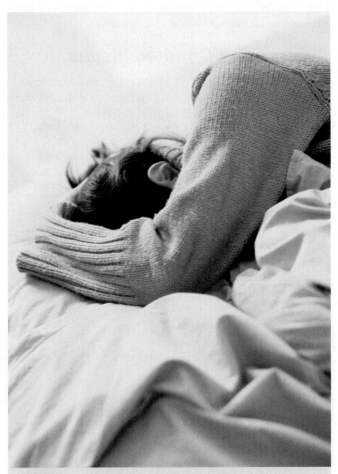

It may feel as if there is no end to the sorrow, anger, and guilt that often accompany a difficult breakup, but time is a miraculous healer. Acknowledging your feelings and finding healthful ways to express them will help you deal with the end of a romantic relationship.

## LO 5 | MARRIAGE, PARTNERING, AND SINGLEHOOD

Compare and contrast the types of committed relationships and lifestyle choices.

Commitment in a relationship means that one intends to act over time in a way that perpetuates the well-being of the other person, oneself, and the relationship. Polls show that the majority of Americans strive to develop a committed relationship whether in the form of marriage, cohabitation, or partnerships, but an increasing number of Americans choose to remain single.[47]

## Marriage

In many societies, traditional committed relationships take the form of marriage. In the United States, marriage means entering into a legal agreement that includes shared finances, property, and often the responsibility for raising children. Many Americans also view marriage as a religious sacrament that emphasizes certain rights and obligations for each spouse. Marriage is socially sanctioned and highly celebrated in American culture, so there are numerous incentives for couples to formalize their relationship in this way.

Historically, close to 90 percent of Americans married at least once during their lifetime, and at any given time, about 50 percent of U.S. adults are married (FIGURE 8.3).[48] However, in recent years Americans have become less likely to marry. Since 1960, the annual number of marriages has steadily declined.[49] This decrease may be due to a delay of first marriages, as well as a substitution of cohabitation for marriage. In 1960, the median age for first marriage was 23 years for men and 20 years for women; today, the median age for first marriage has risen to 29 years for men and 27 years for women.[50]

Divorce rates in the United States have been high for multiple decades. Some estimates indicate that approximately 50 percent of first marriages end in divorce, with even higher divorce rates for second and third marriages.[51] Other studies, however, suggest the divorce rate is only 30 percent and that it has been declining since the early 1980s.[52] This decrease is related to an increase in the number of couples who cohabit instead of marry, an increase in the age at which persons first marry, and a higher level of education among those who are marrying.[53] The risk of divorce is lower for college-educated people marrying for the first time; it is lower still for people who wait to marry until their mid-20s and who haven't lived with multiple partners prior to marriage.[54]

Many Americans believe that marriage involves **monogamy**, or exclusive sexual involvement with one partner. However, the lifetime pattern for many Americans appears to be **serial monogamy**, which means a person has a monogamous sexual relationship with one partner before moving on to another monogamous relationship.[55] A small number of couples choose an **open relationship** (or open marriage), in which partners agree that there may be sexual involvement outside their relationship.

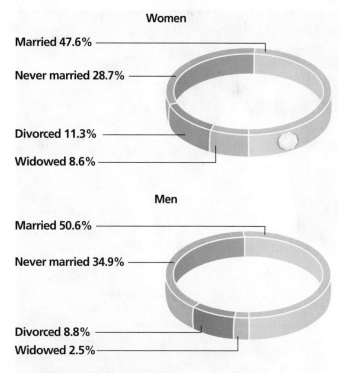

**Women**

Married 47.6%

Never married 28.7%

Divorced 11.3%

Widowed 8.6%

**Men**

Married 50.6%

Never married 34.9%

Divorced 8.8%

Widowed 2.5%

**FIGURE 8.3** Marital Status of the U.S. Population by Sex

Note: The figure does not list the percentages for married men and women with a spouse absent and separated.

**Source:** U.S. Census Bureau, "Table A1, Marital Status of People 15 Years and Over, by Age, Sex, Personal Earnings, Race, and Hispanic Origin: 2014," America's Families and Living Arrangements, 2014, www.census.gov.

A healthy marriage provides emotional support by combining the benefits of friendship with a loving committed relationship. It also provides stability for both the couple and for those involved in their lives. Considerable research indicates that married people live longer, feel happier, remain mentally alert longer, and suffer fewer physical and mental health problems.[56] A new study by the National Bureau of Economic Research confirms the long-lasting benefits of marriage, indicating that friendship is the critical element of these benefits.[57]

Couples in healthy marriages have less stress, which in turn contributes to better overall health. A healthy marriage contributes to lower stress levels in three important ways: less risky personal behaviors, expanded support networks, and financial stability. Risky personal behaviors, including smoking and heavy alcohol use, are lower in married adults. They are about half as likely to be smokers as are cohabitating, divorced, separated, or widowed adults.[58] They are also less likely to be heavy drinkers, more likely to get sufficient sleep, and more likely to utilize preventive health care compared to divorced adults.[59] While it may be that marriage causes the improved behaviors, it may also be that people who engage in healthier behaviors are just more likely to get married.

**monogamy** Exclusive sexual involvement with one partner.

**serial monogamy** Series of monogamous sexual relationships.

**open relationship** A relationship in which partners agree that sexual involvement can occur outside the relationship.

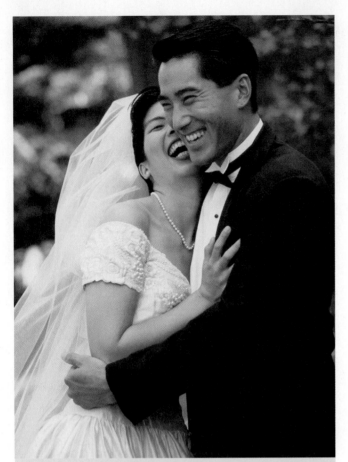

For many, weddings or commitment ceremonies serve as the ultimate symbol of a long-term, exclusive relationship between two people.

**73%**
of Americans list "similar ideas about having and raising children" as the **MOST IMPORTANT TRAIT** when choosing a partner, followed by "a steady job" (63%).

Cohabitation can offer many of the same benefits as marriage: love, sex, companionship, and the opportunity to know a partner better over time. In addition to emotional and physical benefits, some people may live together for practical reasons, such as the opportunity to share bills and housing costs. Over the past 20 years, there has been a large increase in the number of persons who have cohabited. In fact, the majority of young couples now live together before marriage; it is more and more common for cohabitation to be the first coresidential partnership for young adults.[62] On average, the first cohabitation before marriage for people over age 20 lasts about 18 months, with about 40 percent of couples transitioning into marriage within 3 years.[63]

Cohabitation before marriage has been a controversial issue for decades. While some voiced moral objections, other concerns were related to higher divorce rates among couples who cohabited before marriage. However, according to recent research based on more than 7,000 respondents to the National Survey of Family Growth, cohabitation before marriage is no longer a predictor for divorce.[64]

While cohabitation can serve as a prelude to marriage for some people, for others, it is a permanent alternative to marriage. The most likely to cohabit include those of lower socioeconomic status, those who are less religious, people who have been divorced, and those who have experienced parental divorce or high levels of parental conflict during childhood.[65] Although cohabitation has advantages, it also has drawbacks. Perhaps the greatest disadvantage is the lack of societal validation for the relationship, especially if the couple subsequently has children. Many cohabitants must deal with pressure to marry from parents and friends, difficulties in obtaining insurance and tax benefits, and legal issues over property.

## Gay and Lesbian Marriage and Partnerships

The 2014 American Community Survey identified an estimated 783,100 same-sex couples in the United States, 25 percent of whom are legally married.[66] Whether they are gay or straight, male or female, most adults want intimate, committed relationships. Lesbians and gay men seek the same things in primary relationships that heterosexual partners do: love, friendship, communication, validation, companionship, and a sense of stability.

**cohabitation** Intimate partners living together without being married.

**common-law marriage** Cohabitation lasting a designated period of time (usually 7 years) that is considered legally binding in some states.

One negative health indicator for married men is body weight. Married men are far more likely than never-married men to be overweight. Married women, however, are less likely than divorced women to be overweight or obese.[60] Marriage additionally provides the possibility for integration into an existing social network of family and friends to provide assistance and help couples cope when stressors inevitably arise. Finally, marriage is strongly related to economic well-being, which can impact both health status and stress levels.

## Cohabitation

**Cohabitation** is a relationship in which two unmarried people with an intimate connection live together in the same household. For a variety of reasons, more Americans—now more than 6 million couples—are choosing cohabitation.[61] In some states, cohabitation that lasts a designated number of years (usually 7) legally constitutes a **common-law marriage** for purposes of purchasing real estate and sharing other financial obligations.

In addition to facing the same challenges to successful relationships as heterosexual couples, lesbian and gay couples often face discrimination and difficulties dealing with social, religious, and legal issues. For lesbian and gay couples, obtaining the same level of marriage benefits such as tax deductions, power-of-attorney rights, partner health insurance, and child custody rights has been a longstanding challenge. Now, however, with the 5-to-4 Supreme Court ruling in the *Obergefell v. Hodges* case, same-sex marriage is legal in all 50 states.[67]

This was a long-hoped-for decision for many same-sex couples across the country, especially those in the 13 states yet to legalize same-sex marriage. Supreme Court Justice Anthony Kennedy, the deciding vote in the decision, said the Court's decision was based on the acknowledgment of four fundamental principles: that personal choice in marriage is inherent to the concept of individual autonomy, that the right to marry is fundamentally important to committed couples, that it is important for safeguarding the rights of children and families, and that marriage has long been a keystone of social order.[68]

In explaining his opinion, Justice Kennedy stated, "It would misunderstand these men and women to say they disrespect the idea of marriage. Their plea is that they do respect it, respect it so deeply that they seek to find its fulfillment for themselves. Their hope is not to be condemned to live in

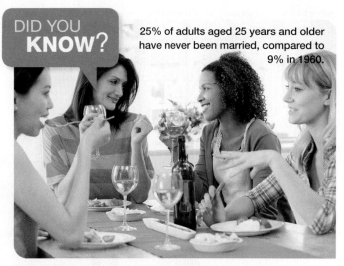

Source: K. Parker, W. Wang, and M. Rohol, "Record Share of Americans Have Never Married," Pew Research, 2014, www.pewsocialtrends.org/files/2014/09/2014-09-24_never-Married-Americans.pdf.

loneliness, excluded from one of civilization's oldest institutions. They ask for equal dignity in the eyes of the law. The Constitution grants them that right."[69]

With this victory, a new era begins for same-sex couples, although challenges remain. Within days of the ruling, the Texas Attorney General said state workers could refuse to grant marriage licenses to same-sex couples if doing so violates their religious beliefs; 3 months after the ruling, a county clerk in Kentucky spent 5 days in jail rather than issue marriage licenses to same-sex couples.[70] These rebuttals indicate that, while same-sex marriage is now the law of the land, homosexual couples still face challenges in being accepted by some.

## Staying Single

Increasing numbers of adults of all ages are choosing to remain single. According to data from the most recent U.S. Census, 57 percent of women aged 20 to 34 had never been married. Likewise, men in this age group postponed marriage in increasing numbers, with 67 percent remaining unmarried.[71] That's more than 5 million people aged 20 to 34 living alone—more than 10 times the number of singles in 1950. This shift toward singlehood is one of the biggest social changes the world has seen in the last half-century.[72]

The single lifestyle allows for rich and productive lives; singles volunteer more, have larger social circles, and go out more than their married peers. Additionally, many singles report enjoying the solitude, self-sufficiency, and the time to pursue what is personally meaningful that singlehood allows.[73]

## Parenthood

Married, single, or cohabiting, homosexual, heterosexual, or bisexual, most adults are parents (74%) or hope to be parents someday (16%).[74] Families in America are changing; about 40 percent of children live in a family structure other than a heterosexual marriage.[75] Single women or lesbian couples

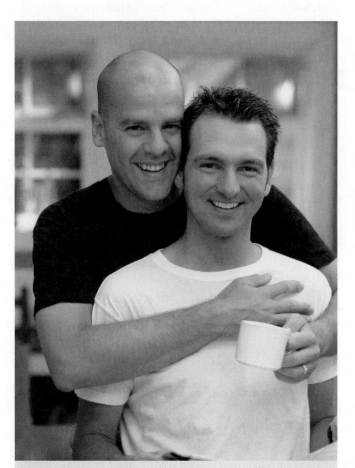

Most adults want to form committed, lasting relationships regardless of their sexual orientation.

can choose adoption or alternative insemination as a way to create a family. Single men or gay couples can choose to adopt or obtain the services of a surrogate mother. Heterosexual couples can choose to cohabit, rather than marry. Regardless of the structure of the family, relationship factors discussed throughout this chapter—social support, nurturance, affirmation, commitment, listening, dependability, communication, and mutual respect—are all important to the well-being of the family unit and are qualities that improve all relationships.

# STUDY **PLAN**

Customize your study plan—and master your health!—in the Study Area of **MasteringHealth.**

## ASSESS YOURSELF

**Do your communication skills need improvement?** Want to find out? Take the **How Well Do You Communicate?** assessment available on MasteringHealth.™

## CHAPTER **REVIEW**

To hear an MP3 Tutor Session, scan here or visit the Study Area in **MasteringHealth.**

### LO 1 | The Value of Relationships

- All types of relationships can bolster our health. Social support, in the form of emotional, instrumental, informational, and appraisal support, helps to reduce our stress and strengthen our resolve.
- In addition to our need for feeling close to family and friends, collective connectedness, the feeling of being part of a group, widens our social network and increases our social capital.

### LO 2 | Intimate Relations: When Connecting Gets Personal

- Characteristics of intimate relationships include behavioral interdependence, need fulfillment, emotional attachment, and emotional availability. Relationships help us fulfill our needs for intimacy, social integration, nurturance, assistance, and affirmation. Family, friends, and romantic partners provide the most common opportunities for intimacy. Each relationship may include healthy and unhealthy characteristics that can affect daily functioning.

### LO 3 | Building Communication Skills

- To improve our communication with others, we need to develop our skills related to self-disclosure, listening effectively, conveying and interpreting nonverbal communication, and managing and resolving conflicts.
- Digital communication allows us to keep in contact like at no other time in history, but there are concerns about its relationship to envy and a lack of nonverbal cues.

### LO 4 | Relationships: For Better and Worse

- There are many strategies for building better relationships. Examining one's own behaviors to determine what to change and how to change is an important ingredient of success. Characteristics of successful relationships include good communication, intimacy, friendship, and trust.
- Factors that can cause problems in romantic relationships include breakdowns in communication, erosion of mutual respect, jealousy, difficulty sharing power and responsibility, and unmet expectations. Before relationships fail, warning signs often appear. By recognizing these signs and taking action to change behaviors, partners may save and enhance their relationship.

### LO 5 | Marriage, Partnering, and Singlehood

- For most people, commitment is an important part of a successful relationship. Types of committed relationships include marriage, partnership, and cohabitation.
- Remaining single is more common than ever before. For some, singlehood is a precursor to a committed relationship; for many, it is a long-term lifestyle choice.

# POP QUIZ

## LO 1 | The Value of Relationships

1. When Neil received a midterm report saying he had a D in his chemistry course, Mariah told him about the tutors available. This is an example of
   a. appraisal support.
   b. emotional support.
   c. informational support.
   d. instrumental support.

2. The power of all the people who could come to your aid with their resources is your
   a. social support.
   b. social potential.
   c. social network.
   d. social capital.

## LO 2 | Intimate Relations: When Connecting Gets Personal

3. Intimate relationships fulfill our psychological need for someone to listen to our worries and concerns. This is known as our need for
   a. dependence.
   b. social integration.
   c. enjoyment.
   d. spontaneity.

4. According to anthropologist Helen Fisher, attraction and falling in love follow a pattern based on
   a. lust, attraction, and attachment.
   b. intimacy, passion, and commitment.
   c. imprinting, attraction, attachment, and the production of a cuddle chemical.
   d. fascination, exclusiveness, sexual desire, giving the utmost, and being a champion.

## LO 3 | Building Communication Skills

5. Sharika sits quietly while listening to her sister, not providing her with any nonverbal feedback as she speaks. This is an example of:
   a. competitive listening.
   b. passive listening.
   c. active listening.
   d. reflective listening.

6. The goal of conflict resolution is to
   a. constructively resolve points of contention.
   b. declare a winner and a loser.
   c. ensure that couples argue as little as possible.
   d. set a time limit on discussion of difficult issues.

## LO 4 | Relationships: For Better and Worse

7. Predictability, dependability, and faith are three fundamental elements of
   a. trust.
   b. friendship.
   c. attraction.
   d. attachment.

8. All of the following are typical causes of jealousy *except*
   a. overdependence on the relationship.
   b. low self-esteem.
   c. a past relationship that involved deception.
   d. belief that relationships can easily be replaced.

## LO 5 | Marriage, Partnering, and Singlehood

9. A relationship in which two unmarried people with an intimate connection share the same household is known as
   a. monogamy.
   b. cohabitation.
   c. common-law household.
   d. civil union.

10. Sofia is 30 years old, and she decides to stay single rather than get married. Which of the following is *true* regarding Sofia's decision?
    a. Sofia should feel pressured to marry by her family and friends.
    b. Sofia is unique as staying single is becoming less common.
    c. Sofia is in the minority of women aged 20 to 34, as most are married.
    d. Sofia can obtain intimacy through relationships with family and friends.

*Answers can be found on page A-1. If you answered a question incorrectly, review the section identified by the Learning Outcome. For even more study tools, visit* **MasteringHealth**.

# THINK ABOUT IT!

## LO 1 | The Value of Relationships

1. What are the four types of social support? What are examples of social support you give and receive in your life?

2. How can people increase the social capital in their lives? How does social capital impact health status?

## LO 2 | Intimate Relations: When Connecting Gets Personal

3. What are the characteristics of intimate relationships? What are behavioral interdependence, need fulfillment, emotional attachment, and emotional availability, and why is each important in relationship development?

4. What problems can form barriers to intimacy? What actions can you take to reduce or remove these barriers?

## LO 3 | Building Communication Skills

5. What is nonverbal communication, and why is it important to develop skills in this area? Give examples of some things you do to communicate without words.

6. Why might Facebook users report more social support in their lives? How can Facebook affect social capital?

## LO 4 | Relationships: For Better and Worse

7. What are common elements of good relationships? What are some warning signs of trouble? What actions can you take to improve your own interpersonal relationships?

8. How can you tell the difference between a love relationship and one that is based primarily on attraction? What characteristics do love relationships share?

9. What are some of the common warning signs that a relationship is going to fail? What are some actions people can take to change behaviors to save or even enhance a troubled relationship?

## LO 5 | Marriage, Partnering, and Singlehood

10. What are the different types of committed relationships? How are they different? What does it take for any kind of committed relationship to succeed?

11. What are some of the benefits of singlehood?

# ACCESS YOUR HEALTH ON THE INTERNET

Visit **MasteringHealth** for links to the websites and RSS feeds.

The following websites explore further topics and issues related to relationships.

**National Center for Health Statistics.** This division of the Centers for Disease Control and Prevention has up-to-date statistics on trends in marriage, divorce, and cohabitation. **www.cdc.gov/nchs**

**The Gottman Institute.** This organization helps couples directly and provides training to therapists. The website includes research information, self-help tips for relationship building, and a relationship quiz. **www.gottman.com**

**The National Gay and Lesbian Task Force.** This organization works toward lesbian, gay, bisexual, and transgender (LGBT) equality and provides research and policy analysis to create social change. **www.thetaskforce.org**

**National Healthy Marriage Resource Center.** A clearinghouse for news and research related to healthy marriages. **www.healthymarriageinfo.org**

**The Hotline.** This site provides information about domestic violence, including how to recognize abuse and how to get help in your local area. Phone support is available 24/7 at 1-800-799-SAFE (7233). **www.thehotline.org**

# 9 Understanding Your Sexuality

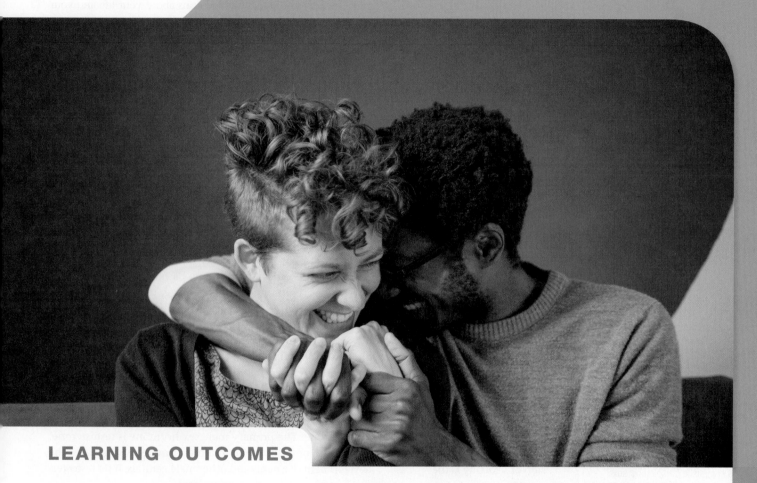

## LEARNING OUTCOMES

**LO 1** Define *sexual identity* and discuss its major components, including biology, gender identity, gender roles, and sexual orientation.

**LO 2** Identify the primary structures of male and female sexual and reproductive anatomy and explain the functions of each.

**LO 3** List and describe the stages of the human sexual response and what factors may influence them.

**LO 4** Discuss the variety of sexual expression and their implications for sexual health and safety.

D o you see yourself as a sexual person? Do you identify as gay, straight, bisexual, pansexual, or something else? Are you comfortable in your own skin? Do you know enough about anatomy and physiology to maximize your sexual pleasure and control your fertility? Human sexuality is complex and involves beliefs, values, attitudes, and knowledge. It includes our anatomy and physiology, biochemistry, sexual response cycle, body image, sexual orientation, and personality.[2] **Sexuality** is so much more than sexual feelings or intercourse. Rather, it includes thoughts and behaviors, experiencing attraction, being in love, and building relationships. A broad view of sexuality includes biological, psychological, cultural, and ethical dimensions that are separate yet influence each other, such as:[3]

- **Biology.** Sexuality is a natural part of our functioning as humans, and although biology is what people often think of when they think about sexuality, it is only one aspect of our sexuality. Biology includes biological sex assignment, physical appearance, growth and development, sexual arousal, and response.
- **Psychology.** Starting at a very young age, attitudes, behaviors, and emotions are modeled for us—all of which can impact our expressiveness and self-concept related to sexuality. This may affect our willingness and comfort to communicate openly about sexuality, as well as our feelings toward our own and others' sexuality.
- **Culture.** The cultural dimension of sexuality is the combination of influences from family, peers, places of worship, school, dating and marriage practices, laws, customs, media and advertising, and technology. The present culture affects us, as well as the cultural norms of the past.
- **Ethics.** Our ideals, values, moral opinions, and religious beliefs impact our behavior, decision making, and how we treat others.

**sexuality** Thoughts, feelings, and behaviors associated with being masculine or feminine, experiencing attraction, being in love, and being in relationships that include sexual intimacy.

**sexual identity** Recognition of oneself as a sexual being; a composite of biological sex characteristics, gender identity, gender roles, and sexual orientation.

**gonads** Reproductive organs that produce germ cells and sex hormones; in males, the testes, and in females, the ovaries.

**intersexuality** Not exhibiting exclusively male or female sex characteristics; also known as disorders of sexual development (DSD).

**puberty** Period of sexual maturation.

**pituitary gland** Endocrine gland that controls the release of hormones from the gonads.

Our sexuality is central to who we are as humans. Having a comprehensive understanding of your sexuality will help you make healthy and satisfying decisions about your life and your interpersonal relationships.

## LO 1 | **YOUR** SEXUAL IDENTITY: MORE THAN BIOLOGY

Define *sexual identity* and discuss its major components, including biology, gender identity, gender roles, and sexual orientation.

**Sexual identity** is a combination of the sex assigned at birth, the gender one identifies as, and who one is attracted to, both physically and emotionally. The beginning of sexual identity occurs at conception with the combining of chromosomes that determine sex. All eggs carry an X chromosome; sperm may carry either an X or a Y chromosome. If a sperm carrying an X chromosome fertilizes an egg, the resulting combination of sex chromosomes (XX) produces a female. If a sperm carrying a Y chromosome fertilizes an egg, the XY combination produces a male.

The genetic instructions included in the sex chromosomes lead to the development of male and female **gonads** (reproductive organs) at about the eighth week of fetal life. Once the male gonads (testes) and the female gonads (ovaries) develop, they play a key role in all future sexual development because the gonads are responsible for the production of sex hormones. The primary female sex hormones are estrogen and progesterone. The primary male sex hormone is testosterone. The release of testosterone in a maturing fetus stimulates the development of a penis and other male genitals. If no testosterone is produced, female genitals form.

On rare occasions, chromosomes are added, lost, or rearranged in this process and the sex of the offspring is not clear. For example, a baby girl may have a large clitoris, but not have a vaginal opening. This condition is known as **intersexuality**. *Disorders of sexual development* (*DSDs*) is a less confusing term that has been recommended to refer to intersex conditions, which occur in an estimated 1 in 4,500 live births (see the **Health in a Diverse World** box).[4]

At the time of **puberty**, sex hormones again play major roles in development. Hormones released by the **pituitary gland**, called *gonadotropins*,

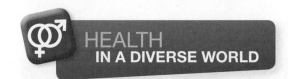
# DISORDERS OF SEXUAL DEVELOPMENT

At the 2016 Summer Olympics in Rio, the South African flag was carried into the Closing Ceremonies by middle-distance runner Caster Semenya, one of the fastest women on Earth. Her gold medal finish was impressive, but most news reports focused on her sex, not her achievements.

Previously, after Semenya won the gold medal in the 800-meter race at the 2009 World Championships, she was required to undergo gender testing and was subsequently barred from competition. Officials at the International Association of Athletics Federations (IAAF) wanted to determine whether Semenya has a disorder of sexual development (DSD) resulting in testosterone levels that give her an unfair athletic advantage over other female competitors. In July 2010, the IAAF announced that Semenya was again eligible to compete. The decision of the IAAF council was the culmination of an 18-month-long review by an expert working group that has studied issues relating to the participation of female athletes with hyperandrogenism, a condition involving overproduction of male sex hormones. The ruling by the IAAF stated a female with hyperandrogenism who is recognized as a female by law will be eligible to compete in women's competition in athletics, provided that she has androgen levels below the male range (measured by reference to testosterone

**Many people considered it an invasion of privacy when runner Caster Semenya was required to submit to gender testing before being allowed to return to competition.**

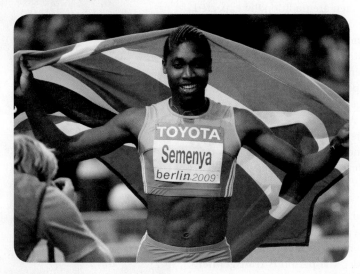

levels in serum) or, if she has androgen levels within the male range, she also has an androgen resistance such that she derives no competitive advantage from such levels. This ruling has since been suspended, pending further research. In the meantime, however, multiple athletes have turned to surgery or drug treatment to reduce androgen levels in order to remain eligible for competition.

Semenya's case highlights the challenges facing people with DSDs. People with DSDs are born with various levels of male and female biological characteristics, ranging from different chromosomal arrangements to altered hormone production to variation in primary and secondary sex characteristics. While most people are born with either XX or XY chromosomes,

some are born with XXY or XO chromosomes (where O signifies a missing or damaged chromosome). In some people, gonads do not develop fully into ovaries or testicles, although there may be no external signs to indicate this, and in others, external genitalia may be ambiguous.

Many, but not all, DSDs require some degree of medical intervention, whether hormonal or surgical, to ensure a person's physical health. It is also necessary to "assign" a gender to all children as early as possible to ensure their psychological health. If this assignment is later found to be inconsistent with the child's own sense of gender, he or she may choose to adopt a different gender identity. Most people born with DSDs today are allowed to grow up, establish their own gender identity, and choose as adults whether to have additional surgeries to alter any sexual tissues they feel are incongruent with their gender. To find out more about DSDs, visit the website of Accord Alliance at www.accordalliance.org.

**Sources:** Peter Lee et al., "Consensus Statement on Management of Intersex Disorders," *Pediatrics* 118 (2006): e488–e500; "IAFF Approves New Rules on Hyperandrogenism," *The Guardian,* April 12, 2011, www.guardian.co.uk/sport/2011/apr/12/iaaf-athletics-rules-hyperandrogenism-caster-semenya; J. Ellison, "Caster Semenya and the IOC's Olympics Gender Bender," *The Daily Beast*, July 26, 2012, www.thedailybeast.com/articles/2012/07/26/caster-semenya-and-the-ioc-s-olympics-gender-bender.html.

stimulate the testes and ovaries to make appropriate sex hormones. Increased estrogen production in females and testosterone production in males lead to the development of **secondary sex characteristics**. Male secondary sex characteristics include deepening of the voice, development of facial and body hair, and growth of the skeleton and musculature. Female characteristics include growth of the breasts, widening of the hips, and the development of pubic and underarm hair.[5]

In addition to a person's biological status as a male or female (or assigned status in the case of a DSD), another important component of sexual identity is gender. **Gender** refers to the interaction between one's biological sex and one's internal sense and external presentation of characteristics and actions typically associated with men (masculine) or women (feminine) as defined by the culture in which one lives. **Gender roles**, then, are socially constructed behavioral norms we use to express masculinity or femininity in ways that conform to society's expectations. Our sense of masculine and feminine

**secondary sex characteristics** Characteristics associated with sex but not directly related to reproduction, such as vocal pitch, amount of body hair, breasts, and location of fat deposits.

**gender** Characteristics and actions associated with being feminine or masculine as defined by the society or culture in which one lives.

**gender roles** Expression of maleness or femaleness in everyday life that conforms to society's expectations.

traits is largely a result of **socialization** during our childhood. For example, your parents may have influenced your perception of gender roles by the toys they gave you (trucks vs. dolls) or chores they assigned you (cooking vs. yard work).[6]

For some, gender roles can be confining when they lead to stereotypes. Boundaries established by **gender-role stereotypes** can make it difficult to express one's true sexual identity. In the United States, men are traditionally expected to be independent, aggressive, logical, and always in control of their emotions, while women are traditionally expected to be passive, nurturing, intuitive, sensitive, and emotional.[7] **Androgyny** refers to the combination of traditional masculine and feminine traits in a single person. Androgynous people do not always follow traditional gender roles, but instead choose behaviors based on a given situation.

Whereas gender roles are an expression of cultural expectations for behavior, **gender identity** is a person's perception of their being male/masculine or female/feminine, including choice of gender pronouns (i.e., *he*, *she*, or *they*).[8]

When the sex assigned at birth (male or female) does not match a person's gender identity-based on cultural expectations of gender, the person is **transgender**. When a person's gender identity matches the sex assigned at birth, this is called **cisgender**.[9]

There is a broad spectrum of *gender expression* among transgender persons. Some transgender persons work to align their outward appearance with their internal gender identity via haircuts or clothing. Some use a different name to be recognized as the gender with which they identify. Others opt to use permanent therapeutic interventions, such as sex reassignment surgery and hormones to physically become another sex. It is important to note that a person's gender identity does not determine to whom they are attracted sexually or emotionally.[10] For more, see the **Health in a Diverse World** box.

## Sexual Orientation

**Sexual orientation** refers to a person's enduring emotional, romantic, or sexual attraction to others. You may be primarily attracted to members of the opposite sex (**heterosexual**), the same sex (**homosexual**),

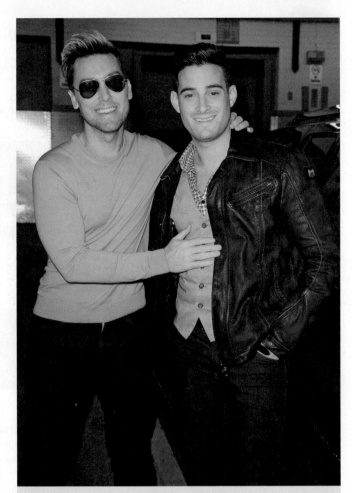

The presence of gay and lesbian celebrities in the media—such as singer Lance Bass and Michael Turchin—contributes to the increasing acceptance of gay relationships in everyday life. The couple made history as the first gay couple to marry on network television on the special, *Lance Loves Michael: The Lance Bass Wedding.*

both sexes (**bisexual**), or neither (**asexual**). Many homosexuals prefer the terms **gay** and **lesbian** to describe their sexual orientation. *Gay* and *queer* can apply to both men and women, but *lesbian* refers specifically to women.[11] Most researchers today agree that sexual orientation is best understood using a model that incorporates biological, psychological, and socioenvironmental factors. Biological explanations focus on research into genetics, hormones, and differences in brain anatomy. Psychological and socioenvironmental explanations examine parent–child interactions, sex roles, and early sexual and interpersonal interactions. Collectively, this growing body of research suggests that the origins of sexual orientation are complex.[12] To diminish the complexity of sexual orientation to a "choice" is a clear misrepresentation of current research. Homosexuals do not "choose" their sexual orientation any more than heterosexuals do.

To better understand sexual orientation as a continuum rather than discreet categories, psychiatrist Fritz Klein developed the Sexual Orientation Grid. This scale takes into account not only who you are attracted to and actually have

**socialization** Process by which a society communicates behavioral expectations to its members.

**gender-role stereotypes** Generalizations concerning how men and women should express themselves and the characteristics each possess.

**androgyny** Combination of traditional masculine and feminine traits in a single person.

**gender identity** Personal sense or awareness of being masculine or feminine, a male or a female.

**transgender** Having a gender identity that does not match one's assigned biological sex.

**cisgender** Having a gender identity that matches the biological sex an individual is assigned at birth.

**sexual orientation** A person's enduring emotional, romantic, or sexual attraction to other persons.

**heterosexual** Experiencing primary attraction to and preference for sexual activity with people of the opposite sex.

**homosexual** Experiencing primary attraction to and preference for sexual activity with people of the same sex.

**bisexual** Experiencing attraction to and preference for sexual activity with people of both sexes.

**asexual** A person who does not experience sexual attraction.

**gay** Sexual orientation involving primary attraction to people of the same sex.

**lesbian** Sexual orientation involving attraction of women to other women.

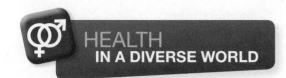
# LIVING BETWEEN GENDERS

For most people, the checkbox on forms asking "male or female" is easy to complete. For people who are transgender, this is just one of many challenges: which box to check on forms, which bathroom or locker room to use, or which college dormitory to sign up for.

Recent policy progress, some forced on institutions by law and some adopted by choice, are efforts to make these choices easier, such as the following:

■ A federal directive telling public schools to allow transgender students to use the bathroom that matches their gender identity or risk facing lawsuits or loss of federal funding.

■ A California law requiring public schools to allow transgender K–12 students access to the restroom and locker room of their choice and the choice to play boys' or girls' sports based on their self-perception of gender regardless of birth gender.

■ Facebook now provides more than 50 gender identity options rather than just male or female, including transgender male, transgender female, gender questioning, and two spirit.

■ More than 200 colleges and universities have gender-inclusive housing in which students can have a roommate of any gender.

Where do you stand?

■ How do you feel about these accommodations for transgender persons? What do you think motivates your feelings?

■ How do you think it feels to be a person who doesn't neatly fit in the male/female categories?

■ What are the risks in public restrooms with/without such policies?

■ How can society protect the dignity of transgender persons while also protecting the privacy of people who may feel uncomfortable with these policy changes?

**Sources:** J. Hirschfield and M. Apuzzo, "U.S. Directs Public Schools to Allow Transgender Access to Restrooms," *New York Times*, May 12, 2016, http://www.nytimes.com/2016/05/13/us/politics/obama-administration-to-issue-decree-on-transgender-access-to-school-restrooms.html?_r=0; ABC10 Staff, "California's Gender-Neutral Restroom Rules," *ABC News*, February 17, 2016, http://www.abc10.com/news/local/california/californias-gender-neutral-restroom-rules/45541071; ReadWrite Editors, "Facebook Provides 56 New Gender Identity Options," February 13, 2014, http://readwrite.com/2014/02/13/facebook-provides-50-new-gender-identity-options#awesm=~oCGUpaYfdpSNmP; Campus Pride, "Campus Pride Trans Policy Clearinghouse," 2016, www.campuspride.org/tpc.

---

sex with, but also factors such as which individuals you feel close to emotionally, who you enjoy socializing with, and in which "community" you feel most comfortable. It then places you on a continuum from exclusively opposite-sex attraction to exclusively same-sex attraction. This questionnaire is available as the **Assess Yourself** activity "What Are Your Sexual Attitudes?" in **MasteringHealth**. Completing the questionnaire may help you understand that there are not just two static sexual orientations, but a whole range of complex, interacting, and fluid factors that influence sexuality over time.

While support of gay rights and marriage equality continues to increase each year in the United States, gay and bisexual people are still often targets of **sexual prejudice**.[13] Sexual prejudice involves negative attitudes and hostile actions directed at people based on their sexual orientation. Hate crimes, discrimination, and hostility toward sexual minorities are evidence of ongoing sexual prejudice.[14] Recent data from the Department of Justice indicates that prejudice related to sexual orientation is the motivation for 19 percent of all hate crimes in the United States.[15]

> **sexual prejudice** Negative attitudes and hostile actions directed at those with a different sexual orientation.
>
> **vulva** External female genitalia.

## LO 2 | SEXUAL AND REPRODUCTIVE ANATOMY AND PHYSIOLOGY

Identify the primary structures of male and female sexual and reproductive anatomy and explain the functions of each.

Understanding the functions of sexual and reproductive anatomy and physiology can help you derive pleasure and satisfaction from sexual relationships, be sensitive to a partner's wants and needs, and make responsible choices regarding your own sexual health.

### Female Sexual and Reproductive Anatomy and Physiology

The female reproductive system includes two major groups of structures, the external genitals and the internal organs (**FIGURE 9.1** on page 244). The external female genitals are collectively known as the **vulva** and include all structures that are outwardly visible: the mons pubis, the labia minora and majora,

# 1%

of college students report currently questioning what their **SEXUAL ORIENTATION** is.

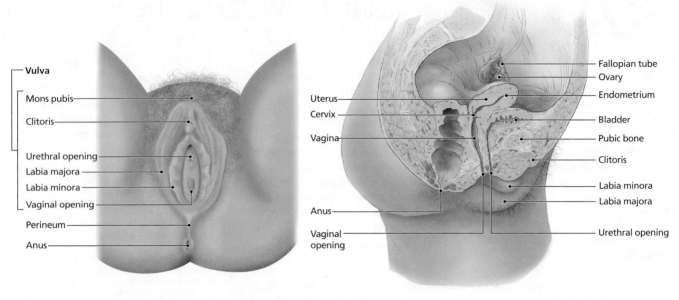

**External Anatomy**

**Internal Organs**

FIGURE 9.1 Female Sexual and Reproductive Anatomy

---

**mons pubis** Fatty tissue covering the pubic bone in females; in physically mature women, the mons is covered with coarse hair.

**labia majora** "Outer lips," or folds of tissue covering the female sexual organs.

**labia minora** "Inner lips," or folds of tissue just inside the labia majora.

**clitoris** Pea-sized nodule of tissue located at the top of the labia minora; central to sexual arousal and pleasure in women.

**urethral opening** Opening through which urine is expelled.

**hymen** In some women, a thin tissue covering the vaginal opening.

**perineum** Tissue that forms the "floor" of the pelvic region, found between the vulva and the anus.

**vagina** Muscular, tube-shaped organ in females that serves as a passageway connecting the vulva to the uterus.

**uterus (womb)** Hollow, pear-shaped muscular organ whose function is to house a developing fetus.

**endometrium** Soft, spongy matter that makes up the uterine lining.

**cervix** Lower end of the uterus that opens into the vagina.

**ovaries** Almond-sized organs that house developing eggs and produce hormones.

**fallopian tubes** Tubes that extend from near the ovaries to the uterus; site of fertilization and passageway for fertilized eggs.

the clitoris, the urethral and vaginal openings, and the vestibule of the vagina and its glands. The **mons pubis** is a pad of fatty tissue covering and protecting the pubic bone; after the onset of puberty, it becomes covered with coarse hair. The **labia majora** are folds of skin and erectile tissue that enclose the urethral and vaginal openings; the **labia minora**, or inner lips, are folds of mucous membrane found just inside the labia majora.

The **clitoris** is located at the upper end of the labia minora and beneath the mons pubis, and its only known function is to provide sexual pleasure. Directly below the clitoris is the **urethral opening** through which urine is expelled from the body. Below the urethral opening is the vaginal opening. In some women, the vaginal opening is covered by a thin membrane called the **hymen**. It is a myth that an intact hymen is proof of virginity, as the hymen is not present in all women and is sometimes stretched or torn by physical activity.

The **perineum** is the area of smooth tissue found between the vulva and the anus. Although not technically part of the external genitalia, the tissue in this area has many nerve endings and is sensitive to touch; it can play a part in sexual excitement.

The internal female genitals include the vagina, uterus, fallopian tubes, and ovaries. The **vagina** is a muscular, tube-shaped organ that serves as a passageway from the uterus to the outside of the body. This passage allows menstrual flow to exit from the uterus during a woman's monthly cycle, receives the penis during intercourse, and serves as the birth canal during childbirth. The **uterus (womb)** is a hollow, muscular, pear-shaped organ. Hormones acting on the inner lining of the uterus (the **endometrium**) either prepare the uterus for implantation and development of a fertilized egg or signal that no fertilization has taken place, in which case the endometrium deteriorates and becomes menstrual flow.

The lower end of the uterus, the **cervix**, extends downward into the vagina. The **ovaries**, almond-sized organs suspended on either side of the uterus, have two main functions: producing hormones (estrogen, progesterone, and small amounts of testosterone) and serving as the reservoir for immature eggs. All the eggs a woman will ever have are present in her ovaries at birth. Eggs mature and are released from the ovaries in response to hormone levels. Extending from the upper end of the uterus are two thin, flexible tubes called the **fallopian tubes**. The fallopian tubes, which do not actually touch the ovaries, capture eggs as they are released from the ovaries during ovulation, and they are the site where sperm and egg meet and fertilization takes place. The fallopian tubes then serve as the passageway to the uterus, where the fertilized egg becomes implanted and development continues.

## The Onset of Puberty and the Menstrual Cycle
With the onset of puberty, the female reproductive system matures, and the development of secondary sex

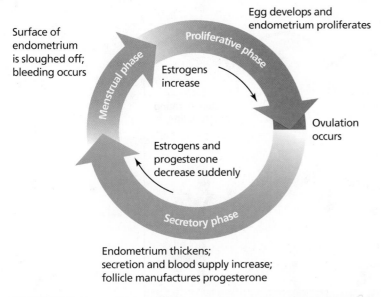

Surface of endometrium is sloughed off; bleeding occurs

Egg develops and endometrium proliferates

Menstrual phase

Proliferative phase

Estrogens increase

Ovulation occurs

Estrogens and progesterone decrease suddenly

Secretory phase

Endometrium thickens; secretion and blood supply increase; follicle manufactures progesterone

**FIGURE 9.2** The Three Phases of the Menstrual Cycle

**Source:** Rathus et al., *Human Sexuality in a World of Diversity*, 6th ed., © 2009. Figure "The Three Phases of the Menstrual Cycle," © 2005 Allyn & Bacon. Reproduced with permission of Pearson Education, Inc.

characteristics transforms young girls into young women. The first sign of puberty is the beginning of breast development, which generally occurs around age 10.[16] The pituitary gland, the **hypothalamus**, and the ovaries all secrete hormones that act as chemical messengers. Working in a feedback system, hormonal levels in the bloodstream act as the trigger mechanism for releasing a certain type or amount of hormone.

Around age 9½ to 11½ the hypothalamus receives the message to begin secreting *gonadotropin-releasing hormone* (*GnRH*). The release of GnRH in turn signals the pituitary gland to release hormones called *gonadotropins*. Two gonadotropins, *follicle-stimulating hormone* (*FSH*) and *luteinizing hormone* (*LH*), signal the ovaries to start producing **estrogen** and **progesterone**. Estrogen regulates the menstrual cycle, and increased estrogen levels assist in the development of female secondary sex characteristics. Progesterone helps the endometrium develop in preparation for nourishing a fertilized egg and helps maintain pregnancy.

The normal age range for the onset of the first menstrual period, or **menarche**, is 10 to 18 years, with the average age falling between 12 and 13 years.[17] Body fat heavily influences the onset of puberty, and increasing rates of obesity in children may account for the fact that girls are reaching puberty earlier than in the past.[18] Other theories attempting to explain early menarche include family disruption, high stress levels, and endocrine disruptors in the food supply.[19]

The average menstrual cycle lasts 28 days and consists of three phases: the proliferative phase, the secretory phase, and the menstrual phase (**FIGURE 9.2**). The *proliferative phase* begins with the end of menstruation. During this time, the endometrium develops or "proliferates." How does this process work? By the end of menstruation, the hypothalamus senses very low levels of estrogen and progesterone in the blood. In response, it increases its secretions of GnRH, which in turn

triggers the pituitary gland to release FSH. When FSH reaches the ovaries, it signals several **ovarian follicles** to begin maturing. Normally, only one of the follicles, the **graafian follicle**, reaches full maturity in the days preceding ovulation. While the follicles mature, they begin producing estrogen, which in turn signals the endometrial lining of the uterus to proliferate. If fertilization occurs, the endometrium will become a nesting place for the developing embryo. High estrogen levels signal the pituitary gland to slow down FSH production and increase release of LH. Under the influence of LH, the ovarian follicle ruptures and releases a mature **ovum** (plural: *ova*), a single mature egg cell, near a fallopian tube (around day 14). This is the process of **ovulation**. The other ripening follicles degenerate and are reabsorbed by the body. Occasionally, two ova mature and are released during ovulation. If both are fertilized, fraternal (nonidentical) twins develop. Identical twins develop when one fertilized ovum (called a *zygote*) divides into two separate zygotes.

The phase following ovulation is called the *secretory phase*. The ruptured graafian follicle, which has remained in the ovary, is transformed into the **corpus luteum** and begins secreting large amounts of estrogen and progesterone. These hormone secretions peak around day 20 or 21 of the average cycle and cause the endometrium to thicken. If fertilization and implantation take place, cells surrounding the developing embryo release a hormone called *human chorionic gonadotropin* (*HCG*), increasing estrogen and progesterone secretions that maintain the endometrium and signal the pituitary gland not to start a new menstrual cycle. If no implantation occurs, the hypothalamus responds by signaling the pituitary to stop producing FSH and LH, thus causing the levels of progesterone in the blood to peak. The corpus luteum begins to decompose, leading to rapid declines in estrogen and progesterone levels. These hormones are needed to sustain the lining of the uterus. Without them, the endometrium is sloughed off in the menstrual flow, and this begins the *menstrual phase*. The low estrogen levels of the menstrual phase signal the hypothalamus to release GnRH, which acts on the pituitary gland to secrete FSH, and the cycle (shown in **FIGURE 9.3** on page 246) begins again.

**hypothalamus** Area of the brain located near the pituitary gland; works in conjunction with the pituitary gland to control reproductive functions.

**estrogen** Hormone secreted by the ovaries that controls the menstrual cycle and assists in the development of female secondary sex characteristics.

**progesterone** Hormone secreted by the ovaries; helps the endometrium develop and helps maintain pregnancy.

**menarche** The first menstrual period.

**ovarian follicles** Areas within the ovary in which individual eggs develop.

**graafian follicle** Mature ovarian follicle that contains a fully developed egg (ovum).

**ovum** Single mature egg cell.

**ovulation** The point of the menstrual cycle at which a mature egg ruptures through the ovarian wall.

**corpus luteum** Cells that form from the remains of the graafian follicle following ovulation; it secretes estrogen and progesterone during the second half of the menstrual cycle.

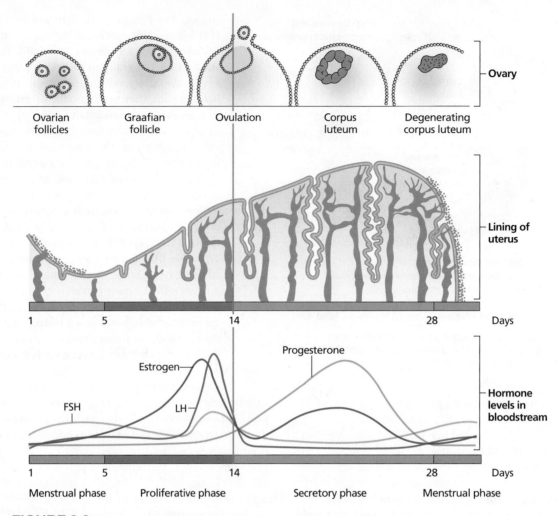

Ovary

Ovarian follicles | Graafian follicle | Ovulation | Corpus luteum | Degenerating corpus luteum

Lining of uterus

1    5    14    28    Days

Progesterone

Estrogen

FSH    LH

Hormone levels in bloodstream

1    5    14    28    Days

Menstrual phase | Proliferative phase | Secretory phase | Menstrual phase

**FIGURE 9.3** Hormonal Control and Phases of the Menstrual Cycle

## Menstrual Problems

**Premenstrual syndrome (PMS)** is a term used for a collection of physical, emotional, and behavioral symptoms that many women experience 7 to 14 days prior to their menstrual period. The most common symptoms are tender breasts, bloating, food cravings, fatigue, irritability, and depression. It is estimated that 85 percent of menstruating women experience at least one symptom of PMS each month.[20] For the majority of women, these disappear as their period begins, but for a small subset of women (5 to 8 percent), their symptoms are severe enough to affect their daily routines and activities to the point of being disabling. This severe form of PMS has its own diagnostic category in the *DSM-5*, **premenstrual dysphoric disorder (PMDD)**, with symptoms that include severe depression, hopelessness, anger, anxiety, low self-esteem, difficulty concentrating, irritability, and tension.[21]

There are several natural approaches to managing PMS that can also help PMDD. These strategies include eating more whole grains, fruits, and vegetables; reducing caffeine and salt intake; exercising regularly; and taking measures to reduce stress.[22] Recent investigation into methods of controlling severe emotional swings has led to the use of antidepressants for treating PMDD, primarily selective serotonin reuptake inhibitors (SSRIs; e.g., Prozac, Paxil, and Zoloft).[23]

**Dysmenorrhea** is a medical term for menstrual cramps, the pain or discomfort in the lower abdomen that many women experience just before or during menstruation. Along with cramps, some women experience nausea and vomiting, loose stools, sweating, and dizziness. Menstrual cramps can be classified as primary or secondary dysmenorrhea. Primary dysmenorrhea doesn't involve any physical abnormality and usually begins 6 months to a year after a woman's first period, while secondary dysmenorrhea has an underlying physical cause such as endometriosis or uterine fibroids.[24] You can reduce the discomfort of primary dysmenorrhea by using over-the-counter nonsteroidal anti-inflammatory drugs (NSAIDs) such as aspirin, ibuprofen (Advil or Motrin), or naproxen (Aleve). Other self-care strategies, such as soaking in a hot bath or using a heating pad on your abdomen, may also ease your cramps. For severe cramping, your health care provider may recommend a low-dose oral contraceptive to prevent ovulation. Without ovulation, there are fewer **prostaglandins** to

**premenstrual syndrome (PMS)** Mood changes and physical symptoms that occur in some women prior to menstruation.

**premenstrual dysphoric disorder (PMDD)** Group of symptoms similar to but more severe than PMS, including severe mood disturbances.

**dysmenorrhea** Condition of pain or discomfort in the lower abdomen just before or during menstruation.

**prostaglandin** Hormone-like substance associated with muscle contraction and inflammation.

trigger muscle contractions, thus reducing the severity of the cramps caused by the muscle contractions. Managing secondary dysmenorrhea involves treating the underlying cause.

Although rare, *toxic shock syndrome* (*TSS*) is a life-threatening complication caused by toxins produced by a bacterial infection. It usually follows skin wounds, injury, or the use of super absorbent tampons, diaphragm, cervical cap, or contraceptive sponge during a woman's period (see Chapter 10 for more on these contraceptive methods). Due to their link to TSS, super absorbent tampons were recalled and modified to decrease risk and provide instructions for safe use. TSS symptoms include a sudden high fever, vomiting, diarrhea, dizziness, muscle aches, or a rash that looks like sunburn. If you have symptoms such as a high fever and vomiting, and have been using a tampon or one of the previously mentioned contraceptive devices, remove it immediately, then contact a health care provider. Proper treatment usually ensures recovery in 2 to 3 weeks.[25]

**Menopause** Just as menarche signals the beginning of a woman's potential reproductive years, **menopause**—the permanent cessation of menstruation—signals the end. *Perimenopause* refers to the 4 to 6 years preceding menopause when hormonal changes take place and menstrual cycles and flow can become irregular. Menopause generally occurs after age 45 among U.S. women.[26] Menopausal changes result in decreased estrogen levels, which may produce troublesome symptoms in some women, such as hot flashes, night sweats, decreased vaginal lubrication, headaches, dizziness, and joint pain.[27]

From the 1970s to the 2000s, women commonly relieved these symptoms with synthetic forms of estrogen and progesterone known as **hormone replacement therapy** (HRT), also called *menopausal hormone therapy*. This therapy was believed to relieve menopausal symptoms and simultaneously reduce the risk of heart disease and osteoporosis. However, research later revealed that HRT increased the risk for heart disease, stroke, blood clots, and breast cancer in some women.[28]

Today, instead of routinely prescribing HRT for women, doctors only prescribe it when menopause symptoms are severe, when women are under age 60, and when women are free of heart disease, diabetes, high cholesterol, high blood pressure, and a history of breast, ovarian, or uterine cancer.[29] Women are now encouraged to manage mild symptoms by changing lifestyle habits such as exercising regularly, sleeping in a cooler room, and limiting caffeine and alcohol intake.[30]

Conflicting research reports highlight the need for all people to discuss the risks and benefits of any therapy with their health care provider in order to make an informed decision. Also, adopting a lifestyle including regular exercise, a healthy diet, and good self-care can help prevent diseases or limit symptoms.

**menopause** Permanent cessation of menstruation; generally occurs after age 45.

**hormone replacement therapy (menopausal hormone therapy)** Use of synthetic estrogens and progesterone to compensate for hormonal changes in a woman's body during menopause.

# Male Sexual and Reproductive Anatomy and Physiology

The structures of the male reproductive system are divided into external and internal genitals (**FIGURE 9.4**). The external genitals are the penis and the scrotum. The internal male genitals include the testes, epididymides, vasa deferentia, ejaculatory ducts, urethra, and other structures—the seminal vesicles, the

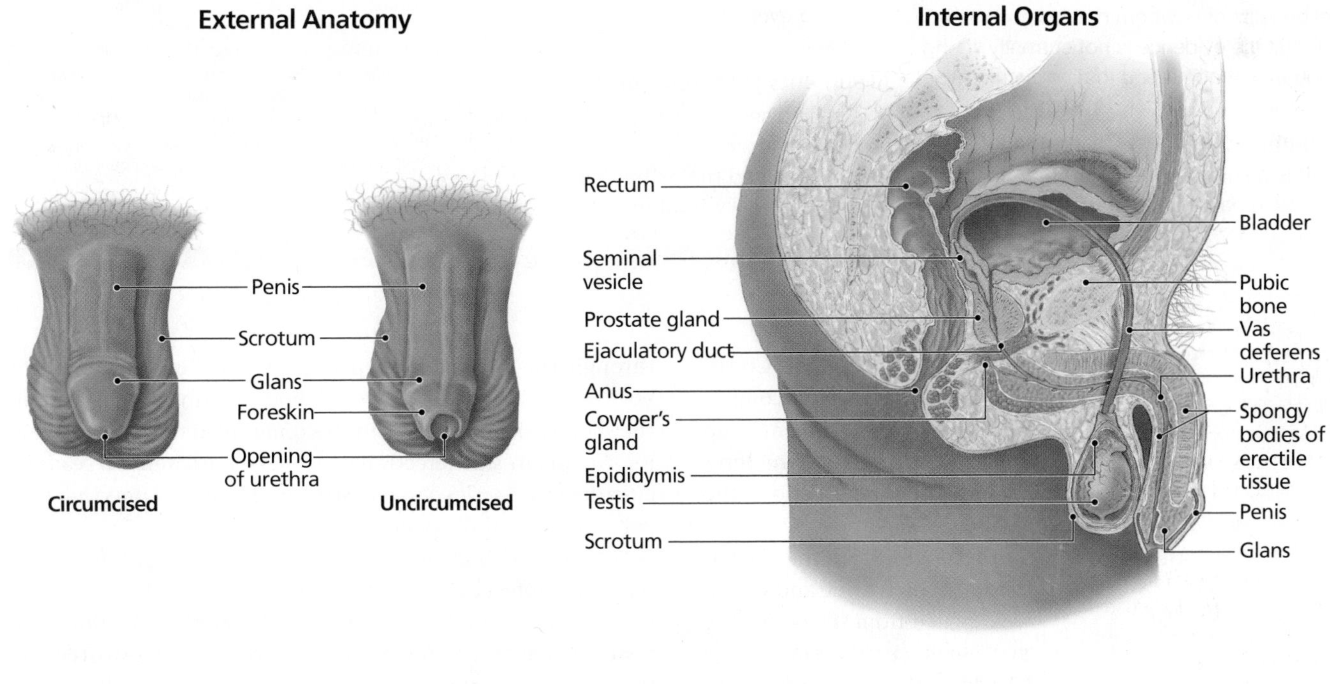

**External Anatomy**

**Internal Organs**

FIGURE 9.4 Male Sexual and Reproductive Anatomy

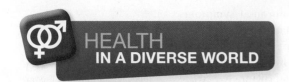

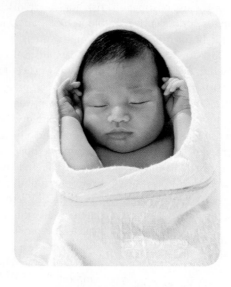

# CIRCUMCISION
*Risk versus Benefit*

Debate continues over the practice of *circumcision*, the surgical removal of a fold of skin, known as the *foreskin*, covering the end of the penis. While nearly universal in the United States decades ago, only about 55 percent of baby boys are now circumcised, mostly for religious or cultural reasons or because of hygiene concerns.

While prescribed in Jewish and Muslim faiths worldwide, circumcision is not required in the Christian faith. Only in the United States do Christians regularly circumcise, although they do so with less frequency today.

Recent research supports claims that circumcision yields medical benefits, including decreased risk of urinary tract infections in the first year, decreased risk of penile cancer (although cancer of the penis is very rare), and decreased risk of sexual transmission of human papillomavirus (HPV) and human immunodeficiency virus (HIV).

However, strong arguments against circumcision include a lack of medical necessity, a possible reduction in sexual sensitivity, and the possibility of bleeding, infection, and surgical complications. The American Academy of Pediatrics recently took a stand on the issue, stating that scientific evidence shows potential medical benefits of newborn male circumcision, but that the evidence is not currently strong enough to recommend routine circumcision.

### Arguments against Circumcision

- It is a surgical procedure that may cause pain to the infant, and there are potential complications such as bleeding, infection, improper healing, or cutting the foreskin too long or too short.
- Much of the research on the relationship between circumcision and sexually transmitted infections was done in developing countries and may not be indicative of outcomes in developed nations.
- Men lose a degree of sexual pleasure and stimulation when the foreskin is removed. Many unique nerve endings—found only in the foreskin—are lost forever.

### Arguments for Circumcision

- Circumcised males have a lower risk of penile cancer.
- Circumcised males have a lower risk of urinary tract infections during their first year, easier genital hygiene, and a lower risk of foreskin infections.
- In developing countries, circumcision has been shown to have a protective effect against human immunodeficiency virus (HIV), herpes simplex virus 2 (HSV-2), and human papillomavirus (HPV) transmission in males.
- Families may have religious or cultural reasons for wishing to circumcise their sons (in the Jewish faith, for example, circumcision is performed in a ceremony called a *bris*, and it represents the covenant God made with the patriarch Abraham).

### Where Do You Stand?

- If you had a son, what decision would you make regarding circumcising him?
- What factors—religious, cultural, aesthetic, or health-related—would have the most influence on your decision?
- If your faith requires circumcision, how do you weigh the medical factors against the religious and cultural factors?

**Sources:** M. Owings and S. Uddin, "Trends in Circumcision for Male Newborns in U.S. Hospitals: 1979–2010," National Center for Health Statistics, 2013, www.cdc.gov/nchs/data/hestat/circumcision_2013/circumcision_2013.htm; Mayo Clinic Staff, "Circumcision (Male): Why It's Done," February 2015, www.mayoclinic.com; American Academy of Pediatrics, "2012 Technical Report, Male Circumcision," *Pediatrics* 130, no. 3 (2012): e756–e785, DOI: 10.1542/peds.2012-1990.

---

**penis** Male organ through which urine and semen are expelled from the body.

**ejaculation** Propulsion of semen from the penis.

**scrotum** External sac of tissue that encloses the testes.

**testes** Male sex organs that manufacture sperm and produce hormones.

**testosterone** Male sex hormone manufactured in the testes.

prostate gland, and the Cowper's glands—that secrete components that, with sperm, make up semen. These three structures are sometimes referred to as the *accessory glands*.

The **penis** is the organ through which urine and semen are expelled from the body. (See the **Health in a Diverse World** for a discussion of circumcision.) The urethra, a tube that passes through the center of the penis, acts as the passageway for both semen and urine to exit the body. During sexual arousal, the spongy tissue in the penis becomes filled with blood, making the organ stiff (erect). Further sexual excitement leads to **ejaculation**, a series of rapid, spasmodic contractions that propel semen out of the penis.

Situated behind the penis is a sac called the **scrotum**. The scrotum protects the testes and helps control their internal temperature, which is vital to proper sperm production. The **testes** (singular: *testis*) manufacture sperm and **testosterone**, the hormone responsible for the development of male secondary sex characteristics.

The development of sperm is referred to as **spermatogenesis**. Like the maturation of eggs in the female, this process is governed by the pituitary gland. FSH is secreted into the bloodstream to stimulate the testes to manufacture sperm. Immature sperm are released into a comma-shaped structure on the back of each testis called the **epididymis** (plural: *epididymides*), where they ripen and reach full maturity. Each epididymis contains coiled tubules that gradually straighten out to become the **vas deferens** (plural: *vasa deferentia*). These make up the tubular transportation system whose sole function is to store and move sperm. Along the way, the **seminal vesicles** provide sperm with nutrients and other fluids that comprise **semen**.

The vasa deferentia eventually connect each epididymis to the **ejaculatory ducts**, which pass through the prostate gland and empty into the urethra. The **prostate gland** contributes more fluids to the semen, including chemicals that help the sperm fertilize an ovum and neutralize the acidic environment of the vagina to make it more conducive to sperm motility (ability to move) and potency (potential for fertilization). Just below the prostate gland are two pea-shaped nodules called the **Cowper's glands**. The Cowper's glands secrete a preejaculatory fluid that lubricates the urethra and neutralizes any acid that may remain in the urethra after urination. In this process, urine and semen never come into contact with each other, as during ejaculation of semen, a small valve closes off the tube to the urinary bladder.

### Andropause

Whether or not men actually go through a form of male menopause, known as *andropause*, is the subject of much debate. While testosterone levels in men vary greatly, men do experience a gradual decline in testosterone levels as they age, similar to the declining hormone levels in women, particularly if they are obese or smoke cigarettes.[31] Men do not, however, experience a rapid hormone decline in middle age that affects their reproductive capacity as women do during menopause. Instead, men typically experience a gradual decline in testosterone levels throughout adulthood, about 1 percent a year on average after age 30.[32] Many doctors use the term *andropause* to describe age-related hormone changes in men. Some men with lowered testosterone levels do not experience signs and symptoms. Those who do may experience the following:[33]

- **Changes in sexual function.** These may include reduced sexual desire, fewer spontaneous erections—such as during sleep—and infertility. Testes may become smaller, as well.
- **Changes in sleep patterns.** Low testosterone may cause insomnia or other sleep disturbances.
- **Physical changes.** Various physical changes may occur, including increased body fat, reduced muscle bulk and strength, and decreased bone density. Abnormal enlargement of the male breasts (gynecomastia) and hair loss are possible.
- **Emotional changes.** Low testosterone levels may contribute to a decrease in motivation or self-confidence, cause sadness or depression, or interfere with concentration or memory.[34]

Treatment is available for age-related low testosterone levels, but it is not without controversy. For some men, testosterone therapy relieves the symptoms. For others, especially older men, the benefits aren't clear. And there are risks; testosterone therapy may increase the risk of prostate cancer or other health problems.[35]

## LO 3 | HUMAN SEXUAL RESPONSE

List and describe the stages of the human sexual response and what factors may influence them.

Many factors, both physical and psychological, influence sexual response and sexual desire. Thus, a person's sexual response may be vastly different from one sexual experience to another or from one partner to another.

Sexual response is a physiological process that generally follows a pattern that can be roughly divided into four stages: excitement/arousal, plateau, orgasm, and resolution (**Figure 9.5** on page 250). Regardless of the type of sexual activity (stimulation by a partner or self-stimulation), the response stages are the same; however, researchers agree that each individual has a personal response pattern that may or may not exactly conform to these phases. And while sexual response is a physiological process, do not underestimate the role of the brain in the process. The brain is involved in each phase including visual stimulation, inhibition reduction, and hormone release.[36]

During the first stage, *excitement/arousal*, **vasocongestion** (increased blood flow that causes swelling in the genitals) stimulates male and female genital responses. The vagina begins to lubricate, and the penis becomes partially erect. Both sexes may exhibit a "sex flush" or light blush all over their bodies. Excitement/arousal can be generated through fantasy or by touching parts of the body, kissing, viewing erotic images, or reading erotic literature.

During the *plateau phase*, the initial responses intensify. Voluntary and involuntary muscle tensions increase. A woman's nipples become erect, as does a man's penis. The penis secretes a few drops of preejaculatory fluid, which may contain sperm.

During the *orgasmic phase*, vasocongestion and muscle tensions reach their peak, and rhythmic contractions occur through the genital regions.

**spermatogenesis** The development of sperm.

**epididymis** Duct system atop the testis where sperm mature.

**vas deferens** Tube that transports sperm from the epididymis to the ejaculatory duct.

**seminal vesicles** Glandular ducts that secrete nutrients for the semen.

**ejaculatory duct** Tube formed by the junction of the seminal vesicle and the vas deferens that carries semen to the urethra.

**semen** Fluid containing sperm and nutrients that increase sperm viability and neutralize vaginal acid.

**prostate gland** Gland that secretes chemicals that help sperm fertilize an ovum and secretes neutralizing fluids into the semen.

**Cowper's glands** Glands that secrete a preejaculatory fluid that lubricates the urethra and neutralizes any acid remaining in the urethra after urination.

**vasocongestion** Engorgement of the genital organs with blood.

**Male**

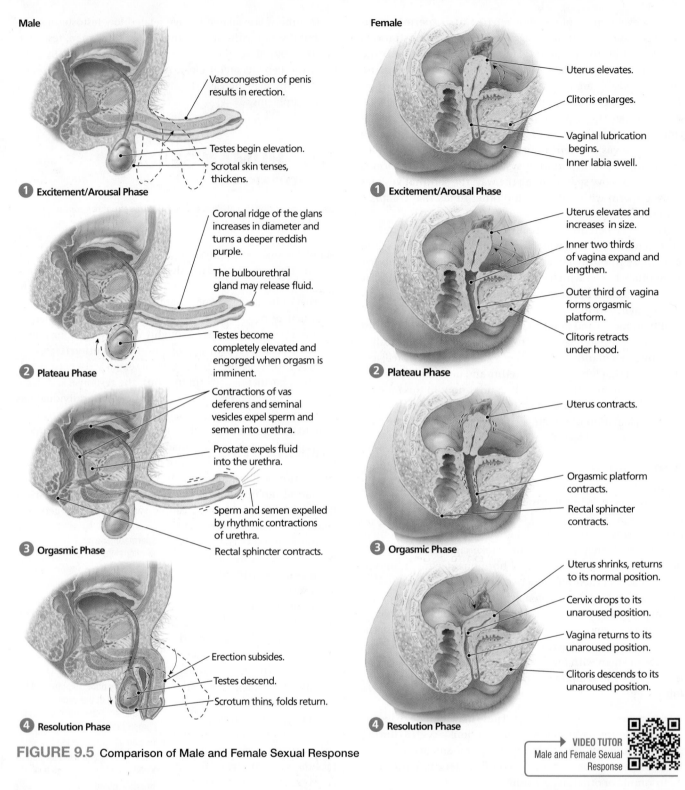

**Female**

Vasocongestion of penis results in erection.

Testes begin elevation.

Scrotal skin tenses, thickens.

**①** Excitement/Arousal Phase

Coronal ridge of the glans increases in diameter and turns a deeper reddish purple.

The bulbourethral gland may release fluid.

Testes become completely elevated and engorged when orgasm is imminent.

**②** Plateau Phase

Contractions of vas deferens and seminal vesicles expel sperm and semen into urethra.

Prostate expels fluid into the urethra.

Sperm and semen expelled by rhythmic contractions of urethra.

Rectal sphincter contracts.

**③** Orgasmic Phase

Erection subsides.

Testes descend.

Scrotum thins, folds return.

**④** Resolution Phase

Uterus elevates.

Clitoris enlarges.

Vaginal lubrication begins.

Inner labia swell.

**①** Excitement/Arousal Phase

Uterus elevates and increases in size.

Inner two thirds of vagina expand and lengthen.

Outer third of vagina forms orgasmic platform.

Clitoris retracts under hood.

**②** Plateau Phase

Uterus contracts.

Orgasmic platform contracts.

Rectal sphincter contracts.

**③** Orgasmic Phase

Uterus shrinks, returns to its normal position.

Cervix drops to its unaroused position.

Vagina returns to its unaroused position.

Clitoris descends to its unaroused position.

**④** Resolution Phase

**FIGURE 9.5** Comparison of Male and Female Sexual Response

▶ VIDEO TUTOR
Male and Female Sexual Response

In women, these contractions are centered in the uterus, outer vagina, and anal sphincter. In men, the contractions occur in two stages. First, contractions within the prostate gland begin propelling semen through the urethra. In the second stage, the muscles of the pelvic floor, urethra, and anal sphincter contract. Semen is usually, but not always, ejaculated from the penis. In both sexes, spasms in other major muscle groups also occur, particularly in the buttocks and abdomen. Feet and hands may also contract, and facial features often contort.

Muscle tension and congested blood subside in the *resolution phase* as the genital organs return to their prearousal states. Both sexes usually experience deep feelings of well-being and profound relaxation. Many women can experience multiple orgasms during the orgasmic phase. Some men experience a refractory period, during which their systems are incapable of subsequent arousal. This refractory period may last from a few minutes to several hours and tends to lengthen with age.

Men and women experience the same stages in the sexual response cycle; however, the length of time spent in any one stage varies. Thus, one partner may be in the plateau phase while the other is in the excitement or orgasmic phase. Such variations in response rates are entirely normal. Some couples believe that simultaneous orgasm is desirable for sexual satisfaction. Although simultaneous orgasm is pleasant, so are orgasms achieved at different times. Sexual pleasure and satisfaction are also possible without orgasm or even intercourse. Expressing sexual feelings for another person involves many pleasurable activities, of which intercourse and orgasm may be only a part.

## Sexuality and Aging

Older adults are sometimes stereotyped as being uninterested or incapable of sexual relations. The truth is, though we do experience some physical changes as we age, the changes generally do not cause us to stop enjoying sex.

In women, the most significant physical changes follow menopause. Skin becomes less elastic; most internal sexual organs, including the uterus and cervix, shrink somewhat; the vaginal walls become thinner; and vaginal lubrication during sexual arousal may decrease. The resulting increased friction during penetration can be painful, although the use of artificial lubricants usually resolves this problem.[37]

Although men do not experience menopause, their bodies do change as a result of the aging process. They often require more direct and prolonged stimulation to achieve an erection, their erections become less firm, and they are more likely

# 23%
of college students report having had **MORE THAN ONE** sex partner in the past 12 months.

to experience erectile dysfunction. They are slower to reach orgasm, and their refractory periods are longer. Men also experience a decrease in the intensity of ejaculation, as semen is expelled with less force as men age.[38]

The majority of healthy older men and women can enjoy a regular and satisfying sex life. In fact, among the advantages experienced by adults at this stage of life are a level of comfort with and appreciation of their bodies, and more time and privacy for sex than when younger. Many older people also no longer need contraception to prevent pregnancy (although protection from sexually transmitted infections [STIs] is still necessary if there are new or multiple partners). To maintain a healthy sex life in the later years, it is important to take care of your body while young. Avoiding tobacco, eating a healthy diet, and exercising regularly will help to prevent heart disease, diabetes, and obesity, all of which increase the risk of sexual dysfunction later in life.[39]

## Sexual Dysfunction

**Sexual dysfunction**, the term used to describe problems that can hinder sexual functioning, can be divided into four categories: desire disorders, arousal disorders, orgasmic disorders, and pain disorders. (See **TABLE 9.1.**) The good news is that all types can be treated successfully.

**sexual dysfunction** Problems associated with achieving sexual satisfaction.

## TABLE **9.1** | Type of Sexual Dysfunction

| Desire Disorders | Description |
|---|---|
| Inhibited sexual desire | Lack or interest in sexual activity |
| Sexual aversion disorder | Phobias (fears) or anxiety about sexual contact |
| **Arousal Disorders** | |
| Erectile dysfunction | Inability to maintain an erection |
| Female sexual arousal disorder | Inability to remain sexually aroused |
| **Orgasmic Disorders** | |
| Premature ejaculation | Reaching orgasm rapidly or prematurely |
| Delayed ejaculation | Difficulty reaching orgasm despite normal desire and stimulation |
| Female orgasmic disorder | Inability to have an orgasm or difficulty or delay in reaching orgasm |
| **Pain Disorders** | |
| Dyspareunia | Pain during or after sex |
| Vaginismus | Forceful contraction of the vaginal muscles that prevents penetration from occurring |

Both men and women can experience **sexual performance anxiety** when they anticipate some sort of problem during a sexual experience. A man may become anxious and unable to maintain an erection (an arousal disorder), or he may experience premature ejaculation (an orgasmic disorder). A woman may be unable to achieve orgasm (an arousal disorder) or to allow penetration because of the involuntary contraction of vaginal muscles (a pain disorder). Both men and women can overcome sexual performance anxiety by learning to focus on immediate sensations and pleasures rather than on orgasm.

### Sexual Desire Disorders

**Libido** is a person's sexual drive or desire. A common reason people seek out a sex therapist is **inhibited sexual desire**, or the lack of interest and pleasure in sexual activity. A low sex drive (decreased libido) may be caused by hormonal imbalances in women or by low testosterone in both men and women. Fatigue, stress, and common conditions such as depression and anxiety can cause decreased libido. Antidepressant medications (e.g., Prozac, Zoloft, Paxil) are well known for reducing sexual desire in both men and women.[40] **Sexual aversion disorder** is another type of desire dysfunction, characterized by sexual phobias (unreasonable fears) and anxiety about sexual contact. The psychological stress related to a punitive upbringing, a rigid religious background, or a history of physical or sexual abuse may be sources of desire disorders. Women experiencing low sex drive can possibly boost sex drive by a daily pill, Addyi, which increases desire in some women.[41]

### Sexual Arousal Disorders

One common sexual arousal disorder is **erectile dysfunction (ED)**—difficulty in achieving or maintaining an erection sufficient for intercourse. At some time in his life, every man experiences erectile dysfunction. The majority of arousal disorders are caused by the same lifestyle issues that increase the risk of high cholesterol, hypertension, and chronic diseases such as cardiovascular disease and diabetes—in turn affecting blood flow.[42] Other risks for ED include certain medical conditions, treatments, and medications; using tobacco; being overweight; injuries; psychological conditions; drug and alcohol use; and prolonged bicycling.[43] Some 30 million men in the United States, half of them under age 65, suffer from ED.[44] The condition generally becomes more of a problem as men age, affecting 1 in 5 men in their 60s.[45] Seeing a doctor to determine possible causes is essential. Lifestyle changes are usually key to risk reduction. The FDA has also approved several drugs, such as Viagra (sildenafil citrate), Levitra (vardenafil hydrochloride), and Cialis (tadalafil) to treat ED. These drugs work by relaxing the smooth muscle cells in the penis, allowing for increased blood flow to the erectile tissues.[46] However, the best prevention for ED is to maintain overall physical and mental health.

### Orgasmic Disorders

**Premature ejaculation** (also known as *early ejaculation*)—ejaculation that occurs prior to or very soon after the insertion of the penis into the vagina—affects up to 70 percent of men at some time in their lives.[47] Treatment first involves a physical examination to rule out physiological causes. If the cause is not physiological, therapy is available to help a man learn how to control the timing of his ejaculation. **Delayed ejaculation** is persistent difficulty in reaching orgasm despite normal desire and stimulation. Fatigue, stress, performance pressure, and alcohol use can all contribute to orgasmic disorders in men.

In a woman, the inability to achieve orgasm is called **female orgasmic disorder**. A woman with this disorder often

**sexual performance anxiety** Sexual difficulties caused by anticipating some sort of problem during a sex act.

**libido** Sexual drive or desire.

**inhibited sexual desire** Lack of sexual appetite or lack of interest and pleasure in sexual activity.

**sexual aversion disorder** Desire dysfunction characterized by sexual phobias and anxiety about sexual contact.

**erectile dysfunction (ED)** Difficulty in achieving or maintaining an erection sufficient for intercourse.

**premature ejaculation** Ejaculation that occurs prior to or almost immediately following penile penetration of the vagina; also known as *early ejaculation*.

**delayed ejaculation** Persistent difficulty in reaching orgasm despite normal desire and stimulation.

**female orgasmic disorder** A woman's inability to achieve orgasm.

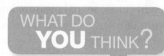

**WHAT DO YOU THINK?**

Why do we find it so difficult to discuss sexual dysfunction?

- Do you think it is more difficult for men than for women? Or vice versa?

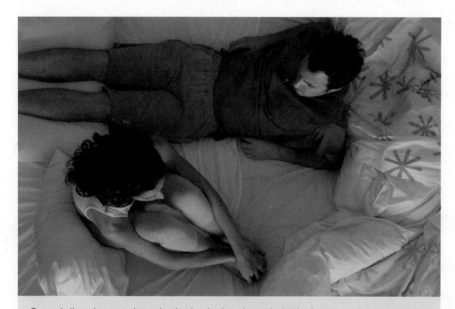

Sexual disorders can have both physical and psychological roots and can occur as a result of stress, fatigue, depression, or anxiety. They frequently have a physiological origin, such as overall poor health, chronic disease, or the use of alcohol or drugs.

learns to fake orgasm to avoid embarrassment or to preserve her partner's ego. Contributing factors include performance anxiety, a conservative upbringing, lack of trust, relationship issues, and difficulty seeing oneself as a sexual being.[48] Again, the first step in treatment is a physical exam to rule out physiological causes.[49] Often the problem is solved by simple self-exploration to learn more about what forms of stimulation are arousing enough to produce orgasm.[50] Through masturbation, a woman can learn how her body responds to various types of touch.[51] Once she has become orgasmic through masturbation, she can then learn to communicate her needs to her partner.[52]

## Sexual Pain Disorders

Two common disorders in this category are dyspareunia and vaginismus. **Dyspareunia** is pain experienced by a woman during intercourse that may be caused by conditions such as endometriosis, uterine tumors, chlamydia, gonorrhea, or urinary tract infections. Childbirth trauma and insufficient lubrication during intercourse may also cause discomfort. Dyspareunia can also be psychological in origin. **Vaginismus** is the involuntary contraction of vaginal muscles, making penile insertion painful or impossible. Vaginismus can be caused by a variety of physical issues (such as endometriosis, vaginal dryness, or pain from injury) or nonphysical causes (such as fear of pain during intercourse, fear of pregnancy, anxiety or guilt about sex, or unresolved sexual conflicts with a current or past partner).[53]

## Seeking Help for Sexual Dysfunction

While sexual dysfunction can happen at any age, the incidence of dysfunction increases during the menopause years in women and after age 50 in men.[54] Many treatment models can help people with sexual dysfunction. It is important not to be afraid to talk to a sex educator, counselor, or health care provider. If you are looking for a qualified professional, the American Association of Sex Educators, Counselors, and Therapists (AASECT) can help. AASECT has been in the forefront of establishing criteria for certifying sex therapists. Their website provides information on how to locate a certified professional in your community.

## Drugs and Sex

Because psychoactive drugs affect the body's overall physiological functioning, it is only logical that they also affect sexual behavior. Promises of increased pleasure make drugs tempting to people seeking greater sexual satisfaction. But if drugs are necessary to increase sexual feelings, it is likely that partners are being dishonest about their feelings for each other. Good sex should not depend on chemical substances. Also, alcohol is notorious for reducing inhibitions and promoting feelings of well-being and desirability. But at the same time, alcohol inhibits sexual response; thus, the mind may be willing, but not the body.

## Recreational Use of ED Medications

An emerging issue is the recreational use of drugs intended to

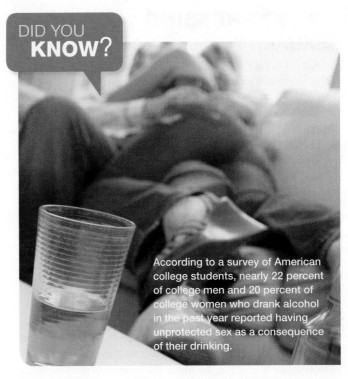

According to a survey of American college students, nearly 22 percent of college men and 20 percent of college women who drank alcohol in the past year reported having unprotected sex as a consequence of their drinking.

**Source:** Data from American College Health Association, *American College Health Association—National College Health Assessment II (ACHA-NCHA II) Reference Group Data Report, Fall 2015* (Baltimore: American College Health Association, 2015).

treat erectile dysfunction (e.g., Viagra). Young men who take this type of medication report they hope to increase their sexual stamina or counteract performance anxiety or the effects of alcohol or other drugs.[55] However, these drugs probably have only a placebo effect in men with normal erections, and combining them with other drugs, such as ketamine, amyl nitrate (poppers), or methamphetamine, can lead to potentially fatal drug interactions.[56]

## Date Rape Drugs

"Date rape drugs" such as Rohypnol or gamma-hydroxybutyrate (GHB) are used to limit an individual's ability to consent to sexual activity. Most often introduced to an unsuspecting person through alcoholic drinks, these drugs make it easier for a perpetrator to commit sexual assault because the victim is less able to resist. Victims often wake with little or no memory of what occurred.[57] (See more detail on these drugs in chapters covering drugs and violence— Chapters 13 and 20, respectively.)

If a person suspects drug-induced sexual assault, evidence should be preserved quickly, as the drugs can leave the body in 12 to 72 hours. You can call the National Sexual Assault Hotline at 800-656-HOPE (4673) to locate a hospital or clinic that can help.[58] While college students should be alert to "date rape drugs," it is important to recognize that alcohol is far more commonly associated with sexual assault than are Rohypnol or GHB.[59]

**dyspareunia** Pain experienced by women during intercourse.

**vaginismus** State in which the vaginal muscles contract so forcefully that penetration cannot occur.

## LO 4 | EXPRESSING YOUR SEXUALITY

Discuss the variety of sexual expression and their implications for sexual health and safety.

Finding healthy ways to express yourself is an important part of sexuality. Many avenues of sexual expression are available. Find behaviors that are satisfying, safe, consensual, and allow you to express who you are, sexually.

### Sexual Behavior: Is There a "Normal"?

What exactly is sexual behavior? It encompasses many things, including if we have sex, who we have sex with, and what sex acts we engage in. You may be asking yourself what sexual behaviors are considered normal? Or is there such a thing as normal? And if there is, is it important to be normal?

Every society sets standards and attempts to normalize sexual behavior. Boundaries arise that distinguish good from bad or acceptable from unacceptable and result in what is viewed as normal or abnormal. Some of the common standards for sexual behavior in Western culture today include:[60]

- **The coital standard.** Penile–vaginal intercourse (coitus) is viewed as the ultimate sex act.
- **The orgasmic standard.** Sexual interaction should lead to orgasm.
- **The two-person standard.** Sex is an activity to be experienced by two people.
- **The romantic standard.** Sex should be related to love.
- **The safer-sex standard.** If we choose to be sexually active, we should act to prevent unintended pregnancy or disease transmission.

These are not laws or rules, but rather social scripts that have been adopted over time. Sexual standards often shift through the years, and some people choose to ignore them altogether. They can also feel limiting, as they do not fit everyone; for example, a lesbian couple cannot participate in penile–vaginal intercourse and those who enjoy "hooking up" may disagree with the romantic standard. Rather than making blanket judgments about normal versus abnormal, we might consider the CERTS Model for Healthy Sexuality. The acronym stands for:[61]

- **Consent:** A person freely chooses to engage in the sexual activity, and can stop the activity at any time.
- **Equality:** Neither partner is dominant; both feel equal power in the relationship.
- **Respect:** You accept and respect your partner and yourself.

- **Trust:** You trust your partner with your body physically and emotionally. You can each be vulnerable together.
- **Safety:** You feel safe from STIs, unintended pregnancy, and violence, and feel comfortable with where, when, and what sexual activity takes place. You are not making decisions under the power of drugs and alcohol.

> **celibacy** State of not engaging in sexual activity.

Using the CERTS model, rather than societal standards for "normal," all behaviors can be evaluated as either healthy or unhealthy for an individual. As you read about the options for sexual expression in the section ahead, use the CERTS model to explore your feelings about what is right for you.

### Options for Sexual Expression

The range of human sexual expression is virtually infinite. What you find enjoyable may not be an option for someone else (see the **Health in a Diverse World** box for a discussion of sexuality and disability). Your sexual needs and the ways you choose to meet them today may be very different from what they were 2 weeks ago or will be 2 years from now. Accepting yourself as a sexual person with individual desires and preferences is the first step in achieving sexual satisfaction.

**Celibacy and Abstinence** While celibacy and abstinence are related terms, they aren't synonymous. **Celibacy** can refer to abstention from all sexual activities whatsoever, including masturbation (complete celibacy) or abstention from sexual activities with another person (partial celibacy).[62] Some individuals choose celibacy for religious or moral reasons. Others may be celibate for a period of time because of illness, a breakup, or lack of an acceptable partner. For some, celibacy is a lonely, agonizing state, but others find

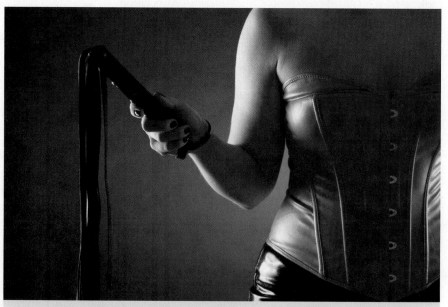

As with any other human behavior, the idea of "normal" sexual behavior varies from person to person and from society to society, usually along a spectrum of perceived acceptability or appropriateness.

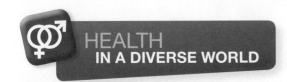

# CAN SOMEONE WHO IS PARALYZED HAVE SEX?

The short answer is yes, people who are paralyzed can have sex. Just as with people who aren't paralyzed, you can't tell by looking at a person who may struggle with sexual dysfunction or what will satisfy a person sexually.

Today, one in five Americans has a disability, either in mobility, cognition, independent living, vision, or self-care. Impairments in mobility, from difficulty walking to complete paralysis, are the most common, affecting 13% of Americans. Two percent of Americans have some form of paralysis necessitating the use of a wheelchair. A person who uses a wheelchair may face frequent challenges, such as buildings that are not accessible, difficulty using public transportation, and stereotypes and stigma, including cultural standards of beauty and misconceptions about what disabled people can and can't do sexually.

People who are paralyzed have a wide range of sexual function and ability to feel sensation depending on their specific injury or diagnosis. Erections

**We are all sexual beings capable and deserving of intimacy and fulfilling sexual relationships.**

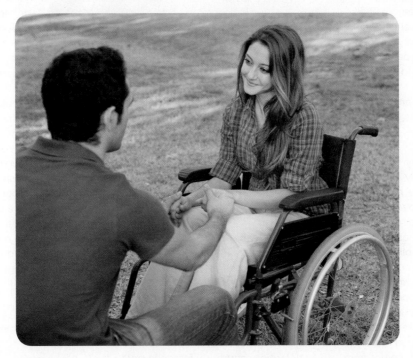

and ejaculation are still possible for many males, as are vaginal lubrication and orgasm for females. For some, erections may need to be enhanced with Viagra or other aid, or lubrication may be needed. There are many sexual positions that work well for both partners whether using a wheelchair, bed, or other surface. A wide variety of aids for stimulation and positioning are available.

If a person has recently become paralyzed, counseling or therapy to deal with sexuality issues is available. Cognitive therapy and sex therapy—the treatment of sexual dysfunction, lack of sexual confidence, and other sexual problems—may help, or the person may want to see a certified sex surrogate. Surrogates offer therapeutic exercises to help the patient. These may include relaxation techniques, intimate communication, social skills, and sexual touching. One or a combination of these methods may help disabled people who want to explore the sexual side of their life.

**Sources:** E. A. Courtney-Long et. al., "Prevalence of Disability and Disability Type Among Adults-United States, 2013," *Morbidity and Mortality Weekly Report* 64, no. 29 (2015): 777–83; Centers for Disease Control and Prevention, "Common Barriers to Participation Experienced by People with Disabilities," March 17, 2016, http://www.cdc.gov/ncbddd/disability-andhealth/disability-barriers.html; Christopher and Dana Reeve Foundation, "Sexual Health for Men," Accessed May 2016, https://www.christopher-reeve.org/living-with-paralysis/health/sexual-health/sexual-health-for-men; International Professional Surrogates Association, "What Is Surrogate Partner Therapy?," Accessed May 2016, www.surrogateth-erapy.org/what-is-surrogate-partner-therapy.

---

it an opportunity for introspection, values assessment, and personal growth.

**Abstinence** usually refers to the avoidance of intercourse: oral, vaginal, or anal. People who are abstinent may engage in other sexual behaviors, such as kissing, touching, or masturbation. So, while celibate people are abstinent, people can be abstinent without being celibate. While no good estimates of celibacy exist, 34 percent of college students report being abstinent (no oral, vaginal, or anal sex) for the past 12 months.[63]

## Autoerotic Behaviors  Autoerotic behaviors involve self-stimulation. The two most common are sexual fantasy and masturbation.

**Sexual fantasies** are sexually arousing thoughts and dreams. Fantasies may reflect real-life experiences, forbidden desires, or the opportunity to practice new or anticipated sexual experiences. The fact that you fantasize about a particular sexual experience does not necessarily mean that you want to, or have to, act out that experience. Sexual fantasies are just that—fantasy. Fantasies are often aided by the use of magazines or videos. (For more on pornography, see Health Headlines on page 256; for more on sexting, see Tech & Health on page 257.)

**Masturbation** is self-stimulation of the genitals. Although many people are uncomfortable discussing masturbation, it is a common sexual practice across the lifespan. Masturbation

**abstinence** The avoidance of intercourse, but not other sexual behaviors.

**autoerotic behaviors** Sexual self-stimulation.

**sexual fantasies** Sexually arousing thoughts and dreams.

**masturbation** Manual stimulation of genitals.

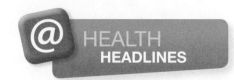

# PORNOGRAPHY
*Helpful, Harmful, or Neither?*

Throughout history, sex has been a prominent theme in art, literature, and the media. But when do depictions of the human body and human sexual behaviors cross the line from story to exploitation or from art to pornography? It can be hard to tell sometimes.

Pornography refers to any visual or literary depictions of sexual activity intended to be sexually arousing. Availability of pornography has increased dramatically with the growth of the Internet; pornographic websites now account for 4 percent of all Web searches, with the most popular porn website logging 4.4 billion page views per month. The pornography industry—including magazines, websites, videos, pay-per-view, phone sex, cable, computer games, and exotic dance clubs—generates annual revenue of more than $10 billion in the United States, the biggest piece of which comes from online revenue. Clearly, pornography is a booming industry supported by many millions of consumers. Why, then, is it so controversial?

People fear that viewing pornographic materials leads to negative attitudes toward women, sexual aggression, and sexual violence. However, current evidence suggests that pornography does not lead to

**Internet pornography is a large part of the multibillion-dollar porn industry.**

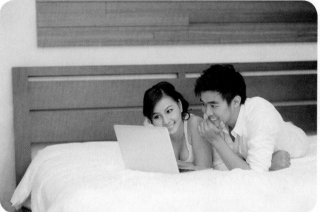

sexual violence, predatory behavior, or major changes in individuals' sexual behaviors in normal, healthy adults, unless individuals have preexisting negative attitudes toward women. Other concerns include preliminary research showing that pornography may have a negative impact on relationships, sexual satisfaction, and body image in both males and females. Specifically, women voice concerns that pornography affects how they are expected to look and sets unrealistic expectations for how sexually adventurous they should be. Others worry that viewing pornography causes emotional withdrawal from relationships; what's unclear is if people sometimes turn to pornography because they are in an

unsatisfying relationship. It's hard to know which might come first.

Whether porn is helpful or harmful is specific to an individual. What's important for you to know is that you should only engage in the use of pornography you feel comfortable with and you should have an open dialogue with your partner about his or her use also. Also, like movie stars, do not compare yourself to people you see on screen. The sex you see in pornography is their job; it's a performance. It's not about connecting with another person and enjoying sex with them. In that respect, your sex life is likely better than the average porn star's!

**Sources:** M. Hussey, "Who are the Biggest Consumers of Online Porn?," *The Next Web*, March 24, 2015, http://thenextweb.com/market-intelligence/2015/03/24/who-are-the-biggest-consumers-of-online-porn/#gref; K. Weir, "Is Pornography Addictive?," *APA Monitor* 45 no. 4 (2014): 46; D. M. Szymanski and D. N. Stewart-Richardson, "Psychological, Relational, and Sexual Correlates of Pornography Use on Young Adult Heterosexual Men in Romantic Relationships," *Journal of Men's Studies* 22, no. 1 (2014): 64–82; T. L. Tylka, "No Harm in Looking, Right?: Men's Pornography Consumption, Body Image, and Well-Being," *Psychology of Men and Masculinity* 16, no. 1 (2015): 97; T. L. Tylka and A. M. Kroom Van Diest, "You Looking at Her 'Hot' Body May Not Be 'Cool' for Me: Integrating Male Partners' Use of Pornography into Objectification Theory for Women," *Psychology of Women Quarterly* 39, no. 1 (2015): 67–84.

---

is a natural pleasure-seeking behavior that begins in infancy. It is a valuable and important means for adolescents, as well as adults, to explore sexual feelings and responsiveness.

**Kissing and Erotic Touching** Kissing and erotic touching are two very common forms of nonverbal sexual communication. Both men and women have **erogenous zones**, areas of the body that, when touched, lead to sexual arousal. Erogenous zones may include genital and nongenital areas, such as the earlobes, mouth, nipples, and inner thighs.

Almost any area of the body can be conditioned to respond erotically to touch. Spending time with your

partner to explore and learn about his or her erogenous areas is another pleasurable, safe, and satisfying means of sexual expression.

## Manual Stimulation

Both men and women can be sexually aroused and achieve orgasm through manual stimulation of the genitals by a partner (masturbation). *Sex toys* include a wide variety of objects that can be used for sexual stimulation alone or with a partner.

**erogenous zones** Areas of the body that, when touched, lead to sexual arousal.

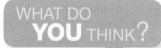

**What do you think about autoerotic behaviors?**

- Could they be a good way to reduce STIs?
- Is there a stigma associated with masturbation? If so, why?

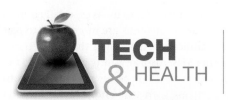

# TECH & HEALTH | CONSENSUAL TEXTS

Actress Jennifer Lawrence was livid. "I can't even describe to anybody what it feels like to have [pictures of] my naked body shoot across the world like a news flash against my will. It just makes me feel like a piece of meat." Photos on her phone, in various states of nudity, were hacked from the Cloud and posted online. "I didn't tell you that you could look at my naked body," she said. She worried it would impact her career. She was mad that her friends looked at the pictures. She said she would rather give back the money from *The Hunger Games* than tell her dad about the pictures.

But wait, this wasn't a case of paparazzi stalking her and secretly taking a picture. She willingly shot the selfies and sent them to her boyfriend. What she didn't consent to was the pictures being hacked, then shared with the world.

What lessons can we take from Ms. Lawrence's story? One, once a photo has been taken, we have limited control over its future. In fact, a recent Kinsey Institute study found that nearly a quarter of adults who receive provocative pictures on their phone share them with three people, on average. Two, "consent," a concept we usually associate with sexual activity, should apply to sexting, too. A few months after the photos were hacked, Ms. Lawrence posed nude with a boa constrictor for the same magazine where the above quotes were published. So when she said, "I didn't tell you that you could look at my naked body,"

**Once a photo of us is taken, we sometimes have limited control over what happens next.**

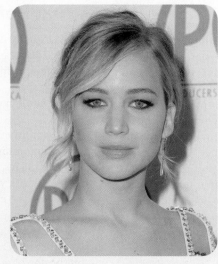

it seems her concern was less about being naked and more that she did not consent for those photos to be shared.

According to popular sex educator Laci Green, there are three times consent can never be truly given: when a person is underage, drunk, or under pressure from a person in power. Perhaps we need to consider similar rules for texting.

1. Never take or send a sexy image of a person under age 18. It is illegal.
2. When you are under the influence, you may regret any pictures you post. Wait to sober up before posting.

3. If you feel pressured to send a pic to someone, don't. While the vast majority of people report no negative outcomes of sexting, people who reported feeling pressured to send a sext were more likely to have a negative outcome. We even have a new word in our vocabulary, "sextortion," to describe when people use the threat of sharing pictures as a way to coerce more pictures or money from another person.

Perhaps the same rule we use for sex, "Yes means yes," could be applied to sharing photos too. Did the person who willingly sent you this photo say you could share it? Yes? Then go ahead. No? Then it was meant for you only; keep it that way.

Think about it: Do you engage in any sexting activity that could cause you future hurt or embarrassment? Do males and females face the same threat of embarrassment from shared photos or videos? Why or why not? If you receive a sexy photo from a person you barely know, what is your responsibility to protect his or her privacy?

**Sources:** S. Kashner, "Both Huntress and Prey," *Vanity Fair* 56, no. 11, November 2014, Available at www.vanityfair.com/hollywood/2014/10/jennifer-lawrence-photo-hacking-privacy; K. Smith, "Girl Meets Boa," *Vanity Fair* 57 no. 3, March 2015; L. Green, "Wanna Have Sex: Consent 101," Video, www.youtube.com/watch?v=TD2EooMhqRI, March 2014; E. Englander, "Coerced Sexting and Revenge Porn Among Teens," *Bullying, Teen Aggression and Social Media* 1, no. 2 (2015): 19–21; S. Harris-Lovett, "In Survey, 88% of U.S. Adults Said They Had Sexted and 96% of Them Endorsed It," *Los Angeles Times,* May 22, 2016, http://www.latimes.com/science/sciencenow/la-sci-sn-sexting-sexual-satisfaction-20150807-story.html.

---

Vibrators and dildos are two common types of toys and can be found in a variety of shapes, styles, and sizes. Sex toys can be used both to enhance the sexual experience and also as therapeutic devices to help with issues such as orgasmic difficulty and erectile dysfunction. For women who may not reach orgasm through intercourse, sex toys can provide another option for sexual satisfaction.[64] Note that all sex toys must be sanitized with soap and water after each use to remove bacteria.[65]

**Oral–Genital Stimulation** **Cunnilingus** refers to oral stimulation of a woman's genitals and **fellatio** to oral stimulation of a man's genitals. Many partners find oral stimulation intensely pleasurable. In the most recent National College Health Assessment (NCHA), 42 percent of all college students (64% of sexually active students) reported having oral sex in the past month.[66]

> **cunnilingus** Oral stimulation of a woman's genitals.
> **fellatio** Oral stimulation of a man's genitals.

**vaginal intercourse** Insertion of the penis into the vagina.

**anal intercourse** Insertion of the penis into the anus.

For some people, oral sex is not an option because of moral or religious beliefs. Remember, HIV and other STIs can be transmitted via unprotected oral–genital sex just as they can through intercourse. Use of an appropriate barrier device is strongly recommended if either partner's disease status is unknown. (See Chapter 15 for more about safer sex.)

**Vaginal Intercourse** The term *intercourse* generally refers to **vaginal intercourse** (*coitus*, or insertion of the penis into the vagina), which is the most frequently practiced form of sexual expression. In the latest NCHA survey, 47 percent of college students (70% of sexually active students) reported having vaginal intercourse in the past month.[67] Coitus can involve a variety of positions, including the missionary position (man on top facing the woman), woman on top, side by side, or man behind (rear entry). Many partners enjoy experimenting with different positions. Knowledge of yourself and your body, along with your ability to communicate effectively, will play a large part in determining the enjoyment and meaning of intercourse for you and your partner. Also, it is easier to relax and enjoy sex when you know that you are protected from disease and unintended pregnancy.

**Anal Intercourse** The anal area is highly sensitive to touch, and some couples find pleasure in stimulation. **Anal intercourse** is the insertion of the penis into the anus. Research indicates that 5 percent of college students (8% of sexually active students) have had anal sex in the past month.[68] Stimulation of the anus by mouth, fingers, or sex toys is also practiced. As with all forms of sexual expression, anal stimulation or intercourse is not for everyone. If you enjoy this form

of sexual expression, note that condom use is especially important, as the delicate tissues of the anus are more likely to tear than vaginal tissues, significantly increasing the risk of transmission of HIV and other STIs. Also, anything inserted into the anus (finger, penis, toys) should not be directly inserted into the vagina without sanitizing with soap and water, as bacteria commonly found in the anus can cause vaginal infections.

## Responsible and Satisfying Sexual Behavior

Healthy sexuality is a product of assimilating information and building skills, of exploring values and beliefs, and of making responsible and informed choices. In addition to Consent, Equality, Respect, Trust, and Safety, healthy and responsible sexuality should include the following:[69]

- **Good communication as the foundation.** Open and honest communication with your partner is the basis for establishing respect, trust, and intimacy. Do you communicate with your partner in caring and respectful ways? Can you express love and intimacy appropriately? Can you share your thoughts and emotions freely with your partner? Can you discuss your sexual history with your partner? Do you agree on contraception and disease prevention? Are you able to communicate what you like and don't like? These are all components of the open communication that is necessary for healthy, responsible sexuality. (See Chapter 8 for more on good communication.)

- **Acknowledging that you are a sexual person.** People who can see and accept themselves as sexual beings are more likely to make informed decisions and take responsible actions. If you see yourself as a potentially sexual person, you will plan ahead for contraception and disease prevention. If you are comfortable being a sexually active person, you will not need or want your sexual experiences to be clouded by alcohol or other drug use. If you choose not to be sexually active, you do so consciously, as a personal decision. Even if you are not sexually active, it is important to acknowledge that sex is a natural aspect of our lives and to recognize that you are in charge of your own decisions about your sexuality.

- **Understanding sexual functions and safety.** If you understand how the human body works, sexual pleasure and response will not be mysterious events. You will be better able to pleasure yourself and communicate to your partner how best to pleasure you. You will understand how pregnancy and STIs can be prevented. You will be able to recognize sexual dysfunction and take responsible actions to address the problem.

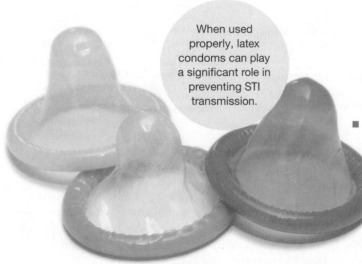

When used properly, latex condoms can play a significant role in preventing STI transmission.

- **Choosing healthy relationships.** Engaging in sexual behaviors within a healthy relationship improves intimacy. Do you value meaningful relationships? Are you steering clear of relationships that might be manipulative, or exploit you? Do you exhibit skills that enhance personal relationships? While some sexual behavior occurs outside relationships, the ability to form strong relationships is an important task in life.
- **Accepting and embracing your gender identity and your sexual orientation.** "Being comfortable in your own skin" is an old saying that is particularly relevant when it comes to sexuality. It is difficult to feel sexually satisfied if you are conflicted about your gender identity or sexual orientation. If you are confident in your sexuality, you can identify your values and live according to them. You should explore and address questions and feelings you may have. Good communication skills, acknowledging that you are a sexual person, understanding your sexual anatomy and its functions, and building strong relationships will help you to complete this task.
- **Becoming an advocate for others.** You can make your community more sexually healthy by advocating for others in a variety of ways. You can work to prevent sexual abuse. You can reject stereotypes and demonstrate tolerance for sexually diverse populations. You can vote for elected officials that will support legislation dealing with sexual issues. Know that you have a lot of power to make positive changes in the lives of those around you.

### Health Benefits of Sexual Behavior

If you asked a classmate what the benefits of engaging in sexual behaviors are, you might hear that "it feels good." But there is more to sex than just feeling good. Sex, especially within an intimate relationship, has health benefits too powerful to ignore:[70]

- **Stress and pain relief.** Being physically intimate can trigger the release of certain brain chemicals, including oxytocin (the "cuddle chemical"), endorphins, and prolactin, which leads to a relaxed feeling
- **Exercise.** In an average sexual encounter, men burn about 200 calories, and women about 70. Those burned calories can add up over a lifetime.
- **Brain activity.** In females, climax carries nutrient-filled blood and oxygen to 30 areas of the brain, far more than other brain-boosters like crossword puzzles.
- **Sleep.** The hormone oxytocin, released during orgasm, promotes better sleep, which is linked to both a stronger immune system and a longer lifespan.
- **Prostate cancer.** There is some evidence that frequent orgasm (more than 21 a month)—whether by masturbation, intercourse, or nocturnal emission—reduces a man's risk for prostate cancer.

- **Blood pressure.** Research shows a link between regular sex (not masturbation) and lowered systolic blood pressure in males. This is likely because sex is good aerobic exercise that uses the big muscles of the body in rhythmic and continuous motion.

## Variant Sexual Behavior

Although attitudes toward sexuality have changed substantially, some behaviors are still considered to be outside the norm. People who study sexuality prefer to use the neutral term **variant sexual behavior** to describe less common sexual behaviors, for example:

- **Group sex.** Sexual activity involving more than two people. Participants in group sex run a higher risk of exposure to HIV and other STIs than that associated with a sexual encounter with only one partner.
- **Swinging.** Also known as partner-swapping, swinging increases the risk of exposure to HIV and other STIs.
- **Fetishism.** Using inanimate objects to heighten sexual arousal. Objects of fetishes often enhance one of the senses, such as silky clothing or lingerie, food with pleasant smells, or fancy shoes.

Some variant sexual behaviors can be harmful to the individual, to others, or to both. Some of the following activities are illegal in certain states:

- **Exhibitionism.** Exposing one's genitals to strangers in public places. Most exhibitionists are seeking a reaction of shock or fear. Exhibitionism is a minor felony in most states.
- **Voyeurism.** Observing other people for sexual gratification. Most voyeurs are men who attempt to watch women undressing or bathing. Voyeurism is an invasion of privacy and is illegal in most states.
- **Sadomasochism.** Sexual activities in which gratification is achieved by inflicting pain (verbal or physical abuse) on a partner or by being the object of such infliction. A sadist is a person who enjoys inflicting pain, and a masochist enjoys experiencing pain. These activities are legal when they involve consenting partners.
- **Pedophilia.** Sexual activity or attraction between an adult and a child. Any sexual activity involving a minor, including possession of child pornography, is illegal in all states.
- **Autoerotic asphyxiation.** The practice of reducing or eliminating oxygen to the brain, usually by tying a cord around one's neck while masturbating to orgasm. Tragically, deaths have occurred when individuals unintentionally strangle themselves.

**variant sexual behavior** A sexual behavior that is not commonly practiced.

# STUDY **PLAN**

Customize your study plan—and master your health!—in the Study Area of **MasteringHealth.**

## **ASSESS** YOURSELF

**How well do you understand your sexuality?** Take the **What Are Your Sexual Attitudes?** assessment available on **MasteringHealth.™**

## CHAPTER **REVIEW**

To hear an MP3 Tutor Session, scan here or visit the Study Area in **MasteringHealth.**

### LO **1** Your Sexual Identity: More than Biology

- *Sexual identity* is determined by the interaction of genetic, physiological, and environmental factors. Biological sex, gender identity, gender roles, and sexual orientation are all blended into our sexual identity.
- *Sexual orientation* refers to a person's enduring emotional, romantic, or sexual attraction to others. Gay, lesbian, and bisexual persons are repeatedly the targets of sexual prejudice. *Sexual prejudice* refers to negative attitudes and hostile actions directed at members of a particular social group.

### LO **2** Sexual and Reproductive Anatomy and Physiology

- The major structures of female sexual anatomy include the mons pubis, labia minora and majora, clitoris, vagina, uterus, cervix, fallopian tubes, and ovaries. The major structures of male sexual anatomy are the penis, scrotum, testes, epididymides, vasa deferentia, ejaculatory ducts, urethra, and the accessory glands (seminal vesicles, prostate gland, and Cowper's glands).

### LO **3** Human Sexual Response

- Physiologically, both males and females experience four stages of sexual response: excitement/arousal, plateau, orgasm, and resolution.
- The processes of aging, sexual dysfunction, and drugs and alcohol can impact the sexual response cycle.

### LO **4** Expressing Your Sexuality

- People can express themselves sexually in a variety of ways, including celibacy, abstinence, autoerotic behaviors, kissing and erotic touch, manual stimulation, oral–genital stimulation, vaginal intercourse, and anal intercourse. Variant sexual behaviors are those that are less common. Some variant sexual behaviors are potentially harmful to others and are therefore illegal in some states.
- Responsible and satisfying sexuality involves good communication, acknowledging yourself as a sexual being, understanding sexual structures and functions, choosing healthy relationships, and accepting your gender identity and sexual orientation. Advocating for others' sexual health is an additional way we can demonstrate our own sexual health.
- There are many health benefits to engaging in sexual behavior, including stress relief, burned calories, better sleep after orgasm, and for men, lowered blood pressure and risk for prostate cancer.

## POP **QUIZ**

Visit **MasteringHealth** to personalize your study plan with Chapter Review Quizzes and Dynamic Study Modules.

### LO **1** Your Sexual Identity: More than Biology

1. Your personal inner sense of maleness or femaleness is known as your
   a. sexual identity.
   b. sexual orientation.
   c. gender identity.
   d. gender.

2. Individuals who are sexually attracted to both men and women are identified as
   a. heterosexual.
   b. bisexual.
   c. homosexual.
   d. intersex.

### LO **2** Sexual and Reproductive Anatomy and Physiology

3. The most sensitive part of the female genital region is the
   a. mons pubis.
   b. vagina.
   c. clitoris.
   d. labia.

4. When a woman is ovulating,
   a. she has released an egg.
   b. she is experiencing menstrual bleeding.
   c. an egg has been fertilized and she is pregnant.
   d. she is experiencing PMS.

5. What is the role of testosterone in the male reproductive system?
   a. It is used to produce sperm for reproduction.
   b. It is the hormone that stimulates development of secondary male sex characteristics.
   c. It allows the penis to harden during sexual arousal.
   d. It secretes the seminal fluid preceding ejaculation.

### LO 3 | Human Sexual Response

6. Which of the following is *true* regarding the first stage of the human sexual response?
   a. In men, testes become completely engorged.
   b. In men and women, the rectal sphincter contracts.
   c. In men, the Cowper's gland may release fluid.
   d. In men and women, vasocongestion occurs.

### LO 4 | Expressing Your Sexuality

7. Fellatio is the oral stimulation of the
   a. male genitals.
   b. female genitals.
   c. anal region.
   d. mouth and tongue.

8. The pain that a woman may experience during sexual intercourse due to involuntary contraction of vaginal muscles is called
   a. dysmenorrhea.
   b. amenorrhea.
   c. dyspareunia.
   d. vaginismus.

9. What is the effect of alcohol on sex?
   a. It promotes feelings of aversion.
   b. It promotes greater sexual satisfaction.
   c. It inhibits sexual response.
   d. It inhibits pregnancy.

10. Benefits of sexual activity include all except:
    a. improved sleep.
    b. lowered blood pressure in males.
    c. reduced breast cancer in females.
    d. increased brain activity.

*Answers to the Pop Quiz can be found on page A-1. If you answered a question incorrectly, review the section identified by the Learning Outcome. For even more study tools, visit MasteringHealth.*

# THINK ABOUT IT!

### LO 1 | Your Sexual Identity: More than Biology

1. How have gender roles changed over your lifetime? Do you view the changes as positive for both men and women?

2. If scientists are able to establish the combination of factors that interact to produce homosexual, heterosexual, or bisexual orientation, will that put an end to prejudice against people who are gay? Why or why not?

### LO 2 | Sexual and Reproductive Anatomy and Physiology

3. Have you ever discussed with your friends what it was like going through puberty? Did you understand what was happening to you physically and emotionally and why?

### LO 3 | Human Sexual Response

4. What makes a person's sexual response to one human vastly different from that to another human or from one sexual experience to another with the same partner?

### LO 4 | Expressing Your Sexuality

5. What criteria do you use to determine "normal" sexual behavior? What criteria should we use to determine healthy sexual practices?

6. How can we remove the stigma that surrounds sexual dysfunction so that individuals feel more comfortable seeking help? Are men and women affected differently by sexual dysfunction?

7. What is the role of alcohol in the sex lives of your peers? How does it both improve and lessen the sexual experience?

# ACCESS YOUR HEALTH ON THE INTERNET

Visit **MasteringHealth** for links to the websites and RSS feeds.

The following websites explore further topics and issues related to sexuality.

**American Association of Sex Educators, Counselors, and Therapists (AASECT).** AASECT is a professional organization that provides standards of practice for treatment of sexual issues and disorders and provides referrals to local counselors and clinics. **www.aasect.org**

**SmarterSex.org.** This site, created by the peer education group BACCHUS network, presents user-friendly information on sexual health targeted at 18- to 24-year-olds. **www.smartersex.org**

**Go Ask Alice.** Columbia University Health Services provides this interactive question-and-answer resource. "Alice" is available to answer questions about any health-related issues, including relationships, nutrition and diet, exercise, drugs, sex, alcohol, and stress. **www.goaskalice.columbia.edu**

**Sexuality Information and Education Council of the United States (SIECUS).** SIECUS provides information, guidelines, and materials for advancement of healthy and proper sex education. **www.siecus.org**

**Advocates for Youth.** Here you can find current news, policy updates, research, and other resources about the sexual health and choices particular to high school and college students. **www.advocatesforyouth.org**

**Rape, Abuse, and Incest National Network (RAINN).** This antisexual assault organization provides information on a variety of topics and live anonymous support via phone (800-656-4673) or a Web-based crisis chatline. **www.rainn.org**

# 10 Considering Your Reproductive Choices

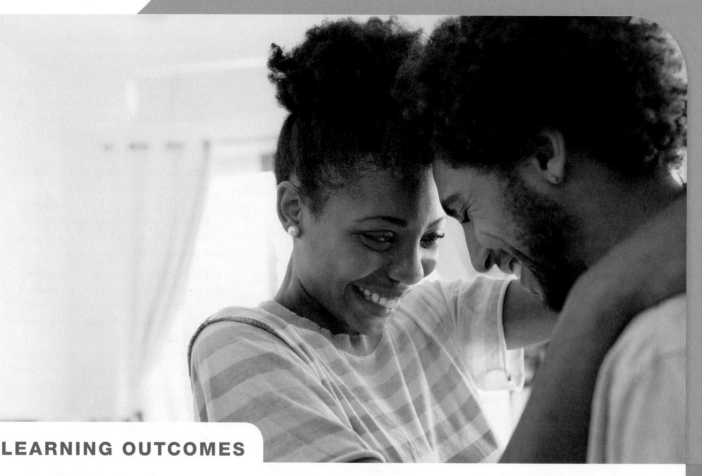

## LEARNING OUTCOMES

LO **1** Discuss key issues to consider when planning a pregnancy, describe the process of pregnancy and fetal development, and explain the importance of prenatal care.

LO **2** Explain the basic stages of childbirth and complications that can arise during pregnancy, labor, and delivery.

LO **3** Review primary causes of and possible solutions for infertility.

LO **4** Explain the process of conception and describe how the effectiveness of contraception is measured.

LO **5** Compare and contrast the advantages, disadvantages, and effectiveness of different types of contraception in preventing pregnancy and sexually transmitted infections, and describe emergency contraception and its use.

LO **6** List and explain factors that you should consider when choosing a method of contraception.

LO **7** Summarize the political issues surrounding abortion and the various types of abortion procedures.

## LO 1 | PREGNANCY

**Discuss key issues to consider when planning a pregnancy, describe the process of pregnancy and fetal development, and explain the importance of prenatal care.**

Pregnancy is an important event in a woman's life, and in the life of her partner. The actions taken before as well as behaviors engaged in during pregnancy can significantly affect the health of both infant and mother.

## Planning for Pregnancy and Parenthood

Today, sexually active people are able to choose if and when they want to have children. As you approach the decision of whether or not to have children, or when to do so, take the time to evaluate your emotions, finances, and physical health. If you decide to remain childless, you will be part of a growing number of Americans remaining child-free. See the **Health in a Diverse World** box on page 264 for more information.

**Emotional Health** Before becoming pregnant, consider first and foremost why you may want to have a child. To fulfill an inner need to carry on the family? To share love? To give your parents grandchildren? To have a close tie or friendship? Then, consider the responsibilities involved with becoming a parent. Are you ready to make all the sacrifices necessary to bear and raise a child? Can you care for this new human being in a loving and nurturing manner? Do you have a strong social support system? This emotional preparation for parenthood can be as important as the physical preparation.

**WHAT DO YOU THINK?**

Have you thought about whether or when to have children?

- Is there a certain age at which you feel you will be ready to be a parent?
- What are your biggest concerns about parenthood?
- What are some common misconceptions about people who choose not to have children?

**Financial Evaluation** Finances are another important consideration. Can you afford to give your child the life you would like him or her to enjoy? The U.S. Department of Agriculture estimates that it will cost an average of $245,340 to raise a child born today to age 18, not including college tuition.[1]

It is important to check whether your medical insurance provides maternity benefits. If not, you can expect to pay, on average, $18,000 for a normal delivery and up to $28,000 for a cesarean section, including prenatal care.[2] Both partners should investigate their employers' policies concerning parental leave, including length of leave available and conditions for returning to work.

**Maternal Age** The average age at which a woman has her first child has been creeping up (from 21 in 1970 to 26 today), so a woman who becomes pregnant in her 30s has plenty of company.[3] In fact, births to women in their 20s are declining, the rate of first births to women between the ages of 30 and 39 is the highest reported in four decades, and births to women over age 39 have continued to increase slightly over the years.[4]

Statistically, the chances of having a baby with birth defects rise after the age of 35. Researchers believe this is due to a decline in the quality of eggs after this age. Two specific age-related risks are **Down syndrome** and miscarriage. The risk of miscarriage nearly doubles for women 35 to 45 compared to women under 35.[5] Another concern is that a woman's fertility begins to decline as she ages. A gradual decline in fertility begins around age 32 and fertility decreases more rapidly after age 37 because of the reduction in the number and quality of eggs in the ovaries.[6] While some risks increase with age, many doctors note that older mothers bring some advantages to their pregnancies: They tend to follow medical advice during pregnancy more thoroughly, are more mature psychologically, are better prepared financially, and are generally more ready to care for an infant than are some younger women.

**Physical Health: Maternal Health** The birth of a healthy baby depends in part on the mother's **preconception care**. The fetus is most susceptible to developing certain problems in the first 4 to 10 weeks after conception, before prenatal care is normally initiated. Since many women don't realize they are pregnant until later, they often can't reduce health risks unless intervention begins before conception.[7] Maternal factors that can affect a fetus or infant include drug use (illicit, prescription, or over-the-counter), alcohol consumption, tobacco use, or obesity. To promote preconception health, get the best medical care you can, practice healthy behaviors,

**Down syndrome** A genetic disorder caused by the presence of an extra chromosome that results in mental disabilities and distinctive physical characteristics.

**preconception care** Medical care received prior to becoming pregnant that helps a woman assess and address potential health issues.

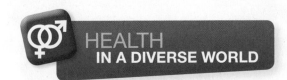
build a strong support network, and encourage safe environments at home and at work.[8]

Nutrition counseling is an important part of preconception care. Among the many important nutrition issues is folic acid (folate) intake. When consumed the month before conception and during early pregnancy, folate reduces the risk of spina bifida, a congenital birth defect resulting from failure of the spinal column to close. A woman also needs to make sure her immunizations are up-to-date before becoming pregnant. If, for example, she has never had rubella (German measles), a woman needs to be immunized prior to becoming pregnant. A rubella infection can kill the fetus or cause blindness or hearing disorders in the infant.

For suggestions on preparing for a healthy pregnancy, see the Making Changes Today box on page 267.

### Physical Health: Paternal Health

Fathers-to-be are recommended to practice the same healthy habits as mothers-to-be because, by one route or another, dozens of chemicals studied so far (from occupational exposures to by-products of cigarette smoke) appear to harm sperm.[9] A fathers' age may also play a role; recent research shows a relationship between older fathers and autism, attention-deficit/hyperactivity disorder, bipolar disorder, and schizophrenia.[10]

### Contingency Planning

A final consideration is how to provide for your child should something happen to you and your partner. If both of you were to die, do you have relatives or close friends who could raise your child? If you have more than one child, would they have to be split up or could they be kept together? Although unpleasant to think about, this sort of contingency planning is crucial. Children who lose their parents are heartbroken and confused. A prearranged plan of action can smooth their transition into new families; without one, a judge will usually decide who will raise them.

## The Process of Pregnancy

The process of pregnancy begins the moment a sperm fertilizes an ovum in the fallopian tubes (**FIGURE 10.1**). From there, the single fertilized cell, now called a *zygote*, multiplies and becomes a sphere-shaped cluster of cells called a *blastocyst* that travels toward the uterus, a journey that may take 3 to 4 days. Upon arrival, the embryo burrows into the thick, spongy endometrium (implantation) and is nourished from this carefully prepared lining.

### Pregnancy Testing

A pregnancy test scheduled with your health care provider or at a local family-planning clinic will confirm a pregnancy. Women who wish to know immediately can purchase home pregnancy test kits sold over-the-counter in drugstores. A positive test is based on the secretion of **human chorionic gonadotropin (HCG)**, which is found in the woman's urine.

Home pregnancy tests vary, but some can be used as early as a week after conception and many are 99 percent reliable.[11] If the test is done too early in the pregnancy, it may show a false negative. Other causes of false negatives are unclean testing devices, ingestion of certain drugs, and vaginal or urinary tract

**human chorionic gonadotropin (HCG)** Hormone detectable in blood or urine samples of a mother within the first few weeks of pregnancy.

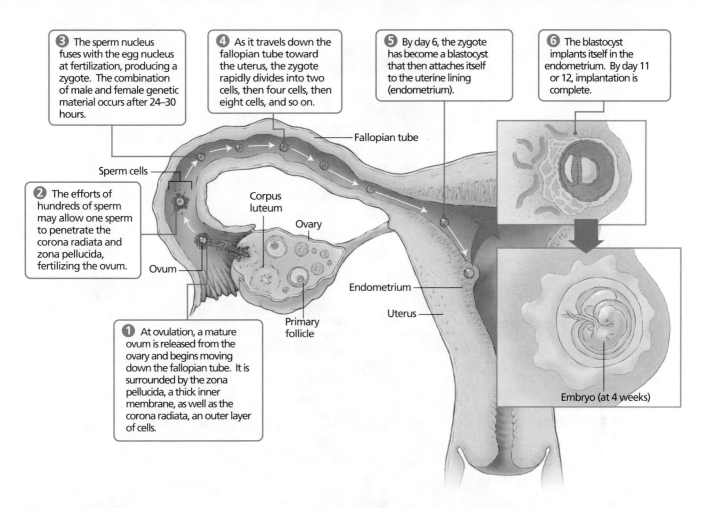

**3** The sperm nucleus fuses with the egg nucleus at fertilization, producing a zygote. The combination of male and female genetic material occurs after 24–30 hours.

**4** As it travels down the fallopian tube toward the uterus, the zygote rapidly divides into two cells, then four cells, then eight cells, and so on.

**5** By day 6, the zygote has become a blastocyst that then attaches itself to the uterine lining (endometrium).

**6** The blastocyst implants itself in the endometrium. By day 11 or 12, implantation is complete.

Fallopian tube

Sperm cells

**2** The efforts of hundreds of sperm may allow one sperm to penetrate the corona radiata and zona pellucida, fertilizing the ovum.

Corpus luteum

Ovary

Ovum

Primary follicle

Endometrium

Uterus

**1** At ovulation, a mature ovum is released from the ovary and begins moving down the fallopian tube. It is surrounded by the zona pellucida, a thick inner membrane, as well as the corona radiata, an outer layer of cells.

Embryo (at 4 weeks)

**FIGURE 10.1** Fertilization usually occurs in the upper third of the fallopian tube, and implantation in the uterus takes place about 6 days later.

infections. Blood tests administered and analyzed in a doctor's office are more accurate than home urine tests.

## Early Signs of Pregnancy

A woman's body undergoes substantial changes during a pregnancy (**FIGURE 10.2** on page 266). The first sign of pregnancy is usually a missed menstrual period (although some women "spot" in early pregnancy, which may be mistaken for a period). Other signs include breast tenderness, emotional upset, extreme fatigue, sleeplessness, nausea, and vomiting (especially in the morning).

Pregnancy typically lasts 40 weeks and is divided into three phases, or **trimesters**, of approximately 3 months each. The due date is calculated from the expectant mother's last menstrual period.

## The First Trimester

During the first trimester, few noticeable changes occur in the mother's body. She may urinate more frequently and experience morning sickness, swollen breasts, or undue fatigue. These symptoms may not be frequent or severe, so women often do not realize they are pregnant right away. During the first 2 months after conception, the **embryo** differentiates and develops its various organ systems, beginning with the nervous and circulatory systems. At the start of the third month, the embryo is called a **fetus**,

indicating that all organ systems are in place. For the rest of the pregnancy, growth and refinement occur in each body system so that at birth they can function independently, yet in coordination with all the others. The photos in **FIGURE 10.3** on page 267 illustrate physical changes during fetal development.

## The Second Trimester

At the beginning of the second trimester, the fourth through sixth months of pregnancy, physical changes in the mother become more visible. Her breasts swell and her waistline thickens. During this time, the fetus makes greater demands on the mother's body. In particular, the **placenta**, the network of blood vessels that carries nutrients and oxygen to the fetus and fetal waste products to the mother, becomes well established.

## The Third Trimester

The end of the sixth month through the ninth mark the third trimester. This is the period of greatest fetal growth. The growing fetus depends entirely on its mother for nutrition and

**trimester** A 3-month segment of pregnancy.

**embryo** Fertilized egg from conception through the eighth week of development.

**fetus** Developing human from the ninth week until birth.

**placenta** Network of blood vessels connected to the umbilical cord that transports oxygen and nutrients to a developing fetus and carries away fetal wastes.

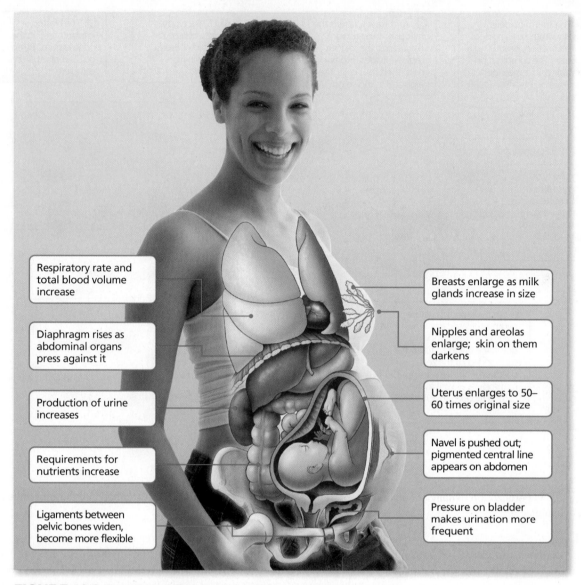

Respiratory rate and total blood volume increase

Diaphragm rises as abdominal organs press against it

Production of urine increases

Requirements for nutrients increase

Ligaments between pelvic bones widen, become more flexible

Breasts enlarge as milk glands increase in size

Nipples and areolas enlarge; skin on them darkens

Uterus enlarges to 50–60 times original size

Navel is pushed out; pigmented central line appears on abdomen

Pressure on bladder makes urination more frequent

**FIGURE 10.2** Changes in a Woman's Body during Pregnancy

must receive large amounts of calcium, iron, and protein from the mother's diet. Although the fetus may survive if it is born during the seventh month, it needs the layer of fat it acquires during the eighth month and time for the organs (especially the respiratory and digestive organs) to develop fully. Infants born prematurely usually require intensive medical care.

**Emotional Changes** Of course, the process of pregnancy involves much more than the changes in a woman's body and the developing fetus. Many important emotional changes occur from the time a woman learns she is pregnant through the postpartum period (the first 6 weeks after her baby is born). Throughout pregnancy, women may experience fear of complications, anxiety about becoming a parent, and wonder and excitement over the developing baby.

## Prenatal Care

A successful pregnancy depends on a mother who takes good care of herself and her fetus. Good nutrition and exercise; avoiding drugs, alcohol, and other harmful substances; and regular medical checkups from the beginning of pregnancy are all essential. Early detection of fetal abnormalities, identification of high-risk mothers and infants, and screening for possible complications are the major purposes of prenatal care. See **TABLE 10.1** on page 268 for tips on choosing a prenatal care provider.

Ideally, a woman should begin prenatal appointments in the first trimester. On the first visit, the practitioner should obtain a complete medical history of the mother and her family and note any hereditary conditions that could put a woman or her fetus at risk. Regular checkups to measure weight gain and blood pressure and to monitor the fetus's size and position should continue throughout the pregnancy.

**Nutrition and Exercise** Despite "eating for two," pregnant women only need about 300 additional calories a day. Special attention should be paid to getting enough folic acid (found in dark leafy greens, citrus fruits, and beans), iron (dried fruits, meats, legumes, liver, egg yolks), calcium (nonfat or low-fat dairy

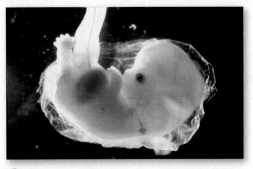

**a** A human embryo during the first trimester. The embryonic period lasts from the third to the eighth week of development. By the end of the embryonic period, all organs have formed.

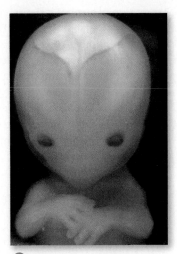

**b** A human fetus during the second trimester. Growth during the fetal period is very rapid.

products and some canned fish), and fluids. While vitamin supplements can correct some deficiencies, there is no substitute for a well-balanced diet. Babies born to poorly nourished mothers run high risks of substandard mental and physical development.

Weight gain during pregnancy helps nourish a growing baby. For a woman of normal weight before pregnancy, the recommended gain during pregnancy is 25 to 35 pounds.[12] For overweight women, weight gain of 15 to 25 pounds is recommended, and for obese women, 11 to 20 pounds is recommended.[13] Underweight women should gain 28 to 40 pounds, and women carrying twins should gain about 35 to 45 pounds.[14] Gaining too much or too little weight can lead to complications. With higher weight gains, women may develop gestational diabetes, hypertension, or increased risk of delivery complications. Gaining too little increases the chance of a low birth weight baby.

As in all other stages of life, exercise is an important factor in overall health during pregnancy. Regular exercise is recommended for pregnant women; however, they should consult with their health care provider before starting any exercise program. Exercise can help control weight, make labor easier,

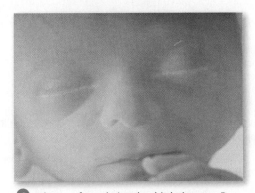

**c** A human fetus during the third trimester. By the end of the fetal period, the growth rate of the head has slowed relative to the growth rate of the rest of the body.

**FIGURE 10.3** Fetoscopic Photographs Showing Development in the First, Second, and Third Trimesters of Pregnancy

and help with a faster recovery due to increased strength and endurance. Women can usually maintain their customary level of activity during most of the pregnancy, although there are some cautions: Pregnant women should avoid exercise that puts them at risk of falling or having an abdominal injury, and in the third trimester, exercises that involve lying on the back should be avoided as they can restrict blood flow to the uterus.

## Avoiding Drugs, Alcohol, Tobacco, and Other Teratogens

A woman should consult with a health care provider regarding the safety of any drugs she might use during pregnancy. Even too much of common over-the-counter medications such as aspirin can damage a developing fetus. During the first 3 months of pregnancy, the fetus is especially subject to the **teratogenic** (birth defect–causing) effects of drugs, environmental chemicals, X-rays, or diseases. The fetus can also develop an addiction to or tolerance for drugs that the mother is using.

Maternal consumption of alcohol is detrimental to a growing fetus. Birth defects associated with **fetal alcohol syndrome (FAS)** include developmental disabilities, neural and cardiac impairments, and cranial and facial deformities. The exact amount of alcohol that causes FAS is not known; therefore, the American Congress of Obstetricians and Gynecologists recommends completely avoiding alcohol during pregnancy.[15]

Women who smoke during pregnancy have a greater chance of miscarriage, complications,

**teratogenic** Causing birth defects; may refer to drugs, environmental chemicals, radiation, or diseases.

**fetal alcohol syndrome (FAS)** Pattern of birth defects, learning, and behavioral problems in a child caused by the mother's alcohol consumption during pregnancy.

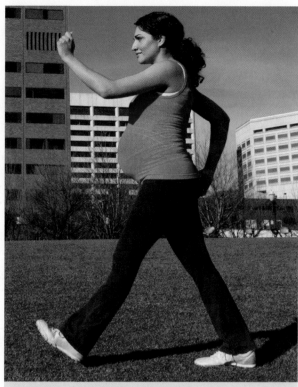

A doctor-approved exercise program during pregnancy can help control weight, make delivery easier, and have a healthy effect on the fetus.

## TABLE 10.1 | Choosing a Prenatal Care Provider

| Provider/Description | Advantages | Disadvantages |
|---|---|---|
| *Obstetrician/gynecologist:* MD who specializes in obstetrics (care of a woman and child during pregnancy, birth, and the postpartum period) and gynecology (care of the reproductive system of women) | Trained to handle all types of pregnancy- and delivery-related emergencies. | Generally can perform deliveries only in a hospital setting. Cannot serve as the baby's physician after birth. |
| *Family practitioner:* MD or nurse practitioner who provides comprehensive care for people of all ages | No need to change physicians; can refer to a specialist if necessary, can serve as the baby's physician after birth. | Some provide pregnancy care only to low-risk pregnancies; rarely perform home births. |
| *Midwife:* Experienced practitioner who can assist with pregnancies and deliveries. Midwives can oversee delivery of babies in nonhospital birthing sites, such as home deliveries or birthing centers. Most strive to help women have a natural childbirth experience. | | |
| *Certified nurse midwife:* RN or NP with specialized training in pregnancy and delivery; most work in private practice or in conjunction with physicians. | Certified nurse midwives have formal training and accreditation. They may work with physicians and have access to traditional medical facilities, but are often able to offer more personal attention than a MD could. | RNs cannot provide medication without physician approval, but NPs can in many states; need to refer to physician when the pregnancy is deemed high risk. |
| *Lay midwives:* Uncertified or unlicensed midwife who was educated through informal routes such as self-study or apprenticeship rather than through a formal program. | Lay midwives tend to view pregnancy and childbirth as a family event. They usually offer low-intervention, highly personalized birth plans. Home birth can lower costs. | Cannot administer any medication; would need to refer to a physician. May not have extensive training in handling an emergency. Women should carefully evaluate the credentials of a prospective lay midwife and seriously consider the risks related to delivery outside a hospital. |

premature births, low birth weight infants, stillbirth, and infant mortality specifically due to **sudden infant death syndrome**.[16] Smoking restricts the blood supply to the developing fetus and thus limits oxygen and nutrition delivery and waste removal. Tobacco use also appears to be a significant factor in the development of cleft lip and palate.[17]

A pregnant woman should avoid exposure to X-rays, toxic chemicals, heavy metals, pesticides, gases, and other hazardous compounds. She should also avoid cleaning litter boxes, if possible, because cat feces can contain organisms that cause **toxoplasmosis**. If a pregnant woman contracts this disease, the baby may be stillborn or suffer mental disabilities or other birth defects. Pregnant women should also avoid traveling to areas with the Zika virus, a mosquito-borne virus associated with children being born with microcephaly—a small head, compared to babies of the same age and sex—as well as eye defects, hearing loss, and some severe brain defects.[18]

**Prenatal Testing and Screening** Modern technology enables medical practitioners to detect health defects in a fetus as early as the 14th to 18th weeks of pregnancy. One common test is **ultrasonography** or **ultrasound**, which uses high-frequency sound waves to create a *sonogram*, or visual image, of the fetus in the uterus. The sonogram is used to determine the fetus's size and position, which can help to safely deliver the infant. Sonograms can also detect birth defects in the nervous and digestive systems.

**Chorionic villus sampling (CVS)** involves snipping tissue from the developing fetal sac. Chorionic villus sampling can be used at 10 to 12 weeks of pregnancy. This is an attractive option for couples who are at high risk for having a baby with Down syndrome or a debilitating hereditary disease.

The **triple marker screen** (often called the TMS or AFT [alpha-fetoprotein] test) is a commonly used maternal blood test that is optimally conducted between the 16th and 18th weeks of pregnancy. The TMS is a screening test, not a diagnostic tool; it can detect susceptibility for a birth defect or genetic abnormality, but it is not meant to confirm a diagnosis of any condition. A *quad screen test* (or AFP-plus test), which screens for an additional protein in maternal blood, is more accurate than the triple marker screen. Even more precise is the *integrated screen*, which uses the quad screen, plus results from an earlier blood test, plus ultrasound, to screen for abnormalities.

**Amniocentesis** is a common testing procedure that is strongly recommended for women over age 35. This test involves inserting a long needle through the mother's abdominal and uterine walls into the **amniotic sac**, the protective pouch surrounding the fetus. The needle draws out 3 to 4 teaspoons of fluid, which is analyzed for genetic information about the baby (**FIGURE 10.4**). Amniocentesis can be performed between weeks 14 and 18.

If any of these tests reveals a serious birth defect, parents are advised to undergo genetic counseling. In the case of a chromosomal abnormality such as Down syndrome, the parents are usually offered the option of a therapeutic abortion. Some parents choose this option; others research the condition and decide to continue the pregnancy.

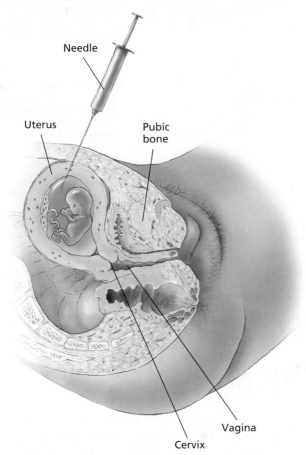

**FIGURE 10.4 Amniocentesis** The process of amniocentesis, in which a long needle is used to withdraw a small amount of amniotic fluid for genetic analysis, can detect certain congenital problems as well as the fetus's sex.

**sudden infant death syndrome (SIDS)** Sudden death of an infant under 1 year of age for no apparent reason.

**toxoplasmosis** Disease caused by an organism found in cat feces that, when contracted by a pregnant woman, may result in stillbirth or birth defects.

**ultrasonography (ultrasound)** Common prenatal test that uses sound waves to create a visual image of a developing fetus.

**chorionic villus sampling (CVS)** Prenatal test that involves snipping tissue from the fetal sac to be analyzed for genetic defects.

**triple marker screen (TMS)** Common maternal blood test that can be used to identify certain birth defects and genetic abnormalities in a fetus.

**amniocentesis** Medical test in which a small amount of fluid is drawn from the amniotic sac to test for Down syndrome and other genetic abnormalities.

**amniotic sac** Protective pouch surrounding the fetus.

## LO 2 | CHILDBIRTH

Explain the basic stages of childbirth and complications that can arise during pregnancy, labor, and delivery.

Prospective parents need to make several key decisions before the baby is born. These include where to have the baby, whether to use pain medication during labor and delivery, which childbirth method to choose, and whether to breastfeed or use formula. Answering these questions in advance will help to smooth the passage into parenthood.

# Labor and Delivery

During the final weeks preceding delivery, the baby normally shifts to a head-down position, and the cervix begins to dilate (widen). The junction of the pubic bones loosens to permit expansion of the pelvic girdle during birth. The exact mechanisms that initiate labor are unknown. A change in the hormones in the fetus and mother cause strong uterine contractions to occur, signaling the beginning of labor. Another common early signal is the breaking of the amniotic sac, which causes a rush of fluid from the vagina (commonly referred to as "water breaking").

The birth process has three stages, shown in **FIGURE 10.5**, which can last from several hours to more than a day. In some cases, toward the end of the second stage, the attending health care provider may perform an *episiotomy*, a straight incision in the mother's perineum (the area between the vulva and the anus) to prevent the baby's head from tearing vaginal tissues and to speed the baby's exit from the vagina. After delivery, the attending provider assesses the baby's overall condition, clears the baby's mucus-filled breathing passages, and ties and severs the umbilical cord. The mother's uterus continues to contract in the third stage of labor until the placenta is expelled.

**Managing Labor** Pain medication given to the mother during labor can cause sluggish responses in the newborn and other complications. For this reason, some women choose a drug-free labor and delivery—but it is important to keep a flexible attitude about pain relief because each labor is different. One person is not a "success" for delivering without medication or another a "failure" for using medical measures.

The Lamaze method is the most popular technique of childbirth preparation in the United States. It discourages the use of pain medication. Prelabor classes teach the mother to control her pain through special breathing patterns, focusing exercises, and relaxation. The partner (or labor coach) assists by giving emotional support, physical comfort, and coaching for proper breath control during contractions.

**Cesarean Section** If labor lasts too long or if a baby is in physiological distress or is about to exit the uterus any way but headfirst, a **cesarean section (C-section)** may be necessary. This surgical procedure involves making an incision across the mother's abdomen and through the uterus to remove the baby. A C-section may also be performed if labor is extremely difficult, maternal blood pressure falls rapidly, the placenta separates from the uterus too soon, the mother has diabetes, or other problems occur. Risks are the same as for any major abdominal surgery, and recovery from birth takes considerably longer after a C-section.

The rate of delivery by C-section in the United States has increased from 5 percent in the mid-1960s to nearly one-third of all births today.[19] Although this procedure is necessary in certain cases, some doctors and critics, including the Centers for Disease Control and Prevention (CDC), feel that C-sections

**cesarean section (C-section)** Surgical birthing procedure in which a baby is removed through an incision made in the mother's abdominal wall and uterus.

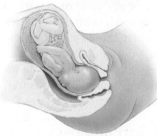

**1** **Stage I: Dilation of the cervix** Contractions in the abdomen and lower back push the baby downward, putting pressure on the cervix and dilating it. The first stage of labor may last from a couple of hours to more than a day for a first birth, but it is usually much shorter during subsequent births.

**2** **End of Stage I: Transition** The cervix becomes fully dilated, and the baby's head begins to move into the vagina (birth canal). Contractions usually come quickly during transition, which generally lasts 30 minutes or less.

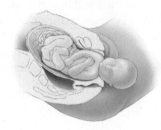

**3** **Stage II: Expulsion** Once the cervix has become fully dilated, contractions become rhythmic, strong, and more intense as the uterus pushes the baby headfirst through the birth canal. The expulsion stage lasts 1 to 4 hours and concludes when the infant is finally pushed out of the mother's body.

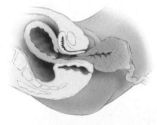

**4** **Stage III: Delivery of the placenta** In the third stage, the placenta detaches from the uterus and is expelled through the birth canal. This stage is usually completed within 30 minutes after delivery.

**FIGURE 10.5 The Birth Process** The entire process of labor and delivery usually takes from 2 to 36 hours. Labor is generally longer for a woman's first delivery and shorter for subsequent births.

are performed too frequently in this country. Natural birth advocates suggest that hospitals, driven by profits and worried about malpractice, are too quick to intervene in the birth process. Some doctors say that the increase is due to maternal demand: busy mothers want to schedule their deliveries.[20]

## Complications of Pregnancy and Childbirth

Pregnancy carries the risk for potential complications and problems that can interfere with the proper development of the fetus or threaten the health of the mother and child. Some complications may result from a preexisting health condition of the mother, such as diabetes or an STI, and others can develop during pregnancy and may result from physiological problems, genetic abnormalities, or exposure to teratogens.

## Preeclampsia and Eclampsia

**Preeclampsia** is a condition characterized by high blood pressure, protein in the urine, and edema (fluid retention), which usually causes swelling of the hands and face. Symptoms may include sudden weight gain, headache, nausea or vomiting, changes in vision, racing pulse, mental confusion, and stomach or right shoulder pain. If preeclampsia is not treated, it can cause strokes and seizures, a condition called *eclampsia*. Potential problems can include liver and kidney damage, internal bleeding, poor fetal growth, and fetal and maternal death.

Preeclampsia tends to occur in the late second or third trimester. The cause is unknown; however, the incidence is higher in first-time mothers; women over 40 or under 18 years of age; women carrying multiple fetuses; and women with a history of chronic hypertension, diabetes, kidney disorder, or previous history of preeclampsia.[21] Family history of preeclampsia is also a risk factor. Treatment for preeclampsia ranges from bedrest and monitoring for mild cases to hospitalization and close monitoring for more severe cases.

## Miscarriage

Even when a woman does everything "right," not every pregnancy ends in a healthy delivery. In fact, in the United States, between 15 to 20 percent of known pregnancies end in **miscarriage** (also referred to as *spontaneous abortion*).[22] Most miscarriages occur during the first trimester.

Reasons for miscarriage vary. In some cases, the fertilized egg has failed to divide correctly. In others, genetic abnormalities, maternal illness, or infections are responsible. Maternal hormonal imbalance may also cause a miscarriage, as may a weak cervix, toxic chemicals in the environment, or physical trauma to the mother. In most cases, the cause is not known.

## Rh Factor

A rare blood incompatibility between mother and fetus can cause Rh factor problems, sometimes resulting in miscarriage. Rh is a blood protein, and problems occur when the mother is Rh-negative and the fetus is Rh-positive.[23] During a first birth, some of the baby's blood passes into the mother's bloodstream. An Rh-negative mother may manufacture antibodies to destroy the Rh-positive blood introduced into her bloodstream at the time of birth.[24] Her first baby will be unaffected, but subsequent babies with positive Rh factor will be at risk for a severe anemia called *hemolytic disease* because the mother's Rh antibodies will attack the fetus's red blood cells.[25] Prevention is preferable to treatment. Women with Rh-negative blood should be injected with a medication called RhoGAM within 72 hours after any birth, miscarriage, or abortion.[26] The injection prevents the mother from developing Rh antibodies.

## Ectopic Pregnancy

The implantation of a fertilized egg outside the uterus, usually in the fallopian tube or occasionally in the pelvic cavity, is called an **ectopic pregnancy**. Because these structures are not capable of expanding and nourishing a developing fetus, the pregnancy must be terminated surgically or a miscarriage will occur. If an ectopic pregnancy progresses undiagnosed and untreated, the fallopian tube will rupture, which puts the woman at great risk of hemorrhage, peritonitis (infection in the abdomen), and even death. Ectopic pregnancy occurs in about 2 percent of pregnancies in North America and is a leading cause of maternal mortality in the first trimester.[27]

## Stillbirth

**Stillbirth** is the death of a fetus *after* the 20th week of pregnancy but before delivery. A stillborn baby is born dead, often for no apparent reason. Each year in the United States, there is about 1 stillbirth in every 160 births.[28] Birth defects, placental problems, poor fetal growth, infections, and umbilical cord accidents are known contributing factors.

# The Postpartum Period

The postpartum period lasts 6 weeks after delivery. During this period, many women experience fluctuating emotions. Many new mothers experience what is called the "baby blues," characterized by periods of sadness, anxiety, headache, sleep disturbances, and irritability. About 1 in 7 new mothers experience **postpartum depression**, a more disabling syndrome characterized by mood swings, lack of energy, crying, guilt, and depression any time within the first year after childbirth.[29] Mothers who experience postpartum depression should seek professional treatment. Counseling is the most common type of treatment, but sometimes medication is recommended.[30]

## Breastfeeding

Although the new mother's milk will not begin to flow for 2 or more days after delivery, her breasts secrete a yellow fluid called *colostrum* beginning immediately after birth. Because colostrum contains vital antibodies to help fight infection and boost the baby's immune system, all newborns should be allowed to suckle at the breast.

The American Academy of Pediatrics strongly recommends that infants be exclusively breast-fed for 6 months and breast-fed as a supplement until 12 months of age.[31] Scientific findings indicate there are many advantages to breast-feeding. Breast milk is perfectly matched to babies' nutritional needs as they grow. Breast-fed babies have fewer illnesses and a much lower hospitalization rate because breast milk contains maternal antibodies and immunological cells that stimulate the infant's immune system. When breast-fed babies do get sick, they recover more quickly. They are also less likely to be obese later in life than are babies fed formula, and they have fewer allergies. They may even be more intelligent: A recent study found that the longer a baby was breast-fed, the higher the IQ in adulthood.[32]

**preeclampsia** Pregnancy complication characterized by high blood pressure, protein in the urine, and edema.

**miscarriage** Loss of the fetus before it is viable; also called *spontaneous abortion*.

**ectopic pregnancy** Dangerous condition that results from the implantation of a fertilized egg outside the uterus, usually in a fallopian tube.

**stillbirth** Death of a fetus after the 20th week of pregnancy but before delivery.

**postpartum depression** Mood disorder experienced by women who have given birth; involves depression, fatigue, and other symptoms and may last for weeks or months.

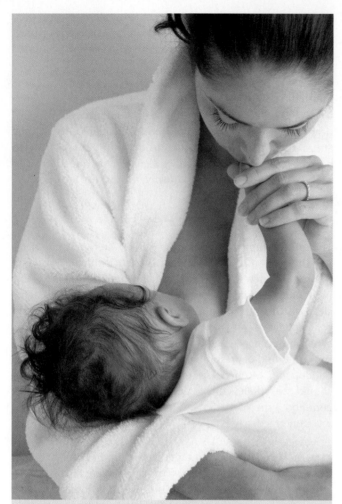

In addition to its numerous health benefits, breastfeeding enhances the development of intimate bonds between mother and child.

Breastfeeding has the added benefit of helping mothers lose weight after birth because the production of milk burns hundreds of calories a day. Breastfeeding also causes the hormone oxytocin to be released, which makes the uterus return to its normal size faster.

Breast milk is not the only way to nourish a baby. Some women are unable or unwilling to breast-feed; women with certain medical conditions or taking certain medications are advised not to breast-feed. Prepared formulas can provide nourishment that allows a baby to grow and thrive. Both feeding methods can supply the physical and emotional closeness essential to the parent–child relationship.

**Infant Mortality** After birth, infant death can be caused by birth defects, low birth weight, injuries, or unknown causes. In the United States, the unexpected death of a child under 1 year of age, for no apparent reason, is called sudden infant death syndrome (SIDS). SIDS is responsible for about 1,500 deaths a year.[33] It is the leading cause of death for children age 1 month to 1 year and most commonly occurs in babies less than 6 months old.[34] It is not a specific disease; rather, it is ruled a cause of death after all other possibilities are ruled out. A SIDS death is sudden and silent; death occurs quickly, often during sleep, with no signs of suffering. The exact cause of SIDS is unknown, but a few risk factors are known. For example, babies placed to sleep on their stomachs are more likely to die from SIDS than those placed on their backs, as are babies who are placed on or covered by soft bedding; however, breastfeeding and avoiding exposure to tobacco smoke are known protective factors.[35]

**Birthweight** When a baby is born weighing less than 5½ pounds, it is considered low birthweight. About 1 in 12 babies in the United States is low birth weight.[36] While some low-birth-weight babies are born healthy despite their size, others develop serious health problems. Low-birth-weight babies are more likely than babies with normal weight to have respiratory distress syndrome, bleeding in the brain, vision loss, and heart problems.

## LO 3 | INFERTILITY

Review primary causes of and possible solutions for infertility.

An estimated 1 in 10 American couples experience **infertility**, usually defined as the inability to conceive after trying for a year or more.[37] Although the focus is often on women, in about one-third of cases, infertility is due to a cause involving only the male partner, and in another third of cases, infertility is due to causes involving both partners or an unknown origin.[38] Because of this, it is important for both partners to be medically evaluated.

## Causes in Women

The most common cause for female infertility is *polycystic ovary syndrome (PCOS)*. A woman's ovaries have follicles, which are tiny, fluid-filled sacs that hold the eggs. When an egg is mature, the follicle breaks open to release the egg so it can travel to the fallopian tubes for fertilization. In women with PCOS, immature follicles bunch together to form large cysts or lumps. The eggs mature within the bunched follicles, but the follicles don't break open to release them. As a result, women with PCOS often don't have menstrual periods, or they have periods infrequently. Researchers estimate that 5 to 10 percent of women of childbearing age—as many as 5 million women in the United States—have PCOS.[39] It also increases the level of estrogen in the body and can cause ovulatory disorders, both of which interfere with getting pregnant.[40] In some women, the ovaries stop functioning before natural menopause, a condition called *premature ovarian failure*. Other causes of infertility include **endometriosis**. With this very painful disorder, parts of the lining of the uterus implant outside the uterus, blocking the fallopian tubes.

**infertility** Inability to conceive after a year or more of trying.

**endometriosis** Disorder in which endometrial tissue establishes itself outside the uterus.

**Pelvic inflammatory disease (PID)** is a serious infection that scars the fallopian tubes and blocks sperm migration. Infection-causing bacteria (chlamydia or gonorrhea) can invade the fallopian tubes, causing normal tissue to turn into scar tissue. This scar tissue blocks or interrupts the normal movement of eggs into the uterus. About 1 in 10 women with PID becomes infertile, and if a woman has multiple episodes of PID, her chance of becoming infertile increases.[41]

## Causes in Men

Among men, the single largest fertility problem is **low sperm count**.[42] Although only one viable sperm is needed for fertilization, research has shown that all the other sperm in the ejaculate aid in the fertilization process. There are normally at least 40 million sperm per milliliter of semen. When the count drops below 20 million, fertility declines.[43]

Low sperm count may be attributable to environmental factors (such as exposure of the scrotum to intense heat or cold, radiation, certain chemicals, or altitude), being overweight, or wearing excessively tight underwear or clothing. Other factors, such as the mumps virus, can damage the cells that make sperm, or varicocele (enlarged veins on a man's testicle) can heat the testicles and damage the sperm.[44]

## Infertility Treatments

Medical procedures can identify the cause of infertility in about 90 percent of cases.[45] Once the cause has been determined and an appropriate treatment has been instituted, the chances of becoming pregnant range from 30 to 70 percent, depending on the reason for infertility.[46]

### Fertility Drugs
Fertility drugs stimulate ovulation in women who are not ovulating. Of women who use these drugs, 60 to 80 percent will begin to ovulate; of those who ovulate, about half will conceive.[47] Fertility drugs can have many side effects, including headaches, depression, fatigue, fluid retention, and abnormal uterine bleeding. Women using fertility drugs are also at increased risk of developing multiple ovarian cysts and liver damage. The drugs sometimes trigger the release of more than one egg. As many as 1 in 3 women treated with fertility drugs will become pregnant with more than one child.[48]

> **pelvic inflammatory disease (PID)** Inflammation of the female genital tract that may cause scarring or blockage of the fallopian tubes, resulting in infertility.
>
> **low sperm count** Sperm count below 20 million sperm per milliliter of semen.
>
> **alternative insemination** Fertilization procedure accomplished by depositing semen from a partner or donor into a woman's vagina via a thin tube.
>
> **in vitro fertilization (IVF)** Fertilization of an egg in a nutrient medium and subsequent transfer back to the mother's body.

### Alternative Insemination and Assistive Reproductive Technology
Another treatment option is **alternative insemination** (also known as *artificial insemination*) of a woman with her partner's sperm. The couple may also choose insemination by an anonymous donor through a sperm bank. Donated sperm are medically screened, classified according to the donor's physical characteristics (such as hair and eye color), and then frozen for future use.

*Assisted reproductive technology (ART)* includes several different medical procedures. The most common is **in vitro fertilization (IVF)**. During IVF, eggs and sperm are mixed in a laboratory dish to fertilize, and some of the fertilized eggs (zygotes) are then transferred to the woman's uterus. Other types of assisted reproductive technologies include:

- *Intracytoplasmic sperm injection (ICSI)*, which involves the injection of a single sperm into an egg. The fertilized egg is then placed in the woman's uterus or fallopian tube. Used with IVF, ICSI is often a successful treatment for men with impaired sperm.
- *Gamete intrafallopian transfer (GIFT)*, which involves collecting eggs from the ovaries then placing them into a thin flexible tube with the sperm. This mixture is then injected into the woman's fallopian tubes, where fertilization takes place.
- *Zygote intrafallopian transfer (ZIFT)*, which combines IVF and GIFT. Eggs and sperm are mixed outside the body. The fertilized eggs (zygotes) are then returned to the fallopian tubes, through which they travel to the uterus.

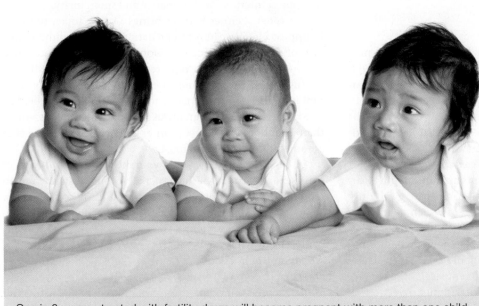

One in 3 women treated with fertility drugs will become pregnant with more than one child.

**Source:** American Society for Reproductive Medicine, "Fertility Drugs and the Risk for Multiple Births," Accessed March 2016, www.asrm.org/uploadedFiles/ASRM_Content/Resources/Patient_Resources/Fact_Sheets_and_Info_Booklets/fertilitydrugs_multiplebirths.pdf

### Other Infertility Treatments
In nonsurgical embryo transfer, a donor egg is fertilized by the man's sperm and implanted in the woman's uterus. In embryo transfer, an ovum from a donor is artificially inseminated by the man's sperm, allowed to stay in the donor's body for a time, and then transplanted into the woman's body. Infertile couples have another alternative—embryo adoption programs. Fertility treatments such as IVF often produce excess fertilized eggs that couples may choose to donate for other infertile couples to adopt.

In addition to helping infertile couples, these technologies can also help young women who are not yet ready to have a baby, but who are concerned about future infertility. A woman can have her eggs frozen to be fertilized in the future when she is ready for a child.

There are many ethical and moral questions surrounding infertility treatments. Before deciding on a treatment, you must ask yourself important questions: Has infertility been confirmed? Have all alternatives and potential risks been considered? Have you examined your attitudes, values, and beliefs about conceiving a child in this manner? Finally, will you tell your child about the method of conception and, if so, how?

## Surrogate Motherhood

Infertile couples who still cannot conceive after treatment may choose to live without children, or they may decide to pursue surrogate motherhood or adoption. With surrogacy, a woman is hired to carry another person's pregnancy to term, at which point the intended parents gain custody. In traditional surrogacy, the gestational carrier is also the biological mother of the child. In gestational surrogacy, the surrogate is not the biological mother; instead, an embryo is created via IVF using the couple's own (or donor) egg and sperm. In the United States, an estimated 750 children a year are born via surrogates.[49]

## Adoption

Adoption provides a way for individuals and couples who may not be able to have a biological child to form a legal parental relationship with a child who needs a home. As such, it benefits children whose birth parents are unable or unwilling to raise them and provides adults who are unable to conceive or carry a pregnancy to term a means to create a family. Approximately 2 percent of U.S. children are adopted.[50]

There are two types of adoption: *confidential* and *open*. In confidential adoption, the birth parents and the adoptive parents never know each other. Adoptive parents are given only basic information about the birth parents, such as medical background that they need to care for the child. In open adoption, birth parents and adoptive parents know some information about each other. There are different levels of openness. Both parties must agree to this plan, and it is not available in every state.

Increasingly, couples are choosing to adopt children from other countries. Each year, U.S. families adopt more than 5,000 foreign-born children.[51] The cost of overseas adoption varies widely, but can cost more than $30,000, including agency fees, dossier and immigration-processing fees, travel, and court costs.[52] Some families find it beneficial to serve as foster parents prior to deciding to adopt, and others choose to adopt older children from the foster system in the United States rather than wait for an infant placed through international adoption.

## LO 4 | BASIC PRINCIPLES OF CONTRACEPTION

Explain the process of conception and describe how the effectiveness of contraception is measured.

Today, we both understand the intimate details of reproduction and possess technologies that can enhance or control our **fertility**. Along with this information and our technological advances comes choice, which goes hand in hand with responsibility. Every time a person has sex, they put themselves at some risk of pregnancy. This choice, of whether and when to have children, is one of our greatest responsibilities. Children transform people's lives. They require a lifelong personal commitment of love and nurturing. Before having children, a person should ask: Am I mature enough physically and emotionally, and do I have the resources to care for another human being for the next 18 years? If you are not ready yet, you may want to postpone or pause sexual activity until you are.

One measure of maturity is the ability to discuss reproduction and birth control with your sexual partner before engaging in sexual activity. Men often assume their partners are taking care of birth control. Women sometimes feel that broaching the topic implies promiscuity. Both may feel that bringing up the subject interferes with romance and spontaneity.

Too often, neither partner brings up the topic, resulting in unprotected sex. In a recent national survey, only 82 percent of sexually active college women and 78 percent of sexually active college men reported having used a method of contraception the last time they had vaginal intercourse.[53] Ambivalence toward contraception has serious consequences, as 51 percent of all pregnancies in the United States—more than 3 million a year—are unintended, and the highest rates are among women ages 18 to 24.[54]

Discussing this topic with your health care provider or your sexual partner will be easier if you understand human reproduction and contraception and honestly consider your attitudes toward these matters. Here we discuss information to consider as you contemplate your own sexual and reproductive choices.

The term **contraception** refers to methods of preventing conception. **Conception** occurs when a sperm fertilizes an egg.

---

**fertility** A person's ability to reproduce.

**contraception** Methods of preventing conception.

**conception** Fertilization of an ovum by a sperm.

---

# 78%

of college students report using a **CONTRACEPTIVE METHOD** the last time they had intercourse.

This usually takes place in a woman's fallopian tube. The following conditions are necessary for conception:

1. **A viable egg.** A sexually mature woman will release one egg (sometimes more) from one of her two ovaries every 28 days, on average. Eggs remain viable for 24 to 36 hours after their release into the fallopian tube.

2. **A viable sperm.** Each ejaculation contains between 200 and 500 million sperm cells. Once sperm reach the fallopian tubes, they survive an average of 48 to 72 hours—and can survive up to a week.

3. **Access to the egg by the sperm.** To reach the egg, sperm must travel up the vagina, through the cervical opening into the uterus, and from there, to the fallopian tubes.

Contraceptive methods prevent conception by interfering with one of these three conditions. While the terms contraceptives and **birth control** are commonly used interchangeably, contraceptives refer to devices, behaviors, or drugs that prevent conception, while birth control includes any method reducing the likelihood of pregnancy or childbirth, including contraceptives, contragestion (e.g., the morning-after pill), and abortion.

Without contraceptives, 85 percent of sexually active women would become pregnant within 1 year.[55] Society has searched for a simple, infallible, and risk-free way to prevent pregnancy since people first associated sexual activity with pregnancy. Outside of abstinence, we have not yet found one.

**birth control** Methods that reduce the likelihood of conception or childbirth.

**perfect-use failure rate** The number of pregnancies (per 100 users) likely to occur in the first year of use of a particular birth control method if the method is used consistently and correctly.

**typical-use failure rate** The number of pregnancies (per 100 users) likely to occur in the first year of use of a particular birth control method if the method's use is not consistent or always correct.

**barrier methods** Contraceptive methods that block the meeting of egg and sperm by means of a physical barrier (such as a condom), a chemical barrier (such as a spermicide), or both.

**hormonal methods** Contraceptive methods that introduce synthetic hormones into a woman's system to prevent ovulation, thicken cervical mucus, or prevent a fertilized egg from implanting.

**intrauterine methods** Contraceptive methods that insert a device into the uterus to either introduce synthetic hormones or interfere with sperm movement or egg fertilization.

**behavioral methods** Temporary or permanent abstinence or planning intercourse in accordance with fertility patterns.

**permanent methods** Surgically altering a man's or woman's reproductive system to permanently prevent pregnancy.

To evaluate the effectiveness of a particular contraceptive method, you must be familiar with two concepts: perfect-use failure rate and typical-use failure rate. **Perfect-use failure rate** refers to the number of pregnancies that are likely to occur in the first year of use (per 100 users of the method) if the method is used absolutely perfectly—without any error. The **typical-use failure rate** refers to the number of pregnancies likely to occur in the first year of typical use—that is, with the normal number of errors, memory lapses, and incorrect or incomplete use. The typical-use failure rate is always higher. Since it reflects how people actually use the method, it is more practical in helping people make informed decisions about contraceptive methods. (To aid discussion of method effectiveness in this chapter, failure rates are converted to effectiveness rates by subtracting failure rates from 100.)

## LO 5 | TYPES OF CONTRACEPTIVES

Compare and contrast the advantages, disadvantages, and effectiveness of different types of contraception in preventing pregnancy and sexually transmitted infections, and describe emergency contraception and its use.

Present methods of contraception fall into several categories. **Barrier methods** block the egg and sperm from joining. **Hormonal methods** prevent ovulation, thicken cervical mucus, or prevent a fertilized egg from implanting. **Intrauterine methods** interfere with sperm movement and egg fertilization. **Behavioral methods** may involve temporary or permanent abstinence or planning intercourse around fertility patterns. **Permanent methods** surgically block the sperm's ability to fertilize the egg. Contraceptive methods could also be categorized by whether they are available with or without a visit to a health care provider or by the length of time it takes fertility to return after ending use.

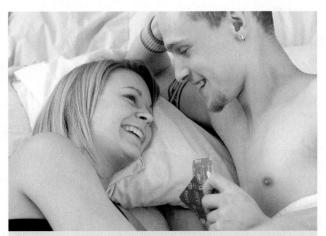

Different methods of birth control on the market include: barrier methods, hormonal methods, and other options (including surgery as a permanent option). When you choose a method, consider the cost, your comfort level, convenience, and health risks.

# TABLE 10.2 | Contraceptive Effectiveness, STI Protection, Frequency of Use, Cost, Advantages, and Disadvantages

| Method | Effectiveness | | STI/HIV Protection | Frequency of Use | Cost |
| | Typical Use | Perfect Use | | | |
| --- | --- | --- | --- | --- | --- |
| **Continuous abstinence** | 100 | 100 | Yes | N/A | None |
| **Nexplanon/Implanon** | 99.95 | 99.95 | No | Inserted every 3 years | $0–800/exam, device, and insertion; $0–$300 for removal |
| **Male sterilization (vasectomy)** | 99.85 | 99.9 | No | Done once | $0–1,000/interview, counseling, examination, operation, and follow-up sperm count |
| **Female sterilization (tubal ligation)** | 99.5 | 99.5 | No | Done once | $0–6,000/interview, counseling, examination, operation, and follow-u |
| **IUD (intrauterine device)** | | | | | |
| **Mirena/Skyla/Liletta** | 99.8 | 99.8 | No | Inserted every 3–5 years | $0–1,000/exam, insertion, and follow-up visit |
| ParaGard (copper T) | 99.2 | 99.4 | No | Inserted every 12 years | $0–1,000/exam, insertion, and follow-up visit |
| Depo-Provera | 94 | 99.8 | No | Injected every 12 weeks | $0–150/3-month injection; $0–250 for initial exam |
| **Oral contraceptives (combined pill and progestin-only pill)** | 91 | 99.7 | No | Take daily | $0–50 monthly pill pack at drugstores, often less at clinics; check fc family-planning programs in your student health center, $0–250 for initial exam |
| **Xulane patch** | 91 | 99.7 | No | Applied weekly | $0–80/month at drugstores; often less at clinics, $0–250 for initial exam |
| **NuvaRing** | 91 | 99.7 | No | Inserted every 4 weeks | $0–80/month at drugstores, often less at clinics; $0–250 for initial exam |
| **Diaphragm (with spermicidal cream or jelly)** | 88 | 94 | No | Used every time | $0–75 for diaphragm; $0–250 for initial exam; $0–17/supplies of spermicide jelly or cream |
| **Today Sponge** | | | | | |
| Women who have never given birth | 88 | 91 | No | Used every time | $0–15/package of three sponges. Available at family-planning centers, drugstores, online, and in some supermarkets |
| Women who have given birth | 76 | 80 | No | Used every time | |
| **Cervical cap (FemCap) (with spermicidal cream or jelly)** | | | | | |
| Women who have never given birth | 86 | 96 | No | Used every time | $0–75 for cap; $0–200 for initial exam; $0–17/supplies of spermicide jelly or cream |
| Women who have given birth | 68 | No data | No | Used every time | |
| **Male condom (without spermicides)** | 82 | 98 | Some | Used every time | $0–1.00 and up per condom—some family-planning or student health centers give them away or charge very little. Available in drugstores, family planning clinics, some supermarkets, and from vending machine |
| **Female condom (without spermicides)** | 79 | 95 | Some | Used every time | $2–4/condom. Available at family-planning centers, drugstores, and in some supermarkets |
| **Withdrawal** | 78 | 96 | No | Used every time | None |
| **Fertility awareness–based methods** | 76 | 95–99 | No | Followed every month | $10–12 for temperature kits. Charts and classes often free in health centers and churches |
| **Spermicides (foams, creams, gels, vaginal suppositories, and vaginal film)** | 72 | 82 | No | Used every time | $8/applicator kits of foam and gel ($4–8 refills). Film and suppositories are priced similarly. Available at family-planning clinic drugstores, and some supermarkets |
| **No method** | 15 | 15 | No | N/A | None |
| **Emergency contraceptive pill** | Treatment initiated within 72–120 hours after unprotected intercourse reduces the risk of pregnancy by 75–89% (with no protection against STIs). Costs depend on what services are needed: $30–65 for over-the-counter pills. Not meant for frequent use. Many women report nausea and vomiting. | | | | |

Note: "Effectiveness" refers to the number of women not experiencing unintended pregnancies during the first year of use per 100 users. "Typical Use" refers to failure rates fo those whose use is not consistent or always correct. "Perfect Use" refers to failure rates for those whose use is consistent and always correct.
Some family planning clinics charge for services and supplies on a sliding scale according to income. Cost varies based on insurance coverage, many are supplied at no cost

| Advantages | Disadvantages |
|---|---|
| ...omen who abstain until their 20s have fewer partners in their lifetimes and are less ...ely to get STIs, become infertile, or develop cervical cancer. | Can be difficult to maintain. Partners must decide together on a definition of abstinence. |
| ...hree years of continuous protection. The ability to get pregnant returns quickly. ...othing to remember to take or use. For most women, periods become fewer and ...hter. May be used while breastfeeding. | Minor surgery is required for insertion. Pain during insertion and removal. Irregular bleeding is common in the first 6 to 12 months. |
| ...ermanent. No long-term side effects. Allows for privacy. Allows men to be actively ...volved in their fertility. | Difficult to reverse if you change your mind in the future. |
| ...ermanent. No long-term side effects. Allows for privacy. | Difficult to reverse if you change your mind in the future. |
| ...ontinuous protection for 3 to 5 years. Ability to get pregnant returns quickly. Nothing ... remember to take or use. Reduces cramps and menstrual flow by 90%. Many ...omen report no period after first few months. May be used while breastfeeding. | Minor surgery is required for insertion. Pain during insertion and removal. |
| ...ontinuous protection for 12 years. Ability to get pregnant returns quickly. Nothing to ...member to take or use. No hormones. May be used while breastfeeding. | Some women report heavier periods and more cramping. Minor surgery is required for insertion. Pain during insertion and removal. Not a good choice for women with multiple partners. |
| ...othing to remember daily. Private, no evidence of use. Can help prevent endometrial ...ancer. Most women stop having periods in the first year of use. May be used while ...eastfeeding. | Prescription is required. Irregular bleeding in first months. Some women have longer, heavier periods. No way to stop side effects until shot wears off. May have some weight change, moodiness or headaches. May reduce bone density over time. May delay return of fertility. Even though that is already very full. |
| ...othing to remember right before sex. Reduces PMS symptoms; makes periods ...ghter. Protects against bone thinning and PID. Lowers risks of ovarian and ...ndometrial cancer. | Prescription is required. In first months, there can be breast tenderness and nausea. Some brands have high risks for blood clots. Not good for women over age 35 who smoke. Must take at the same time each day. May delay return of fertility for a few months. |
| ...othing to remember daily. Lighter, shorter periods. Like the pill, some benefits ...gainst cramps, PID, and PMS. | Prescription is required. Similar to the pill, but must remember weekly, not daily. Higher risks for blood clots, heart attacks, and strokes than with pills. |
| ...othing to remember daily. Lighter, shorter periods. Like the pill, some benefits ...gainst cramps, PID, and PMS. | Prescription is required. Similar to the pill, but must remember monthly. Higher risks for blood clots, heart attacks, and strokes than with pills. |
| ...o hormones. Immediately effective and reversible. Can be inserted hours in advance ... sex. | Doctor visit is required. Takes practice to insert correctly. Must be used every time. Can be dislodged with deep thrusting during sex. Cannot be used with silicone or spermicide sensitivity/allergy. |
| ...milar benefits as diaphragm. No doctor visit required. | Cannot be used during period. Do not leave in more than 30 hours or risk for toxic shock syndrome. Must be used every time. Can be difficult to insert and remove for beginners. Cannot be used with spermicide sensitivity/allergy. |
| ...milar benefits as diaphragm. Good for those with a latex allergy. | Doctor visit is required. Cannot be used during menstruation, or risk of TSS. Must be used every time. Can be difficult to insert and remove for beginners. Cannot be used with silicone or spermicide sensitivity/allergy. Can be dislodged with deep thrusting during sex. |
| ...o doctor visit required. Easily reversible. Helps protect against STIs and HIV. Can ...e used in conjunction with other forms of birth control. No side effects. No effect on ...ormones. Safe with water-based lubricants. This is the only temporary option for men. | Have to use every time. Have to have on hand. Can be disruptive to sex. Can reduce sensitivity during intercourse. Rare allergies to latex require use of condoms made from materials other than latex. |
| ...o doctor visit required. Easily reversible. Helps protect against STIs and HIV. Can ...e used in conjunction with other forms of birth control. No side effects. No effect on ...ormones. Safe with oil or water-based lubricants. Latex-free, so no allergy issues. ...an be inserted in advance of sex. | Have to use every time. Have to have on hand. Can cause irritation. Can reduce sensitivity during intercourse. Takes practice to insert. |
| ...o side effects. Easily reversible. No effect on hormones. Can be used when no other ...ethod is available. Can improve the effectiveness of other methods. | Requires strong self-control and trust. Not good for sexually inexperienced or premature ejaculators. |
| ...o side effects. Easily reversible. Consistent with the Roman Catholic Church. ...ctively involves males. | Both partners must be willing to abstain for 10 days per month. Requires a regular cycle. |
| ...o doctor visit required. Easily reversible. No side effects. No effect on hormones. ...an improve the effectiveness of other methods. | Can be messy or leak. Some risk related to frequent use of non-oxynol-9. Must be applied shortly before sex. |
| ...o hormones, no prescription. | N/A |

...urces: Adapted from R. Hatcher et al., *Contraceptive Technology*, 20th rev. ed. (New York: Ardent Media, 2011); R. Hatcher et al., *Contraceptive Technology*, 19th rev.
Copyright © 2007 Contraceptive Technology Communications, Inc. Reprinted by permission of Ardent Media, LLC; Planned Parenthood, "Birth Control," 2014, www.
...nnedparenthood.org.

A few contraceptive methods can also protect, to some degree, against **sexually transmitted infections (STIs)**. **TABLE 10.2** summarizes the effectiveness, STI protection, frequency of use, cost, advantages, and disadvantages of various contraceptive methods.

## Barrier Methods

Barrier methods work on the simple principle of preventing sperm from ever reaching the egg by use of a physical or chemical barrier. Some barrier methods prevent semen from contacting the woman's body and others prevent sperm from going past the cervix. Many barrier methods contain or are used in combination with a substance that kills sperm.

**Male Condom** The **male condom** is a thin sheath designed to cover the erect penis and prevent semen from entering the vagina. It is one of only two forms of contraception that offer some protection against STIs and HIV. Most male condoms are made of latex, although condoms made of polyurethane, polyisoprene, or lambskin are available. While lambskin condoms can prevent pregnancy, they are not effective protection against HIV and STIs. Condoms come in a wide variety of styles and may be purchased in pharmacies, supermarkets, some public bathrooms, and many health clinics. A new condom must be used for each act of vaginal, oral, or anal intercourse.

A condom must be rolled onto the penis before the penis touches the vagina, and it must be held in place when removing the penis from the vagina after ejaculation to prevent slippage (see **FIGURE 10.6**). Uncircumcised males should retract the foreskin slightly before putting on a condom. In condoms without a reservoir tip, a ½-inch

**sexually transmitted infections (STIs)** Infectious diseases caused by pathogens transmitted through some form of sexual contact.

**male condom** Single-use sheath of thin latex or other material designed to fit over an erect penis and to catch semen upon ejaculation.

**spermicide** Substance designed to kill sperm.

space should be left to catch the ejaculate. To do so, the user can pinch the tip to remove air while unrolling the condom down the shaft of the penis.

Condoms come with or without lubrication. If desired, users can lubricate their own condoms with contraceptive foams, creams, and jellies or other water-based lubricants. Never use products such as baby oil, cooking oils, petroleum jelly, vaginal yeast infection medications, or body lotion with a condom. These products contain substances that will cause the latex to disintegrate.

Condoms are available with or without **spermicide**. Recent research indicates that the most commonly used spermicide, nonoxynol-9 (N-9), can cause irritation and increase the

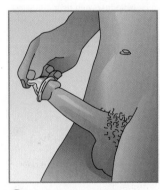 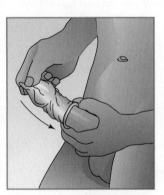 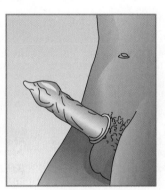 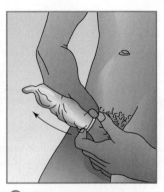

❶ Pinch the air out of the top half-inch of the condom to allow room for semen.

❷ Holding the tip of the condom with one hand, use the other hand to unroll it onto the penis.

❸ Unroll the condom all the way to the base of the penis, smoothing out any air bubbles.

❹ After ejaculation, hold the condom around the base until the penis is totally withdrawn to avoid spilling any semen.

**FIGURE 10.6** How to Use a Male Condom

→ VIDEO TUTOR
Choosing Contraception

likelihood of infection, including HIV infection, when used multiple times per day.[56] The current recommendation is that users purchase condoms without spermicide and lubricate the condom themselves with water-based lubricants. Of course, the use of condoms with N-9 is safer than using no condom at all.

Condom options are seemingly endless. If a couple is unhappy with one type, they should try another. Couples should note that not all condoms are labeled for contraceptive and STI-prevention purposes. Some novelty condoms, such as flavored, glow-in-the-dark, or ticklers, may only be for pleasure enhancement, so be sure check the label.

Condoms are less effective and more likely to break during intercourse if they are old or improperly stored. To maintain effectiveness, store them in a cool place (not in a wallet or glove compartment). Lightly squeeze the package before opening to feel that air is trapped inside and the package has not been punctured. Discard all condoms that have passed their expiration date.

Many people choose condoms because they are inexpensive and readily available without a prescription, and their use is limited to times of sexual activity, with no negative health effects. However, there is considerable potential for user error with the condom and, as a result, the effectiveness rate of condoms is only 82 percent.[57] Improper use of a condom can lead to breakage, leakage, or slippage, potentially exposing the users to STI transmission or unintended pregnancy. For example, if the penis is not removed from the vagina before it becomes flaccid (soft), semen may leak out of the condom. Even when used perfectly, a condom doesn't protect against STIs that may have external areas of infection (e.g., herpes).

## Female Condom
The **female condom** is a single-use, soft, lubricated, loose-fitting sheath meant for internal vaginal use. The newest, improved version, called FC2, is made from nitrile rather than polyurethane, so there is very little risk of allergy. The sheath has a flexible ring at each end. One ring lies inside the sheath to serve as an insertion mechanism and holds the condom in place over the cervix. The other ring remains outside the vagina once the condom is inserted and protects the labia and the base of the penis from exposure to STIs. **FIGURE 10.7** shows the proper use of the female condom.

Used consistently and correctly, female condoms are one of only two forms of contraception that offer some protection from HIV and other STIs, including those transmitted by external genital contact (e.g., herpes). The female condom can be inserted in advance, so its use doesn't have to interrupt lovemaking. Some women choose the female condom because it gives them more personal control over pregnancy prevention and STI protection or because they cannot rely on their partner to use a male condom. Because the nitrile material is thin and pliable, there is less loss of sensation with the female condom than there is with the latex male condom. The female condom is relatively inexpensive, readily available without a prescription, and causes no negative health effects.

**female condom** Single-use nitrile sheath for internal use during vaginal intercourse to catch semen upon ejaculation.

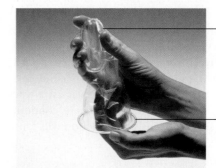
Inner ring is used for insertion and to help hold the sheath in place during intercourse.

Outer ring covers the area around the opening of the vagina.

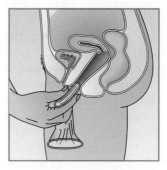
❶ Grasp the flexible inner ring at the closed end of the condom, and squeeze it between your thumb and second or middle finger so it becomes long and narrow.

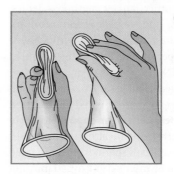
❷ Choose a comfortable position for insertion: squatting, with one leg raised, or sitting or lying down. While squeezing the ring, insert the closed end of the condom into your vagina.

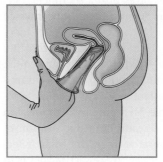
❸ Placing your index finger inside of the condom, gently push the inner ring up as far as it will go. Be sure the sheath is not twisted. The outer ring should remain outside of the vagina.

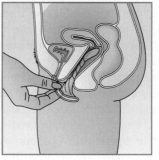
❹ During intercourse, be sure that the penis is not entering on the side, between the sheath and the vaginal wall. When removing the condom, twist the outer ring so that no semen leaks out.

**FIGURE 10.7** How to Use a Female Condom

As with the male condom, there is potential for user error with the female condom, including possible slipping or leaking, both of which could lead to STI transmission or an unintended pregnancy. Because of the potential problems, the typical-use effectiveness rate of the female condom is 79 percent.[58] As with the male condom, a new condom is required for each act of intercourse, so users must always have them on hand. Finally, male and female condoms should never be used simultaneously; the friction will cause breakage.

## Jellies, Creams, Foams, Suppositories, and Film

Like condoms, some other barrier methods—jellies, creams, foams, suppositories, sponges, and film—do not require a prescription. They are referred to as spermicides—substances designed to kill sperm. The active ingredient in most of them is nonoxynol-9 (N-9).

*Jellies and creams* are packaged in tubes, and *foams* are available in aerosol cans. All have applicators designed for insertion into the vagina. They must be inserted far enough to cover the cervix, thus providing both a chemical barrier that kills sperm and a physical barrier that keeps sperm from an egg. Jellies and creams usually need to be inserted at least 10 minutes before intercourse and remain effective for about 1 hour after insertion.

*Suppositories* are waxy capsules inserted deep into the vagina, where they melt. They must be inserted 10 to 20 minutes before intercourse, but no longer than 1 hour prior to intercourse, or they lose their effectiveness. An additional suppository or other spermicide must be inserted for each act of intercourse.

**Vaginal contraceptive film** is another method of spermicide delivery. A thin film infused with spermicidal gel is inserted into the vagina so that it covers the cervix 15 minutes before intercourse. The film dissolves into a spermicidal gel that is effective for up to 3 hours. A new film must be inserted for each act of intercourse.

Like condoms, spermicides are inexpensive, do not require a prescription or pelvic examination, and are readily available. They are simple to use, and their use is limited to the time of sexual activity. The most effective way to use spermicides is in conjunction with another barrier method; used alone their typical-use effectiveness rate is 72 percent.[59] Spermicides can be messy and must be reapplied for each act of intercourse. Some people experience irritation or allergic reactions to spermicides, and recent studies indicate that while spermicides containing N-9 are effective at preventing pregnancy, they are not effective in preventing transmission of HIV, chlamydia, or gonorrhea.[60] Frequent use (multiple times a day) of N-9 spermicides has been shown to cause irritation and breaks in the mucous layer or skin of the genital tract, creating a point of entry for viruses and bacteria that cause disease. Spermicides containing N-9 have also been associated with increased risk of urinary tract infection.[61] Contragel, popular in Europe, and Amphora, currently undergoing testing in the United States, are spermicides that use lactic acid to create an environment hostile to sperm. These and others will, it is hoped, provide future N-9 alternatives.

## Diaphragm with Spermicidal Jelly or Cream

Invented in the mid-nineteenth century, the **diaphragm** was the first widely used birth control method for women. The device is a soft, shallow cup made of thin latex rubber. Its flexible, rubber-coated metal ring is designed to fit snugly behind the pubic bone in front of the cervix and over the back of the cervix on the other side so it blocks access to the uterus. Because diaphragms come in different sizes, they must be fitted by a trained health care provider.

Spermicidal cream or jelly must be applied to the inside of the diaphragm before it is inserted, up to 6 hours before intercourse. The diaphragm holds the spermicide in place, creating a physical and chemical barrier against sperm; without spermicide, the diaphragm is ineffective (**FIGURE 10.8**). Although the diaphragm can be left in place for multiple acts of intercourse, additional spermicide must be applied each time. The diaphragm must then stay in place for 6 to 8 hours after intercourse. After removal, diaphragms should be cleaned, inspected for damage, and stored safely.

Because a diaphragm can be inserted up to 6 hours in advance, some users find it less disruptive than other barrier methods. Diaphragms have a higher typical-use effectiveness rate (88%) than other barrier methods.[62] The diaphragm does require a visit to a health care provider; however, after the initial prescription and fitting, the only ongoing expense is spermicide. The U.S. Food and Drug Administration (FDA) has recently approved a new one-size-fits-most diaphragm, Caya. It is not yet widely available, but your health care provider or pharmacy should be able to order it. One-size-fits-most means that women will not have to be fitted to use it or refitted for a different size if they gain or lose weight.

Some women find inserting a diaphragm awkward at first. When inserted incorrectly, diaphragms are much less effective. It is also possible for a diaphragm to slip out of place due to heavy thrusting during sex. Like other barrier methods, supplies must be kept on hand as additional spermicide is required for each act of intercourse. The device cannot be used during the menstrual period or for longer than 48 hours because of the risk of **toxic shock syndrome (TSS)**.

## Cervical Cap with Spermicidal Jelly or Cream

One of the oldest methods used to prevent pregnancy, early **cervical caps** were made from beeswax, silver, or copper. The only cervical cap available in the United States, the *FemCap,* is a clear silicone cup that fits snugly over the entire cervix

**vaginal contraceptive film** A thin film infused with spermicidal gel that is inserted into the vagina so that it covers the cervix.

**diaphragm** Latex, cup-shaped device designed to cover the cervix and block access to the uterus; should always be used with spermicide.

**toxic shock syndrome (TSS)** Rare, potentially life-threatening disease that occurs when specific bacterial toxins multiply and spread to the bloodstream, most commonly through improper use of tampons, diaphragms, or cervical caps.

**cervical cap** Small cup made of silicone that is designed to fit snugly over the entire cervix; should always be used with spermicide.

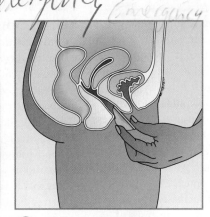

**①** Place spermicidal jelly or cream inside the diaphragm and all around the rim.

**②** Fold the diaphragm in half and insert dome-side down (spermicide-side up) into the vagina, pushing it along the back wall as far as it will go.

**③** Position the diaphragm with the cervix completely covered and the front rim tucked up against your pubic bone; you should be able to feel your cervix through the rubber dome.

**FIGURE 10.8** Proper Use and Placement of a Diaphragm

and has a ring on the back to assist with removal. It comes in three sizes and must be fitted by a health care provider. The FemCap is designed for use with spermicidal jelly or cream. It is held in place by suction created during application and works by blocking sperm from the uterus. The FemCap can be inserted up to 6 hours prior to intercourse. The device must be left in place for 6 to 8 hours after sex, using additional spermicide for any additional intercourse. After removal, the cervical cap should be cleaned, inspected for damage, and stored safely.

With a typical-use effectiveness rate of 86 percent,[63] cervical caps are reasonably effective. They are relatively inexpensive, as the only ongoing cost is the spermicide, and they last for 2 years.[64] Some users find FemCap less disruptive than other barrier methods because like the diaphragm it can

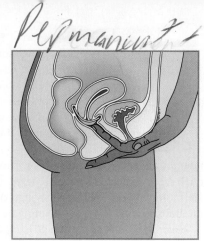

FemCap is used in conjunction with spermicide and is positioned to cover the cervix. It is shaped like a sailor's cap and has a loop to aid in removal.

be inserted up to 6 hours prior to intercourse and used for multiple acts of intercourse.

The FemCap is somewhat more difficult to insert than a diaphragm because of its smaller size. Like a diaphragm, it requires an initial fitting by a physician and may require subsequent refitting if a woman's cervix size changes (e.g., after giving birth). Because the FemCap can become dislodged during intercourse, placement must be periodically checked. The device cannot be used during the menstrual period or for longer than 48 hours because of the risk of TSS. Some women report unpleasant vaginal odors after use. Like other barrier methods, users must keep a supply of spermicidal cream or jelly on hand.

**Contraceptive Sponge** The **contraceptive sponge** (sold in the United States as the *Today Sponge*) is a small, round pillow of polyurethane foam with a loop on the back to assist with removal and a dimple on the front to help it fit closely to the cervix. Prior to insertion, the sponge must be moistened with water to activate the infused spermicide. It is then folded and inserted deep into the vagina, where it fits over the cervix and creates a barrier against sperm. Protection begins immediately upon insertion and lasts for up to 24 hours.[65] The sponge must be left in place for at least 6 hours after the last intercourse.[66] Unlike other barrier methods, there is no need to reapply spermicide or insert a new sponge for any subsequent acts of intercourse within the same 24-hour period. After use, it is thrown away.

The main advantage of the sponge is convenience because it does not require a trip to a health care provider for fitting. The sponge allows for more spontaneity than some other barrier methods because

**contraceptive sponge** Contraceptive device containing nonoxynol-9 and made of polyurethane foam that fits over the cervix to create a barrier against sperm.

**oral contraceptives** Pills containing synthetic hormones that prevent ovulation by regulating hormones.

protection begins immediately upon insertion and lasts for 24 hours without reapplication of spermicide for additional intercourse.

The sponge is similarly effective as the diaphragm for women who have never given birth (88% typical-use effectiveness rate), but less effective for women who have previously given birth (76% typical-use effectiveness rate).[67] Allergic reactions are more common with the sponge than with other barrier methods. Should the vaginal lining become irritated, the risk of yeast infections and other STIs may increase. The sponge should not be used during menstruation. Some cases of TSS have been reported in women using the sponge, thus the same precautions should be taken as with the diaphragm and cervical cap. Finally, the sponge is infused with nonoxynol-9, thus users should be aware of related risks.

## Hormonal Methods

The term *hormonal contraception* refers to birth control that contains synthetic estrogen, progestin (synthetic progesterone), or both—similar to the hormones estrogen and progesterone that a woman's ovaries produce naturally for the process of ovulation and the menstrual cycle. Synthetic estrogen works to prevent the ovaries from releasing an egg. If no egg is released, there is nothing to be fertilized by the sperm and pregnancy cannot occur. Progestin thickens the cervical mucus, which hinders the movement of the sperm, inhibits the egg's ability to travel through the fallopian tubes, and suppresses the sperm's ability to unite with the egg. Progestin also thins the uterine lining, making it unlikely for a fertilized egg to implant in the uterine wall.

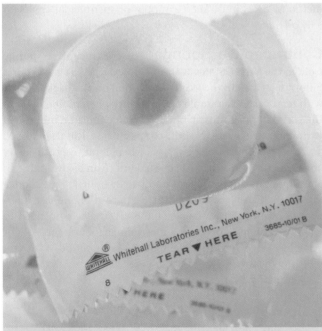

The Today Sponge is a barrier method infused with spermicide that is most effective when inserted correctly and used in conjunction with male condoms.

## Oral Contraceptives

**Oral contraceptive pills** were first marketed in the United States in 1960. Today, oral contraceptives are a commonly used birth control method among college women (57% of sexually active women report using pills, second only to condoms at 59%).[68] Birth control pills are highly effective at preventing pregnancy (91% with typical use).[69] It is easier for a motivated user to approach perfect use with hormonal methods than with barrier contraceptives, as most errors are due to user error, not method failure.

Much of the pill's popularity is due to its convenience and ability to be used discreetly. Users tend to like the fact that the pill doesn't interrupt lovemaking, potentially leading to greater sexual enjoyment. The challenge to successful use of oral contraceptives is that they must be taken every day at the same time, without fail (see the **Tech & Health** box). If a woman misses a pill, she should use a backup method of contraception for the remainder of that cycle. After discontinuing use of the pill, return of fertility may be delayed, but the pill is not known to cause infertility. Other drawbacks are that the pill does not protect against HIV and STIs, and its effectiveness may be affected by certain medications, including St. John's wort and the antibiotic rifampin, as well as some treatments for seizures, HIV, and yeast infections.

More than 40 brands of pills exist, fitting into two categories: combination pills and progestin-only pills.

*Combination pills* work through the combined effects of synthetic estrogen and progestin and are taken in a cycle. At the end of each 3-week cycle, the user stops taking pills or takes placebo pills for 1 week. The resultant drop in hormone level causes the uterine lining to shed, and the user will have a menstrual period, usually within 1 to 3 days. Menstrual flow is generally lighter than it is for women who don't use the pill because the hormones in the pill prevent thick endometrial buildup.

Several newer brands of combination pills have *extended cycles*, such as the 91-day *Seasonale* and *Seasonique*.[70] A woman using this regimen takes active pills for 12 weeks, followed by 1 week of placebos.[71] On this cycle, women can expect a menstrual period every 3 months.[72] *Lybrel*, another extended-cycle pill, supplies an active dose of hormones every day for 365 days, eliminating menstruation completely during use.[73] While the idea of not having a period for a year may be unsettling, there is no known physiological need for a woman to have a monthly period, and there are no known risks associated with avoidance.

In addition to effectively preventing pregnancy, the combination pill may lessen menstrual difficulties, such as cramps and premenstrual syndrome (PMS), and lower the risk of several health conditions, including endometrial and ovarian cancers, noncancerous breast disease, osteoporosis, ovarian cysts, pelvic inflammatory disease (PID), and iron-deficiency

**SEE IT!** VIDEOS

Concerned about the health effects of contraception? Watch **Newer Birth Control Pills May Have Increased Risks of Blood Clots**, available on MasteringHealth.™

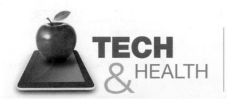

# TECH & HEALTH

# REPRODUCTIVE HEALTH APPS

The difference between the "perfect-use" failure rates and "typical-use" failure rates is most often human error. It is easy to leave your pills at home when you go out of town, to run out of condoms, or to forget to schedule an appointment to get your shot. Apps can help reduce this error and provide other resources for pregnancy and parenting.

Reminder apps, such as myPill and iPill, send text messages or sound discreet alarms to remind you to take your pill, schedule your shot, or visit the pharmacy to buy more pills. Cycle-tracking apps like Clue help you get a sense for what your normal cycle is like, giving you an idea of when your most fertile window is, as well as when your period is likely to begin.

For women trying to get pregnant, Maybe Baby and FemiCycle help predict fertility cycles based on fertility awareness methods. While not perfect, because ovulation is not always predictable, they do simplify charting basal temperatures and predicting fertile times.

Once pregnant, there are many apps to choose from, such as I'm Expecting and Baby Bump. These apps provide many great tools, such as pregnancy countdowns, week-by-week information about fetal growth and development, and details on what you can expect from each week of pregnancy.

When the baby arrives, you can download all kinds of apps to chart growth, play white noise, and track nursing times and diaper changes. Just don't forget to put down your phone and cuddle the baby!

anemia.[74] Many different brands of combination pills are on the market, some of which contain progestins that offer additional benefits, such as reducing acne, minimizing fluid retention, or relieving cramps. Users of extended-cycle pills also like that they don't need to remember when to stop or start a cycle of pills or when to use placebos.

Although estrogen in combination pills is associated with increased risk of several serious health problems among older women, the risk is low for most healthy, nonsmoking women under age 35.[75] Problems include increased risk for blood clots and higher risk for increased blood pressure, thrombotic stroke, and myocardial infarction. These risks increase with age and cigarette smoking. Early warning signs of complications associated with oral contraceptives include severe abdominal, chest, or leg pain; severe headache; and/or eye problems.[76]

Different brands of pills have varying minor side effects. Some of the most common are spotting between periods, breast tenderness, moodiness, and nausea. With most pills, side effects clear up within a few months. Other, less common side effects include acne, hair loss or growth, and a change in sexual desire. With so many brands available, most women who wish to use the pill are able to find one without unpleasant side effects.

*Progestin-only pills* (or minipills) contain small doses of progestin and no estrogen. These pills are available in 28-day packs of active pills (menstruation usually occurs during the fourth week even though the active dose continues through the entire month). Ovulation may occur, but the progestin prevents pregnancy by thickening cervical mucus and interfering with implantation of a fertilized egg. Progestin-only pills are a good choice for women who are at high risk for estrogen-related side effects or who cannot take estrogen-containing pills because of diabetes, high blood pressure, or other cardiovascular conditions. They can also be used safely by women who are older than age 35 and by women who are currently breastfeeding.

Like combination pills, progestin-only pills are highly effective at preventing pregnancy: 91 percent with typical use.[77]

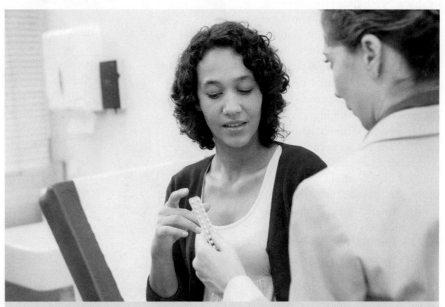

Studies show that college-age women are most familiar with the birth control pill and the male condom; talk to your health care provider about other options available to you and your partner.

Progestin-only pills share many of the health benefits of combination pills, but unlike combination pills, they carry no estrogen-related cardiovascular risks. Also, some of the typical side effects of combination pills, including nausea and breast tenderness, usually do not occur with progestin-only pills. With progestin-only pills, women's menstrual periods generally become lighter or stop altogether.

Because of the lower dose of hormones in progestin-only pills, it is especially important to take them at the same time each day. If a woman takes a pill 3 or more hours later than usual, she will need to use a backup method of contraception for the next 48 hours.[78] The most common side effect of progestin-only pills is irregular menstrual bleeding or spotting. Less common side effects include mood changes, changes in sex drive, and headaches.

### Contraceptive Skin Patch
**Xulane** (a generic form of Ortho Evra, which has been removed from the market) is a square transdermal (through the skin) adhesive patch less than 2 inches wide, as thin as a plastic strip bandage. It is worn for 1 week and replaced on the same day of the week for 3 consecutive weeks; during the fourth week, no patch is worn. Xulane works by delivering continuous levels of estrogen and progestin into the bloodstream. The patch can be worn on the buttocks, abdomen, upper torso (front or back, excluding the breasts), or upper outer arm. It should not be used by women over age 35 who smoke cigarettes and is less effective in women who weigh more than 198 pounds.[79]

Xulane is anticipated to have the same level of effectiveness with typical use (91%) as the brand-name patch Ortho Evra.[80] Women who choose to use the patch often do so because they find it easier to remember to replace it weekly than to take a daily pill. Xulane is not yet shown to, but likely offers, similar potential health benefits as combination pills (reduction in risk of certain cancers and diseases, lessening of PMS symptoms, etc.). Like other hormonal methods, the patch regulates a woman's menstrual cycle. Because the user only has to think about her birth control once a week, it may increase convenience and spontaneity.

Similar to other hormonal birth control methods, the patch offers no protection against HIV or other STIs. Some women experience minor side effects like those associated with combination pills. Rarely, women report the patch falling off or irritation at the site of application. The estrogen in the patch is associated with cardiovascular risks, particularly in women who smoke and women over the age of 35.[81] Amid evidence that the patch may increase the risk of life-threatening blood clots in women of all ages, the FDA mandated an additional warning label explaining that patch use exposes women to about 60 percent more estrogen than a typical combination pill.[82] There may be some delay in return of fertility with the patch, especially if a woman had irregular menstrual cycles before beginning use. As with oral contraceptives, some medications can make Xulane less effective.

### Vaginal Contraceptive Ring
**NuvaRing** is a soft, flexible plastic hormonal contraceptive ring about 2 inches in diameter. The user inserts the ring into the vagina, leaves it in place for 3 weeks, then removes it for 1 week, during which she will have a menstrual period. Once the ring is inserted, it releases a steady flow of estrogen and progestin.

The ring is 91 percent effective with typical use.[83] Advantages of NuvaRing include lower risk of user error, as there is no pill to take daily or patch to change weekly, no need to be fitted by a health care provider, and rapid return of fertility when use is stopped. It also exposes the user to a lower dosage of estrogen than do the patch and some combination pills, and may have fewer estrogen-related side effects. It likely offers some of the same potential health benefits as combination pills and regulates the menstrual cycle.

Like other hormonal methods, the ring provides no protection against STIs or HIV. Like combination pills, the ring poses rare but potentially serious health risks for some women. Possible side effects unique to the ring include increased vaginal discharge and vaginal irritation or infection.

### Contraceptive Injections
**Depo-Provera** (injected intramuscularly) and the newer **Depo-subQ Provera** (injected just below the skin in a lower dose) are long-acting progestins injected every 3 months by a health care provider. Both prevent ovulation, thicken cervical mucus, and thin the uterine lining, all of which prevent pregnancy.

Xulane is an adhesive patch that delivers estrogen and progestin through the skin for 1 week. Patches are changed weekly and worn for 3 out of 4 weeks.

## Contraceptive Implants

A single-rod implantable contraceptive, **Nexplanon** (formerly called **Implanon**) is a small, soft plastic capsule (about the size of a matchstick) that is inserted just beneath the skin on the inner side of a woman's upper underarm by a health care provider. Nexplanon continually releases a low, steady dose of progestin for up to 3 years, suppressing ovulation during that time.

After insertion, Nexplanon is generally not visible, making it a discreet method of birth control. It is highly effective, allowing no user error, and has a more than 99 percent typical-use effectiveness rate.[86] It has benefits similar to other progestin-only forms of contraception, including the lightening or cessation of menstrual periods, the lack of estrogen-related side effects, and safety for use by breastfeeding women. Fertility usually returns quickly after removal of the implant.

Potential minor side effects include irritation, allergic reaction, and swelling or scarring around the area of insertion, and there is a possibility of infection or complications with removal. As with all hormonal methods, Nexplanon offers no protection against STIs or HIV.[87]

## Intrauterine Contraceptives

The **intrauterine device (IUD)** is a small plastic, flexible device, with a nylon string attached. It is placed in the uterus through the cervix and provides protection from pregnancy for 3 to 12 years. The exact mechanism by which it works is not completely understood, but researchers believe that IUDs affect the way sperm and eggs move, thereby preventing fertilization, and/or affect the lining of the uterus to prevent a fertilized ovum from implanting.

The IUD was once extremely popular in the United States; however, in the 1970s most brands were removed from the market because of serious complications, such as pelvic inflammatory disease and infertility. Redesigned for safe use, the IUD is again very popular with women around the world and is experiencing a resurgence of popularity among U.S. women.[88]

### ParaGard, Mirena, Skyla, and Liletta

Four IUDs are currently available in the United States. *ParaGard* is a T-shaped plastic device with copper around the shaft. It does not contain any hormones and can be left in place for 12 years. *Mirena* is effective for 5 years and releases small amounts of progestin. *Skyla* is a lower-dose and smaller-sized version of Mirena. It was tested with and is designed for women who have not yet had a baby, and it is effective for 3 years. Newest to the market is *Liletta*, effective for at least 3 years, and designed to be a more affordable choice.

A health care provider must insert an IUD. One or two strings extend from the IUD into the vagina so the user can periodically check to make sure that the device is in place. While IUDs were initially not recommended

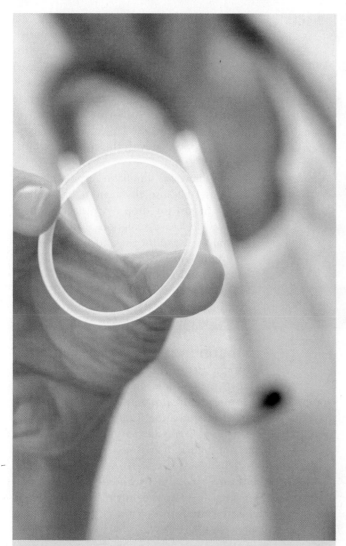

NuvaRing is inserted into the vagina, where it releases estrogen and progestin for 3 weeks. Be sure to ask your doctor for information about possible side effects.

Depo-Provera and Depo-subQ Provera take effect within 24 hours of the first shot, so there is usually no need for a backup method. There is little room for user error as a health care provider administers the injection every 3 months. With typical use it is 94 percent effective.[84] With continued use, a woman's menstrual periods become lighter and may eventually cease. There are no estrogen-related health risks associated with Depo-Provera and Depo-subQ Provera, and it offers the same potential health benefits as progestin-only pills. Unlike estrogen-containing hormonal methods, this method can be used by women who are breastfeeding.

The main disadvantage of this method is irregular bleeding, which can be troublesome at first, but within a year, most women are amenorrheic (have no menstrual periods). Also, it offers no protection against STIs or HIV. Prolonged use of Depo-Provera has been linked to loss of bone density and some medications can make contraceptive injections less effective.[85] A disadvantage for women who want to get pregnant is that fertility may not return for up to 1 year after the final injection.

> **Nexplanon (Implanon)** A plastic capsule inserted in a woman's upper arm that releases a low dose of progestin to prevent pregnancy.
>
> **intrauterine device (IUD)** A device, often T-shaped, that is inserted in the uterus to prevent pregnancy.

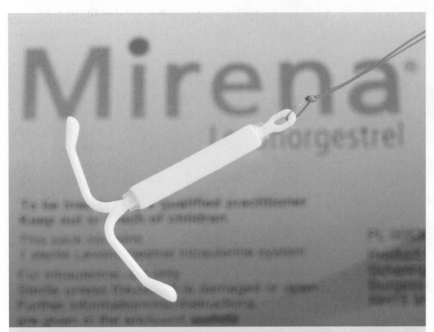

The Mirena IUD is a flexible plastic device inserted by a health care provider into a woman's uterus, where it releases progestin for up to 5 years.

National College Health Assessment (ACHA-NCHA), 33 percent of respondents reported that withdrawal was the method of birth control (or one of the methods) they used the last time they had sexual intercourse.[91] This statistic is startlingly high, considering the high risk of both STI transmission and pregnancy (only 78% effective with typical use) associated with this method of birth control.[92]

Withdrawal is unreliable, even with "perfect" use, because there are a half-million sperm in just the drop of preejaculate fluid released *before* ejaculation. Timing withdrawal is also difficult, and males concentrating on accurate timing may not be able to relax and enjoy intercourse. Withdrawal offers no protection against STIs or HIV and requires a high degree of self-control, experience, and trust.

## Abstinence and "Outercourse"

Strictly defined, *abstinence* means avoiding oral, vaginal, and anal sex. This definition would allow one to engage in forms of sexual intimacy such as massage, kissing, and masturbation. Couples who go beyond fondling and kissing to activities such as oral sex and mutual masturbation, but not vaginal or anal sex, are sometimes said to be engaging in "outercourse."

Abstinence is the only method of avoiding pregnancy that is 100 percent effective. It is also the only method that is 100 percent effective against transmitting and contracting STIs or HIV. Like abstinence, outercourse can be 100 percent effective for birth control as long as the male does not ejaculate near the vaginal opening. Unlike abstinence, however, outercourse is not 100 percent effective against STIs. Oral–genital contact can transmit disease, although the practice can be made safer by using a condom on the penis or a latex barrier, such as a **dental dam**, over the vulva. Both abstinence and outercourse require discipline and commitment for couples to sustain over long periods of time. Thirty-four percent of college students report being abstinent for the past 12 months. Thirty-five percent report having never engaged in vaginal sex, 32 percent never in oral sex, and 76 percent never in anal sex.[93]

**withdrawal** Contraceptive method that involves withdrawing the penis from the vagina before ejaculation; also called *coitus interruptus.*

**dental dam** A square of latex used as a barrier between the mouth and a woman's genitals to protect from vaginal fluids.

**fertility awareness methods (FAMs)** Several types of birth control that require alteration of sexual behavior rather than chemical or physical intervention in the reproductive process.

for women who had never had a baby, the American Congress of Obstetricians and Gynecologists now supports their use for women of all ages.[89]

The IUD is a safe, discreet, and highly effective method that is more than 99% effective.[90] ParaGard has the benefit of containing no hormones and so has none of the potential negative health impacts of hormonal contraceptives. Skyla, Mirena, and Liletta, on the other hand, likely offer some of the same potential health benefits as other progestin-only methods. IUDs are fully reversible, meaning after removal there is usually no delay in return of fertility. Although they are effective for 3 to 12 years, a health care provider can remove the IUD at any time if a woman decides to become pregnant.

Some disadvantages of IUDs include possible discomfort during insertion and removal and potential complications, such as expulsion. Also, the IUD does not protect against HIV and STIs.

## Behavioral Methods

Some methods of contraception rely on one or both partners altering their sexual behavior. In general, these methods require more self-control, diligence, and commitment, making them more prone to user error than hormonal and barrier methods.

**Withdrawal** **Withdrawal**, also called *coitus interruptus*, involves removing the penis from the vagina just before ejaculation. In the 2015 *American College Health Association's*

**Fertility Awareness Methods** Fertility awareness methods (FAMs) of birth control, sometimes referred to as periodic abstinence, natural family planning, or the "rhythm" method, rely on altering sexual behavior during certain times of the month (**FIGURE 10.9**).

Fertility awareness methods are rooted in an understanding of basic physiology. A released ovum can survive about 36 hours after ovulation, and sperm can live for about 7 days in the reproductive tract. These techniques require observing female fertile periods and abstaining from sexual intercourse (or any penis–vagina contact) during the times

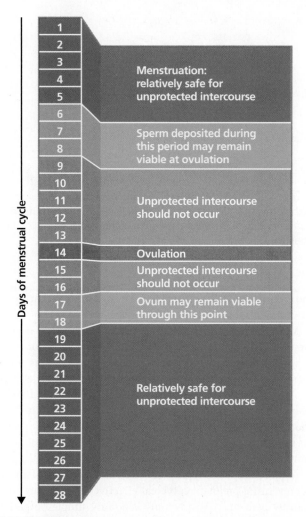

**FIGURE 10.9** **The Fertility Cycle** Fertility awareness methods (FAMs) can combine the use of a calendar, the cervical mucus method, and body temperature measurements to identify the fertile period. It is important to remember that most women do not have a consistent 28-day cycle.

when a sperm and egg could meet. Some of the more common forms include:

- **Cervical mucus method.** This method requires women to examine the consistency of their normal vaginal secretions. Prior to ovulation, vaginal mucus becomes slippery, thin, and stretchy, and normal vaginal secretions may increase. To prevent pregnancy, partners must avoid sexual activity involving penis–vagina contact while this mucus is present and for several days afterward.
- **Body temperature method.** This method relies on the fact that a woman's basal (resting) body temperature rises between 0.4 and 0.8 degrees after ovulation has occurred. For this method to be effective, a woman must chart her temperature for several months to learn to recognize her body's temperature fluctuations. To prevent pregnancy, partners must abstain from penis–vagina contact before the temperature rise until several days after the temperature rise is observed.

- **Calendar method.** This method requires the woman to record the exact number of days in her menstrual cycle. Because few women menstruate with complete regularity, this method involves keeping a record of the menstrual cycle for 12 months, during which time some other method of birth control must be used. This method assumes that ovulation occurs during the midpoint of the cycle. To prevent pregnancy, the couple must abstain from penis-vagina contact during the fertile time.

Fertility awareness methods are the only forms of birth control that comply with certain religious teachings, including those of the Roman Catholic Church. The effectiveness of FAMs depends on diligence, commitment, and self-discipline; they have a 76 percent effectiveness rate with typical use.[94] Women who attempt to use these methods without proper training run a high risk of unintended pregnancy; anyone interested in using them is advised to take a class, often offered for free by health centers and churches. These methods offer no STI protection, and they may not work for women with irregular menstrual cycles.

## Permanent Methods of Birth Control

In the United States, **sterilization** has become the second leading method of contraception for women of all ages and the leading method of contraception among women over age 35.[95] Because sterilization is permanent, anyone considering it should think through possibilities such as divorce and remarriage or a future improvement in financial status that might make pregnancy realistic or desirable.

### Female Sterilization
One method of sterilization for women is **tubal ligation**, a surgical procedure in which the fallopian tubes are cut or tied shut to block the sperm's access to released eggs (see **FIGURE 10.10** on page 288). The operation is usually done laparoscopically (via a half-inch incision in the abdomen) on an outpatient basis. The procedure usually takes less than an hour, is performed under local or general anesthesia, and the patient is usually allowed to return home within a short time. A tubal ligation does not affect ovarian and uterine function. The woman's menstrual cycle continues; released eggs simply disintegrate and are absorbed by the lymphatic system.

A newer sterilization procedure, *Essure*, involves the placement of small microcoils into the fallopian tubes via the vagina. The entire procedure takes about 35 minutes and can be performed in a physician's office, usually under local anesthetic. Once in place, the metallic microcoils expand to the shape of the fallopian tubes. The coils promote the growth of scar tissue around the coils and lead to a blockage in the fallopian tubes. Like traditional forms of tubal

> **sterilization** Permanent fertility control achieved through surgical procedures.
>
> **tubal ligation** Sterilization of a woman that involves cutting and tying off or cauterizing the fallopian tubes.

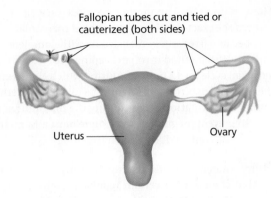

**FIGURE 10.10** Female Sterilization: Tubal Ligation In a tubal ligation, both fallopian tubes are cut and tied or sealed shut. The procedure is usually performed laparoscopically.

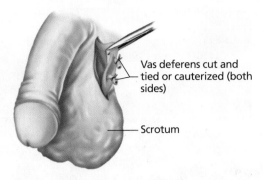

**FIGURE 10.11** Male Sterilization: Vasectomy In a vasectomy, the surgeon makes an incision in the scrotum, then locates and cuts the vasa deferentia, either sealing or tying both sides shut.

**hysterectomy** Surgical removal of the uterus.

**vasectomy** Male sterilization procedure that involves cutting and tying off the vasa deferentia.

ligation, Essure is permanent. It is recommended for women who cannot have a tubal ligation because of chronic health conditions such as obesity or heart disease; however, Essure has been under review by the FDA due to concerns about its safety and effectiveness, so if a person is interested in this method it is important to be informed of potential risks.[96]

A **hysterectomy**, or removal of the uterus, is a method of sterilization requiring major surgery. It is usually done only when a woman's uterus is diseased or damaged, not as a primary means of female sterilization.

The main advantage to female sterilization is that it is highly effective (more than 99% effective) and permanent.[97] After the one-time expense of the procedure, there is no other cost or ongoing action required. Sterilization has no negative effect on a woman's sex drive. These methods require no use of hormones, are discreet, and require no ongoing purchase or thought about supplies, thus allowing sex with full spontaneity.

As with any surgery, there are risks involved with a tubal ligation. Although rare, possible complications include infection, pulmonary embolism, hemorrhage, anesthesia complications, and ectopic pregnancy. Of course, sterilization offers no protection against STIs and is not effective immediately. A backup method of birth control is needed for 3 months. While the permanent nature of this method is considered an advantage, people need to seriously consider if they may want children later; reversal is possible in some instances, but the procedure should be considered permanent.

### Male Sterilization
Sterilization in men is less complicated than it is in women. A **vasectomy** is frequently done on an outpatient basis, using a local anesthetic (see **FIGURE 10.11**). This procedure involves making a small incision in the side of the scrotum to expose a vas deferens, cutting the vas deferens

and either tying off or cauterizing the ends, then repeating the procedure on the other side.

Many men are reluctant to consider sterilization because they fear the operation will affect their sexual performance or sex drive. However, a vasectomy in no way affects sexual response. The testes continue to produce sperm, but the sperm can no longer enter the ejaculatory duct. Any sperm that are manufactured disintegrate and are absorbed into the lymphatic system. Because sperm constitute only a small part of the semen (about 2%), the amount of ejaculate is not changed significantly.

A vasectomy is a highly effective and permanent means of preventing pregnancy; typical effectiveness rates are more than 99 percent.[98] A vasectomy is a fairly simple outpatient procedure requiring minimal recovery time, and after the one-time expense, there is no other cost or ongoing action required. It is discreet, uses no hormones, allows for spontaneity, and is one of the few methods that allow men to be in charge of fertility. Of course, men don't have to make permanent body alterations to be more involved with birth-control choices. See **Student Health Today** for more ideas on male involvement.

Male sterilization offers no protection against STI transmission. Also, a vasectomy is not immediately effective in preventing pregnancy. Because sperm are stored in other areas of the reproductive system besides the vasa deferentia, couples must use alternative birth control methods for at least 1 month after the vasectomy. A physician will do a semen analysis to determine when unprotected intercourse can take place. As with any surgery, there are some risks involved with a vasectomy. In a small percentage of cases, serious complications occur, such as formation of a blood clot in the scrotum, infection, or inflammatory reactions. Very infrequently, the vasa deferentia may create a new path, cancelling out the procedure. While the permanent nature of this method is considered an advantage, people need to seriously consider if they may want children later if their circumstances change. While vasectomies can be reversed in some

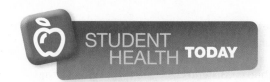
# HOW CAN MEN BE MORE INVOLVED IN BIRTH CONTROL?

The sexual health needs of young men have been largely overlooked in the field of reproductive health. Most of the research and outreach related to preventing unintended pregnancy is focused on women, leading to missed opportunities to emphasize the importance of shared responsibility for sexual health.

There are many reasons for the disparity: Men seek health care less often; it is sometimes incorrectly assumed that men are not interested in sexual health issues; and since women carry the baby, they are often seen as having a bigger stake in pregnancy prevention. Male contraceptive methods are also more medically challenging, as you need to suppress up to 500,000 sperm per ejaculation, only one of which is needed for fertilization—as opposed to one egg per month in women.

However, healthy sexual relationships and ongoing reproductive health require that both partners be stakeholders. So, how can men be more involved in responsible sexual decision making?

- Initiate discussions with your partner about contraception and your sexual health histories.
- Take an active role in discussing and deciding what type of contraception is best for you and your partner.
- Buy and use condoms every time you have sex.
- Help pay for contraceptive costs.

**Don't let embarrassment put your health at risk! Talking about safe sex may be uncomfortable, but it is worth the effort.**

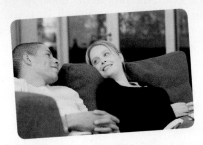

- If an unintended pregnancy occurs, share in the responsibility and decision making about the best way to handle the situation.

---

instances, the reversal procedure is costly and is not guaranteed to work.

## Emergency Contraception

Emergency contraception is the use of a contraceptive to prevent pregnancy after unprotected intercourse, a sexual assault, or the failure of another birth control method. Combination estrogen–progestin pills and progestin-only pills are two common types of **emergency contraceptive pills (ECPs)**, sometimes referred to as "morning-after pills." ECPs contain the same type of hormones as regular birth control pills and are used after unprotected intercourse, but before a woman misses her period. A woman taking ECPs does so to prevent

pregnancy; the method will not work if she is already pregnant, nor will it harm an existing pregnancy.

Multiple types of ECPs are available in the United States without a prescription. They must be taken within 72 hours (3 days) of intercourse. The FDA has more recently approved *ella*, which is available only by prescription, and can prevent pregnancy when taken up to 120 hours (5 days) after unprotected intercourse. ECPs use the same hormones that other hormonal contraceptives do and prevent pregnancy in the same way: by delaying or inhibiting ovulation, inhibiting fertilization, or blocking implantation of a fertilized egg, depending on the phase of the woman's menstrual cycle. When taken within 24 hours, ECPs reduce the risk of pregnancy by up to 95 percent; when taken 2 to 5 days later, ECPs reduce the risk of pregnancy by 88 percent.[99]

In the past, only people age 17 and older could purchase emergency contraception, and it was only available by asking a pharmacist for it because it was kept behind the pharmacy counter. Today, anyone of any age can purchase ECPs, and it is kept on the regular store shelves, usually near other family-planning supplies. According to a recent national survey, about 1 in 11 sexually active college students reported using (or their partner using) emergency contraception within the past year.[100] Although ECPs are no substitute for taking proper precautions before having sex (such as using a condom), widespread availability of emergency contraception has the potential to significantly reduce the rates of unintended pregnancies and abortions, particularly among young women.

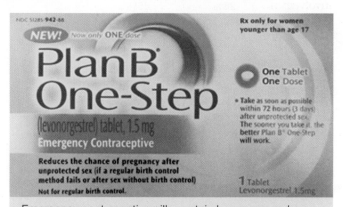

Emergency contraceptive pills contain hormones and are used after an act of unprotected intercourse. When taken within 24 hours of unprotected intercourse, ECPs reduce the risk of pregnancy by up to 95 percent.

**emergency contraceptive pills (ECPs)** Drugs taken within 3 to 5 days after unprotected intercourse to prevent pregnancy.

# LO 6 | CHOOSING A METHOD OF CONTRACEPTION

List and explain factors that you should consider when choosing a method of contraception.

With all the options available, how does a person or a couple decide what method of contraception is best? Take some time to research the various methods, ask questions of your health care provider, and be honest with yourself about your own preferences. TABLE 10.3 lists the most popular forms of contraception among sexually active college students. Questions to ask yourself and discuss with your partner are included below. Also see the **Student Health Today** box.

- **How comfortable would I be using a particular method?** If you aren't at ease with a method, you may not use it consistently, and it probably will not be a reliable choice for you. Consider your own comfort level with touching your body or whether the method may cause discomfort for you or your partner.

- **Will this method be convenient for me and my partner?** Some methods require more effort than others. Be honest with yourself about how likely you are to use the method consistently. Are you willing to interrupt lovemaking, to abstain from sex during certain times of the month, or to take a pill at the same time every day?

- **Am I at risk for the transmission of STIs?** If you have multiple sex partners or are uncertain about the sexual history or disease status of your current sex partner, then you are at risk of contracting HIV or other STIs. Next to abstinence, condoms (male and female) are the best defense against STIs and HIV.

- **Do I want to have a biological child in the future?** If you are unsure about your plans for future childbearing, you should use a temporary birth control method rather than a permanent one such as sterilization. If you know you want to have children in the future, consider how soon that will be, as some methods, such as Depo-Provera, will cause a delay in return to fertility.

- **How would an unplanned pregnancy affect my life?** If an unplanned pregnancy would be a potentially devastating event for you or would have a serious impact on your plans for the future, then you should choose a highly effective birth control method. If, however, you are in a stable relationship, have a reliable source of income, are planning to have children in the future, and would embrace a pregnancy should it occur now, then you may be comfortable with a less reliable method.

## TABLE 10.3 | Contraception Methods Used by College Students or Their Partners the Last Time They Had Sex

| Method | Male | Female | Total |
|---|---|---|---|
| Male condom | 67% | 59% | 61% |
| Birth control pills (monthly or extended cycle) | 61% | 57% | 58% |
| Withdrawal | 28% | 35% | 33% |
| Intrauterine device | 8% | 9% | 9% |
| Fertility awareness (calendar, mucus, basal body temperature) | 6% | 9% | 8% |
| NuvaRing/ring | 3% | 3% | 3% |
| Depo-Provera/shots | 5% | 4% | 4% |
| Spermicide (foam, jelly, cream) | 6% | 3% | 4% |
| Nexplanon/implant | 6% | 5% | 5% |
| Sterilization | 2% | 4% | 3% |
| Xulane/patch | 1% | 1% | 1% |
| Female condom | 1% | 0% | 1% |
| Diaphragm/cervical cap | 0% | 0% | 0.2% |
| Sponge | 0% | 0% | 0.1% |

**Note:** Survey respondents could select more than one method.

**Source:** Data from American College Health Association, *American College Health Association—National College Health Assessment II: Reference Group Data, Fall 2015* (Hanover, MD: American College Health Association, 2015).

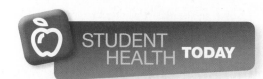
# LET'S TALK ABOUT (SAFER) SEX!

Communication is key to a healthy relationship, especially for those who are sexually intimate. It can be challenging to talk to your partner about using protection, but don't let embarrassment put your health at risk. The person that you're thinking about having sex with may or may not initially agree about using a condom or dental dam, so it's helpful to be prepared to discuss your concerns ahead of time. Remember: Communicating about sex is all about getting the most from your sex life and doing so safely.

## Why Communicating about Sex Is Essential

Open communication about sexual health is a sign of care and respect for your own body and your partner's. It empowers both of you to be assertive about your needs, likes, limits, and desires in the sexual relationship. Open communication also creates a safe environment to ask about your partner's sexual history, STI testing, and expectations.

If you are concerned that talking about sex beforehand is going to make your partner think you don't trust him or her, take some time to examine the strength of your relationship. Trust is about being open and honest. If you're afraid to talk with your partner, is it possible that you lack trust in him or her? If so, you might want to examine if this is a healthy relationship for you.

## Finding the Time and Place for Sexual Communication

Find a convenient time and a place where you are both comfortable and free of distractions. It's generally better to have this conversation outside of the bedroom, so that you're not pressured by the heat of the moment to skip the conversation. And remember, you need to think about both preventing pregnancy and avoiding STIs.

## Finding the Words for Condom/ Dental Dam Negotiation

The table below lists some examples of how you can address potential excuses from your partner when you talk about using a condom or dental dam. While there is no perfect response for every situation, these may provide some helpful suggestions.

| Excuse | Response |
|---|---|
| Don't you trust me? | It's not an issue of trust; people can have sexually transmitted infections and not know it. |
| It doesn't feel as good with a condom/dental dam. | I'll feel more relaxed; if I'm more relaxed, I can make it feel better for you. We can also use lubricant to increase sensation for both of us. |
| I don't have a condom with me. | I do. |
| It's up to you. | It's your health too, so it should be your decision, too. |
| I'm on the pill; you don't need a condom. | I'd like to use one anyway. It will help to protect us from infections that we may not know we have. |
| Putting it on interrupts everything. | Not if we put it on together. |
| I guess you don't really love me. | I do, but I'm not willing to risk our futures to prove it. |
| I will pull out in time. | Preejaculate can still cause pregnancy and spread STIs. |
| I'm allergic to latex. | No problem, Student Health Services has a selection of nonlatex condoms and dental dams that we can get for free. |
| But I love you. | Then you'll help us protect ourselves. |
| Just this once. | Once is all it takes. |

- **What are my religious and moral values?** If your beliefs prevent you from considering other birth control methods, FAMs are a good option. When both partners are motivated to use these methods, FAMs are more successful preventing unintended pregnancy. If you are considering this option, sign up with your partner for a class to get specific training for using the method effectively.
- **How much will the birth control method cost?** Some contraceptive methods involve an initial outlay of money and few continuing costs (e.g., sterilization, IUD), whereas others are fairly inexpensive but must be purchased repeatedly (e.g., condoms, spermicides, monthly pills). You should consider whether a method will be cost-effective for you in the long run. Remember that any prescription

methods require routine checkups, which may involve some cost to you. Be sure to check your health insurance to determine if the Affordable Care Act's requirement to cover "preventive services" makes hormonal contraceptives available to you at no cost. (See **Money & Health** on page 292 for more information.) The provision lets many women upgrade their method of birth control to a more reliable (and more expensive) hormonal method or IUD for no extra cost. If uninsured, your local family planning clinic or campus health center may offer low-cost options. (See **Health Headlines** on page 293 for discussion of funding for family planning clinics.)
- **Do I have any health factors that could limit my choice?** Hormonal birth control methods can pose potential health risks to women with certain preexisting

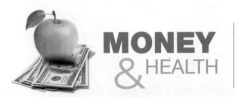

# MONEY & HEALTH | HEALTH CARE REFORM AND CONTRACEPTIVES

The Patient Protection and Affordable Care Act requires new private health insurance plans to cover "preventive services" with no co-payments or deductibles. Preventive services include birth control, yearly "wellness visits" (physical exams), breastfeeding counseling and supplies, and screening for domestic violence and sexually transmitted infections. Abortions are not included, but emergency contraception is.

Family-planning experts anticipate that in coming years the law will significantly impact unintended pregnancy and abortion rates in two ways. One, women who have been unable to afford birth control will now have access. Half of all young adult women report having been unable to afford birth control consistently at some point, and when women have to choose between paying the heat bill and paying for birth control, birth control usually loses. Two, this coverage will enable women to "upgrade" their birth control to a more reliable method. Women who

would prefer to use an IUD or implant to reduce the risk of "user error," but have been unable to because of the high upfront costs (about $1,000), will now be able to get one. The CHOICE study offered ACA-like benefits in St. Louis, Missouri, in advance of the implementation of the Affordable Care Act, and researchers found significant reductions in unplanned pregnancies, first abortions, and repeat abortions when women were given their choice of birth control method at no cost.

The law requires insurance companies to cover all contraceptive methods that have been approved by the FDA, but there are a few exceptions you might encounter:

1. This birth control benefit applies to all new plans. "New plan" doesn't mean you have to switch plans; it just means that the plan has changed since the passing of the health care law. Plans that have not made changes do not have to comply with the law.

2. If your insurance is provided by a religious organization, it does not have to comply.

3. Insurance companies must cover all types of contraceptive methods, but not all brands. This may mean that while many oral contraceptives are covered, your brand may not be.

If your insurance plan doesn't seem to be following the law, contact the National Women's Law Center. They will help you figure it out for free. Call the toll-free hotline (1-866-745-5487), email CoverHer@nwlc.org, or visit CoverHer.org to get started.

**Sources:** U.S. Centers for Medicaid and Medicare Services, "What Are My Birth Control Benefits?," Accessed April 2016, www.healthcare.gov/what-are-my-birth-control-benefits/; Planned Parenthood, "Key Facts on Birth Control Coverage," Accessed March 2016, https://www.plannedparenthood.org/files/6813/9611/6794/Myth_V_Fact_on_Birth_Control_coverage.pdf; Planned Parenthood, "The Affordable Care Act," Accessed April 2016, https://www.plannedparenthood.org/about-us/newsroom/the-affordable-care-act; National Women's Law Center, "CoverHer," Accessed April 2016, www.coverher.org.

conditions, such as high blood pressure, a history of stroke or blood clots, liver disease, migraines, or diabetes. In addition, women who smoke or are over age 35 are at risk from complications of combination hormonal contraceptives. Breastfeeding women can use progestin-only methods, but should avoid methods containing estrogen. Men and women with latex allergies can use barrier methods made of polyurethane, polyisoprene, silicone, or other materials, rather than latex condoms.

■ **Are there any additional benefits I'd like from my contraceptive?** Hormonal birth control methods may have desirable secondary effects, such as the reduction of acne or the lessening of premenstrual symptoms. Some hormonal birth control methods have been associated with reduced risks of certain cancers. Extended-cycle pills and some progestin-only methods cause menstrual periods to be less frequent or to stop altogether, which some women find desirable. Condoms carry the added health benefit of protecting against STIs.

**abortion** Termination of a pregnancy by expulsion or removal of an embryo or fetus from the uterus.

## LO 7 | ABORTION

**Summarize the political issues surrounding abortion and the various types of abortion procedures.**

Women obtain **abortions** for a variety of reasons. The vast majority of abortions occur because of unintended pregnancies, as even the best birth control methods can fail.[101] In addition, some pregnancies are terminated because they are a consequence of rape or incest. Other reasons commonly cited are not being ready financially or emotionally to care for a child.[102] When an unintended pregnancy does occur, a woman must decide whether to terminate the pregnancy, carry to term and keep the baby, or carry to term and give the baby up for adoption. This is a personal decision that each woman must make based on her personal beliefs, values, and resources and after carefully considering all alternatives.

In 1973, the landmark U.S. Supreme Court decision in *Roe v. Wade* stated that the "right to privacy . . . founded on the Fourteenth Amendment's concept of personal liberty . . . is broad enough to encompass a woman's decision whether or not to terminate her pregnancy."[103] The decision maintained

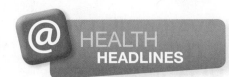

# YOU DECIDE
### Should Taxpayers Fund Planned Parenthood?

Defunding Planned Parenthood has made major headlines recently. For some, it would be a major victory to defund the country's largest abortion provider. For others it would be devastating, as Planned Parenthood is the source of their health care. The opinions and half-truths of media personalities can make it difficult to sift through to the truth, so let's look at some facts:

- Planned Parenthood receives about $500 million a year in government funding (the majority of which is in the form of Medicaid payments for services provided to clients). That's about 40 percent of its funding, its largest source. So, Planned Parenthood would struggle to stay open without federal funding.
- Seventy-six percent of Planned Parenthood services are related to either screening for or treating STIs or providing contraception. These services are targeted at low- to middle-income Americans, those who have the most limited access to health care services.
- Defunding Planned Parenthood doesn't save tax dollars. The tax dollars would

be redistributed to other women's health care providers. The problem with this is that "other providers" can't be built overnight, so in the meantime, some patients would not have access to care.

- Family planning is cost-effective. It's estimated that for each tax dollar spent on family planning, $7.09 is saved in public expenditures that would have been spent on health care and other social benefits for children whose births would have been prevented.
- Family-planning clinics provide abortions, but they prevent far more. About 2 million unintended births are prevented each year by the contraceptives received at a family-planning clinic. Of these, nearly 700,000 would have ended in abortion. And while Planned Parenthood is the largest single provider of abortions in the United States, abortions are a very small part of what Planned Parenthood does. Only about 3 percent of its services are abortion related. It has been argued that there is a difference between "services" and "patients." In that case, it's estimated that about 12 percent of their patients receive abortions.

- Federal law prohibits federal funds from being spent on abortions in nearly all circumstances. Title X money cannot be spent on abortions, and Medicaid money can only be spent on abortions in the case of rape, incest, or to protect the life of the mother.

**What do you think?** Based on these facts, does it make sense to spend tax dollars on Planned Parenthood? If yes, are there changes that could be made to alleviate concerns? If no, how can we meet the reproductive health care needs of patients in need without Planned Parenthood? And if we don't meet those needs, how do we fund the costs of care for the unintended pregnancies that will result?

**Sources:** A. Flynn, "The Economic Case for Funding Planned Parenthood," *The Atlantic,* September 17, 2015, http://www.theatlantic.com/business/archive/2015/09/planned-parenthood-economic-benefits/405922/; D. Kurtzleben, "Fact Check: How Does Planned Parenthood Spend that Government Money?" National Public Radio, August 5, 2015, http://www.npr.org/sections/itsallpolitics/2015/08/05/429641062/fact-check-how-does-planned-parenthood-spend-that-government-money.

---

that during the first trimester of pregnancy a woman and her health care provider have the right to terminate the pregnancy through abortion without legal restrictions. It allowed individual states to set conditions for second-trimester abortions. Third-trimester abortions were ruled illegal unless the mother's life or health was in danger. Prior to the legalization of abortions, women wishing to terminate a pregnancy had to travel to a country where the procedure was legal, consult an illegal abortionist, or perform their own abortions. These procedures sometimes led to infertility from internal scarring or death from hemorrhage or infection.

## The Abortion Debate

Abortion is a highly charged and politically thorny issue in American society. In a recent national poll, 53 percent of people reported that *Roe v. Wade* should be kept in place, 29 percent felt it should be overturned, and 18 percent had no opinion.[104] Pro-choice individuals feel that it is a woman's right to make decisions about her own body and health, including the decision to continue or terminate a pregnancy.

On the other side of the issue, pro-life individuals believe that the embryo or fetus is a human being with rights that must be protected.

In the 40 years since *Roe v. Wade* legalized abortion nationwide, hundreds of laws have been passed at the state and federal level to narrow or expand its limits. In 2015 alone, 47 new abortion-related laws were passed in the United States, most of which focused on regulation of abortion providers or facilities, limitations on provision of medication abortions, or forcing women to make two in-person visits to a clinic instead of one.[105] These types of laws make abortions more difficult and costly to provide, consequently reducing the number of clinics and providers

# 47%
of Americans describe themselves as "PRO-CHOICE," 46% as "PRO-LIFE."

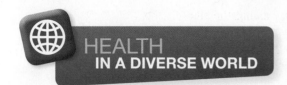

# CONTRACEPTIVE AVAILABILITY AND ABORTION IN THE DEVELOPING WORLD

While American women wrestle with the choice of which birth control to use, women in developing countries often struggle to access contraceptives at all. One-quarter of the 225 million women in developing countries are unable to access modern birth control methods; thus, unintended pregnancies in the developing world take a great toll. If contraceptive needs were to be met, unintended pregnancies would decline by 70 percent from 74 million to 22 million, unsafe abortions would drop 74 percent from 20 million to 5 million, maternal deaths would drop from 290,000 to 96,000, and newborn deaths would drop from 2.9 million to 660,000.

Unintended pregnancy is the primary driver of abortion in the United States and around the world, but whether abortion is legal or not has little to do with its overall incidence. The abortion rate in Africa, where abortion is illegal in most countries, is higher than the rate in Western Europe, where abortion is generally legal (29 per 1,000 women of childbearing age in Africa

vs. 12 per 1,000 women of childbearing age in Western Europe). Not only are abortions more frequent in the developing world, they are less safe. Fifty-six percent of all abortions in developing countries are defined as "unsafe," compared with just 6 percent in the developed world. An estimated 47,000 women died from unsafe abortions last year, nearly all in developing nations where abortion is illegal. To put that risk in perspective, worldwide, women are 350 times more likely to die from unsafe abortions than from a legal abortion in the United States. When abortion is legalized, it becomes safer. After the legalization of abortion in 1997, South Africa experienced a 91 percent reduction in abortion-related deaths.

When contraceptives are unavailable, women often turn to abortion to end an unwanted pregnancy, even when death is a potential risk. Access to voluntary family-planning services, including contraception, is essential in helping to reduce the number of unintended pregnancies and

the incidence of abortion—and save the lives of mothers and babies in the developing world. Contraceptive availability for the developing world is not only essential, is is cost effective. For every additional dollar invested in contraception, the cost of pregnancy-related care is reduced by $1.47. Providing modern contraception to all is probably less expensive than you might imagine. For $25 per woman, or $7 per person in the developing world, we could fully satisfy the need for modern contraception. Amazingly, the key to reducing unintended pregnancies, and thus decreasing unsafe abortions, maternal deaths, and infant deaths, could be had by all for the price of one movie ticket per person!

**Sources:** S. Singh and J. E. Darroch, "Adding It Up: Investing in Sexual and Reproductive Health" (New York, NY: Guttmacher Institute, November 2015), https://www.guttmacher.org/fact-sheet/adding-it-investing-sexual-and-reproductive-health; Guttmacher Institute, "Facts on Induced Abortion Worldwide," November 2015, https://www.guttmacher.org/fact-sheet/facts-induced-abortion-worldwide.

---

**suction curettage** Abortion technique that uses gentle suction to remove fetal tissue from the uterus; also called vacuum aspiration or dilation and curettage (D&C).

willing and able to provide abortion services. Thus, while abortion remains legal in all 50 states, for many women, due to difficulty accessing abortion services, abortion availability is severely limited.

For a discussion of contraception and abortion access in developing countries, see the **Health in a Diverse World** box.

## Emotional Aspects of Abortion

The best scientific evidence available indicates that among adult women who have an unplanned pregnancy, the risk of mental health problems is no greater if they have an abortion than if they deliver the baby. Although a variety of feelings such as regret, guilt, sadness, relief, and happiness are normal, evidence does not show that having an abortion causes an increase in anxiety, mood or impulse control disorders, or suicidal ideation.[106] Researchers have found that the best predictor of a woman's emotional well-being following an abortion was her emotional well-being prior to the procedure.[107] The factors that place a woman at higher risk for negative psychological responses following an abortion include perception of stigma, need for secrecy, low levels of social support for the

abortion decision, prior history of mental health issues, low self-esteem, and avoidance and denial coping strategies.[108]

## Methods of Abortion

The choice of abortion procedure is determined by how many weeks the woman has been pregnant. Length of pregnancy is calculated from the first day of her last menstrual period.

**Surgical Abortions** The majority of abortions performed in the United States today are surgical. If performed during the first trimester, abortion presents a relatively low health risk to the mother. About 89 percent of abortions occur during the first 12 weeks of pregnancy and most are in women in their 20s (see **FIGURE 10.12**).[109] The most commonly used method of first-trimester abortion is **suction curettage**, also called *vacuum aspiration* or *dilation and curettage (D&C)* (**FIGURE 10.13**). The vast majority of abortions in the United States are done using this procedure, which is usually performed under local anesthesia. The cervix is dilated with instruments or by placing laminaria, a sterile seaweed product, in the cervical canal. The laminaria is left in place for a few hours or overnight and slowly dilates the cervix. After the laminaria is removed, a long tube is inserted

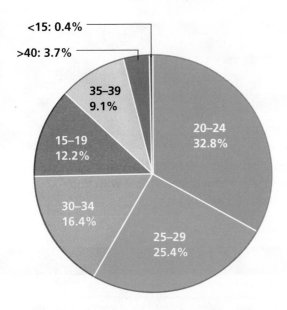

<15: 0.4%
>40: 3.7%
35–39
9.1%
15–19
12.2%
20–24
32.8%
30–34
16.4%
25–29
25.4%

**FIGURE 10.12** Age at which Women Have Abortions

Source: K. Pazol et al., "Abortion Surveillance—United States 2012," *Surveillance Summaries* 64, no. SS10 (2014): 1–40.

through the cervix and into the uterus, and gentle suction removes fetal tissue from the uterine walls.

Pregnancies that progress into the second trimester (after week 12) are usually terminated through **dilation and evacuation (D&E)**. For this procedure, the cervix is dilated for 1 to 2 days, and a combination of instruments and vacuum aspiration is used to scrape and suck fetal tissue from the uterus. The D&E can be performed on an outpatient basis (usually in a physician's office), usually under general anesthesia. This procedure may cause moderate to severe uterine cramping and blood loss. After a D&E, a return visit to the clinic is an important follow-up.

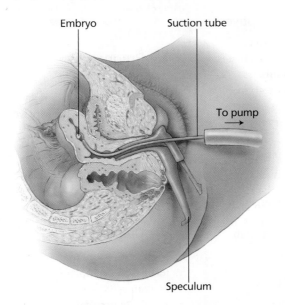

Embryo    Suction tube

To pump →

Speculum

**FIGURE 10.13** Suction Curettage Abortion
This procedure, in which a long tube with gentle suction is used to remove fetal tissue from the uterine walls, can be performed until the 12th week of pregnancy.

Abortions during the third trimester are very rare (fewer than 2% of abortions in the United States).[110] When they are performed, a D&E is the most commonly utilized procedure. The much-debated **intact dilation and extraction (D&X)**, often referred to as "partial birth abortion," is no longer legal in the United States.

The risks associated with surgical abortion include infection, incomplete abortion (when parts of the placenta remain in the uterus), excessive bleeding, and cervical and uterine trauma. Follow-up and attention to danger signs decrease the chances of long-term problems.

The mortality rate for women undergoing first-trimester abortions in the United States averages 3 deaths for every 1 million procedures at 8 or fewer weeks.[111] The risk of death increases with the length of pregnancy. At 18 weeks or later, the mortality rate is 7 per 100,000.[112] This higher rate later in the pregnancy is due to the increased risk of uterine perforation, bleeding, infection, and incomplete abortion; these complications occur because the uterine wall becomes thinner as the pregnancy progresses.

### Medical Abortions
Unlike surgical abortions, a **medical abortion** (also called *medication abortion*) is performed without entering the uterus. Mifepristone, formerly known as RU-486 and currently sold in the United States under the brand name Mifeprex, is a steroid hormone that induces abortion by blocking the action of progesterone, the hormone produced by the ovaries and placenta that maintains the uterine lining. As a result, the lining and embryo are expelled from the uterus, terminating the pregnancy. Medical abortions must be performed early in the pregnancy, no later than 9 weeks after a woman's last menstrual period.

Mifepristone's nickname, "the abortion pill," may imply an easy process; however, this treatment actually involves more steps than a suction curettage abortion, which takes approximately 15 minutes followed by a physical recovery of about 1 day. With mifepristone, an initial visit to the clinic involves a physical exam and a dose of mifepristone and antibiotics, which may cause minor side effects such as nausea, headaches, weakness, and fatigue. The patient returns 2 to 3 days later for a dose of prostaglandins (misoprostol), which causes uterine contractions that expel the fertilized egg. The patient is required to stay under observation at the clinic for 4 hours and to make a follow-up visit within 2 weeks.[113]

More than 99 percent of women who use mifepristone early in pregnancy will experience a complete abortion.[114] The side effects are similar to those reported during heavy menstruation and include cramping, minor pain, and nausea. Less than 1 percent have more serious outcomes requiring a blood transfusion because of severe bleeding or the administration of intravenous antibiotics.[115]

**dilation and evacuation (D&E)** Abortion technique that uses a combination of instruments and vacuum aspiration.

**intact dilation and extraction (D&X)** Late-term abortion procedure in which the body of the fetus is extracted up to the head and then the contents of the cranium are aspirated.

**medical abortion** Termination of a pregnancy during the first 9 weeks using hormonal medications that cause the embryo to be expelled from the uterus.

# STUDY **PLAN**

Customize your study plan—and master your health!—in the Study Area of **MasteringHealth.**

## ASSESS YOURSELF

**Is your current method of contraception right for you?**
Want to find out? Take the **Are You Comfortable with Your Contraception?** assessment available on

# MasteringHealth.™

## CHAPTER **REVIEW**

To hear an MP3 Tutor Session, scan here or visit the Study Area in **MasteringHealth.**

### LO **1** | Pregnancy

- Prospective parents must consider emotional health, maternal and paternal health, and financial resources. Full-term pregnancy has three trimesters. Prenatal care includes a complete physical exam within the first trimester, follow-up checkups throughout the pregnancy, healthy nutrition and exercise, and avoidance of all substances that could have teratogenic effects on the fetus. Prenatal tests—including ultrasonography, chorionic villus sampling, triple marker screen, and amniocentesis—can be used to detect birth defects.

### LO **2** | Childbirth

- Childbirth occurs in three stages. Partners should jointly choose a labor method early in the pregnancy to be better prepared when labor occurs. Possible complications of pregnancy and childbirth include preeclampsia and eclampsia, miscarriage, ectopic pregnancy, and stillbirth.

### LO **3** | Infertility

- Infertility in women may be caused by polycystic ovary syndrome (PCOS), pelvic inflammatory disease (PID), or endometriosis. In men, it

may be caused by low sperm count. Treatments may include fertility drugs, alternative insemination, in vitro fertilization (IVF), assisted reproductive technology (ART), embryo transfer, and embryo adoption programs. Surrogate motherhood and adoption are also options.

### LO **4** | Basic Principles of Contraception

- Contraception, commonly called birth control, prevents conception, the fertilization of an egg by sperm. Types of contraception include barrier, hormonal, intrauterine, behavioral, and permanent methods.

### LO **5** | Types of Contraceptives

- There are many types of birth control, which vary widely in effectiveness, advantages, disadvantages, costs, reversibility, STI protection, and health benefits. There is a birth control method to fit every lifestyle, body, and budget.

- Emergency contraception may be used up to 5 days after unprotected intercourse or the failure of another contraceptive method. Emergency contraception can only prevent pregnancy; it cannot end an established pregnancy.

### LO **6** | Choosing a Method of Contraception

- Choosing a method of contraception involves taking time to research the various options, asking

questions of your health care provider, being honest with yourself, and having open conversations with potential partners.

### LO **7** | Abortion

- Abortion is legal in the United States, but strongly opposed by many Americans. Abortion methods include suction curettage, dilation and evacuation (D&E), and medical abortions.

## POP **QUIZ**

Visit **MasteringHealth** to personalize your study plan with Chapter Review Quizzes and Dynamic Study Modules.

### LO **1** | Pregnancy

1. What is the recommended pregnancy weight gain for a woman who is at a healthy weight before pregnancy?
   a. 15 to 20 pounds
   b. 20 to 30 pounds
   c. 25 to 35 pounds
   d. 30 to 45 pounds

### LO **2** | Childbirth

2. In an ectopic pregnancy, the fertilized egg implants in the woman's:
   a. fallopian tube.
   b. uterus.
   c. vagina.
   d. ovaries.

3. The number of American couples who experience infertility is:
   a. 1 in 10.
   b. 1 in 24.
   c. 1 in 60.
   d. 1 in 100.

LO **4** | Basic Principles of Contraception

4. What is meant by the *failure rate* of contraceptive use?
   a. The number of times a woman fails to get pregnant when she wanted to
   b. The number of times a woman gets pregnant when she did not want to
   c. The number of pregnancies that occur in women using a particular method of birth control
   d. The number of times a couple fails to use birth control

LO **5** | Types of Contraceptives

5. Mariana and David want to practice a method of avoiding pregnancy that is 100 percent effective. What method would you recommend?
   a. Abstinence
   b. Calendar method
   c. NuvaRing
   d. Condoms

6. Which type of lubricant could you safely use with a latex condom?
   a. Coconut oil
   b. Water-based lubricant
   c. Body lotion
   d. Petroleum jelly

7. Benjamin wants to be sterilized. The male sterilization process his health care provider will perform is called:
   a. suction curettage
   b. tubal ligation
   c. hysterectomy
   d. vasectomy

8. Emergency contraception is up to 88 percent effective when used within how many days of unprotected intercourse?
   a. 1
   b. 2–5
   c. 5–7
   d. 7–14

LO **6** | Choosing a Method of Contraception

9. Emily wants to use a contraception method that also protects against STIs. Her best option is:
   a. Xulane.
   b. condoms.
   c. a contraceptive sponge.
   d. an IUD.

LO **7** | Abortion

10. What is the most commonly used method of first-trimester abortion?
    a. Suction curettage
    b. Dilation and evacuation (D&E)
    c. Medical abortion
    d. Induction abortion

*Answers to the Pop Quiz can be found on page A-1. If you answered a question incorrectly, review the section identified by the Learning Outcome. For even more study tools, visit* **MasteringHealth***.*

# THINK ABOUT IT!

LO **1** | Pregnancy

1. Discuss the growth of the fetus through the three trimesters. What medical checkups or tests should be done during each trimester?

LO **2** | Childbirth

2. What are some of the complications that can occur during pregnancy and childbirth? What actions can we take to prevent these complications?

LO **3** | Infertility

3. If you and your partner are unable to have children, what alternative methods of conception would you consider? Would you consider adoption?

LO **4** | Basic Principles of Contraception

4. How, in general, do contraceptives work? What is the difference between perfect-use and typical-use failure rates? Which do you think is a better predictor of effectiveness?

LO **5** | Types of Contraceptives

5. What are the options for different birth control methods? What are their major advantages and disadvantages? What makes one more appealing than others?

6. Can you imagine using ECPs if you had a contraceptive failure? What do you think about ECPs being available to people of all ages without a prescription?

LO **6** | Choosing a Method of Contraception

7. List the most effective contraceptive methods. What are their drawbacks? What medical conditions would keep a person from using each one? Which methods do you think would be most effective for you? Why?

LO **7** | Abortion

8. What are the various methods of abortion? What are the two opposing viewpoints concerning abortion? What is *Roe v. Wade*, and what impact has it had on the abortion debate in the United States?

# ACCESS YOUR HEALTH ON THE INTERNET

Visit **MasteringHealth** for links to the websites and RSS feeds.

Use the following websites to further explore topics and issues related to reproductive health.

**Guttmacher Institute**. This is a nonprofit organization focused on sexual and reproductive health research, policy analysis, and public education. **www.guttmacher.org**

**Association of Reproductive Health Professionals**. This organization was originally founded by Alan Guttmacher as the educational arm of Planned Parenthood. Now an independent organization, it provides education for health care professionals and the general public. The *Patient Resources* portion of the website includes information on various methods of birth control and an interactive tool to help you choose a method that will work for you. **www.arhp.org**

**Planned Parenthood**. This site offers a range of up-to-date information on sexual health issues, such as birth control, the decision of when and whether to have a child, sexually transmitted infections, abortion, and safer sex. **www.plannedparenthood.org**

**Bedsider**. This easy-to-read and humorous website offers up-to-date and thorough information on contraceptives. **www.bedsider.org**

The American Pregnancy Association. This is a national organization offering a wealth of resources to promote reproductive and pregnancy wellness. The website includes educational materials and information on the latest research. **www.americanpregnancy.org**

**Sexuality Information and Education Council of the United States**. Information, guidelines, and materials for the advancement of sexuality education are all found here. The site advocates the right of individuals to make responsible sexual choices. **www.siecus.org**

**International Council on Infertility Information Dissemination**. This site includes current research and information on infertility. **www.inciid.org**

# FOCUS ON Recognizing and Avoiding Addiction

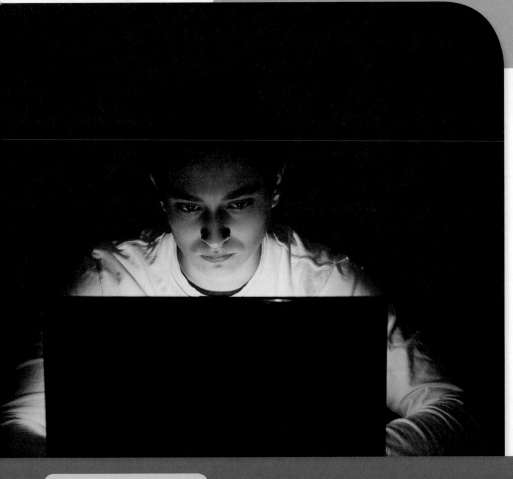

## LEARNING OUTCOMES

**LO 1** Define *addiction*, identify the signs of addiction, and describe the impact of addiction on friends and family.

**LO 2** Discuss the addictive process, the physiology of addiction, and the biopsychosocial model of addiction.

**LO 3** Describe types of addictions, including disordered gambling, compulsive buying, compulsive Internet or technology use, work addiction, compulsive exercise, and sexual addiction.

**LO 4** Evaluate treatment and recovery options for addicts, including intervention, individual therapy, group therapy, family therapy, and 12-step programs.

## WHY SHOULD I CARE?

Addictions of any kind limit your ability to make good decisions and maintain your focus, making it hard to meet your full potential as a student and a community member. A seemingly harmless habit may actually be progressing into an addiction that prevents you from attending classes, meeting new people, participating in other activities that you might find enjoyable or help you meet career goals.

These days, it's easy to find high-profile cases of compulsive and destructive behavior. Stories of celebrities, athletes, and politicians struggling with addictions to alcohol and drugs fill headlines and TV news programs. Heroin deaths in youth have been epidemic in some regions of the United States. But millions of people—young and old, rich and poor—from a wide range of socioeconomic conditions throughout the world are waging their own battles with addiction as well. People with addictions can sometimes be unaware that they have a problem because many potentially addictive activities may appear to enhance the lives of those who engage in them moderately. In addition to alcohol and drugs, the most commonly recognized addictions include food, sex, relationships, shopping, work, exercise, gambling, and using technology and the Internet.

# LO 1 | WHAT IS ADDICTION?

Define *addiction*, identify the signs of addiction, and describe the impact of addiction on friends and family.

**Addiction** is defined as continued involvement with a substance or activity despite its ongoing negative consequences. It is classified by the American Psychiatric Association (APA) as a mental disorder. Addictive behaviors initially provide a sense of pleasure or stability that is difficult for some individuals to achieve in other ways.

Some researchers speak of two types of addictions: *substance addictions* (e.g., alcoholism, drug abuse, and smoking) and *process addictions* (e.g., gambling, spending, shopping, eating, and sexual activity). Many addicts, such as *polydrug abusers*, are those addicted to more than one substance or process.

In this text, *addiction* is used interchangeably with *physiological addiction*. However, **physiological dependence**, the adaptive state that occurs with regular addictive behavior and results in withdrawal syndrome, is only one indicator of addiction. Psychological dynamics play an important role too,

---

**addiction** Persistent, compulsive dependence on a behavior or substance, including mood-altering behaviors or activities, despite ongoing negative consequences.

**physiological dependence** The adaptive state that occurs with regular addictive behavior and results in withdrawal syndrome.

**compulsion** Preoccupation with a behavior and an overwhelming need to perform it.

**obsession** Excessive preoccupation with an addictive object or behavior.

**loss of control** Inability to reliably predict whether a particular instance of involvement with the addictive substance or behavior will be healthy or damaging.

**negative consequences** Severe problems associated with addiction, such as physical damage, legal trouble, financial problems, academic failure, or family dissolution.

**denial** Inability to perceive or accurately interpret the self-destructive effects of the addictive behavior.

---

which explains why behaviors may also be addictive.

To be addictive, a behavior must have the potential to produce a positive mood change. In many ways, addiction is a form of *operant conditioning* in which people do a drug or shop incessantly and it "feels good." Before they know it, they crave that pleasurable experience. Repeating the drug or the shopping reactivates the pleasure center in the brain. Before long, they lose control and would rather shop or do drugs to feel that pleasure than almost anything else in their lives. Chemicals are responsible for the most profound addictions because they produce dramatic mood changes and cause cellular changes to which the body adapts so well that it eventually requires the chemical in order to function normally. Yet other behaviors, such as gambling, working, and sex, also create changes at the cellular level along with positive mood changes.[1] A person with an intense, uncontrollable urge to continue engaging in a particular activity is said to have developed a psychological dependence. In fact, psychological and physiological dependence are so intertwined that it is not really possible to separate the two. Although the mechanism is not well understood, all forms of addiction probably reflect dysfunction of certain biochemical systems in the brain.[2]

Most drugs of abuse directly or indirectly target the brain's reward system by flooding the circuit with *dopamine*. Dopamine is a neurotransmitter present in regions of the brain that regulate movement, emotion, cognition, motivation, and feelings of pleasure. The overstimulation of this system, which rewards our natural behaviors, produces the euphoric effects sought by people who abuse drugs and teaches them to repeat the behavior.

## Common Characteristics of Addiction

Our brains are wired to ensure that we will repeat life-sustaining activities by associating them with reward or pleasure. Whenever the reward circuit is activated, the brain notes that

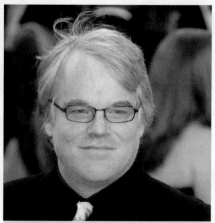

Addiction affects all kinds of people. Academy Award–winning actor Philip Seymour Hoffman, widely respected for his work, was found dead in his New York apartment with a needle in his arm. A mix of cocaine, heroin, and other drugs ultimately proved fatal.

something important is happening and needs to be remembered, and teaches us to do it again and again. Because drugs stimulate the same reward circuit as a satisfying meal or sexual encounter, we learn to abuse drugs.[3] We all engage in potentially addictive behaviors to some extent because some are essential to our survival and are highly reinforcing, such as eating, drinking, and sex. At some point along the continuum, however, some individuals are not able to engage in these or other behaviors moderately—they become addicted and face a nearly uncontrollable urge to act on them 24/7.

Addiction has five common characteristics: (1) **compulsion**, which is characterized by **obsession**, or excessive preoccupation, with the behavior and an overwhelming need to perform it; (2) **loss of control**, the inability to reliably predict whether any isolated occurrence of the behavior will be healthy or damaging; (3) **negative consequences**, such as physical damage, legal trouble, financial problems, academic failure, and family dissolution, which do not occur with healthy involvement in any behavior; (4) **denial**, the inability to perceive that the behavior is self-destructive; and the (5) inability to abstain. These five components are present in all addictions, whether chemical or behavioral.[4]

## Addiction Affects Family and Friends

The family and friends of an addicted person can suffer many negative consequences. Often they struggle with **codependence**, a self-defeating relationship pattern in which a person is controlled by an addict's addictive behavior.

Codependence is often the result of growing up in an environment of addiction. Codependents find it hard to set healthy boundaries and often live in the chaotic, crisis-oriented mode that occurs around addicts. They assume responsibility for meeting others' needs to the point that they subordinate or even cease being aware of their own needs. They may be unable to perceive their needs because they have been taught that their needs are inappropriate or less important than someone else's. Although the word *codependent* is used less frequently today, treatment professionals still recognize the importance of helping addicts see how their behavior affects those around them and of working with family and friends to establish healthier relationships.

Family and friends can play an important role in getting an addict to seek treatment. They are most helpful when they refuse to be enablers. **Enablers** are people who knowingly or unknowingly protect addicts from the natural consequences of their behavior. If they don't have to deal with the consequences, addicts cannot see the self-destructive nature of their behavior. Codependents are the primary enablers of their addicted loved ones, although anyone who has contact with an addict can be an enabler and contribute to continuation of the addictive behavior. Enablers are generally unaware that their behavior has this effect. In fact, enabling is rarely conscious and certainly not intentional.

## LO 2 | HOW ADDICTION DEVELOPS

**Discuss the addictive process, the physiology of addiction, and the biopsychosocial model of addiction.**

Addiction is a process that evolves over time. It begins when a person repeatedly seeks the illusion of relief to avoid unpleasant feelings or situations. This pattern is known as *nurturing through avoidance* and is a maladaptive way of meeting emotional needs. As a person becomes increasingly dependent on the addictive behavior, there is a corresponding deterioration in relationships with family, friends, and coworkers; in performance at work or school; and in personal life. Eventually, addicts do not find the addictive behavior pleasurable but consider it preferable to the unhappy realities they are seeking to escape. **FIGURE 1** on page 302 illustrates the cycle of psychological addiction.

## The Physiology of Addiction

Today, scientists view addiction as a chronic disease that involves disruption of the brain's system related to reward, motivation, and memory. Virtually all intellectual, emotional, and behavioral functions occur as a result of biochemical interactions between nerve cells in the body. Biochemical messengers, called **neurotransmitters**, exert their influence at specific receptor sites on nerve cells. Drug use and chronic stress can alter these receptor sites and cause the production and breakdown of neurotransmitters. Some people's bodies naturally produce insufficient quantities of these neurotransmitters, predisposing them to seek out chemicals, such as alcohol, as substitutes or pursue behaviors, such as exercise, that increase natural production. Thus, some people may be more susceptible to addiction, "wired" to seek substances or experiences that increase pleasure or reduce discomfort.

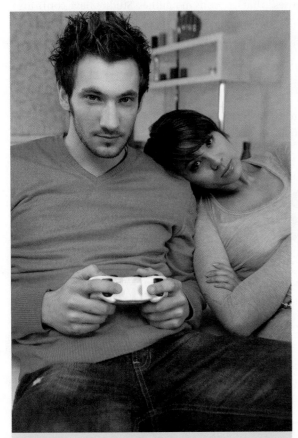

Addiction can be difficult to recognize or acknowledge. Symptoms to look for are an obsession or compulsion with a behavior or activity, a loss of control, and negative consequences as a result of the behavior. Another symptom, denial of a problem, may be easy to see in another person but difficult to recognize in yourself.

**codependence** A self-defeating relationship pattern in which a person is controlled by an addict's addictive behavior.

**enablers** People who knowingly or unknowingly protect addicts from the natural consequences of their behavior.

**neurotransmitters** Biochemical messengers that bind to specific receptor sites on nerve cells.

**tolerance** Phenomenon in which progressively larger doses of a drug or more intense involvement in a behavior is needed to produce the desired effects.

**withdrawal** A series of temporary physical and biopsychosocial symptoms that occurs when an addict abruptly abstains from an addictive chemical or behavior.

**biopsychosocial model of addiction** Theory of the relationship between an addict's biological (genetic) nature and psychological and environmental influences.

Mood-altering substances and experiences produce **tolerance**, a phenomenon in which progressively larger doses of a drug or more intense involvement in an experience are needed to obtain the desired effects. All of us develop some degree of tolerance to any mood-altering experience. Because addicts tend to seek intense mood-altering experiences, they eventually increase their amount and intensity to the point of causing negative side effects.

An addictive substance or activity replaces or causes an effect that the body should normally provide on its own. If the experience is repeated often enough, the body adjusts: It starts requiring the experience to obtain that effect. Stopping the behavior will cause **withdrawal** because the body can no longer create the same effect naturally. Mood-altering chemicals, for example, fill up the receptor sites for the body's natural neurotransmitters (dopamine), and nerve cells shut down production of these substances temporarily. When the drug use stops, those receptor sites sit empty, resulting in uncomfortable feelings that remain until the body resumes normal neurotransmitter production or the person consumes more of the drug.

Withdrawal symptoms of chemical dependencies are generally the opposite of the effects of the drugs. For example, a cocaine addict who feels a high while using will experience a characteristic "crash" (depression and lethargy) upon stopping. Conversely, a heroin addict experiences drowsiness, slowed speech and reactions, and uninhibited behavior while using the drug. When withdrawing from heroin, the addict experiences anxiety, elevated heart rate, trembling, irritability, insomnia, and convulsions. Withdrawal symptoms for addictive behaviors are usually less dramatic. They typically involve psychological discomfort such as anxiety, depression, irritability, guilt, anger, and frustration, with an underlying preoccupation with or craving for the behavior. Withdrawal syndromes range from mild to severe. The most severe form is delirium tremens (DTs), which can last from 1 day to 1 week and occur in approximately 5 to 10 percent of dependent individuals withdrawing from alcohol.[5] DTs can be life-threatening; 1 to 2 percent of addicts die while withdrawing from alcohol.[6]

## The Biopsychosocial Model of Addiction

The most effective treatment today is based on the **biopsychosocial model of addiction**, which proposes that addiction is caused by a variety of factors operating together. The biopsychosocial model was developed to explain the complex interaction between the biological, psychological, and social aspects of addiction. Although one factor may play a larger role than another in a specific individual, it is rarely sufficient to explain an addiction. **FIGURE 2** lists risk factors for addiction.

### Biological Influences

For many people, addiction is thought to be based in the brain and involves memory, motivation, and emotional state. The processes that control these aspects of brain function are thus logical subjects for genetic research into a biologically based risk for addiction, particularly to mood-altering substances. Studies show that drug addicts metabolize these substances differently than do nonaddicted people. Genes affecting the activity of the neurotransmitters serotonin and GABA (gamma-aminobutyric acid) are likely involved in the risk for alcoholism.[7]

Research also supports a genetic influence on addiction. It has been known for centuries that alcoholism runs in families. Studies have confirmed that identical twins, who share the same genes, are about twice as likely as fraternal twins, who share an average of 50 percent of their genes, to resemble each other in terms of the presence of alcoholism. Studies also show that half of the likelihood a person will develop an addiction is due to genetic factors.[8]

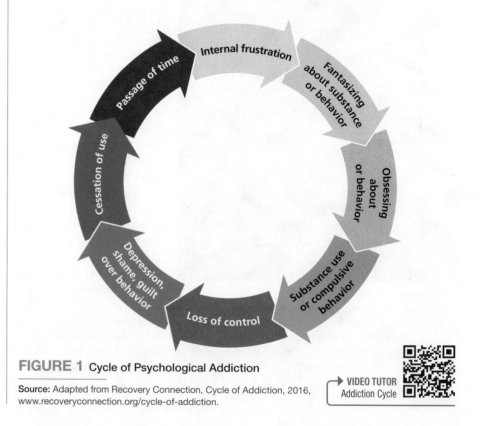

**FIGURE 1** Cycle of Psychological Addiction

**Source:** Adapted from Recovery Connection, Cycle of Addiction, 2016, www.recoveryconnection.org/cycle-of-addiction.

VIDEO TUTOR
Addiction Cycle

## Psychological Factors

A person's psychological makeup also factors into the potential for addiction. People with low self-esteem, a tendency toward risk-taking behavior, or poor coping skills are more likely to develop addictive patterns. Individuals who consistently look outside themselves for solutions and explanations for life events (who have an external locus of control) are more likely to experience addiction.

## Environmental Influences

Culture also plays a role in how an addiction begins. Social expectations and mores help determine whether people engage in certain behaviors. For example, although many Italians use alcohol abundantly, there is a low incidence of alcoholism in this culture. Low rates of alcoholism typically exist in countries and cultures where children are gradually introduced to alcohol in diluted amounts, on special occasions, and within a strong family group. There is deep disapproval of intoxication, which is not viewed as socially acceptable, stylish, or funny.[9] Such cultural traditions and values are less widespread in the United States, where the incidence of alcohol addiction and alcohol-related problems is very high.

Societal attitudes and messages also influence addictive behavior. The media's emphasis on appearance and the ideal body plays a significant role in exercise addiction. Societal glorification of money and material achievement can lead to work addiction, which is often admired. Societal changes, in turn, influence individual norms. People living in cities characterized by rapid social change or social disorganization often feel less connected to civic and religious institutions. The resulting disenfranchisement leads to increased destructive behaviors, including addiction.[10]

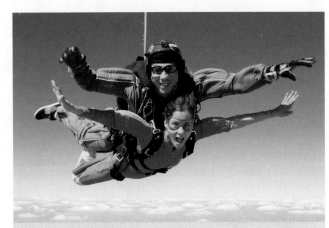

A tendency toward risk-taking behavior, as well as other psychological factors such as low self-esteem and poor coping skills, may put you at higher risk of developing an addiction than someone without these traits.

**Social learning theory** proposes that people learn behaviors by watching role models—parents, caregivers, and significant others. The effects of modeling, imitation, and identification with behavior from early childhood on are well documented.[11] Modeling is especially influential when it involves behavior that is mood altering.

On an individual level, major stressful life events—such as divorce, change in work status, or death of a loved one—may trigger addictive behaviors as traumatized people seek to medicate their pain. Addictive behaviors reliably alleviate personal pain for a short time. However, over the long term, addictive behaviors actually cause more pain than they relieve.

Family members whose needs for love, security, and affirmation are not consistently met; who are refused permission to express their feelings; and who frequently submerge their personalities to "keep the peace" are prone to addiction. Children whose parents are not consistently available to them (physically or emotionally); who are subjected to sexual abuse, physical abuse, neglect, or abandonment; or who receive inconsistent or disparaging messages about their self-worth may experience psychosocial or physical illness and addiction in adulthood.

**Environmental factors**
- Ready access to the substance or experience
- Abusive or neglectful home environment
- Peer norms
- Membership in an oppressed or marginalized group
- Chronic or acute stressors

**Psychological factors**
- Low self-esteem
- External locus of control (looking outside oneself for solutions)
- Passivity
- Post-traumatic stress disorders (victims of abuse or other trauma)

**Biological factors**
- Unusual early response to the substance or experience
- Attention-deficit/hyperactivity disorder and other learning disabilities
- Biologically based mood disorders
- Addiction among biological family members

**FIGURE 2** Risk Factors for Addiction

**social learning theory** Theory that people learn behaviors by watching role models—parents, caregivers, and significant others.

## LO 3 | ADDICTIVE BEHAVIORS

Describe types of addictions, including disordered gambling, compulsive buying, compulsive Internet or technology use, work addiction, compulsive exercise, and sexual addiction.

Traditionally, the word *addiction* has been used mainly with alcohol and other psychoactive substances. However, new knowledge about the brain's reward system suggests that, as far as the brain is concerned, a reward is a reward, whether brought on by a chemical or a behavior.[12] **Process addictions** are those behaviors known to be addictive because they are mood altering. Examples of process addictions include disordered gambling, compulsive buying, compulsive Internet or technology use, work addiction, compulsive exercise, and sexual addiction.

## Gambling Disorder

Gambling is a form of recreation and entertainment for millions of Americans. Most people who gamble do so casually and moderately to experience the excitement of anticipating a win. In the United States, more than 5 million people meet the criteria for having a gambling addiction; many others are directly or indirectly impacted by the gambling behavior of friends or relatives.[13] The APA, which previously used the term *pathological gambling*, now uses the term **gambling disorder** and recognizes it as an addictive disorder. In fact, gambling addiction is the only nonsubstance condition listed as an addiction in the DSM-5. According to the APA's *Diagnostic and Statistical Manual of Mental Disorders*, 5th edition (DSM-5), characteristic behaviors associated with gambling disorder include a preoccupation with gambling, unsuccessful efforts to cut back or quit, gambling when feeling distressed, and lying to family members to conceal the extent of gambling.[14] Where casual gamblers can stop and are capable of seeing the necessity to do so, individuals with gambling disorder are unable to control the urge to gamble even in the face of devastating consequences such as high debt or the loss of homes, families, jobs, health—even their lives.

There is strong evidence that disordered gambling has a biological component. Gambling addiction has come to be viewed as a disorder of the dopamine neurotransmitter system, coupled with decreased blood flow to a key section of the brain's reward system. It is thought that individuals with gambling disorder, like people who abuse drugs, compensate for this deficiency in their brain's reward system by overdoing it and getting hooked.[15] Most individuals with a gambling disorder seek excitement even more than money, living from fix to fix, placing increasingly large bets to obtain the desired level of excitement. Like drug abusers, people with a gambling disorder show tolerance in their need to increase the amount of their bets; and they experience highs rivaling those brought on by drugs. Those with a gambling disorder show withdrawal symptoms similar to a mild form of drug withdrawal, including sleep disturbance, sweating, irritability, and craving.[16]

Men are more likely to have gambling problems than are women. Women, however, tend to begin gambling later than do men, but they develop gambling problems more rapidly. Gambling disorder prevalence is also higher among racial and ethnic minorities, individuals with a family history of gambling, veterans, and individuals with disabilities.[17] If they are regularly exposed to gambling, family members of those with gambling disorder are more susceptible to developing gambling disorder themselves than are individuals with family members who don't have gambling disorder.

Individuals with gambling disorder are much more likely to have mental disorders and/or substance use disorders than are those without gambling disorder. It is not uncommon for gamblers to suffer from mood disorders such as depression, anxiety, or posttraumatic stress disorder.[18] A significant number of those with gambling disorder are more likely to be alcoholics, drug abusers, and/or smokers.[19]

Distorted thinking is one of the characteristics associated with gambling disorder. Similar to other addictions, denial is common. Gambling disorder differs from other addictions in the prevalence of superstitions, which serve to reinforce addictive behaviors. Another disordered thinking pattern is frequent and long-term chasing of one's losses.

Although gambling is illegal for anyone under the age of 21, college students have easier access to gambling opportunities than ever before. The percentage

**process addictions** Behaviors such as disordered gambling, compulsive buying, compulsive Internet or technology use, work addiction, compulsive exercise, and sexual addiction that are known to be addictive because they are mood altering.

**gambling disorder** Compulsive gambling that cannot be controlled.

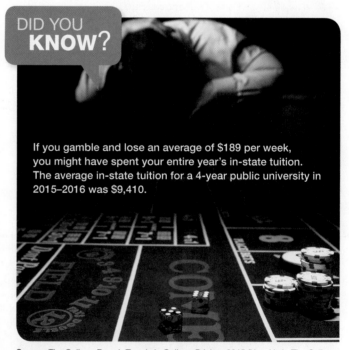

**DID YOU KNOW?**

If you gamble and lose an average of $189 per week, you might have spent your entire year's in-state tuition. The average in-state tuition for a 4-year public university in 2015–2016 was $9,410.

**Source:** The College Board, *Trends in College Pricing, 2015* (New York: The College Board, 2015), Available at http://trends.collegeboard.org/sites/default/files/trends-college-pricing-web-final-508-2.pdf.

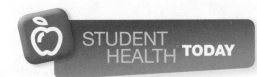
# GAMBLING AND COLLEGE STUDENTS

Although many people gamble occasionally without it ever becoming a problem, even model students can find themselves caught up in it. Disordered gambling on college campuses has become a big concern.

It is anticipated that each year approximately 70 million (about one in five) Americans are expected to participate in some form of tournament gambling, with nearly 40 million involved in bracket activity. A good example is what happens on campuses and across the country each year during March Madness, the National Collegiate Athletic Association men's college basketball tournament. An estimated $80–90 million is taken in legal wagers over the 3 weeks during which the tournament takes place—more than is wagered on the Super Bowl. While over $2.5 billion of the money wagered is from office pools, more and more of these dollars come from the pockets of college students. In a recent survey, approximately 75 percent of students reported they had gambled during the past year, whether legally or illegally. College students give three main reasons for gambling: risk, excitement, and the chance to make money. Consider the following:

- Almost 53 percent of college students have participated in most forms of gambling, including casino gambling, lottery tickets, racing, and sports betting, in the past month.
- At least 78 percent of youths have placed a bet by the age of 18.
- An estimated 10 percent of college students can be classified as problem gamblers.
- Although most college students who gamble are able to do so without developing a problem, warning signs of disordered gambling include:
  - Frequent talk about gambling; encouraging or challenging others to gamble
  - Spending more time or money on gambling than he or she can afford
  - Borrowing money, using financial aid money or other money, or committing crimes to finance gambling
  - "Chasing" losses with more gambling
  - Secrecy about gambling habits and being defensive when confronted
  - Possessing gambling paraphernalia such as lottery tickets or poker items
  - Missing or being late for school, work, or family activities due to gambling
  - Feeling sad, anxious, fearful, or angry about gambling losses

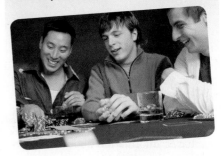

**Call, fold, or raise? For increasing numbers of college students, gambling and the debts it can incur are becoming serious problems.**

If any of these warning signs apply to you, consider talking with a counselor to get help.

**Sources:** D. Nowak and A. Aloe, "The Prevalence of Pathological Gambling Among College Students: A Meta-Analytic Synthesis, 2005–2013," *Journal of Gambling Studies* 30, no. 4 (2014): 819–43; N.W. Shead et al., "Trends in Gambling Behavior among College Student-Athletes: A Comparison of 2004 and 2008 NCAA Survey Data," *Journal of Gambling Issues* 29 (2014): 1–21; M. Henderson, "March Madness: A Big Deal (and Threat) for Gamblers," Elements Behavioral Health, March 19, 2015, https://www.elementsbehavioralhealth.com/featured/march-madness-a-big-deal-and-threat-for-gamblers/; National Council on Problem Gambling, "College Gambling Facts and Statistics," Accessed March 2016, www.ncpgambling.org/files/NPGAWcollegefactsheet.pdf.

---

of college students who gamble—close to 75 percent (legally or illegally)—is consistent with these growing opportunities.[20] Nearly 18 percent of those students reported gambling once a week or more.[21] With the advent of online gambling, televised poker tournaments, and a growing number of casinos, scratch tickets, lotteries, and sports-betting networks, there are many opportunities for college students to gamble. It is estimated

## SEE IT! VIDEOS

How do you battle compulsive shopping? Watch **Woman's Shopping Addiction Revealed**, available on **MasteringHealth.™**

that 6 percent of college students in the United States have a serious gambling problem, which can result in psychological difficulties, debt, and failing grades.[22] The **Student Health Today** box discusses student gambling in more detail.

## Compulsive Buying Disorder

In the United States today, many people often use shopping as a way to make themselves feel better. However, **compulsive** buyers are preoccupied with shopping and spending and exercise little control over their impulses to buy. Shopping actually makes them feel worse, not better. Compulsive buying is estimated to afflict up to 6 percent of

adults.[23] The vast majority of compulsive buyers are women.[24]

Compulsive buying has many of the same characteristics as alcoholism, gambling, and other addictions. Symptoms that signal that a person has crossed the line into compulsive buying include preoccupation with shopping and spending, buying more than one of the same item, shopping for longer periods than intended, repeatedly buying much more than he or she needs or can afford, and buying to the point that it interferes with social activities or work and creates financial problems (e.g., indebtedness

**compulsive buying disorder** Compulsive shopping and spending disorder that cannot be controlled.

# $25,000

is the average amount of **DEBT** a compulsive shopper owes.

or bankruptcy). Compulsive buying frequently results in psychological distress, such as depression and feelings of guilt, as well as conflict with friends and between couples.[25]

In addition, the Internet provides instant access to millions of tempting purchases, information about the newest fashions, and continuous alerts about new products. The Internet enables a compulsive buyer to be alone with their addiction, and permits little to no social interaction, absent direct, face-to-face

contact. Ashamed of their uncontrolled behavior, many compulsive buyers prefer buying online to real stores. Compulsive buyers often do not want others (including family members) to see what, how frequently, and how much they buy. Nevertheless, some compulsive buyers admit that they buy alone because they don't want to be interfered with.[26]

Compulsive buying disorders are reported to begin in a person's late teens and early 20s, coinciding with the age that people first establish credit and independence from their parents. A recent study found approximately 3.5 percent of college students surveyed met the criteria for compulsive buying.[27] Access to student loans and financial aid may provide new financial resources not previously available.[28]

In addition to financial problems, college students experience personal distress, lower grade point averages,

family and social problems, higher perceived stress, and poorer physical health. Students also report more depression, anxiety, and problems with impulse control disorders.[29]

## Technology Addictions

Have you ever hopped online to check something quickly, and an hour later found yourself still Snapping or checking Facebook? Do you have friends who seem more concerned with texting or Tweeting than eating, going out, studying, or having a face-to-face conversation? These behaviors are not unusual; many experts suggest that technology addiction is real and can present serious problems.

Recent data indicate over 84 percent of adult Americans use the Internet, and 18- to 29-year-olds compose the largest group of users (with 96% using).[30] Overall, 73 percent of Americans 18 years and older go online daily.[31] Twenty-one percent of adults go online almost constantly, and another 42 percent sign on several times a day.[32] Young adults are the most constantly connected, with 36 percent of 18-29 year olds almost constantly online.[33] Sixty-five percent of adults in the United States use social networking sites.[34] Overall, young adults (18- to 29-year-olds) are most likely to use social media (90 percent).[35] Women are more likely than men to be on these sites.[36] This type of use does not come without risk: An estimated 1 in 8 Internet users will likely experience **Internet addiction**.[37] Younger people are more likely to be addicted to the Internet than are middle-aged users.[38] Approximately 12 percent of college students report that Internet use and computer games have interfered with their academic performance.[39] To read about the experiences of students taking part in an "unplug from technology day," see the **Tech & Health** box.

For compulsive buyers, shopping is an exhilarating experience.

**Internet addiction** Compulsive use of the computer, personal digital device, cell phone, or other forms of technology to access the Internet for activities such as e-mail, games, shopping, social networking, or blogging.

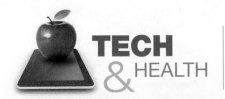

# MOBILE DEVICES, MEDIA, AND THE INTERNET *Could You Unplug?*

If someone asked you to give up your mobile devices, media, and the Internet for 24 hours, how hard would it be? Judging from the results of a study with participants hailing from 37 different countries on six continents—extremely hard. All students followed the same assignment: give up Internet, newspapers, magazines, TV, radio, phones, iPods/MP3 players, movies, Facebook, chat, Twitter, video games, and any other form of electronic or social media for 24 hours.

Students around the world repeatedly used the term *addiction* to speak about their dependence on media and likened their reactions to feelings of a drug withdrawal. "Media is my drug; without it I was lost," said one student from the United Kingdom. A student from the United States noted: "I was itching, like a crackhead, because I could not use my phone." A student from Argentina observed: "Sometimes I felt 'dead,'" and a student from Slovakia simply noted: "I felt sad, lonely, and depressed."

Students also reported that media—especially their mobile phones—have virtually become an extension of themselves. Going without media, therefore, made it seem like they had lost part of themselves.

Despite the withdrawal symptoms, many students found there were definite benefits to being unplugged for 24 hours. Some students found they had more time to talk, listen, and share with others. Students also reported feeling liberated. They took time to do things they normally would not do, such as visiting relatives, playing board games, or having face-to-face conversations.

How do you "unplug" from texting and Twitter for 24 hours (or more) without the anxiety of ignoring your friends online? Smartphone and computer apps can actually helpAvailable apps can post automatic status updates to Facebook and Twitter, send you reminders before scheduled technology breaks, or temporarily lock out your access to the Internet for a set interval. Here are a few suggested apps:

BRB. (Free: iPhone) www.brbapp.com

Unplug and Reconnect. (Free: Android) http://unplugreconnect.com

Freedom. (Modest cost: Windows, Mac, Android) https://macfreedom.com

**Source:** "The World Unplugged, Going 24 Hours Without Media," Accessed March 8, 2016, https://theworldunplugged.wordpress.com/about.

So how important is technology to college students? A reported 91 percent of college students own at least one small mobile device.[40] Students own on average 6.9 electronic devices.[41] Over 85 percent of students own laptops and rely on them for schoolwork; 70 percent use them for research and coursework, and 47 percent use them for note taking in a classroom.[42] However, these devices are also used frequently outside of schoolwork. The average time a day a college student spends texting on a cell phone is 3.5 hours, followed by over 5 hours on a laptop, 1.3 hours a day using a gaming console, roughly 1 hour per day with an e-reader or handheld gaming device, and approximately 3 hours per week watching TV.[43] Some online activities, such as gaming and cybersex, seem to be more potentially addictive than others.

Technology addicts typically exhibit symptoms such as general disregard for their health, sleep deprivation, depression, neglecting family and friends, lack of physical activity, euphoria when online, lower grades in school, and poor job performance. Internet addicts may

## 50%

of Americans would give up chocolate, alcohol, and caffeine for a week before parting temporarily with their **PHONES**.

feel moody or uncomfortable when they are not online. They may be using their behavior to compensate for loneliness, marital or work problems, a poor social life, or financial problems.

## Work Addiction

To understand work addiction, we must first understand the concept of healthy work. Healthy work provides a sense of identity; helps develop our strengths; and is a means of satisfaction, accomplishment, and mastery of problems. Healthy workers may work passionately for long hours. Although they have occasional projects that keep them away from family, friends, and personal interests for short periods of time, they generally maintain balance in their lives and full control of their schedules. Healthy work does not "consume" the worker.

Conversely, **work addiction** is the compulsive use of work and the work persona to fulfill needs of intimacy, power, and success. Work addicts usually set an intense work schedule, are unable to set boundaries regarding work, and feel driven to work even when they are away from work. Work addiction can be defined as a person's need for work becoming excessive to the point that it interferes with a person's physical health, personal happiness, interpersonal relationships, and the ability to maintain social relationships with others.[44] The disorder is characterized by excessive time spent working; difficulty disengaging from work; going above and beyond what the job calls for; a compulsive work style; high levels of

**work addiction** The compulsive use of work and the work persona to fulfill needs for intimacy, power, and success.

stress; low life satisfaction; marital conflict; and work burnout.[45] Work addicts may feel too busy to take care of their health, and there is some evidence work addiction may cause physical symptoms such as sleep problems and exhaustion, high blood pressure, anxiety and depression, weight gain, ulcers and chest pain, or more chronic health conditions such as heart disease and asthmatic attacks.[46] FIGURE 3 identifies other signs of work addiction.

Work addiction is found among all age, racial, and socioeconomic groups, but it typically develops in people in their 40s and 50s. Male work addicts outnumber female work addicts, but this is changing as women gain equality in the workforce.[47] Most work addicts come from homes in which one or more parents were work addicts, rigid, violent, or otherwise dysfunctional.[48] While work addiction can bring admiration from society at large, as addicts often excel in their professions, the negative effects on individuals and those around them may be far-reaching.[49]

## Exercise Addiction

Generally speaking, most Americans get too little physical activity, not too much. However, exercise, when taken to extremes, can become addictive due to its powerful mood-enhancing effects. **Exercise addicts** use exercise compulsively to try to meet needs— for nurturance, intimacy, self-esteem, and self-competency—that an object or activity cannot truly meet. Consequently, addictive or compulsive exercise results in negative consequences similar to those found in other addictions: alienation of family and friends, injuries from overdoing it, and a craving for more. Warning signs of exercise addiction include injuring and reinjuring the body through excessive exercise or lack of proper rest; difficulty concentrating; a feeling of restlessness; adhering to a rigid workout plan; becoming fixated on burning calories or losing

**exercise addicts** People who exercise compulsively to try to meet needs of nurturance, intimacy, self-esteem, and self-competency.

**sexual addiction** Compulsive involvement in sexual activity.

weight; cancelling social plans, skipping work, or missing class to exercise; or working out beyond the point of pain.[50]

## Compulsive Sexual Behavior

Everyone needs love and intimacy, but the sexual practices of people addicted to sex involve neither. **Sexual addiction** is compulsive involvement in sexual activity.

Compulsive sexual behavior may involve a normally enjoyable sexual experience that becomes an obsession, or it may involve fantasies or activities outside the bounds of culturally, legally, or morally acceptable sexual behavior.[51] In fact, people with compulsive sexual behavior do not necessarily seek partners to obtain sexual arousal; they may be satisfied by masturbation, whether alone, during phone sex, or while reading or watching erotica. They may participate in a wide range of sexual activities, including affairs, sex with strangers, prostitution, voyeurism, exhibitionism, rape, incest, or pedophilia. People with compulsive sexual behavior frequently experience crushing episodes of depression and anxiety, fueled by the fear of discovery. The toll that compulsive sexual behavior exacts is most clearly seen in loss of intimacy

WHAT DO **YOU** THINK?

Do you think any behavior can be addictive?

- Can one be a chocolate addict, a study addict, or a shoe addict? Why or why not?
- What dangers lie in using the word addiction too loosely?

with loved ones, which frequently leads to family disintegration and a host of health-related problems.

Compulsive sexual behaviors affect men and women of all ages, although it is more common in men, whether married or single, and it can affect anyone, regardless of sexual preference. Compulsive sexual behavior often occurs in people who experience other psychological conditions such as a mood disorder, impulse control disorder, or who have alcohol or drug abuse problems. Many have a history of physical, emotional, and/or sexual abuse or a history of trauma.[52]

## Multiple Addictions

Addicts often depend on more than one chemical or behavior. Although they tend to have a favorite drug or

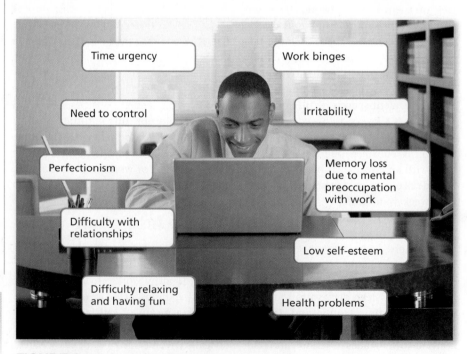

**FIGURE 3** Signs of Work Addiction

behavior—one that is most effective at meeting their needs—it is not uncommon for people to be in treatment for more than one drug. For example, alcohol addiction and eating disorders are commonly paired in women. Individuals trying to break a chemical dependency frequently resort to compulsive eating to keep themselves from taking drugs. Although multiple addictions complicate recovery, they do not make it impossible. As with single addictions, recovery begins with recognizing that there is a problem.

## Costs of Addiction

Addiction affects approximately 8 to 10 percent of the United States population ages 12 and older; 22 to 29 million people are addicted to alcohol or other drugs.[53] Addiction and risky use constitute the largest preventable and most costly health problem facing the U.S. today. It is estimated that more than 20 percent of deaths in the United States are attributable to tobacco, alcohol, and other drug use. Addiction and risky use cause or contribute to more than 70 other conditions requiring medical care, including cancer, respiratory disease, cardiovascular disease, HIV/AIDS, pregnancy complications, cirrhosis, ulcers, and trauma. They also drive and contribute to a wide range of costly social consequences, including crime, accidents, suicide, child neglect and abuse, family dysfunction, unplanned pregnancies, and lost productivity. Costs of addiction and risky substance use to the government alone total at least $700 billion each year.[54]

## LO 4 | RECOVERING FROM ADDICTION

Evaluate treatment and recovery options for addicts, including intervention, individual therapy, group therapy, family therapy, and 12-step programs.

Recovery from addiction is a lifelong process. Before treatment can begin, the individual must recognize the addiction. This can be difficult because denial—the inability to see the truth—is the hallmark of addiction. Denial can be so powerful that intervention is sometimes necessary to break down the addict's defenses.

## Intervention

**Intervention** is a planned process of confrontation by people who are important to the addict, including spouses, parents, children, bosses, and friends. Its purpose is to break down the denial compassionately so that the person can see the addiction's destructive nature. Getting addicts to admit they have a problem is not enough. They must perceive that the behavior is destructive and requires treatment.

Individual confrontation is difficult and often futile. However, an addict's defenses generally crumble when significant others collectively share their observations and concerns. Effective intervention includes (1) emphasizing care and concern for the addicted person; (2) describing the behavior that is the cause for concern; (3) expressing how the behavior affects the addict, each person taking part in the intervention, and others; and (4) outlining specifically what those participating in the intervention would like to see happen.

It is critical that those involved in the intervention clarify how they plan to end their enabling. In addition, persons contemplating interventions must choose consequences they are ready to stick to if the addict refuses treatment. Significant others must also be ready to give support if the addict is willing to begin a recovery program.

Intervention is a serious step that should be well planned and rehearsed.

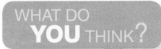

WHAT DO **YOU** THINK?

Why might addicts resist seeking treatment, even when they may admit they have a problem?

■ What factors need to be considered in helping prevent relapse?

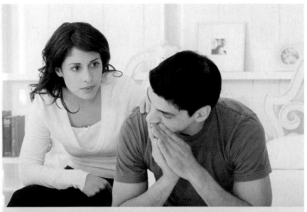

The process of acknowledging and overcoming an addiction is a long and difficult journey for everyone involved.

Most addiction treatment centers have specialists on staff who can help plan an intervention. In addition, books and Internet resources are available.

## Treatment for Addiction

Treatment and recovery for any addiction generally begin with **abstinence**—refraining from the addictive behavior. For people addicted to behaviors such as work and sex, abstinence means restoring balance to their lives through non-compulsive engagement in the behaviors. See the Making Changes Today box on page 310 for tips for dealing with your own potentially addictive behaviors.

**Detoxification** refers to an early abstinence period during which an addict adjusts physically and cognitively to being free from the addiction's influence. It occurs in virtually every recovering addict. While it is uncomfortable for all addicts, it can be dangerous for some—primarily those addicted to chemicals—as early abstinence may involve profound withdrawal symptoms that require medical supervision. Therefore, most inpatient treatment programs provide a pre-treatment component of supervised

**intervention** A planned process of confronting an addict carried out by close family, friends, and significant others.

**abstinence** Refraining from a behavior.

**detoxification** The early abstinence period during which an addict adjusts physically and cognitively to being free from the influences of the addiction.

detoxification to achieve abstinence safely before treatment begins.

Abstinence alone does little to change the psychological, biological, and environmental dynamics that underlie the addictive behavior. Without treatment, an addict is apt to relapse repeatedly or simply change addictions. Treatment involves learning new ways of looking at oneself, others, and the world. It may require exploring a traumatic past so that psychological wounds can be healed. It also involves developing communication skills and new ways of having fun.

## Finding a Quality Treatment Program

For a large number of addicts, recovery begins with a period of formal treatment. The best programs provide a combination of therapies (behavioral therapy, medications, or both) and other services to meet an addict's needs. A good treatment program includes the following:

- Professional staff familiar with the specific addictive disorder for which help is being sought
- A flexible schedule of inpatient and outpatient services
- Access to medical personnel who can assess the addict's health and treat all medical concerns as needed, including complicated detoxification
- Involvement of family members in the treatment process
- A coordinated team approach to treating addictive disorders (e.g., medical staff, counselors, psychotherapists, social workers, clergy, educators, dietitians, and fitness counselors)
- Both group and individual therapy options
- Peer-led support groups that encourage the addict to continue involvement after treatment ends
- Structured aftercare and relapse-prevention programs
- Accreditation by The Joint Commission (a national organization that accredits and certifies health care organizations and programs) and a license from the state in which the program operates

Most programs apply a combination of family, individual, and group counseling, supplemented with attendance at a 12-step support group. Individuals may also wish to explore alternatives to 12-step groups. Organizations such as Rational Recovery and the Secular Organization for Sobriety provide support without the spiritual emphasis of 12-step groups such as Alcoholics Anonymous.

## Relapse

**Relapse** is a return to an addictive behavior after a period of abstinence. It is one of the defining characteristics of addiction. A person who does not relapse or have powerful urges to do so was probably not addicted in the first place. Addicts are set up to relapse long before they actually do so because of their tendency to meet change and stress with the same kind of denial they once used to justify their addictive behavior (e.g., thinking, "I don't have a problem; I can handle this"). This sets off a series of events involving immediate or gradual abandonment of structured recovery plans. For example, the addict may quit attending support group meetings and slip into situations that previously triggered the addictive behavior.

Because those who facilitate treatment programs recognize this strong tendency to relapse, they routinely teach clients and significant others to recognize the signs of imminent relapse and develop a plan for responding to these signs. Without such a plan, recovering addicts are likely to relapse more frequently, more completely, and perhaps permanently.

Relapse should not be interpreted as failure to change or lack of desire to stay well. The appropriate response to relapse is to remind addicts that they are addicted and to redirect them to the strategies that have previously worked for them. In addition to teaching skills, relapse prevention may involve aftercare planning such as connecting the recovering person with support groups, career counselors, or community services.

**relapse** The tendency to return to the addictive behavior after a period of abstinence.

# STUDY **PLAN**

Customize your study plan—and master your health—in the Study Area of **MasteringHealth**.

## ASSESS YOURSELF

**Are you affected by addiction?** Want to find out?
Take the **Are You Addicted?** assessment available on
**MasteringHealth.™**

## CHAPTER **REVIEW**

To head an MP3 Tutor Session, scan here or visit the Study Area in **MasteringHealth**.

### LO **1** | What is Addiction?

- Addiction is the continued involvement with a substance or activity despite ongoing negative consequences of that involvement. Addiction is behavior resulting from compulsion; without the behavior, the addict experiences withdrawal. All addictions share four common signs: compulsion, loss of control, negative consequences, and denial.
- Codependents are typically friends or family members who are controlled by an addict's behavior. Enablers are people who knowingly protect addicts from the consequences of their behavior.

### LO **2** | How Addiction Develops

- Addiction is a process that occurs over time. It begins when a person repeatedly seeks relief to avoid unpleasant feelings.
- Addiction is a chronic disease that involves the disruption of the brain's system related to reward, motivation, and memory.
- Neurotransmitters can be influenced by drug use or the body's naturally

insufficient supply, causing people to pursue alcohol or other behaviors as a way to increase the body's natural production.

- The biopsychosocial model was developed to explain the complex interaction between the biological, psychological, and social aspects of addiction.

### LO **3** | Addictive Behaviors

- Behaviors known to be addictive because they are mood altering are called process addictions.
- Process addictions include disordered gambling, compulsive buying, compulsive Internet or technology use, work addiction, compulsive exercise, and sexual addiction.

### LO **4** | Recovering from Addiction

- Recovery from addiction is a lifelong process. Before a person can be treated for addiction, the individual must recognize they have an addiction.
- An intervention is a planned process of confrontation by people who are important to an addict including family, children, friends, and bosses. Treatment for addiction includes abstinence.
- Recovery options for addicts include individual therapy, group therapy, family therapy, and 12-step programs.

## POP **QUIZ**

Visit **MasteringHealth** to personalize your study plan with Chapter Review Quizzes and Dynamic Study Modules.

### LO **1** | What is Addiction?

1. Which of the following is not a characteristic of addiction?
   a. Denial
   b. Acknowledgment of self-destructive behavior
   c. Loss of control
   d. Obsession with a substance or behavior

2. A self-defeating relationship pattern in which a person is controlled by an addict's behavior is called:
   a. an obsessive ideation
   b. an enabler
   c. a child
   d. a codependent

### LO **2** | How Addiction Develops

3. A phenomenon in which progressively larger doses of a drug are needed to produce the desired effect is called:
   a. withdrawal
   b. antagonism
   c. tolerance
   d. synergism

## LO 3 | Addictive Behaviors

4. The only nonsubstance addiction listed in the DSM-5 is:
   a. exercise addiction
   b. disordered gambling
   c. Internet addiction
   d. compulsive exercise

## LO 4 | Recovering from Addiction

5. The hallmark of addiction is:
   a. loss of control
   b. denial
   c. relapse
   d. attempted suicide

*Answers to the Pop Quiz questions can be found on page A-1. If you answered a question incorrectly, review the section identified by the Learning Outcome. For even more study tools, visit **MasteringHealth**.*

# THINK ABOUT IT!

## LO 1 | What is Addiction?

1. Discuss the signs of addiction. What signs might you look for in a friend or family member?

2. Discuss how addiction affects family and friends. What role do family and friends play in helping the addict get help and maintain recovery?

## LO 2 | How Addiction Develops

3. Describe and discuss each of the stages of psychological addiction. How do you think this cycle influences relapse?

## LO 3 | Addictive Behaviors

4. What differentiates a process addiction from a substance abuse addiction?

## LO 4 | Recovering from Addiction

5. Does your campus have treatment and recovery programs for students with addictions? What type of treatment programs do you think would be effective for treating college students with process addictions and substance abuse addictions?

# 11 Drinking Alcohol Responsibly

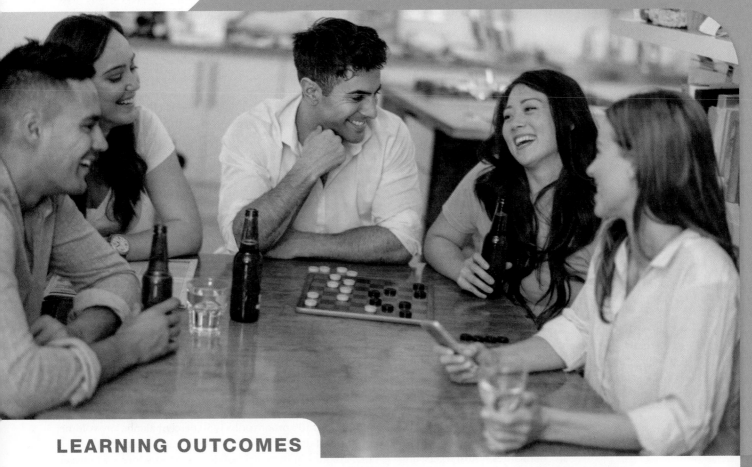

## LEARNING OUTCOMES

**LO 1** Explain the physiological and behavioral effects of alcohol, including absorption, metabolism, and blood alcohol concentration.

**LO 2** Identify short-term and long-term effects of alcohol consumption.

**LO 3** Describe alcohol use patterns of college students, practical strategies for drinking responsibly, and ways to cope with campus and societal pressures to drink.

**LO 4** Describe the impact of drinking and driving on society.

**LO 5** Compare the differences in alcohol consumption and abuse among various ethnic and racial minority groups.

**LO 6** Describe alcohol use disorder (AUD), its risk factors, causes, and costs to society, and discuss options for treatment.

**LO 7** Describe the various types of treatment programs for alcoholism and their effectiveness and explore the concepts of relapse and recovery.

Going out drinking may be fun at the time, but excessive alcohol consumption can result in a hangover that ruins the day after you overindulge—leading you to skip class and to miss out on other activities—as well as a number of negative long-term effects. More than just hangovers, alcohol use increases the likelihood of risky sexual behaviors, violence, and accidental injury and death. While it may seem that this is what most college students do to socialize and have fun, it can seriously impact your academic and personal success.

Throughout history, humans have used alcohol for everything from social gatherings to religious ceremonies. The consumption of alcoholic beverages is interwoven with many traditions, and moderate use of alcohol can enhance celebrations or special times. Research even shows that very low levels of alcohol consumption, particularly red wine, may actually lower some health risks in older adults.[1] Potential benefits include reduced risks of cardiovascular diseases and osteoporosis, though some critics of these studies argue that confounding factors, such as socioeconomic status, may account for the apparent benefits.[2] While alcohol can sometimes play a positive role in some people's lives, it is first and foremost a chemical substance that affects both physical and mental functions. Alcohol is a drug, and if it is not used responsibly, it can be dangerous.

## LO 1 | ALCOHOL: AN OVERVIEW

**Explain the physiological and behavioral effects of alcohol, including absorption, metabolism, and blood alcohol concentration.**

It is estimated that half of Americans consume alcoholic beverages regularly, and about 21 percent abstain from drinking alcohol altogether.[3] Among those who drink, consumption patterns vary. More men are regular drinkers, and men typically drink more than women.[4] White drinkers are more likely to drink daily or nearly daily than are nonwhites.[5] Abstainers are more likely to be women, Asian American or African American, and employed.[6] Adults in poor families are more than twice as likely to be lifetime abstainers as adults in nonpoor families.[7]

New estimates also show that **binge drinking**—a pattern of drinking alcohol that brings blood alcohol concentration (BAC) to 0.08 gram-percent or above—is a bigger problem now than previously thought. More than 38 million U.S. adults binge-drink (or approximately 1 in 6)

about four times a month, and the largest number of drinks per binge is on average eight.[8] More than 50% of the alcoholic beverages American adults consume are binge drinks.[9] Binge drinking is most common among young adults aged 18 to 34.[10] Those households with incomes over $75,000 had the highest drinking prevalence.[11] Men are twice as likely to binge-drink as women.[12]

Learning about the metabolism and absorption of alcohol can help you understand how it affects each person differently and how it is possible to drink safely. It is also key to understanding how to avoid life-threatening alcohol-related circumstances such as alcohol poisoning.

## The Chemistry and Potency of Alcohol

The intoxicating substance found in beer, wine, liquor, and liqueurs is **ethyl alcohol**, or **ethanol**. It is produced during a process called **fermentation**, in which yeast organisms break down plant sugars, yielding ethanol and carbon dioxide. For beers, ales, and wines, the process ends with fermentation. Hard liquor is produced through further processing called **distillation**, during which alcohol vapors are condensed and mixed with water to make the final product.

The **proof** of an alcoholic drink is a measure of the percentage of alcohol in the beverage and therefore the strength of the drink. Alcohol percentage is half of the given proof. For example, 80 proof whiskey or scotch is 40 percent alcohol by volume, and 100 proof vodka is 50 percent alcohol by volume. Lower-proof drinks will produce fewer alcohol effects than the same amount of higher-proof drinks. Most wines are between 12 and 15 percent alcohol, and most beers are between 2 and 8 percent, depending on state laws and the type of beer.

When discussing alcohol consumption, researchers usually talk in terms of "standard drinks." As defined by the National Institute on Alcohol Abuse and Alcoholism (NIAAA), a **standard drink** is any drink that contains about 14 grams of pure alcohol (about 0.6 fluid ounce or 1.2 tablespoons; see FIGURE 11.1). The actual size of a standard drink depends on the proof: A 12-ounce can of beer and a 1.5-ounce shot of vodka are both considered one standard drink because they contain the same amount

**binge drinking** A pattern of drinking alcohol that brings BAC to 0.08 gram-percent or above; corresponds to consuming five or more drinks (adult male) or four or more drinks (adult female) in 2 hours.

**ethyl alcohol (ethanol)** Addictive drug produced by fermentation that is the intoxicating substance in alcoholic beverages.

**fermentation** Process in which yeast organisms break down plant sugars to yield ethanol.

**distillation** Process in which alcohol vapors are condensed and mixed with water to make hard liquor.

**proof** Measure of the percentage of alcohol in a beverage; the proof is double the percentage of alcohol in the drink.

**standard drink** Amount of any beverage that contains about 14 grams of pure alcohol.

**HEAR IT! PODCASTS**

Want a study podcast for this chapter? Download the podcast on Alcohol, available on **MasteringHealth.™**

| Standard drink equivalent (and % alcohol) | Approximate number of standard drinks in: |
|---|---|
| Beer = 12 oz (~5% alcohol) | 12 oz = 1<br>16 oz = 1.3<br>22 oz = 2<br>40 oz = 3.3 |
| Malt liquor = 8.5 oz (~7% alcohol) | 12 oz = 1.5<br>16 oz = 2<br>22 oz = 2.5<br>40 oz = 4.5 |
| Table wine = 5 oz (~12% alcohol) | 750-mL (25-oz) bottle = 5 |
| 80 proof spirits (gin, vodka, etc.) = 1.5 oz (~40% alcohol) | mixed drink = 1 or more*<br>pint (16 oz) = 11<br>fifth (25 oz) = 17<br>1.75 L (59 oz) = 39 |

**FIGURE 11.1** What is a Standard Drink?

\*Note: It can be difficult to estimate the number of standard drinks in a single mixed drink made with hard liquor. Depending on factors such as the type of spirits and the recipe, a mixed drink can contain from one to three or more standard drinks. For example, a typical margarita may contain two shots (3-oz) of tequila, or two standard drinks.

Source: Adapted from National Institute on Alcohol Abuse and Alcoholism, *Rethinking Drinking: Alcohol and Your Health* (NIH Publication No. 10-3770) (Bethesda, MD: National Institutes of Health, 2010), http://pubs.niaaa.nih.gov/publications/Tips/tips.htm.

of alcohol—about 0.6 fluid ounce. If you are estimating your blood alcohol concentration using standard drinks as a measure (see the following sections), you need to keep in mind the size of your drinks as well as their proof. For example, you may have bought only one beer while you were at the ballpark last weekend, but if that beer came in a 22-ounce cup, then you actually consumed two standard drinks.

## Absorption and Metabolism

Unlike the molecules found in most foods and drugs, alcohol molecules are sufficiently small and fat soluble to be absorbed throughout the entire gastrointestinal system. Approximately 20 percent of ingested alcohol diffuses through the stomach lining into the bloodstream, and nearly 80 percent passes through the lining of the upper third of the small intestine. A negligible amount of alcohol is absorbed through the lining of the mouth.

Several factors influence how quickly your body will absorb alcohol: the alcohol concentration in your drink, the amount of alcohol you consume, the amount of food in your stomach,

your metabolism, your weight, your body mass index, and your mood. The higher the concentration of alcohol in your drink, the more rapidly it will be absorbed. As a rule, wine and beer are absorbed more slowly than distilled beverages.

"Fizzy" alcoholic beverages—such as champagne and carbonated wines—are absorbed more rapidly than those containing no carbonation. Carbonated beverages and drinks served with mixers cause the pyloric valve—which controls passage of stomach contents into the small intestine—to relax, thereby emptying stomach contents more rapidly into the small intestine. Because the greatest absorption of alcohol occurs in the small intestine, carbonated beverages increase the rate of absorption. In drinkers of high concentrations of alcohol, the pyloric valve can become stuck in the closed position—a condition called *pylorospasm*. During pylorospasm, alcohol becomes trapped in the stomach, causing irritation and often inducing vomiting. The Health Headlines box on page 316 discusses the effects of mixing energy drinks with alcohol.

The more alcohol you consume, the longer absorption takes. Alcohol also takes longer to absorb if there is food in your stomach because the surface area exposed to alcohol is smaller and because a full stomach retards the emptying of alcoholic beverages into the small intestine.

Mood is another factor because emotions affect how long it takes for the stomach's contents to empty into the intestine. Powerful moods like stress and tension are likely to cause the stomach to dump its contents into the small intestine more rapidly, meaning alcohol is absorbed much faster when people are tense than it is when they are relaxed.

Once it has been absorbed into the bloodstream, alcohol circulates throughout the body and is metabolized in the liver, where it is converted to *acetaldehyde*—a toxic chemical that can cause nausea and vomiting as well as long-term effects like liver damage—by the enzyme *alcohol dehydrogenase*. It is then rapidly oxidized to *acetate*, converted to carbon dioxide and water, and eventually excreted from the body. A very small portion of alcohol is excreted unchanged by the kidneys, lungs, and skin.

Alcohol contains 7 calories (kcal) per gram. This means that the average regular beer contains about 150 calories. Mixed drinks may contain more if they are combined with sugary

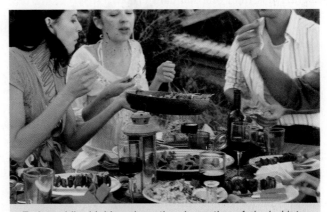

Eating while drinking slows the absorption of alcohol into your bloodstream. Other factors that influence how rapidly a person's body absorbs alcohol include gender, body weight, body composition, and mood.

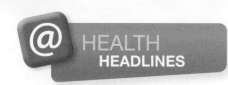

# @ HEALTH HEADLINES

# ALCOHOL AND ENERGY DRINKS
## A Dangerous Mix

Energy drinks are aggressively marketed on college campuses, with manufacturers often giving away samples to promote them. The success of these products is based on claims that they provide a burst of energy from caffeine and other plant-based stimulants and vitamins. Thirty-four percent of 18- to 24-year-olds are regular energy drink consumers.

The alcohol industry has used the popularity of energy drinks to promote its own products, introducing premixed alcohol and energy drink products (no longer sold in the U.S.) such as Sparks, Rockstar 21, and Tilt. In addition, energy drink companies promote mixing energy drinks with alcohol products. Red Bull, for example, promotes a top drinks list suggesting "Jaegerbombs" and "Tucker Death mix." Drinkers who mix alcohol with energy drinks are three times as likely to binge-drink than drinkers who do not.

Both college men and women are equally likely to consume alcohol-mixed energy drinks (AmED). Students involved in fraternities/sororities, students living

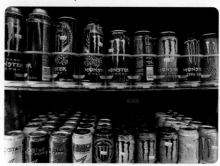

**Mixing alcohol with energy drinks can have serious consequences.**

off-campus, and athletes report great use of AmED than their fellow students. The increased risk for fraternity and sorority use of AmED could be related to the practice of energy-drink manufacturers sponsoring fraternities by supplying them products in exchange for their endorsement. Those students who had greater fun/social motivations for drinking were most likely to use AmED.

Students often mix energy drinks with alcohol, and these drinks can be particularly dangerous. Students report not noticing the signs of intoxication (dizziness,

fatigue, headache, or lack of coordination) when they had consumed alcohol-mixed energy drinks. Caffeine may delay the onset of normal sleepiness, increasing the amount of time a person would normally stay awake and drink. The caffeine in energy drinks also reduces the subjective feeling of drunkenness without actually reducing alcohol-related impairment.

Studies indicate that students who report drinking alcohol-mixed energy drinks are more likely to consume large amounts of alcohol, have unprotected sex or sex under the influence of alcohol or drugs, pass out, be hurt or injured, and meet criteria for alcohol dependency.

**Sources:** M. Patrick et al., "Who Uses Alcohol Mixed with Energy Drinks?: Characteristics of College Student Users," *American Journal of College Health* 64, no.1 (2016): 74–9; Centers for Disease Control and Prevention, "Caffeine and Alcohol," November 12, 2015, http://www.cdc.gov/alcohol/fact-sheets/caffeine-and-alcohol.htm; C. Cobb, "The Role of Caffeine in the Alcohol Consumption Behaviors of College Students," *Substance Abuse* 36, no. 1 (2015): 90–8; J. Verster et al., "Motives for Mixing Alcohol with Energy Drinks and Other Nonalcoholic Beverages and Consequences for Overall Alcohol Consumption," *International Journal of Internal Medicine* 7 (2014): 285–93.

---

soda or fruit juice. The body uses the calories in alcohol in the same manner it uses those found in carbohydrates: for immediate energy or for storage as fat if not immediately needed.

The breakdown of alcohol occurs at a fairly constant rate of 0.5 ounce per hour (slightly less than one standard drink). This amount of alcohol is approximately equivalent to 12 ounces of 5 percent beer, 5 ounces of 12 percent wine, or 1.5 ounces of 40 percent (80 proof) liquor. Unmetabolized alcohol circulates in the bloodstream until enough time passes for the body to break it down.

## Blood Alcohol Concentration

Blood alcohol concentration (BAC) is the ratio of alcohol to total blood volume. It is the factor used to measure the physiological and behavioral effects of alcohol. Despite individual differences,

| Blood Alcohol Concentration (BAC) | Psychological and Physical Effects |
|---|---|
| **Not Impaired** | |
| <0.01% | Negligible |
| **Sometimes Impaired** | |
| 0.01–0.04% | Slight muscle relaxation, mild euphoria, slight body warmth, increased sociability and talkativeness |
| **Usually Impaired** | |
| 0.05–0.07% | Lowered alertness, impaired judgment, lowered inhibitions, exaggerated behavior, loss of small muscle control |
| **Always Impaired** | |
| 0.08–0.14% | Slowed reaction time, poor muscle coordination, short-term memory loss, judgment impaired, inability to focus |
| 0.15–0.24% | Blurred vision, lack of motor skills, sedation, slowed reactions, difficulty standing and walking, passing out |
| 0.25–0.34% | Impaired consciousness, disorientation, loss of motor function, severely impaired or no reflexes, impaired circulation and respiration, uncontrolled urination, slurred speech, possible death |
| 0.35% and up | Unconsciousness, coma, extremely slow heartbeat and respiration, unresponsiveness, probable death |

**FIGURE 11.2** The Psychological and Physical Effects of Alcohol

alcohol produces some general behavioral effects, depending on BAC (see FIGURE 11.2).

At a BAC of 0.02 percent, a person feels slightly relaxed and in a good mood. At 0.05 percent, relaxation increases, there is some motor impairment, and a willingness to talk becomes apparent. At 0.08 percent, a person feels euphoric, and there is further motor impairment. The legal limit for driving a motor vehicle is a 0.08 percent BAC in all states and the District of Columbia. At 0.10 percent, the depressant effects of alcohol become apparent, drowsiness sets in, and motor skills are further impaired, followed by a loss of judgment. Thus, a driver may not be able to estimate distance or speed, and some drinkers may do things they would not do when sober. As BAC increases, the drinker suffers increasingly negative physiological and psychological effects.

A drinker's BAC depends on weight and percentage of body fat, the water content in body tissues, the concentration of alcohol in the beverage consumed, the rate of consumption, and the volume of alcohol consumed. Heavier people have larger body surfaces through which to diffuse alcohol; therefore, they have lower concentrations of alcohol in their blood than do thin people after drinking the same amount. Because alcohol does not diffuse as rapidly into body fat as it does into water, alcohol concentration is higher in a person with more body fat. Because women tend to have more body fat and less water in their tissues than men of the same weight, they will become more intoxicated after drinking the same amount of alcohol.

Body fat is not the only contributor to the differences in alcohol's effects on men and women. Compared to men, women have half as much *alcohol dehydrogenase*, the enzyme that breaks down alcohol in the stomach before it reaches the bloodstream and the brain. So if a man and a woman drink the same amount of alcohol, the woman's BAC will be approximately 30 percent higher than the man's. Hormonal differences can also play a role: Certain points in the menstrual cycle and the use of oral contraceptives are likely to contribute to longer periods of intoxication. This prolonged peak appears to be related to a woman's estrogen levels. FIGURE 11.3 compares blood alcohol levels in men and women by weight and number of drinks consumed.

Both breath analysis (breathalyzer test) and urinalysis are used to determine whether an individual is legally intoxicated, but blood tests are more accurate measures of BAC. An increasing number of states require blood tests for people suspected of driving under the influence of alcohol. In some states, refusal to take the breath, urine, or blood test results in immediate revocation of the person's driver's license.

People can develop physical and psychological tolerance of the effects of alcohol through regular use. The nervous system adapts over time, so greater amounts of alcohol are required to produce the same physiological and psychological effects. Though BAC may be quite high, some individuals learn to modify their behavior to appear sober. This ability is called **learned behavioral tolerance**.

## LO 2 | ALCOHOL AND YOUR HEALTH

Identify short-term and long-term effects of alcohol consumption.

The immediate and long-term effects of alcohol consumption can vary greatly (FIGURE 11.4). Whether you experience any immediate or long-term consequences as a result of your alcohol use depends on you as an individual, the amount of alcohol you consume, and your circumstances.

## Short-Term Effects of Alcohol

The most dramatic effects produced by ethanol occur within the central nervous system (CNS). Alcohol depresses CNS functions, which decreases respiratory rate, pulse rate, and blood pressure. As CNS depression deepens, vital functions

> **blood alcohol concentration (BAC)** The ratio of alcohol to total blood volume; the factor used to measure the physiological and behavioral effects of alcohol.
>
> **learned behavioral tolerance** The ability of heavy drinkers to modify behavior so they appear to be sober even when they have high BAC levels.

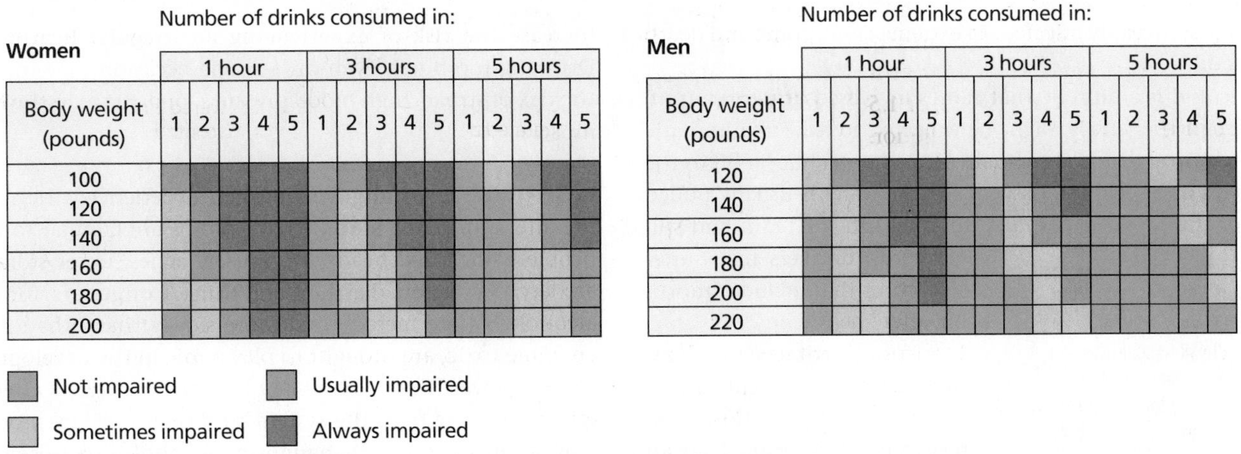

Number of drinks consumed in:

**Women**

| Body weight (pounds) | 1 hour | | | | | 3 hours | | | | | 5 hours | | | | |
|---|---|---|---|---|---|---|---|---|---|---|---|---|---|---|---|
| | 1 | 2 | 3 | 4 | 5 | 1 | 2 | 3 | 4 | 5 | 1 | 2 | 3 | 4 | 5 |
| 100 | | | | | | | | | | | | | | | |
| 120 | | | | | | | | | | | | | | | |
| 140 | | | | | | | | | | | | | | | |
| 160 | | | | | | | | | | | | | | | |
| 180 | | | | | | | | | | | | | | | |
| 200 | | | | | | | | | | | | | | | |

Number of drinks consumed in:

**Men**

| Body weight (pounds) | 1 hour | | | | | 3 hours | | | | | 5 hours | | | | |
|---|---|---|---|---|---|---|---|---|---|---|---|---|---|---|---|
| | 1 | 2 | 3 | 4 | 5 | 1 | 2 | 3 | 4 | 5 | 1 | 2 | 3 | 4 | 5 |
| 120 | | | | | | | | | | | | | | | |
| 140 | | | | | | | | | | | | | | | |
| 160 | | | | | | | | | | | | | | | |
| 180 | | | | | | | | | | | | | | | |
| 200 | | | | | | | | | | | | | | | |
| 220 | | | | | | | | | | | | | | | |

■ Not impaired   ■ Usually impaired
■ Sometimes impaired   ■ Always impaired

**FIGURE 11.3 Approximate Blood Alcohol Concentration (BAC) and the Physiological and Behavioral Effects** Remember that there are many variables that can affect BAC, so this is only an estimate of what your BAC would be.

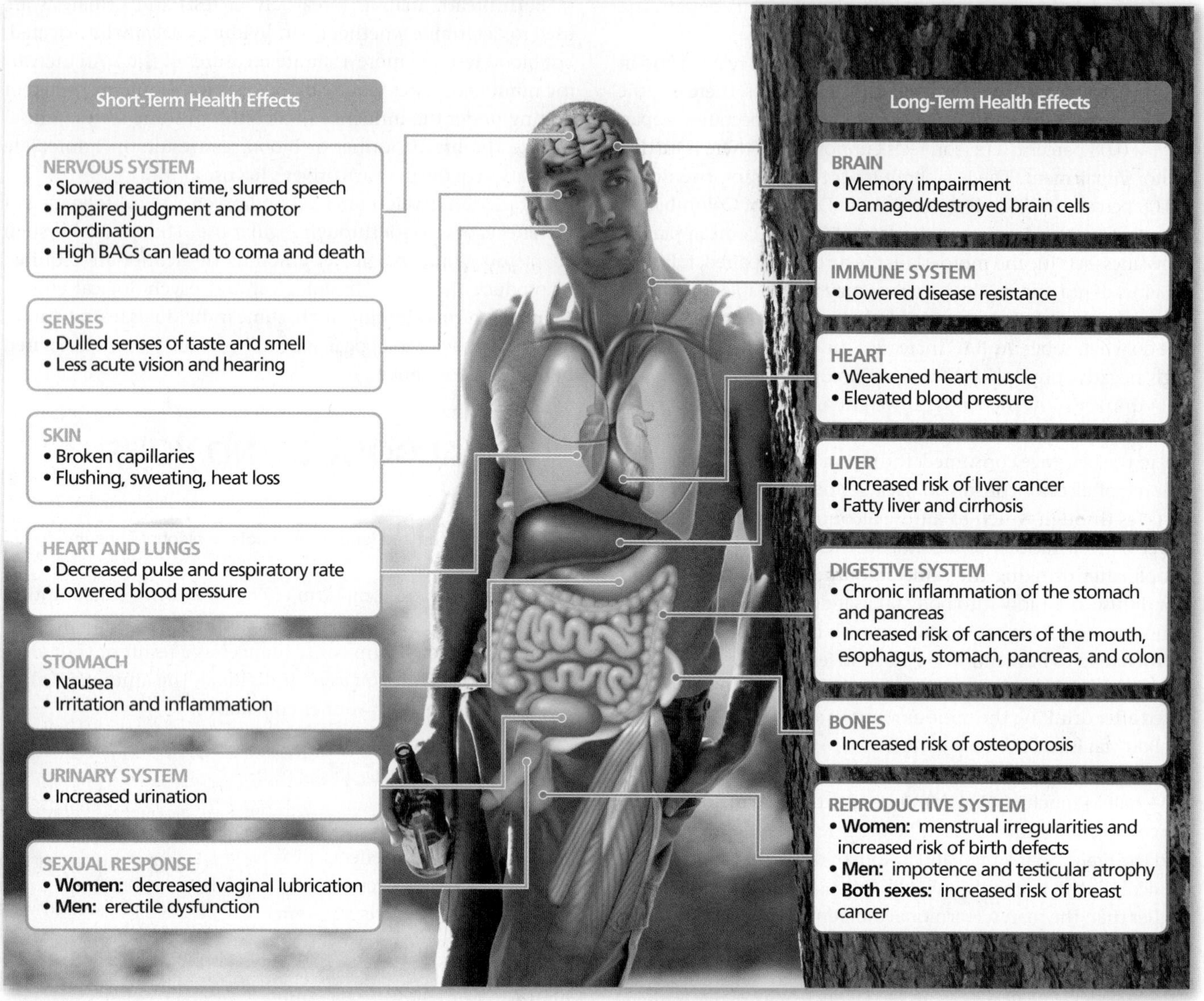

## Short-Term Health Effects

**NERVOUS SYSTEM**
- Slowed reaction time, slurred speech
- Impaired judgment and motor coordination
- High BACs can lead to coma and death

**SENSES**
- Dulled senses of taste and smell
- Less acute vision and hearing

**SKIN**
- Broken capillaries
- Flushing, sweating, heat loss

**HEART AND LUNGS**
- Decreased pulse and respiratory rate
- Lowered blood pressure

**STOMACH**
- Nausea
- Irritation and inflammation

**URINARY SYSTEM**
- Increased urination

**SEXUAL RESPONSE**
- **Women:** decreased vaginal lubrication
- **Men:** erectile dysfunction

## Long-Term Health Effects

**BRAIN**
- Memory impairment
- Damaged/destroyed brain cells

**IMMUNE SYSTEM**
- Lowered disease resistance

**HEART**
- Weakened heart muscle
- Elevated blood pressure

**LIVER**
- Increased risk of liver cancer
- Fatty liver and cirrhosis

**DIGESTIVE SYSTEM**
- Chronic inflammation of the stomach and pancreas
- Increased risk of cancers of the mouth, esophagus, stomach, pancreas, and colon

**BONES**
- Increased risk of osteoporosis

**REPRODUCTIVE SYSTEM**
- **Women:** menstrual irregularities and increased risk of birth defects
- **Men:** impotence and testicular atrophy
- **Both sexes:** increased risk of breast cancer

**FIGURE 11.4** Effects of Alcohol on the Body and Health

**VIDEO TUTOR**
Long- and Short-Term Effects of Alcohol

---

become noticeably affected. In extreme cases, coma and death can result.

Alcohol is a diuretic that causes increased urinary output. Although this effect might be expected to lead to automatic **dehydration**, the body actually retains water, most of it in the muscles or in cerebral tissues. Because water is usually pulled out of the *cerebrospinal fluid* (fluid within the brain and spinal cord), drinkers may suffer symptoms that include "morning-after" headaches.

Alcohol irritates the gastrointestinal system and may cause indigestion and heartburn if consumed on an empty stomach. In addition, people who drink as little as one to three drinks a day may

increase the risk of experiencing an irregular heartbeat.[13] Drinking too much even on a single occasion may increase the risk of stroke, high blood pressure, or damage to the heart muscle.[14]

**Hangover** A **hangover** is often experienced the morning after a drinking spree. Its symptoms are familiar to most people who drink: headache, muscle aches, upset stomach, anxiety, depression, diarrhea, and thirst. **Congeners**, forms of alcohol that are metabolized more slowly than ethanol and are more toxic, are thought to play a role in the development of a hangover. The body metabolizes the congeners after the ethanol is gone from the system, and their toxic by-products may contribute to the hangover. Alcohol also upsets the water balance in the body, which results in excess urination, dehydration, and thirst the next day. Increased production of hydrochloric acid can irritate the stomach lining and cause

**dehydration** Loss of water from body tissues.

**hangover** Physiological reaction to excessive drinking, including headache, upset stomach, anxiety, depression, diarrhea, and thirst.

**congeners** Forms of alcohol that are metabolized more slowly than ethanol and produce toxic by-products.

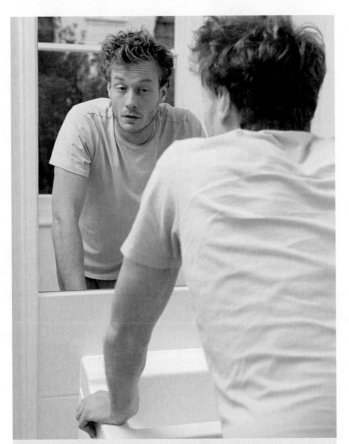

Although there are rumors about a cure for the hangover, the best advice is to refrain from drinking too much!

nausea. Recovery from a hangover usually takes 12 hours. Bedrest, solid food, plenty of water, and aspirin or ibuprofen may help relieve a hangover's discomforts, but the only sure way to avoid one is to abstain from excessive alcohol use in the first place.

There is good news for those suffering from a hangover. The FDA has approved the only over-the-counter hangover drug called *Blowfish*. The tablet is a combination of aspirin, an antacid, and caffeine, to fight headache, fatigue, and upset stomach after a night of drinking.[15]

## Alcohol and Injuries
Alcohol use plays a significant role in the types of injuries people experience. The relationship between alcohol and a variety of accidents, such as automobile crashes, falls, and fires, has long been established. Approximately 70 percent of fatal injuries during activities such as swimming and boating involve alcohol.[16] Drinking affects psychomotor skills and cognitive skills; in other words, drinking can have an adverse effect on a person's reaction time, as well as judgment, meaning people under the influence of alcohol often set themselves up for injury.[17]

Alcohol use is also a key risk factor for suicide—playing a role in approximately 20 percent of suicides in the United States.[18] Alcohol may increase the risk for suicide by intensifying depressive thoughts or feelings of hopelessness, lowering inhibitions to hurt oneself, and interfering with the ability to assess future consequences of one's actions.[19]

## Alcohol and Sexual Decision Making
Because it lowers inhibitions, alcohol has a clear influence on one's ability to make good decisions about sex. Intoxicated people are less likely to use safer sex practices and are more likely to engage in high-risk sexual activity.[20] About 1 in 5 college students reports engaging in sexual activity, including having sex with someone they just met and having unprotected sex, after drinking.[21] The chance of acquiring a sexually transmitted infection or experiencing unplanned pregnancy also increases as students drink more heavily.[22]

## Alcohol and Rape, Sexual Assault, and Dating Violence
In a recent survey, almost 20 percent of undergraduate women and 5 percent of undergraduate men reported being sexually assaulted by physical force or while incapacitated while in college.[23] Various drugs are used to facilitate rape. Alcohol is by far the drug most commonly used.[24] Among the women who experienced a sexual assault or unwanted sexual contact, 61 percent had been drinking alcohol and 88 percent reported not taking or using any drug other than alcohol prior to the incident.[25] Alcohol use by women makes them more vulnerable to sexual assault.[26] While men, when drinking, are also at increased risk of victimization, they are also more likely to engage in coercive sexual behaviors, including sexual assault.[27] Alcohol is sometimes used as an excuse for unacceptable behavior. When a man sexually assaults an acquaintance, he is often viewed as bearing less responsibility for his actions if he was drunk. The double standard in our society often places blame for the assault on the victim if she was intoxicated. No one deserves to be raped. Rape is a violent crime; choosing to imbibe alcohol is not volunteering to be sexually assaulted.

## Alcohol and Weight Gain
Alcohol has 7 calories per gram—nearly as much as fat (9 calories per gram) and more than carbohydrates or protein (4 calories per gram)—and the calories from alcohol provide few nutrients. A standard drink contains 12–15 grams of alcohol, meaning a single drink can add about 100 empty calories to your daily intake. By drinking an extra 150 calories a day more than you need, you can gain 1 pound a month and up to 12 pounds a year.[28] In addition, alcohol stimulates the appetite, so when you drink you are likely to eat more.

## Alcohol Poisoning
Alcohol poisoning (also known as *acute alcohol intoxication*) occurs much more frequently than people realize—and it can be fatal. Alcohol, used alone or with other drugs, is responsible for more toxic overdose deaths than any other substance. According to the CDC, alcohol poisoning kills 2,200 Americans each year.[29] About three in four are men most often between the ages of 35 and 64.[30] Alcohol poisoning varies by gender and race.

The amount of alcohol that causes a person to lose consciousness—0.35 percent BAC for most (see Figure 11.3)—is dangerously close to the lethal dose. Death from alcohol poisoning can be caused by central nervous system

**alcohol poisoning (acute alcohol intoxication)** Potentially lethal BAC that inhibits the brain's ability to control consciousness, respiration, and heart rate; usually occurs as a result of drinking a large amount of alcohol in a short period of time.

**LAST CALL! WHAT'S THE HARM IN HAVING ONE MORE DRINK?**

WHICH **PATH** WOULD YOU TAKE?

Scan the QR code to play Which Path Would You Take? and see where decisions like these lead you!

**cirrhosis** The last stage of liver disease associated with chronic heavy alcohol use, during which liver cells die and damage becomes permanent.

**alcoholic hepatitis** Condition resulting from prolonged use of alcohol in which the liver is inflamed; can be fatal.

and respiratory depression or by inhaling vomit or fluid into the lungs. Alcohol depresses the nerves that control involuntary actions such as breathing and the gag reflex (which prevents choking). As BAC levels reach higher concentrations, eventually these functions can be completely suppressed. If a drinker becomes unconscious and vomits, there is a danger of asphyxiation through choking to death on the vomit.

Blood alcohol concentration can continue rising even after a drinker becomes unconscious because alcohol in the stomach and intestine continues to empty into the bloodstream. Signs of alcohol poisoning include inability to be roused; a weak, rapid pulse; an unusual or irregular breathing pattern; and cool (possibly damp), pale, or bluish skin. If you are with someone who has been drinking heavily and who exhibits these symptoms, or if you are unsure about the person's condition, call your local emergency number (9-1-1 in most areas) for immediate assistance.

## Long-Term Effects of Alcohol

Alcohol is distributed throughout most of the body and may affect many organs and tissues. Problems associated with long-term, habitual alcohol abuse include diseases of the nervous system, cardiovascular system, and liver, as well as some cancers.

### Effects on the Nervous System
The nervous system is especially sensitive to alcohol. Even people who drink moderately experience shrinkage in brain size and weight and a loss of some degree of intellectual ability.

Research suggests that developing brains in adolescents are much more prone to damage than was previously thought. Alcohol appears to damage the frontal areas of the adolescent brain, which are crucial for controlling impulses and thinking through consequences of intended actions.[31] In addition, researchers suggest that people who begin drinking at an early age are at much higher risk of experiencing alcohol abuse or dependence, drinking five or more drinks per occasion, and driving under the influence of alcohol at least weekly.[32]

### Cardiovascular Effects
Several studies have associated light to moderate red wine consumption (no more than two drinks a day) with a reduced risk of coronary artery disease.[33] Several mechanisms have been proposed to explain how this might happen. The strongest evidence points to an increase in high-density lipoprotein (HDL) cholesterol—"good" cholesterol—among moderate drinkers.[34] Alcohol's effects on blood clotting, insulin sensitivity, and inflammation are also thought to play a role in protecting against heart disease. However, alcohol consumption is not a preventive measure against heart disease—it causes many more hazards than benefits. Regular or heavy drinking is a major cause of degenerative disease of the heart muscle called *cardiomyopathy* and *heart arrhythmias* (irregular heartbeats).[35] Drinking too much alcohol also contributes to high blood pressure, increasing the risk of a stroke and heart attack in some people.[36] Combining the use of alcohol with tobacco and other drugs increases the likelihood of damage to the heart.[37]

### Liver Disease
One result of heavy drinking is that the liver begins to store fat—a condition known as *fatty liver*. If there is insufficient time between drinking episodes, this fat cannot be transported to storage sites, and the fat-filled liver cells stop functioning. Continued drinking can cause a further stage of liver deterioration called *fibrosis*, in which the damaged area of the liver develops fibrous scar tissue. Cell function can be partially restored at this stage with proper nutrition and abstinence from alcohol. However, if the person continues to drink, **cirrhosis** of the liver results (**FIGURE 11.5**). Among the top 10 causes of death in the United States, cirrhosis occurs as liver cells die and damage becomes permanent. **Alcoholic hepatitis** is another serious condition resulting from prolonged alcohol use. A chronic inflammation of the liver develops, which may be fatal in itself or progress to cirrhosis.

### Cancer
Many consider craft beers, wine, and cocktails tools for celebration; no one wants to know that alcohol causes cancer. But, in its Report on Carcinogens, the U.S. Department of Health and Human Services lists alcoholic beverages as known carcinogens.[38] Two recent studies have indicated that

# 42%
of college students in Collegiate Recovery Programs cite **ALCOHOL** as their primary lifetime problem.

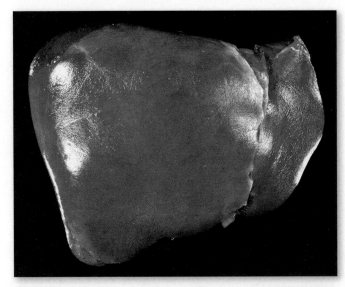

**a** A normal liver

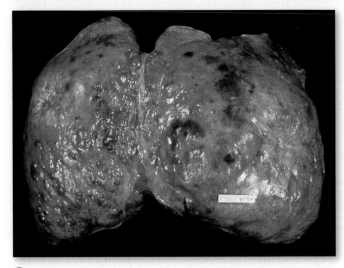

**b** A liver with cirrhosis

**FIGURE 11.5 Comparison of a Healthy Liver with a Cirrhotic Liver** In cirrhosis, healthy liver cells are replaced with scar tissue that interferes with the liver's ability to perform its many vital functions.

alcohol use is strongly associated with the risk of cancer in both women and men.[39] For women, the increased cancer risk appears at lower levels of alcohol consumption then in men, and the total amount of alcohol consumption rather than the regularity of drinking or binge drinking seem to have greatest effect.[40] Alcohol use has been linked to cancers of the esophagus, colon, rectum, breast, stomach, oral cavity, and liver. The leading alcohol-related cancer in women is breast cancer and for men it is colorectal cancer.[41]

There is substantial evidence to suggest that women who consume even low levels of alcohol have a higher risk of breast cancer than those who abstain. A recent study found that women who consumed 0.5–1.5 drinks per day had a 6 percent increased risk of breast cancer compared to those that drank up to half a drink a day.[42] The risk was elevated for those who have a family history of breast cancer.[43]

**Sleep** People who suffer from insomnia are much more likely to develop drinking problems, and individuals with alcohol dependence are more likely to suffer from sleep problems. These sleep problems can persist for months or years after abstinence. A single drink has the potential to increase snoring and worsen sleep apnea. In young adults, binge drinking increases the frequency and severity of sleep problems.[44] For both young men and women, drinking alcohol significantly increases trouble with both falling asleep and staying asleep.

**Immune System** Drinking excessively can weaken your immune system by lowering the body's white blood cell count.[45] The lower the number of white blood cells, the more difficult it is to fight off disease.[46] Alcohol also inhibits the body's ability to produce red blood cells—cells that transport needed oxygen to the body's tissues and organs.[47] If you have a cold or the flu and drink alcohol it will interfere with the body's ability to recover.

**Other Effects** Alcohol abuse is a major cause of chronic inflammation of the pancreas, the organ that produces digestive enzymes and insulin. Chronic alcohol abuse inhibits enzyme production, which further inhibits the absorption of nutrients. Drinking alcohol can block the absorption of calcium, a nutrient that strengthens bones. This should be of particular concern to women because of their risk for osteoporosis.

## Alcohol and Pregnancy

*Teratogenic* substances cause birth defects. Of the 30 known teratogens in the environment, alcohol is one of the most dangerous. If a woman ingests alcohol while pregnant, it will pass through the placenta and enter the growing fetus's bloodstream. In the United States, more than 1 in 5 pregnant women report alcohol use during early pregnancy.[48] Fetal development can be disrupted by alcohol at any point during a woman's pregnancy, even before she is aware that she is pregnant. When pregnant, no amount of alcohol is known to be safe to drink.[49] Alcohol consumed during the first trimester poses the greatest threat to organ development; exposure during the last trimester, when the brain is developing rapidly, is most likely to affect CNS development.[50]

A disorder called **fetal alcohol syndrome (FAS)** is associated with alcohol consumption during pregnancy. FAS is the third most common birth defect and the second leading cause of mental retardation in the United States, with an estimated incidence of 0.2 to 1.5 cases in every 1,000 live births.[51] It is the most common preventable cause of mental impairment in the Western world. Among the symptoms of FAS are mental retardation; small head size; tremors; and abnormalities of the face, limbs, heart, and brain. Children with FAS may experience problems such as poor memory and impaired learning, reduced attention span, impulsive behavior, and poor problem-solving abilities, among others.

**fetal alcohol syndrome (FAS)** Birth defect involving physical and mental impairment that results from the mother's alcohol consumption during pregnancy.

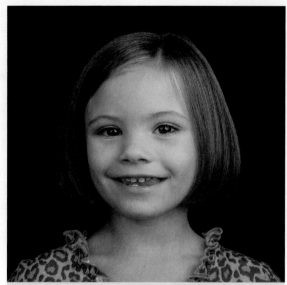
Characteristic facial features of FAS include a small, upturned nose with a low bridge and a thin upper lip.

2 hours. Binge drinking is especially dangerous because it can lead to extreme intoxication, unconsciousness, alcohol poisoning, and even death. Drinking competitions, celebrations, or games and hazing rituals encourage this type of drinking.

College is a critical time to become aware of and responsible for drinking. Many students are away from home, often for the first time, and are excited by their newfound independence. For some students, this rite of passage into college culture is symbolized by alcohol use. Many students say they drink to have fun. "Having fun," which often means drinking simply to get drunk, may really be a way of coping with stress, boredom, anxiety, or pressures created by academic and social demands.

A significant number of students experience negative consequences as a result of their alcohol consumption (FIGURE 11.6). About 29 percent of college students who drank reported doing something they later regretted; 25 percent forgot where they were or what they did; approximately 12 percent accidentally injured themselves; and 20 percent had unprotected sex.[59] Nearly 2 percent reported having sex with someone without giving consent, and 0.3 percent reported having sex with

Some children may have fewer than the full physical or behavioral symptoms of FAS and may be diagnosed with disorders such as partial fetal alcohol syndrome (PFAS) or alcohol-related neurodevelopmental disorder (ARND); all of these disorders (including FAS) fall under the umbrella term *fetal alcohol spectrum disorder* (FASD). An estimated 40,000 infants in the United States are affected by FASD each year—more than those affected by spina bifida, Down syndrome, and muscular dystrophy combined.[52] Infants whose mothers binge-drink when pregnant are at higher risk for FASD.[53] Risk levels for babies whose mothers consume smaller amounts are uncertain.[54] To avoid any chance of harming her fetus, any woman of childbearing age who is or may become pregnant is advised to refrain from consuming any amount of alcohol.

## LO 3 | ALCOHOL USE IN COLLEGE

Describe alcohol use patterns of college students, practical strategies for drinking responsibly, and ways to cope with campus and societal pressures to drink.

Alcohol is the most popular drug on college campuses: 60 percent of students report having consumed alcoholic beverages in the past 30 days.[55] On college campuses, the gap between men and women's alcohol consumption is closing. In 1992, 36 percent of men and 20 percent of women engaged in binge drinking one or more times per week; in 2015, 37 percent of men and 27 percent of women did so.[56]

Approximately 35 percent of all college students engage in binge drinking.[57] For a typical adult, this means consuming five or more drinks (men) or four or more drinks (women) in about 2 hours.[58] Students who drink only once a week are considered binge drinkers if they consume these amounts within

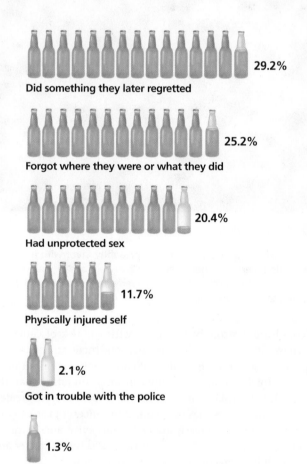

**29.2%**
Did something they later regretted

**25.2%**
Forgot where they were or what they did

**20.4%**
Had unprotected sex

**11.7%**
Physically injured self

**2.1%**
Got in trouble with the police

**1.3%**
Physically injured another person

**FIGURE 11.6** Prevalence of Negative Consequences of Drinking among College Students, Past Year

Source: Data from American College Health Association, *American College Health Association—National College Health Assessment II (ACHA-NCHA II) Reference Group Data Report Fall 2015* (Linthicum, MD: American College Health Association, 2015).

**SEE IT! VIDEOS**

Heavy drinking during spring break can lead to bad decisions, or worse. Watch **Sloppy Spring Breaker**, available on **MasteringHealth.**™

someone without getting consent.[60] A recent study found students who played intramural sports, were in abusive relationships, had high stress levels, belonged to a fraternity or sorority, or were depressed reported higher levels of drinking and negative alcohol-related effects.[61]

Alcohol use among college students also has consequences related to academic performance. Alcohol consumption tends to disrupt sleep, particularly the second half of the night's sleep. These disruptive effects increase daytime sleepiness and decrease alertness, which negatively impacts students' academic performance.[62]

Fortunately, many college students report practicing protective behaviors when consuming alcohol to reduce the risk of negative consequences as a result of their alcohol use. In a recent survey, 81 percent of students reported eating before or during drinking, about 88 percent said they usually or always stayed with the same group of friends the entire time they drank, 87 percent reported using a designated driver most or all of the time, and 69 percent always or usually kept track of how many drinks they consumed.[63] The Making Changes Today box provides additional strategies for drinking responsibly.

## High-Risk Drinking and College Students

According to one study, 1,825 college students die each year because of alcohol-related unintentional injuries, including car accidents.[64] Consumption of alcohol is the number one cause of preventable death among undergraduate college students in the United States today.[65]

**Who Drinks?** It's likely that students who enter college will drink at some point, but there are groups of students who are more likely to drink more and more often. For example, students who believe that their parents approve of their drinking are more likely to drink.[66] Students who drank heavily in high school are also at risk for heavy drinking in college.[67] Many students have tried alcohol in high school. By their senior year, 17 percent of high school students report engaging in binge drinking, 20 percent report having been drunk, and 35 percent report consuming some alcohol in the past month.[68]

**Why Do College Students Drink So Much?** Although everyone who drinks is at some risk for alcohol-related problems, college students are particularly vulnerable for the following reasons:

- Alcohol exacerbates their already high risk for suicide, automobile crashes, and falls.
- Some university celebrations encourage certain dangerous practices and patterns of alcohol use.
- The alcoholic beverage industry heavily targets university campuses with promotions and ads.
- Drink specials enable students to consume large amounts of alcohol cheaply.
- College students are particularly vulnerable to peer influence.
- College administrators often deny that alcohol problems exist on their campuses.

**Pre-gaming, Binge Drinking, and Calorie "Saving"** College students are more likely than their noncollegiate peers to drink recklessly, play drinking games, and engage in other dangerous practices.[69] One such practice is **pregaming** (also called *preloading* or *front-loading*), which involves planned heavy drinking in a compressed time frame, usually in someone's home, apartment, or residence hall, prior to going out to a bar, nightclub, or sporting event. In a recent study, 44 percent of students reported pregaming in the past month.[70] College men are more likely than women to pregame.[71] Some of the motivations for pregaming are to avoid

**WHAT DO YOU THINK?**

Why do some college students drink excessive amounts of alcohol?

- Are there particular traditions or norms related to when and why students drink on your campus?
- Have you ever had your sleep or studies interrupted or have you had to babysit a friend because he or she had been drinking?

**pregaming** Drinking heavily at home before going out to an event or other location.

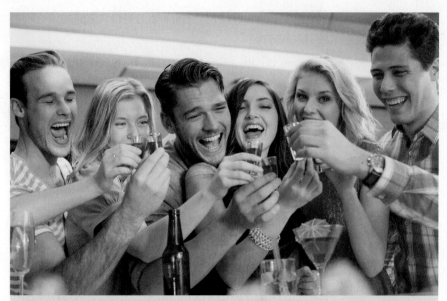

While about 60 percent of college students drink only occasionally, and 25.3 percent don't drink at all, college students have high rates of binge drinking. Take control of when you drink and how much.

**Source:** American College Health Association, *American College Health Association—National College Health Assessment II (ACHA-NCHA II) Reference Group Data Report Fall 2015* (Linthicum, MD: American College Health Association, 2016).

paying for high-cost drinks, to socialize with friends, to reduce social anxiety, and to enhance male bonding. Pregaming can result in higher alcohol consumption during the evening and increase the risk for negative consequences such as blackouts, hangovers, passing out, and alcohol poisoning.

Binge drinking is especially dangerous because it involves drinking a lot of alcohol in a very short period of time. Two-thirds of college students engage in drinking games that involve binge drinking.[72] Those who participate in drinking games are much less likely to monitor or regulate how much they are drinking and are at risk for extreme intoxication. Students participating in drinking games tend to consume the most alcohol, and are most likely to experience consequences such as memory loss and spending large amounts of money.[73] Men more often than women participate in drinking games to consume larger amounts of alcohol.[74] Drinking games have been associated with alcohol-related injuries and deaths from alcohol poisoning. Easy access to alcohol also contributes to higher rates of binge drinking.

Some college students use extreme measures to control their eating and/or exercise excessively so that they can save calories, consume more alcohol, and become intoxicated faster.[75] **Drunkorexia** is a colloquialism currently being used to describe the combination of two dangerous behaviors: disordered eating and heavy drinking. Early studies have found that college students who restrict the number of calories they consume prior to drinking are more likely to drink heavily.[76] One study found that 28 percent of women and 8 percent of men surveyed "saved" calories for drinking by restricting normal caloric intake.[77] The same study found 29 percent of those surveyed engaged in drunkorexia before all drinking occasions.[78] Similarly, another study found that highly physically active

**drunkorexia** A colloquial term to describe the combination of disordered eating, excessive physical activity, and heavy alcohol consumption.

college students are more likely to binge-drink than their nonactive peers.[79] Motivations for drunkorexia include preventing weight gain, getting drunk faster, and saving money that would be spent on food to buy alcohol. Potential risks of drunkorexia include risk of blackouts, forced sexual activity, unintended sexual activity, and alcohol poisoning.

**A Dangerous Alternative: Alcohol Inhalation** Some students are trying new ways to get drunk. Motivated by wanting to get drunk faster, or get drunk without the calories, some students have begun "vaping" alcohol. One recent study found that a very small number of students actually participate in consuming alcohol as vapor; the risks for those that do are very high.[80] Alcohol is turned into vapor by using nebulizers, carbon dioxide pills, or by pouring alcohol over dry ice and inhaling with a straw. The ability to turn liquid alcohol into an alcohol-rich cloud creates an opportunity for quick intoxication with almost no calories. However, inhaling alcohol is extremely dangerous. When alcohol is inhaled it goes directly from the lungs to the brain and bloodstream, getting the drinker drunk very quickly. Bypassing the stomach and liver, inhaled alcohol isn't metabolized—meaning it doesn't lose any potency. When alcohol is absorbed into the bloodstream so quickly, the body's natural defense against alcohol overdose, the gag reflex, is bypassed and the body cannot expel the alcohol.[81] Risks include liver and brain damage.

## What is the Impact of Student Drinking?

People who drink and drink heavily cause problems not only for themselves, but also for those around them. Approximately 3 percent of college men and 1 percent of college women report injuring another person in the past year after consuming alcohol.[82] The laws regarding sexual consent are clear: A person who is drunk or passed out cannot consent to sex. Anyone who has sex with a person who is drunk or unconscious is committing rape. Claiming you were also drunk when you had sex with someone who was intoxicated or unconscious does not absolve you of your legal and moral responsibility for this crime.

Some students report sleep disruptions and academic problems related to alcohol. The more students drink, the more likely they are to miss class, do poorly on tests and papers, have lower grade point averages, and fall behind on assigned work. Some students even drop out of school as a result of their drinking.

## Efforts to Reduce Student Drinking

Some colleges are implementing strong policies against drinking to curb binge drinking and alcohol abuse. University

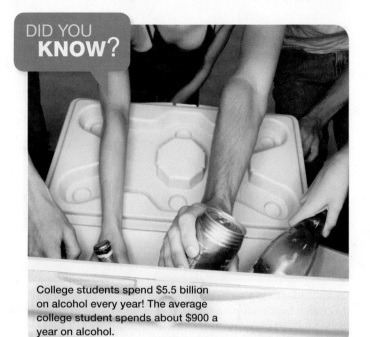

## DID YOU KNOW?

College students spend $5.5 billion on alcohol every year! The average college student spends about $900 a year on alcohol.

**Source:** Banyan Treatment Center, "How Much Are College Students Really Spending on Alcohol?" March 23, 2015, https://www.banyantreatmentcenter.com/college-binge-drinking-alcohol-abuse-florida-alcoholism-rehab-young-adult/.

policies include banning alcohol on campus or at university events, as well as banning advertising of alcohol in campus newspapers. Many fraternities have elected to have "dry" houses. At the same time, schools are making more help available to students with drinking problems. Today, most campuses offer both individual and group counseling and are directing more attention toward preventing alcohol abuse.

Programs that have proven particularly effective include cognitive-behavioral skills training with *motivational interviewing*, a nonjudgmental approach to working with students to change behavior. The NIAAA has recognized Brief Alcohol Screening and Intervention for College Students (BASICS) as an effective program for students who drink heavily and have experienced or are at risk for alcohol-related problems.

A recent study found that both male and female students significantly decreased their alcohol consumption as a result of participating in this program.[83] E-interventions—electronically based alcohol education interventions using text messages, e-mails, and podcasts—and Web interventions such as the Alcohol e-Check Up to Go (e-Chug) have shown promise in reducing alcohol-related problems among first-year students.

Web-based education for first-year students has become an increasingly important intervention. Because first-year students are at increased risk for alcohol-related problems, schools ensure that students are made aware of risks and effects of alcohol. Colleges and universities have been using a *social norms* approach to reducing alcohol consumption, sending a consistent message to students about actual drinking behavior on campus. Many students perceive that their peers drink more than they actually do, which may cause students to feel pressured to drink more themselves. This misperception includes inaccurately estimating the frequency and amount that students drink and the actual consequences of students' drinking (see **FIGURE 11.7** for a comparison of perceived and actual drinking habits). As a result of social norms campaigns, binge drinking has declined at campuses across the country. For example, Michigan State University, Florida State University, and the University of Arizona all reported 20–30 percent reductions in heavy episodic alcohol consumption within 3 years of implementing social norms campaigns, while Hobart and William Smith Colleges saw a 40 percent reduction in 5 years and Northern Illinois University saw a 44 percent reduction in 10 years.[84]

## LO 4 | DRINKING AND DRIVING

Describe the impact of drinking and driving on society.

Traffic accidents are the leading cause of accidental death for all age groups from 1 to 25 years old.[85] In the United States, adults drink too much and get behind the wheel approximately 121 million times (based on self-reports) in a year.[86] Alcohol-impaired drivers are involved in about 1 in 3 crash

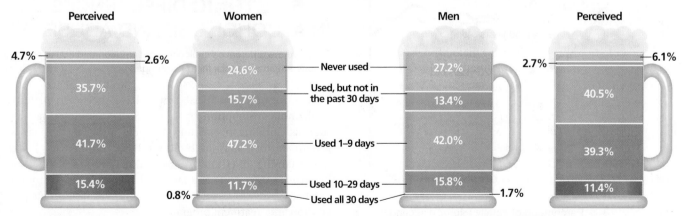

| Perceived | Women | | Men | Perceived |
|---|---|---|---|---|
| 4.7% — 2.6% | 24.6% | Never used | 27.2% | 2.7% — 6.1% |
| 35.7% | 15.7% | Used, but not in the past 30 days | 13.4% | 40.5% |
| 41.7% | 47.2% | Used 1–9 days | 42.0% | 39.3% |
| 15.4% | 11.7% | Used 10–29 days | 15.8% | 11.4% |
| | 0.8% | Used all 30 days | 1.7% | |

**FIGURE 11.7** Percentage of Alcohol Use in Past 30 Days among College Men and Women versus the Perceived Percentage of Alcohol Use

**Source:** Data from American College Health Association, *American College Health Association—National College Health Assessment II: Reference Group Executive Summary, Fall 2015* (Hanover, MD: American College Health Association, 2015).

deaths, resulting in nearly 10,000 deaths a year—roughly one traffic fatality every 53 minutes.[87] Some groups are more likely to drink and drive than others. Men were responsible for 81 percent of the drinking and driving episodes, and 85 percent of people drinking and driving were reportedly binge drinking.[88] Unfortunately, college students are overrepresented in alcohol-related crashes. A recent survey reported that 23 percent of college students have driven after drinking, and about 2 percent said they had driven after drinking five or more drinks in the past 30 days.[89]

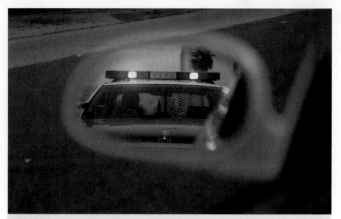

Getting behind the wheel after drinking alcohol is a dangerous choice, with serious legal consequences.

# 0.06

is the **AVERAGE BAC** for college students (both men and women) who drink alcohol.

Over the past 20 years, the percentage of intoxicated drivers involved in fatal crashes decreased for all age groups (**FIGURE 11.8**). Several factors probably contributed to these reductions in fatalities: laws that raised the drinking age to 21, stricter law enforcement, laws prohibiting anyone under 21 from driving with any detectable BAC, increased automobile safety, and educational programs designed to discourage drinking and driving. Furthermore, all states have zero-tolerance laws for driving while intoxicated. Penalties for driving under the influence (DUI) include driving restrictions, fines, mandatory counseling, revoking your license, and jail time. In many states three DUI convictions make you a felon, meaning that you lose your right to vote and own a weapon, and you may also be permanently banned from driving. If you are involved

in a drunk-driving accident in which someone dies, you may be charged with manslaughter or second-degree murder.

Despite all these measures, the risk of being involved in an alcohol-related automobile crash remains substantial. Laboratory and test track research shows that the vast majority of drivers are impaired even at 0.08 BAC with regard to critical driving tasks. The likelihood of a driver being involved in a fatal crash rises significantly with a BAC of 0.05 percent and even more rapidly after 0.08 percent.[90]

Alcohol-related fatal car crashes occur more often at night than during the day, and the hours between 9:00 P.M. and 6:00 A.M. are the most dangerous.[91] Sixty-five percent of fatally injured drivers involved in nighttime single-vehicle crashes had BACs at or above 0.08 percent.[92] The risk of being involved in an alcohol-related crash increases not only with the time of day, but also with the day of the week; 25 percent of all fatal crashes during the week were alcohol related, compared with 44 percent on weekends.[93] For information on phone apps that claim to help you estimate your blood alcohol level, presumably so you can judge whether it is safe to drive after drinking, see the **Tech & Health** box.

## LO **5** | **ETHNIC** DIFFERENCES IN ALCOHOL USE AND ABUSE

Compare the differences in alcohol consumption and abuse among various ethnic and racial minority groups.

Different ethnic and racial groups have their own patterns of alcohol consumption and abuse. Social or cultural factors, such as drinking norms and attitudes and, in some cases, genetic factors, may account for those differences. Better understanding of ethnic and racial differences in alcohol use patterns (**TABLE 11.1**) and factors that influence alcohol use can help guide the development of culturally appropriate prevention and treatment programs.

Among Native American populations, alcohol is the most widely used drug; the rate of alcoholism in this population is two to three times higher than the national average, and the death rate from alcohol-related causes is eight times higher

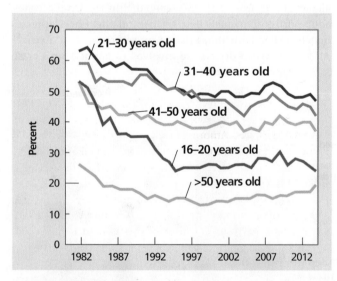

**FIGURE 11.8** Percentage of Fatally Injured Passenger Vehicle Drivers with BACs At or Above 0.08 Percent, by Driver Age, 1982–2014.

**Source:** Insurance Institute for Highway Safety, "Alcohol Impaired Driving 2014: Alcohol," Copyright 2016. Reprinted with permission.

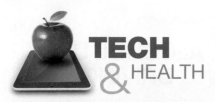

# TECH & HEALTH

## SMARTPHONE BREATHALYZERS
### Better Than BAC Apps?

Some smartphone applications can estimate a person's blood alcohol concentration (BAC) to help them decide if they should avoid driving after drinking. Enter how many drinks you've consumed along with weight, gender, and total number of hours spent drinking, and the apps estimate your BAC. Some even provide the phone number of a local taxi if a person has exceeded the legal BAC limit.

It is important to realize that these apps give general estimates, not your actual BAC. Many apps don't take into consideration elements such as food consumption, medication, general health, psychological conditions, and the time it takes for the body to fully absorb a drink.

With over 100 models now on the market, breathalyzer sales in the United States are soaring. Breathalyzers for smartphones come with many of the same features as BAC apps, and are better indicators of your actual BAC. BAC breathalyzers allow you to enter your body weight, age, and sex, all of which

can influence your BAC readings. Like standard breathalyzers, these products work by measuring the amount of alcohol in your breath. It is also suggested that you wait 15–20 minutes after you finish your last drink before you use the breathalyzer. This reduces the chance of the alcohol vapors in your mouth, making the BAC reading too high.

While smartphone breathalyzer attachments cost more than BAC apps, they give more accurate information about your level of intoxication. Here are examples of three of the many smartphone breathalyzers that are available:

■ **Breathometer Breeze.** ($80: Android, iPhone)
Small size, FDA-registered device that ensures accuracy from 0.000 to 0.25 percent BAC. Provides an estimated return to 0.00 percent BAC. Uses Bluetooth technology.
■ **BACtrack Mobile Pro Breathalyzer.** ($99.99: Android, iPhone).
Small size, professional-grade device that senses BAC as low as 0.001

percent. Estimates when your BAC will return to 0.00 percent. Connects to the phone using Bluetooth technology, and the battery is rechargeable with a USB cord.
■ **BACtrack-Vio Smartphone Keychain Breathalyzer.** (39.99: Apple and most Android devices)
A keychain breathalyzer that uses Bluetooth technology to pair with your smartphone, rapidly estimating BAC and tracking results. Will also estimate when your BAC will return to 0.00 percent.

Remember, it isn't safe to rely on a BAC app or breathalyzer alone to decide if it's okay to drive after a night out. It's much better to arrange for a designated driver ahead of time or plan to take the bus or a taxi.

**Sources:** J. Jolly, "Turning Your Smartphone into a Breathalyzer," *The New York Times*, December 21, 2015, http://well.blogs.nytimes.com/2015/12/21/turning-your-smartphone-into-a-breathalyzer/?_r=0; K. Dohney, "Smartphone Breathalyzers Hit the Market," Edmunds.com, March 16, 2015, http://www.edmunds.com/car-safety/smartphone-breathalyzers-hit-the-market.html.

## TABLE 11.1 | Prevalence of Heavy Alcohol Use* by Ethnicity

| Ethnic Group | Percent of Total Population |
|---|---|
| Whites | 7.3 |
| African Americans | 4.5 |
| Latinos | 5.8 |
| Native Americans/Alaska Natives | 8.9 |
| Asian Americans | 2.0 |
| Persons reporting two or more races | 7.5 |

*"Heavy alcohol use" is defined by the Substance Abuse and Mental Health Services Administration as five or more drinks on at least 5 days within the past month.

**Source:** Substance Abuse and Mental Health Services Administration, *Results from the 2013 National Survey on Drug Use and Health: Summary of National Findings* (NSDUH Series H-48, HHS Publication No. [SMA] 14-4863) (Rockville, MD: Substance Abuse and Mental Health Services Administration, 2014).

than the national average.[94] When comparing other racial or ethnic groups, Native Americans have the highest alcohol-related motor vehicle crash and pedestrian fatalities, suicide,

and falls.[95] Poor economic conditions and the cultural belief that alcoholism is a spiritual problem, not a physical disease, may partially account for high alcoholism rates.

African American and Latino populations also exhibit distinct patterns of abuse. On average, African Americans drink less than white Americans; however, those who do drink tend to be heavy drinkers, and twice as many African Americans die of cirrhosis of the liver.[96] Alcohol also contributes to high rates of hypertension, esophageal cancer, and homicide in African Americans. Among Latino populations, men have a higher than average rate of alcohol abuse and alcohol-related health problems.[97] In contrast, in many Latino cultures, women typically do not drink alcohol, and therefore many Latinas abstain; however, this cultural norm is changing. Recent evidence shows drinking rates among Latina women matching or surpassing those of young Latino men.[98] A key factor in predicting drinking patterns in the Hispanic community is the level of an individual's acculturation—drinking increases with acculturation into American culture.[99] Drinking trends among Hispanics also vary by country of origin; Cuban men tend to drink the least, Puerto Rican men the most.[100] Among women, Mexican Americans and Puerto Ricans are generally more relaxed about drinking than are Cuban women.[101]

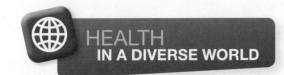

# GLOBAL HEALTH, ALCOHOL USE, AND DRINKING AND DRIVING

Alcohol consumption comes with many serious social and developmental issues, including violence, child neglect and abuse, and absenteeism in the workplace. Throughout the world, alcohol is a factor in 60 types of diseases and injuries and a component cause in 200 others. Almost 4 percent of all deaths worldwide are attributed to alcohol, greater than deaths caused by HIV/AIDS, violence, or tuberculosis. Worldwide, the impact of alcohol use follows:

- Alcohol use results in 3.3 million deaths each year.
- 7.6 percent of male deaths and 4.0 percent of female deaths worldwide are attributable to alcohol consumption.
- Early alcohol use (before the age of 14) is positively correlated with harmful behaviors later in life, including alcohol addiction and drunk driving.
- At the same level of alcohol consumption, men are more likely to become injured and women are more likely to experience negative health outcomes such as cancer (particularly breast cancer), cardiovascular disease, and gastrointestinal problems.

A large variation exists in adult per capita consumption. The highest consumption levels can be found in the developed world, including Europe and the Americas. Intermediate consumption levels can be found in regions of the Western Pacific and Africa. Low consumption levels can be found in Southeast Asia and the Eastern Mediterranean regions. Many factors, including culture, economic development, and socioeconomic status, contribute to these differences.

### Drinking and Driving Laws Around the World

Much of the progress around American drinking and driving laws has come from comparisons with laws in other countries. The illegal BAC limits vary widely by country, with the lowest illegal BAC level in Sweden (.02). There are many countries—Russia, Yemen, Uzbekistan, and the United Arab Emirates, to name a few—that have zero tolerance for drinking and diving. The legal limit in most countries is .05. A number of countries have other, lower BAC limits for younger, less experienced drivers, as well as for professional drivers. Depending on the countries, punishments can be severe. In Brazil, for example, the fine is based on the BAC—the higher the BAC the larger the fine. In some cases the driver faces suspension, and a driver that causes an accident, injury, or death may also face jail time.

**BAC across Countries**

| Country | BAC | Country | BAC |
|---|---|---|---|
| United States | .08 | Japan | .03 |
| Australia | .05 | Mexico | .08 |
| Austria | .05 | South Africa | .05 |
| Brazil | zero tolerance | Sweden | .02 |
| Italy | .05 | United Kingdom and Wales | .08 |

**Sources:** World Health Organization, "Global Status Report on Alcohol and Health," 2014, www.who.int/substance_abuse/publications/global_alcohol_report/en; Drinking and Driving.org, "Worldwide Blood Alcohol Concentration," January 2016, http://www.drinkdriving.org/worldwide_drink_driving_limits.php#bac_limits.

---

Asian Americans have a very low rate of alcohol use compared to other ethnic communities.[102] Social and cultural influences, such as strong kinship ties, are thought to discourage heavy drinking in Asian American groups. Asians also have a genetic predisposition that might influence their low risk for alcohol abuse: Many possess a variant of the gene that codes for the enzyme aldehyde dehydrogenase, which plays a key role in the metabolism of alcohol.[103] People with this variant gene experience unpleasant side effects from consuming alcohol, making drinking a less pleasurable experience.

The **Health in a Diverse World** box discusses global patterns of alcohol use and abuse.

**alcohol abuse** Use of alcohol in a way that interferes with work, school, or personal relationships or that entails violations of the law.

**alcoholism (alcohol dependence)** Condition in which personal and health problems related to alcohol use are severe, and stopping alcohol use results in withdrawal symptoms.

**alcohol use disorder** Refers to problem drinking so severe that at least two or more alcohol-related issues are present, such as engaging in risky behaviors, having problems at work or school, or issues with relationships.

## LO 6 | ABUSE AND DEPENDENCE

Describe alcohol use disorder (AUD), its risk factors, causes, and costs to society, and discuss options for treatment.

The new edition of the *Diagnostic and Statistical Manual of Mental Disorders (DSM-5)* has integrated **alcohol abuse** and **alcohol dependence** into a single disorder: **alcohol use disorder (AUD)**. Any person who meets two or more of the new criteria would receive a diagnosis of AUD. Severity of AUD falls along a spectrum from mild, to moderate, to severe, according to the number of criteria a person meets (**FIGURE 11.9**). For example, if a student shares having a strong desire or craving to use alcohol and a high tolerance for alcohol with a counselor or clinician, he would meet the criteria for mild AUD.

### Identifying an Alcoholic

As with other drug addictions, craving, loss of control, tolerance, psychological dependence, and withdrawal symptoms must be present to qualify a drinker as an addict (see

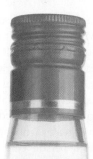

**Answer each of these questions for the past year:**

Do you ever drink more or for longer periods of time than you'd planned?

Do you have a strong desire to cut down, or are you unable to control your alcohol use?

At times, are you unable to think of anything other than your next drink?

Do you spend considerable time in activities related to drinking or recovering from drinking?

Have you reduced your involvement in pleasurable social, occupational, or recreational activities?

Have you neglected responsibilities at work, school, and/or at home?

Do you continue drinking despite knowing that physical/psychological problems are caused or exacerbated by your drinking? Or after a memory blackout?

Have you more than once physically endangered yourself during or after drinking?

Have you continued to use alcohol despite social or interpersonal problems caused or aggravated by use?

Do you meet the definition of having developed tolerance based on these criteria?
1) You need increasingly greater amounts of alcohol to get the same desired effect.
2) Over time, you experience fewer effects from alcohol when you drink the same amount.

Do you experience characteristic signs of alcohol withdrawal when you stop drinking or do you use another substance to relieve or avoid withdrawal?

If you answered yes to two or more of the questions, you are considered someone with an alcohol use disorder (AUD). The level of AUD is defined as: **mild**: 2–3 items; **moderate**: 4–5 items; and **severe**: 6 or more items.

**FIGURE 11.9** Alcohol Use Disorder (AUD) Criteria

**Source:** National Institutes of Health, *Alcohol Use Disorder: A Comparison between DSM-IV and DSM-5* (National Institute on Alcohol Abuse and Alcoholism NIH Publication No.13-7999, July 2015), http://pubs.niaaa.nih.gov/publications/dsmfactsheet/dsmfact.htm.

**Focus On: Recognizing and Avoiding Addiction** on page 299). Irresponsible and problem drinkers, such as people who get into fights or embarrass themselves or others when they drink, are not necessarily alcoholics. Alcoholics can be found at all socioeconomic levels and in all professions, ethnic groups, geographical locations, religions, and races. Data indicate that about 15 percent of people in the United States are problem drinkers, and about 5 to 10 percent of male drinkers and 3 to 5 percent of females would be diagnosed as alcohol dependent.[104]

Recognizing and admitting the existence of an alcohol problem is often extremely difficult. Alcoholics often deny their problem, making statements such as, "I can stop any time I want to. I just don't want to right now." The fear of being labeled a "problem drinker" often prevents people from seeking help. People who recognize alcoholic behaviors in themselves may wish to seek professional help to determine whether alcohol has become a controlling factor in their lives.

AUD is not uncommon among college students; in fact, about 1 in 5 college students meet the criteria.[105] College students at highest risk for AUD drank to facilitate socializing with peers or to have a good time, drank in a parked car, or drank to bolster their confidence to talk to or have sex with someone.[106] In a recent study, the progression to alcohol dependency based on college students' drinking patterns when they entered college indicated that 1.9 percent of nondrinkers, 4.3 percent of light drinkers, 12.8 percent of moderate drinkers, and 19 percent of heavy drinkers developed alcohol dependency.[107]

**Functional Alcoholics** Most of us picture an alcoholic as someone who drinks too much, too often, with obviously negative impact on their life. However, not all alcoholics fit that stereotype. Functional alcoholics are typically educated, have a steady job, have a family, and have made it to middle age.[108] By all outward appearances, functional alcoholics seem to have their personal and professional lives in order. Functional alcoholics also suffer from denial. Having a job, being able to pay bills, and having a lot of friends might keep the functional alcoholic from thinking they have a problem. However, no one can drink heavily and maintain major responsibilities; over time, drinking catches up.

## The Causes of Alcohol Use Disorders

We know that alcohol use disorder (formerly known as *alcoholism*) is a disease with biological and social/environmental components, but we do not yet know what role each component plays.

**Biological and Family Factors** Research into the hereditary and environmental causes of alcoholism has found higher rates of alcoholism among children of alcoholics than in the general population. Alcoholism among individuals with a family history of alcoholism is about four to eight times

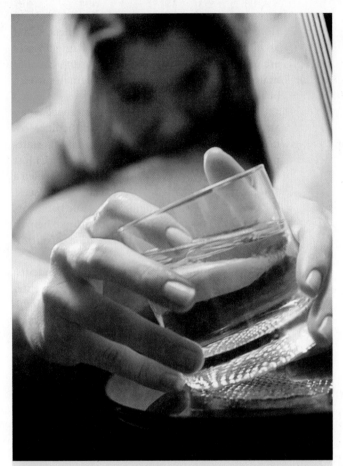

Drinking alone or in secret and using alcohol to cope with stress and emotional problems are all potential signs of alcohol dependency.

Family attitudes toward alcohol also seem to influence whether a person will develop a drinking problem. It has been clearly demonstrated that people who are raised in cultures where drinking is a part of religious or ceremonial activities or part of the family meal are less prone to alcohol dependence. In contrast, societies where alcohol purchase is carefully controlled and drinking is regarded as a rite of passage to adulthood appear to have greater tendency for abuse.

The amount of alcohol a person consumes seems to be directly related to the drinking habits of that individual's social group. Friends and relatives who drink heavily are more likely to drink heavily themselves. Even having friends of friends who drank heavily appeared to influence individual alcohol consumption. The opposite is also true, that people with abstinent friends or family members were less likely to drink themselves. This is especially important for individuals who are in treatment or have been in treatment and their need to sever ties with heavy drinkers to successfully maintain their abstinence.

## AUD in Women

Women tend to become alcoholics at later ages and after fewer years of heavy drinking than do men. Women also get addicted faster with less alcohol use. With greater risks for cirrhosis; excessive memory loss and shrinkage of the brain; heart disease; and cancers of the mouth, throat, esophagus, liver, and colon than male alcoholics, women suffer the consequences of alcoholism more profoundly.[113]

The highest risks for alcoholism occur among women who are unmarried but living with a partner, are in their 20s or early 30s, or have a husband or partner who drinks heavily. Other risk factors for women include a family history of drinking problems, pressure to drink from a peer or spouse, depression, and stress.

## Alcohol and Prescription Drug Abuse

When alcohol and prescription drugs are taken together, severe medical problems can result, including alcohol poisoning, unconsciousness, respiratory depression, and death. The greatest risks from drug mixing occur when alcohol is mixed with prescription painkillers. Both drugs slow breathing rates in unique ways and inhibit the coughing reflex; when combined, they can stop breathing altogether. Alcohol also interacts with antianxiety medications, antipsychotics, antidepressants, sleep medications, and muscle relaxants, causing dizziness and drowsiness and making falls and unintentional injuries more likely. The prescription drugs that are most commonly combined with alcohol include opioids (e.g., Vicodin,

more common than it is among individuals with no such family history.[109]

Despite evidence of heredity's role in alcoholism, scientists do not yet understand the precise role of genes and increased risk for alcoholism, nor have they identified a specific "alcoholism" gene. Alcohol use disorders are approximately 60 percent heritable.[110] Adoption studies demonstrate a strong link between biological parents' substance use and their children's risk for addiction.[111] Research has found that alcohol stimulates the production of dopamine, which activates the pleasure center of the brain. In alcoholics, the dopamine response to alcohol is diminished, leading them to drink more alcohol to feel the same pleasurable effects.[112] Alcohol gives individuals with the gene a stronger sense of reward from alcohol, making it more likely for them to be heavy drinkers. However, there is nothing deterministic about the genetic basis for addiction. Although no single gene causes addiction, multiple genes can affect the ability to develop addiction.

**Social and Cultural Factors** Some people begin drinking as a way to dull the pain of an acute loss or an emotional or social problem. Unfortunately, they become even sadder as the depressant effect of alcohol begins to take its toll, sometimes causing them to antagonize friends and other social supports. Eventually, the drinker becomes physically dependent on the drug.

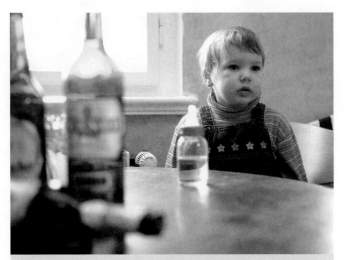

Children of alcoholics can have trouble developing social attachments and suffer low self-esteem and other problems from lack of parental nurturing. Fortunately, as they mature, many children of alcoholics can also develop resiliency in response to their families' problems.

OxyContin, Percocet); stimulants (e.g., Ritalin, Adderall, Concerta); sedative/anxiety medications (e.g., Ativan, Xanax); and sleeping medications (e.g., Ambien, Halcion).

## Effects on Family and Friends

In addition to harming themselves, people who abuse alcohol cause tremendous harm to their family and friends. Everyone close to an addicted person—including family, friends, and roommates—suffers and becomes a part of the dynamics of addiction.

Approximately 1 in 4 children in the United States live in families with a parent addicted to alcohol.[114] These children are at increased risk for a range of problems, including physical illness, emotional disturbances, behavioral problems, lower educational performance, and susceptibility to alcoholism or other addictions later in life.

In dysfunctional families, children learn certain rules from an early age: Don't talk, don't trust, and don't feel. These unspoken rules allow the family to avoid dealing with real problems and issues as family members adapt to the alcoholic's behavior by adjusting their own behavior. Unfortunately, these behaviors enable the alcoholic to keep drinking. Children in such dysfunctional families generally assume at least one of the following roles:

- **Family hero.** Tries to divert attention from the problem by being too good to be true
- **Scapegoat.** Draws attention away from the family's primary problem through misbehavior
- **Lost child.** Becomes passive and quietly withdraws from upsetting situations
- **Mascot.** Disrupts tense situations by providing comic relief

For children in alcoholic homes, life is a struggle. They have to deal with constant stress, anxiety, and embarrassment.

Because the alcoholic is the center of attention, the child's needs are often ignored. It is not uncommon for these children to be victims of violence, abuse, neglect, or incest.

Living with a family member (or friend or roommate) who is an alcoholic can be extremely stressful. People in close proximity to alcoholics can find themselves in codependent relationships that are often emotionally destructive or abusive and that enable the alcoholic's addiction. Codependents try to cover up for the addicted person: They may make excuses for the drinker's behavior or lie to others to cover for him or her. (For more information on how addiction can affect families and friends, see **Focus On: Recognizing and Avoiding Addiction** on page 299.)

## Costs to Society

Alcohol-related costs to society are estimated to be well over $249 billion when health insurance, criminal justice costs, treatment costs, and lost productivity are considered.[115] These costs break down to a 72 percent loss in workplace productivity, 11 percent related to health care expenses for treating problems caused by excessive drinking, 10 percent criminal justice costs, and 5 percent related to losses from motor vehicle crashes.[116] Binge drinking alone accounts for the majority (77%) of the economic cost. Excessive drinking cost $807 per person, or $2.05 for each drink consumed.[117] Alcoholism is directly or indirectly responsible for more than 25 percent of the nation's medical expenses and lost earnings.[118] Emotional, mental, and physical costs are impossible to measure; however, the toll that alcohol takes from loss of loved ones in drunk-driving accidents, as a result of alcohol-related violence and abuse in homes, and the costs to families and relationships is likely to be huge.

### The Cost of Underage Drinking

Underage drinking plays a role in a large number of social and health-related problems, including automobile accidents, self-injury, unintentional injury, interpersonal violence, risky sexual behavior, brain damage, academic struggles, and addiction treatment. Underage drinking also results in tremendous economic costs. Each year it is estimated that $24.6 billion of excessive alcohol consumption was related to underage drinking.[119] The costs largely result from lost work productivity (58%), law enforcement and criminal justice costs (19%), health care expenses caused by excessive drinking (15%) and costs related to automobile accidents resulting from impaired driving (6%).[120]

## LO 7 | TREATMENT AND RECOVERY

Describe the various types of treatment programs for alcoholism and their effectiveness and explore the concepts of relapse and recovery.

- - - - - - - - - - - - - - - - - - - - - - - - - - - - - - - - - - - - - - -

Despite growing recognition of our national alcohol problem, only a very small percentage of those with alcohol use disorder ever seek and undergo treatment.[121] Numerous factors contribute to this low treatment utilization, including an inability

## MAKING **CHANGES** TODAY

### Thinking and Talking About Alcohol Use

The following questions can help gauge whether you or someone you know has an alcohol problem. The more "yes" answers, the more likely a problem exists.

Does the person you are concerned about:

- ⦿ Lose time from classes, studying, or work because of drinking?
- ◎ Feel embarrassed about his or her behavior after sobering up?
- ◎ Drink to get drunk?
- ◎ Do dangerous things or get injured while drunk?
- ◎ Drink to cope with problems or stress?

Use these tips to talk to someone about alcohol abuse:

- ⦿ Talk when he or she is sober. Avoid lecturing.
- ◎ Restrict comments to what you have experienced of the person's behavior.
- ◎ Use concrete examples: "You started a fight" or "You were hung over and failed an exam."
- ◎ Contrast sober and drunk behavior: "You have the most wonderful sense of humor, but when you drink it turns into cruel sarcasm."
- ◎ Distinguish between the person you like and the behavior you don't.
- ◎ Encourage him or her to consult a professional. Offer to go along for support.

## Family's and Friends' Roles in Recovery

Members of an alcoholic's family sometimes take action before the alcoholic does. An effective method of helping an alcoholic confront the disease is a process called **intervention**—a planned confrontation with the alcoholic that involves family members and friends assisted by professional substance abuse counselors. See the Making Changes Today box for tips on confronting someone about alcohol abuse.

## Treatment Programs

The alcoholic who is ready for help has several avenues of treatment: psychologists and psychiatrists specializing in the treatment of alcoholism, private treatment centers, hospitals specifically designed to treat alcoholics, community mental health facilities, and support groups.

**Private Treatment Facilities** Upon admission to a private treatment facility, the patient receives a complete physical exam to determine whether underlying medical problems will interfere with treatment. Shortly after detoxification, alcoholics begin their treatment for psychological addiction. Most treatment facilities keep their patients from 3 to 6 weeks. Treatment at private facilities can cost several thousand dollars, but some insurance programs or employers will assume most of this expense.

**Therapy** Several types of therapy—including family therapy, individual therapy, and group therapy—are commonly used in alcoholism recovery programs. In family therapy, the person and family members examine the psychological reasons underlying the addiction and the environmental factors enabling it. In individual and group therapy, alcoholics learn positive coping skills for situations that have regularly caused them to turn to alcohol.

While there are many recovery management strategies for adults, developing an appropriate recovery support system for college students has received less attention. In particular, there has been a lack of campus-based services for recovering students. The high prevalence of alcohol and other drug use on college campuses makes attending college a threat to sobriety. However, many campuses are beginning to recognize the need to create recovery-friendly space and supportive environments for students engaged in recovery. Common features of such programs include a designated campus meeting space, drug-free housing options, individual or group counseling, relapse prevention, and sober leisure activities; peer support and 12-step tenets are typically emphasized.[123]

**Pharmacological Treatment** Disulfiram (trade name Antabuse) is a drug commonly used for treating alcoholism. It is given to deter drinking, as it causes an individual to become acutely ill when he or she consumes alcohol. Disulfiram inhibits the breakdown of acetaldehyde from the liver. If individuals taking this drug drink alcohol or consume any foods with alcohol content, acetaldehyde will build up in

or unwillingness to admit to an alcohol problem, the social stigma, seeking treatment would require abstinence, and desire to deal with alcohol problems on one's own.[122] Most problem drinkers who seek help have experienced a turning point when the person recognizes that alcohol controls his or her life.

Alcoholics who quit drinking will experience *detoxification*, the process by which addicts end their dependence on a drug. Withdrawal symptoms include hyperexcitability, confusion, agitation, sleep disorders, convulsions, tremors, depression, headaches, and seizures. For a small percentage of people, alcohol withdrawal results in a severe syndrome known as **delirium tremens (DTs)**, characterized by confusion, delusions, agitated behavior, and hallucinations.

**delirium tremens (DTs)** State of confusion, delusions, and agitation brought on by withdrawal from alcohol.

**intervention** A planned confrontation with an alcoholic led by a professional counselor in which family members and/or friends try to get the alcoholic to face the reality of his or her problem and to seek help.

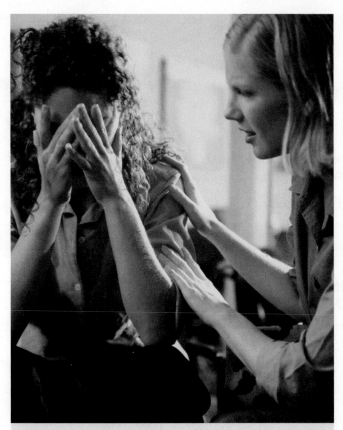

Most alcohol-dependent people need the help of others during their recovery, whether through support groups or individual, family, or group therapy.

their struggles and talk about the devastating effects alcoholism has had on their personal and professional lives. AA established the concept of the 12-step program for recovery from addiction, and its guiding principles are now used by other recovery organizations. The 12 steps ask members to address recovery one step at a time and to place their faith and control of their habit into the hands of a "Higher Power."

Alcoholics Anonymous also has auxiliary groups to help spouses or partners, friends, and children of alcoholics. *Al-Anon* is the group dedicated to helping adult relatives and friends of alcoholics understand the disease and how they can contribute to the recovery process. *Alateen* helps adolescents living with alcoholic parents by teaching that they are not at fault for their parents' problems. They develop their self-esteem to overcome their guilt and function better socially.

Other self-help groups include *Women for Sobriety* and *Secular Organizations for Sobriety (SOS)*. Women for Sobriety addresses the specific needs of female alcoholics, who often have more severe problems than do males. Unlike AA meetings, where attendance can be quite large, each group has no more than 10 members. These meetings focus on behavioral changes through positive reinforcement, cognitive strategies, relaxation techniques, meditation, diet, exercise, and dynamic group involvement. SOS was founded to help people who are uncomfortable with AA's spiritual emphasis. It is a self-empowerment approach to recovery and maintains that sobriety is a separate issue from all else. Like AA, SOS holds confidential meetings, celebrates sobriety anniversaries, and views recovery as a one-day-at-a-time process.

the liver and cause nausea and vomiting. Other unpleasant effects—such as headache, bad breath, drowsiness, and temporary impotence—discourage drinking. Because disulfiram does not reduce the cravings for alcohol, this treatment works best in conjunction with ongoing psychotherapy and support groups.

*Naltrexone* is used to reduce the craving for alcohol and decrease the pleasant reinforcing effects of alcohol without making the user ill. It also works most effectively with counseling and other forms of psychotherapy. Another pharmaceutical treatment for alcoholism approved by the U.S. Food and Drug Administration (FDA) is called *acamprosate (Campral)*. Acamprosate helps stabilize the resulting chemical imbalance in the brain. It also helps to reduce the physical and emotional distress associated with the attempt to stay alcohol free. As with other pharmacological treatments, acamprosate should be used in conjunction with psychotherapy and support groups.

## Support Groups

The support gained from talking with others who have similar problems is one of the greatest benefits derived from self-help/support groups. **Alcoholics Anonymous (AA)** is a private, nonprofit, self-help organization founded in 1935. The organization, which relies on group support to help people stop drinking, currently has branches all over the world and more than 1 million members. At meetings, participants do not give their last names and no one is forced to speak. Members are taught that alcoholism is a lifetime problem and that they can never drink alcohol again. They share

## Relapse

Success in recovery varies with the individual. Treating an addiction requires more than getting the addict to stop using a substance; it also requires getting the person to break a pattern of behavior that has dominated his or her life. Many alcoholics refer to themselves as "recovering" throughout their lifetime rather than "cured." In fact, only about a third of people who are abstinent less than a year will remain abstinent.[124]

People seeking to regain a healthy lifestyle must not only confront their addiction but also guard against the tendency to relapse. Treatment programs focus on relapse prevention to help their clients develop coping strategies and techniques to make it much more likely they will remain sober. For alcoholics, it is important to identify situations that could trigger a relapse, such as becoming angry or frustrated, being bored, and being around others who drink. Some specific issues that can lead to relapse include loss of a loved one, major financial changes, change in employment, change in marital status, or health issues. During the initial recovery period, it can help to join a support group, maintain stability (resisting the urge to relocate, travel, take a new job, or make other drastic life changes), set aside time each day for reflection, and maintain a pattern of assuming responsibility for one's own actions. To be effective, recovery programs must offer alcoholics ways to increase self-esteem and resume personal growth.

**Alcoholics Anonymous (AA)**
Organization whose goal is to help alcoholics stop drinking; includes auxiliary branches such as Al-Anon and Alateen.

# STUDY PLAN

## ASSESS YOURSELF

**Are you at risk of alcohol abuse?** Want to find out? Take the **What is Your Risk of Alcohol Abuse?** assessment available on

### MasteringHealth.™

## CHAPTER REVIEW

To hear an MP3 Tutor Session, scan here or visit the Study Area in **MasteringHealth**.

### LO 1 | Alcohol: An Overview

- Alcohol is a central nervous system (CNS) depressant used by about half of all Americans. Alcohol's effect on the body is measured by the blood alcohol concentration (BAC). The higher the BAC, the greater the drowsiness and impaired judgment and motor function.

### LO 2 | Alcohol and Your Health

- Excessive alcohol consumption can cause long-term damage to the nervous system and cardiovascular system, liver disease, and increased risk for cancer. Drinking during pregnancy can cause fetal alcohol spectrum disorders (FASD).

### LO 3 | Alcohol Use in College

- Large numbers of college students report drinking in the past 30 days. Negative consequences associated with alcohol use among college students include academic problems, traffic accidents, unplanned sex, hangovers, alcohol poisoning, injury to self or others, and dropping out of school.

### LO 4 | Drinking and Driving

- Alcohol-impaired drivers are responsible for about 1 in 3 car crash deaths. College students have high rates of alcohol-related crashes.

### LO 5 | Ethnic Differences in Alcohol Use and Abuse

- Rates of alcohol consumption and abuse vary among different racial and ethnic groups. African Americans, Latinos, and Native Americans have high rates of heavy alcohol use.

### LO 6 | Abuse and Dependence

- Alcohol use becomes alcohol use disorder when it interferes with school, work, or social and family relationships or entails violations of the law. Causes of alcoholism include biological, family, social, and cultural factors. Alcoholism has far-reaching effects on families and children, who may take those problems into adulthood.

### LO 7 | Treatment and Recovery

- Most alcoholics do not admit to having a problem until reaching a major life crisis or until their families intervene. Treatment options include detoxification at private medical facilities, therapy (family, individual, or group), and self-help programs. Most recovering alcoholics relapse (over half within 3 months) because alcoholism is a behavioral addiction as well as a chemical addiction.

## POP QUIZ

Visit **MasteringHealth** to personalize your study plan with Chapter Review Quizzes and Dynamic Study Modules.

### LO 1 | Alcohol: An Overview

1. If a man and a woman drink the same amount of alcohol, the woman's BAC will be approximately
   a. the same as the man's BAC.
   b. 60 percent higher than the man's BAC.
   c. 30 percent higher than the man's BAC.
   d. 30 percent lower than the man's BAC.

2. BAC is the
   a. concentration of plant sugars in the bloodstream.
   b. percentage of alcohol in a beverage.
   c. level of alcohol content in the blood.
   d. ratio of alcohol to the total blood volume.

### LO 2 | Alcohol and Your Health

3. Drinking large amounts of alcohol in a short period of time that leads to passing out is known as
   a. learned behavioral tolerance.
   b. alcoholic unconsciousness.
   c. alcohol poisoning.
   d. acute metabolism syndrome.

4. Which of the following is typical of a child born with fetal alcohol syndrome?
   a. Deafness
   b. Impaired learning
   c. Cirrhosis
   d. Osteoporosis

## LO 3 | Alcohol Use in College

5. When Amanda goes out with her friends on the weekends, she usually has four or five beers in a row. This type of high-risk drinking is called
   a. tolerance.
   b. alcoholic addiction.
   c. alcohol overconsumption.
   d. binge drinking.

6. Which is a strategy you could take to avoid drinking too much alcohol at a party?
   a. Pregame before going out
   b. Drink only carbonated alcoholic beverages
   c. Don't eat before or during the party
   d. Alternate alcoholic and nonalcoholic drinks

## LO 4 | Drinking and Driving

7. A BAC as low as _____ increases the likelihood of a driver being involved in a fatal car crash.
   a. 0.02
   b. 0.05
   c. 0.07
   d. 0.08

## LO 5 | Ethnic Differences in Alcohol Use and Abuse

8. Which of the following ethnic groups has the lowest rates of alcoholism?
   a. Asian Americans
   b. African Americans
   c. Latinos
   d. Native Americans

## LO 6 | Abuse and Dependence

9. Jake was raised in an alcoholic family. To adapt to his father's alcoholic behavior, he played the good, obedient son. Which role did Jake assume?
   a. Family hero
   b. Mascot
   c. Scapegoat
   d. Lost child

## LO 7 | Treatment and Recovery

10. The alcohol withdrawal syndrome that results in confusion, delusion, agitated behavior, and hallucination is known as
    a. automatic detoxification.
    b. delirium tremens.
    c. acute withdrawal.
    d. transient hyperirritability.

*Answers to the Pop Quiz can be found on page A-1. If you answered a question incorrectly, review the section identified by the Learning Outcome. For even more study tools, visit MasteringHealth.*

# THINK ABOUT IT!

## LO 1 | Alcohol: An Overview

1. Would a person be more intoxicated after having four gin and tonics instead of four beers? Why or why not?

## LO 2 | Alcohol and Your Health

2. At what point in your life should you start worrying about the long-term effects of alcohol abuse?

## LO 3 | Alcohol Use in College

3. What are some of the most common negative consequences college students experience as a result of drinking? Why do students tolerate the negative behaviors of students who have been drinking?

## LO 4 | Drinking and Driving

4. When it comes to drinking alcohol, how much is too much to drive? How can you avoid drinking amounts that will affect your judgment and impair your ability to safely operate a vehicle? If you see a friend having too many drinks at a party, what actions could you take to make sure he or she makes it home safely?

## LO 5 | Ethnic Differences in Alcohol Use and Abuse

5. In what ways do genetics influence ethnic differences in alcohol use and abuse? How much of the differences between ethnic groups in terms of alcohol use and abuse can be attributed to cultural or social differences?

## LO 6 | Abuse and Dependence

6. Describe the difference between a problem drinker and an alcoholic. What factors can cause someone to become an alcoholic? What effect does alcoholism have on an alcoholic's family?

## LO 7 | Treatment and Recovery

7. Does anyone ever permanently recover from alcoholism? Why or why not? Do you think society's views on drinking have changed over the years? Explain your answer.

# ACCESS YOUR HEALTH ON THE INTERNET

Visit **MasteringHealth** for links to the websites and RSS feeds.

The following websites explore further topics and issues related to alcohol abuse.

**Alcoholics Anonymous (AA).** This website provides general information about AA and the 12-step program. **www.aa.org**

**College Drinking: Changing the Culture.** This resource center targets three audiences: the student population as a whole, the college and its surrounding environment, and the individual at risk or alcohol-dependent drinker. **www. collegedrinkingprevention.gov**

**Students against Destructive Decisions.** SADD is an organization of students dedicated to raising awareness about the dangers of underage drinking, drug use, and impaired driving, among other destructive decisions. **www.sadd.org**

# 12 Ending Tobacco Use

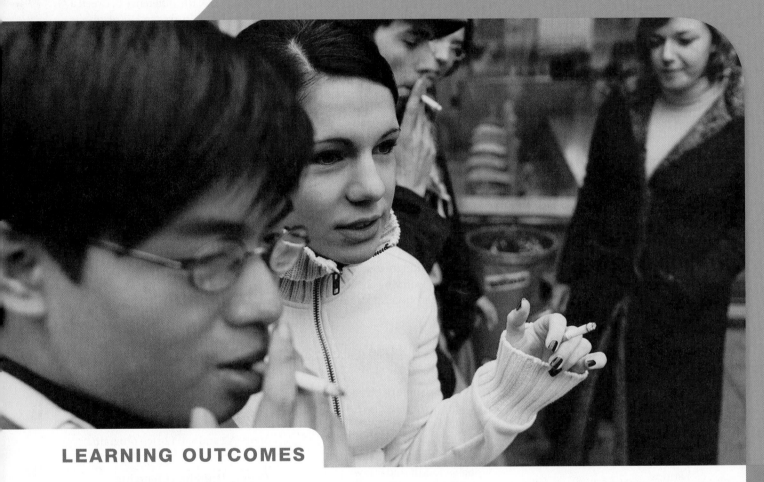

## LEARNING OUTCOMES

LO **1** Describe the rate of tobacco use in the United States, and explain the social and political issues involved in tobacco use.

LO **2** Discuss the use of tobacco by college students, and identify some of the reasons college students smoke.

LO **3** Describe how the chemicals in tobacco products affect the body.

LO **4** Explain the health risks of smoking and using smokeless tobacco.

LO **5** Explain the dangers created by environmental tobacco smoke.

LO **6** Discuss prevention policies enacted by the U.S. government to curb tobacco use.

LO **7** Describe various quitting strategies, including those aimed at ending the body's addiction to nicotine.

The prevalence of cigarette smoking among adults has declined significantly over the last 50 years.[1] However, tobacco use is still the single most preventable cause of death in the United States: Nearly 480,000 Americans die each year from tobacco-related diseases. Moreover, another 16 million people will suffer from health disorders caused by tobacco. To date, tobacco is known to cause more than 20 diseases, and about half of all regular smokers die of smoking-related causes. Smoking kills more Americans than alcohol, motor vehicle accidents, suicide, AIDS, homicide, and illegal drugs combined.[2] Any contention by the tobacco industry that tobacco use is not dangerous completely ignores the overwhelming scientific evidence to the contrary.

## LO 1 | TOBACCO USE IN THE UNITED STATES

Describe the rate of tobacco use in the United States, and explain the social and political issues involved in tobacco use.

Approximately 70 million Americans age 12 and older report using tobacco products (cigarettes, cigars, smokeless tobacco, and pipe tobacco) at least once in the past month.[3] Declines in cigarette smoking over the past two decades have slowed compared with earlier periods. In 2014, 18.8 percent of men and 14.8 percent of women were current cigarette smokers. Nearly 17 percent of adults aged 18 to 24 are cigarette smokers, yet adults aged 25 to 44 had the highest percentage of current cigarette smoking (24 percent); then the percentage continues to decrease with age, with 18 percent of adults aged 45 to 64 and 9 percent of adults aged 65 years and older reported to be current smokers.[4]

The rate of past-month cigarette use among those 12 to 17 years old declined from 13 percent in 2002 to 7 percent in 2014. The rate of past-month smokeless tobacco use among those 12 to 17 years old stayed the same—at 2 percent in 2002 and 2 percent in 2014. In addition, every day over 3,000 teens under the age of 18 smoke their first cigarette, and approximately 1,000 of them become daily smokers.[5]

## Why People Smoke

More than 20 percent of Americans are former smokers, and about 60 percent have never smoked. The most commonly used tobacco product is cigarettes, more common among men (19%) than women (15.0%), followed by cigars (8.2% of men and 2.0% of women) and smokeless tobacco (3.6 percent of people age 12 and older).[6] But why do people smoke at all? Here are a few of the more common reasons.

**Addiction** Similar to other addictive drugs such as cocaine and heroin, nicotine increases levels of the neurotransmitter dopamine, which affects the brain pathways that control reward and pleasure. For many tobacco users, long-term brain changes induced by continued nicotine exposure result in addiction—a condition of compulsive drug-seeking and use, even in the face of negative consequences.[7] Of adult smokers, 80 percent started by age 21, and half became regular smokers by age 18.[8] Tobacco companies target children and teens with tobacco products that are candy, fruit, or alcohol-flavored, thus making them more palatable to young people.[9]

**Advertising** The tobacco industry spends an estimated $26 million per day on advertising and promotional material.[10] With the number of smokers declining by about 1 million each year, the industry must actively recruit new smokers.[11] Studies have found that kids are three times as susceptible to advertising run by tobacco companies as are adults, are more likely to actually smoke as a result of cigarette marketing than peer pressure, and that tobacco company advertising and promotion can be cited as the culprit for a third of underage experimentation with smoking.[12]

Tobacco products are heavily advertised to specific populations. In women's magazines, it is implied that smoking is the key to financial success, desirability, beauty, weight control, independence, social acceptance, and being "cool." These ads have apparently been working. From the mid-1970s through the early 2000s, cigarette sales to women increased dramatically. Not coincidentally, by 1987, cigarette-induced lung cancer had surpassed breast cancer as the leading cancer killer among women and has remained the leading cancer killer in every year since.[13]

# 100 MILLION

**DEATHS** have been caused worldwide by tobacco during the twentieth century.

Women are not the only targets of gender-based cigarette advertisements. Men are depicted in locker rooms, charging over rugged terrain in off-road vehicles, or riding stallions into the sunset in blatant appeals to a need to feel and appear masculine. Minorities are also often the targets of heavy marketing. Tobacco advertising, particularly menthol cigarettes, is much more common in magazines aimed at African Americans, such as *Jet* and *Ebony*, than in similar magazines aimed at broader audiences, such as *Time* and *People*. Billboards and posters spreading the cigarette message have dotted the landscape in Hispanic communities for many years, especially in low-income areas. Tobacco companies also sponsor community-based events such as festivals and annual fairs.

## Limited Education
Cigarette use is closely linked to education. Adults with a bachelor's degree or higher education are two times *less* likely to smoke than are those with less than a high school education.[14] Cigarette smoking also varies by ethnicity; the highest rates of smoking are found among American Indian and Alaska Natives, with a prevalence of 21.8 percent.[15] TABLE 12.1 shows the percentage of Americans who smoke by demographic group.

## Behavioral Dependence
People who smoke are not just physically dependent on nicotine, they are also psychologically dependent. Nicotine "tricks" the brain into creating pleasurable memory associations between sensory stimuli or environmental cues that may trigger the urge for a cigarette.[16] Even those who smoke only occasionally may find it hard to quit because of associations between smoking and a behavior like having a drink or a morning cup of coffee.

Many smokers have a difficult time imagining not smoking. They often describe their cigarette as their friend. For some smokers, simply holding a cigarette provides comfort and can have a calming effect. Some former smokers remain vulnerable to sensory and environmental cues, such as the smell of tobacco or driving a car, for years after they quit.

## Weight Control
People who start smoking often lose weight. Nicotine is an appetite suppressant and slightly increases the smoker's *basal metabolic rate* (the rate of energy expended by the body at complete rest). After smoking, a smoker's metabolism increases right away and then returns to a normal level. Heavy smokers have surges in metabolism throughout the day. As a result, they experience less appetite than do those who smoke less or not at all. When a smoker quits, the metabolic rate slows down and appetite returns. People tend to eat more (sweets in particular) when they stop smoking, and have a tendency to gain weight if they don't watch what they eat. Fear of gaining weight is one of the biggest reasons smokers are reluctant to quit. Ways to avoid weight gain after quitting include avoiding crash diets, keeping low-calorie treats handy, and drinking plenty of water.

## Genetics
Studies have found genetic factors to be significantly influential in smoking initiation and nicotine

### TABLE 12.1 | Percentage of Population That Smokes (Age 18 and Older) among Select Groups in the United States

| | Percentage |
|---|---|
| United States overall | 20.9 |
| **Race** | |
| Asian | 13.3 |
| Black | 21.5 |
| Hispanic | 16.2 |
| American Indian/Alaska Native | 32.0 |
| White, non-Hispanic | 21.9 |
| **Age** | |
| 18–24 | 24.4 |
| 25–44 | 24.1 |
| 45–64 | 21.9 |
| 65+ | 8.6 |
| **Gender** | |
| Male | 18.8 |
| Female | 14.8 |
| **Education** | |
| Undergraduate | 10.7 |
| High school | 24.6 |
| GED diploma | 43.2 |
| Less than 12 years (no diploma) | 26.0 |
| Postgraduate | 7.1 |
| **Income Level** | |
| Below poverty level | 29.9 |
| At or above poverty level | 20.6 |

**Source:** Centers for Disease Control and Prevention, "Current Cigarette Smoking Status—United States 2005–2014," *Morbidity and Mortality Weekly Report* 64, no. 44 (2015): 1233–40.

dependence. Specifically, one study found that teenagers carrying variants in two genes were three times more likely to become regular smokers in adolescence and twice as likely to be persistent smokers in adulthood compared to noncarriers.[17] These two specific genes may influence smoking behavior by affecting the action of dopamine, a brain chemical.[18] Understanding the influence of genetics on nicotine addiction could be crucial to developing more effective smoking-cessation treatments.

## Parent Role Models
The relationship between parents smoking and their children smoking is clear.[19] Children who start smoking are more likely to have a parent who smokes. The risk of a child becoming a smoker increases with the intensity of the parents' smoking behavior and the amount of exposure children have to their parents smoking.

The greater the exposure to the smoking parent, the increased risk there is for the child to become a smoker.

## Mental Disorders

People with mental illness make up a large percentage of American cigarette smokers. It is estimated about 50 percent of those with a mental illness or substance abuse disorder smoke cigarettes.[20] The prevalence of smoking increases with the severity of the mental illness. Half of all deaths in the severely mentally ill (schizophrenia, bipolar disorder, and major depressive disorder) can be attributed to smoking.[21]

## Stress

Many people smoke when they feel stressed.[22] People with high levels of stress are more likely to smoke. A recent study on college students found that stress smokers are more likely to smoke at a specific time (e.g., while studying for a test) when they are under stress.[23] Students reported they were also more likely to smoke in social situations that were stressful, such as at a party or in other stressful social situations.[24]

# U.S. Tobacco: Political and Economic Issues

The production and distribution of tobacco products involve many political and economic issues. Tobacco-growing states derive substantial income from tobacco production, and federal, state, and local governments benefit enormously from cigarette taxes.

Estimates show annual costs attributed to smoking in the United States are between \$289 and \$333 billion.[25] The economic burden of tobacco use totals more than \$170 billion in direct medical expenditures and \$156 billion in lost productivity.[26] It is estimated that smoking-related health costs and productivity losses are \$19.16 per pack of cigarettes sold.[27]

## LO 2 | COLLEGE STUDENTS AND TOBACCO USE

Discuss the use of tobacco by college students, and identify some of the reasons college students smoke.

College students are the targets of heavy tobacco marketing and advertising campaigns. The tobacco industry has set up aggressive marketing promotions at bars, music festivals, and other events specifically targeted at the 18- to 24-year-old age group. Being placed in a new, often stressful social and academic environment

There is no safe form of tobacco. Nicotine is nicotine and is addictive. Tobacco companies know that once a person starts smoking, chances are good that he or she will get hooked, so they cleverly offer options designed to start the habit.

makes college students especially vulnerable to outside influences. Peer influence can prompt students to start or continue smoking, and many colleges and universities still sell tobacco products in campus stores. However, cigarette smoking among U.S. college students has decreased in recent years (see **FIGURE 12.1** on page 340). In a 2015 survey, about 11 percent of college students reported having smoked cigarettes in the past 30 days.[28] College men have slightly higher rates of smoking (14%) compared to women (9%).[29] Men also use more cigars and smokeless tobacco.[30]

Among those aged 18 to 22, full-time college students are less likely to smoke than their peers who are not enrolled full time in college.[31] In 2014, cigarette use in the past month was reported by 22.6 percent of full-time college students, less than the rate of 34.7 percent for those not enrolled full time.[32] Among males age 18 to 22 who were full-time college students in 2014, cigarette use declined from 31.7 percent in 2009 to 24.5 percent.[33]

## Social Smoking

Many college-age smokers identify themselves as "social smokers"—those who engage in occasional smoking in social situations or as a social activity. Social smokers typically smoke on weekends, at night, at social events, or just hanging out with friends. Often, social smokers smoke to fit in with groups and to help social interactions.[34] However, occasional smoking is not without risks of damaging health effects. Social smoking in college can lead to a complete dependence on nicotine and thus to all the same health risks as smoking regularly. Not surprisingly, there is a strong belief held by social smokers that they are not addicted to cigarettes.[35] Whether that is true or not remains to be seen.

Smoking less than a pack of cigarettes a week has been shown to damage blood vessels and to increase the risk of heart disease and cancer.[36] In women taking birth control pills, even a few cigarettes a week can increase the likelihood of heart disease, blood clots, stroke, liver cancer, and gallbladder disease.[37]

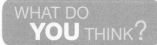

**WHAT DO YOU THINK?**

Have you noticed a change in the number of your friends who smoke?

- How many smoked prior to college compared to now?
- What are their reasons for smoking?
- What keeps your friends from quitting?

## Most Student Smokers Want to Quit

Unlike social smokers, most students who smoke regularly and are nicotine dependent do want to stop smoking, but in spite of their efforts or desire to

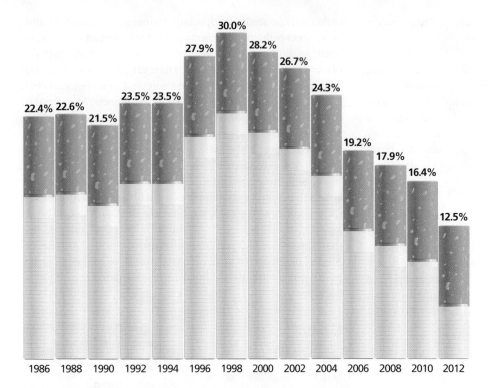

**FIGURE 12.1** Trends in Prevalence of Cigarette Smoking in the Past Month among College Students

**Source:** Data from L. D. Johnston et al., *Monitoring the Future National Survey Results on Drug Use, 1975–2014, Volume II, College Students and Adults Ages 19–50* (Ann Arbor: Institute for Social Research, University of Michigan, 2015).

quit, they continue to smoke throughout college. To reduce the incidence of smoking among students, colleges and universities need to engage in antismoking efforts, control tobacco advertising, provide smoke-free residence halls, and offer greater access to smoking-cessation programs.

## LO 3 | EFFECTS OF TOBACCO

Describe how the chemicals in tobacco products affect the body.

Smoking, the most common form of tobacco use, delivers a strong dose of nicotine along with 7,000 other chemical substances, including arsenic, formaldehyde, and ammonia, directly to the lungs.[38] Among these chemicals are at least 69 known or suspected carcinogens.[39] Some of the chemicals contained in tobacco smoke can also be found in chemical weapons, household cleaners, car exhaust, and embalming fluid (see **TABLE 12.2**). Inhaling toxic gases exposes sensitive mucous membranes to irritating chemicals that weaken the tissues and contribute to cancers of the mouth, larynx, and throat. The heat from tobacco smoke is also harmful to tissues.

**nicotine** Primary stimulant chemical in tobacco products that is highly addictive.

**nicotine poisoning** Symptoms often experienced by beginning smokers, including dizziness, diarrhea, lightheadedness, rapid and erratic pulse, clammy skin, and nausea and vomiting.

**tar** Thick, brownish sludge condensed from particulate matter in smoked tobacco.

## Nicotine

The highly addictive chemical stimulant **nicotine** is the major psychoactive substance in all tobacco products. In its natural form, nicotine is a colorless liquid that turns brown upon exposure to air. When tobacco leaves are burned in a cigarette, pipe, or cigar, nicotine is released and inhaled into the lungs. Sucking or chewing tobacco releases nicotine into the saliva, which is then absorbed through the mucous membranes in the mouth.

Nicotine is a powerful central nervous system stimulant that produces a variety of physiological effects. In the cerebral cortex, it produces an aroused, alert mental state. Nicotine stimulates the adrenal glands, which increases the production of adrenaline. It also increases heart and respiratory rates, constricts blood vessels, and, in turn, increases blood pressure because the heart must work harder to pump blood through the narrowed vessels.

Beginning smokers usually feel the effects of nicotine with their first puff. These symptoms, called **nicotine poisoning**, can include dizziness, lightheadedness, rapid and erratic pulse, clammy skin, nausea and vomiting, and diarrhea. These unpleasant effects cease as tolerance develops, which happens almost immediately in new users, perhaps after the second or third cigarette. In contrast, tolerance to most other drugs, such as alcohol, develops over a period of months or years. Regular smokers generally do not experience a "buzz" from smoking. They continue to smoke simply because quitting is so difficult.

## Tar and Carbon Monoxide

Cigarette smoke is a complex mixture of chemicals and gases produced by the burning of tobacco and its additives. Particulate matter condenses in the lungs to form a thick, brownish sludge called **tar**, which contains various carcinogenic agents, such as benzopyrene, and chemical irritants, such as phenol. Phenol has the potential to combine with other chemicals that contribute to developing lung cancer.

In healthy lungs, millions of tiny hairlike projections (*cilia*) on the surfaces lining the upper respiratory passages sweep away foreign matter, which is expelled from the lungs by coughing. However, the cilia's cleansing function is impaired in smokers' lungs by nicotine, which paralyzes the cilia for up to 1 hour following a single cigarette. This allows tars and other solids in tobacco smoke to accumulate and irritate sensitive lung tissue. **FIGURE 12.2** illustrates how tobacco smoke damages the lungs.

## TABLE 12.2 | What Exactly Are You Inhaling?

| Chemical in Tobacco Smoke | Where Else Can You Find It? |
|---|---|
| Acetic acid | Vinegar |
| Acetone | Nail polish remover |
| Ammonia | Floor/toilet cleaner |
| Arsenic | Rat poison |
| Butane | Lighter fluid |
| Cadmium | Rechargeable batteries |
| Carbon monoxide | Car exhaust |
| DDT/dieldrin | Insecticides |
| Ethanol | Alcohol |
| Hexamine | Barbecue lighter |
| Hydrogen cyanide | Gas chamber poison, chemical weapons |
| Methane | Swamp gas, cow flatulence |
| Methanol | Rocket fuel |
| Naphthalene | Mothballs |
| Nicotine | Insecticide/addictive drug |
| Stearic acid | Candle wax |
| Toluene | Industrial solvent, paint thinner |

**Source:** U.S. Food and Drug Administration, "Harmful and Potentially Harmful Constituents in Tobacco Products and Tobacco Smoke: Established List," December 2015, http://www.fda.gov/TobaccoProducts/GuidanceComplianceRegulatoryInformation/ucm297786.htm.

intended; (2) persistent desire and unsuccessful efforts to cut down or quit; (3) spending a large amount of time getting or using tobacco; (4) craving tobacco; (5) tobacco use interfering with work, school, or social obligations; (6) reoccurring social or personal relationship issues caused by smoking; (7) giving up or reducing important activities; (8) persistent tobacco use in physically hazardous situations, such as smoking in bed; (9) continued tobacco use despite a persistent or reoccurring physical or psychological problem resulting from tobacco use; (10) increasing tolerance, such as smoking an increasing number of cigarettes to obtain the desired effect; and (11) withdrawal symptoms related to reducing or quitting tobacco use.[41]

## Tobacco Products

Tobacco comes in several forms. Cigarettes, cigars, pipes, and bidis are used for burning and inhaling tobacco. Smokeless tobacco is sniffed or placed in the mouth. Electronic cigarettes are an increasingly popular vehicle for nicotine, with their own health risks.

**Cigarettes** *Filtered cigarettes* are the most common form of tobacco available today. Almost all manufactured cigarettes have filters designed to reduce levels of gases such as hydrogen cyanide and carbon monoxide, but these products may actually deliver more hazardous gases to the user than nonfiltered brands. Some smokers use low-tar and low-nicotine products as an excuse to smoke more cigarettes,

> **carbon monoxide** Gas found in cigarette smoke that reduces the ability of blood to carry oxygen.

Cigarette smoke also contains poisonous gases, the most dangerous of which is **carbon monoxide**, the deadly gas emitted in car exhaust. Carbon monoxide reduces the oxygen-carrying capacity of the red blood cells by binding with the receptor sites for oxygen, causing oxygen deprivation in many body tissues. It is at least partly responsible for the increased risk of heart attacks and strokes in smokers.

## Tobacco Use Disorder

The American Psychiatric Association defines tobacco use disorder as a "problematic pattern of tobacco use leading to clinically significant impairment or distress"[40] that is characterized by at least two of these signs and symptoms in a 12-month period: (1) use of tobacco in larger amounts or over a longer period of time than

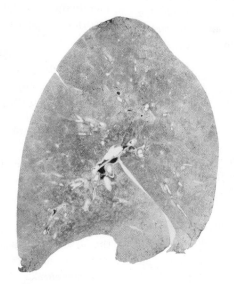

 **a** A healthy lung

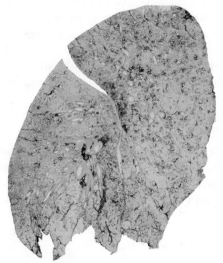

**b** A smoker's lung permeated with deposits of tar

**FIGURE 12.2 Lung Damage from Chemicals in Tobacco Smoke** Smoke particles irritate lung pathways, causing extra mucus production, and nicotine paralyzes the cilia that normally function to keep the lungs clear of excess mucus. The result is difficulty breathing, "smoker's cough," and chronic bronchitis. At the same time, tar collects within the alveoli (air sacs), ultimately causing their walls to break, leading to emphysema. Tar and other carcinogens in tobacco smoke also cause cellular mutations that lead to cancer.

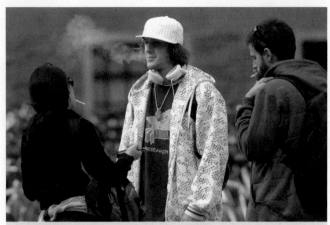

An occasional puff once in a while when you are out with friends can't hurt, right? Wrong! There is no "safe" amount of tobacco use—any smoking or exposure to smoke increases your risks for negative health effects such as heart disease and lung cancer. And even if you smoke only once or twice a week and consider yourself a social smoker, chances are you're on the road to dependence and a more frequent smoking habit.

**bidis** Hand-rolled flavored cigarettes.

but wind up exposing themselves to more harmful substances than they would with a smaller number of regular-strength cigarettes.

*Clove cigarettes* contain about 40 percent ground cloves (a spice) and about 60 percent tobacco. Many users mistakenly believe that these products are made entirely of ground cloves and that smoking them eliminates the risks associated with tobacco. In fact, clove cigarettes contain higher levels of tar, nicotine, and carbon monoxide than do regular cigarettes—and the numbing effect of eugenol, an ingredient in cloves, allows smokers to inhale more deeply. The same effect is true of *menthol cigarettes*: The throat-numbing effect of the menthol allows for deeper inhalation. Menthol cigarettes also have higher carbon monoxide concentrations than regular cigarettes.

**E-Cigarettes** Electronic cigarettes (also called *e-cigarettes* or *electronic nicotine delivery systems*) are battery-operated devices designed to deliver nicotine with flavorings (mint, chocolate, candy) and other chemicals to users as vapor instead of smoke. They are often made to look like regular cigarettes, cigars, pipes, or other small items like memory sticks or writing utensils. More than 460 different e-cigarette brands are currently on the market.[42]

# 1,483

SMOKE-FREE CAMPUSES are present in the United States.

In a recent survey of college students, about 29 percent of college students reported using e-cigarettes in the past, with 14 percent reporting usage in the past 30 days.[43] Students who use e-cigarettes are more likely to be heavy drinkers. While many campuses and many student apartments and rental houses have become tobacco or smoke free, the availability of e-cigarettes—and their barely detectable odor—may have allowed students to work around those bans and be able to more easily co-use alcohol and nicotine.[44]

Despite the fact that e-cigarettes are marketed as a safer choice than cigarettes, there is still very little known in terms of their health risks (see the **Health Headlines** box).

**Cigars** While cigarette use has declined in recent years, the sale of large cigars has more than tripled.[45] Many people believe that cigars are safer than cigarettes, when in fact the opposite is true. Cigars have higher levels of cancer-causing substances, more tar per gram of tobacco smoked, and higher levels of toxins than do cigarettes.[46] In addition, smoking cigars causes many of the same diseases as cigarette smoking and smokeless tobacco. Regular cigar smokers are at risk for developing cancers of the lung, oral cavity, larynx, esophagus, and possibly pancreas. Cigar smokers have 4 to 10 times the risk of dying from lung, laryngeal, oral, or esophageal cancer compared to those who have never smoked.[47] Most cigars contain as much nicotine as several cigarettes, and when cigar smokers inhale, nicotine is absorbed as rapidly as it is with cigarettes. For those who don't inhale, they still expose vulnerably body parts, like the lips, tongue, throat, and larynx, to a number of toxic chemicals contained in tobacco smoke. Even if smoke is not inhaled, high levels of nicotine are still absorbed through the mouth's mucous membranes. A single cigar can potentially provide as much nicotine as a pack of cigarettes.[48]

**Pipes and Hookahs** Pipes have a long history of use throughout the world, including ritualistic and ceremonial use in many cultures. Often thought to be safer than cigarettes or cigars, pipes are not risk-free options. According to the National Cancer Institute and the American Cancer Society, pipe smoking carries risks similar to cigar smoking. Of concern in recent years is the increasing prevalence, particularly among college students, of the use of hookahs, or water pipes. Hookah smoking originated in the Middle East and involves burning flavored tobacco in a water pipe and inhaling the smoke through a long hose. Hookahs are marketed as a safe alternative to cigarettes because they reduce the risks from hazardous chemicals by filtering the smoke through water before it is inhaled. While water pipes may cool the smoke, they do not eliminate or filter out harmful substances.[49] In addition to the health risks associated with all tobacco products, risks associated with hookah use include the possibility of infectious disease transmission by sharing a pipe.

**Bidis** Generally made in India or Southeast Asia, **bidis** are small, hand-rolled cigarettes that come in a variety of flavors, such as vanilla, chocolate, and cherry. They have become

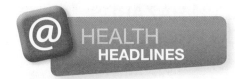 

# E-CIGARETTES
## Health Risks and Concerns

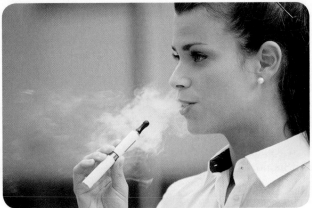

**Electronic cigarette, or e-cigarette.**

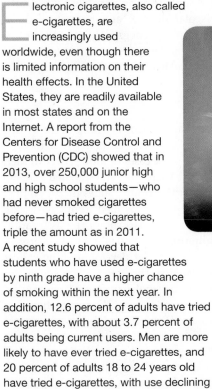

Electronic cigarettes, also called e-cigarettes, are increasingly used worldwide, even though there is limited information on their health effects. In the United States, they are readily available in most states and on the Internet. A report from the Centers for Disease Control and Prevention (CDC) showed that in 2013, over 250,000 junior high and high school students—who had never smoked cigarettes before—had tried e-cigarettes, triple the amount as in 2011. A recent study showed that students who have used e-cigarettes by ninth grade have a higher chance of smoking within the next year. In addition, 12.6 percent of adults have tried e-cigarettes, with about 3.7 percent of adults being current users. Men are more likely to have ever tried e-cigarettes, and 20 percent of adults 18 to 24 years old have tried e-cigarettes, with use declining as age increases.

Most e-cigarettes consist of a battery, a charger, an atomizer, and a cartridge containing nicotine and propylene glycol. When a smoker draws air through an e-cigarette, an airflow sensor activates the battery and heats the atomizer to vaporize the propylene glycol and nicotine. Upon inhalation, the aerosol vapor delivers a dose of nicotine into the lungs of the smoker, after which residual aerosol is exhaled into the environment. Nothing is known, however, about the chemicals present in the aerosolized vapors emanating from e-cigarettes.

Although manufacturers claim that electronic cigarettes are a safe alternative to conventional cigarettes, the FDA analyzed samples of two popular brands and found variable amounts of nicotine and traces of toxic chemicals, including known cancer-causing substances (carcinogens). These carcinogens included an ingredient used in antifreeze and formaldehyde, which was present in higher amounts when higher-voltage charges are used. This prompted the FDA to issue a warning about potential health risks associated with electronic cigarettes. There is no quality control in the manufacturing of the product. Many e-cigarettes are manufactured in China under no controlled conditions.

Furthermore, New York City, Chicago, and Los Angeles have banned e-cigarette use in public places. Many employers are struggling with employees wanting to "vape" indoors on break. Some corporations such as Exxon allow vaping, while Starbucks Corp. and Wal-Mart Stores, Inc. do not. UPS charges nonunion e-cigarette and tobacco users a higher price for their insurance premiums.

With various colors, fruity flavors, clever designs, and other options, e-cigarettes may hold too much appeal for young people, critics warn, offering an easy gateway to nicotine addiction. Currently, e-cigarettes do not contain any health warnings comparable to FDA-approved nicotine-replacement products or conventional cigarettes. They are often marketed as a method to quit smoking, but health professionals recommend using FDA-approved medications and aids that have been shown to be safe and effective for this purpose. A recent study found no merit to the claim that e-cigarettes are better in terms of helping people quit smoking over the nicotine patch.

As e-cigarettes have increased in popularity, a new health risk has emerged for those who do not smoke. The CDC has reported a dramatic increase in calls to poison control centers regarding e-cigarettes and liquid nicotine poisoning. Over 51 percent of these calls involved children under 5 years of age. The cartridges are not required to be childproof and feature flavors such as spearmint, banana, and bubble gum, making them appealing to children.

As a result, health professionals continue to urge for more action to regulate these products.

**Sources:** N. A. Rigotti, "e-Cigarette Use and Subsequent Tobacco Use by Adolescents: New Evidence about a Potential Risk of E-cigarettes," *Journal of the American Medical Association* 314, no. 7 (2015): 673–4; C. A. Schoenborn and R. M. Gindi, "Electronic Cigarette Use Among Adults: United States, 2014," *NCHS Data Brief* No. 217 (Hyattsville, MD: National Center for Health Statistics, 2015); D. Barboza, "China's E-Cigarette Boom Lacks Oversight for Safety," *New York Times,* December 13, 2014, http://www.nytimes.com/2014/12/14/business/international/chinas-e-cigarette-boom-lacks-oversight-for-safety-.html?_r=0; Centers for Disease Control and Prevention, "Smoking & Tobacco Use: Electronic Cigarettes," 2014, www.cdc.gov/tobacco/basic_information/e-cigarettes/youth-intentions/index.htm; Centers for Disease Control and Prevention, "Key Findings: Trends in Awareness and Use of Electronic Cigarettes among U.S. Adults, 2010–2013, 2014, www.cdc.gov/tobacco/basic_information/e-cigarettes/adult-trends/index.htm; American Lung Association, "American Lung Association Statement on E-Cigarettes," March 2015, www.lung.org/stop-smoking/tobacco-control-advocacy/federal/e-cigarettes.html; M. Hug, "Health-Related Effects Reported by Electronic Cigarette Users in Online Forums," *Journal of Medical Internet Research* 15, no. 4 (2014): e59; L. M. Dutra and S. A. Glanz, "Electronic Cigarettes and Conventional Cigarette Use among US Adolescents: A Cross-Sectional Study," *JAMA Pediatrics* (2014), doi:10.1001/jamapediatrics.2013.5488 (Epub ahead of print); L. Weber et al., "E-Cigarette Rise Poses Quandary for Employers," *Wall Street Journal,* January 16, 2014, 41–2; K. Chatham-Stephens et al., "Notes from the Field: Calls to Poison Centers for Exposures to Electronic Cigarettes—United States, September 2010–February 2014," *Morbidity and Mortality Weekly Report* 63, no. 13 (2014): 292–3; Centers for Disease Control and Prevention, "Youth and Tobacco Use," Smoking and Tobacco Use, February 2014, www.cdc.gov/tobacco/data_statistics/fact_sheets/youth_data/tobacco_use.

**chewing tobacco** Stringy form of tobacco that is placed in the mouth and then sucked or chewed.

**dipping** Placing a small amount of chewing tobacco between the lower lip and teeth for rapid nicotine absorption.

**snuff** Powdered form of tobacco that is sniffed or absorbed through the mucous membranes in the nose or placed inside the cheek and sucked.

**leukoplakia** Condition characterized by leathery white patches inside the mouth, which is produced by contact with irritants in tobacco juice.

increasingly popular with college students because they are viewed as safer and cheaper than cigarettes. However, they are far more toxic than cigarettes. Smoke from a bidi contains three to five times more nicotine than do cigarettes.[50] The leaf wrappers are nonporous, which means that smokers must suck harder to inhale and must inhale more to keep the bidi lit. During testing, it took an average of 28 puffs to smoke a bidi, compared to only 9 puffs for a regular cigarette. This results in increased exposure to higher amounts of tar, nicotine, and carbon monoxide. Bidi smoking increases the risk for oral, lung, stomach, and esophageal cancer and is also associated with emphysema and chronic bronchitis.[51]

### Smokeless Tobacco

There are two types of smokeless tobacco: chewing tobacco and snuff.

**Chewing tobacco** comes in three forms—loose leaf, plug, or in a pouch—and contains tobacco leaves treated with molasses and other flavorings. The user dips the tobacco by placing a small amount between the lower lip and teeth to stimulate the flow of saliva and release the nicotine. **Dipping** rapidly releases nicotine into the bloodstream. While cigarette smoking has been on the decline in the United States among youth, use of smokeless tobacco by youth held steady since 1999.[52]

**Snuff** is a finely ground form of tobacco that can be inhaled, chewed, or placed against the gums. It comes in dry or moist powdered form or sachets (tea bag–like pouches). In 2009, "snus" became the latest form of smokeless tobacco to hit the market in the United States. Popular for more than 100 years in Sweden, these small sachets of tobacco are placed inside the cheek and sucked. Some people prefer snus to chewing tobacco because it doesn't require the user to spit frequently.

Smokeless tobacco is just as addictive as cigarettes and actually contains more nicotine—holding an average-sized dip or chew in the mouth for 30 minutes delivers as much nicotine as smoking four cigarettes. A two-can-a-week snuff user gets as much nicotine as a ten-pack-a-week smoker.

Dental problems are common among users of smokeless tobacco. Contact with tobacco juice causes receding gums, tooth decay, bad breath, and discolored teeth. Damage to both the teeth and jawbone can contribute to loss of teeth.

### WHAT DO **YOU** THINK?

Should nicotine be regulated as a controlled substance?

- Should more resources be used for research into nicotine addiction?
- Why or why not?

Explain the health risks of smoking and using smokeless tobacco.

Each day, cigarettes contribute to approximately 1,200 deaths from cancer, cardiovascular disease, and respiratory disorders.[53] In addition, tobacco use can negatively affect the health of almost every system in your body. **FIGURE 12.3** summarizes some of the physiological and health effects of smoking.

## Cancer

Lung cancer is the leading cause of cancer deaths in the United States. The American Cancer Society estimates that tobacco smoking causes 90 percent of all cases of lung cancer in men and 78 percent in women.[54] There were an estimated 224,390 *new* cases of lung cancer in the United States in 2016 alone, and an estimated 158,080 Americans died from the disease in 2016.[55] **FIGURE 12.4** on page 346 shows the association between tobacco consumption rates and lung cancer deaths.

If you are a smoker, your risk of developing lung cancer depends on several factors. First, the amount you smoke per day is important. The more you smoke, the more likely you are to develop lung cancer. A second factor is the age at which you started smoking; if you started in your teens, you have a greater chance of developing lung cancer than do people who start later. And a third risk factor is whether you inhale deeply when you smoke. Smokers are also more susceptible to the cancer-causing effects of exposure to other irritants, such as asbestos and radon, than are nonsmokers.

A major risk of chewing tobacco is **leukoplakia**, a condition characterized by leathery white patches inside the mouth, produced by contact with irritants in tobacco juice. While the majority of leukoplakia cases do not develop into cancer, some are precancerous and can eventually progress to cancer without proper treatment, or are already cancerous on initial sighting.[56]

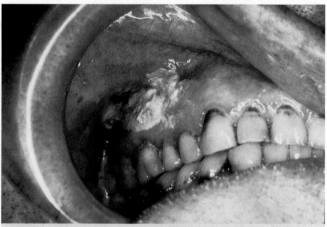

Yellow teeth, bad breath, and gum disease are just part of the problems smokers experience. Leukoplakia can appear on the tongue or in the mouth, as shown here.

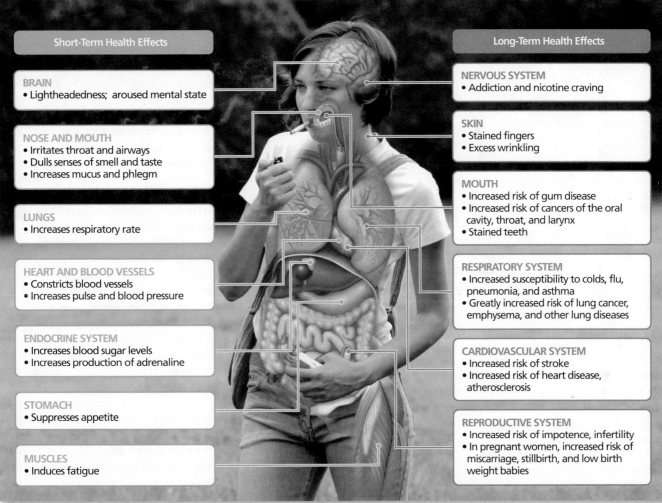

| Short-Term Health Effects | Long-Term Health Effects |
|---|---|

**Short-Term Health Effects**

**BRAIN**
• Lightheadedness; aroused mental state

**NOSE AND MOUTH**
• Irritates throat and airways
• Dulls senses of smell and taste
• Increases mucus and phlegm

**LUNGS**
• Increases respiratory rate

**HEART AND BLOOD VESSELS**
• Constricts blood vessels
• Increases pulse and blood pressure

**ENDOCRINE SYSTEM**
• Increases blood sugar levels
• Increases production of adrenaline

**STOMACH**
• Suppresses appetite

**MUSCLES**
• Induces fatigue

**Long-Term Health Effects**

**NERVOUS SYSTEM**
• Addiction and nicotine craving

**SKIN**
• Stained fingers
• Excess wrinkling

**MOUTH**
• Increased risk of gum disease
• Increased risk of cancers of the oral cavity, throat, and larynx
• Stained teeth

**RESPIRATORY SYSTEM**
• Increased susceptibility to colds, flu, pneumonia, and asthma
• Greatly increased risk of lung cancer, emphysema, and other lung diseases

**CARDIOVASCULAR SYSTEM**
• Increased risk of stroke
• Increased risk of heart disease, atherosclerosis

**REPRODUCTIVE SYSTEM**
• Increased risk of impotence, infertility
• In pregnant women, increased risk of miscarriage, stillbirth, and low birth weight babies

**FIGURE 12.3** **Effects of Smoking on the Body and Health** While some smoking effects are immediate, others occur within a short time, and others occur later in life. Not smoking is your best means of preventing all risks to health.

➡ **VIDEO TUTOR**
Long- and Short-Term Effects of Tobacco

There were over 48,330 cases of oral cancer diagnosed in 2016—the vast majority of which were caused by smokeless tobacco or cigarettes.[57] Smokeless tobacco users have significantly higher rates of oral cancer than nonusers. Warning signs include lumps in the jaw or neck; color changes or lumps inside the lips; white, smooth, or scaly patches in the mouth or on the neck, lips, or tongue; a red spot or sore on the lips or gums or inside the mouth that does not heal in 2 weeks; repeated bleeding in the mouth; and difficulty or abnormality in speaking or swallowing.

The lag time between first use and contracting cancer is shorter for smokeless tobacco users than for smokers because absorption through the gums is the most efficient route of nicotine administration. Many smokeless tobacco users eventually "graduate" to cigarettes and increase their risk for developing additional problems.

Tobacco is linked to other cancers as well. The rate of pancreatic cancer is more than twice as high for smokers as for nonsmokers. Typically, the prognosis for people with pancreatic cancer is not good—the 5-year survival rate is 7 percent.[58] Smokers are at increased risk to develop cancers of the

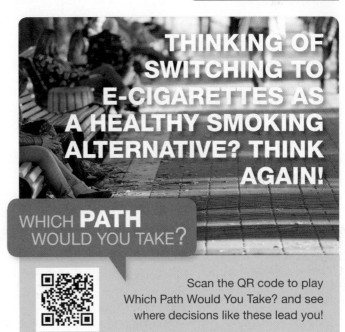

**THINKING OF SWITCHING TO E-CIGARETTES AS A HEALTHY SMOKING ALTERNATIVE? THINK AGAIN!**

WHICH **PATH** WOULD YOU TAKE?

Scan the QR code to play Which Path Would You Take? and see where decisions like these lead you!

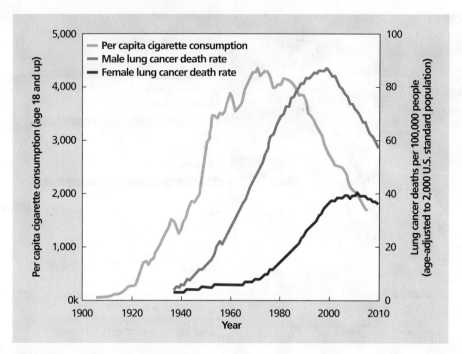

**FIGURE 12.4** Correlation between Tobacco Consumption and Lung Cancer Deaths in the United States  A dramatic rise in lung cancer death rates echoed the rise in popularity of cigarettes and other tobacco products in the last century. After tobacco use and smoking rates began to decline in the 1980s, the lung cancer death rates began to decline as well.

**Source:** E. Mendes, "The Study That Helped Spur the U.S. Stop-Smoking Movement," American Cancer Society, January 2014, www.cancer.org/research/acsresearchupdates/the-study-that-helped-spur-the-us-stop-smoking-movement.

lip, tongue, salivary glands, and esophagus. A growing body of evidence suggests that long-term use of smokeless tobacco increases the risk of cancers of the larynx, esophagus, nasal cavity, pancreas, colon, kidney, and bladder. For more on various cancers, see Chapter 17.

## Cardiovascular Disease

Over a third of all tobacco-related deaths occur from heart disease.[59] Smoking poses as great a risk for developing heart disease as high blood pressure and high cholesterol do.

Smoking contributes to heart disease by aging the arteries.[60] This occurs because smoking and exposure to environmental tobacco smoke (ETS; see the definition on page 000) encourage and accelerate the buildup of fatty deposits (plaque) in the heart and major blood vessels (*atherosclerosis*). Smokers can experience a 50 percent increase in plaque accumulation in the arteries as compared with ex-smokers. Nonsmokers regularly exposed to ETS can have a 20 to 25 percent increase in plaque buildup.[61] For unknown reasons, smoking decreases blood levels of high-density lipoproteins (HDLs), the "good" cholesterol that helps protect against heart attacks.

Smoking also contributes to **platelet adhesiveness**, the

**platelet adhesiveness** Stickiness of red blood cells associated with blood clots.

**emphysema** Chronic lung disease in which the tiny air sacs in the lungs are destroyed, making breathing difficult.

sticking-together of red blood cells associated with blood clots. The oxygen deprivation associated with smoking decreases the oxygen supplied to the heart and can weaken tissues. Smoking also contributes to irregular heart rhythms, which can trigger a heart attack. Both carbon monoxide and nicotine can precipitate angina attacks (chest pain due to the heart muscle not getting the blood supply it needs).

Smokers are two to four times as likely to suffer strokes as nonsmokers.[62] A stroke occurs when a small blood vessel in the brain bursts or is blocked by a blood clot, denying oxygen and nourishment to vital portions of the brain. Depending on the area of the brain affected, stroke can result in paralysis, loss of mental functioning, or death. Smoking contributes to strokes by raising blood pressure, which increases the stress on vessel walls. Platelet adhesiveness contributes to blood clot formation.

If a person quits smoking, the risk of dying from a heart attack falls by half after only 1 year and declines steadily thereafter. After about 15 years without smoking, an ex-smoker's risk of coronary heart disease is similar to that of people who have never smoked.[63]

## Respiratory Disorders

Smoking quickly impairs the respiratory system. Smokers can feel its impact in a relatively short period of time—they are more prone to breathlessness, chronic cough, and excess phlegm production than are nonsmokers of the same age. Over time, cumulative lung damage can lead to chronic obstructive pulmonary disease (COPD), including chronic bronchitis and emphysema. Ultimately, smokers are up to 25 times more likely to die of lung disease than are nonsmokers.[64]

*Chronic bronchitis* may develop in smokers because their inflamed lungs produce more mucus, which they constantly try to expel along with foreign particles. This results in the persistent cough known as "smoker's hack." Smokers are also more prone to respiratory ailments such as influenza, pneumonia, and colds. Smokers tend to miss work one-third more often than nonsmokers, primarily because of respiratory conditions.

**Emphysema** is a chronic disease in which the alveoli (the tiny air sacs in the lungs) are destroyed, impairing the lungs' ability to obtain oxygen and remove carbon dioxide. As a result, breathing becomes difficult. While healthy people expend only about 5 percent of their energy in breathing, people with advanced emphysema expend nearly 80 percent. Because the heart has to work harder to do even the simplest tasks, it may become enlarged, and death from heart damage may result. There is no known cure for emphysema, and the damage is irreversible. Approximately 80 to 90 percent of all cases of emphysema are related to cigarette smoking.[65]

## Sexual Dysfunction and Fertility Problems

Despite attempts by tobacco advertisers to make smoking appear sexy, research shows that it can actually cause impotence in men. Studies have found that male smokers are much more likely to experience erectile dysfunction than are nonsmokers.[66] Toxins in cigarette smoke damage blood vessels, reducing blood flow to the penis and leading to an inadequate erection. Impotence may indicate oncoming cardiovascular disease.

In women, smoking can lead to infertility and problems with pregnancy. Women who smoke increase their risk for infertility, ectopic pregnancy, miscarriage, and stillbirth. Smoking also increases the risk of sudden infant death syndrome and the chances of a baby being born with a cleft lip or cleft palate.[67] Smoking during pregnancy increases the chance of premature birth and the risk of low birth weight (less than 5.5 pounds), which in turn increases the likelihood of illness or death of an infant.[68] For information on specific health risks faced by women smokers, see the **Health in a Diverse World** box on page 348.

**WHAT DO YOU THINK?**

Should smokeless tobacco be banned wherever smoking is forbidden?

■ Why do you think smokeless tobacco is popular with many athletes and young men?

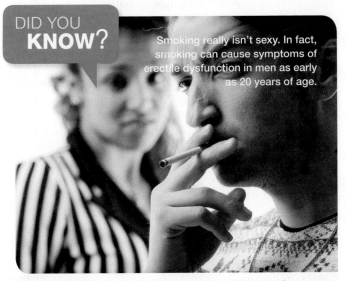

**DID YOU KNOW?**

Smoking really isn't sexy. In fact, smoking can cause symptoms of erectile dysfunction in men as early as 20 years of age.

**Source:** U.S. Department of Health and Human Services, "The Health Consequences of Smoking: 50 Years of Progress. A Report of the Surgeon General," Atlanta, GA: U.S. Department of Health and Human Services, Centers for Disease Control and Prevention, National Center for Chronic Disease Prevention and Health Promotion, Office on Smoking and Health, 2014. Printed with corrections, January 2014.

## Other Health Effects

Studies have shown tobacco use to be a serious risk factor in the development of gum disease.[69] In addition, smoking increases the risk of macular degeneration, one of the most common causes of blindness in older adults. It also causes premature skin wrinkling, staining of the teeth, yellowing of the fingernails, and bad breath. Nicotine speeds up the process by which the body uses and eliminates drugs, making medications less effective. In addition, research suggests that smoking significantly increases the risk of Alzheimer's disease.[70]

> **environmental tobacco smoke (ETS)** Smoke from tobacco products, including secondhand and mainstream smoke.
>
> **mainstream smoke** Smoke that is drawn through tobacco while inhaling.
>
> **sidestream smoke** Smoke from the burning end of a cigarette, pipe, or cigar or exhaled by smokers, commonly called *secondhand smoke*.

## LO 5 | ENVIRONMENTAL TOBACCO SMOKE

Explain the dangers created by environmental tobacco smoke.

Although fewer Americans smoke than in the past, air pollution from smoking in public places continues to be a problem. **Environmental tobacco smoke (ETS)** is divided into two categories: mainstream and sidestream smoke. **Mainstream smoke** refers to smoke drawn through tobacco while inhaling; **sidestream smoke** (commonly called *secondhand smoke*)

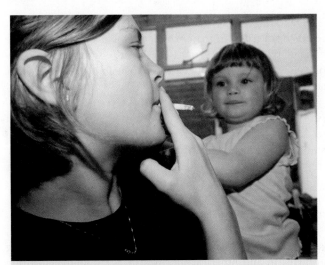

Every year, ETS is responsible for thousands of deaths from lung cancer and heart disease in nonsmoking adults, as well as hundreds of infant deaths from SIDS among babies who live with smokers. Because their bodies and brains are still developing, infants and children are particularly vulnerable to the toxins in secondhand smoke: It can cause respiratory problems, including lower respiratory infections and increased frequency and severity of asthma attacks, and other health concerns, such as greater risk of ear infections.

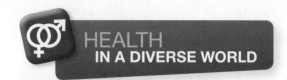
# WOMEN AND SMOKING
*Unique Health Risks*

Today, 14.8 percent of women—slightly more than 1 in 6—smoke, compared with 18.8 percent of men. Women who smoke now are just as likely to die of cancer and other smoking-related diseases as men, and both active and passive smoking increase chances of breast cancer. Accordingly, women have assumed a much larger burden of smoking-related diseases than they did in the past, and the prevalence of tobacco-related disease continues to increase. Consider the following:

■ Women are 25 times more likely to die from lung cancer than nonsmoking women compared to 30 years ago.

■ Smoking reduces a woman's life expectancy on average by at least 10 years.

■ Women who smoke have two to four times the risk of heart disease and stroke.

■ Women who smoke (particularly those who also use oral contraceptives) are

Cigarette companies have become adept at marketing to women using "glamorous" packaging and ad campaigns borrowed from the cosmetic, perfume (such as the famous Chanel scents evoked by this Camel No. 9 brand), and fashion industries.

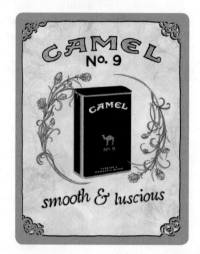

at increased risk for blood clots, as well as heavier menstrual bleeding, longer duration of cramps, and less predictable length of menstrual cycle.

■ Postmenopausal women who smoke have lower bone density than do women who never smoked, putting these women at increased risk for osteoporosis.

**Sources:** M. Thun et al., "50-Year Trends in Smoking-Related Mortality in the United States," *New England Journal of Medicine* 368 (2013): 351–64, doi: 10.1056/NEJMsa1211127; American Cancer Society, "Women and Smoking: An Epidemic of Smoking-Related Cancer and Disease in Women," revised February 2014, www.cancer.org/Cancer/CancerCauses/TobaccoCancer/WomenandSmoking/women-and-smoking-intro; Current Cigarette Smoking Status—United States 2005–2014," *Morbidity and Mortality Weekly Report* 64, no. 44 (2015): 1233–40; Go Red for Women Editors, "Smoking and Heart Disease," *American Heart Association,* Accessed April 2016, https://www.goredforwomen.org/know-your-risk/factors-that-increase-your-risk-for-heart-disease/smoking-heart-disease/; P. Jha et al., "21st-Century Hazards of Smoking and Benefits of Cessation in the United States," *New England Journal of Medicine* 368, no. 4 (2013): 341–50; M. Thun et al., "50-Year Trends in Smoking-Related Mortality in the United States," *New England Journal of Medicine* 368, no. 4 (2013): 351–64.

refers to smoke from the burning end of a cigarette or smoke exhaled by a smoker. People who breathe smoke from someone else's smoking product are said to be *involuntary* or *passive* smokers.

Between 1988 and 2008, detectable levels of nicotine exposure in nonsmoking Americans decreased from 87.9 percent to 25.3 percent.[71] The decrease in exposure to secondhand smoke is due to the growing number of laws that ban smoking in workplaces and other public areas. As of 2016, 41 states and the District of Columbia had laws in effect requiring workplaces, restaurants, and bars to be 100 percent smoke-free.[72] There are 22,578 municipalities—82 percent of the U.S. population—that are covered by either state, commonwealth, territorial, or local law.[73] Groups such as Action on Smoking and Health and Americans for Nonsmokers' Rights continue to push for policies and laws in support of smoke-free public places.[74]

## Risks from Environmental Tobacco Smoke

Although involuntary smokers breathe less tobacco than active smokers do, they still face risks from exposure. According to the American Lung Association, secondhand smoke contains hundreds of chemicals known to be toxic or carcinogenic, including formaldehyde, benzene, vinyl chloride, arsenic ammonia, and hydrogen cyanide.[75] Every year, ETS is estimated to be responsible for approximately 3,400 lung cancer deaths in nonsmoking adults, 46,000 coronary and heart disease deaths in nonsmoking adults who live with smokers, and higher risk of death in newborns from sudden infant death syndrome.[76]

The Environmental Protection Agency has designated secondhand smoke as a known carcinogen. There are more than 70 cancer-causing agents found in secondhand smoke.[77] There is also strong evidence that secondhand smoke interferes with normal functioning of the heart, blood, and vascular systems, significantly increasing the risk for heart disease. Studies indicate that nonsmokers exposed to secondhand smoke were far more likely to have coronary heart disease and stroke than nonsmokers not exposed to smoke.[78]

**Children and ETS** Exposure to ETS increases children's risk of lower respiratory tract infections. Chemicals in tobacco smoke also show up in breast milk, and breastfeeding may pass more chemicals to the infant of a smoking mother than direct exposure to ETS. In addition, children exposed to secondhand smoke have a greater chance of developing other respiratory problems such as coughing, wheezing, asthma, and chest colds, along with a decrease in lung function. ETS is also linked to fluid buildup in the middle ear, a contributing factor in middle ear infections, a leading reason for childhood surgery. Children exposed to secondhand smoke daily in the home miss more school days and have more colds and acute respiratory infections than do those not exposed.[79] Disparities in ETS also occur along ethnic, racial, and economic lines. Mexican American children have been found to have higher levels of exposure to ETS than whites and Latinos.[80] ETS exposure is also higher among low-income persons.[81]

Secondhand smoke affects not only children's physical health, but also their cognitive abilities and academic success. Children exposed to high levels of secondhand smoke are more likely to develop learning disabilities, conduct disorders, and other behavioral disorders.[82]

**ETS and Additional Health Problems** ETS in enclosed areas presents other hazards; it can cause allergic reactions such as itchy eyes, difficulty in breathing, headaches, nausea, and dizziness. Environmental tobacco smoke may also increase the risk of breast cancer in women; cancer of the nasal sinus cavity and of the pharynx in adults; and leukemia, lymphoma, and brain tumors in children.[83] The level of carbon monoxide in cigarette smoke in enclosed spaces is 4,000 times higher than that allowed in the clean-air standard recommended by the EPA.

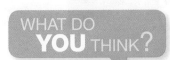

**WHAT DO YOU THINK?**

Why do most smokers continue despite knowing long-term hazards?

■ What strategies might be effective in reducing the number of people who begin smoking?

## LO 6 | TOBACCO USE AND PREVENTION POLICIES

Discuss prevention policies enacted by the U.S. government to curb tobacco use.

It has been more than 40 years since the U.S. government began warning that tobacco use was hazardous to health. Despite all the education on the health hazards of tobacco use, health care spending and lost productivity associated with smoking costs between $289 and $333 billion each year.[84]

In 1998, the tobacco industry reached the Master Settlement Agreement with 46 states. The agreement requires tobacco companies to pay out more than $206 billion over 25 years. The agreement includes a variety of measures to support antismoking education and advertising and to fund research to determine effective smoking-cessation strategies. The agreement also curbs certain advertising and promotions directed at youth.

Unfortunately, most of the money designated for tobacco control and prevention at the state level has not been used for this purpose. Facing budget woes, many states have drastically

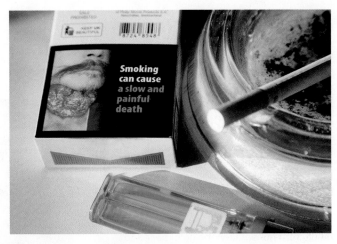

**FIGURE 12.5 Pictorial Health Warnings in Europe** In Europe, warnings like "Smoking Kills" are required to be printed on tobacco products. Since 2005, the European Commission for Public Health has also required graphic labels like this one to be printed on cigarette packs. In fact, the Commission has adopted an entire library, made up of 42 different images, so that countries can choose pictorial warnings most effective for their populations.

**Source:** European Commission for Public Health, "Pictorial Health Warnings," June 18, 2014, http://ec.europa.eu/health/tobacco/law/pictorial/index_en.htm.

cut spending on antismoking programs. In the few states that have spent the settlement money on smoking-cessation programs, there has been some success in decreasing cigarette use.[85] The Family Smoking Prevention and Tobacco Control Act of 2009 allows the U.S. Food and Drug Administration (FDA) to forbid advertising geared toward children, to lower the amount of nicotine in tobacco products, to ban sweetened cigarettes that appeal to young people, and to prohibit labels such as "light" and "low tar."[86] The FDA recently ordered four tobacco products (bidis) to be taken off the market when the company that created them was unwilling to provide ingredient information—the first time since being given the authority in 2009.

One of the most significant impacts of the law is that it requires more prominent health warnings on advertising of tobacco products. Smokeless tobacco ads must contain a warning that fills 20 percent of the advertising space. The FDA attempted to require cigarette packages and advertising to have larger, graphical warnings depicting the negative consequences of smoking, but a federal judge declared the requirement unconstitutional in 2012. In Europe, though, graphic and text-based warnings are required (**FIGURE 12.5**).

Outside of legal action, there are a number of things that can be done to reduce societal smoking rates. See the **Health in a Diverse World** box on page 350 for more on this.

## LO 7 | QUITTING SMOKING

Describe various quitting strategies, including those aimed at ending the body's addiction to nicotine.

Smokers who want to quit must break both the physical addiction to nicotine and the psychological habit of lighting up at certain times or in certain situations. Approximately 70

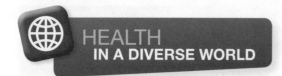
Tobacco is an epidemic. In fact, it kills nearly 6 million people each year and is one of the largest public health threats facing the world. Approximately one person dies from a tobacco-related disease every 6 seconds. More than 5 of every 6 deaths caused by tobacco result from direct tobacco use, while at least another 600,000 of them result from nonsmokers being exposed to secondhand smoke.

Of the more than 1 billion smokers in the world, almost 80 percent of them live in low- and middle-income countries—countries with the heaviest burden of tobacco-related illness and death. When tobacco users die young; they make it harder for their families to get by because of lack of income; they contribute to rising health care costs, and they stifle economic development.

In some countries, young people from households of low socioeconomic status often work in tobacco farming to help make money for their families. Children working in tobacco fields are particularly susceptible to what is called "green tobacco sickness"—an illness caused by the nicotine absorbed through the skin when handling wet tobacco leaves. What can be done to curtail the damage done by tobacco? Here are a few ideas:

**Graphic media campaigns.** Focused antitobacco ads and packs featuring graphic warnings lower the number of children who smoke, as well as raise the number of quitters. More than 80 countries require graphic warning labels to be conspicuously placed on packs of cigarettes and some other tobacco products. Not only do these warnings reduce the number of smokers, but they are also effective in convincing smokers to respect the health of those around them by not smoking inside the home or near children.

**Taxes.** Tobacco taxes are the most cost-effective way to reduce tobacco use, especially among young and poor people. Despite taxes being the least expensive way to reduce the use of

tobacco products—and clear evidence that it works—more than 80 percent of countries still don't tax tobacco. And not only does taxation cost governments little to implement, it actually increases government revenues.

**Stop illicit tobacco trade.** Illegal trading of tobacco products causes serious health, security, and economic concerns across the globe. In fact, nearly 10 percent of tobacco products consumed globally are from illegal markets. Putting an end to illicit tobacco trading will cut harmful consumption of tobacco in two ways: by reducing the availability of cheap, unregulated options and by driving up tobacco prices overall. Eliminating or curtailing

illegal trading of tobacco products will lower the numbers of premature deaths caused by tobacco use, as well as increase the amount of tax revenue raised by governments.

**Sources:** World Health Organization, "Tobacco" Fact Sheet No. 339, July 2015, http://www.who.int/mediacentre/factsheets/fs339/en/; V. L. Costa e Silva, "World No Tobacco Day 2015: Time to Act Against Illicit Tobacco," May 2015, http://www.who.int/mediacentre/commentaries/illicit-tobaco/en/; World Health Organization, "WHO Report on the Global Tobacco Epidemic, 2015: Raising Taxes on Tobacco, Executive Summary," Accessed April 2016, http://apps.who.int/iris/bitstream/10665/178577/1/WHO_NMH_PND_15.5_eng.pdf?ua=1&ua=1; Campaign for Tobacco Free Kids, "International Issues: Warning Labels," April 2016, http://global.tobaccofreekids.org/en/solutions/international_issues/warning_labels#pictorial.

---

A TIP ABOUT
SECONDHAND
SMOKE

## SECONDHAND SMOKE TRIGGERS SEVERE ASTHMA ATTACKS.

Jamason
High School Student
Kentucky

When Jamason was 16, secondhand smoke triggered such a severe asthma attack, he was hospitalized for four days. If you or someone you know wants free help to quit smoking, call **1-800-QUIT-NOW.**
#CDCTips

CDC | U.S. Department of Health and Human Services Centers for Disease Control and Prevention www.cdc.gov/tips

percent of U.S. adult smokers want to quit smoking, and up to 48 percent make a serious attempt to quit each year.[87] Quitting is often a lengthy process involving several unsuccessful attempts before success is finally achieved. Even successful quitters suffer occasional slips. For those smokers unable to quit, they can expect to lose at least one decade of life compared to those who do not smoke.

## Benefits of Quitting

Many body tissues damaged by smoking can repair themselves. As soon as smokers stop, the body begins the repair process. Within 12 hours, carbon monoxide levels return to normal, and "smoker's breath" disappears.[88] Often, within a month of quitting, the mucus that clogs airways is broken up and eliminated. Circulation and the senses of taste and smell improve within weeks. Many ex-smokers say that they have more energy, sleep better, and feel more alert.

After 1 year, the risk for heart disease decreases.[89] Women are less likely to bear babies of low birth weight.[90] After 10 smoke-free years, the risk of developing cancer of the lung, larynx, pancreas, kidney, bladder, or cervix is considerably reduced.[91] See **FIGURE 12.6** for a timeline of how the body recuperates after a smoker quits.

Another significant benefit of quitting smoking is the money saved. A single pack of cigarettes ranges from about $5.00 (including tax) to as much as $11.00 to $13.50 in the most expensive states, so a pack-a-day smoker who lives in an area where cigarettes cost $8.00 per pack spends $56.00 per week, or $2,912 per year.[92] That is money that could have gone toward school expenses, a down payment on a car, or a vacation. See the **Money & Health** box on page 352 for more on the cost of smoking versus quitting.

## How Can You Quit?

A person who wishes to quit smoking has several options. Most people who are successful quit "cold turkey"—that is, they simply decide not to smoke again. Others focus on gradual reduction in smoking levels, which can reduce risks over time. Some rely on short-term programs, such as those offered by the American Cancer Society, which are based on behavior modification and a system of self-rewards. Still others turn to treatment centers, community outreach programs, or a telephone helpline. Finally, some people work privately with their physicians to reach their goal. Programs that combine several approaches have shown the most promise. Financial considerations, personality, and level of addiction are all factors to consider in deciding on a method.

## Breaking the Nicotine Addiction

Nicotine addiction may be one of the toughest addictions to overcome. Symptoms of **nicotine withdrawal** include irritability, restlessness, nausea and vomiting, and intense cravings for tobacco (see **TABLE 12.3** on page 353). The evidence is strong that consistent pharmacological treatments can help a smoker quit: An estimated 25 percent of people who have used nicotine replacement therapy or

**nicotine withdrawal** Symptoms including nausea, headaches, irritability, and intense tobacco cravings suffered by nicotine-addicted individuals who stop using tobacco.

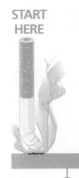

**START HERE**

**8 hours**
- Carbon monoxide level in blood drops to normal.
- Oxygen level in blood increases to normal.

**48 hours**
- Nerve endings start regrowing.
- Ability to smell and taste is enhanced.

**1 to 9 months**
- Coughing, sinus congestion, fatigue, shortness of breath decrease.
- Cilia regrow in lungs, which increases ability to handle mucus, clean the lungs, reduce infection.
- Body's overall energy increases.

**5 years**
- Lung cancer death rate for average former smoker (one pack a day) decreases by almost half.

**15 years**
- Risk of coronary heart disease is the same as that of a nonsmoker.

**20 minutes**
- Blood pressure drops to normal.
- Pulse rate drops to normal.
- Body temperature of hands and feet increases to normal.

**24 hours**
- Chance of heart attack decreases.

**2 weeks to 3 months**
- Circulation improves.
- Walking becomes easier.
- Lung function increases up to 30%.

**1 year**
- Excess risk of coronary disease is half that of a smoker.

**10 years**
- Lung cancer death rate similar to that of nonsmokers.
- Precancerous cells are replaced.
- Risk of cancers of the mouth, throat, esophagus, bladder, kidney, and pancreas decreases.

**FIGURE 12.6 When Smokers Quit** Within 20 minutes of smoking that last cigarette, the body begins a series of changes that continues for years. However, by smoking just one cigarette a day, the smoker loses all of these benefits of quitting smoking, according to the American Cancer Society.

**Source:** American Cancer Society, "When Smokers Quit—What Are the Benefits Over Time?," February 2014, www .cancer.org/healthy/stayawayfromtobacco/guidetoquittingsmoking/guide-to-quitting-smoking-benefits.

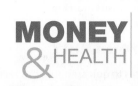

# MONEY & HEALTH | THE COST OF QUITTING VERSUS SMOKING

The cost of smoking cessation can add up, especially if you're relying on many stop-smoking aids, but there are many things to consider when comparing the cost of smoking to the cost of quitting.

### The Costs of Quitting

Using a combination of aids such as the nicotine patch and gum can be pricey. A 12-week supply of the patches would cost approximately $180, and a 12-week supply of the gum would cost about $240. The total for both aids would be estimated at $420 for less than 3 months of nicotine replacement treatment.

However, smoking-cessation experts state that it's important to keep these stop-smoking costs in perspective. Let's say that the average cost of a pack of cigarettes is $7.00. That means that over the span of a year, a pack-a-day smoker will pay more than $2,555. That's more than enough savings to buy 3 or 6 months' worth of nicotine replacement or other medications, or to pay for a class or a few counseling sessions.

In other states, the costs of smoking are even higher. In Rhode Island, Alaska, Illinois, and Hawaii, a pack of cigarettes costs anywhere from $9 to $12, and in New York it is more than $14 a pack. When comparing this to a supply of smoking-cessation aids, it is clear that quitting smoking is less costly than smoking.

In addition, these numbers don't take into account the potential future health care costs of continuing to smoke. Smokers cost employers more to employ because smokers take more sick time, use more insurance dollars, and lose about 1 month of work time per year related to their smoking behaviors. Quitting smoking or not smoking in the car or home can increase their resale value. It is estimated that the resale value of smokers' homes can be reduced anywhere from 10 to 29 percent. Nonsmokers have lower insurance premiums and increased wellness benefits, as some employers incentivize employees who do not smoke.

### The Bottom Line

Add it all up, and the answer is evident. Even if you paid full price for all your smoking-cessation aids, it's still going to be less expensive in the long run than smoking. Even if someone needed to take medications for longer than 6 months, the reduced health care costs down the road would likely result in substantial savings.

Furthermore, people who want to quit smoking also have a number of resources at their disposal that can reduce the cost of quitting. The national smoking quit line, 1-800-QUIT-NOW, can transfer you to your local quit-smoking hotline. The therapy and counseling sessions offered by the over-the-phone counselors are completely free, and in a number of studies, they have been shown to be very effective.

You can also ask your counselor if you can get free nicotine replacement products mailed to you. Many quit lines offer a starter kit of nicotine replacement products, such as free patches, to help the smoker get their quit attempt started.

If you're looking for other ways to save on quitting, there are many generic versions of medication or the generic or store versions of nicotine replacement products. These generics are usually as good as the brand-name products, but at a more affordable price.

As a part of the Affordable Care Act, insurance companies now are required to cover tobacco cessation treatment with no cost to the smoker. This makes it clear: It doesn't pay to continue to smoke.

**Sources:** M. Kofman, S. Craig, "Smoking Can Diminish the Value of Your Home by 30%—Word of Caution for Homeowners," *My Reality Times,* December 23, 2015, http://opinions.realtytimes.com/advicefromagents1/item/41135-smoking-can-diminish-the-value-of-your-home-by-30-word-of-caution-for-homeowners; American Lung Association, "Tobacco Cessation Treatment: What is Covered?" Accessed April 2016, http://www.lung.org/our-initiatives/tobacco/cessation-and-prevention/tobacco-cessation-treatment-what-is-covered.html; HealthCare.gov, "What Are My Preventive Care Benefits?" 2014, www.healthcare.gov/what-are-my-preventive-care-benefits/; W. Myers, "Is It Cheaper to Smoke or Quit?," 2011, *Everyday Health,* www.everydayhealth.com/stop-smoking/is-it-cheaper-to-smoke-or-quit.aspx; quitnowca, "Smoking Cost Calculator," Accessed April 2016, https://www.quitnow.ca/tools-and-resources/calculate-your-savings; H. Holmes, "What a Pack of Cigarettes Costs Now, State by State," *The Awl,* August 28, 2015, www.theawl.com/2013/07/what-a-pack-of-cigarettes-costs-now-state-by-state.

---

smoking-cessation medications continue to abstain from cigarettes for more than 6 months.[93]

### Nicotine Replacement Products

Nontobacco products that replace depleted levels of nicotine in the bloodstream have helped some people stop using tobacco. The two most common are nicotine chewing gum and the nicotine patch, both of which are available over the counter.

The FDA has also approved nicotine lozenges, a nicotine nasal spray, and a nicotine inhaler.

Nicotine gum is available without a prescription. The user chews up to 20 pieces of gum a day for 1 to 3 months. Nicotine gum delivers about the same amount of nicotine as a cigarette, but because it is absorbed through the mucous membrane of the mouth, it doesn't produce the same rush. Users experience no withdrawal symptoms and fewer cravings for

# TABLE 12.3 | Coping Strategies for Common Smoking Withdrawal Problems

| Withdrawal Challenge | Estimated Length of Symptoms | Coping Strategies* |
|---|---|---|
| Anger, frustration, and irritability | Peaks in first week after quitting but can last 2–4 weeks | Avoid caffeine, which can amp up an already agitated mood. Get a massage, try deep breathing or exercise. |
| Anxiety | Builds over the first 3 days and may last up to 2 weeks | Same strategies as above. Also remind yourself that the symptoms usually pass by themselves over time. |
| Mild depression | One month or less | Be with supportive friends, increase physical activity, make a list of things that are upsetting you and write down possible solutions. If depression lasts longer than a month, seek medical advice. |
| Weight gain | Usually begins in the early weeks and continues through the first year after quitting | Studies show nicotine replacement products such as gum and lozenges can help counter weight gain. You may also ask your doctor about the drug bupropion (brand names Wellbutrin or Zyban), which has also been shown to counter weight gain. |

*Asking your doctor for nicotine replacement products or other medications is a valid coping strategy for any of the withdrawal challenges listed here.

**Sources:** Adapted from National Cancer Institute, National Institutes of Health, "Handling Withdrawal Symptoms and Triggers When You Decide to Quit Smoking," Accessed July 2016, http://www.cancer.gov/about-cancer/causes-prevention/risk/tobacco/withdrawal-fact-sheet; Centers for Disease Control and Prevention, "Quitting Smoking," Accessed April 2016, http://www.cdc.gov/tobacco/data_statistics/fact_sheets/cessation/quitting/index.htm#overview; WebMD, "Quitting Tobacco: Help for the First Hard Days," March 2015, http://www.webmd.com/smoking-cessation/understanding-nicotine-withdrawal-symptoms.

## WHAT DO YOU THINK?

**Do you know anyone who has tried to quit smoking?**

- Why did they do so?
- What was their experience like?
- Were they successful?
- If not, what will they do differently the next time?

## SEE IT! VIDEOS

What are the hidden dangers of liquid nicotine? Watch **GMA investigates liquid nicotine**, available on MasteringHealth.™

nicotine as the dosage is reduced until they are completely weaned. Nicotine-containing lozenges are available in two strengths, and a 12-week program of use is recommended to allow users to taper off the drug.

The nicotine patch is generally used in conjunction with a comprehensive smoking-cessation program. A small, thin patch placed on the smoker's upper body delivers a continuous flow of nicotine through the skin, helping to relieve cravings. Patches can be bought with or without a prescription and are available in different dosages. It is recommended that those using the patch as a part of their smoking-cessation program use it for 9 to 10 weeks.[94] During this time, the dose of nicotine is gradually reduced until the smoker is fully weaned from the drug. The patch costs less than a pack of cigarettes—about $4—and some insurance plans will pay for it.[95]

The nicotine nasal spray, which requires a prescription, is much more powerful and delivers nicotine to the bloodstream faster than gum, lozenges, or the patch.

Patients are warned to be careful not to overdose; as little as 40 mg of nicotine taken at once could be lethal. The FDA has advised that the spray should be used for no more than 3 months and never for more than 6 months so that smokers don't find themselves as dependent on nicotine in spray form as they were on cigarettes. The FDA also advises that no one who experiences nasal or sinus problems, allergies, or asthma should use it.

The nicotine inhaler, which also requires a prescription, consists of a mouthpiece and cartridge. By puffing on the mouthpiece, the smoker inhales air saturated with nicotine, which is absorbed through the lining of the mouth, not the lungs, entering the body much more slowly than does the nicotine in cigarettes. Using the inhaler mimics the hand-to-mouth actions used in smoking and causes the back of the throat to feel as it would when inhaling tobacco smoke.

**Smoking-Cessation Medications** Bupropion (brand name Zyban), an antidepressant, is FDA approved as a smoking-cessation aid. Varenicline (brand name Chantix) reduces nicotine cravings and the urge to smoke and blocks the effects of nicotine at nicotine receptor sites in the brain. Both drugs may cause changes in behavior such as hostility, agitation, depressed mood, and suicidal thoughts or actions. People taking one of these drugs who experience any unusual changes in mood are advised to stop taking the drug immediately and contact their health care professional.[96]

See **TABLE 12.4** for a summary of recommended smoking-cessation therapies. Additionally, see the **Tech & Health** box on page 354 for information on smoking apps.

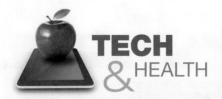

# TECH & HEALTH | CAN SMOKING APPS HELP YOU QUIT?

With the thousands of smartphone apps available for quitting smoking, it may seem like all you need to stop smoking is to start downloading. But users should proceed with caution: A recent study that examined popular smoking apps in 2012 found that most apps did not adhere to known cessation methods, meaning they may not be based on evidence or established behavior change strategies.

However, several research-based smoking apps available from reputable institutions may actually help you stop smoking:

- **QuitGuide.** (Free: iPhone) http://smokefree.gov/apps-quitguide

Developed by the National Cancer Institute, QuitGuide allows users to track smoking habits, mood, and cravings, as well as access other features to stay motivated to quit.

- **QuitForLife.** (Free: iPhone, Android) www.quitforlifeapp.com The American Cancer Society developed this app with resources including a savings calculator, daily motivational tips, and a 24-hour coaching phone line and online community (for eligible individuals).

- **UCSF/SFGH Stop Smoking.** (Modest cost: iPhone) https://itunes.apple.com/us/app/ucsf-sfgh-stop-smoking/id393637213?mt=8 The University of California, San

Francisco's app is a self-help tool that tracks your mood and triggers for smoking and helps you plan healthier activities.

Remember that these apps alone may not be enough to help you quit. Determining what works best for you is an individual process, and programs that combine multiple methods (behavior modification, telephone hotlines, etc.) are usually your best bet.

**Sources:** Abroms et al., "A Content Analysis of Popular Smartphone Apps for Smoking Cessation," *American Journal of Preventive Medicine* 45, no. 6 (2013): 732–36; J. Choi et al., "Smoking Cessation Apps for Smartphones: Content Analysis with the Self-Determination Theory," *Journal of Medical Internet Research* 16, no. 2 (2014): e44.

## Breaking the Smoking Habit

For some smokers, the road to quitting includes antismoking therapy. Two common techniques are operant conditioning and self-control therapy. Pairing the act of smoking with an external stimulus is a typical example of an operant strategy. For example, one technique requires smokers to carry a timer that sounds like a buzzer at various intervals. When the buzzer sounds, the patient is required to smoke a cigarette. Once the smoker is conditioned to associate the sound of the buzzer with smoking, the buzzer is eliminated, and, one hopes, so is the smoking.

Self-control strategies view smoking as a learned habit associated with specific situations. Therapy aims to identify these situations and teach smokers the skills necessary to resist smoking. The Making Changes Today box presents one of the American Cancer Society's approaches to quitting.

## MAKING CHANGES TODAY

### Tips for Quitting Smoking

Ready to quit tobacco? These strategies can help:

- ◉ Ask smokers who live with you to keep cigarettes out of sight and not offer you any.

- ◎ Use the four Ds: deep breaths, drink water, do something else, and delay (tell yourself you'll smoke in 10 minutes when the urge hits).

- ◎ Keep "mouth toys" handy: Hard candy, chewing gum, toothpicks, or carrot or celery sticks can help.

- ◎ Ask your doctor about nicotine gum, patches, nasal sprays, inhalers, or lozenges.

- ◎ Make an appointment with your dental hygienist to have your teeth cleaned.

- ◎ Examine those associations that trigger your urge to smoke.

- ◎ Spend your time in places that don't allow smoking.

- ◎ Take up a new sport, exercise program, hobby, or organizational commitment. This will help shake up your routine and distract you from smoking.

# TABLE 12.4 | Recommended Therapies for Smoking Cessation

| Therapy | Duration |
|---|---|

### Bupropion (Zyban)

A non-nicotine-based antidepressant that helps reduce nicotine withdrawal symptoms and the urge to smoke. Common side effects are dry mouth, difficulty sleeping, dizziness, and skin rash. Contraindicated if smoker has a history of seizures. Zyban can also cause changes in behavior such as hostility, agitation, depression, and suicidal thoughts or actions.

*Availability:* Prescription only with a doctor consultation

*Cost:* Approximately $2–$4 per day

**Duration:** 7–12 weeks; maintenance up to 6 months; start 1–2 weeks before the quit date

### Varenicline (Chantix)

A non-nicotine-based prescription medicine developed for the sole purpose of helping people stop smoking. Interferes with nicotine receptors in the brain to lessen the pleasurable physical effects from smoking and to reduce symptoms of nicotine withdrawal. Usually well tolerated, but reported side effects have included headaches, nausea, vomiting, difficulty sleeping, flatulence, changes in taste, and depressed mood. Chantix may change how you react to alcohol, and you should drink less alcohol until you know whether Chantix affects your tolerance for alcohol.

*Availability:* Prescription only with a doctor consultation

*Cost:* Approximately $2–$4 per day

**Duration:** 12 weeks; maintenance of 12 weeks after successfully quitting; start 1–2 weeks in advance

### Nicotine Gum

A chewing gum that releases nicotine into the bloodstream through the lining of the mouth; might not be appropriate for people with temporomandibular joint disease or those with dentures or other dental work. Up to 2 mg dose if less than 25 cigarettes/day; 4 mg dose if more than 25 cigarettes/day.

*Availability:* Over the counter (OTC)

*Cost:* Varies upon usage, ranging from $5 to $10 a day

**Duration:** Up to 12 weeks

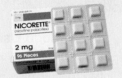

### Nicotine Lozenges

The lozenges are available in two strengths as part of a 12-week program. Doses can be regularly lowered as treatment progresses. Users should not eat or drink 15 minutes before using lozenges.

*Availability:* OTC

*Cost:* Depending on frequency of usage, ranges from $6 to $12 per day

**Duration:** The recommended dose is one lozenge every 1–2 hours for 6 weeks, then one lozenge every 2–4 hours for weeks 7–9, and one lozenge every 4–8 hours for weeks 10–12.

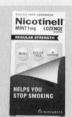

### Nicotine Patch

Patch supplies a steady amount of nicotine to the body through the skin. It is sold in varying strengths as an 8-week smoking-cessation treatment. Doses can be regularly lowered as treatment progresses or given as a steady dose during treatment. May not be a good choice for people with skin problems or allergies to adhesive tape.

*Availability:* Either OTC or by prescription with a doctor consultation

*Cost:* Approximately $4 per day.

**Duration:** 4 weeks; then 2 weeks; then 2 weeks (8 weeks total)

### Nicotine Nasal Spray

Comes in a pump bottle containing nicotine that tobacco users can inhale when they have an urge to smoke. Not recommended for people with nasal or sinus conditions, allergies, or asthma, or for young tobacco users.

*Availability:* Prescription only with a doctor consultation

*Cost:* Approximately $5–$15 per day, depending on frequency of use

**Duration:** 3–6 months

### Nicotine Inhaler

This device delivers a vaporized form of nicotine to the mouth through a mouthpiece attached to a plastic cartridge. Nicotine travels to the mouth and throat and is absorbed through the mucous membranes. Common side effects include throat and mouth irritation and coughing. Anyone with bronchial problems should use caution.

*Availability:* Prescription only with a doctor consultation

*Cost:* Ranges from $40 to $60 per package

**Duration:** Up to 6 months

**Sources:** Adapted from the Federal Food and Drug Administration, "FDA: Smoking 101," February 2016, http://www.fda.gov/ForConsumers/ConsumerUpdates/ucm198176.htm#learn; Drugs.com "Smoking Cessation Agents," April 1, 2016, http://www.drugs.com/drug-class/smoking-cessation-agents.html.

# STUDY **PLAN**

Customize your study plan—and master your health!—in the Study Area of **MasteringHealth**.

## **ASSESS** YOURSELF

**Are you a smoker?** Take the **Tobacco: Are Your Habits Placing You at Risk?** assessment available on

# MasteringHealth.™

## CHAPTER **REVIEW**

To hear an MP3 Tutor Session, scan here or visit the Study Area in **MasteringHealth**.

### LO **1** | Tobacco Use in the United States

- Tobacco use involves many social and political issues, including advertising targeted at youth and women, the fastest-growing populations of smokers. Smoking costs the United States between $289 and $333 billion per year.

### LO **2** | College Students and Tobacco Use

- While smoking has decreased in college students in recent years, students are heavily targeted by tobacco marketing and advertising campaigns. Social smoking, common among college students, significantly increases the smoker's risks for heart disease and cancer.

### LO **3** | Effects of Tobacco

- Smoking delivers more than 7,000 chemicals to the lungs. Tobacco comes in smoking and smokeless forms; both contain nicotine, an addictive psychoactive substance.

### LO **4** | Health Hazards of Tobacco Products

- Health hazards include markedly higher rates of cancer, heart and circulatory disorders, respiratory diseases, sexual dysfunction, fertility problems, low birth weight babies, and gum diseases. Smokeless tobacco increases risks for oral cancer and other oral problems.

### LO **5** | Environmental Tobacco Smoke

- Environmental tobacco smoke puts nonsmokers at risk for cancer, heart disease, allergies, asthma, and other respiratory illnesses.

### LO **6** | Tobacco Use and Prevention Policies

- The FDA requires prominent health warnings on tobacco products and enacts other policies to prevent young people from using tobacco products.

### LO **7** | Quitting Smoking

- To quit, smokers must kick a chemical addiction and a behavioral habit. Nicotine-replacement products or drugs such as Zyban and Chantix can help wean smokers off nicotine. Various types of psychotherapy and alternative methods can also help.

## POP **QUIZ**

Visit **MasteringHealth** to personalize your study plan with Chapter Review Quizzes and Dynamic Study Modules.

### LO **1** | Tobacco Use in the United States

1. Smoking rates are highest among which of the following education levels?

   a. Undergraduate
   b. High school
   c. GED diploma
   d. Postgraduate

### LO **2** | College Students and Tobacco Use

2. Which age group is most targeted by tobacco advertisers?

   a. Teenagers age 14 to 17
   b. Young adults age 18 to 24
   c. Adults age 25 to 30
   d. Married men age 31 to 35

### LO **3** | Effects of Tobacco

3. What is the major psychoactive ingredient in tobacco products?

   a. Carbon monoxide
   b. Tar
   c. Formaldehyde
   d. Nicotine

4. What does nicotine do to cilia in the lungs?

   a. Instantly destroys them
   b. Thickens them
   c. Paralyzes them
   d. Accumulates on them

5. What effect does carbon monoxide have on a smoker's body?

   a. It accumulates on alveoli in lungs, making breathing difficult.
   b. It increases heart rate.
   c. It interferes with the ability of red blood cells to carry oxygen.
   d. It dulls taste and smell.

6. Which tobacco product contains eugenol, which allows smokers to inhale smoke more deeply?
   a. Bidis
   b. Cigars
   c. Snuff
   d. Clove cigarettes

## LO 4 | Health Hazards of Tobacco Products

7. A major health risk of chewing tobacco is
   a. lung cancer.
   b. leukoplakia.
   c. heart disease.
   d. emphysema.

## LO 5 | Environmental Tobacco Smoke

8. What is sidestream smoke?
   a. Smoke inhaled by a smoker
   b. Smoke released from the burning end of a cigarette
   c. Smoke from a low-tar cigarette
   d. Smoke from a pipe or hookah

## LO 6 | Tobacco Use and Prevention Policies

9. Which federal policy allows the FDA to regulate the amount of nicotine in tobacco products and to require health warnings on tobacco products?
   a. The Family Smoking Prevention and Tobacco Control Act
   b. The Master Settlement Agreement
   c. The Child Smoking Prevention and Anti-Tobacco Act
   d. The Environmental Assessment for Tobacco Products Act

## LO 7 | Quitting Smoking

10. How quickly will an individual begin to see health benefits after quitting smoking?
    a. Within 8 hours
    b. Within a month
    c. Within a year
    d. Never

*Answers to the Pop Quiz can be found on page A-1. If you answered a question incorrectly, review the section identified by the Learning Outcome. For even more study tools, visit* **MasteringHealth**.

# THINK ABOUT IT!

## LO 1 | Tobacco Use in the United States

1. What tactics do tobacco companies use to target different groups of people?

## LO 2 | College Students and Tobacco Use

2. What are some of the main reasons college students choose to use tobacco?

## LO 3 | Effects of Tobacco

3. Discuss the various ways that tobacco is used. Is any method less addictive or less hazardous to health than another?

## LO 4 | Health Hazards of Tobacco Products

4. Discuss the health hazards associated with tobacco. Who should be responsible for the medical expenses of smokers? Insurance companies? Smokers themselves?

## LO 5 | Environmental Tobacco Smoke

5. How is sidestream smoke dangerous?

## LO 6 | Tobacco Use and Prevention Policies

6. Do you think restrictions on smoking are fair? Why or why not?

## LO 7 | Quitting Smoking

7. Describe the various methods of tobacco cessation. Which would be most effective for you? Why?

# ACCESS YOUR HEALTH ON THE INTERNET

Visit **MasteringHealth** for links to the websites and RSS feeds.

Use the following websites to further explore topics and issues related to ending tobacco use.

**American Lung Association.** This site offers a wealth of information regarding smoking trends, environmental smoke, and advice on smoking cessation. **www.lungusa.org**

**Action on Smoking and Health (ASH).** The nation's oldest and largest antismoking organization, ASH works to fight smoking and protect nonsmokers' rights. **www.ash.org**

**Tobacco Information and Prevention Source (TIPS).** This site provides information regarding tobacco use in the United States, with specific information for young people. **www.cdc.gov/tobacco**

**The Tobacco Atlas.** This book and website, produced by the World Lung Foundation and the American Cancer Society, cover a range of topics including the history of tobacco use, prevalence of use, youth smoking, secondhand smoke, quitting, and more. **www.tobaccoatlas.org**

**Americans for Nonsmokers' Rights (ANR).** This site provides information about smoke-free communities across the United States and tips for taking action to ban smoking in workplaces and other public areas. **www.no-smoke.org**

**Tobacco-Free College Campus Initiative.** Serves as a clearinghouse of key information to assist educational communities to establish their own tobacco-free environments. The site includes news updates, state-specific information, links to a wide range of external resources, and referrals to national experts. **www.tobaccofreecampus.org**

# 13 Avoiding Drug Misuse and Abuse

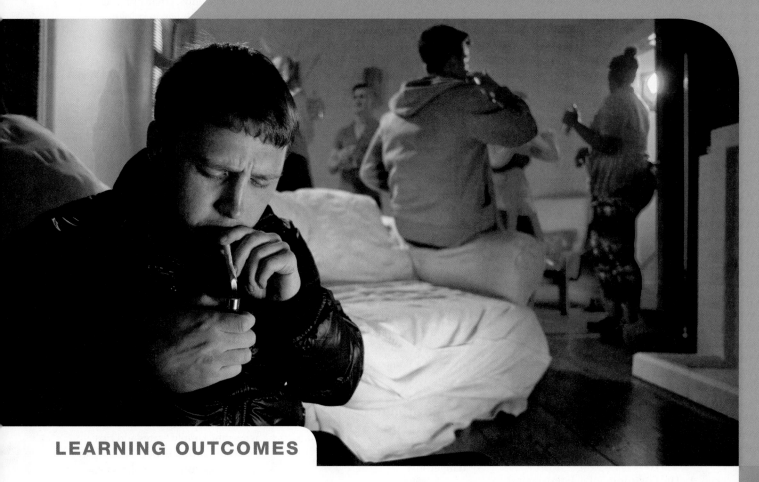

## LEARNING OUTCOMES

LO **1** Explain how drugs affect physical functions and activate the brain's pleasure circuit.

LO **2** List and describe the six categories of drugs and their routes of administration.

LO **3** Review problems relating to the misuse and abuse of prescriptions drugs, including the use of illicit drugs among college students.

LO **4** Discuss the use and abuse of controlled substances, including cocaine, amphetamines, marijuana, opioids, hallucinogens, club drugs, inhalants, and steroids.

LO **5** Provide examples of treatment and recovery options for addicts and their effectiveness.

LO **6** Profile illicit drug use in the United States, including who uses illicit drugs, financial impact, and impact on college campuses and the workplace.

You may think drugs are helping you relax, improving your concentration, or enhancing your social enjoyment, but those effects are transient—and often illusory—and they are nothing compared to the many negative effects those same drugs can have on your life and health. Sooner or later, drug misuse and abuse is likely to catch up with you and cause problems—be they academic, social, career, legal, financial, or health related. Are a few moments of excitement really worth a lifetime of trouble?

Consciousness can be altered in many ways: Children spinning until they become dizzy and adults enjoying the thrill of extreme sports are two examples. To change our awareness, some of us listen to music, ski, read, daydream, meditate, pray, or have sexual relations. Others turn to drugs to alter consciousness.

Drug misuse and abuse are problems of staggering proportions in our society. Whether it is the meth addict who has lost everything in a fall into dependence and crime or the high-functioning executive who gets prescribed OxyContin or Vicodin for back pain and then gets hooked, drug addiction wreaks havoc on individuals, families, businesses, and society. The use and abuse of drugs occurs at all income levels, among all ethnic groups, and at all ages. Approximately 10 percent of Americans report being current (defined as use during the past month) users of illicit drugs.[1] By senior year in high school, 49 percent of American students report having used illicit drugs in their lifetime.[2] Approximately 13 percent of high school students have taken prescription drugs without a doctor's supervision.[3]

# 4.4%

of adults aged 18 to 25 report having abused **PRESCRIPTION PAINKILLERS** such as codeine, Vicodin, and OxyContin in the past year.

Recently, the overall rate of drug use in the United States rose to its highest level in almost a decade, mostly driven by an increase in the use of marijuana.[4] Drug abuse costs taxpayers more than $193 billion annually in health care costs, public costs related to crime, and lost productivity.[5] It's impossible to put a dollar amount on the pain, suffering, and dysfunction that drugs cause in our everyday lives.

Why do people use drugs? There are no simple answers. For some, drugs help them escape from their current situations—help them to face disappointments, failure, fear, or enable coping; for others, drugs numb very real physical pain or mental/emotional problems. In some cases, drugs help people "fit in." For a while, they bring pleasure and excitement, and help

people feel comfortable in their skin, until they eventually no longer do. Others get hooked by accident and suddenly find their bodies need that drug high. Whatever the underlying reason, the net effect is the same. In this chapter, we look at these net effects—on individuals and on society. First, let's take a look at how drugs affect the brain.

## LO 1 | DRUG DYNAMICS

**Explain how drugs affect physical functions and activate the brain's pleasure circuit.**

**Drugs** work because they physically resemble chemicals produced naturally within the body. Most bodily processes result from chemical reactions or from changes in electrical charge. Because drugs possess an electrical charge and chemical structure similar to those of chemicals that occur naturally in the body, they can affect physical functions in many ways.

## How Drugs Affect the Brain

Pleasure, which scientists call *reward*, is a powerful biological force for survival. If you do something that feels pleasurable, the brain is wired in such a way that you tend to want to do it again. Life-sustaining activities, such as eating, activate a circuit of specialized nerve cells devoted to producing and regulating pleasure. One important set of these nerve cells, which uses a chemical neurotransmitter called *dopamine*, sits at the very top of the brainstem in the *ventral tegmental area (VTA)*. These dopamine-containing neurons relay messages about pleasure through their nerve fibers to nerve cells in the limbic system, structures in the brain regulating emotions. Still other fibers connect to a related part of the frontal region of the cerebral cortex, the area of the brain that plays a key role in memory, perception, thought, and consciousness. Thus, this "pleasure circuit," known as the *mesolimbic dopamine system*, spans the survival-oriented brainstem, the emotional limbic system, and the thinking frontal cerebral cortex.

All drugs that are addicting—in fact, all addictive substances and behaviors—can activate the brain's pleasure circuit. Drug addiction is a biological, pathological process that alters the way in which the pleasure center, as well as other parts of the brain, functions. Almost all

> **drugs** Nonfood, non-nutritional substances that are intended to affect the structure or function of the mind or body through chemical action.

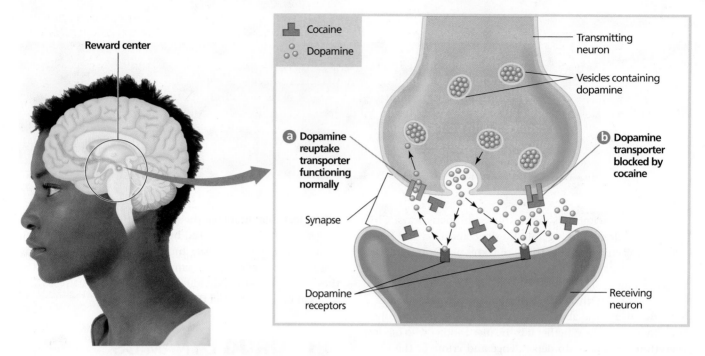

**Reward center**

Cocaine

Dopamine

Transmitting neuron

Vesicles containing dopamine

**ⓐ Dopamine reuptake transporter functioning normally**

Synapse

**ⓑ Dopamine transporter blocked by cocaine**

Dopamine receptors

Receiving neuron

**FIGURE 13.1** **The Action of Cocaine at Dopamine Receptors in the Brain** (a) In normal neural communication, dopamine is released into the synapse between neurons. It binds temporarily to dopamine receptors on the receiving neuron and is then recycled back into the transmitting neuron by a transporter. (b) When cocaine molecules are present, they attach to the dopamine transporter and block the recycling process. Excess dopamine remains active in the synaptic gaps between neurons, creating feelings of excitement and euphoria.

**Source:** Adapted from NIDA "Cocaine—How the Brain Responds to Cocaine," February 2016, Available at https://www.drugabuse.gov/videos/reward-circuit-how-brain-responds-to-cocaine.

▶ VIDEO TUTOR
Psychoactive Drugs Acting on the Brain

---

**psychoactive drugs** Drugs that affect brain chemistry and have the potential to alter mood or behavior.

**psychoactive drugs** (those that change the way the brain works) do so by affecting chemical neurotransmission by enhancing it, suppressing it, or interfering with it. Some drugs, such as heroin and lysergic acid diethylamide (LSD), mimic the effects of a natural neurotransmitter. Others, such as phenylcyclidine (PCP), block receptors and thereby prevent neuronal messages from getting through. Still others, such as cocaine, block the *reuptake* of neurotransmitters by neurons, thus increasing the concentration of the neurotransmitters in the synaptic gap, the space between individual neurons (**FIGURE 13.1**). Finally, some drugs, such as methamphetamine, cause neurotransmitters to be released in greater amounts than is normal.

## LO 2 | TYPES OF DRUGS

**List and describe the six categories of drugs and their routes of administration.**

Scientists divide drugs into six categories: prescription, over-the-counter (OTC), recreational, herbal preparations, illicit, and commercial drugs. These classifications are based primarily on drug action, although some are based on the source of the chemical in question. Each category includes some drugs

that stimulate the body, some that depress body functions, and others that produce hallucinations (sounds, images, or other sensations that are perceived but are not real). Each category also includes psychoactive drugs.

- **Prescription drugs.** These drugs can be obtained only with a prescription from a licensed health practitioner. Approximately 59 percent of Americans have reported using at least one prescription medication in the past month.[6] The percentage of people taking five or more prescription drugs is 15 percent.[7]

- **Over-the-counter (OTC) drugs.** These can be purchased without a prescription in many locations such as grocery, drug, and convenience stores. OTC drugs, used to treat everything from headaches to pain, cold, stomach upsets, and athlete's foot, provide an important access to medicine. They create substantial savings for the health care system through decreased visits to health care providers and decreased use of prescription medications.[8] However, there is a risk of OTC drugs being used improperly or misused.[9] (See Chapter 19 for more information on OTC drugs.)

- **Recreational drugs.** These belong to a somewhat vague category whose boundaries depend on how the term *recreation* is defined. Generally, recreational drugs contain chemicals used to help people relax or socialize. Most of them are legal even though they are psychoactive. Alcohol, tobacco, and caffeine products are included in this category.

- **Herbal preparations.** Herbals encompass approximately 750 substances, including herbal teas and other products of botanical (plant) origin that are believed to have medicinal properties. (See Chapter 19 for more on herbal preparations.)
- **Illicit (illegal) drugs.** These are the most notorious type of drug. Although laws governing their use, possession, cultivation, manufacture, and sale differ from state to state, illicit drugs are generally recognized as harmful. All of them are psychoactive.
- **Commercial drugs.** These are drugs found in commercially sold products. More than 1,000 of them exist, including those used in seemingly benign items such as perfumes, cosmetics, household cleansers, paints, glues, inks, dyes, and pesticides.

## Routes of Drug Administration

*Route of administration* refers to the way in which a given drug is taken into the body. The route largely determines the rapidity of the drug's effect on the body (**FIGURE 13.2**). The most common method is by swallowing a tablet, capsule, or liquid (**oral ingestion**). Drugs taken in this manner don't reach the bloodstream as quickly as do drugs introduced to the body by other means. A drug taken orally may not reach the bloodstream for as long as 30 minutes.

Drugs can also enter the body through the respiratory tract via sniffing, snorting, smoking, or inhaling (**inhalation**). Drugs that are inhaled and absorbed by the lungs travel the most rapidly compared to all the routes of drug administration.

Another rapid form of drug administration is by **injection** directly into the bloodstream (intravenously), muscles (intramuscularly), or just under the skin (subcutaneously). Intravenous injection, which involves inserting a hypodermic needle directly into a vein, is the most common method of injection for drug users owing to the rapid speed (within seconds in most cases) with which a drug's effect is felt. It is also the most

**oral ingestion** Intake of drugs through the mouth.

**inhalation** The introduction of drugs through the respiratory tract.

**injection** The introduction of drugs into the body via a hypodermic needle.

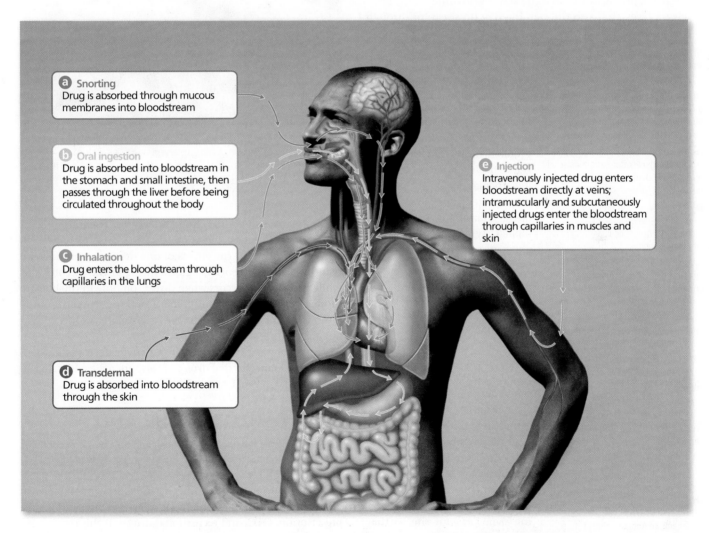

**a Snorting**
Drug is absorbed through mucous membranes into bloodstream

**b Oral ingestion**
Drug is absorbed into bloodstream in the stomach and small intestine, then passes through the liver before being circulated throughout the body

**c Inhalation**
Drug enters the bloodstream through capillaries in the lungs

**d Transdermal**
Drug is absorbed into bloodstream through the skin

**e Injection**
Intravenously injected drug enters bloodstream directly at veins; intramuscularly and subcutaneously injected drugs enter the bloodstream through capillaries in muscles and skin

**FIGURE 13.2 Routes of Drug Administration** Drugs are most commonly swallowed, inhaled, or injected. They can also be absorbed through the skin or mucous membranes (as in snorting) and through suppository use (not shown here).

dangerous method of administration because of the risk of damaging blood vessels and contracting HIV (human immunodeficiency virus) and hepatitis B.

Drugs can also be absorbed through the skin or tissue lining (**transdermal**)—the nicotine patch is a common example of a drug that is administered in this manner—or through the mucous membranes, such as those in the nose (snorting) or in the vagina or anus (**suppositories**). Suppositories are typically mixed with a waxy medium that melts at body temperature, releasing the drug into the bloodstream.

However the drug enters the system, it eventually finds its way to the bloodstream and circulates throughout the body to various **receptor sites** where chemicals, enzymes, and other substances interact. Psychoactive drugs are able to cross the blood–brain barrier to reach receptor sites in the brain, where they can affect cognition, emotions, and physiological functioning. Once a drug reaches receptor sites in the brain and other body organs, it may remain active for several hours before it dissipates and is carried by the blood to the liver where it is metabolized (broken down by enzymes). The products of enzymatic breakdown, called metabolites, are then excreted, primarily through the kidneys (in urine) or the bowels (in feces), but also through the skin (in sweat) or through the lungs (in expired air).

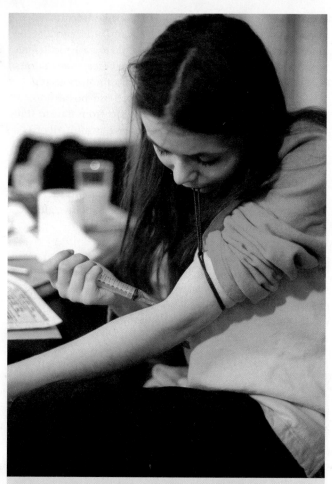

Using a needle to inject drugs poses health threats beyond the effects of the drugs themselves, such as risk of transmission of potentially deadly infections such as HIV and hepatitis B and C.

**transdermal** The introduction of drugs through the skin.

**suppositories** Mixtures of drugs in a waxy medium designed to melt at body temperature after being inserted into the anus or vagina.

**receptor sites** Specialized areas of cells and organs where chemicals, enzymes, and other substances interact

**polydrug use** Use of multiple medications, vitamins, recreational drugs, or illicit drugs simultaneously.

**synergism** Interaction of two or more drugs that produces more profound effects than would be expected if the drugs were taken separately; also called *potentiation*.

**antagonism** A type of interaction in which two or more drugs work at the same receptor site so that one blocks the action of the other.

**inhibition** A drug interaction in which the effects of one drug are eliminated or reduced by the presence of another drug at the same receptor site.

**intolerance** A type of interaction in which two or more drugs produce extremely uncomfortable reactions.

**cross-tolerance** Development of a tolerance to one drug that reduces the effects of another, similar drug.

**drug misuse** Use of a drug for a purpose for which it was not intended.

## Drug Interactions

**Polydrug use**—taking several medications, vitamins, recreational drugs, or illegal drugs simultaneously—can lead to dangerous health problems. Alcohol in particular frequently has dangerous interactions with other drugs. Hazardous interactions include synergism, inhibition, antagonism, intolerance, and cross-tolerance.

**Synergism**, also called *potentiation*, is an interaction of two or more drugs in which the effects of the individual drugs are multiplied beyond what would normally be expected if they were taken alone. You might think of synergism as 2 + 2 = 10. A synergistic reaction can be very dangerous and even deadly.

**Antagonism**, although usually less serious than synergism, can also produce unwanted and unpleasant effects. In an antagonistic reaction, drugs work at the same receptor site so that one drug blocks the action of the other. The blocking drug occupies the receptor site and prevents the other drug from attaching, thus altering its absorption and action.

With **inhibition**, the effects of one drug are eliminated or reduced by the presence of another drug at the receptor site, while **intolerance** occurs when drugs combine in the body to produce extremely uncomfortable reactions. The drug Antabuse, used to help alcoholics give up drinking, works by producing this type of interaction.

**Cross-tolerance** occurs when a person develops a physiological tolerance to one drug that also increases tolerance to other substances that act similarly on the body.

## LO 3 | DRUG MISUSE AND ABUSE

Review problems relating to the misuse and abuse of prescriptions drugs, including the use of illicit drugs among college students.

Although drug abuse is usually referred to in connection with illicit psychoactive drugs, many people also abuse and misuse prescription, OTC, and recreational drugs. In this section, we discuss these drug-related behaviors and focus, in particular, on college students' drug use. **Drug misuse** involves using a drug for a purpose for which it was not intended. For example, taking a friend's high-powered prescription painkiller for your headache is a misuse of that drug. This is not too far removed from **drug abuse**, or the excessive use of any drug, and may cause serious harm. The misuse and abuse of any drug may lead to addiction, the habitual reliance on a substance or a behavior to produce a desired mood. (See **Focus On: Recognizing and Avoiding Addiction** on page 299 for more on addiction.)

## Abuse of Over-the-Counter Drugs

Over-the-counter medications come in many different forms, including pills, liquids, nasal sprays, and topical creams. Although many people assume that no harm can come from legal nonprescription drugs, OTC medications can be abused, with resultant health complications and potential addiction. People who appear to be most vulnerable to abusing OTC drugs are teenagers, young adults, and people over the age of 65.

OTC drug abuse can involve taking more than the recommended dosage, combining it with other drugs, or taking it over a longer period of time than is recommended. Abuse of and addiction to OTC drugs can be accidental. A person may develop tolerance from continued use, creating an unintended dependence. However, teenagers and young adults sometimes intentionally abuse OTC medications in search of a cheap high—by drinking large amounts of cough medicine, for instance. The following are a few types of OTC drugs that are subject to misuse and abuse:

- **Caffeine pills and energy drinks.** Energy drinks, OTC caffeine pills, and pain relievers containing caffeine are commonly abused for the energy boost they provide. Caffeine in large doses can result in tremors/shaking, restlessness and edginess, insomnia, dehydration, panic attacks, heart irregularities, and other symptoms. We look more closely at caffeine later in the chapter.
- **Cold medicines (cough syrups and tablets).** There are many different ingredients in cough and cold medicines, but one of particular concern is dextromethorphan (DXM), which is present in many types of OTC cold and cough medications. As many as 5 percent of high school seniors report taking drugs containing DXM to get high.[10] Large doses of products containing DXM can cause hallucinations, loss of motor control, and "out-of-body" (dissociative) sensations. In combination with alcohol or other drugs, large doses can be deadly. Other possible side effects of DXM abuse include confusion, impaired judgment, blurred vision, dizziness, paranoia, excessive sweating, slurred speech, nausea, vomiting, abdominal pain, irregular heartbeat, high blood pressure, headache, lethargy, numb fingers and toes, facial redness, and dry and itchy skin. In extreme cases,

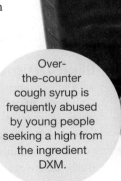

Over-the-counter cough syrup is frequently abused by young people seeking a high from the ingredient DXM.

DXM abuse can lead to loss of consciousness, brain damage, and even death. Some states have passed laws limiting the amount of products containing DXM that a person can purchase or prohibiting sale to individuals under age 18.[11]

**drug abuse** Excessive use of a drug.

- **Pseudoephedrine** is another cold and allergy medication ingredient that is frequently abused, most commonly in the illegal manufacture of methamphetamine (discussed later). United States law limits the number of products containing this drug that an individual may purchase in a month and requires that it be sold "behind the counter" (i.e., without a prescription, but only through a pharmacist) and that photo identification be presented and recorded. Pharmacists are required to keep a record of purchasers for at least 2 years.[12]
- **Diet pills.** Some teens use diet pills as a way of getting high, whereas other people use these drugs in an attempt to lose weight. Diet pills often contain a stimulant such as caffeine or an herbal ingredient claimed to promote weight loss, such as *Hoodia gordonii*. Although they can sometimes cause serious side effects, many diet pills are marketed as dietary supplements and so are regulated by the Food and Drug Administration (FDA) as "food," not as "drugs." This means their manufacturers may make unsubstantiated claims of effectiveness or use untested and unsafe ingredients.
- **Sleep aids.** These drugs may be harmful in excess as they can cause problems with the sleep cycle, weaken areas of the body, or induce narcolepsy (a condition of excessive, intrusive sleepiness). Continued use can lead to tolerance and dependence.

## Nonmedical Use or Abuse of Prescription Drugs

In the United States today, the abuse of prescription medications is at an all-time high. Only marijuana is more widely abused.[13] Individuals abuse prescription medications because they are an easily accessible and inexpensive means of altering a user's mental and physical state. Some people also have the mistaken idea that prescription drugs are a "safer high." The latest data available indicate that approximately 6.5 million Americans aged 12 and older used prescription drugs for nonmedical reasons in the past month.[14]

Prescription drug abuse is particularly common among teenagers and young adults. In 2014, 3 percent of teenagers aged 12 to 17 and 4 percent of people aged 18 to 25 reported abusing prescription drugs in the past month.[15] Often these drugs are taken from friends or family members who have prescriptions. The problem may be getting worse, with approximately 13 percent of twelfth-graders reporting abuse of prescription drugs by the time they graduate from high school.[16]

The risks associated with prescription drug abuse vary depending on the drug. Abuse of opioid pain relievers can result in life-threatening respiratory depression (reduced breathing). Overdoses involving prescription painkillers are at epidemic levels; since 1999, deaths from oxycodone, hydrocodone, and methadone have increased by 400%.[17] Individuals who abuse depressants place themselves at risk of seizures, respiratory depression, and decreased heart rate. Stimulant abuse can cause elevated body temperature, irregular heart rate, cardiovascular system failure, and fatal seizures. It can also result in hostility or feelings of paranoia. Individuals who abuse prescription drugs by injecting them expose themselves to additional risks, including contracting HIV, hepatitis B and C, and other bloodborne viruses.

Unfortunately, prescription drugs are often easier to obtain than illegal ones. In some cases, unscrupulous pharmacists or other medical professionals either steal the drugs or sell fraudulent prescriptions. In a process called doctor shopping, abusers visit several doctors to obtain multiple prescriptions. Some may fake or exaggerate symptoms to persuade physicians to write prescriptions. Individuals may also call pharmacies with fraudulent prescriptions. Young people typically obtain prescription drugs from peers, friends, or family members. Some teenagers and college students who have legitimate prescriptions sell or give away their medications to other students or trade them for others. Some abusers order from Internet pharmacies where prescriptions are not always required.

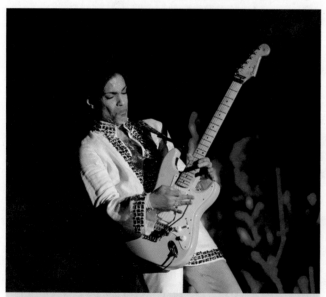

Abusing prescription drugs is no safer than abusing illicit drugs, as tragically demonstrated by the 2016 death of pop star Prince, whose death ultimately stemmed from an overdose of Fentanyl, a narcotic prescribed to treat pain during cancer treatment.

**College Students and Prescription Drug Abuse** Prescription drug abuse among college students has increased dramatically over the past decade. Because drugs are prescribed by doctors and approved by the FDA, many college students seem to perceive prescription drugs as safer and more socially acceptable than illicit drugs, or they believe prescription drugs will enhance their well-being or performance. However, nothing could be further from the truth when these drugs are misused.

According to the 2015 *American College Health Association–National College Health Assessment*, the illicit use of prescription drugs is not uncommon on college campuses. The report shows nearly 11 percent of surveyed students reported illegally using prescription drugs in the last year.[18]

The most commonly abused prescription drugs on college campuses are stimulants—drugs intended to treat attention-deficit/hyperactivity disorder (ADHD) such as Ritalin or Adderall, followed by painkillers (e.g., OxyContin and Vicodin).[19] Approximately 6 percent of students report using stimulants not prescribed to them in the past 12 months, while 5 percent of students report using painkillers that were not prescribed to them in the past 12 months.[20] The **Student Health Today** box discusses OxyContin and Vicodin abuse.

Students who misuse prescription stimulants such as Adderall primarily report using ADHD drugs for academic gain.[21] According to a recent study, students indicate that it is easy or very easy to get prescription medications and friends with prescriptions were the most commonly reported source of prescription stimulants.[22] Users generally believed that the drugs were beneficial, despite frequent reports of adverse reactions. The most commonly reported adverse effects were sleeping difficulties, irritability, and reduced appetite.

## Use and Abuse of Illicit Drugs

The problem of illicit (illegal) drug use touches us all. We may use illicit substances ourselves, watch someone we love struggle with drug abuse, or become the victim of a drug-related crime. At the very least, we pay increasing taxes for law enforcement and drug rehabilitation. When our coworkers use drugs, the effectiveness of our own work is diminished.

Illicit drug users span all age groups, genders, ethnicities, occupations, and socioeconomic groups. The good news about illicit drug use is that it peaked at around 25 million users between 1979 and 1986, then declined until 1992, and has since remained stable at around 27 million users per year.[23] Among youth, however, illicit drug use, notably of marijuana and heroin, has been rising in recent years.[24]

**Illicit Drug Use on Campus** Illicit drug use has seen a resurgence on college campuses in recent years. Close to 50 percent of college-aged students nationwide have tried an illicit drug at some point; the vast majority of them reported using marijuana (see **TABLE 13.1** on page 366).[25]

College administrators, staff, and faculty are concerned about the link between substance abuse and poor academic performance, depression, anxiety, suicide, property damage, vandalism,

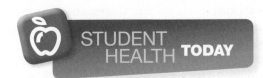
# OXYCONTIN AND VICODIN ABUSE

Since the mid-1990s, there has been a sharp increase in prescription drug abuse among youth. The 2014 Monitoring the Future (MTF) study found that approximately 2.8 percent of college students had used Vicodin and 1.3 percent used OxyContin, both prescription painkillers, without a doctor's prescription in the past year. In addition, 34 percent of college students said pills were "easy" for them to acquire. The easiest source was from parents or friends. According to a study commissioned by the Hazelton Ford Foundation, 22.5 percent of those who have used pain medications (OxyContin or Vicodin) at some point in their lifetime are or were in intercollegiate athletics. As with most other drugs, some of the reasons college students use OxyContin and Vicodin are that they feel young and often invincible; they need to express their new-found independence; they like the excitement of risk-taking; or they feel pressure from their peers. Often, there is the

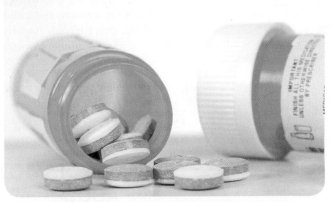

**Addiction to painkillers like Oxycontin and Vicodin have led to a significant rise in heroin addiction as addicts look for less expensive ways of getting high.**

perception that prescription drugs are safer than illicit drugs.

However, painkillers such as OxyContin, Percocet, Percodan, Vicodin, and others are highly addictive; if they are taken daily for several weeks, that is enough time for addiction to develop. OxyContin, in particular, can be a highly addictive and dangerous narcotic when abused. The "rush" is similar to that of heroin. In fact, it's common for people who are addicted

to OxyContin to turn to heroin when they can't afford to buy OxyContin. Chronic use can also result in increasing tolerance, and more of the drug is needed to achieve the desired effect.

Many people who abuse prescription medications are simultaneously abusing illegal drugs. It is not uncommon for those abusing prescription painkillers to also binge-drink. This poses another set of problems, as alcohol in combination with any one of these medications can make a dangerous cocktail. If someone you know seems unusually drunk, drowsy, slurs speech, has trouble moving, or passes out, call for help immediately.

**Sources:** L. D. Johnston et al., *Monitoring the Future: National Survey Results on Drug Use, 1975–2014*, Volume 2, *College Students and Adults Ages 19–50* (Ann Arbor: Institute for Social Research, University of Michigan, 2014), Available at http://monitoringthefuture.org/new.html; Hazelden Betty Ford, "Survey Finds Risky Opioid Use Among College-Age Youth, with Limited Knowledge of Danger or Where to Get Help," June 10, 2015, https://www.hazelden.org/web/public/youth-opioid-survey.page.

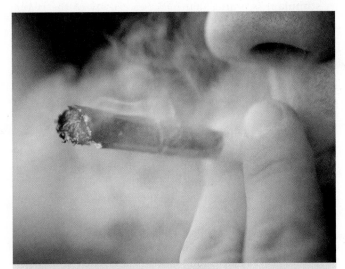

Choosing to use drugs, even on an infrequent or sporadic basis, may decrease your ability to obtain and keep a full time job after you graduate. The more you use, the greater the chances of working only part time or being unemployed.

fights, serious medical problems, and death. Students who use marijuana and/or other illicit drugs are at increased risk for disruptions in college attendance.[26] A longer-term consequence of illicit drug use among college students is a significantly increased chance of unemployment after college. The most recent research shows that 10 percent of people who were persistent drug users during college experienced unemployment after college compared with 1.7 percent of students who did not use drugs and 4.8 percent of those who used drugs sporadically.[27]

## Why Do Some College Students Use Drugs?

Research has identified the following factors in a student's life that increase the risk of substance abuse; the more factors, the greater the risk.

■ **Positive expectations.** As mentioned previously, some students take drugs such as Adderall and Ritalin believing that the drugs will help their ability to study. But the vast majority of students say they take drugs in order to relax, reduce stress, and forget problems.[28]

## TABLE 13.1 | Thirty-Day Drug Use Prevalence, Full-Time College Students versus Respondents 1–4 Years beyond High School

| | Full-Time College (%) | Others (%) |
|---|---|---|
| Any illicit drug | 38.6 | 44.1 |
| Any illicit drug other than marijuana | 20.8 | 24.5 |
| Marijuana | 34.4 | 39.7 |
| Inhalants | 1.3 | 1.2 |
| Hallucinogens | 4.0 | 7.0 |
| LSD | 2.2 | 4.5 |
| Hallucinogens other than LSD | 3.2 | 4.9 |
| Ecstasy (methylene-dioxymethamphetamine, MDMA) | 5.0 | 6.5 |
| Cocaine | 4.4 | 5.1 |
| Crack | 0.8 | 0.3 |
| Other cocaine | 4.1 | 4.4 |
| Heroin | * | 0.6 |
| Narcotics other than heroin | 4.8 | 7.8 |
| Amphetamines, adjusted | 10.1 | 9.2 |
| Crystal methamphetamine | * | 0 8 |
| Sedatives (barbiturates) | 3.1 | 4.7 |
| Tranquilizers | 3.5 | 6.0 |
| Alcohol | 76.1 | 74.5 |
| Been drunk | 60.5 | 58.9 |
| Alcoholic drink containing caffeine | 32.8 | 36.7 |
| Cigarettes | 22.6 | 34.7 |
| Approximate weighted N = | 1,030 | 660 |

*Indicates prevalence less than 0.05%.

**Source:** L. D. Johnston et al., *Monitoring the Future National Survey Results on Drug Use, 1975–2014, Volume 2, College Students and Adults Ages 19–50* (Ann Arbor: Institute for Social Research, University of Michigan, 2015), Available at http://monitoringthefuture.org/new.html.

■ **Genetics and family history.** Genetics and family history play a significant role in the risk for developing an addiction.

■ **Substance use in high school.** Two-thirds of college students who use illicit drugs began doing so in high school.[29]

■ **Curiosity.** College students are learning a lot about themselves, both personally and professionally. Sometimes, that journey of self-discovery includes experimenting with different mind-altering substances.

■ **Social norms.** College students often overestimate the amount of drug use on campus. Surveys conducted on college campuses found students perceived that 83 percent of their peers used marijuana within the last 30 days, when actually 15 percent had used.[30]

■ **Sorority and fraternity membership.** Being a member of a sorority or fraternity increases the likelihood of abusing alcohol and drugs.[31] A few factors that may contribute to more drinking and use of drugs in sororities and fraternities include group living, hazing or initiation rituals, lack of supervision, and social pressure.[32]

■ **Stress.** For some students under academic and social stress, seemingly easy relief comes in the form of drugs or alcohol.[33]

To prepare yourself for a possible offer of drugs on campus and to be ready to make the decision that is best for *you*, see the Making Changes Today box.

# LO 4 | COMMON DRUGS OF ABUSE

Discuss the use and abuse of controlled substances, including cocaine, amphetamines, marijuana, opioids, hallucinogens, club drugs, inhalants, and steroids.

Hundreds of drugs are subject to abuse—some are legal, such as recreational drugs and prescription medications, whereas many others are illegal and classified as "controlled substances." For general purposes, drugs can be divided into the following categories: *stimulants, cannabis products (cannabinoids) including marijuana, narcotics, depressants, hallucinogens, inhalants*, and *anabolic steroids*. These categories are discussed in subsequent sections; **TABLE 13.2** summarizes the categorization, uses, and effects of various drugs of abuse, both legal and illicit.

## Stimulants

A **stimulant** is a drug that increases activity of the central nervous system. Its effects usually involve increased activity, anxiety, and agitation; users often seem jittery or nervous while high. Commonly used illegal stimulants include cocaine, amphetamines, and methamphetamine. Legal stimulants include caffeine and nicotine (see Chapter 12 for a discussion of nicotine, the addictive substance in tobacco products).

**Cocaine** A white crystalline powder derived from the leaves of the South American coca shrub (not related to cocoa plants), *cocaine* ("coke") has been described as one of the most powerful naturally occurring stimulants.

Cocaine can be taken in several ways, including snorting, smoking, and injecting. The powdered form is snorted through the nose, which can damage mucous membranes and cause sinusitis. It can destroy the user's sense of smell, and occasionally it even eats a hole through the septum. When snorted, the drug enters the bloodstream through the lungs in less than 1 minute and reaches the brain in less than 3 minutes. It binds at receptor sites in the central nervous system, producing an intense high that disappears quickly, leaving a powerful craving for more.

**stimulants** Drugs that increase activity of the central nervous system.

through shared needles, but also for skin infections, vein damage, inflamed arteries, and infection of the heart lining.

Cocaine is both an anesthetic and a central nervous system stimulant. In tiny doses, it can slow the heart rate. In larger doses, the physical effects are dramatic: increased heart rate and blood pressure, loss of appetite that can lead to dramatic weight loss, convulsions, muscle twitching, irregular heartbeat, and even death from overdose. Other effects of cocaine include temporary relief of depression, decreased fatigue, talkativeness, increased alertness, and heightened self-confidence. However, as the dose increases, users become irritable and apprehensive, and their behavior may turn paranoid or violent.

### Amphetamines

The **amphetamines** include a large and varied group of synthetic agents that stimulate the central nervous system. Small doses of amphetamines improve alertness, lessen fatigue, and generally elevate mood. With repeated use, however, physical and psychological dependence develops. Sleep patterns are affected (insomnia); heart rate, breathing rate, and blood pressure increase; and restlessness, anxiety, appetite suppression, and vision problems are common. High doses over long time periods can produce hallucinations, delusions, and disorganized behavior.

Certain types of amphetamines or amphetamine-like drugs are used for medicinal purposes. As discussed earlier, drugs prescribed to treat ADHD are stimulants and are increasingly abused on college campuses.

An increasingly common form of amphetamine, *methamphetamine* (commonly called "meth"), is a potent, long-acting, inexpensive drug that strongly motivates the brain's reward center by producing a sense of euphoria. In the short term, methamphetamine produces increased physical activity, alertness, euphoria, rapid breathing, increased body temperature, insomnia, tremors,

> **amphetamines** A large and varied group of synthetic agents that stimulate the central nervous system.

Cocaine alkaloid, or *freebase*, is obtained from removing the hydrochloride salt from cocaine powder. *Freebasing* refers to smoking cocaine by placing it at the end of a pipe and holding a flame near it to produce a vapor, which is then inhaled. *Crack* is identical pharmacologically to freebase, but the hydrochloride salt is still present and is processed with baking soda and water. It is a cheap, widely available drug that is smokable and very potent. Crack is commonly smoked in the same manner as freebase. Because crack is such a pure drug, it takes little time to achieve the desired high, and a crack user can become addicted quickly.

Some cocaine users occasionally inject the drug intravenously, which introduces large amounts into the body rapidly, creating a brief, intense high and a subsequent crash. Injecting users place themselves at risk not only for contracting HIV and hepatitis (a severe liver disease)

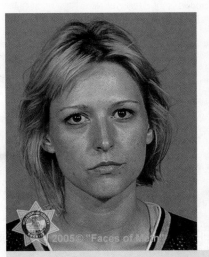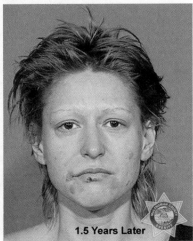

**1.5 Years Later**

The physical consequences of methamphetamine use are often dramatic. The photo at left shows a person before she began using methamphetamine. The photos above show the same person after just 1.5 years of methamphetamine use.

# TABLE 13.2 | Drugs of Abuse: Uses and Effects

| Category | Drugs | Trade or Street Names | Dependence | Usual Method | Possible Effects | Overdose Effects | Withdrawal Syndrome |
|---|---|---|---|---|---|---|---|
| **Stimulants** | Cocaine | Coke, Flake, Snow, Crack, Coca, Blanca, Perico | *Physical:* Possible *Psychological:* High *Tolerance:* Yes | Snorted, smoked, injected | Increased alertness, excitation, euphoria, increased pulse rate and blood pressure, insomnia, loss of appetite | Agitation, increased body temperature, hallucinations, convulsions, possible death | Apathy, long periods of sleep, irritability, depression, disorientation |
| | Amphetamine, methamphetamine | Crank, Ice, Cristal, Crystal Meth, Speed, Adderall, Dexedrine | *Physical:* Possible *Psychological:* High *Tolerance:* Yes | Oral, injected, smoked | | | |
| | Methylphenidate | Ritalin (Illy's), Concerta, Focalin, Metadate | *Physical:* Possible *Psychological:* High *Tolerance:* Yes | Oral, injected, snorted, smoked | | | |
| **Cannabis** | Marijuana | Pot, Grass, Sinsemilla, Blunts, Mota, Yerba | *Physical:* Possible *Psychological:* High *Tolerance:* Yes | Oral, smoked | Euphoria, relaxed inhibitions, increased appetite, disorientation | Fatigue, paranoia, possible psychosis | Hyperactivity, decreased appetite, insomnia |
| | Hashish, hashish oil | Hash, hash oil | *Physical:* Unknown *Psychological:* Moderate *Tolerance:* Yes | Smoked, oral | | | |
| **Narcotics** | Heroin | Diamorphine, Horse, Smack, Black tar, Chiva | *Physical:* High *Psychological:* High *Tolerance:* Yes | Injected, snorted, smoked | Euphoria, drowsiness, respiratory depression, constricted pupils, nausea | Slow and shallow breathing, clammy skin, convulsions, coma, possible death | Watery eyes, runny nose, yawning, loss of appetite, irritability, tremors, panic, cramps, nausea, chills and sweating |
| | Morphine | MS-Contin, Roxanol | *Physical:* High *Psychological:* High *Tolerance:* Yes | Oral, injected | | | |
| | Hydrocodone, oxycodone | Vicodin, OxyContin, Percocet, Percodan | *Physical:* High *Psychological:* High *Tolerance:* Yes | Oral | | | |
| | Codeine | Acetaminophen w/ Codeine, Tylenol w/ Codeine | *Physical:* Moderate *Psychological:* Moderate *Tolerance:* Yes | Oral, injected | | | |
| **Depressants** | Gamma-hydroxybutyrate | GHB, Liquid Ecstasy, Liquid X | *Physical:* Moderate *Psychological:* Moderate *Tolerance:* Yes | Oral | Slurred speech, disorientation, drunken behavior without odor of alcohol, impaired memory of events, interacts with alcohol | Shallow respiration, clammy skin, dilated pupils, weak and rapid pulse, coma, possible death | Anxiety, insomnia, tremors, delirium, convulsions, possible death |
| | Benzodiazepines | Valium, Xanax, Halcion, Ativan, Rohypnol (Roofies, R-2), Klonopin | *Physical:* Moderate *Psychological:* Moderate *Tolerance:* Yes | Oral, injected | | | |
| | Other depressants | Ambien, Sonata, Barbiturates, Methaqualone (Quaalude) | *Physical:* Moderate *Psychological:* Moderate *Tolerance:* Yes | Oral | | | |
| **Hallucinogens** | Methylene-dioxymeth-amphetamine (MDMA), analogs | Ecstasy, XTC, Adam, MDA (Love Drug), MDEA (Eve) | *Physical:* None *Psychological:* Moderate *Tolerance:* Yes | Oral, snorted, smoked | Heightened senses, teeth grinding, dehydration | Increased body temperature, electrolyte imbalance, cardiac arrest | Muscle aches, drowsiness, depression, acne |
| | LSD | Acid, Microdot, Sunshine, Boomers | *Physical:* None *Psychological:* Unknown *Tolerance:* Yes | Oral | Hallucinations, altered perception of time and distance | Longer, more intense "trips" | None |
| | Phencyclidine, analogs | PCP, Angel Dust, Hog, Ketamine (Special K) | *Physical:* Possible *Psychological:* High *Tolerance:* Yes | Smoked, oral, injected, snorted | | Unable to direct movement, feel pain, or remember | Drug-seeking behavior |
| | Other hallucinogens | Psilocybe mushrooms, mescaline, peyote, Dextromethorphan | *Physical:* None *Psychological:* None *Tolerance:* Possible | Oral | | | |
| **Inhalants** | Amyl and butyl nitrite | Pearls, Poppers, Rush, Locker Room | *Physical:* Unknown *Psychological:* Unknown *Tolerance:* No | Inhaled | Flushing, hypotension, headache | Methemo-globinemia | Agitation |
| | Nitrous oxide | Laughing gas, Balloons, Whippets | *Physical:* Unknown *Psychological:* Low *Tolerance:* No | Inhaled | Impaired memory, slurred speech, drunken behavior, slow-onset vitamin deficiency, organ damage | Vomiting, respiratory depression, loss of consciousness, possible death | Trembling, anxiety, insomnia, vitamin deficiency, confusion, hallucinations, convulsions |
| | Other inhalants | Adhesives, spray paint, hairspray, lighter fluid | *Physical:* Unknown *Psychological:* High *Tolerance:* No | Inhaled | | | |
| **Anabolic Steroids** | Testosterone | Depo testosterone, Sustanon, Sten, Cypt | *Physical:* Unknown *Psychological:* Unknown *Tolerance:* Unknown | Injected | Virilization, edema, testicular atrophy, gynecomastia, acne, aggressive behavior | Unknown | Possible depression |
| | Other anabolic steroids | Parabolan, Winstrol, Equipose, Anadrol, Dianabol | *Physical:* Unknown *Psychological:* Yes *Tolerance:* Unknown | Oral, injected | | | |

**Source:** Adapted from U.S. Department of Justice Drug Enforcement Administration, "DEA Drug Fact Sheets," 2015, www.justice.gov.

anxiety, confusion, and decreased appetite. Over 569,000 Americans are regular users of methamphetamine, and it is believed that more than 12 million Americans have tried it.[34] In 2015, about 1 percent of high school seniors reported using methamphetamine in their lifetime.[35] The rate of methamphetamine use may be increasing because it is relatively easy to make. Recipes often include common OTC ingredients such as ephedrine and pseudoephedrine.

Methamphetamine can be snorted, smoked, injected, or orally ingested. When snorted, the effects can be felt in 3 to 5 minutes; if orally ingested, effects occur within 15 to 20 minutes. The pleasurable effects of methamphetamine are typically an intense rush lasting only a few minutes when snorted; in contrast, smoking the drug can produce a high lasting more than 8 hours. Users often experience tolerance after the first use, making methamphetamine highly addictive.

Methamphetamine increases the release of and blocks the reuptake of the neurotransmitter dopamine, leading to high levels of the chemical in the brain. This action occurs rapidly and produces the intense euphoria, or "rush," that many users feel. Over time, meth destroys dopamine receptors, making it impossible to feel pleasure. Researchers have now established that due to the destruction of dopamine receptors, people who abuse methamphetamine (or cocaine) are at increased risk for developing Parkinson's disease later in life.[36]

Other long-term effects of methamphetamine can include severe weight loss, cardiovascular damage, increased risk of heart attack and stroke, hallucinations, extensive tooth decay and tooth loss ("meth mouth"), violence, paranoia, psychotic behavior, and even death. Chronic methamphetamine abusers often demonstrate severe structural and functional changes in areas of the brain associated with emotion and memory, which may account for many of the emotional and cognitive problems observed in chronic methamphetamine abusers. Some of these changes persist after the methamphetamine abuse has stopped. Other changes reverse after sustained periods of abstinence from methamphetamine, lasting typically longer than a year, but problems can remain.[37]

Meth users are at increased risk for transmission of HIV, hepatitis B and C, and other sexually transmitted diseases. Meth can alter judgment, increase libido, and lessen inhibitions, leading users to engage in unsafe behaviors, including risky sexual behavior. Among meth users who inject the drug, HIV and other infectious diseases can be spread through sharing of contaminated needles, syringes, and other injection equipment that is used by more than one person.[38]

### Bath Salts

"Bath salts" are synthetic (human-made) cathinones—drugs chemically related to the stimulant cathinone, occurring naturally in the khat plant.[39] The designer drug is synthetic powder sold legally online and in corner stores and truck stops. These packages contain various amphetamine or cocaine-like substances, such as methylene-dioxypyrovalerone (MPDV), which act much like cocaine does, but are at least 10 times stronger.[40] The powder can be smoked, snorted, injected, and wrapped in pieces of paper and ingested or "bombed." These chemicals cannot be detected by routine drug screening, making them attractive for misuse.[41]

Effects include intense stimulation, alertness, euphoria, elevated mood, and pleasurable rush. Users may describe feelings of closeness, sociability, and moderate sexual arousal. Other symptoms can include tremor, shortness of breath, and loss of appetite. Changes in body temperature regulation are accompanied by hot flashes and sweating, with bleeding from the nose and throat from ulcerations when snorted.[42]

This drug can also have significant effects on the cardiovascular system, resulting in rapid heart rate, increased blood pressure, and chest pain. Psychiatric effects at higher doses consist of anxiety, agitation, hallucinations, paranoia, and erratic behavior. Depression and suicide have also been reported as a result of use. While withdrawal symptoms are reported as minimal, users have often described a strong craving for the drug.[43]

### Caffeine

Unlike cocaine and methamphetamine, **caffeine** is a legal stimulant. More than 85 percent of Americans drink at least one caffeinated beverage per day.[44] Ninety-six percent of caffeine consumed is from coffee, soft drinks, and tea.[45] Beverages like energy drinks, chocolate drinks, and energy shots represent only a small portion of overall caffeine intakes.[46] One of the many reasons coffee, tea, soft drinks, chocolate, and other caffeine-containing products are loved is for their wake-up effects. Caffeine may be commonplace, but excessive consumption is associated with certain health problems.

Caffeine is derived from the chemical family called *xanthines*, which are found in plant products such as coffee, tea, and chocolate. The xanthines are mild central nervous system stimulants that enhance mental alertness, reduce feelings of fatigue, and increase heart muscle contractions, oxygen consumption, metabolism, and urinary output. A person feels these effects within 15 to 45 minutes of ingesting a caffeinated product. It takes 4 to 6 hours for the body to metabolize half of the caffeine ingested, so, depending on the amount of caffeine taken in, it may continue to exert effects for a day or longer. FIGURE 13.3 on page 370 compares the caffeine content of various products.

As the effects of caffeine wear off, frequent users may feel let down—mentally or physically depressed, tired, and weak. To counteract this, they commonly choose to drink another cup of coffee or tea, or another soda. Habitually engaging in this practice leads to tolerance and psychological dependence. Symptoms of excessive caffeine consumption include chronic insomnia, jitters, irritability, nervousness, anxiety, and involuntary muscle twitches. Withdrawing from caffeine may compound the effects and produce severe headaches, fatigue, and nausea. Because caffeine meets the

**caffeine** A stimulant drug that is legal in the United States and found in coffee, tea, chocolate, energy drinks, and certain medications.

### WHAT DO YOU THINK?

How much caffeine do you consume regularly, and why?

- What is your pattern of caffeine consumption?
- Have you ever experienced any ill effects after going without caffeine for a period of time?

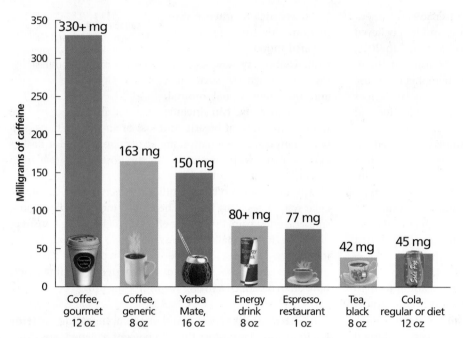

**FIGURE 13.3** Caffeine Content Comparison

**Source:** Caffeine Informer, "Caffeine Content of Drinks," Accessed June 2016, http://www.caffeineinformer.com/the-caffeine-database.

**marijuana** Chopped leaves and flowers of *Cannabis indica* or *Cannabis sativa* plants (hemp); a psychoactive stimulant.

**tetrahydrocannabinol (THC)** The chemical name for the active ingredient in marijuana.

requirements for addiction—tolerance, psychological dependence, and withdrawal symptoms—it can be classified as addictive.

Heavy levels of caffeine use have been suspected of being linked to several serious health problems such as high blood pressure, and arrythmias increased risk of heart attacks among young adults, and increased anxiety and depression.[47] However, no strong evidence exists to suggest that moderate caffeine use (less than 300 mg daily, or approximately three cups of regular coffee) produces harmful effects in healthy, nonpregnant people. For most people, caffeine poses few health risks and may actually have some benefits, such as improving memory, lowering risk of depression among women, helping open airways for those with asthma, lowering risk of prostate cancer among men, and lowering risk of stroke among both men and women.[48]

## Marijuana and Other Cannabinoids

Although archaeological evidence documents the use of **marijuana** ("grass," "weed," or "pot") as far back as 6,000 years, the drug did not become popular in the United States until the 1960s. Today, marijuana is the most commonly used illicit drug in the United States.[49] Some 33 million Americans

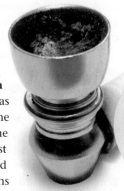

One common way of smoking marijuana is to use a pipe.

have reported using marijuana in the past year, and more than 22 million have reported using marijuana within the past month.[50] Marijuana use is also on the rise on college campuses, with approximately 36% of college students reportedly using marijuana in the past year, following the trends of increased use in the general population, as well as legalization for recreational use in a number of states.[51]

Marijuana is derived from either *Cannabis sativa* or *Cannabis indica*, or from hybrids. The difference between these strains of marijuana is the sativa strains offer an uplifting high whereas the indica high is more relaxing and good for stress relief.[52]

Most of the time, marijuana is smoked, although it can also be ingested. When marijuana is smoked, it is usually rolled into cigarettes (joints), *vaped*, or placed in a pipe or water pipe (bong). Consumption of marijuana by using edibles is becoming an increasingly popular alternative to smoking marijuana. By infusing food items with marijuana, edibles become a way to consume cannabis that can be more convenient and discreet. However, there are challenges with consuming edibles. The effects are hard to predict and can differ between individuals. It also takes longer to feel the effects—sometimes 30 to 60 minutes—and the effects can last longer.[53] The potency of edibles can also be quite a bit stronger, with a single chocolate bar containing as much as 100 milligrams of THC, far too much for consumption at one time.[54]

**Tetrahydrocannabinol (THC)** is the psychoactive substance in marijuana and the key to determining how powerful a high it will produce. More potent forms of the drug can contain up to 27 percent THC, but most average 15 percent.[55] *Hashish*, a potent cannabis preparation derived mainly from the plant's thick, sticky resin, contains high THC concentrations. Smoking THC-rich resin extracts, called *dabbing*, is becoming much more common among marijuana users. These extracts contain high levels of THC and have resulted in people ending up in the emergency room. Another danger is the extraction process, which involves butane lighter fluid; a number of people have suffered burns and explosions or fires in their homes.[56]

The effects of smoking marijuana are generally felt within 30 minutes to an hour and usually wear off within 3 hours.[57] The most noticeable effect of THC is the dilation of the eyes' blood vessels, which gives the smoker bloodshot eyes. Marijuana smokers also exhibit coughing; dry mouth

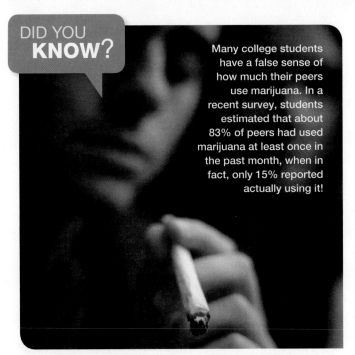

and throat ("cotton mouth"); impaired body movement; increased heart rate; and changes in mood. Users can also experience severe anxiety, panic, paranoia, and psychosis, and may have intensified reactions to various stimuli; colors, sounds, and the speed at which things move may seem altered.[58]

### Marijuana and Driving

Between 2007 and 2014, the number of nighttime drivers on the weekends with marijuana in their systems increased by 50 percent.[59] Marijuana use presents clear hazards for drivers of motor vehicles and others on the road with them. The drug substantially reduces a driver's ability to react and make quick decisions. Perceptual and other performance deficits resulting from marijuana use may persist for some time after the high subsides. Users who attempt to drive, fly, or operate heavy machinery often fail to recognize their impairment. In 2014, in the state of Washington where recreational use of marijuana is legal, 1 in 6 drivers involved in fatal car crashes had recently used marijuana.[60] Recent research indicates you are two and a half times more likely to be involved in a motor vehicle accident if you drive under the influence of marijuana.[61] Combining even a low dose of marijuana and alcohol enhances the impairing effects of both drugs.

# 1 IN 10

Americans over the age of 12 have used **ILLICIT DRUGS** in the past 30 days.

States are exploring different ways to enforce drug-impaired driving by creating legal limits to identify the amount of THC drivers can have in their system. However, a challenge is that, to date, there is no scientific evidence that drivers reliably become impaired with a specific level of marijuana in their blood. Marijuana affects people differently. Frequent users can have THC in the blood for a long period of time after use whereas infrequent users' THC levels decrease more rapidly. States need to explore alternative methods enforcement other than setting legal limits of THC in the blood. It has been suggested that states should use a two-component system that requires a driver to both test positive for recent marijuana use as well as show evidence of behavioral and or physiological impairment.[62]

### Effects of Chronic Marijuana Use

Smoking marijuana is harmful to lung health. The smoke from marijuana has been shown to contain many of the same toxins, irritants, and carcinogens as tobacco smoke.[63] Because marijuana smokers typically inhale more deeply and hold the smoke in their lungs longer than do tobacco smokers, the lungs are exposed to more tar per breath. Likewise, effects from irritation (e.g., cough, excessive phlegm, and increased lung infections) similar to those experienced by tobacco smokers can occur.[64] Lung conditions such as chronic bronchitis, emphysema, and other lung disorders are also associated with smoking marijuana.

Some marijuana users believe that "vaping" marijuana poses fewer health risks than smoking marijuana. Vaporizers heat marijuana to a temperature that releases as much THC, its active compound, without creating smoke. While a small percentage of recreational marijuana users (7.6%) report vaping as a way to use marijuana, the majority still smoke marijuana.[65] Studies report very minimal difference to lungs by vaping instead of smoking.[66]

Frequent and/or long-term marijuana use may significantly increase a man's risk of developing testicular cancer. The risk was particularly elevated (about twice that of those who never smoked marijuana) for those who used marijuana at least weekly or who had long-term exposure to the substance beginning in adolescence.[67]

The link between marijuana and common mental health disorders can be conflicting. A recent study found that using marijuana as an adult is not associated with a variety of mood and anxiety disorders, including depression and bipolar disorder, challenging some previous research.[68] However, use of marijuana is associated with a higher likelihood of drug dependence.[69]

Some research suggests that frequent or heavy use of marijuana during adolescence may be associated developing anxiety disorders in young adulthood.[70] The American Academy of Pediatrics has stated that marijuana is harmful to adolescent health and development.[71] For adolescents, marijuana use can disrupt concentration and memory. It can also cause problems with learning, and is linked to lower rates of high school and college completion.[72] It can also affect motor control, coordination, and judgment, which increase

**depressants** Drugs that slow down the activity of the central nervous and muscular systems and cause sleepiness or calmness.

**benzodiazepines** A class of central nervous system depressant drugs with sedative, hypnotic, and muscle relaxant effects; also called *tranquilizers.*

**barbiturates** Drugs that depress the central nervous system, have sedative and hypnotic effects, and are less safe than benzodiazepines.

the risk of unintentional deaths and injuries.[73]

Chronic or heavy use of marijuana can decrease the quality of sleep. Heavy users may get lower-quality sleep, characterized by fewer hours sleeping both when using and when abstaining from marijuana. One common characteristic for heavy marijuana users is not being able to fall asleep when they are not using marijuana. For marijuana users in recovery, this may eventually lead to relapse.[74]

Recent studies suggest that pregnant women who smoke marijuana may have children who have subtle brain changes that can cause difficulties with problem-solving skills, memory, and attention.[75]

### Legalization of Marijuana and Medicinal Uses

Although classified as a dangerous drug by the U.S. government, marijuana has been legalized for medicinal uses in 24 states and the District of Columbia, and is known to have several medical purposes. It helps control such side effects as the severe nausea and vomiting produced by chemotherapy, the chemical treatment for cancer. It improves appetite and forestalls the loss of lean muscle mass associated with AIDS-wasting syndrome. Marijuana reduces the muscle pain and spasticity caused by diseases such as multiple sclerosis. Opponents of medical marijuana argue that there are FDA-approved drugs that are just as effective in treating the same conditions, and that the potential side effects of marijuana make it inappropriate for FDA approval. Although several states have legalized marijuana for medicinal and/or recreational purposes, its legal status continues to be hotly debated (see the Health Headlines box).

### Synthetic Marijuana (Spice or K2)

Also known as K2 or "Spice," synthetic marijuana is used to describe a diverse family of herbal blends marketed under many names, including K2, fake marijuana, Yucatan Fire, Skunk, Moon Rocks, and others. These products contain dried, shredded plant material and one or more synthetic cannabinoids, with results that mimic marijuana intoxication but with longer duration and poor detection on urine drug screens. K2 is sold legally as herbal-blend incense. However, Spice is smoked by people to gain effects similar to marijuana, hashish, and other forms of cannabis.[76]

Spice is used by nearly 1 in 7 college students and is more commonly used by males and first- and second-year college students.[77] Students who reported using Spice were more likely to have smoked cigarettes, marijuana, and hookahs.[78] It is also gaining more attention among high school seniors, with reports that 1 in every 9, or 11.3 percent, of high school seniors are using this drug.[79]

The most common way of smoking Spice is by rolling it in papers (as with marijuana or handmade tobacco cigarettes).[80] Sometimes it is mixed with marijuana. Some users also make it as an herbal tea for drinking.[81] People smoking Spice may experience several adverse health effects such as hallucinations, severe agitation, extremely elevated heart rate and blood pressure, coma, suicide attempts, and drug dependence, which is not common among cannabis users.[82] Emergency departments are also reporting a significant increase in the numbers of people being treated for Spice use.[83]

## Depressants and Narcotics

Whereas central nervous system stimulants increase muscular and nervous system activity, **depressants** have the opposite effect. These drugs slow down neuromuscular activity and cause sleepiness or calmness. If the dose is high enough, brain function can stop, causing death. Alcohol is the most widely used central nervous system depressant. (For details on alcohol's effect on the body, see Chapter 11.) Other forms include benzodiazepines, barbiturates, and GHB.

### Benzodiazepines and Barbiturates

A *sedative* drug promotes mental calmness and reduces anxiety, whereas a *hypnotic* drug promotes sleep or drowsiness. The most common sedative-hypnotic drugs are **benzodiazepines**, more commonly known as *tranquilizers.*[84] These include prescription drugs such as Valium, Ativan, and Xanax. Benzodiazepines are most commonly prescribed for tension, muscular strain, sleep problems, anxiety, panic attacks, and alcohol withdrawal.[85] **Barbiturates** are sedative-hypnotic drugs such as Amytal and Seconal. Today, benzodiazepines have largely replaced barbiturates, which were used medically in the past for relieving anxiety and inducing relaxation and sleep.

Sedative-hypnotics have a synergistic effect when combined with alcohol, another central nervous system depressant. Taken together, these drugs can lead to respiratory failure and death. All sedative or hypnotic drugs can produce physical and psychological dependence in several weeks. A complication specific to sedatives is cross-tolerance, which occurs when users develop tolerance for one sedative or become dependent on it and develop tolerance for others as well. Withdrawal from sedative or hypnotic drugs may range from mild discomfort to severe symptoms, depending on the degree of dependence.[86]

One benzodiazepine of concern is Rohypnol, a potent tranquilizer similar in nature to Valium but many times stronger. The drug produces a sedative effect, amnesia, muscle relaxation, and slowed psychomotor responses. The most publicized "date rape" drug, Rohypnol has gained notoriety as a growing problem on college campuses. The drug has been added to punch and other drinks at parties, where it is reportedly given to a woman in hopes of incapacitating her so she is unable to resist sexual assault. (See Chapter 20 for more on drug-facilitated rape.)

### GHB

*Gamma-hydroxybutyrate (GHB)* is a central nervous system depressant known to have euphoric, sedative, and anabolic (bodybuilding) effects. It was originally sold over the counter to bodybuilders to help reduce body fat and build muscle. Concerns about GHB led the FDA to ban OTC sales

# MARIJUANA LEGALIZATION

Currently, 24 states and the District of Columbia have chosen to legalize marijuana for medicinal use, and voters in Washington, Colorado, Oregon, and Alaska recently passed ballot initiatives to legalize marijuana for recreational use. The arguments for and against the legalization of marijuana have been very strong over the past few decades.

Proponents of marijuana legalization argue that the plant has medical benefits for individuals dealing with cancer and other chronic diseases. From a public service standpoint, some supporters argue that legalizing marijuana and taxing its sale would bring in revenue for the government. Environmentally, legal government and U.S. Food and Drug Administration (FDA) oversight would allow for standardization of marijuana growth and production and could promote more responsible cultivation methods. From a law enforcement perspective, some argue that legalizing marijuana will result in more effective law enforcement and criminal justice since police officers will have more time and money to pursue criminals for other, more serious crimes. Additionally, having legal outlets for drugs such as marijuana may reduce illegal drug trafficking from off-shore criminal elements and reduce the risk of harmful drug additives.

Of course, not everyone supports treating marijuana much the way we currently treat alcohol. Some individuals

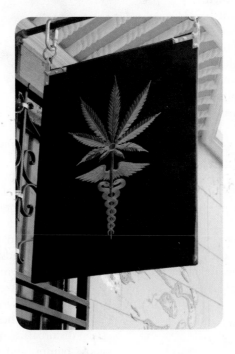

believe that it is morally wrong to consume marijuana, and that legalization could make marijuana more available to children and teenagers. From a health care perspective, marijuana use can cause or worsen respiratory symptoms or conditions such as bronchitis, alter mood and judgment, damage the immune system, and impair short-term memory and motor coordination. These side effects, some say, make it inappropriate for FDA approval. Research indicates that marijuana use impacts young users

the most in the long term, finding that those who used marijuana heavily as teenagers lose an average of 8 IQ points that are not recovered with quitting or aging. Lastly, in terms of public health, opponents of legalization argue that marijuana is known to be addictive; approximately 9 percent of people who experiment with marijuana become addicted.

As the tide seems to shift toward more and more states legalizing marijuana for medical and recreational uses, where do you stand? Do you think marijuana should be legalized by the federal government? What potential problems do you think this would create or solve? What criteria do you think should be used to determine the legality of a particular substance? Who should make those determinations? What are your feelings on drug laws in general—do you think they should be more or less prohibitive? What sorts of policies would you propose to protect individuals and their rights?

This issue is continuing to evolve. Stay tuned!

**Sources:** National Institute on Drug Abuse, "DrugFacts: Is Marijuana Medicine?," July 2014, www.drugabuse.gov; DrugRehab.us, "Pros and Cons of Legalizing Recreational Marijuana," April 2014, www.drugrehab.us/news/pros-cons-legalizing-recreational-marijuana; N. Volkow et al., "Adverse Health Effects of Marijuana Use," *New England Journal of Medicine,* 370 (2014): 2219–27.

---

in 1992, and GHB is now a Schedule I drug. (Schedule I drugs are classified as having a high potential for abuse, with no currently accepted medical use in the United States.)[87] GHB is an odorless, tasteless fluid. Like Rohypnol, GHB has been slipped into drinks without being detected, resulting in loss of memory, unconsciousness, amnesia, and even death. Other dangerous side effects include nausea, vomiting, seizures, hallucinations, coma, and respiratory distress.

### Opioids (Narcotics)
**Opioids** cause drowsiness, relieve pain, and produce euphoria. Also called *narcotics*, opioids are derived from the parent drug **opium**, a dark, resinous substance made from the milky juice of the opium poppy seedpod, and they are all highly addictive. Opium and heroin are both illegal

in the United States, but some opioids are available by prescription for medical purposes: Morphine is sometimes prescribed for severe pain, and codeine is found in prescription cough syrups and other painkillers. Several prescription drugs—including Vicodin, Percodan, OxyContin, Demerol, and Dilaudid—contain synthetic opioids.

Opioids are powerful depressants of the central nervous system. Opioid drugs are derived naturally from the opium plant or created synthetically. Side effects include drowsiness, mental confusion, nausea, and constipation.[88]

> **opioids** Drugs that induce sleep, relieve pain, and produce euphoria; includes derivatives of opium and synthetics with similar chemical properties; also called *narcotics*.
>
> **opium** The parent drug of the opioids; made from the seedpod resin of the opium poppy.

The human body's physiology could be said to encourage opioid addiction. Opioid-like hormones called **endorphins** are manufactured in the body and have multiple receptor sites, particularly in the central nervous system. When endorphins attach themselves at these points, they create feelings of painless well-being; medical researchers refer to them as "the body's own opioids." When endorphin levels are high, people feel euphoric. The same euphoria occurs when opioids or related chemicals are active at the endorphin receptor sites.

Of all the opioids, heroin has the greatest notoriety as an addictive drug. *Heroin* is a white powder derived from morphine. *Black tar heroin* is a sticky, dark brown, foul-smelling form of heroin that is relatively pure and inexpensive. Once considered a cure for morphine dependence, heroin was later discovered to be even more addictive and potent than morphine. Today heroin has no medical use.

Opium is extracted from opium poppy seedpods like this one.

# 6.5 MILLION

**NONMEDICAL USERS** of prescription drugs have been estimated in 2014.

Heroin is a depressant that produces drowsiness and a dreamy, mentally slow feeling. It can cause mood swings, with euphoric highs followed by depressive lows. Chronic heroin users may develop a number of complications, including liver and kidney diseases, collapsed veins, abscesses, constipation, and infection of the heart lining. Symptoms of tolerance and withdrawal can appear within 3 weeks of first use.[89]

In 2014, 435,000 Americans reported using heroin in the past month, a considerable increase since 2002, an increase of nearly 114 percent among whites and up 77 percent in the middle class.[90] Once predominant in urban areas, heroin use is becoming increasingly common in suburban and rural communities, particularly among white men and women.[91] Deaths from heroin overdoses have skyrocketed in recent years, rising from just over 1,800 deaths in 2000 to nearly 10,600 in 2014, particularly among those who are finding that heroin is a cheaper high than prescription opiates that they have become addicted to.[92] This trend appears to be driven largely by 18- to 25-year-olds, among whom there have been the largest increases. However, addicted opiate users of older ages find that these opiates serve as a kind of "gate-keeper" drug for heroin, particular among those who can no longer pay the rapidly rising costs for prescription painkillers.[93] Young and older adults hooked on painkillers

are finding that heroin is cheaper and easier to obtain than prescription opioids.[94]

While heroin is usually injected intravenously ("mainlined"), the contemporary version of heroin is so potent that users can get high by snorting or smoking the drug. This has attracted a more affluent group of users who may not want to inject, for reasons such as the increased risk of contracting diseases such as HIV.

Many users describe the rush they feel when injecting themselves as intensely pleasurable, whereas others report unpredictable and unpleasant side effects. The temporary nature of the rush contributes to the drug's high potential for addiction—many addicts shoot up four or five times a day. Mainlining can cause veins to scar and eventually collapse. Once a vein has collapsed, it can no longer be used to introduce heroin into the bloodstream. Addicts become expert at locating new veins to use: in the feet, the legs, the temples, under the tongue, or in the groin.

Heroin addicts experience a distinct pattern of withdrawal. Symptoms of withdrawal include intense desire for the drug, sleep disturbance, dilated pupils, loss of appetite, irritability, goose bumps, and muscle tremors. The most difficult time in the withdrawal process occurs 24 to 72 hours following last use. All of the preceding symptoms continue, along with nausea, abdominal cramps, restlessness, insomnia, vomiting, diarrhea, extreme anxiety, hot and cold flashes, elevated blood pressure, and rapid heartbeat and respiration. Once the peak of withdrawal has passed, all these symptoms begin to subside.[95]

## Hallucinogens

**Hallucinogens**, or *psychedelics*, are substances that are capable of creating auditory or visual hallucinations and unusual changes in mood, thoughts, and feelings. The major receptor sites for most of these drugs are in the reticular formation (located in the brain stem at the upper end of the spinal cord), which is responsible for interpreting outside stimuli before allowing these signals to travel to other parts of the brain. When a hallucinogen is present at a reticular formation site, messages become scrambled, and the user may see wavy walls instead of straight ones or may "smell" colors and "hear" tastes. This mixing of sensory messages is known as *synesthesia*. Users may also become less inhibited or recall events long buried in the subconscious mind. The most widely recognized hallucinogens are LSD, Ecstasy, PCP, mescaline, psilocybin, and ketamine. All are illegal and carry severe penalties for manufacture, possession, transportation, or sale.

**LSD** First synthesized in the late 1930s by Swiss chemist Albert Hoffman, *lysergic acid diethylamide (LSD)*

**endorphins** Opioid-like hormones that are manufactured in the human body and contribute to natural feelings of well-being.

**hallucinogens** Substances capable of creating auditory or visual distortions and unusual changes in mood, thoughts, and feelings.

received media attention in the 1960s when young people used the drug to "turn on, tune in, drop out." In 1970, federal authorities placed LSD on the list of controlled substances (Schedule I). Today, this dangerous psychedelic drug, known alternately as "acid," has been making a comeback. It is estimated that 9.4 percent of Americans aged 12 or older have used LSD at least once in their lifetime.[96] A national survey of college students showed that less than 4.5 percent had used the drug in their lives.[97]

LSD is one of the most potent hallucinogenic drugs. An odorless, water-soluble material, it is synthesized from lysergic acid, a compound found in rye fungus. A common method for taking LSD is by using blotter acid—small squares of blotter-like paper that have been impregnated with a liquid LSD mixture. The blotter is swallowed or chewed briefly. LSD also comes in tiny thin squares of gelatin called *windowpane* and in tablets called *microdots*, which are less than an eighth of an inch across (it would take 10 or more to equal the size of an aspirin tablet).[98]

The psychological effects of LSD vary. LSD also distorts ordinary perceptions, such as the movement of stationary objects, as well as auditory or visual hallucinations. In addition, the drug shortens attention span, causing the mind to wander. Thoughts may be interposed and juxtaposed, so the user experiences several different thoughts simultaneously. Users become introspective, and suppressed memories may surface, often taking on bizarre symbolism. Many more effects are possible, including decreased aggressiveness and enhanced sensory experiences.[99]

In addition to its psychedelic effects, LSD produces several physical effects, including increased heart rate, elevated blood pressure and temperature, goose bumps (roughened skin), increased reflex speeds, muscle tremors and twitches, perspiration, increased salivation, chills, headaches, and mild nausea. Because the drug also stimulates uterine muscle contractions, it can lead to premature labor and miscarriage in pregnant women.

Although there is no evidence that LSD is addictive, it does produce tolerance, so users may need to take more of the drug to get the same effect. This is a dangerous practice as the drug is unpredictable.[100]

**Ecstasy** *Ecstasy* is a common street name for the drug *methylene-dioxymethamphetamine (MDMA)*, a synthetic compound with both stimulant and mildly hallucinogenic effects. It is one of the most well-known **club drugs** or "designer drugs," a term applied to synthetic analogs of existing illicit drugs popular at nightclubs and all-night parties. Ecstasy creates feelings of extreme euphoria, openness, and warmth; an increased willingness to communicate; feelings of love and empathy; increased awareness; and heightened appreciation for music. Young people may use Ecstasy initially to improve their mood or get energized. Ecstasy can enhance the sensory experience and distort perceptions, but it does not create visual hallucinations. Effects can last for 3 to 6 hours.[101]

Some of the risks associated with Ecstasy use are similar to those of other stimulants. Because of the nature of the drug, Ecstasy users are at greater risk of inappropriate or unintended emotional bonding and have a tendency to say things they might feel uncomfortable about later. Physical consequences of Ecstasy use may include mild to extreme jaw clenching, tongue and cheek chewing; short-term memory loss or confusion; increased body temperature; and increased heart rate and blood pressure. Combined with alcohol, Ecstasy can be extremely dangerous and sometimes fatal. As the effects of Ecstasy wear off, the user can experience mild depression, fatigue, and a hangover that can last from days to weeks. Chronic use appears to damage the brain's ability to think and to regulate emotion, memory, sleep, and pain. Some studies indicate that the drug may cause long-lasting neurotoxic effects by damaging brain cells that produce serotonin.[102]

MDMA in powder or crystal form—called "Molly," short for molecule—has become a popular festival drug. Unlike Ecstasy, which tends to be laced with ingredients like caffeine or methamphetamine, Molly is considered pure MDMA. Still, many powders sold as Molly contain zero actual MDMA. Some typical side effects of using Molly include grinding one's teeth, becoming dehydrated, feeling anxious, having trouble sleeping, fever, and losing one's appetite, as well as elevated blood pressure, high body temperature, and depression; it can occasionally result in liver, kidney, or heart failure and possibly death.[103]

**PCP (Phencyclidine)** The synthetic substance *phencyclidine (PCP)* was originally developed as a dissociative anesthetic—patients administered this drug could keep their eyes open, apparently remain conscious, and feel no pain during a medical procedure. Afterward, they would experience amnesia for the time that the drug was in their system. Such a drug had

> **club drugs** Synthetic analogs that produce similar effects of existing drugs.

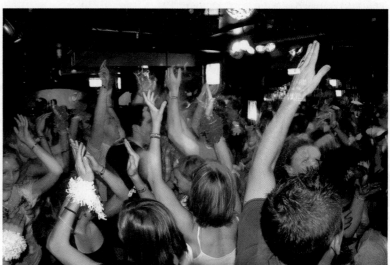

Although users may think so-called *club drugs* (such as Ecstasy, GHB, and ketamine) are harmless, research has shown that they can produce hallucinations, paranoia, amnesia, dangerous increases in heart rate and blood pressure, coma, and, in some cases, death.

obvious advantages as an anesthetic, but its unpredictability and drastic effects (postoperative delirium, confusion, and agitation) caused it to be withdrawn from the legal market.[104]

On the illegal market, PCP is a white, crystalline powder that users often sprinkle onto marijuana cigarettes. It is dangerous and unpredictable regardless of the method of administration. The effects of PCP depend on the dose. A small dose can produce effects similar to those of strong central nervous system depressants—slurred speech, impaired coordination, reduced sensitivity to pain, and reduced heart and respiratory rate. Larger doses can cause fever, salivation, nausea and vomiting, and total loss of sensitivity to pain. PCP can also cause a rise in blood pressure, seizures, violent outbursts, coma and possibly death.[105]

Psychologically, PCP may produce either euphoria or dysphoria. It is also known to produce hallucinations as well as delusions and overall delirium. Some users experience a prolonged state of "nothingness." The long-term effects of PCP use are unknown.

### Mescaline

*Mescaline* is one of hundreds of chemicals derived from the peyote cactus, a small, button-like plant that grows in the southwestern United States and in Latin America. Natives of these regions have long used the dried peyote "buttons" for religious purposes. It is both a powerful hallucinogen and a central nervous system stimulant.

Users typically swallow pieces of the cactus called buttons, which are chewed or soaked in water to create a liquid that is intoxicating. The effects of mescaline include visual hallucinations, altered states of consciousness, and occasionally users feel anxious or have episodes of revulsion. Side effects of mescaline may include vomiting, dizziness, diarrhea, and headache. Effects may persist for up to 12 hours.[106]

Products sold on the street as mescaline are likely to be synthetic chemical relatives of the true drug. Street names of these products include DOM, STP, TMA, and MMDA. Any of these can be toxic in small quantities.

### Psilocybin

*Psilocybin* and *psilocin* are the active chemicals in a group of mushrooms sometimes called "magic mushrooms." *Psilocybe* mushrooms, which grow throughout the world, can be cultivated from spores or harvested wild. When consumed, these mushrooms can cause hallucinations. Because many mushrooms resemble the *Psilocybe* variety, people who harvest wild mushrooms for any purpose should be certain of what they are doing. Mushroom varieties can be easily

Mescaline comes from "buttons" of the peyote cactus, like this one.

Psilocybe mushrooms produce hallucinogenic effects when ingested.

misidentified, and mistakes can be fatal. Psilocybin is similar to LSD in its physical effects, which generally wear off in 6 to 12 hours.[107]

**inhalants** Chemical vapors that are sniffed or inhaled to produce highs.

### Ketamine

The liquid form of *ketamine* ("Special K") is used as an anesthetic in some hospitals and veterinary clinics. Special K causes hallucinations because it inhibits the relay of sensory input; the brain fills the resulting void with visions, dreams, memories, and sensory distortions. The effects of ketamine are similar to those of PCP—confusion, agitation, aggression, and lack of coordination—but even less predictable. Aftereffects of ketamine are less severe than those of Ecstasy, so it has grown in popularity as a club drug.[108]

### Salvia

Native to southern Mexico, salvia is an herb from the mint family.[109] Its main active ingredient, salvinorin A, causes hallucinations by changing brain chemistry.[110] Although associated hallucinatory episodes have been described as intense, they are relatively short lasting, often beginning after a minute and fading after 30 minutes.[111] These brief, but extreme hallucinations often include changes in mood, body sensations, changes to visual perception, emotional swings, feeling detached, and an altered sense of self and reality.[112] Salvia's long-term effects have not been studied.

## Inhalants

**Inhalants** are chemicals whose vapors, when inhaled, can cause hallucinations and create intoxicating and euphoric effects. Not commonly recognized as drugs, inhalants are legal to purchase and widely available, but dangerous. They generally appeal to young people who can't afford or obtain illicit substances. Some misused products include rubber cement, model glue, paint thinner, aerosol sprays, lighter fluid, varnish, wax, spot removers, and gasoline. Most of these substances are sniffed or "huffed" by users in search of a quick, cheap high.

Because they are inhaled, the volatile chemicals in these products reach the bloodstream within seconds. This characteristic, along with the fact that dosages are extremely difficult to control because everyone has unique lung and breathing capacities, makes inhalants particularly dangerous. The effects of inhalants resemble those of central nervous system depressants: dizziness, disorientation, impaired coordination, reduced judgment, and slowed reaction times.[113]

An overdose of fumes from inhalants can cause unconsciousness and even death. Because the effect only lasts a few minutes, users can continue to inhale readily over several hours; by doing this, users can suffer loss of consciousness and death.[114]

**Amyl Nitrite** Sometimes called "poppers" or "rush," *amyl nitrite* is packaged in small, cloth-covered glass capsules that can be crushed to release the active chemical for the user to inhale. The drug is often prescribed to alleviate chest pain in heart patients because it dilates small blood vessels and reduces blood pressure. Dilation of blood vessels in the genital area is thought to enhance sensations or perceptions of orgasm. It also produces fainting, dizziness, warmth, and skin flushing.[115]

**Nitrous Oxide** *Nitrous oxide* is sometimes used as a dental or minor surgical anesthesia. It is also a propellant chemical in aerosol products such as whipped toppings. Users who inhale nitrous oxide experience a state of euphoria, floating sensations, and illusions. Effects also include pain relief and a silly feeling (hence its nickname "laughing gas"). Effects include dizziness, loss of balance, dissociation, and impaired memory and cognition. Sustained inhalation can lead to unconsciousness, coma, and death.[116]

## Anabolic Steroids

**Anabolic steroids** are artificial forms of the male hormone testosterone that promote muscle growth and strength. Steroids are available in two forms: injectable solutions and pills. **Ergogenic drugs** are used primarily by people who believe the drugs will increase their strength, power, bulk (weight), speed, and athletic performance.

It has been estimated that 6.4 percent of males and 1.6 percent of females have used anabolic-androgenic steroids (AAS) in their lifetime. The prevalence of AAS was most common among recreational and competitive athletes and the likelihood that someone would use AAS increased by 91 percent by their participation in at least one sport.[117]

It was once estimated that up to 20 percent of college athletes used steroids.[118] Now that stricter drug-testing policies have been instituted by the National Collegiate Athletic Association (NCAA), reported use of anabolic steroids among intercollegiate athletes has decreased. Currently, less than half of 1

> Common household products, such as aerosol sprays, solvents, and glues, can be inhaled for a quick but risky high.

**anabolic steroids** Artificial forms of the hormone testosterone that promote muscle growth and strength.

**ergogenic drugs** Substances believed to enhance athletic performance.

percent of college athletes surveyed report use of anabolic steroids within the past 12 months.[119] Those who report using anabolic steroids use them less than once per week. Of those, half reported their first experience with anabolic steroids occurred after the age of 18.[120] The use of anabolic steroids on the college campus is very low; approximately 1 percent report using them within the past 30 days.[121] However, the perception of anabolic steroid use on the college campus is much higher than reality.[122]

**Physical Effects of Steroids** Although their primary effects are not psychotropic, anabolic steroids can produce a state of euphoria and diminished fatigue in addition to increased bulk and power in both sexes. These qualities give steroids an addictive quality. When users stop, they can experience psychological withdrawal and sometimes severe depression, in some cases leading to suicide attempts.[123]

Men and women who use steroids experience a variety of adverse effects, including mood swings (aggression and violence, sometimes known as "roid rage"), acne, liver damage,

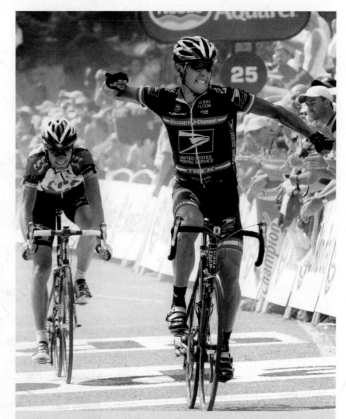

After being stripped of seven Tour de France titles in 2012 and an Olympic medal in 2013, cyclist Lance Armstrong publicly ended his years of denial and admitted to doping. He was banned from cycling for life and has been sued by the U.S. federal government and others for fraud.

elevated cholesterol levels, changes in blood cholesterol, kidney damage, and immune system disturbances.[124] There is also a danger of transmitting HIV and hepatitis through shared needles. In women, large doses of anabolic steroids may trigger the development of masculine attributes such as lowered voice, increased facial and body hair, and male-pattern baldness; they may also result in an enlarged clitoris, smaller breasts, and changes in or absence of menstruation. When taken by healthy men, anabolic steroids shut down the body's production of testosterone, causing men's breasts to grow and testicles to atrophy.

**Steroid Use and Society** The Anabolic Steroids Control Act (ASCA) of 1990 makes it a crime to possess, prescribe, or distribute anabolic steroids for any use other than the treatment of specific diseases. Penalties for their illegal use include up to 1-year imprisonment and/ or a fine of $1,000 for the first offense and a mandatory 15 days and maximum 2-year imprisonment and a $2,500 fine. Federal punishment for intent to distribute steroids is not more than 5-year imprisonment, with 2 years of parole and a $250,000 fine for the first offense.[125]

In recent years, high-profile athletes in sports such as cycling, track and field, swimming, and baseball have garnered media attention for suspected use of steroids or other banned performance-enhancing drugs.

programs involve individual or group drug counseling. *Residential treatment programs* can also be very effective, especially for those with more severe problems. Therapeutic communities (TCs) are highly structured programs in which people looking to get clean remain at a residence, typically for 6 to 12 months, with a focus on resocializing to a drug-free lifestyle.

**12-Step Programs** The first 12-step program was Alcoholics Anonymous (AA), begun in 1935 in Akron, Ohio. The 12-step program has since become the most widely used approach to dealing with not only alcoholism, but also with drug abuse and various other addictive or dysfunctional behaviors. There are more than 130 different recovery programs based on the program, including Narcotics Anonymous, Cocaine Anonymous, Crystal Meth Anonymous, Gamblers Anonymous, and Pills Anonymous.[127]

The 12-step program is nonjudgmental and based on the idea that a program's only purpose is to work on personal recovery. Working the 12 steps includes admitting to having a serious problem, recognizing there is an outside power that could help, consciously relying on that power, admitting and listing character defects, seeking deliverance from defects, apologizing to those individuals one has harmed in the past, and helping others with the same problem. There is no membership cost, and the meetings are open to anyone who wishes to attend.

**Vaccines against Addictive Drugs** A promising new cocaine vaccine is in development. The vaccine does not eliminate the desire for cocaine; instead, it keeps the user from getting high by stimulating the immune system to attack the drug when it's taken. Clinical human trials are expected to begin soon. Vaccines against heroin and methamphetamine are also in development.[128]

## LO 5 | TREATING AND REDUCING DRUG ABUSE

Provide examples of drug treatment and recovery options for addicts and their effectiveness.

An estimated 21.5 million Americans aged 12 or older needed treatment for an illicit drug or alcohol use problem in 2014.[126] Below are some common approaches to treating substance abuse problems (more on this in **Focus On: Recognizing and Avoiding Addiction** on page 299).

## Treatment Approaches

*Outpatient behavioral treatment* encompasses a variety of programs for people with substance abuse problems who visit a clinic at regular intervals. Most of the

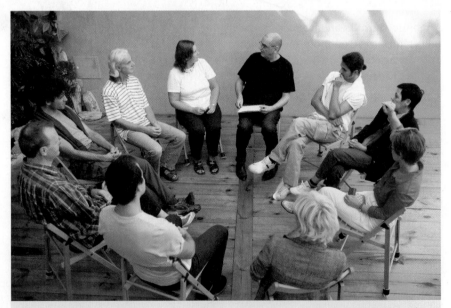

For most addicts, recovery is a long, difficult process—for some people it can be a lifelong journey. Therapy often takes the form of group meetings, such as those held by 12-step programs like Narcotics Anonymous.

**Other Pharmacological Treatments** Methadone maintenance is one treatment available for people addicted to heroin or other opioids. Methadone, a synthetic narcotic, is chemically similar enough to opioids to control the tremors, chills, vomiting, diarrhea, and severe abdominal pains of withdrawal. Methadone dosage is decreased over a period of time until the addict is weaned off it.[129]

Methadone maintenance is controversial because of the drug's own potential for addiction. Critics contend that the program merely substitutes one addiction for another. Proponents argue that people on methadone maintenance are less likely to engage in criminal activities to support their habits than heroin addicts are. For this reason, many methadone maintenance programs are financed by state or federal government and are available free of charge or at reduced cost.

Naltrexone (Trexan), an opioid antagonist, has been approved as a treatment. It is used to treat opioid use disorders and alcohol use disorders. While on naltrexone, recovering addicts do not have the compulsion to use heroin, and, if they do use it, they don't get high, so there is no point in using the drug.[130]

A number of new drug therapies for opioid dependence are emerging. Another new drug therapy, buprenorphine (Temgesic), is a mild, nonaddicting synthetic opioid; it works a lot like methadone by blocking withdrawal symptoms and heroin cravings. One of the advantages of buprenorphine is that it does not require addicts to go to a clinic/pharmacy to get take their medication; rather, it can be taken at home.

## Drug Treatment and Recovery for College Students

For college students who have developed substance or behavioral addictions, early intervention increases the likelihood of successful treatment. Depending on the severity of the abuse or dependence, college students undergoing drug treatment may be required to spend time away from school in a residential drug rehabilitation inpatient facility. The needs of college students seeking drug treatment in rehab do not differ greatly from other adult recovering addicts, but for best results, the community of addicts should include others of a similar age and educational background. Private therapy, group therapy, cognitive training, nutrition counseling, and health therapies can all be used to help with recovery.

A growing number of colleges and universities are promoting recovery in an academic setting. For instance, *Collegiate Recovery Programs (CRPs)* is a campus-based peer support program for students in recovery from substance abuse problems. Currently, over 100 institutions of higher education nationwide are at various stages of providing or developing recovery supports for students. The overarching goal of CRPs is to provide recovering students with support, allowing them to sustain their recovery without having to postpone their educational goals.[131]

A recent study found that over half (53%) indicated that drug addiction (i.e., illegal substances or abuse of prescription medications) was their primary addiction, followed by alcohol (39%).[132] Those enrolled in the CRP programs reported high levels of addiction. Some of their past consequences related to their addictions included homelessness (one-third), one-half had been arrested and charged with a crime, and over a third had been incarcerated. However, most students had no current involvement with the criminal justice system.[133]

There are multiple reasons students enroll in collegiate recovery programs. Some of the most frequently cited reasons are the need for a recovery supportive peer network and a safe place to recover on campus, which help with stress and prevent relapse.

At Kennesaw State University's 4-year-old program, students first enter the Center for Young Adult Addiction and Recovery, where addiction specialists use clinical techniques to support the social and academic success of students while they abstain from substance use. After students have been sober for 6 months, they enter the center's Collegiate Recovery Community, which includes weekly meetings and seminars on relapse prevention and community building and meetings with academic advisers.

Some tuition waivers are available for out-of-state students if they are active members of the CRP. To join CRP, there are a number of requirements, including enrollment in Kennesaw State University, a minimum 6 months of sustained recovery, and either participation in a 12-step program or the ability to describe a recovery program. Recovering students are trained to go back into the classroom and educate their peers who are most at risk of

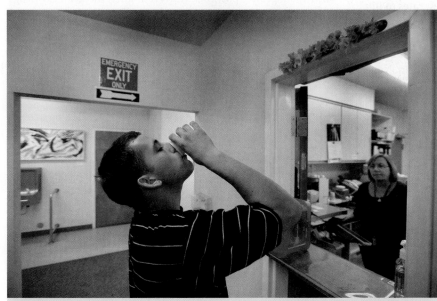

Methadone is a synthetic narcotic that blocks the effects of heroin withdrawal. Although it is still a narcotic and must be administered under the supervision of clinic or pharmacy staff, methadone allows many heroin addicts to lead somewhat normal lives.

developing substance abuse problems, such as fraternity and sorority members and incoming first-year students.[134]

Another campus, Texas Tech University, received a federal grant to create a national model of its students-in-recovery program. The program offers scholarships to students in recovery, as well as on-campus 12-step meetings and academic support.[135]

## LO 6 | ADDRESSING DRUG MISUSE AND ABUSE IN THE UNITED STATES

Profile illicit drug use in the United States, including who uses illicit drugs, financial impact, and impact on college campuses and the workplace.

While stories of people who have tried illegal drugs may tempt you to try them yourself, the risks associated with drug use extend beyond the personal. The decision to try any illicit substance supports illicit drug manufacture and transport, thus contributing to the national drug problem.

Illegal drug use in the United States costs about $193 billion per year.[136] This estimate includes $11 billion in the cost of health care, $120 billion in lost productivity, and $61 billion in the cost of criminal investigation, prosecution, incarceration, and other associated criminal justice costs.[137]

### Drugs in the Workplace

In the United States, 70 percent of all workers who use illicit drugs are employed.[138] Marijuana is the most common drug of choice for employees, with cocaine also popular and prescription drug use steadily on the rise.[139] The highest rates of illicit drug use were found in the hotel and food services industry, with 19 percent of workers reporting having used illicit drugs in the past month.[140] Many companies have instituted drug testing for their employees. Mandatory drug urinalysis is controversial. Critics argue that such testing violates Fourth Amendment rights of protection from unreasonable search and seizure. Proponents believe the personal inconvenience entailed in testing pales in comparison to the problems caused by drug use in the workplace. For more information on drug testing, see the **Tech & Health** box.

### Preventing Drug Use and Abuse on Campus

Strategies that universities should consider to reduce the number of students who become involved in substance use include:

- Changing student expectations that college is a time to party and experiment with drugs
- Engaging parents about substance use on campus and encouraging them to continue open communication with their children

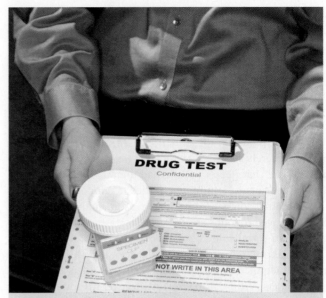

Several court decisions have affirmed the right of employers to test their employees for drug use. Most Americans apparently support drug testing for certain types of jobs.

- Identifying high-risk students through early detection screening programs
- Providing services such as treatment programs specifically tailored for students

The pressure to take drugs is often tremendous, and the reasons for using them are complex. People who develop drug problems generally believe they can control their drug use when they start out. Initially, they view taking drugs as a fun and manageable pastime. However, since most illegal drugs and many prescription drugs produce physical and psychological dependency, it is unrealistic to think that a person can use them regularly without becoming addicted. Peer influence is also a strong motivator, especially among adolescents, who fear not being accepted as part of the group.

### Possible Solutions to the Drug Problem

Americans are alarmed by the persistent problem of illegal drug use. Respondents in public opinion polls feel that the government should focus on treatment for those who use illegal drugs such as heroin or cocaine. There is increased support for moving away from mandatory sentences for nonviolent drug crimes. Many strategies include prevention strategies that focus on helping individuals develop the knowledge, attitudes, and skills to make good decisions. Other approaches encourage use of community prevention strategies to make it easier to act in healthy ways. These strategies involve community leaders, parents, and local officials working together to shift individual attitudes and community norms.[141] To address safety concerns, many employers have instituted mandatory

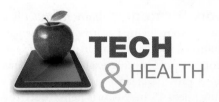

## TECH & HEALTH | TYPES OF DRUG TESTS

Several years ago, Linn State Technical College, a 2-year public institution, made the news when it implemented a mandatory drug-testing program for all students. The policy was later ruled to be a violation of students' right to privacy. But beyond the campus, drug testing is an ever-more-common condition of many employers. There are many types of drug tests.

### Urine Tests

Urine tests are the least expensive test method, with costs varying between $7 and $50 for the home versions. They can be conducted anywhere, but labs must verify results. Urine tests are best at detecting drug use within the past week, although if someone uses a drug over a long period of time the ability of urine tests to detect it outside that effective window increases. There are some problems with this test: Many find giving a urine sample to be embarrassing and intrusive, and if drug users know the date of an upcoming urine test they can abstain for a short period of time to get a clean result and then go back to using afterward.

### Saliva Tests

At $15 to $75 per test, saliva tests are cost effective, easy to administer, and they are not seen by sample givers to be as much of a violation of privacy as urine tests often are. Like urine tests, they can be done at any location, but results must be verified by a lab. Saliva tests are growing in popularity and can detect more recent drug use than other testing methods, especially use in the past few days. They are good at detecting methamphetamine and opiates, but less reliable for THC and cannabinoids found in marijuana.

### Hair Tests

Hair and follicle tests cost about $100 to $150 to perform. They can give information on a person's drug use for the past 90 days rather than for just a few days or weeks, as with saliva or urine tests. These tests have a positive result a little more than twice as often as urine tests. Hair tests also do not have as many false positives for certain substances, such as poppy seed ingestion versus opiate abuse. The tests are also difficult to "game," since shampoos and other follicle-cleansing products have not been shown to reliably remove drug metabolites from hair.

Opiates (codeine, morphine, heroin) lay down on the hair shaft very tightly and are shown not to migrate along the shaft; thus, if a long segment of hair is available, one can draw some "relative" conclusions about when the use occurred. However, cocaine, although very easy to detect, is able to migrate along the shaft, making it very difficult to determine when the drug was used and for how long.

A drawback of hair tests is that they are not good at detecting very recent use, such as in the past week. While hair tests are not considered to be as much of an intrusion of privacy as urine tests, the amount of hair required for a sample is about the diameter of a pencil and 1.5 inches long.

### Blood Tests

Blood tests are the most expensive type of testing, and they are therefore the type least frequently used. They are considered the most intrusive method of testing, but also the most accurate.

The detection period is small— just hours or days, depending on the substance.

**Sources:** N. Koppel, "Suit Claims Public College's Drug Testing Policy is Unconstitutional," *Wall Street Journal*, September 15, 2011, http://blogs.wsj.com/law/2011/09/15/suit-claims-public-collegesdrug-testing-policy-is-unconstitutional/; The Vaults of EROWID, "Drug Testing Basics," September 27, 2012, www.erowid.org/psychoactives/testing/testing_info1.shtml.

---

drug testing. Despite controversies over accuracy of urinalysis tests, this practice is becoming more common.

All of these approaches will probably help up to a point, but they do not offer a total solution to the problem. Drug abuse has been a part of human behavior for thousands of years, and it is not likely to disappear in the near future. For this reason, it is necessary to educate ourselves and to develop the self-discipline necessary to avoid dangerous drug dependence.

For many years, the most popular antidrug strategy has been total prohibition. This approach has proved to be ineffective. Prohibition of alcohol during the 1920s created more problems than it solved, as did prohibition of opioids in 1914. A more recent campaign is commonly referred to as the "War on Drugs," undertaken by the U.S. government and other countries. This campaign includes laws and policies that are intended to discourage the production, distribution, and consumption of illicit substances. However, there are many critics to this program, which began in 1971 under President Richard Nixon.[142] The budget for the program in 1991 was $100 million; now it is 15.6 billion, 150 times the 1991 budget.[143] In 40 years, taxpayers have spent $1 trillion on the "War on Drugs" but it has not stopped the flow of drugs into the United States.[144]

In general, researchers in the field of drug education agree that a multimodal approach is best. Young people should be taught the difference between drug use, misuse, and abuse. Factual information that is free of scare tactics must be presented; lecturing and moralizing have proven not to work.

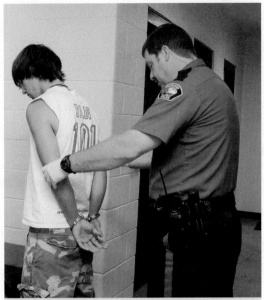

A high percentage of violent and nonviolent crime is linked to drug abuse, affecting not only the abuser but also entire communities.

**Harm Reduction Strategies** *Harm reduction* is a set of practical approaches to reducing negative consequences of drug use, incorporating a spectrum of strategies from safer use to abstinence. For example, needle exchange programs for injection drug users provide clean needles and syringes and bleach for cleaning needles; these efforts help reduce the number of HIV and hepatitis B cases. Harm reduction may also involve changing the legal sanctions associated with drug use, increasing the availability of treatment services to drug abusers, and/or attempting to change drug users' behavior through education. Harm reduction strategies meet drug users "where they're at," addressing conditions of use along with the use itself. This strategy recognizes that people always have and always will use drugs and, therefore, attempts to minimize the potential hazards associated with drug use rather than the use itself. It is an alternative to the moral/criminal and disease models of drug use and acknowledges that while abstinence is the ideal, anything that reduces use and harm to self and others is a positive outcome. It also emphasizes empowering users through helping them meet basic needs for shelter, safety, and food while assisting with least minimal services to provide a better chance for recovery.

# STUDY **PLAN**

Customize your study plan—and master your health!—in the Study Area of **MasteringHealth**.

## ASSESS YOURSELF

**Is your relationship with drugs unhealthy?** Take the **Learn to Recognize Drug Use and Potential Abuse** assessment available on

## MasteringHealth.™

## CHAPTER **REVIEW**

To hear an MP3 Tutor Session, scan here or visit the Study Area in **MasteringHealth**.

### LO **1** | Drug Dynamics

- Mood-altering substances and experiences produce biochemical reactions that make the body feel good; when absent, the person feels the effects of withdrawal.

### LO **2** | Types of Drugs

- The six categories of drugs are prescription drugs, over-the-counter (OTC) drugs, recreational drugs, herbal preparations, illicit drugs, and commercial drugs. Routes of administration include oral ingestion, inhalation, injection (intravenous, intramuscular, and subcutaneous), transdermal, and insertion of suppositories.

### LO **3** | Drug Misuse and Abuse

- OTC medications are drugs that do not require a prescription. Some OTC medications, including sleep aids, cold medicines, and diet pills, can be addictive.

- Prescription drug abuse is at an all-time high, particularly among college students. Only marijuana is more commonly abused. The most commonly abused prescription drugs are opioids/narcotics, depressants, and stimulants.

- People from all walks of life use illicit drugs, although college students report higher usage rates than do the general population. Drug use declined from the mid-1980s to the early 1990s, but has remained steady since then. However, among young people, use of drugs has been rising in recent years.

## LO 4 | Common Drugs of Abuse

- Drugs of abuse (both legal and illegal) include stimulants; cannabis products, including marijuana; narcotics/depressants; hallucinogens; inhalants; and anabolic steroids. Each has its own set of risks and effects.

## LO 5 | Treating and Reducing Drug Abuse

- Treatment begins with abstinence from the drug or addictive behavior, usually instituted through intervention by close family, friends, or other loved ones. Treatment programs may be outpatient or residential and may include individual, group, or family therapy, as well as 12-step programs.

## LO 6 | Addressing Drug Misuse and Abuse in the United States

- The drug problem reaches everyone through crime and elevated health care costs. Public health and governmental approaches to the problem involve regulation, enforcement, education, and harm reduction.

# POP QUIZ

Visit **MasteringHealth** to personalize your study plan with Chapter Review Quizzes and Dynamic Study Modules.

## LO 1 | Drug Dynamics

1. Drugs that have the potential to alter mood or behavior are called
   a. recreational drugs.
   b. psychoactive drugs.
   c. psychotic drugs.
   d. dopamine reactor drugs.

## LO 2 | Types of Drugs

2. Cross-tolerance occurs when
   a. drugs work at the same receptor site so that one blocks the action of the other.
   b. the effects of one drug are eliminated or reduced by the presence of another drug at the receptor site.
   c. a person develops a physiological tolerance to one drug and shows a similar tolerance to selected other drugs as a result.
   d. two or more drugs interact and the effects of the individual drugs are multiplied beyond what normally would be expected if they were taken alone.

3. Rebecca takes a number of medications for various conditions, including Prinivil (an antihypertensive drug), insulin (a diabetic medication), and Claritin (an antihistamine). This is an example of
   a. synergism.
   b. illegal drug use.
   c. polydrug use.
   d. antagonism.

4. The most common method for taking drugs is
   a. injection.
   b. inhalation.
   c. oral ingestion.
   d. transdermal.

## LO 3 | Drug Misuse and Abuse

5. The most commonly reported illicit drug used on college campuses is
   a. Aderall.
   b. marijuana.
   c. Ecstasy.
   d. tranquillizers.

## LO 4 | Common Drugs of Abuse

6. Which of the following is classified as a stimulant?
   a. Methamphetamine
   b. Alcohol
   c. Marijuana
   d. LSD

7. *Freebasing* is
   a. mixing cocaine with heroin.
   b. burning marijuana and inhaling smoke.
   c. injecting a drug into the veins.
   d. heating a drug and inhaling the vapor.

8. The psychoactive drug mescaline is found in what plant?
   a. Mushrooms
   b. Peyote cactus
   c. Marijuana
   d. Belladonna

## LO 5 | Treating and Reducing Drug Abuse

9. Generally, the first step in a drug treatment program is
   a. cognitive therapy.
   b. behavioral therapy.
   c. resocialization.
   d. detoxification.

## LO 6 | Addressing Drug Misuse and Abuse in the United States

10. Which of the following is an example of a *harm reduction strategy*?
    a. Providing clean needles and syringes to a heroin user
    b. Using scare tactics to show the negative consequences of drug use
    c. Enforcing antidrug laws
    d. Favoring longer prison sentences for drug dealers

*Answers to the Pop Quiz can be found on page A-1. If you answered a question incorrectly, review the section identified by the Learning Outcome. For even more study tools, visit* **MasteringHealth**.

# THINK ABOUT IT!

## LO 1 | Drug Dynamics

1. Why and how do drugs work? What are some of the different ways that different types of drugs interact with brain chemistry?

## LO 2 | Types of Drugs

2. Explain the terms *synergism*, *antagonism*, and *inhibition*.

## LO 3 | Drug Misuse and Abuse

3. Do you think there is such a thing as responsible use of illicit drugs? Would you change any of the current laws governing drugs?

How would you determine what is legitimate and illegitimate use?

4. Why do you think so many young people today are abusing prescription drugs? Do you perceive prescription drug abuse as being less dangerous or illegal than illicit drug use? Why? Do you think this is an accurate or biased perception?

### LO 4 | Common Drugs of Abuse

5. What accounts for the fact that some drugs are more addictive than others, chemically, culturally, and psychologically?

### LO 5 | Treating and Reducing Drug Abuse

6. What accounts for the fact that some drugs are more addictive than others, chemically, culturally, and psychologically?

### LO 6 | Addressing Drug Misuse and Abuse in the United States

7. What are the arguments for and against drug testing in the workplace? Would you apply for a job that had drug testing as an interview requirement? Why or why not?

8. What types of programs do you think would be effective in preventing drug abuse among high school and college students? How might programs for high school students differ from those for college students?

## ACCESS YOUR HEALTH ON THE INTERNET

Visit **MasteringHealth** for links to the websites and RSS feeds.

The following websites explore further topics and issues related to drug abuse.

**Club Drugs.** The website provides science-based information about club drugs.
**www.drugabuse.gov/drugs-abuse/club-drugs**

**Join Together.** An excellent site for the most current information related to substance abuse. Also includes information on alcohol and drug policy and provides advice on organizing and taking political action.
**www.drugfree.org/join-together**

**National Institute on Drug Abuse (NIDA).** The home page of this U.S. government agency has information on the latest statistics and findings in drug research.
**www.nida.nih.gov**

**Substance Abuse and Mental Health Services Administration (SAMHSA).** Outstanding resource for information about national surveys, ongoing research, and national drug interventions.
**www.samhsa.gov**

*[Handwritten margin notes:]*

male sperm pathway
- made in testis
- stored in epididymus
- moved to vas deferens
- seminal vesicle secretes liquid to semen
- pushed towards ejaculatory ducts
- prostate secretes and gives the force to ejac.

Male Left
1 bladder
2 pubic bone
3 vas deferens
4 corpus spongous
5 penis
6 urethra
7 glans
8 opening of urethra
9

Right
1 seminal vesicle
2 rectum
3 prostate gland
4 cowper gland
5 anus
6 embididymus
7 testis
8 scrotum

Ovum Pathway
- ovum made in ovary
- to fallopian tube
- sperm fertilizes
- zygote @ day 6
- moves towards uterus
- constantly splitting in ½
- becomes a blastocyst
- attaches to uterine lining
- Day 9/12 fully implanted.

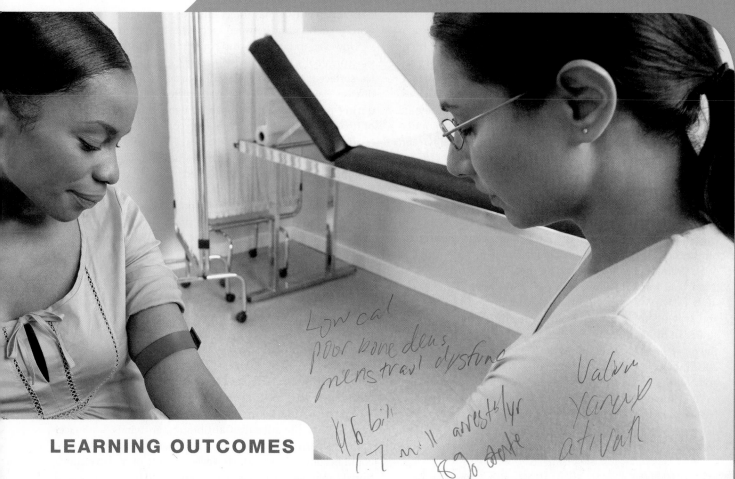

# 14 Protecting against Infectious Diseases

## LEARNING OUTCOMES

**LO 1** Describe the process of infection and the factors that increase your risk for infectious diseases.

**LO 2** Explain how your immune system protects you, factors that diminish its effectiveness, and what you can do to boost its effectiveness.

**LO 3** Describe the most common pathogens infecting humans today, key diseases caused by each, and the threat of growing antimicrobial resistance as well as individual- and community-based strategies for prevention and control of infectious diseases.

**P**athogens—disease-causing agents—are everywhere. We inhale them, swallow them, rub them in our eyes, and are constantly in a hidden, high-stakes battle with them. Although many pathogens have existed as long as there has been life on the planet, new varieties seem to emerge daily. Some infectious diseases, like the common cold, are **endemic**, meaning that they are present at expected prevalence rates in virtually all populations on Earth, with rates that rise and fall predictably each season.

When the number of cases of a disease increases, often suddenly, with higher than projected endemic numbers in a population area, it becomes an **epidemic**. Epidemics such as the *Black Death*, or *bubonic plague*, which killed up to one-third of the population of Europe in the 1300s, have occurred throughout history, and **pandemics**, or global epidemics, continue to cause premature death throughout the world.

In fact, humans have faced wave after wave of infectious diseases, wiping out civilizations, killing the most vulnerable, and leaving their mark on survivors. Particularly powerful strains of influenza have emerged several times in our history, the most notable of which was the "Spanish flu" of 1918–1919, affecting between 20 and 40 percent of the world's population and killing over 50 million people—675,000 of whom died in the United States. Vaccines and other preventive strategies have kept large-scale deaths from influenza strains in check for decades; however, several new strains have emerged—strains that could pose an ominous threat.

H1N1, also known as *swine flu*, became a global threat in 2009. This new version—"novel H1N1"—was notably different from past strains in that it was reported to have killed over 500,000 people globally—mainly young, otherwise healthy adults. Schools were closed, churches canceled services, and people feared the slightest cough or sneeze from others. In recent years, several potential variants of H1N1 have emerged, as well as fears that these typically nonhuman viruses may infect humans. Fortunately, the predictions of such a jump between species has not materialized.

However, in late 2015 and early 2016, reports of the explosive spread of a little-known virus in Central and South America surfaced. Known as the **Zika virus**, this mosquito-borne disease was reported to be transmitted by infected women during pregnancy, resulting in a higher than expected rate of babies born with *microcephaly*, a condition where a baby's head is smaller than others at birth. The World Health Organization estimates that 61 countries have reported infections, 1 million people are already infected in South America, and as many as 5 million additional people might be infected in 2016 as temperatures rise and mosquito populations increase.[1]

Recent concerns over possible sexual transmission of the disease and possible increased risk of *Guillain-Barré syndrome (GBS)*—a disorder in which the body's immune system attacks part of the peripheral nervous system—have surfaced. However, more research is needed before these are confirmed to be Zika related. Although the global community is mobilizing to kill mosquitos, reduce breeding grounds, and protect populations, cases are likely to increase in the months ahead as politicians in the United States stall on funding prevention as of July 2016.

New viruses, resistant bacteria, and resurgence of diseases we thought were controlled have many questioning our progress in preventing, controlling, and treating today's infectious agents. With the advent of antibiotics, antivirals, and vaccinations, many envisioned a world where infectious diseases could become eradicated. However, in spite of massive educational campaigns, changes in sanitation and infection control, major investments in vaccinations, and newer generations of antibiotics, infectious diseases continue to be among the leading causes of death globally.

Fueled by media attention, worry over getting infected from others, from insects, from foods, and from other sources can result in **mysophobia** (or *germophobia*)—an obsessive fear of becoming infected with germs. Sales of masks and antimicrobial wipes, soaps, and cleansers have soared. Is all of this anxiety over germs really necessary? What are the most ominous threats that we currently face? How can we protect ourselves and our loved ones? What policies, agencies, and programs are currently in place to protect us? The old adage is probably the best advice: "To be forewarned (knowledgeable) is to be forearmed (prepared)."

---

**pathogen** A disease-causing agent.

**endemic** Describing a disease that is always present to some degree.

**epidemic** Disease outbreak that affects many people in a community or region at the same time.

**pandemic** Global epidemic of a disease.

**zika virus** Emerging threat from bite of Aedes mosquito in U.S. and globally, particularly for pregnant women.

**mysophobia** (or *germophobia*) An obsessive fear of becoming infected with germs.

# LO 1 | THE PROCESS OF INFECTION

Describe the process of infection and the factors that increase your risk for infectious diseases.

Despite constant bombardment by pathogens, our immune systems are usually adept at protecting us. Millions of *endogenous microorganisms* live in and on our bodies all the time, usually in a symbiotic, peaceful coexistence, and exposure to invading microorganisms helps us build resistance to various pathogens. Generally harmless to someone in good health, these organisms can cause serious health problems in those with weakened immune systems.

*Exogenous microorganisms* are those that do not normally inhabit the body. When these pathogens gain entry into the body, they are apt to produce an infection or illness. The more easily these pathogens can gain a foothold in the body and sustain themselves, the more **virulent**, or aggressive, they may be in causing disease. By keeping your immune system strong, you increase your ability to resist and fight off even the most virulent pathogen.

## Three Conditions Needed for Infection

Most infectious diseases are *multifactorial*, or caused by the interaction of several factors inside and outside the person. For an **infection** to occur, three key conditions known as the **epidemiological triad of disease** (**FIGURE 14.1**), must be met. First, the person, or *host, must come into contact with a pathogen* (infectious agent) able to overcome the body's elaborate defenses and must be capable of sustaining itself long enough to cause an infection.

Second, the *host must be susceptible*, or in some way vulnerable to infection. In other words, the pathogen must be so virulent that it overcomes a typical healthy immune system, or, in an **opportunistic infection**, a normal pathogen overcomes an **immunocompromised** immune system—one that has been weakened or is nonfunctional. As an example, a person on anti-rejection drugs due to an organ transplant may be severely immunocompromised and vulnerable

**virulent** Strong enough to overcome host resistance and cause disease.

**infection** The state of pathogens being established in or on a host and causing disease.

**epidemiological triad of disease** The process explaining how a disease is likely to occur, including characteristics of the host (health of immune system, etc.), the agent (pathogen and its virulence), and the environment (whether conditions are conducive to spread)

**opportunistic infection** An infection that occurs when the immune system is vulnerable and the organism is able to gain a foothold in the body.

**immunocompromised** A condition in which the immune system becomes weakened and vulnerable to pathogens entering and gaining a foothold in the body.

**autoinoculate** Transmit a pathogen from one part of your body to another part.

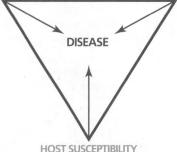

**HOSPITABLE ENVIRONMENT**
- Temperature
- Moisture/humidity
- Light
- Infection control protocols
- Ventilation/materials
- Building design/surface

**AGENT INFECTIVITY**
- Virulence
- Ability to breech body defenses
- Unique pathogen characteristics

**DISEASE**

**HOST SUSCEPTIBILITY**
- Genetics
- Smoking
- Age
- Diabetes
- Stress
- Lack of sleep
- HIV or AIDS
- Presence of other diseases
- Organ transplants
- Nutritional status
- Chemical exposures
- Long-term use of steroids
- Chemotherapy

**FIGURE 14.1 Epidemiological Triad of Disease** For a disease to occur, the agent, host, and environment must be conducive to overcoming the body's elaborate defense systems.

**VIDEO TUTOR**
Chain of Infection

to any number of pathogens, be they lurking in a hospital room or carried in on the hands or cough of well-wishing visitors.

Finally, the *environment must be hospitable* to the pathogen in terms of temperature, light, moisture, and other requirements. Although pathogens pose a threat if they gain entry and begin to grow in your body, the chances that they will do serious, long-term harm are actually quite small.

## Routes of Transmission

Pathogens may enter the body by *direct contact* between infected persons or by *indirect contact*, such as touching an

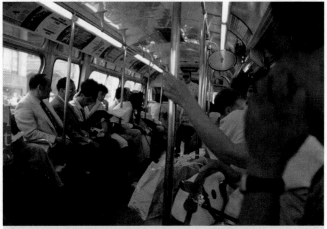

Crowded public transportation, trains, and airplanes are key areas where infectious diseases can be transmitted. Washing your hands and keeping hands from your face will help reduce risks.

## TABLE 14.1 | Routes of Disease Transmission

| Transmission Mode | Description |
|---|---|
| Contact | Either *direct* (e.g., skin or sexual contact) or *indirect* (e.g., infected blood or body fluid) |
| Foodborne or waterborne | Eating, drinking, washing, and unsanitary food preparation |
| Airborne | Infection spreads by inhaling droplets from an infected person's sneezes or coughs |
| Vector-borne | Blood-sucking insects such as mosquitoes, fleas, flies, or ticks pass along pathogens when they bite human victims |
| Perinatal | Similar to contact infection; happens in the uterus, as the baby passes through the birth canal, or through breastfeeding |

object an infected person has touched. **TABLE 14.1** lists common routes of transmission. You may also **autoinoculate** yourself, or transmit a pathogen from one part of your body to another—for example, by touching a herpes sore on your lip and then touching your eye.

Additionally, if you have pets, your "best friend" may be the source of *animal-borne (zoonotic) infections.* Although rare in occurrence, dogs, cats, livestock, and wild animals can directly or indirectly spread viruses, bacteria, parasites, and fungi to each other and to humans. Companion animals like cats and dogs can carry fleas and ticks into homes; when these insects bite humans, diseases such as *Lyme disease* can occur. Untreated puppies and dogs can be infested with worms that can be transmitted to humans via saliva, or through fecal residue on bedding, household carpets, or furniture. In 2015, when a form of influenza struck many dogs in the United States, people worried that they might get the flu from their dogs or transmit flu to their dogs. While some forms of influenza may be transmitted between humans and animals, this strain of influenza was not one of them. Although *interspecies transmission*—transmission between humans and animals— can occur, with rabies being one of the most well-known zoonotic diseases in the United States, vaccination of pets, basic hygiene around pets, and care in contact with animal fluids are all important parts of prevention.[2]

## Risk Factors You Can Control

Surrounded by pathogens, how can you be sure you don't get sick? Too much stress, poor diet, a low fitness level, lack of sleep, misuse or abuse of drugs, poor personal hygiene, and high-risk behavior significantly increase the risk for many diseases. In addition, college students are at higher risk because of their close living conditions; all these factors create higher risk for exposure to pathogens. The Making Changes Today box lists some actions you can take to minimize risk of infection.

## MAKING CHANGES TODAY

### Reduce Your Risk of Infectious Disease

As risks for infectious diseases increase and the threat of resistant pathogens is more likely, taking steps to prevent infection is ever more important. Practice the following on a regular basis to reduce your risk of infection.

- **Limit exposure to pathogens.** Don't drag yourself to classes or work and infect others when you are seriously ill. Also, don't share utensils or drinking glasses, and keep your toothbrush away from those of others. Keep hands away from your mouth, nose, and eyes. Use disposable tissues rather than reusable handkerchiefs.

- **Exercise regularly.** Regular exercise raises core body temperature and kills pathogens, and sweat and oil make the skin a hostile environment for many bacteria.

- **Get enough sleep.** Sleep allows the body time to refresh itself, produce necessary cells, and reduce inflammation. Even a single night without sleep can increase inflammatory processes and delay wound healing.

- **Stress less.** Rest and relaxation, stress management practices, laughter, and calming music have all been shown to promote healthy cellular activity and bolster immune functioning.

- **Optimize eating.** Enjoy a healthy diet, including adequate amounts of water, fruits and vegetables, protein, and complex carbohydrates. Eat more omega-3 fatty acids to reduce inflammation, and restrict saturated fats.

- **Get vaccinated.** Study the immunization schedule included in this chapter, assess your own vaccine history, and make sure you have the recommended shots in a timely manner.

## Risk Factors You Cannot Typically Control

Unfortunately, some risk factors for certain diseases are hard or impossible to control. The following are the most common:

- **Heredity.** Perhaps the single greatest factor influencing disease risk is genetics. It is often unclear whether hereditary diseases are due to inherited genetic traits or to inherited insufficiencies in the immune system. Some believe that we may inherit the quality of our immune system, thus some people are naturally more resistant to disease and infection.

- **Age.** Thinning of the skin, reduced sweating, and other physical changes can make people more susceptible to disease as they age. The very young also tend to be particularly vulnerable to infectious diseases.

- **Environmental conditions.** A growing body of research points to climate change as a major contributor to infectious diseases. As temperatures rise, insect populations may rise, potentially increasing cases of mosquito-borne diseases such as *malaria, dengue fever, chikungunya virus*, and others. *Malaria* infects over 303 million people in the world today, killing as many as 635,000 each year—the majority of whom are children in Africa.[3] *Chikungunya*, a viral disease, is prevalent in many tropical regions of the world. However, an estimated 700 cases are diagnosed in the United States each year.[4] *Dengue fever*—caused by any one of four mosquito-borne viruses that can result in severe flu-like symptoms and death—has increased dramatically in the global community, with up to 100 million new cases per year, primarily in Asian and Latin American countries.[5] Although cases have been reported in Hawaii, Puerto Rico, and the southernmost areas of the United States, most cases are contracted by travelling to tropical areas where the disease is endemic.[6]

  Dwindling water supplies, or areas where there is little water turnover or flow, contribute to more concentrated pathogen growth. When animals move to new environments in search of water and congregate near water sources, they are exposed to new species of animals with a new set of pathogens. In these environments, disease spreads quickly, as animals may have no acquired resistance to these particular pathogens. Scientists argue that changing environmental conditions—such as hurricanes, drought, flooding, fires, and other events—may increase the rate of disease spread, lead to newer variants of pathogens, and hasten interspecies transmission potential for humans.[7]

  Chronic exposure to toxic chemicals found in pesticides, herbicides, mercury, and lead and other threats such as radiation exposure can damage the immune system and lead to one becoming immunocompromised. Toxic substances can lead to immune system malfunction, hypersensitivity, and other reactions that can increase risks of infection. When the immune system begins to lose effectiveness, infectious disease rates can rise dramatically.[8]

- **Organism virulence and resistance.** Even tiny numbers of a particularly virulent organism may make the hardiest of us ill. Other organisms have mutated and become resistant to the body's defenses and to medical treatments. This kind of **drug resistance** occurs when pathogens grow and proliferate in the presence of chemicals that would normally slow growth or kill them. See the Health Headlines box on page 390 for more on antibiotic and antimicrobial resistance and superbugs.

## LO 2 | YOUR BODY'S DEFENSES AGAINST INFECTION

**Explain how your immune system protects you, factors that diminish its effectiveness, and what you can do to boost its effectiveness.**

To gain entry into your body, pathogens must overcome barriers that prevent them from entering, mechanisms that weaken organisms, and substances that counteract the threat that these organisms pose. **FIGURE 14.2** on page 391 summarizes some of the body's defenses against invasion and disease.

## Physical and Chemical Defenses

Our most critical early defense system is the skin. Layered to provide an intricate web of barriers, the skin allows few pathogens to enter. Enzymes in body secretions such as sweat provide additional protection, destroying microorganisms on skin surfaces by producing inhospitable pH levels. Only through cracks or breaks in the skin can pathogens gain easy access to the body.

The internal linings, structures, and secretions of the body provide another layer of protection. Mucous membranes in the respiratory tract, for example, trap and engulf invading organisms. Cilia, hairlike projections in the lungs and respiratory tract, sweep invaders toward body openings, where they are expelled. Nose hairs trap airborne invaders with a sticky film. Tears, earwax, and other secretions contain enzymes that destroy or neutralize pathogens.

## How the Immune System Works

*Immunity* is a condition of being able to resist a particular disease by counteracting the substance that produces the disease. Humans have two major forms of immune system activity: innate immunity and adaptive immunity. What are they and how do they work?

Essentially when a pathogen invades, *innate immunity* is the first line of defense. It is a fast, *nonspecific*, and generic attempt to prevent or knock out an invader. It goes to work within minutes and responds to common characteristics of an invader. Physical and chemical defenses, described previously, as well as cells that disable or kill invaders are all spurred to action.

*Adaptive immunity* takes more time to kick into action (2 to 3 days, for example), but is *more specific* to the threat. Lymphocytes and B and T cells target aspects of the invading organism and work to knock it out. A person who gets sufficient sleep (see Chapter 4) and prevents or controls stress (see Chapter 3) is more likely

**drug resistance** The ability of pathogens to resist the effects of drugs, meaning the germs grow and proliferate.

**WHAT DO YOU THINK?**

What are your current risks for infectious disease? Do you have any health risks that might make your risk of contracting an infectious disease more likely? Do you have any that are the result of your lifestyle?

- What infectious diseases are you concerned about getting right now on campus? What actions can you take to reduce your risks?
- Do you know where you can go to be tested for infectious diseases? What behaviors do you or your friends engage in that might make you more susceptible to various infections?
- Are your risks greater today than before you entered college? Why or why not?

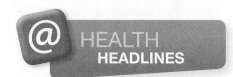

# ANTIBIOTIC RESISTANCE
*Bugs versus Drugs*

Bacteria evolve and develop ways to survive drugs that previously killed them. Some microorganisms that were easily dealt with a few decades ago are becoming "superbugs" that cannot be stopped with existing medications.

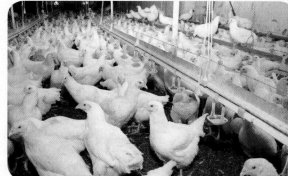

Widespread use of antibiotics in industrial food production (factory farms) has been a key factor in antibiotic resistance.

## Why is Antibiotic Resistance on the Rise?

- **Overuse of antibiotics in food production.** About 70 percent of antibiotic production today is ingested by animals or fish living in crowded feedlots or fish farms to encourage their growth and fight off disease. Water runoff and sewage from feedlots can contaminate the water in rivers and streams with antibiotics. Antibiotic-resistant bacteria may also spread beyond farms via dried particles of animal manure that disperse in the wind.

- **Improper use of antibiotics by people** In the past, doctors were more inclined to give a patient antibiotics for ear infections, colds, and other ailments without verifying that bacteria was the true cause of the complaint and therefore a useful treatment. The Centers for Disease Control and Prevention (CDC) estimates that one-third of the 150 million antibiotic prescriptions written each year are unnecessary, resulting in bacterial strains that are tougher than the drugs used to fight them. As resistance has become more widespread, many more doctors are asking patients to hold off on antibiotics to see if the problem will clear up without them.

- **Misuse and overuse of antibacterial soaps and other cleaning products.** Preying on the public's fear of germs and disease, the cleaning industry adds antibacterial ingredients to many soaps and household products. Just how much these products contribute to overall resistance is difficult to assess; as with antibiotics, the germs these products do not kill may become stronger than before.

## What Can You Do?

- **Be responsible with medications.** Don't pressure your provider to give you something to fix an ailment when they may not be sure about the cause. Use antibiotics only when prescribed for you and for the disease for which they are intended. Antibiotics are often specific and what might treat one illness may have no effect on another. Ask your doctor if there is an older-generation antibiotic that still works to treat the illness and save the newer drugs for the most difficult problems.

- **If you get a prescription, complete the full treatment as prescribed, even though you may not note any symptoms.** Antibiotic regimens are designed to kill entire colonies of bacteria if taken exactly as prescribed. If you stop early, the hardiest may survive, leading to increased chances of drug-resistant pathogens. Don't dump unused drugs down the toilet or sink or give to friends. If you don't know where to take them, talk to your local pharmacist or waste disposal company

- **Use regular soap when washing your hands.** Research suggests that antibacterial agents contained in soaps actually may kill normal bacteria found on the skin that does not cause disease, thus creating an environment for resistant, mutated bacteria that are impervious to antibacterial cleaners and antibiotics to colonize the skin.

- **Avoid food treated with antibiotics.** Know where your food comes from. Buy organic meat and poultry, particularly those products that say that they have not been fed antibiotics or hormones. Look for farmed fish grown in U.S. coastal waters, where there is less likelihood of questionable fish-feeding practice and less chance of contaminated water and antibiotics or growth hormones.

**Sources:** CDC, "Fast Facts: Get Smart about Antibiotics," March 2016. www.cdc.gov/getsmart/community/about/index.html; WHO, "WHO's First Global Report on Antibiotic Resistance Reveals Serious, Worldwide Threat to Public Health," April 2014, http://www.who.int/mediacentre/news/releases/2014/amr-report/en/; CDC, "About Antimicrobial Resistance," September 8, 2015, http://www.cdc.gov/drugresistance/about.html.

---

**antigen** Substance capable of triggering an immune response.

**antibodies** Substances produced by the body that are individually matched to specific antigens.

**humoral immunity** Aspect of immunity that is mediated by antibodies secreted by white blood cells.

**toxins** Poisonous substances produced by certain microorganisms that cause various diseases.

to have an immune system primed to resist disease, even when bombarded with pathogens 24/7.

Any substance capable of triggering an immune response—a virus, a bacterium, a fungus, a parasite, a toxin, or a tissue or cell from another organism, or even chemicals from the environment—is called an **antigen**. When a pathogen breaches initial, outer defenses, the body first analyzes the antigen, verifying that it isn't part of the body itself. It then responds by forming **antibodies** specific to that antigen, much as a key is matched to a lock. Specific to each antigen, antibodies are designed to destroy or weaken the antigen. This process is part of a system called *humoral immune responses*. **Humoral immunity** uses antibodies to inactivate an antigen and is the body's major defense against many bacteria and the poisonous substances—**toxins**—they produce.

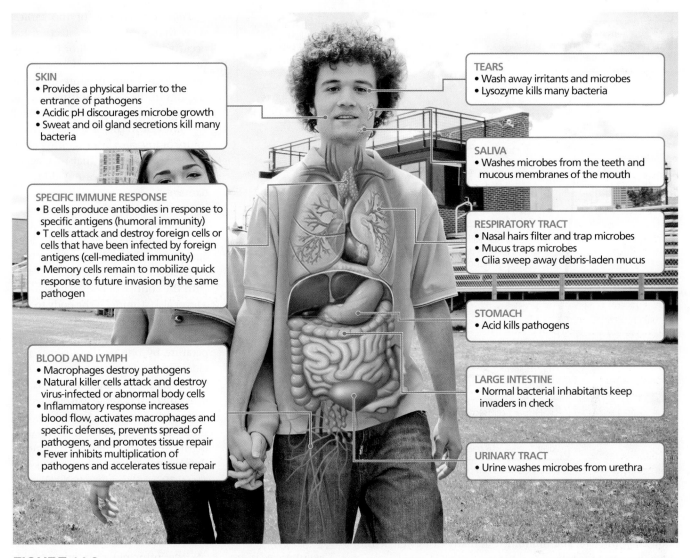

**SKIN**
- Provides a physical barrier to the entrance of pathogens
- Acidic pH discourages microbe growth
- Sweat and oil gland secretions kill many bacteria

**SPECIFIC IMMUNE RESPONSE**
- B cells produce antibodies in response to specific antigens (humoral immunity)
- T cells attack and destroy foreign cells or cells that have been infected by foreign antigens (cell-mediated immunity)
- Memory cells remain to mobilize quick response to future invasion by the same pathogen

**BLOOD AND LYMPH**
- Macrophages destroy pathogens
- Natural killer cells attack and destroy virus-infected or abnormal body cells
- Inflammatory response increases blood flow, activates macrophages and specific defenses, prevents spread of pathogens, and promotes tissue repair
- Fever inhibits multiplication of pathogens and accelerates tissue repair

**TEARS**
- Wash away irritants and microbes
- Lysozyme kills many bacteria

**SALIVA**
- Washes microbes from the teeth and mucous membranes of the mouth

**RESPIRATORY TRACT**
- Nasal hairs filter and trap microbes
- Mucus traps microbes
- Cilia sweep away debris-laden mucus

**STOMACH**
- Acid kills pathogens

**LARGE INTESTINE**
- Normal bacterial inhabitants keep invaders in check

**URINARY TRACT**
- Urine washes microbes from urethra

**FIGURE 14.2** The Body's Defenses against Disease-Causing Pathogens. To protect against a steady onslaught by pathogens, the body has developed an elaborate defense system to keep invaders out!

In **cell-mediated immunity**, specialized white blood cells called **lymphocytes** attack and destroy the foreign invader. Lymphocytes constitute the body's main defense against viruses, fungi, parasites, and some bacteria, and they are found in the blood, lymph nodes, bone marrow, and certain glands. Another key player in this immune response are **macrophages** (a type of phagocytic, or cell-eating, white blood cell).

Two forms of lymphocytes in particular, the *B lymphocytes* (B cells) and *T lymphocytes* (T cells), are involved in the immune response. *Helper T cells* are essential for activating B cells to produce antibodies. They also activate other T cells and macrophages. *Killer T cells* directly attack infected or malignant cells. *Suppressor T cells* turn off or suppress the activity of B cells, killer T cells, and macrophages. After a successful attack on a pathogen, some attacker T and B cells are preserved as *memory T and B cells*, enabling the body to recognize and respond quickly to subsequent attacks by the same kind of organism. Once people have survived certain infectious diseases, they will likely not develop them again. **FIGURE 14.3** provides a summary of the cell-mediated immune response.

## When the Immune System Misfires: Autoimmune Diseases

Sometimes the process for recognizing (and ignoring) the body's own cells goes awry, and the immune system targets its own tissues. This is known as **autoimmune disease** (*auto* means "self"). Common autoimmune disorders include *rheumatoid arthritis*, *lupus*, *type 1 diabetes*, and *multiple sclerosis*. However, there are over 80 different types of autoimmune diseases that affect humans, with millions of new cases occurring each year. In these cases, people's *autoantibodies*—proteins made by the immune system—fail to recognize "self"

**cell-mediated immunity** Aspect of immunity that is mediated by specialized white blood cells that attack pathogens and antigens directly.

**lymphocyte** A type of white blood cell involved in the immune response.

**macrophage** A type of white blood cell that ingests foreign material.

**autoimmune disease** Disease caused by an overactive immune response against the body's own cells.

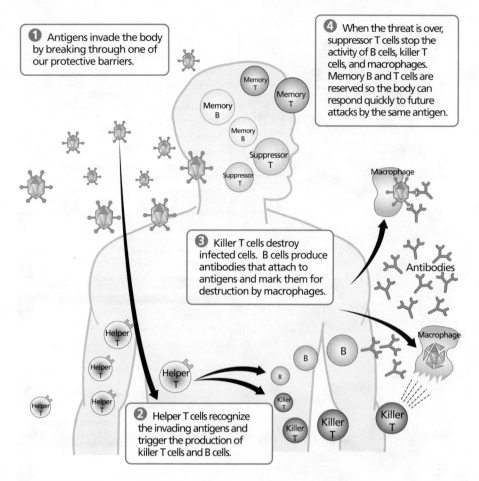

① Antigens invade the body by breaking through one of our protective barriers.

④ When the threat is over, suppressor T cells stop the activity of B cells, killer T cells, and macrophages. Memory B and T cells are reserved so the body can respond quickly to future attacks by the same antigen.

③ Killer T cells destroy infected cells. B cells produce antibodies that attach to antigens and mark them for destruction by macrophages.

② Helper T cells recognize the invading antigens and trigger the production of killer T cells and B cells.

Memory T
Memory T
Memory B
Memory B
Suppressor T
Suppressor T
Macrophage
Antibodies
Macrophage
Helper T
Helper T
Helper T
Helper T
Helper T
Helper T
B
B
B
Killer T
Killer T
Killer T
Killer T

**FIGURE 14.3** The Cell-Mediated Immune Response

and attack the body's own tissues. The presence of autoantibodies can indicate autoimmunity, in many cases well before the symptoms of autoimmune diseases actually begin.[9]

Many autoimmune diseases can be chronic, debilitating, and life-threatening. They can affect virtually any part of the body and cause disability and death. Although the above diseases are among the most common, other serious autoimmune diseases include psoriasis, Graves' disease, multiple sclerosis, Guillain-Barré syndrome, celiac disease, Crohn's disease, and inflammatory and irritable bowel syndrome. Many people do not realize that autoimmune diseases are among the leading causes of death in female children and women under the age of 65 in the United States.[10] (See Chapter 18.)

## Inflammatory Response, Pain, and Fever

If an infection is localized, pus formation, redness, swelling, and irritation often occur. These symptoms are components of the body's inflammatory response and indicate the invading organisms are being fought. The four cardinal signs of inflammation are *redness, swelling, pain, and heat.*

**vaccination** Inoculation with killed or weakened pathogens or similar, less dangerous antigens, in order to prevent or lessen the effects of some disease.

*Pain* is often one of the earliest signs that an injury or infection has occurred. Pathogens kill or injure tissue at the site of infection, causing swelling that puts pressure on nerve endings in the area, resulting in pain. Although pain is unpleasant, it plays a valuable role in the body's response to injury or invasion by prompting a person to avoid activity that may aggravate the injury and cause additional damage.

In addition to *inflammation,* another frequent indicator of infection is *fever,* or a body temperature above the average norm of 98.6°F. Caused by toxins secreted by pathogens that interfere with the control of body temperature, a fever also stimulates the body to produce more white blood cells. A mild fever is protective; raising body temperature by one or two degrees provides an environment that destroys some disease-causing organisms. As fever increases, more pathogens are destroyed. However, for babies and small children, when a fever goes higher than 101°F, medical attention should be sought. When fevers rise above 103°F for adults, medical attention is warranted.

## Vaccines Bolster Immunity

**Vaccination** is based on the principle that once people have been exposed to a specific pathogen and had a successful immune response, subsequent attacks will activate their "immune memory" and allow them to fight the pathogen off in the future.

A vaccine consists of killed or weakened versions of a disease-causing microorganism or an antigen that is similar to but less dangerous than the disease antigen. The dose given produces antibodies against future attacks—without actually causing the disease (or by causing a very minor case of it). Vaccines typically are given orally or by injection, and this form of immunity is termed *artificially acquired active immunity,* in contrast to *naturally acquired active immunity* (which is obtained by exposure to antigens in the normal course of daily life) or

**75%**
of the 50 million Americans living and coping with **AUTOIMMUNE DISEASE** are women.

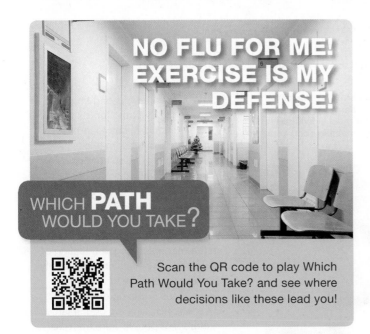

NO FLU FOR ME! EXERCISE IS MY DEFENSE!

WHICH **PATH** WOULD YOU TAKE?

Scan the QR code to play Which Path Would You Take? and see where decisions like these lead you!

*naturally acquired passive immunity* (as occurs when a mother passes immunity to her fetus via their shared blood supply or to an infant via breast milk).

Concern about the safety of vaccines among certain Americans has led to a drop in vaccination rates and subsequent outbreaks of serious diseases such as the measles and pertussis—diseases that have rarely been seen in the United States since vaccines first became available beginning in the 1950s and 1960s (see the **Health Headlines** box on page 394).

Specific vaccination schedules have been established for various population groups. See **TABLE 14.2** for recommended vaccines for teens and college students aged 19 to 26. **FIGURE 14.4** on page 395 shows the recommended vaccination schedule for the general adult population. Childhood vaccine schedules are available at the Centers for Disease Control and Prevention (CDC) website, as are requirements that vary by state.

## TABLE **14.2** | Recommended Vaccinations for Teens and College Students

- Tetanus-diphtheria-pertussis vaccine (Td/Tdap)
- Meningococcal vaccine (booster at age 16)
- HPV vaccine series
- Hepatitis B vaccine series
- Polio vaccine series
- Measles-mumps-rubella (MMR) vaccine series
- Varicella (chickenpox) vaccine series
- Influenza vaccine
- Pneumococcal polysaccharide (PPV) vaccine
- Hepatitis A vaccine series (for high-risk groups)

**Source:** CDC, "Preteen and Teen Vaccines," July 2014, www.cdc.gov/vaccines/who/teens/vaccines/index.html; CDC, "Vaccine Information for Adults," September 2014, www.cdc.gov/vaccines/adults/rec-vac/index.html.

Because of their close living quarters, high stress levels, poor sleep habits, increased alcohol consumption, and possible sexual interactions, college students face a higher-than-average risk of infection from largely preventable diseases. Some of these are vaccine preventable and need to be updated annually, such as the flu vaccine; others require boosters because their effectiveness may begin to fade over time. Sometimes, newer vaccines are available that were not available when you or your parents were children. Also, as you age, you may become more susceptible to certain diseases, such as the flu, pneumococcus, and shingles. If you have questions or think someone you know should have a particular vaccine, talk with your doctor or encourage them to talk to their doctor. Vaccines that should be a high priority among 20-somethings and college students include *tetanus-diphtheria-pertussis vaccine (Tdap)*, *meningococcal conjugate vaccine (MenACWY)*, *human papillomavirus (HPV)*, and the yearly *influenza vaccine.*[11]

Although vaccines are generally safe for most people, there are some special situations where vaccines may not be advisable, such as an allergy to a vaccine component. Before getting any vaccine, be sure to talk with your doctor about potential complications.

Additionally, if you are traveling to certain regions of the world, you may need additional vaccines to stay safe. Some campuses have travel docs who will provide this key information. The CDC website also has current advisories around vaccinations recommended and required when traveling to different regions.

## LO **3** | **TYPES** OF PATHOGENS AND THE DISEASES THEY CAUSE

Describe the most common pathogens infecting humans today, key diseases caused by each, and the threat of growing antimicrobial resistance as well as individual- and community-based strategies for prevention and control of infectious diseases.

Pathogens fall into six categories: *bacteria, viruses, fungi, protozoans, parasitic worms,* and *prions.* **FIGURE 14.5** on page 395 shows several examples. Each has a particular route of transmission and characteristic elements that make it unique. In the following pages, we discuss each of these categories and give an overview of some diseases they cause that have a significant impact on public health.

### Bacteria

**Bacteria** (singular: *bacterium*) are single-celled organisms that are found on virtually every surface of the earth. They cover plants and animals and are found in the deepest parts of the oceans, in the most remote forests, and in ice caps formed millions of years ago. They can live in frozen foods, survive high temperatures, and your body is teeming with them. While most are necessary and beneficial to life on the planet, some (over

**bacteria (singular: bacterium)** Simple, single-celled microscopic organisms; about 100 known species of bacteria cause disease in humans.

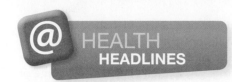

# VACCINE CONTROVERSY
## Should Parents be Allowed to Opt Out?

In 2000, the United States claimed victory over the measles, indicating that measles was no longer of concern on U.S. soil. In California last year, nearly 4 percent of children were allowed to skip measles vaccines. However, when a particularly nasty bout of measles was contracted in Disneyland, 169 people from over 20 states became ill. Most of those who got sick were unvaccinated. A 2014 outbreak of measles in Ohio among unvaccinated Amish children and the Disneyland outbreak has raised major concerns in many states.

In response, in 2015, California passed one of the strictest laws in the country, mandating vaccinations of all school-age children. Several other states are examining their own policies about exemptions as rates of unvaccinated children in Washington, Oregon, Colorado, Wisconsin, and other states have grown with corresponding increases in vaccine-preventable diseases. Washington State passed a law requiring a doctor's signature to opt out of vaccinations. As rates of measles, pertusssis, and other vaccine-preventable diseases skyrocket and large numbers of unvaccinated individuals travel to the United States, putting people at all ages and stages of life at risk, more states are considering the rights of parents versus rights of the population as a whole. In fact, vaccination percentages in 2015 were actually up in the United States overall, coming closer to the Healthy People 2020 national goal of a 95 percent vaccination rate. We still have a way to go until these rates reach this goal.

Immunizations against widespread infectious diseases are one of the greatest public health success stories of all time—so successful, in fact, that most people have never seen or heard of anyone having diseases such as smallpox that once wiped out entire populations. Today, fear of the old "killer" diseases has waned and been replaced with distrust of the vaccines themselves, leading to a growing trend for parents to opt out of vaccinations for their children, even though failure to vaccinate puts children and communities at risk.

**Some parents have concerns over vaccination safety, but research shows that vaccines are safe and effective for most individuals, as well as crucial for maintaining good community health.**

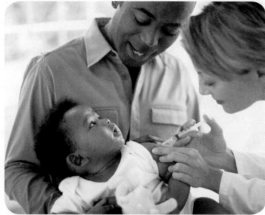

So why do people opt out? Typical reasons for vaccine exemptions include religious beliefs, personal beliefs, and medical reasons, while others consider vaccinations to be a government intrusion into their individual rights. In some states, exemptions have been as easy to get as checking a box on a form. With the proliferation of misleading information about supposed dangers of vaccination, many mistakenly believe that they are doing the right thing by avoiding some or all vaccines.

Undervaccination rates are particularly high in non-Hispanic, college-educated white families, with incomes above $75,000 a year and with health insurance. Although all 50 states require vaccinations, 48 states have religious or medical exemptions and several have personal belief options.

Much initial anxiety was fueled by an article in the medical journal *Lancet* in 1998, linking the MMR vaccine to increased risk of autism and bowel disease. The article prompted many to refuse the vaccine in the United States and elsewhere, and the resulting dropoff in immunizations led to increased cases of measles in many parts of the world. Over 10 years later, after a thorough investigation of ethical and factual issues with the research, *Lancet* retracted the article as being false. The lead author of the paper was later fired from his research position and had his license to practice revoked.

While research is ongoing, the Centers for Disease Control and Prevention (CDC) has found *no* evidence to substantiate claims that vaccines lead to conditions like autism, multiple sclerosis, or sudden infant death syndrome. Virtually all medical and public health organizations support vaccinations, pointing to stringent safety controls in the manufacturing and testing of vaccines, as well as ongoing safety monitoring and the long history of vaccines in wiping out killer diseases across the globe. If large numbers of people were to avoid vaccinations, old killers would be likely to reemerge, and those people who were already sick or weak from other conditions would be extremely vulnerable.

Today, the CDC's Immunization Safety Office monitors complaints and investigates potential problems with vaccines as they occur. Still, the danger of major complications from getting vaccinations is extremely low and generally pales in comparison to the effects of contracting the diseases that the vaccinations protect against. For an interactive and updated comparison of how your state compares to others on vaccine exemptions, see http://www.nvic.org/vaccine-laws/state-vaccine-requirements.aspx.

**Sources:** CDC, "Vaccine Coverage in the United States," February 2016, http://www.cdc.gov/vaccines/imz-managers/coverage/imz-coverage.html; R Seither et al., "Vaccination Coverage among Children in Kindergarten—United States, 2013–14 School Year," *Morbidity and Mortality Weekly Report* 63, no. 41 (2014): 913–20; CDC, "National Health Interview Survey," June 11, 2015, www.cdc.gov/nchs/nhis.htm; S. Omer et al., "Legislative Challenges to School Immunization Mandates, 2009–2012," *Journal of the American Medical Association* 3111, no. 6 (2014): 620–1; The Editors of the *Lancet*, "Retraction—Ileal-Lymphoid-Nodular Hyperplasia, Non-specific Colitis, and Pervasive Development Disorder in Children," *Lancet* 375, no. 9713 (2010): 445; S. Bean, "Vaccine Beliefs of Complementary and Alternative Medical (CAM) Providers in Oregon," Doctoral dissertation, Oregon State University, May 2014; CDC, "State School and Childcare Vaccination Laws," March 2015, http://www.cdc.gov/phlp/publications/topic/vaccinations.html.

| Vaccine | 19–21 years | 22–26 years | 27–49 years | 50–59 years | 60–64 years | 65+ years |
|---|---|---|---|---|---|---|
| Influenza (Flu)[1] | Get a flu vaccine every year | | | | | |
| Tetanus, diphtheria, pertussis (Td/Tdap)[2] | Get a Tdap vaccine once, then a Td booster vaccine every 10 years | | | | | |
| Varicella (Chickenpox)[3] | 2 doses | | | | | |
| HPV Vaccine for Women[3,4] | 3 doses | | | | | |
| HPV Vaccine for Men[3,4] | 3 doses | 3 doses | | | | |
| Zoster (Shingles)[5] | | | | | 1 dose | |
| Measles, mumps, rubella (MMR)[3] | 1 or 2 doses | | | | | |
| Pneumococcal (PCV13)[7] | 1 dose | | | | | 1 dose |
| Pneumococcal (PPSV23)[7] | 1 or 2 doses | | | | | 1 dose |
| Meningococcal | 1 or more doses | | | | | |
| Hepatitis A[3] | 2 or 3 doses | | | | | |
| Hepatitis B[3] | 3 doses | | | | | |
| *Haemophilus influenzae* type b (Hib) | 1 or 3 doses | | | | | |

1. Influenza vaccine: There are several flu vaccines available—talk to your health care professional about which flu vaccine is right for you.

2. Td/Tdap vaccine: Pregnant women are recommended to get tdap vaccine with each pregnancy in the third trimester to increase protection for infants who are too young for vaccination, but at highest risk for severe illness and death from pertussis (whooping cough). People who have not had Tdap vaccine since age 11 should get a dose of Tdap followed by TD booster doses every 10 years.

3. Varicella, HPV, MMR, hepatitis A, hepatitis B vaccine: These vaccines are needed for adults who didn't get these vaccines when they were children.

4. HPV vaccine: There are two HPV vaccines, but only one, HPV (Gardasil), should be given to men. Gay men or men who have sex with men who are 22 through 26 years old should get HPV vaccine if they haven't already started or completed the series.

5. Zoster vaccine: You should get the zoster vaccine even if you've had shingles.

6. MMR vaccine: If you were born in 1957 or after, and don't have a record of being vaccinated or having had these infections, talk to your health care professional about how many doses you may need.

7. Pneumococcal vaccine: There are two different types of pneumococcal vaccines: PCV13 and PPSV23. Talk with your health care professional to find out if one or both pneumococcal vaccines are recommneded for you.

**If you travel outside of the United States, you may need additional vaccines. Ask your health care professional which vaccines you may need.**
**For more information, call toll free 1-800-CDC-INFO (1-800-232-4636) or visit http://www.cdc.gov/vaccines**

Recommended for all adults who have not been vaccinated, unless your health care professional tells you that you cannot safely receive the vaccine or that you do not need it.

Recommended for adults with certain risks related to their health, job or lifestyle that put them at higher risk for serious diseases. Talk to your halth care professional to see if you are at higher risk.

No recommendation

**FIGURE 14.4** Recommended Adult Immunization Schedule, by Vaccine and Age Group, 2016

**Source:** Centers for Disease Control and Prevention, "Recommended Adult Immunization Schedule—United States, 2016," Updated February 2016, http://www.cdc.gov/vaccines/schedules/downloads/adult/adult-schedule.pdf.

**Note:** Important explanations and additions to these recommendations should be checked by consulting the latest schedule at *www.cdc.gov*.

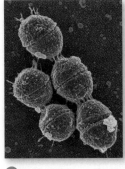 **a** Bacteria
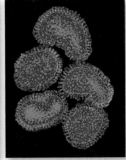 **b** Viruses
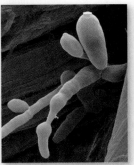 **c** Fungi
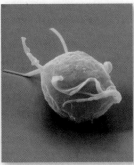 **d** Protozoan
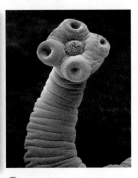 **e** Parasitic worm

**FIGURE 14.5** **Examples of Major Types of Pathogens** (a) Color-enhanced scanning electron micrograph (SEM) of *Streptococcus* bacteria, magnified 40,000×. (b) Colored transmission electron micrograph (TEM) of influenza (flu) viruses, magnified 32,000×. (c) Color SEM of *Candida albicans*, a yeast fungus, magnified 50,000×. (d) Color TEM of *Trichomonas vaginalis*, a protozoan, magnified 9,000×. (e) Color-enhanced SEM of a tapeworm, magnified 50×.

**antibiotics** Medicines used to kill microorganisms, such as bacteria.

**antibiotic/antimicrobial resistance** The ability of microbes to resist the effects of drugs, meaning the germs grow and proliferate.

**staphylococci** A group of round bacteria, usually found in clusters, that cause a variety of diseases in humans and other animals.

100 are known) are dangerous or deadly to humans. These unfriendly bacteria are the ones we focus on here.

There are three major types of bacteria, classified by shape: *cocci*, *bacilli*, and *spirilla*. Often it is not actually the bacteria themselves that cause disease symptoms, but rather the toxins they produce.

## Antibiotic and Antimicrobial Resistance

Since the development of penicillin in 1928 by Alexander Fleming, bacteria were in a losing battle with their enemy: **antibiotics**. With each decade thereafter, newer, more potent, and more specialized antibiotics decimated generation after generation of bacterial diseases. Because many doctors prescribed antibiotics for things they were not designed to treat, and because patients didn't take others as they were instructed, generations of bacteria survived weaker than necessary antibiotic treatments.

They mutated, changed, and developed into "superbugs" that could overcome many of the drugs originally used to fight them. These resistant pathogens have grown stronger with each generation.

Today **antibiotic/antimicrobial resistance**—the ability of microbes to resist the effects of drugs, to grow and proliferate, even in the face of our best weapons—is one of the world's most pressing problems.[12] It is estimated that primary care doctors, physician assistants, nurse practitioners, and dentists provide over 215 courses of antibiotic prescriptions in outpatient settings each year, making up nearly 60 percent of all antibiotics prescribed.[13] Our current arsenal of antibiotics is becoming less effective and our supply of weapons declines each year. FIGURE 14.6 outlines the ways that antibiotic resistance spreads.

## Staphylococcal Infections
Staphylococci are present on the skin or in the nostrils of up to 30 percent of us at any given time and usually cause no problems for otherwise healthy persons. The presence of bacteria on or in a person without infection is called **colonization**. A colonized person

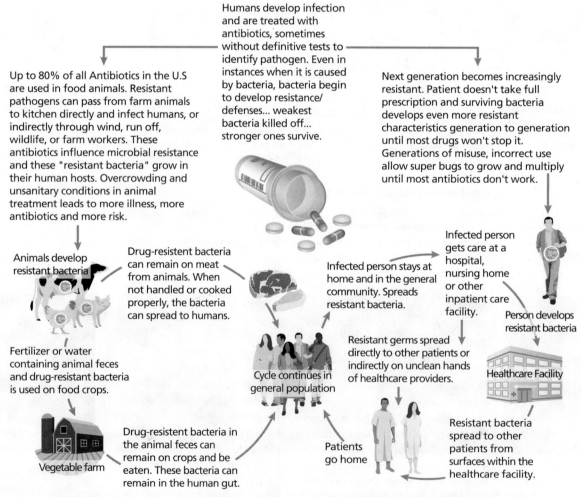

Humans develop infection and are treated with antibiotics, sometimes without definitive tests to identify pathogen. Even in instances when it is caused by bacteria, bacteria begin to develop resistance/ defenses... weakest bacteria killed off... stronger ones survive.

Up to 80% of all Antibiotics in the U.S are used in food animals. Resistant pathogens can pass from farm animals to kitchen directly and infect humans, or indirectly through wind, run off, wildlife, or farm workers. These antibiotics influence microbial resistance and these "resistant bacteria" grow in their human hosts. Overcrowding and unsanitary conditions in animal treatment leads to more illness, more antibiotics and more risk.

Next generation becomes increasingly resistant. Patient doesn't take full prescription and surviving bacteria develops even more resistant characteristics generation to generation until most drugs won't stop it. Generations of misuse, incorrect use allow super bugs to grow and multiply until most antibiotics don't work.

Animals develop resistant bacteria

Drug-resistent bacteria can remain on meat from animals. When not handled or cooked properly, the bacteria can spread to humans.

Infected person stays at home and in the general community. Spreads resistant bacteria.

Infected person gets care at a hospital, nursing home or other inpatient care facility.

Person develops resistant bacteria

Fertilizer or water containing animal feces and drug-resistant bacteria is used on food crops.

Cycle continues in general population

Resistant germs spread directly to other patients or indirectly on unclean hands of healthcare providers.

Healthcare Facility

Vegetable farm

Drug-resistent bacteria in the animal feces can remain on crops and be eaten. These bacteria can remain in the human gut.

Patients go home

Resistant bacteria spread to other patients from surfaces within the healthcare facility.

FIGURE 14.6 **How Antibiotic Resistance Spreads** Adapted from CDC, "About Antimicrobial Resistance: Examples of How Antibiotic Resistance Spreads," September 8, 2015, http://www.cdc.gov/drugresistance/about.html.

may spread the bacteria to others, some of whom may develop infections, yet never develop the disease. For example, colonized persons can inadvertently touch their nose without a tissue and spread those bacteria on a door handle or steering wheel, potentially infecting the next person who touches these spots. Likewise, when the pathogen is present on the skin surface, a cut or break in the skin can allow it to gain entry to the body, where infection develops. If you have ever suffered from acne, boils, sties (infections of the eyelids), or infected wounds, you have probably had a "staph" infection. If you pick at pimples and don't wash your hands, you can transmit those same bacteria to your eyes and autoinocculate yourself, or you can pass those bacteria on to other people. If you floss your teeth and don't wash your hands afterward, your hands may be teeming with bacteria and other organisms that could infect others. Simple changes in your personal hygiene, such as limiting tooth flossing to the bathroom only and having a ready supply of hand soap available, can make a huge difference in reducing risk.

One form of staph, **methicillin-resistant** *Staphylococcus aureus* (MRSA), has come under intense international scrutiny as numerous cases have arisen around the world, especially in the United States. As the name implies, this bacteria has grown resistant to the class of drugs normally used to treat staph infections. Symptoms of MRSA infection often start with a rash or pimple-like skin irritation. Within hours, early symptoms may progress to redness, inflammation, pain, and deeper wounds. If untreated, MRSA may invade the blood, bones, joints, surgical wounds, heart valves, and lungs, and it can be fatal.

In the last decade, *health care–associated* or *health care–acquired MRSA* has been one of the leading **health care–associated infections (HAIs)** in the United States, being found in significant numbers in hospitals, nursing homes, and clinics where invasive treatments, infectious pathogens, and weakened immune systems converge. Today, significant numbers of patients continue to get HAIs while in treatment; many suffer costly, prolonged stays due to these illnesses; and over 75,000 die.[14] Common HAI infections include pneumonia, urinary tract infections, *sepsis* (bloodstream infections), surgical site infections, and gastrointestinal infections.[15] Many of the deaths related to HAIs were among patients with HA-MRSA, even though rates are on the decline due to intensive infection control methods.[16] While HA-MRSA is on the decline, *community-acquired MRSA (CA-MRSA)* is on the rise in the home, workplace, and other communities. Although the exact number of persons with CA-MRSA is not known, studies show that about 1 in 3 people carry staph in their nose, usually without any illness. Two in 100 people carry MRSA.[17]

Often, CA-MRSA appears as a skin infection that becomes red, inflamed, painful and may be filled with pus or fluids. The initial irritated spot is often mistaken for a spider bite or boil, or an infection due to some type of injury, such as a cut or infected hair follicle. Although it can occur anywhere, irritation often appears in the groin area, beard, buttocks, underarm areas, or on the scalp. Because the initial site of infection may look like other things, many delay treatment until later in the infection process and unknowingly infect others.

Prevention of CA-MRSA involves keeping the hands away from the nose (since the nose often harbors the staph organism) and not touching areas such as gym equipment, towels, the skin of others, and other places where these pathogens may be deposited. Handwashing, good personal hygiene, not sharing razors, hankies, towels, pillows, or other personal products in the home, sanitizing gym equipment, and careful attention to unusual sores on the body are all part of risk reduction. Additionally, be sure to wash clothing that comes in contact with seats in high-use athletic facilities with each visit, and wash your hands thoroughly before leaving the facility.

Another type of MRSA appears to be spread among people who work closely with livestock in many regions of the world and is known as *livestock-associated MRSA*, or LA-MRSA.

*Clostridium Difficile* Another highly resistant bacterial pathogen that causes significant problems is *C-diff* or *C. difficile*. Symptoms commonly include major inflammation of the colon, complete with watery diarrhea, fever, pain, bloating, and nausea. Ironically, the antibiotics used to treat bacterial infection are the major cause of *C. diff* development; when long-term antibiotic use occurs, some of the good bacteria that help keep the system running smoothly are often killed. Older adults, particularly those suffering from chronic conditions or living in nursing home or long-term care facilities, are at particular risk, with over 500,000 new cases annually. As such, *C. diff* is the most common cause of health care–associated infections in the United States. Unnecessary antibiotic use and poor infection control are key culprits in *C. diff* spread.[18] Discontinuing antibiotic treatment and working to bolster the immune system are a key part of treatment.

*Streptococcal Infections* At least five types of the *Streptococcus* microorganism are known to cause bacterial infections. *Group A streptococci (GAS)* cause the most common diseases, such as streptococcal pharyngitis ("strep throat") and scarlet fever. One particularly virulent group of GAS can lead to a rare but serious disease called *necrotizing fasciitis* ("flesh-eating strep"). *Group B streptococci* can cause illness in newborn babies, pregnant women, older adults, and adults with illnesses such as diabetes or liver disease. Since about 1 in 4 pregnant women have group B strep in their rectum or vagina, the CDC recommends testing for it in the last weeks of pregnancy.[19] Expectant mothers who are group B positive can be treated with antibiotics to prevent problems in their newborn.

**SEE IT! VIDEOS**

How can a South Korean MERS outbreak affect the U.S.? Watch **CDC Issuing New Alert on MERS**, available on **MasteringHealth.**™

**colonization** The process of bacteria or some other infectious organisms establishing themselves in a host without causing infection.

**methicillin-resistant** *Staphylococcus aureus* **(MRSA)** Highly resistant form of staph infection that is growing in international prevalence.

**health care–associated infections (HAIs)** Infections that arise in patients while in treatment for other conditions.

**Streptococcus** A round bacterium, usually found in chain formation.

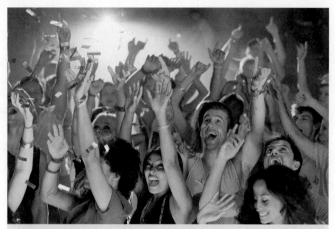

Crowded events like athletic contests and concerts are prime breeding grounds for some contagious diseases such as the flu, colds, and meningitis.

The species *Streptococcus pneumoniae* is responsible for thousands of cases of bacterial meningitis and pneumonia each year and is the primary culprit in most ear infections. While antibiotic treatments are still effective, an increasing number of cases are becoming resistant.

**Meningitis** is an inflammation of the *meninges*, the membranes that surround the brain and spinal cord. There are a variety of causes, including bacterial, viral, parasitic, and fungal infections, as well as noninfectious causes such as trauma to the brain, cancer, lupus, drugs, or brain surgery.

One virulent form of bacterial meningitis prevalent on college campuses, *meningococcal meningitis*, is the most serious infectious form. Spread through contact with saliva, nasal discharge, feces, or respiratory and throat secretions, it is highly contagious, particularly in close living conditions such as dormitories. Globally, it results in deaths for between 5 and 10 percent of those infected—despite treatment, within 24–48 hours; up to 20 percent of those infected are left with neurological issues.[20] There were slightly over 500 cases of meningococcal disease in the United States last year.[21] Adolescents and young adults between 16 and 23 years old are among the most likely to contract the disease and have serious complications.[22]

A suspected student death from bacterial meningitis at San Diego State University and over 31 cases of viral meningitis at the University of Maryland in 2014 caused significant concern on college campuses throughout the country. *Bacterial meningitis* progresses rapidly, is life-threatening, and needs immediate medical attention. *Viral meningitis* is much less dangerous and symptoms usually diminish in 3 to 5 days in otherwise healthy people. There is no vaccine or treatment for this form.

Fortunately, vaccines exist for *pneumococcal meningitis*, the most common form of bacterial meningitis, and *meningococcal meningitis*. The other vaccine-preventable form of bacterial meningitis is *Haemophilus influenzae* type b (Hib). Check your immunization table for information regarding vaccination.

Typical signs of many forms of meningitis are sudden fever, severe headache, and a stiff neck, particularly stiffness that causes difficulty touching your chin to your chest. Persons who are suspected of having meningitis should receive immediate, aggressive medical treatment. Talk to the medical or health education staff at your local student health center to see if they have the vaccine most likely to protect you in your area.

Prevention of meningitis involves common-sense infection control procedures such as frequent handwashing; using recommended cough/sneeze protocols such as sneezing into your arm and using disposable tissues rather than reusable hankies; keeping your hands away from your nose; and keeping "high-touch" surfaces, such as phones, doorknobs, and remote controls, clean.

**Pneumonia** Pneumonia is a general term for a wide range of conditions that result in inflammation of the lungs and difficulty breathing. It is characterized by chronic cough, chest pain, chills, high fever, fluid accumulation, and eventual respiratory failure. Although bacterial and viral pathogens are the most common culprits, pneumonia can also be caused by fungi, occupational exposure to chemicals, or trauma.

Bacterial pneumonia responds readily to antibiotic treatment in early stages, but can be deadly in more advanced stages. Forms of pneumonia caused by other organisms are more difficult to treat. Although medical advances have reduced the overall incidence of pneumonia, it continues to be a major threat in the United States and throughout the world.

**Tuberculosis** Only HIV/AIDS is a greater infectious agent killer than **tuberculosis (TB)** in the global population.[23] With over 9.6 million new cases and 1.5 million deaths in 2014, an astounding one-third of the world's population is infected with TB.[24] Although infection rates decreased dramatically in the United States since the 1950s, there were still over 9,400 cases in 2014.[25] Tuberculosis is the number one infectious killer of women of reproductive age worldwide, as well as the leading cause of death among HIV-positive patients. Poverty and lack of access to treatment are also key risk factors.

Historically, people used the term *consumption* to refer to a bacterial respiratory disease with symptoms that include wasting/weight loss, fever, chronic cough and blood-streaked sputum, fluid- and blood-filled lungs, and eventual spread throughout the body. The term is still used in some parts of the world today; however, TB is now widely recognized for these same symptoms.

**meningitis** An infection of the meninges, the membranes that surround the brain and spinal cord.

**pneumonia** Inflammatory disease of the lungs characterized by chronic cough, chest pain, chills, high fever, and fluid accumulation; may be caused by bacteria, viruses, fungi, chemicals, or other substances.

**tuberculosis (TB)** A disease caused by bacterial infiltration of the respiratory system.

# 1.5 MILLION

people were killed globally by **TB**. The toll comprised 890,000 men, 480,000 women, and 140,000 children.

Airborne transmission via the respiratory tract is the primary mode of infection. Infected people can be contagious without showing symptoms and can transmit the disease while talking, coughing, sneezing, or singing.

The current recommended treatment for TB involves taking four drugs for 6 to 9 months; however, a new 12-dose regimen is available for high-risk populations.[26] Medications may cause side effects, ranging from minor stomach irritation to liver failure. Newer combination drug treatments, and use of turmeric and other natural substances, are currently being investigated for effectiveness.[27] The side effects, lengthy treatment, and barriers to obtaining drugs and care in many developing areas lead to missed doses and treatments that end before the cure. This, in turn, breeds drug-resistant tuberculosis. **Multidrug-resistant TB (MDR-TB)** is currently resistant to at least two of the best anti-TB drugs in use today, and **extensively drug-resistant TB (XDR-TB)** is resistant to nearly all current TB drugs. These newer strains of tuberculosis are reaching epidemic proportions in over 58 countries.[28]

### Tick-Borne Bacterial Diseases

In the past few decades, certain tick-borne diseases have become major health threats in the United States. The most noteworthy include two bacterially caused diseases. **Lyme disease** is a tick-borne disease present in many regions of the United States, particularly the upper Midwest. Symptoms of Lyme disease may range from none, to a rash or bull's-eye lesion and flu-like symptoms, to chronic arthritis, blindness, and long-term disability.

**Babesiosis** is a tick-borne disease garnering increased attention in the upper Midwest and northeastern United States. When symptoms occur, they often mimic flu-like aches, headache, fatigue, and nausea. Because the babesiosis parasite attacks and destroys red blood cells, anemia may result. Older adults and those whose immune systems are weakened are at greatest risk of complications.

Another tick-borne disease, *ehrlichiosis*, also has flu-like symptoms that may progress quickly to respiratory difficulties, and even death.

Fortunately, antibiotics given early in the disease course are effective in preventing any serious threats from these diseases. The bottom line is, if you have flu-like symptoms in the typical nonflu months of the year, particularly if you have been in areas where ticks live, get yourself checked out.

**Rickettsia** are a small form of bacteria that produce toxins and multiply within small blood vessels, causing vascular blockage and tissue death. Rickettsia require an insect vector (carrier) for transmission to humans. Two common forms of human rickettsial disease are *Rocky Mountain spotted fever*, carried by a tick, and *typhus*, carried by a louse, flea, or tick. These diseases produce similar symptoms, including high fever, weakness, rash, and coma, and both can be life-threatening.

The best protection against insect-borne diseases is to stay indoors at dusk and early morning to avoid hours of high insect activity. To prevent tick-borne diseases, remember to stay out of grass and woods during the times ticks are most active, from late spring to fall. Use insect repellents that contain 20 to 30 percent DEET, natural oils, or pyrethrins that you put on your clothing. Wear long sleeves and pants and tuck pants into socks. Do tick checks by examining genitals, buttocks, hair, and other body parts where ticks like to hide. Bathe or shower as soon as possible after coming indoors (within 2 hours) to wash off ticks. Also, do pet checks to make sure ticks don't crawl off your pets and onto you!

If you are traveling in areas of the world where insect-borne diseases such as malaria or the Zika virus are prevalent, then bed nets, EPA-registered insect products (those having "EPA Reg" on the label), and sprays containing *deet*, a chemical called *IR3535*, and those containing the chemically synthesized, though plant-like, *lemon eucalyptus and picaridin* are recommended.[29] Consult a travel doctor; they may prescribe you with preventive medications.

*Tick-borne diseases such as Lyme disease, Rocky Mountain spotted fever, and babesiosis are on the rise in many parts of the United States. Protect yourself with bug sprays and protective clothing.*

### Escherichia coli O157:H7

*Escherichia coli* O157:H7 is one of over 170 types of *E. coli* bacteria that can infect humans. Most *E. coli* organisms are harmless and live in the intestines of healthy animals and humans. *E. coli* O157:H7, however, produces a lethal toxin and can cause severe illness or death. You can get it from eating ground beef that is undercooked, drinking unpasteurized milk or juice, or swimming in sewage-contaminated water. Outbreaks in the United States have been caused by foods like frozen pizza and quesadillas, organic spinach and spring mix lettuce, raw clover sprouts, romaine lettuce, bologna, cheese, and poultry.

A symptom of infection is nonbloody diarrhea, usually 2 to 8 days after exposure; however, asymptomatic cases have been noted. Children, older adults, and people with weakened immune systems are particularly vulnerable to serious side effects such as kidney failure, intestinal damage, or death.

Strengthened regulations on chlorine levels in pools and the cooking of meat have helped reduce *E. coli* infections. Difficulties in isolating the source of infections have prompted a close examination of labeling and distribution of food products. The U.S. Department of Agriculture (USDA) as well as the Environmental Protection Agency (EPA), Food and Drug Administration, and others are all involved in developing food and transportation policies designed to keep the food supply safe.

**multidrug-resistant TB (MDR-TB)** Form of TB that is resistant to at least two of the best antibiotics available.

**extensively drug-resistant TB (XDR-TB)** Form of TB that is resistant to nearly all existing antibiotics.

**Lyme disease** Tick-borne disease whose symptoms may range from none, to a rash or bull's-eye lesion and flu-like symptoms, to chronic arthritis, blindness, and long-term disability

**Babesiosis** A tick-borne disease whose parasite attacks and destroys red blood cells

**rickettsia** A small form of bacteria that live inside other living cells.

# Viruses

**Viruses** are the smallest known pathogens, approximately 1/500th the size of bacteria, and hundreds of viruses are known to cause diseases in humans. Essentially, a virus consists of a protein structure that contains either *ribonucleic acid (RNA)* or *deoxyribonucleic acid (DNA)*. Viruses are incapable of carrying out any life processes on their own. To reproduce, they must invade and inject their own DNA or RNA into a host cell and force it to make copies of themselves. The new viruses then erupt out of the host cell and seek other cells to invade.

Viral diseases can be difficult to treat because many viruses can withstand heat, formaldehyde, and large doses of radiation with little effect on their structure. Some viruses have **incubation periods** (the length of time required to develop fully and cause symptoms in their hosts) that last for years, which delays diagnosis. Drug treatment for viral infections is also limited. Drugs powerful enough to kill viruses generally kill the host cells, too, although some medications block stages in viral reproduction without damaging the host cells.

## The Common Cold
Some experts claim there may be over 200 different viruses responsible for the common cold. Colds are the main reason for missed work and missed school in the United States, with millions of cases each year.[30] Although most colds occur in the winter and spring, you can actually get a cold anytime. Adults have an average of two to three colds per year, and children have even more.[31] If you get a cold, the most likely cause is the rhinovirus, which causes 10 to 40 percent of all colds, followed by the coronavirus, responsible for 20 percent of all colds.[32] Colds are endemic (always present to some degree) throughout the world, with increasing prevalence in colder weather as people spend more time indoors. Otherwise healthy people carry cold viruses in their noses and throats most of the time, held in check until immune defenses are weakened. It is possible to "catch" a cold—through airborne transmission, touching skin-to-skin, or mucous membrane contact—and the hands are the greatest avenue for transmitting colds and other viruses. Obviously, then, covering your nose and mouth with a tissue, handkerchief, or even the crook of your elbow when sneezing is better than using your bare hand. Contrary to popular belief, you cannot catch a cold from getting a chill or being in the cold, but the chill may lower your immune system's resistance to a virus if one is present.

## Influenza
**Influenza**, or flu, is a contagious respiratory illness that includes fever and chills along with other cold symptoms. While death rates from the flu are only estimates since influenza is not a reportable disease, common estimates range from 3,000 per year to 49,000.[33] Although a rapid-diagnosis flu test is available, doctors typically diagnose influenza based on symptoms.

Although many people don't realize it, there are actually many different types of influenza, including the most common *seasonal variety* and some other less common types. Fortunately, most types of flu in the world are not readily transmitted to humans.

For seasonal flu, although symptoms are always more serious than a cold, most adolescents and adults recover after a week or two. However, seasonal flu can be deadly to the very young, people over age 65, and those who have weakened immune systems. Occasionally, a particularly deadly strain of influenza evolves and spreads rapidly, killing many.

Five to 20 percent of Americans get the flu each year, and of these, 200,000 will need hospitalization.[34] Once a person gets the flu, treatment is *palliative*—focused on relief of symptoms rather than a cure.

The best way to avoid the flu is to get an annual vaccination against it. Since there are numerous and constantly mutating flu strains, vaccines are formulated for the few strains most likely to be prevalent in an upcoming season. If researchers correctly predict strains, vaccines are thought to be 70 to 90 percent effective in healthy adults for about a year; if the prediction is off, a shot is less beneficial.[35]

In spite of minor risks, the CDC now recommends everyone over the age of 6 months get a seasonal flu vaccine annually. Unfortunately, only about 170 million people are projected to have had vaccinations for the 2015–2016 flu season.[36] Flu shots take 2 to 3 weeks to become effective, so it's best to get shots in the fall, before the flu season begins. Today, you have options for vaccination, including a standard shot, a high-dose shot if you are over age 65 or at risk, or the *Flublok* shot if you are allergic to the eggs used to produce vaccines. Another popular vaccine option, *FluMist*, is a nasal spray used by those who opt out of the shot vaccination. Unfortunately, in June 2016, the CDC recommended that *FluMist* not be given for the next flu season as its effectiveness has been called into question until more research has been conducted.[37]

## Hepatitis
One of the most highly publicized viral diseases is **hepatitis**, a virally caused inflammation of the liver. Symptoms include fever, headache, nausea, loss of appetite, skin rashes, pain in the upper right abdomen, dark yellow (with brownish tinge) urine, and jaundice. Internationally, viral hepatitis is a major contributor to liver disease and accounts for high morbidity and mortality. Currently, there are several known forms (A, B, C, D, and E), with hepatitis A, B, and C having the highest rates of incidence.

*Hepatitis A (HAV)* is contracted by eating food or drinking water contaminated with human feces. Since vaccinations became available, HAV rates had been steadily declining until 2013, when they again began to increase. In 2013, there were nearly 1,800 reported new cases of HAV.[38] Hepatitis A can also be spread through sexual contact with HAV-positive individuals or through the use of contaminated needles. Fortunately, individuals infected with HAV do not become chronic carriers, and vaccines for the disease are available. Many who contract HAV are asymptomatic (symptom-free).

**viruses** Minute microbes consisting of DNA or RNA that invade a host cell and use the cell's resources to reproduce themselves.

**incubation period** The time between exposure to a disease and the appearance of symptoms.

**influenza** A common viral disease of the respiratory tract.

**hepatitis** A viral disease in which the liver becomes inflamed, producing symptoms such as fever, headache, and possibly jaundice.

*Hepatitis B (HBV)* is spread through body fluid exchange during unprotected sex, sharing needles when injecting drugs, through needlesticks on the job, or, in the case of a newborn baby, from an infected mother during birth. Hepatitis B can lead to chronic liver disease or liver cancer. Since vaccines became available in 1981, numbers of HBV cases have declined rapidly. Globally, HBV infections are on the decline, but over 240 million are chronically infected, with complications of hepatitis B, like cirrhosis and liver cancer, killing over 780,000 people each year.[39] Needle exchange programs are believed to be an important part of risk reduction for HBV, HCV, and HIV infection in the last decade.[40]

Rates are also on the decline in the United States; however, an estimated 20,000 cases are reported each year, and nearly 1.4 million people are chronic carriers.[41] The highest rates of infection are among males aged 30 to 39 and black non-Hispanics; the lowest rates are among Asian Pacific Islanders and Hispanics.[42] Because the hepatitis B virus is considered 50 to 100 times more virulent than HIV, efforts to increase global vaccination rates have become a major priority.

*Hepatitis C (HCV)* infections are on an epidemic rise in many regions of the world as resistant forms emerge. Some cases can be traced to blood transfusions or organ transplants. An estimated 29,718 cases of HCV occurred in 2013, and the estimated number of chronic cases of HCV may be as high as 3.5 million.[43] Of those infected with the hepatitis C virus, 75 to 85 percent will develop chronic hepatitis C, and 60–70 percent will develop chronic liver disease.[44] Of those who develop chronic liver disease, between 5 and 20 percent will develop cirrhosis of the liver.[45] One in 5 people will die from cirrhosis or liver cancer.[46] Several new drugs are being tested to treat HCV. New drugs such as Harvoni, a combination pill produced by Gilead Pharmaceuticals, have been approved. Initial results appear promising.[47]

To prevent the spread of HBV and HCV, use latex condoms correctly every time you have sex; don't share personal-care items that might have blood on them, such as razors or toothbrushes; get a blood test for HBV so you know your status; never share needles; and if you are having body art done, go only to reputable artists or piercers who follow established sterilization and infection-control protocols.

### Herpes Viruses: Chickenpox, Shingles, and Herpes Gladiatorum

From cold sores to the chickenpox, herpes-caused diseases are known for painful, blistering rashes and are easily transmitted via physical contact. They can become chronic problems for the person infected. (Genital herpes is covered in Chapter 15.)

Caused by the herpes varicella zoster virus (HVZV), *chickenpox* produces characteristic symptoms of fever and fatigue 13 to 17 days after exposure, followed by skin eruptions that itch, blister, and produce a clear fluid. The virus is present in these blisters for approximately 1 week. Although a vaccine for chickenpox is available, many parents incorrectly assume that the vaccine is not necessary and that contracting the disease will ensure lifelong immunity.

For a small segment of the population, the chickenpox virus reactivates later in life during times of high stress or when the immune system is taxed by other diseases. This painful, blistering rash, extreme pain, and other possible complications is called *shingles*. The disease shingles affects over 1 million people in the United States, most of whom are over the age of 60. The best way to prevent shingles is to get vaccinated.

Another form of herpes-caused disease that is increasing on college campuses is *herpes gladiatorum*, which shows itself as a blistered rash on the face, neck, or torso. Caused by the herpes simplex type 1 virus, herpes gladiatorum is also referred to as "mat pox" or "wrestler's herpes," as it's highly contagious via mats used in a yoga studio or gym, or through body-to-body contact.

## Other Pathogens

While bacteria and viruses account for many common diseases, other organisms can also infect people. Among these are fungi, protozoans, parasitic worms, and prions.

### Fungi

Hundreds of species of **fungi** exist. While many of these multi- or unicellular organisms are beneficial—edible mushrooms, penicillin, and yeast used in bread—*candidiasis* (the cause of vaginal yeast infections, discussed later), athlete's foot, ringworm, jock itch, and toenail fungus are examples of common fungal diseases. With most fungal diseases, keeping the affected area clean and dry and treating it promptly with appropriate medications will generally bring relief. Fungal diseases typically transmit via physical contact, so avoid going barefoot in public showers, hotel rooms, and other areas where fungus may be present, and use care in choosing where you go for pedicures. Another key fungal disease that is increasing in the United States is *Valley fever*—a potentially life-threatening respiratory disease common in the desert Southwest. Others may be spread to humans and pets via breathing in fungal spores found in dirt and in dusty conditions.

### Protozoans

**Protozoans** are single-celled organisms that cause diseases such as malaria and African sleeping sickness and are largely controlled in the United States. A common waterborne protozoan disease in many regions of the country is *giardiasis*. Persons who drink contaminated water may be exposed to the *giardia* pathogen and will suffer intestinal pain and discomfort weeks after initial infection. Protection of water supplies is the key to prevention.

### Parasitic Worms

**Parasitic worms** are the largest pathogens. Ranging in size from small pinworms typically found in children to large tapeworms that can take up large portions of the human intestines, most are more nuisance than threat. Of special note are the worm infestations associated with eating raw fish (as in some forms of sushi). You can prevent worm infestations by cooking fish and

**fungi** A group of multicellular and unicellular organisms that obtain their food by infiltrating the bodies of other organisms, both living and dead; several microscopic varieties are pathogenic.

**protozoans** Microscopic single-celled organisms that can be pathogenic.

**giardiasis** A common waterborne protozoan disease.

**parasitic worms** The largest of the pathogens, most of which are more a nuisance than a threat.

other foods to temperatures sufficient to kill the worms and their eggs. Other preventive measures you can take include getting your pets checked and dewormed regularly; washing pet beds or your own bedding and blankets, where worm eggs may be lurking; being careful while swimming in international areas known for these infections; and wearing shoes in parks or places where animal feces are present.

**Prions** A **prion** is a self-replicating, protein-based agent that can infect humans and other animals. One such prion is believed to be the underlying cause of spongiform diseases such as *bovine spongiform encephalopathy (BSE)*, or "mad cow disease". If humans eat contaminated meat from cattle with BSE, they may develop a mad cow–like disease known as *variant Creutzfeld-Jakob disease (vCJD)*. Symptoms of vCJD include loss of memory, tremors, and muscle spasms or "ticks." Over time, depression, difficulty walking, seizures, and severe dementia can ultimately lead to death in both cows and humans. An increasing number of infected cattle have been found in the United States and globally; however, to date, there have been no confirmed human infections from U.S. beef.

# Emerging and Resurgent Diseases

Although our immune systems are adept at responding to challenges, microbes and other pathogens constantly evolve and try to gain an edge. Within the past decade, rates for many infectious diseases have increased. This trend can be attributed to a combination of widely recognized factors. *Economic development and land use* (humans encroaching on delicate ecosystems and upsetting microbial balances established over the centuries); *human behaviors* that overuse, pollute, overfish, and overconsume natural resources, upsetting species balances, the earth's ability to regenerate and heal, and contributing to climate change; and the *proliferation of international travel* contributing to the transport and intermingling of microbes that have been protected by natural barriers over the centuries all are factors in emergent and resurgent diseases. In addition, overpopulation, inadequate health care, increasing poverty, loss of habitat, microbial mutation and change, and antibiotic resistance all lead to assaults on our immune systems.

Significant increases in vaccine-preventable disease cases for pertussis, meningococcal meningitis, measles, chickenpox, hepatitis A, and other childhood diseases, as well as increases in persons opting out of vaccinations in recent years are causing concern throughout the country. Increased hospitalizations and deaths of children from vaccine-preventable diseases and more families using the "personal belief exemption" from vaccination prompted California to reinstate mandatory vaccinations of school-age children in May 2015.[48] Stay tuned as other states move to protect the population through similar vaccine mandates in schools.

## Measles and Mumps

The most well-known symptom of **mumps** is swelling of the salivary glands. In severe cases it can cause hearing loss or male sterility. **Measles**, known for its high fever and itchy red rash, is increasingly common—particularly on college campuses. Increased incidences of these and other vaccine-preventable diseases between 2013 and 2014 are reason for significant concern in many regions of the country. A growing number of children and young adults have not been vaccinated against measles or mumps because their parents believe the diseases are gone and the risk of a vaccine is greater than the risk of contracting the disease. Refer back to the Health Headlines box on page 394 for more on the vaccine controversy.

## West Nile Virus (WNV)

Several thousand cases of West Nile virus occur in the United States each year. For most, symptoms are flu-like and can include a form of encephalitis (inflammation of the brain). There were 2,060 cases of WNV in the United States in 2015, with 119 deaths and hundreds disabled.[49] Older adults and those with impaired immune systems bear the brunt of the disease burden. Today, only Alaska and Hawaii remain free of the disease in the United States. Spread by infected mosquitoes, the best way to avoid infection is through mosquito eradication programs, wearing mosquito repellant, and avoiding mosquito-infested areas altogether, especially at peak mosquito feeding times. There is no vaccine or specific treatment.

## Avian (Bird) Flu and Swine (Pig) Flu

**Avian influenza** is an infectious disease of birds. Birds infect other

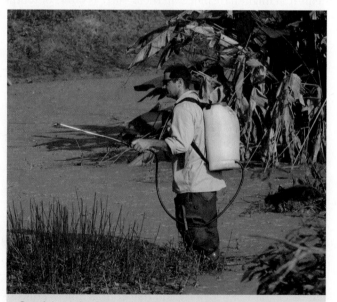

Careful monitoring and control of mosquito and other insect populations is important to combat emerging and resurging diseases such as the Zika and West Nile viruses.

**prion** A recently identified self-replicating, protein-based pathogen.

**mumps** A once common viral disease that is controllable by vaccination.

**measles** A viral disease that produces symptoms such as an itchy rash and a high fever.

**avian influenza** An infectious disease of birds with some strains capable of crossing the species barrier and causing severe illness in humans that come in contact with bird droppings or fluids.

**swine flu** A respiratory infection initially believed to be found primarily in pigs; also referred to as H1N1 or one of its variants.

birds during migratory patterns, spreading the disease internationally as they fly among locations. Strains capable of crossing the species barrier can cause severe illness in humans who come in contact with bird droppings or fluids. Bird flu appears to have originated in Asia and spread via migrating bird populations.[50] Although the virus has yet to mutate into a form highly infectious to humans, outbreaks in rural areas of the world (where people live in close proximity to poultry and other animals) have occurred. By the end of 2015, the World Health Organization had recorded 846 cumulative cases of bird flu in humans, with 449 deaths, an indication of the severity of this disease.[51]

**Swine flu**, also referred to as H1N1 or one of its variants, is a respiratory infection initially believed to be found primarily in pigs. In 2009, an outbreak of a virus that combined elements of a human flu virus and the pig virus occurred. Twelve cases were reported in the United States initially, primarily among people who had touched pigs or were in close proximity to them.[52] Today, H1N1 is one of the many possible viruses that humans can contract.

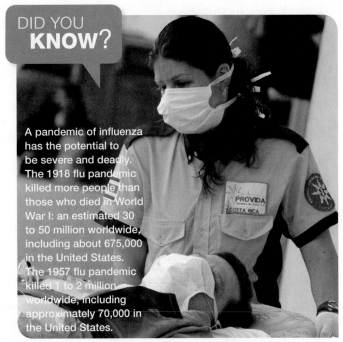

## DID YOU KNOW?

A pandemic of influenza has the potential to be severe and deadly. The 1918 flu pandemic killed more people than those who died in World War I: an estimated 30 to 50 million worldwide, including about 675,000 in the United States. The 1957 flu pandemic killed 1 to 2 million worldwide, including approximately 70,000 in the United States.

**Source:** Flu.gov, "Pandemic Flu History," Accessed April 2016, www.flu.gov/pandemic/history.

# STUDY PLAN

Customize your study plan—and master your health!—in the Study Area of **MasteringHealth.**

## ASSESS YOURSELF

**How much do you really know about infectious diseases?** Take the **Myth or Fact? Test Your Infectious Diseases IQ** assessment available on **MasteringHealth.™**

# CHAPTER REVIEW

To hear an MP3 Tutor Session, scan here or visit the Study Area in **MasteringHealth.**

### LO 1 | The Process of Infection

- For a person to become infected with a disease, he or she must come into contact with a pathogen, and the pathogen must get past the body's immune system defenses to establish infection.

### LO 2 | Your Body's Defenses against Infection

- The skin is the body's major barrier against infection, helped by enzymes and body secretions.
- Innate immunity, adaptive immunity, and cell-mediated and humoral immunity play unique roles in

- The agent, host, and environment must be conducive for disease to occur. Knowing your risk factors can help you remain free of disease.

the elaborate human response to infection.
- Autoimmune diseases are the result of an immune system that becomes hypersensitive and misfires. If pathogens get inside the body, the immune system finds the foreign cells or particles and creates antibodies to destroy them. Inflammation and fever also play a role in defending the body against infections.
- Vaccines bolster the body's immune system against specific diseases.

## Types of Pathogens and the Diseases they Cause

LO **3**

- The major classes of pathogens are bacteria, viruses, fungi, protozoans, parasitic worms, and prions. Bacterial infections include staphylococcal infections, streptococcal infections, meningitis, pneumonia, tuberculosis, and tick-borne diseases. Major viral infections include the common cold, influenza, and hepatitis.
- Emerging and resurgent diseases such as West Nile virus and avian flu potentially pose significant threats for future generations. Many factors contribute to these risks.
- Strategies for preventing infectious diseases include getting enough sleep, reducing stress, engaging in behaviors that reduce risks, being vaccinated, and working to enhance environmental and health-care related infections.

## POP QUIZ

Visit **MasteringHealth** to personalize your study plan with Chapter Review Quizzes and Dynamic Study Modules.

LO **1** | **The Process of Infection**

1. Fernando catches a cold after his roommate Jason sneezes and coughs near Fernando in their shared dorm room. The likely mode of transition for Fernando's cold was
   a. waterborne.
   b. airborne.
   c. vector-borne.
   d. perinatal.

2. Jennifer touched her viral herpes sore on her lip and then touched her eye. She ended up with the herpes virus in her eye as well. This is an example of
   a. acquired immunity.
   b. passive spread.
   c. autoinoculation.
   d. self-vaccination.

3. Which of the following would put a 70-year-old person at a greater risk for infectious diseases?
   a. Vaccinations from birth wearing off or not as effective
   b. Thickening of the skin
   c. Losing sense of smell
   d. Getting "chilled" from a drafty room.

LO **2** | **Your Body's Defenses against Infection**

4. Which of the following do not assist the body in fighting disease?
   a. Antigens
   b. Antibodies
   c. Lymphocytes
   d. Macrophages

5. Which of the following is NOT an example of adaptive immunity?
   a. Body defenses such as sweat, tears, and mucous
   b. Getting a vaccine to protect against a virus
   c. Cell-mediated immunity, lymphocytes, and T cells
   d. Getting a disease and developing resistance to that disease due to antibodies

6. A disease that occurs when the bodies defense mechanisms turn against the body's own cells is a(n)
   a. allergy.
   b. opportunistic infection.
   c. autoimmune disease.
   d. vaccination.

LO **3** | **Types of Pathogens and the Diseases they Cause**

7. Which of the following diseases is caused by a prion?
   a. Shingles
   b. Listeria
   c. Mad cow disease
   d. Trichomoniasis

8. Which of the following is a viral disease?
   a. Giardiasis
   b. Measles
   c. Malaria
   d. Streptococcal infection

9. Because colds are always present to some degree throughout the world, they are said to be
   a. globally acquired.
   b. vector-borne.
   c. endemic.
   d. resistant to antibiotics.

10. For which of the following diseases can you reduce your risk by using mosquito repellent when outdoors?
    a. Candidiasis
    b. West Nile virus
    c. Rubella
    d. *E. coli* O157:H7

*Answers to the Pop Quiz can be found on page A-1. If you answered a question incorrectly, review the section identified by the Learning Outcome. For even more study tools, visit* **MasteringHealth**.

## THINK ABOUT IT!

LO **1** | **The Process of Infection**

1. What are three lifestyle changes you could make right now that would reduce your risk of developing an infectious disease? What could you do to help protect your friends, partner, and family members? Discuss noncontrollable and controllable risk factors that can make you more or less susceptible to infectious pathogens.

LO **2** | **Your Body's Defenses against Infection**

2. What are pathogens, antigens, and antibodies? What does it mean if someone says a pathogen is particularly *virulent*? What is the difference between *antigens* and *antibodies*?

3. What is the difference between active and passive immunity? How do they compare to natural and acquired immunity? What type of immunity do vaccines provide?

## Types of Pathogens and the Diseases they Cause

LO **3**

4. What are some differences between bacteria and viruses? How do certain pathogens develop drug resistance? What policies and programs should be enacted to protect us from drug resistant pathogens?

# ACCESS YOUR HEALTH ON THE INTERNET

Visit **MasteringHealth** for links to the websites and RSS feeds.

The following websites explore further topics and issues related to infectious diseases.

**Centers for Disease Control and Prevention (CDC).** This government agency is dedicated to disease intervention and prevention. The site links to all the latest data and publications put out by the CDC. **www.cdc.gov**

Specialized CDC sites. These sites focus on infectious diseases:

**National Center for Immunization and Respiratory Diseases.** **www.cdc.gov/ncird/index.html**

**National Center for Emerging and Zoonotic Infectious Diseases.** **www.cdc.gov/ncezid**

**ArboNET.** A national surveillance system for arboviral (arthropod-caused) diseases in the United States, ARboNET monitors West Nile disease, eastern equine encephalitis, dengue, and other mosquito and tick-borne diseases. **www.cdc.gov/westnile/resource pages/survResources.html**

**Association for Professionals in Infection Control and Epidemiology (APIC).** Excellent resource for health professionals and consumers covering a wide range of infectious disease issues in health care, workplaces, schools, and personal environments. **www.apic.org**

**World Health Organization (WHO).** You'll gain access to the latest information on world health issues and direct access to publications and fact sheets at WHO's site. **www.who.int**

# 15 Protecting against Sexually Transmitted Infections

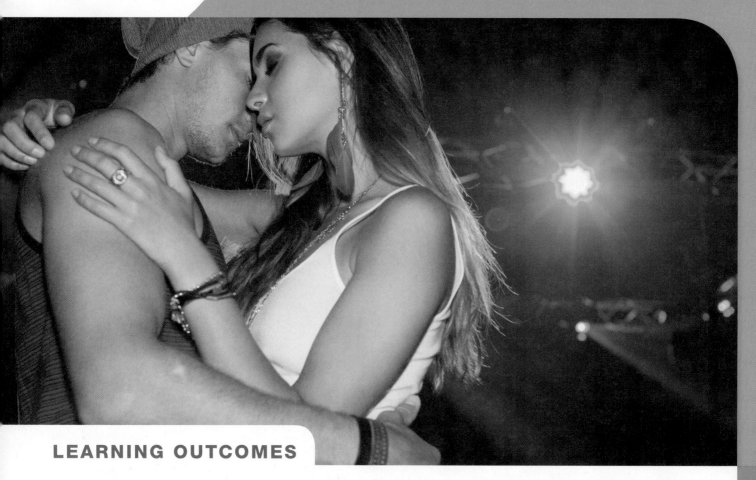

## LEARNING OUTCOMES

LO **1** Explain the risk factors for sexually transmitted infections and actions that can prevent their spread.

LO **2** Describe common types of sexually transmitted infections, including their symptoms and treatment methods.

LO **3** Discuss human immunodeficiency virus (HIV) and acquired immune deficiency syndrome (AIDS), trends in infection and treatment, and the impact of these diseases on special populations.

Nearly half of the 20 million new cases of sexually transmitted infections (STIs) diagnosed each year occur in 15- to 24-year-olds.[1] While some STIs are treatable, others result in painful and debilitating problems like pelvic inflammatory disease, infertility, tubal scarring, ectopic pregnancy, and chronic sterility in women, as well as a variety of negative effects in men. Being savvy about sexual intimacy means acting responsibly to keep you and your partner sexually safe—now and in the future.

A though more than 20 million cases of **sexually transmitted infections (STIs)** are reported each year, many others are never diagnosed or reported, often because they are *asymptomatic*.[2] Some STIs, particularly *chlamydia*, *gonorrhea*, and *syphilis*, are increasing at alarming rates, particularly among young adults.[3] Huge disparities in rates exist by age, race, income, and gender.[4]

Sexually transmitted infections affect people of all backgrounds and socioeconomic levels, but they disproportionately affect women, minorities, and infants.[5] Barriers to prevention and treatment—such as lack of knowledge about risks, disease symptoms, and options for treatment, access to affordable health care, issues of stigma and confidentiality, transportation issues, peer norms and media influences, risk-taking behaviors, and social and cultural norms that promote and influence sexual interest and activity—are examples of some of the factors that put adolescents and young adults at risk.[6]

make up 80 percent of HIV diagnoses.[7] Shame and embarrassment, denial, and perceived stigma often keep infected people from seeking treatment. Unfortunately, they usually continue to be sexually active, thereby infecting unsuspecting partners. People uncomfortable discussing sexual issues may also be less likely to use condoms to protect against STIs and pregnancy. But your sexual health is too important to not talk about. See the **Student Health Today** box on page 408 for more on having "the conversation."

Ignorance—about the infections, their symptoms, and the fact that someone can be asymptomatic but still be infected—is also a factor. A person who is infected but asymptomatic can unknowingly spread an STI to others. By the time anyone seeks medical help, several others may already be infected. In

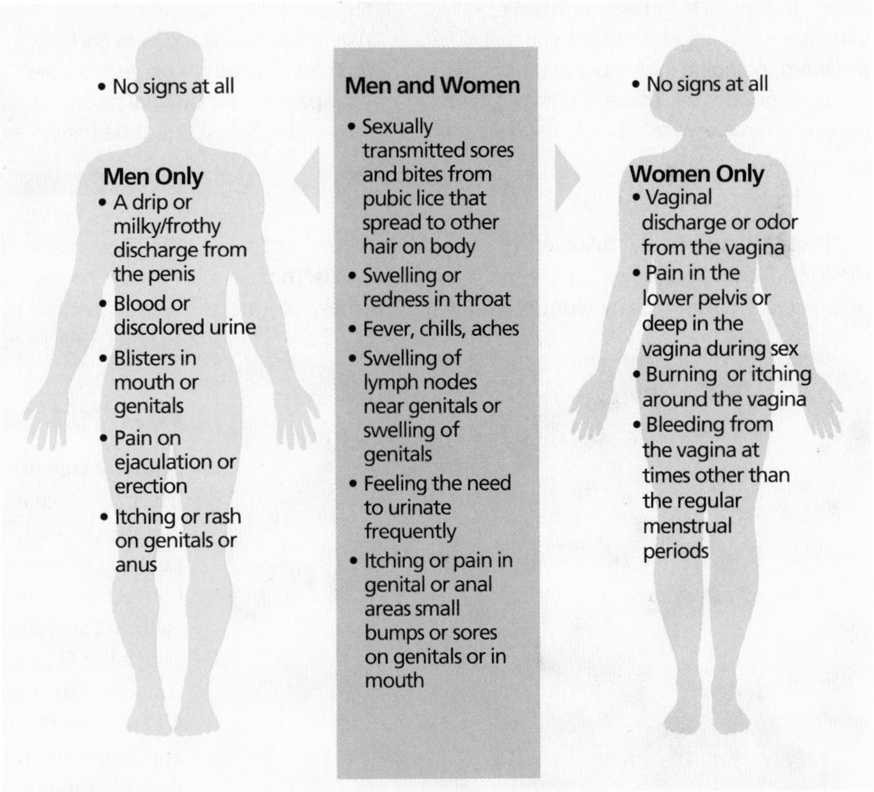

> **sexually transmitted infections (STIs)** Infections transmitted through some form of intimate, usually sexual, contact.

## LO **1** | **SEXUALLY TRANSMITTED INFECTIONS**

Explain the risk factors for sexually transmitted infections and actions that can prevent their spread.

Early STI symptoms are often mild and unrecognizable (see **FIGURE 15.1**). Left untreated, some STIs can result in sterility, blindness, central nervous system destruction, disfigurement, and even death. Infants born to mothers carrying these infections are at risk for a variety of health problems.

### What's Your Risk?

Generally, the more sexual partners a person has, the greater the risk for contracting an STI. Adolescents aged 15 to 24 account for nearly half of the new cases of STIs each year in America. Four out of 10 sexually active teen girls have been infected with an STI and while rates of HIV are low among adolescents, males aged 13 to 19

**• No signs at all**

**Men Only**
• A drip or milky/frothy discharge from the penis
• Blood or discolored urine
• Blisters in mouth or genitals
• Pain on ejaculation or erection
• Itching or rash on genitals or anus

**Men and Women**
• Sexually transmitted sores and bites from pubic lice that spread to other hair on body
• Swelling or redness in throat
• Fever, chills, aches
• Swelling of lymph nodes near genitals or swelling of genitals
• Feeling the need to urinate frequently
• Itching or pain in genital or anal areas small bumps or sores on genitals or in mouth

**• No signs at all**

**Women Only**
• Vaginal discharge or odor from the vagina
• Pain in the lower pelvis or deep in the vagina during sex
• Burning or itching around the vagina
• Bleeding from the vagina at times other than the regular menstrual periods

**FIGURE 15.1** Signs or Symptoms of Sexually Transmitted Infections (STIs) In their early stages, many STIs may be asymptomatic or have such mild symptoms that they are easy to overlook.

→ VIDEO TUTOR
Signs and Symptoms of STIs

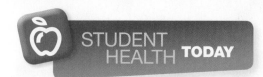

# HAVE THE CONVERSATION
*Reduce Your Risks of STIs*

Millions of people have one or more STIs and rates of disease are growing at epidemic rates globally. Many don't know they are infected—and others don't care if they are. When you meet someone you are attracted to and think they look clean-cut and disease free, remember this: *The most common symptom of an STI is no symptom at all!* Young and old, rich and poor, well kempt or grubby, anyone can be infected. You can't tell by looking at them!

If all this makes you nervous, think about how you will feel if you have that amazing hookup and days or weeks later, you discover you have symptoms. Or, worse yet, you give someone you care about an STI you didn't know you had! Try explaining your way out of that one.

The bottom line is that in today's sexual marketplace, one-night stands with strangers should be a big "NO" on your list of possible behaviors. Sex should be reserved for people you know and with whom you've had "the conversation" about STI risks. Regardless of whether it makes you uncomfortable or you feel awkward, plunging in and being up-front is always a good idea. These simple pointers may help reduce your risks of infection:

1. *Don't beat around the bush.* Ask your partner or potential partner if they have had an STI in the past. Were they treated? Have they been tested recently? Remember, people are not always honest in their responses, so don't be gullible. Ask them what they think about testing. Is it something they would consider before becoming intimate?
2. *Be yourself and use language you are comfortable with.* Don't be accusing or apologetic. Stay calm and matter of fact, even though you might feel awkward and nervous.
3. *Stress that you are asking because you care about them and yourself* and don't want either of you to be at risk.
4. *Have the conversation sober,* and when you can have a private, comfortable, and serious conversation. Don't ask at dinner with friends or in a group. "Hey John, have you had any STIs lately?" Take it seriously and be firm.
5. *Ask the right questions to find out their feelings about prevention.* Ask your partner or potential partner if they would be willing to be tested, to

wait until test results are in, and then be monogamous after the test.
6. *Share a bit of your recent history, especially if you have an infectious disease that cannot be cured, like genital herpes.* They deserve to know what the implications of this might be long term.
7. *Share information about what you have already done to be safe and what you are willing to do.* Have you been vaccinated for HPV? Do you carry condoms or protective devices?
8. *Do your homework and talk about where you might go for treatment, confidentiality, resources on campus, possible prevention strategies, and so on.*
9. *Don't worry about whether a conversation like this might cause someone to walk away.* If they refuse or are more interested in *sex now,* let them walk. Anyone who would do that is not a very responsible person and may not ever have your best interests at heart.
10. *Plan ahead.* If you are going out with someone and the sparks begin to fly, make sure you're prepared. Never have unprotected sex.

---

addition, many people mistakenly believe that certain sexual practices—oral sex, for example—carry no risk for STIs. In fact, oral sex practices among young adults may be responsible

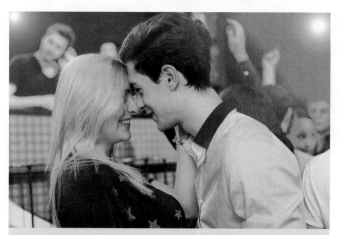

When considering sex, think about your own past history as well as the history of your potential partner. Many of these diseases are asymptomatic, meaning that you may have no clue that you are a carrier.

for increases in herpes, genital warts, and other infections. **FIGURE 15.2** shows the continuum of disease risk for various sexual behaviors, and the Making Changes Today box offers tips for ways to practice safer sex.

## Routes of Transmission

Sexually transmitted infections are generally spread through intimate sexual contact such as vaginal intercourse, oral–genital contact, hand–genital contact, and anal intercourse. Less likely modes of transmission include mouth-to-mouth contact or contact with fluids from body sores. Although each STI is a different infection caused by a different pathogen, all STI pathogens prefer dark, moist places, especially the mucous membranes lining reproductive organs. Most are susceptible to light, extreme temperature, and dryness, and many die quickly on exposure to air. Like other communicable infections, STIs have both pathogen-specific *incubation periods* and *periods of communicability*—times during which transmission is most likely. See the Health Headlines box on page 410 for info on sexual transmission of the Zika virus.

# MAKING CHANGES TODAY

## Safe is Sexy

Practicing the following behaviors will help you reduce your risk of contracting a sexually transmitted infection (STI) when considering a sexual encounter:

- *Avoid multiple sexual encounters*, which increase your risks.

- *Just say NO to casual sex.* Prepare ahead of time and know what you will say. An example might be, "No. Sorry. I'm attracted to you, but I don't have sex with anyone I don't know well and when I'm not sure about their history. The risks are too great."

- *Insist on using a latex condom or a dental dam* (a sensitive latex sheet, about the size of a tissue, that can be placed over the female genitals to form a protective layer) during vaginal, oral, or anal sex. Many an unsuspecting female has contracted genital warts in the mouth due to oral sex without a condom or vaginal sex with someone who has highly infectious "flat warts"—which are nearly impossible to see—on their penis. Remember that condoms do not provide 100 percent protection against all STIs.

- *Know in advance where you or your partner can go to be tested for an STI*, including costs and what you need to do. If you've ever been sexually active without protection, you should be tested first. When talking with a partner, try something like, "I'm going for testing and I'd like you to go, too. That way we can both stay safe."

- *Avoid injury to body tissue, including abrasions and microscopic tears during sexual activity*. Anal sex is particularly risky as the anus tears easily. However, any rough sex increases risks. Don't be afraid to say, "That hurts. Stop."

- Make handwashing a habit, *insisting that both of you wash hands prior to sex/petting and afterward*. Herpes or genital warts can easily be spread by someone touching the sore on their mouth or their genitals and then touching yours. If you masterbate, wash your hands, too. As a rule, use soap and water and count to 20 before and after sexual encounters. Urinate after sexual relations and, if possible, wash your genitals.

- Total abstinence is the only absolute way to prevent the transmission of STIs, but abstinence can be a difficult choice to make. If you have any doubt about the potential risks of having sex, consider other means of intimacy (at least until you can assure your safety)—massage, dry kissing, hugging, holding and touching, and masturbation (alone or with a partner).

- Get vaccinated for HPV, hepatitis B, and hepatitis C.

- If you contract an STI, ask your health care provider for advice on notifying past or potential partners.

**Sources:** American College of Obstetricians and Gynecologists, *How to Prevent Sexually Transmitted Diseases,* Frequently Asked Questions. FQ009 (Washington, DC: American College of Obstetricians and Gynecologists, 2015), Available at: http://www.acog.org/~/media/For%20Patients/faq009.pdf?dmc=; American Sexual Health Association, "Reduce Your Risk," Accessed March 2016, http://www.ashasexualhealth.org/stdsstis/reduce-your-risk/.

| High-risk behaviors | Moderate-risk behaviors | Low-risk behaviors | No-risk behaviors |
| --- | --- | --- | --- |
| Unprotected vaginal, anal, and oral sex—any activity that involves direct contact with bodily fluids, such as ejaculate, vaginal secretions, or blood—are high-risk behaviors. | Vaginal, anal, or oral sex with a latex or polyurethane condom and a water-based lubricant used properly and consistently can greatly reduce the risk of STI transmission. Dental dams used during oral sex can also greatly reduce the risk of STI transmission. | Mutual masturbation, if there are no cuts on the hand, penis, or vagina, is very low risk. Rubbing, kissing, and massaging carry low risk, but herpes can be spread by skin-to-skin contact from an infected partner. | Abstinence, phone sex, talking, and fantasy are all no-risk behaviors. |

**FIGURE 15.2 Continuum of Disease Risk for Various Sexual Behaviors** There are different levels of risk for various behaviors and various sexually transmitted infections (STIs); however, no matter what, any sexual activity involving direct contact with blood, semen, or vaginal secretions is high risk.

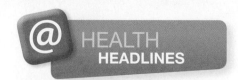
## ZIKA VIRUS
### *New Sexually Transmitted Threat?*

Zika, a mosquito-borne virus, hit the news media in 2015, just as images of babies with Zika-related birth defects became widely available. Although Zika has been present in tropical regions of the world for decades, no known cases were recorded in the United States. However, as of March 2016, nearly 300 cases were recorded on U.S. soil, presumably among those who had been infected in regions where Zika thrives.

Zika itself is usually a fairly mild disease; persons infected may have symptoms including fever, rash, joint pain, and conjunctivitis (red, itchy eyes) that last for a week or so. So why all the worry? Recently, concerns over sexual transmission have emerged. Although experts are sifting through the accumulated data to determine specific risks, as of July 2016, these are the facts the Centers for Disease Control and Prevention is providing:

- Men with Zika can pass it to sexual partners (male or female) via vaginal, anal, or oral (mouth to penis) sex without a condom.
- Unlike many other viruses, Zika can be passed from a man with symptoms to his sex partners before his symptoms start, while he has symptoms, and after his symptoms end.
- Men with Zika who never develop symptoms may also be able to pass the virus to their sex partners.
- Zika virus can stay in semen longer than in blood, but we don't know exactly how long Zika stays in semen or how long it can be passed to the sex partner.

- It is unknown whether Zika is passed on through deep kissing.
- Check CDC's website below to find out specific recommendations for males and females traveling to Zika endemic regions to find out how long you should refrain from sex after returning.
- Check CDC's website below to find continual updates of Zika-related recommendations.

If the partner is pregnant, she can pass it on to her fetus, risking potential birth defects. Whether infected women might spread it via body fluids remains unknown. Stay tuned!

**Source:** Centers for Disease Control and Prevention, "Zika and Sexual Transmission," July, 2016, http://www.cdc.gov/zika/transmission/sexual-transmission.html.

---

## LO 2 | COMMON TYPES OF SEXUALLY TRANSMITTED INFECTIONS

**Describe common types of sexually transmitted infections, including their symptoms and treatment methods.**

Although 47 percent of sexually active college students report having vaginal sex with at least one partner over the past 30 days, fewer than half of those students used a condom or other protective barrier.[8] Likewise, while 42 percent of sexually active students had oral sex in the last 30 days, only 5.4 percent used condoms or protective barriers most of the time or always.[9] In addition to other risky behaviors, sex without a condom, and oral sex without a dental dam or other form of protection—whether it's with a well-known lover or someone whom you just met—puts you at significantly higher risk for STIs. Add alcohol, and the likelihood of safer sex decreases dramatically.[10] Just one unprotected hookup can expose you to any of the highly infectious organisms that can cause a lifetime of very real risks. How great is that risk?

There are more than 20 known types of STIs. Once referred to as *venereal diseases* and *sexually transmitted diseases*, current terminology (STI) is more reflective of the number and types of infections—as well as the fact they are caused by pathogens. Today's strains are not your grandparent's pathogens! Several have reached *superbug resistance* status, where only a few antibiotics work to slow them down or knock them out. Learning how to protect yourself and

loved ones, reduce risks, and know the options for treatment are key parts of responsible sexual behavior. Here, we focus on the most common forms of STIs and emphasize that your behaviors can either prevent lingering consequences of STIs or put you at greater risk.

### Chlamydia

**Chlamydia**, an infection caused by the bacterium *Chlamydia trachomatis*, is one of the most commonly reported STIs in the United States. In 2014, there were just over 1.4 million chlamydia infections reported in the United States; however, these numbers probably underestimate the nearly 3 million infections that occur annually.[11] Many cases aren't reported because most people have no symptoms and don't seek treatment. Young people aged 15 to 24—particularly young women, non-Hispanic blacks, and men who have sex with men—have the highest rates of infection.[12]

Chlamydia can be transmitted via sexual contact with the penis, vagina, mouth, or anus of a person who is infected. A mother can also transmit infection to her baby during childbirth. Only about 10 percent of infected men and 5 to 30 percent of infected women show symptoms, giving it the distinction of being a "silent infection."[13]

**Signs and Symptoms** In men with symptoms, there may be painful urination, an urge to urinate frequently, or difficult urination, as well as a watery, pus-like discharge from the penis. Women with symptoms may have a yellowish discharge, spotting between periods, and occasional spotting after intercourse.

**chlamydia** Bacterially caused STI of the urogenital tract.

# 4 IN 10

**SEXUALLY ACTIVE TEENAGE** women have had an STD that can cause infertility and even death. Among 13- to 19-year-olds, males account for more than 75% of HIV diagnoses.

**Complications** Men can suffer injury to the prostate gland, seminal vesicles, and bulbourethral glands, as well as arthritis-like symptoms and inflammatory damage to the blood vessels and heart. Men can also experience *epididymitis*—inflammation of the area near the testicles. In women, chlamydia-related inflammation can injure the cervix or fallopian tubes, causing sterility, and it can damage the inner pelvic structure, leading to **pelvic inflammatory disease (PID)**—an infection and inflammation of the uterus, ovaries, and other female reproductive organs. Untreated, PID can lead to infertility, ectopic pregnancy, pain, and scarring of the reproductive organs. Chlamydia is one of the most common causes of PID—one of the most common preventable causes of infertility in the United States.

If an infected woman becomes pregnant, she has a high risk for miscarriage and stillbirth. Women with chlamydia and those who are sexually active with multiple partners are also at greater risk for **urinary tract infections (UTIs)**. Although not all UTIs are sexually transmitted, STIs are one way they can occur. Women are at greater risk for UTIs anatomically. Their urethra is much shorter than a man's, making it easier for bacteria to enter the bladder. In addition, a woman's urethra is closer to her anus than is a man's, allowing bacteria to spread into her urethra and cause an infection. Symptoms of a UTI in women include a burning sensation during urination and lower abdominal pain. A UTI can be diagnosed through a urine test and treated by antibiotics. If left untreated, UTIs can cause kidney damage.

UTIs occur in men, but much less frequently than in women. One form most commonly caused by *Chlamydia trachomatis* is *nongonococcal urethritis*. Infections should be taken seriously—if you have a milky penile discharge and/or burning during urination, contact your health care provider.[14]

Chlamydia may also be responsible for one type of *conjunctivitis*, an eye infection that affects adults who don't wash their hands after intimacy and touch their eyes. It can also be spread to infants, who can contract the disease from an infected mother during delivery. Untreated conjunctivitis can cause blindness.

**Diagnosis and Treatment** A sample of urine or fluid from the vagina or penis is collected and tested to identify the presence of the bacteria. Unfortunately, chlamydia tests are not a routine part of many health clinics' testing procedures.

If detected early, chlamydia is easily treatable with antibiotics such as tetracycline, doxycycline, or erythromycin. It is important that you refrain from all sex while being treated and that your partner get treated and is cured before you have sex to avoid a ping-pong transmission back and forth. You do not develop immunity to chlamydia!

**pelvic inflammatory disease (PID)** Term used to describe various infections of the female reproductive tract.

**urinary tract infections (UTIs)** Infection, more common among women than men, of the urinary tract; causes include untreated STIs.

**gonorrhea** Second most common bacterial STI in the United States; if untreated, may cause sterility.

## Gonorrhea

**Gonorrhea** is on an epidemic rise in the United States, with over 820,000 new gonorrheal infections in the United States each year.[15] Like chlamydia, gonorrhea is also likely largely underreported, with actual estimates approaching double the reported cases. Over two-thirds of reported cases occur in 15- to 24-year-olds.[16] Caused by the bacterial pathogen *Neisseria gonorrhoeae*, gonorrhea primarily infects the linings of the urethra, genital tract, pharynx, and rectum. It may spread to the eyes or other body regions by the hands or through body fluids, typically during vaginal, oral, or anal sex. It most frequently occurs in people in their early 20s.

**Signs and Symptoms** While some men are asymptomatic, a typical symptom is a white, milky discharge from the penis accompanied by painful, burning urination 2 to 9 days after contact (**FIGURE 15.3**). Epididymitis can also occur as a symptom of infection.

Most women do not experience any symptoms, but others may have vaginal discharge or a burning sensation on urinating. The organism can remain in the woman's vagina, cervix, uterus, or fallopian tubes for long periods with no apparent symptoms other than an occasional slight fever. Thus a woman

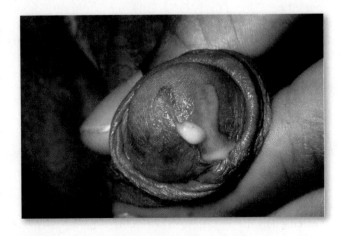

**FIGURE 15.3 Gonorrhea** One common symptom of gonorrhea in men is a milky discharge from the penis, accompanied by burning sensations during urination. Whereas these symptoms will cause most men to seek diagnosis and treatment, women with gonorrhea are often asymptomatic, so they may not be aware they are infected.

can be unaware that she has been infected and that she is infecting her sexual partners.

## Complications
Gonorrhea may spread to the prostate, testicles, urinary tract, kidneys, and bladder in men, and scar tissue may cause sterility. In some cases, the penis develops a painful curvature during erection. If the infection goes undetected in a woman, it can spread to the fallopian tubes and ovaries, causing sterility or severe inflammation and PID. If untreated, the gonorrhea can spread through the blood and cause *disseminated gonococcal infection (DGI)*, which can result in arthritis and problems with bones and joints, as well as cardiovascular and brain issues—problems that can be life-threatening.[17] If an infected woman becomes pregnant, the infection can be transmitted to her baby during delivery, potentially causing blindness, joint infection, or a life-threatening blood infection.

## Diagnosis and Treatment
Diagnosis of gonorrhea requires a sample of either urine or fluid from the vagina or penis to detect the presence of the bacteria. In early stages, gonorrhea is treatable with antibiotics, but it is becoming increasingly resistant to current treatment regimens. It is also important to recognize that chlamydia and gonorrhea often occur at the same time, but different antibiotics are needed to treat each infection.

## Syphilis

**Syphilis** is caused by a bacterium called *Treponema pallidum.* While syphilis used to be a disease that occurred most commonly among heterosexual and certain minority groups, today, 83% of syphilis cases occur in men who have sex with men (MSM) and partners of MSM.[18] There were 63,450 reported new cases of syphilis in 2014, up significantly from the 17,375 cases in 2013.[19] Because it is extremely delicate and dies readily on exposure to air, dryness, or cold, the organism is generally transferred only through direct sexual contact or from mother to fetus. The incidence of syphilis in newborns has continued to increase in the United States.[20]

## Signs and Symptoms
Syphilis is known as the "great imitator" because its symptoms resemble those of several other infections. It should be noted, however, that some people experience no symptoms at all. Syphilis can occur in four distinct stages:[21]

■ **Primary syphilis.** The first stage of syphilis is often characterized by the development of a **chancre** (pronounced "shank-er"), a bacteria-oozing sore located at the infection site that usually appears about a month after initial infection (see **FIGURE 15.4**). In men, the site of the chancre tends to be the penis or scrotum; in women, the site of infection is often internal, on the vaginal wall or high on the cervix where the chancre is not readily apparent, making the

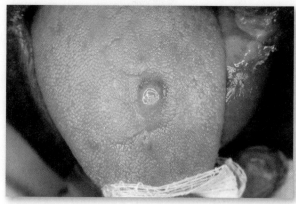

ⓐ Primary syphilis

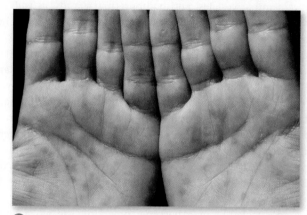

ⓑ Secondary syphilis

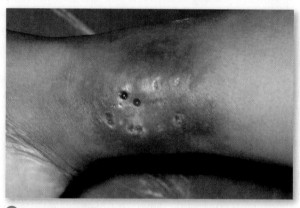

ⓒ Latent syphilis

**FIGURE 15.4** **Syphilis** A chancre on the site of the initial infection is a symptom of primary syphilis (a). A rash is characteristic of secondary syphilis (b). Lesions called *gummas* are often present in latent syphilis (c).

likelihood of detection small. In both men and women, the chancre will disappear in 3 to 6 weeks.

■ **Secondary syphilis.** If the infection is left untreated, a month to a year after the chancre disappears, secondary symptoms may appear, including a rash or white patches on the skin or on the mucous membranes of the mouth, throat, or genitals. Hair loss may occur, lymph nodes may enlarge, and the victim may develop a slight fever or headache. In rare cases, bacteria-containing sores develop around the mouth or genitals.

- **Latent syphilis.** After the secondary stage, if the infection is left untreated, the syphilis spirochetes begin to invade body organs, causing lesions called *gummas*. The infection now is rarely transmitted to others, except during pregnancy, when it can be passed to the fetus.
- **Tertiary/late syphilis.** Years after syphilis has entered the body, its effects become all too evident if still untreated. Late-stage syphilis indications include heart and central nervous system damage, blindness, deafness, paralysis, dementia, and possible death.

**Complications** Pregnant women with syphilis can experience premature births, miscarriages, stillbirths, or transmit the infection to their unborn child. An infected pregnant woman may transmit to her unborn child *congenital syphilis*, which can cause death; severe birth defects such as blindness, deafness, or disfigurement; developmental delays; seizures; and other health problems. Because in most cases the fetus does not become infected until after the first trimester, treatment of the mother during this time will usually prevent infection of the fetus.

**Diagnosis and Treatment** Syphilis can be diagnosed with a blood test or by collecting a sample from the chancre. It is easily treated with antibiotics, usually penicillin, for all stages except the late stage.

## Herpes

*Oral herpes* is a general term for a family of infections characterized by sores or eruptions on the skin usually caused by **herpes simplex virus type 1 (HSV-1)**. Most oral herpes cases are mild and occur in the mouth or lips. They often resurface in times of stress or when the body's immune system has been weakened. Herpes sores often are filled with fluid, teeming with the herpes virus. Have oral sex with someone when you have a HSV-1 lesion, or when no lesion is present but the virus is shedding, and you can transmit HSV-1 to the genitals. Kissing or sharing glasses or eating utensils can transmit the infection to other body parts. Herpes infections range from mildly uncomfortable to extremely serious. **Herpes simplex virus type 2 (HSV-2)**, also referred to as **genital herpes**, affects nearly 16 percent of the population aged 14 to 49 in the United States, with over 776,000 new cases overall each year.[22]

Only about 1 in 6 Americans are believed to have HSV-2; however, exact numbers are difficult to assess.[23] HSV-1 is believed to be much more common, potentially infecting between 50 and 80 percent of all adults.[24] Both types can infect any area of the body (**FIGURE 15.5**).[25]

Many people have the mistaken belief that you can only pass herpes on by contact with herpes sores. In fact, herpes may be spread when no obvious sores are present and there continues to be viral shedding. Assuming many people have this infection is probably a good rule of thumb, even when you don't see a sore. Protection is a smart choice.

**Signs and Symptoms** The precursor phase of a herpes infection is characterized by a burning sensation and redness at the site of infection. By the second phase, a blister filled with a clear fluid teeming with the virus forms. If you pick at this blister or otherwise touch the site, you can autoinoculate other body parts. Particularly dangerous is the possibility of spreading the infection to your eyes, which could result in injury or blindness.

Over a period of days, the unsightly blister will crust over, dry up, and disappear, and the virus will travel to the base of an affected nerve supplying the area and become dormant. Only when the victim becomes overly stressed, when diet and sleep are inadequate, when the immune system is overworked, or when excessive exposure to sunlight or other stressors occur will the virus become reactivated (at the same site every time) and begin the blistering cycle all over again. Each time a sore develops, it casts off (sheds) viruses that can be highly infectious,

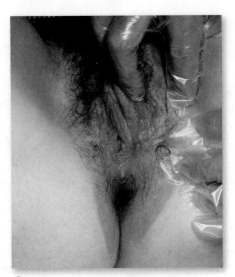

ⓐ Genital herpes is a highly contagious and incurable STI. It is characterized by recurring cycles of painful blisters on the genitalia.

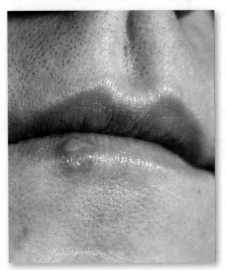

ⓑ Oral herpes is also extremely contagious and can cause painful sores and blisters around the mouth.

**FIGURE 15.5 Herpes** Both genital and oral herpes can be caused by either herpes simplex virus type 1 or type 2.

> **herpes simplex virus type 1 (HSV-1)** A family of infections characterized by sores or eruptions on the skin.
>
> **herpes simplex virus type 2 (HSV-2)** (also called **genital herpes**) STI caused by the herpes simplex virus.

but a herpes site can shed the virus even when no overt sore is present.

## Complications

Many physicians recommend cesarean deliveries for infected pregnant women, as herpes can be passed to the baby during birth. Additionally, women with a history of genital herpes appear to have a greater risk of developing cervical cancer and may have regular flare-ups during the menstrual cycle or in times of high stress.

## Diagnosis and Treatment

Diagnosis of herpes can be determined by collecting a sample from the suspected sore or by performing a blood test. Although there is no cure for herpes at present, antiviral medications can prevent or shorten outbreaks. Certain prescription drugs like *acyclovir* and over-the-counter medications like *Abreva* can be used to treat symptoms. Unfortunately, most only work if the infection is confirmed during the first few hours after contact. Other drugs, such as *famciclovir* (Famvir), may reduce viral shedding between outbreaks—potentially reducing risks to your sexual partners. Although vaccines are being tested, there is currently no commercially available vaccine that is protective against genital herpes.[26]

# Human Papillomavirus (HPV) and Genital Warts

**Human papillomavirus (HPV)** is one of a group of over 150 related viruses—each given a number indicating its type. HPV is the type that causes **genital warts** (also known as *venereal warts* or *condylomas*). It may surprise you to know that about 79 million Americans are currently infected with HPV, with nearly 14 million new infections each year.[27] HPV is the most common of all STIs, with experts reporting that most sexually active men and women will have at least one form of HPV at a time in their lives![28] More than 40 types can actually infect the genital or anal areas of humans via skin-to-skin contact, making vaginal, anal, and oral sex all risky behaviors.[29] While genital warts are the most common result of the infection, HPV can also lead to cancer, particularly cervical cancer; however, cancer of the vulva, penis, anus, vagina, back of the throat, and tongue can occur. Because HPV is often asymptomatic in the early stages, the risk of infection is great, particularly among those who are immunocompromised, such as those with HIV or AIDS.

## Signs and Symptoms

The typical incubation period is 6 to 8 weeks after contact. People infected with low-risk types of HPV may develop genital warts, a series of bumps or growths on the genitals, ranging in size from small pinheads to large cauliflower-like growths (**FIGURE 15.6**). Warts on penis may be flat and difficult to see. Cancer may develop years after sexual contact and be symptomless for years.

## Complications

High-risk types of HPV (HPV-16 and -18) are responsible for an estimated 70 percent of cervical cancer cases.[30] Exactly how high-risk HPV infection leads to cervical cancer is uncertain, though it may lead to *dysplasia*, or changes in cells that may lead to a precancerous condition. It is known that a Pap test done as routine screening for women aged 21 to 65 can help prevent cervical cancer.[31] As part of the Pap test, an HPV test can help forecast cervical cancer risk many years in the future and is currently recommended to be used as part of the Pap test in some women, either as additional screening or when Pap tests are uncertain. These tests can also identify women at risk for rare cervical cancers (adenocarcinomas) that Pap tests may miss.[32] Ask your doctor if your Pap test includes an HPV test and, if not, discuss whether one might be right for you.

Of cases that become precancerous and are left untreated, the majority will eventually result in actual cancer. In addition, HPV may also pose a threat to a fetus that is exposed to the virus during birth. Cesarean deliveries may be considered in serious cases. Human papillomavirus can cause cancers—called *oropharyngeal cancers*—around the tonsils or the base of the tongue. Each year, approximately 9,000 Americans are diagnosed with HPV-caused cancers of the oropharynx, with over 80 percent of sexually active people aged 14 to 44 indicating they have had oral sex with a partner.[33] Men are about four times more likely to develop cancers of the oropharynx

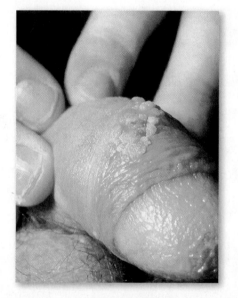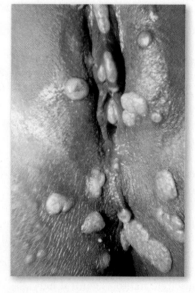

**FIGURE 15.6 Genital Warts** Genital warts are caused by certain types of the human papillomavirus.

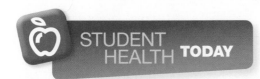

# MAKING ORAL SEX SAFE
## Condoms, Dental Dams, and Abstinence

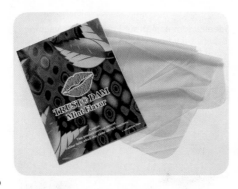

Oral sex refers to orally stimulating the penis (fellatio), vagina and clitoris (cunnilingus), and/or anus (analingus). Many young people tend to believe that oral sex is safe, and while the risks of contracting an STI are lower with oral sex than with vaginal or anal intercourse, the risk is still not zero. It is entirely possible to contract HIV from oral sex, as well as herpes, gonorrhea, syphilis, genital warts, and other diseases. Beyond common STIs, it's also possible to spread or contract intestinal parasites, as well as hepatitis A and B. That being the case, here are a couple things you can do to minimize your risk:

- **Use a condom correctly.** Condom use during oral sex is especially important for HIV prevention. When performing or receiving fellatio, use a new latex condom each time. Check it for holes before using, and discard it after use. Never reuse a condom.
- **Use a dental dam correctly.** A dental dam is essentially a small square of latex. While they were originally developed to be used during dental procedures, they are now commonly used as barriers when performing cunnilingus or analingus. Before using a

dental dam, visually check it for holes, and be sure to use a new one every time. Discard it after use, and never reuse a dental dam.

Lastly, keep in mind that condoms and dental dams provide less protection against STI spread through contact with exposed sores, like HPV or herpes, than for other STIs. Abstinence is the only way to be 100 percent sure you don't transmit or contract an STI.

**Sources:** Centers for Disease Control and Prevention, "Oral Sex and HIV Risk," October 2015. www.cdc.gov/hiv/risk/behavior/oralsex.html; Centers for Disease Control and Prevention, "HIV Prevention," March 2014, www.cdc.gov/hiv/basics/prevention.html; U.S. Department of Veterans Affairs, "Tips for Using Condoms and Dental Dams," www.hiv.va.gov/patient/daily/sex/condom-tips.asp.

---

than are women.[34] The exact means of contracting oropharyngeal cancer is unknown. While some research shows that you can get it by oral sex or french kissing, other research has not shown this. More research is necessary; however, in the interim, erring on the side of caution is a good idea.[35] See the **Student Health Today** box for information on making oral sex safe.

New research has also implicated HPV as a possible risk factor for coronary artery disease, potentially causing an inflammatory response in the artery walls, leading to cholesterol and plaque buildup. (See Chapter 16 for more on the effects of inflammation and plaque buildup on arteries.)

**Diagnosis and Treatment** Diagnosis of genital warts from low-risk types of HPV is determined through a visual examination. High-risk types can be diagnosed in women through microscopic analysis of cells from a Pap smear or by collecting a sample from the cervix to test for HPV DNA. There is currently no HPV DNA test for men.

Treatment is available only for the low-risk forms of HPV that cause genital warts. Most warts can be treated with topical medication or can be frozen with liquid nitrogen and then removed, but large warts may require surgical removal. See the **Student Health Today** box on page 416 for more information about available vaccines for HPV.

## Candidiasis (Moniliasis)

Most STIs are caused by pathogens that come from outside the body; however, the yeast-like fungus *Candida albicans* is a normal inhabitant of the vaginal tract in most women. (See **FIGURE 14.5c** on page 395 for a micrograph of this fungus.) Only when the normal chemical balance of the vagina is disturbed by actions such as taking antibiotics for other ailments will these organisms multiply and cause the fungal disease **candidiasis**, also sometimes called *moniliasis* or a *yeast infection*.

### Signs and Symptoms
Symptoms of candidiasis include severe itching and burning of the vagina and vulva and a white, cheesy vaginal discharge. When this microbe infects the mouth, whitish patches form, and the condition is referred to as *thrush*. Thrush infection can also occur in men and is easily transmitted between sexual partners. Symptoms of candidiasis can be aggravated by contact with soaps, douches, perfumed toilet paper, chlorinated water, and spermicides.

### Diagnosis and Treatment
Diagnosis of candidiasis is usually made by collecting a vaginal sample and analyzing it to identify the pathogen. Antifungal drugs applied on the surface or by suppository usually cure candidiasis in just a few days.

> **candidiasis** Yeast-like fungal infection often transmitted sexually; also called *moniliasis* or *yeast infection*.

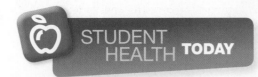
# Q&A ON HPV VACCINES

Most sexually active people will contract some form of human papillomavirus (HPV) at some time in their lives, though they may never even know it. There are about 40 types of sexually transmitted HPV, most of which cause no symptoms and go away on their own. Low-risk types can cause genital warts, but some high-risk types can cause cervical and other cancers. Every year in the United States, about 12,000 women are diagnosed with cervical cancer, and almost 4,000 die from this disease. There are currently two HPV vaccines that can help prevent women from becoming infected with HPV and subsequently developing cervical cancer.

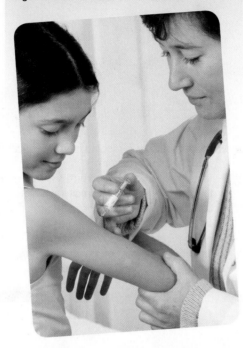

Ideally, females should get an HVP vaccine before they become sexually active. Males aged 9 to 26 can also be vaccinated.

■ **Who should get the HPV vaccine?** There are two vaccines currently available—Cervarix and Gardasil. Human papillomavirus vaccines are recommended for 11- and 12-year-old girls, but can be given to girls as young as 9 years old. It is also recommended for girls and women aged 13 to 26 who have not yet been vaccinated or completed the vaccine series. Ideally, females should get a vaccine before they become sexually active. Females who are sexually active may get less benefit from it because they may have already contracted an HPV type targeted by the vaccines.

One of the HPV vaccines, Gardasil, is also licensed, safe, and effective for males aged 9 to 26. The CDC recommends Gardasil for all boys 11 or 12 years old and for males aged 13 to 21 who did not get

any or all of the three recommended doses when they were younger. All men may receive the vaccine through the age of 26, but it is recommended that they should speak with their doctor to find out if getting vaccinated is right for them.

■ **How are the two HPV vaccines, Cervarix and Gardasil, similar and different?** Both vaccines are very effective against high-risk HPV types 16 and 18, which cause 70 percent of cervical cancer cases. Both vaccines are given as shots and require three doses. But only Gardasil protects against low-risk HPV types 6 and 11.

These HPV types cause 90 percent of cases of genital warts in females and males, so Gardasil is approved for use with males as well as females.

■ **What do the two vaccines *not* protect against?** The vaccines do not protect against all types of HPV, so about 30 percent of cervical cancers will not be prevented by the vaccines. It will be important for women to continue getting screened for cervical cancer through regular Pap tests. Also, the vaccines do not prevent other STIs.

■ **How safe are the HPV vaccines?** The vaccines are licensed by the FDA and approved by the CDC as safe and effective. They have been studied in thousands of females (aged 9 to 26) around the world, and their safety continues to be monitored by the CDC and the FDA.

■ **Are there side effects?** As with most vaccines and medications, side effects are rare, but possible. When they occur, they may include pain, redness and swelling in the arm where the shot was given, fever, headache, fatigue, nausea, or muscle pain. These usually go away within a short time. People with a history of allergies should talk to their doctor before getting the HPV vaccines.

**Sources:** Centers for Disease Control and Prevention, "HPV Vaccine Information for Young Women," March 26, 2015, http://www.cdc.gov/std/hpv/STDFact-HPV-vaccine-young-women.htm; CDC, HPV Vaccine—Questions & Answers," December 2015. http://www.cdc.gov/hpv/parents/questions-answers.html.

## Trichomoniasis

Unlike many STIs, **trichomoniasis** is caused by a protozoan, *Trichomonas vaginalis.* (See **FIGURE 14.5d** on page 395 for a micrograph of this organism.) The "trich" organism can be spread by sexual contact and by contact with items that have

discharged fluids on them. An estimated 3.7 million new cases occur in the United States each year, although only about one-third of people who contract it experience symptoms. The good news is that it is one of the most curable STIs if diagnosed and treated.[36]

### Signs and Symptoms
Symptoms among women include a foamy, yellowish, unpleasant-smelling discharge

**trichomoniasis** Protozoan STI characterized by foamy, yellowish discharge and unpleasant odor.

**pubic lice** Parasitic insects that can inhabit various body areas, especially the genitals.

**acquired immune deficiency syndrome (AIDS)** A disease caused by a retrovirus, the human immunodeficiency virus (HIV), that attacks the immune system, reducing the number of helper T cells and leaving the victim vulnerable to infections, malignancies, and neurological disorders.

**human immunodeficiency virus (HIV)** The virus that causes AIDS by infecting helper T cells.

accompanied by a burning sensation, itching, and painful urination. Most men with trichomoniasis do not have any symptoms, though some men experience irritation inside the penis, mild discharge, and a slight burning after urinating.[37]

**Diagnosis and Treatment** Diagnosis of trichomoniasis is determined by collecting fluid samples from the penis or vagina to test. Treatment includes oral metronidazole, usually given to both sexual partners to avoid the possible "ping-pong" effect of repeated cross-infection.

## Pubic Lice

**Pubic lice**, often called "crabs," are small parasitic insects that are usually transmitted during sexual contact (**FIGURE 15.7**). More annoying than dangerous, they have an affinity for pubic hair and attach themselves to the base of these hairs, where they deposit their eggs (nits). One to 2 weeks later, these nits develop into adults that lay eggs and migrate to other body parts.

**Signs and Symptoms** Symptoms of pubic lice infestation include itchiness in the area covered by pubic hair, bluish-gray skin color in the pubic region, and sores in the genital area.

**Diagnosis and Treatment** Diagnosis of pubic lice involves an examination by a health care provider to

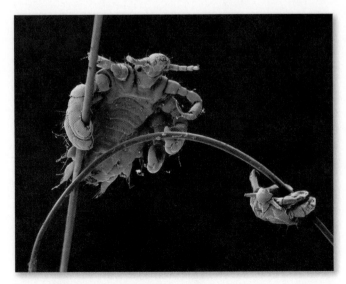

**FIGURE 15.7 Pubic Lice** Pubic lice, also known as "crabs," are small, parasitic insects that attach themselves to pubic hair. Concerns have arisen over "super lice" outbreaks in some states—lice that are resistant to most treatments.

identify the eggs in the genital area. Treatment includes washing clothing, furniture, and linens that may harbor the eggs, and usually takes 2 to 3 weeks to kill all larval forms.

## LO 3 | HIV/AIDS

Discuss human immunodeficiency virus (HIV) and acquired immune deficiency syndrome (AIDS), trends in infection and treatment, and the impact of these diseases on special populations.

Since **acquired immune deficiency syndrome (AIDS)** was first recognized in the 1980s, approximately 78 million people worldwide have become infected with **human immunodeficiency virus (HIV)**, the virus that causes AIDS, and 35 million have died.[38] About 37 million people worldwide are living with HIV, with 2.1 million new infections and 1.1 million deaths in 2015.[39] Approximately 16 million people are on HIV treatment.[40] The vast majority of HIV-infected individuals (25.8 million) are in sub-Saharan Africa, which makes up nearly 70 percent of all new cases in the world.[41] Globally, the numbers of people living with HIV have decreased, the numbers of new infections and deaths have declined, and the numbers of people receiving treatments have increased.[42]

In the United States, there are over 1.2 million people infected with HIV and nearly 1 in 8 of these individuals aren't aware they are infected.[43] There are approximately 50,000 new HIV infections each year, down significantly from the nearly 130,000 new cases per year in the 1980s.[44] Since first discovered, nearly 660,000 people in the United States have died of AIDS, with just over 13,000 deaths each year.[45] Due to improved treatments, more people are living with HIV than ever before.

## How HIV is Transmitted

HIV typically enters the body when another person's infected body fluids (e.g., semen, vaginal secretions, blood) gain entry through a breach in body defenses. If there is a break in mucous membranes of the genitals or anus (as can occur during sexual intercourse, particularly anal intercourse), the virus enters and begins to multiply, invading the bloodstream and cerebrospinal fluid. It progressively destroys helper T cells, weakening the body's resistance to disease.

HIV/AIDS is not highly contagious. It cannot reproduce outside a living host, except in a laboratory, and does not survive well in open air. As a result, HIV cannot be transmitted through casual contact, including sharing food utensils, musical instruments, toilet seats, and so on. Research also provides overwhelming evidence that insect bites do not transmit HIV.

# 1 IN 8

people with **HIV** in the United States do not know they are infected.

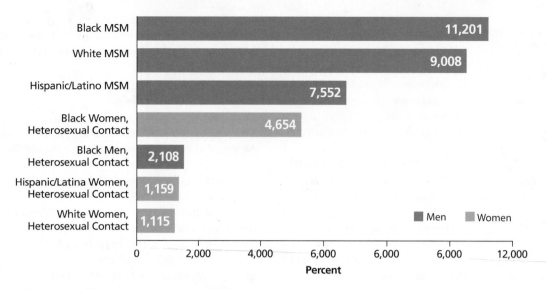

| Subpopulation | Count |
|---|---|
| Black MSM | 11,201 |
| White MSM | 9,008 |
| Hispanic/Latino MSM | 7,552 |
| Black Women, Heterosexual Contact | 4,654 |
| Black Men, Heterosexual Contact | 2,108 |
| Hispanic/Latina Women, Heterosexual Contact | 1,159 |
| White Women, Heterosexual Contact | 1,115 |

■ Men  ■ Women

0    2,000    4,000    6,000    6,000    6,000    12,000

Percent

**FIGURE 15.8** Estimates of New HIV Diagnoses in the United States for Most Affected Subpopulations, 2014

**Source:** CDC, "HIV Among Women," March 16, 2016, http://www.cdc.gov/hiv/group/gender/women/.

---

**Engaging in High-Risk Behaviors** During the early days of the pandemic, it appeared that HIV infected only homosexuals, but it quickly became apparent that the disease was related to certain high-risk behaviors rather than groups of people. **FIGURE 15.8** shows the breakdown of new HIV diagnoses for the most-affected populations.

Men who have sex with men (MSM), particularly young black/African American MSM, are most seriously affected by HIV.[46] Overall, African Americans, Hispanic/Latinos, and white Americans bear the greatest burden of HIV infection in the United States. People of color have poorer HIV/AIDS outcomes than whites due to a number of social and economic barriers and challenges, such as lack of access to early diagnosis and treatment, discrimination, stigma, homophobia, and poverty.

The majority of HIV infections arise from the following:

■ **Exchange of body fluids.** Substantial research indicates that blood, semen, and vaginal secretions are the major fluids of concern. Since the vaginal area is more susceptible to microtears and has a greater surface area, and because a woman is exposed to more semen than a man is to vaginal fluids, they are more likely to become infected. In fact, women are 4 to 10 times more likely than men to contract

HIV through unprotected heterosexual intercourse and 80 percent of HIV in women is through heterosexual contact.[47] In rare instances, the virus has been found in saliva, but most health officials state that saliva is a less significant risk than other shared body fluids.

■ **Contaminated needles.** Although users of illicit drugs are the most obvious members of this category, people with diabetes who inject insulin or athletes who inject steroids may also share needles. Sharing needles and engaging in high-risk sexual activities increases risks dramatically. Tattooing and body piercing can also be risky (see the **Student Health Today** box).

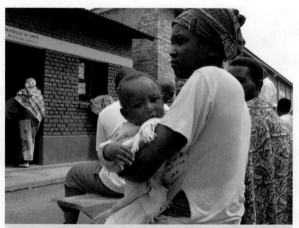

HIV/AIDS remains a devastating problem throughout the world. Over 70 percent of the new cases of HIV globally occur in sub-Saharan Africa. The woman and child shown here await treatment outside a clinic in Rwanda.

**Source:** UNAIDS, "Fact Sheet, 2015," Accessed March 2016, Available at http://www.unaids.org/en/resources/campaigns/HowAIDSchangedeverything/factsheet.

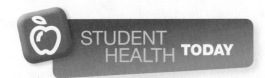

# BODY PIERCING AND TATTOOING
## *Potential Risks*

During body piercing or tattooing, the use of unsterile needles—which can transmit staph, HIV, hepatitis B and C, tetanus, and other diseases—poses a very real risk.

Laws and policies regulating body piercing and tattooing vary greatly by state. Because of the lack of universal regulatory standards and the potential for transmission of dangerous pathogens, anyone who receives a tattoo or body piercing cannot donate blood for 1 year.

If you opt for tattooing or body piercing, take the following safety precautions:

■ Look for clean, well-lighted work areas, and inquire about sterilization procedures. Be wary of establishments that won't answer questions or show you their sterilization equipment.

■ Packaged, sterilized needles should be used only once and then discarded. A piercing gun should not be used, because it cannot be sterilized properly. Watch that the artist uses

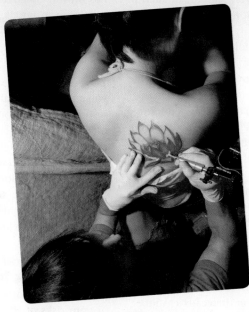

Use caution when selecting a tattoo artist and facility to ensure that proper infection control procedures are in place.

new needles and tubes from a sterile package before your procedure begins. Ask to see the sterile confirmation logo on the bag itself.

■ Immediately before piercing or tattooing, the body area should be carefully sterilized. The artist should wash his or her hands and put on new latex gloves for each procedure. Make sure the artist changes those gloves if he or she needs to touch anything else, such as the telephone, while working.

■ Leftover tattoo ink should be discarded after each procedure. Do not allow the artist to reuse ink that has been used for other customers. Used needles should be disposed of in a "sharps" container, a plastic container with the biohazard symbol clearly marked on it.

Like any activity that involves body fluids, tattooing carries some risk of disease transmission.

**Source:** Mayo Clinic Staff, "Tattoos: Understand Risks and Precautions," March 2015, www.mayoclinic.com.

---

Prior to 1985, blood donations were not checked for HIV, and some people contracted the virus from transfusions. Because of massive screening efforts, the risk of receiving HIV-infected blood is now almost nonexistent in developed countries.

## Mother-to-Child (Perinatal) Transmission

Mother-to-child transmission of HIV can occur during pregnancy, during labor and delivery, or through breastfeeding. Without antiretroviral treatment, approximately 15 to 45 percent of HIV-positive pregnant women will transmit the virus to their infant.[48] With appropriate interventions during pregnancy, labor, birth, and breastfeeding, transmission rates can be lowered to 5 percent.[49]

## Signs and Symptoms of HIV/AIDS

A person may go for months or years after infection before any significant symptoms appear, and incubation time varies greatly from person to person. Without treatment, it takes an average of 8 to 10 years for the virus to cause the slow, degenerative changes in the immune system that are characteristic of

AIDS. During this time, the person may experience *opportunistic infections* (infections that gain a foothold when the immune system is not functioning effectively). Colds, sore throats, fever, tiredness, nausea, night sweats, and other generally non-life-threatening conditions commonly appear and are described as pre-AIDS symptoms. Other symptoms of progressing HIV infection include wasting syndrome, swollen lymph nodes, and neurological problems. A diagnosis of AIDS, the final stage of HIV infection, is made when the infected person has either a dangerously low CD4 (helper T) cell count (below 200 cells per cubic milliliter of blood) or has contracted one or more opportunistic infections characteristic of the disease, such as Kaposi's sarcoma, tuberculosis, recurrent pneumonia, or invasive cervical cancer.

## Testing for HIV

Once antibodies have formed in reaction to HIV, a blood test known as the *ELISA* (enzyme-linked immunosorbent assay) may detect their presence. It can take 3 to 6 months after initial infection for enough antibodies to show a positive test

■ Have you been tested for an
STI? For HIV? Why or why
not? How important is it that
a potential partner be tested
for either of the above? How
would you ask that person to
get tested?

■ If you suddenly found out
that your partner had a rather
obvious herpes sore on his
face, what would you do?
What if you found out that you
were positive for chlamydia
and you had had sex with
two other people in the last
month?

result, and individuals with negative test results should be retested within 6 months. When a person who previously tested *negative* (no HIV antibodies present) has a subsequent test that is *positive*, seroconversion is said to have occurred. In such a situation, the person would typically take another ELISA test, followed by a more precise test known as the *Western blot*, to confirm the presence of HIV antibodies.

A *polymerase chain reaction* (PCR) test detects the genetic material of HIV instead of the antibodies to the virus and can identify HIV within the first few weeks of infection. It is often performed on babies born to mothers who are HIV positive. Rapid HIV tests using blood or oral fluids are also available and can produce results in 20 minutes. However, they require a confirmatory test with positive results, which may take up to several weeks. Home kits are also available, allowing a person to take a blood or saliva sample and anonymously send it to a laboratory. The person then calls a number to find out their results, with professional counselors available to provide support. Health officials distinguish between *reported* and *actual* cases of HIV infection because it is believed that many HIV-positive people avoid being tested for fear of knowing the truth, or recrimination from employers, insurance companies, and medical staff. However, early detection and reporting are important because immediate treatment in early stages is critical.

## New Hope and Treatments

New drugs have slowed the progression from HIV to AIDS and have prolonged life expectancies for most AIDS patients. In fact, since the 1990s, the U.S. death rate from AIDS is down nearly 83 percent.[50] The average cost for antiretroviral therapy (ART) is in excess of $23,000/year, with a lifetime estimated cost in excess of $380,000.[51]

Current treatments combine selected drugs, especially protease inhibitors and reverse transcriptase inhibitors. *Protease inhibitors* (e.g., amprenavir, ritonavir, and saquinavir) act to prevent the production of the virus in chronically infected cells that HIV has already invaded and seem to work best in combination with other therapies. Other drugs—such as AZT, ddI, ddC, d4T, and 3TC—inhibit the HIV enzyme *reverse transcriptase* before the virus has invaded the cell, thereby preventing the virus from infecting new cells. Combination treatments are still experimental, and no combination has proven effective for all people. Today, 44 new medicines, including antivirals, and vaccines are in testing.[52]

## Preventing HIV Infection

The best way to prevent HIV infection is through the choices you make in sexual behaviors and drug use and by taking responsibility for your own health and the health of your loved ones. You can't determine the presence of HIV by looking at a person; you can't tell by questioning the person, unless he or she has been tested recently and is giving an honest answer. So what should you do?

Of course, the simplest answer is abstinence. If you do decide to be intimate, the next best option is to use a condom, and for both individuals to be monogamous.

**Newer Prevention Strategies for Persons at High Risk for HIV Infection** When abstinence, protection, and other prevention strategies are inconsistent—or your risks of HIV are increased with multiple sexual partners, high-risk sexual partners (MSM), and other risks—there are promising new options available. Studies have shown promising results from the use of **preexposure prophylaxis (PrEP) for HIV** called *Truvada*. People who do not currently have HIV, who may be having sex with someone with HIV, and are at high risk themselves take a PrEP pill daily to prevent HIV infection. Used together with other HIV medication and safer sex practices, a significant reduction of infection risk has been shown.[53] The key to its effectiveness is taking it consistently, using condoms and other prevention strategies, and seeing your doctor regularly for checkups.[54]

**Where to Go for Help** If you are concerned about your own risk or that of a close friend, arrange a confidential meeting with the health educator or other health professional at your college health service. He or she will provide you with the information that you need to decide whether you should be tested for HIV antibodies. If the student health service is not an option for you, seek assistance through your local public health department or community STI clinic.

**preexposure prophylaxis (PrEP) for HIV** A daily pill, taken by those having sex with someone with HIV or otherwise at high risk, to help prevent HIV infection.

# STUDY **PLAN**

Customize your study plan—and master your health!—in the Study Area of **MasteringHealth**.

## ASSESS YOURSELF

**Is misinformation about STIs putting your health at risk?** Take the **STIs: Do You Really Know What You Think You Know?** assessment available on **MasteringHealth.**™

## CHAPTER **REVIEW**

To hear an MP3 Tutor Session, scan here or visit the Study Area in **MasteringHealth**.

### LO 1 | Sexually Transmitted Infections

- Sexually transmitted infections (STIs) are spread through vaginal intercourse, oral–genital contact, anal intercourse, hand–genital contact, and sometimes through mouth-to-mouth contact.
- Every year, there are at least 20 million new cases of STIs in the United States. They affect people of all backgrounds and socioeconomic levels, but rates are disproportionately higher among young adults, women, minorities, and infants.
- Reducing sexual contacts and practicing safer sex are key to prevention. Knowledge, good communication skills, and always practicing safer sex are key to staying safe.

### LO 2 | Common Types of Sexually Transmitted Infections

- STIs are spread by many different pathogens, including viruses, bacteria, and parasites. Knowing which one you have will help you understand options for treatment.
- Major STIs include chlamydia, gonorrhea, syphilis, herpes, human papillomavirus (HPV) and genital warts, candidiasis, trichomoniasis, and pubic lice. New diseases like

the Zika virus pose a risk for sexual partners as well as pregnant women. Dramatic increases in infections and resistant strains make chances of infection greater, particularly if you have sex with multiple partners.

### LO 3 | HIV/AIDS

- Acquired immunodeficiency syndrome (AIDS) is caused by the human immunodeficiency virus (HIV). HIV/AIDS is a global pandemic.
- Anyone can get HIV by engaging in unprotected sexual activities or by injecting drugs (or by having sex with someone who does).

## POP **QUIZ**

Visit **MasteringHealth** to personalize your study plan with Chapter Review Quizzes and Dynamic Study Modules.

### LO 1 | Sexually Transmitted Infections

1. Which behavior from the following list is considered the riskiest behavior for a sexually transmitted infection?
   a. Anal sex with a condom
   b. Mutual masturbation
   c. Deep kissing/french kissing
   d. Unprotected oral sex
2. What types of environments do STI pathogens prefer?
   a. Any environment, whether it's dark, light, cold, hot, dry, or moist
   b. Dark, moist places

   c. Light, dry places
   d. Excessively hot and humid places

### LO 2 | Common Types of Sexually Transmitted Infections

3. Which of the following is a common sign of gonorrhea in men?
   a. Whitish patches in the mouth
   b. Itchiness in the pubic hair region
   c. A milky discharge from the penis
   d. Gummas appearing near the penis
4. Which of the following STIs cannot be treated with antibiotics?
   a. Chlamydia
   b. Gonorrhea
   c. Syphilis
   d. Herpes
5. The most widespread sexually transmitted bacterium is
   a. gonorrhea.
   b. chlamydia.
   c. syphilis.
   d. chancroid.

### LO 3 | HIV/AIDS

6. Which of the following is a true statement about HIV?
   a. PrEP is a method of treating HIV among those with resistant forms of the disease.
   b. New cases of HIV have dropped dramatically in the last decade in the United States.

c. You can get HIV from a public restroom toilet seat.

d. HIV symptoms usually appear immediately after initial infection.

*Answers to the Pop Quiz can be found on page A-1. If you answered a question incorrectly, review the section identified by the Learning Outcome. For even more study tools, visit **MasteringHealth**.*

# THINK ABOUT IT!

LO **1** | **Sexually Transmitted Infections**

1. What are the key risk factors for STI infections? How many risk factors do you have? What kinds of behaviors should you avoid to cut down on the risk of contracting a sexually transmitted infection?

LO **2** | **Common Types of Sexually Transmitted Infections**

2. Identify five STIs and their symptoms. Which of these are readily treatable? Curable? How are they transmitted? What are their potential long-term effects?

LO **3** | **HIV/AIDS**

3. What factors have lead to decreasing rates of HIV/AIDS in the United States? Why have rates not fallen as fast in the developing regions of the world? Why are women more susceptible to HIV infection than men? What implication does this have for prevention, treatment, and research?

# ACCESS YOUR HEALTH ON THE INTERNET

Visit **MasteringHealth** for links to the websites and RSS feeds.

The following websites explore further topics and issues related to STIs.

**The U.S. President's Emergency Plan for AIDS Relief (PEPFAR).** A government initiative designed to help save the lives of people suffering from HIV/AIDS globally through a coordinated effort of nations working to create policy, programs, and services to help those most in need. The U.S. has a huge leadership and financial commitment to PEPFAR and reducing HIV/AIDS globally. https://www.aids.gov/federal-resources/around-the-world/pepfar/index.html

**Centers for Disease Control and Prevention (CDC).** This government agency is dedicated to disease intervention and prevention. The site links to all the latest data and publications put out by the CDC. www.cdc.gov

**Association for Professionals in Infection Control and Epidemiology (APIC).** Excellent resource for health professionals and consumers covering a wide range of infectious disease issues in health care, workplaces, schools, and in personal environment. www.apic.org

**World Health Organization (WHO).** You'll gain access to the latest information on world health issues and direct access to publications and fact sheets at WHO's site. www.who.int

**American Sexual Health Association.** This site provides facts, support, and referrals about sexually transmitted infections and diseases. www.ashastd.org

**AVERT.** This is an international site with information on HIV/AIDS, global STI statistics, interactive quizzes, and graphics displaying current statistics for vulnerable populations. www.avert.org

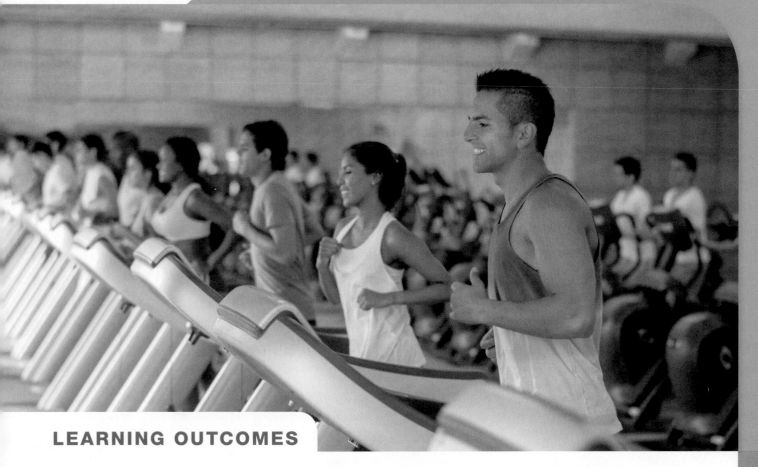

# 16

# Reducing Your Risk of Cardiovascular Disease

## LEARNING OUTCOMES

**LO 1** Discuss the social and economic burden of cardiovascular disease in the United States and the importance of ideal cardiovascular health.

**LO 2** Describe the anatomy and physiology of the heart and circulatory system and the importance of healthy heart function.

**LO 3** Explain the incidence, prevalence, outcomes, and impacts of cardiovascular disease in the United States and globally.

**LO 4** Review major types of cardiovascular disease and their symptoms, as well as at-risk populations.

**LO 5** Describe the modifiable and nonmodifiable risk factors for cardiovascular disease and methods of prevention.

**LO 6** Examine current strategies for diagnosis and treatment of cardiovascular disease.

As a young adult, the lifestyle you choose matters. The best defense against CVD is to reduce your risks and prevent it from developing in the first place. Considerable research points to the fact that the sooner you start, the better![2] Even a few months of effort now can lower your blood pressure, help you lose weight, and reduce CVD risks before they become more difficult to change.[3] In this chapter, we look at CVD causes and risk factors, for individuals and society, as well as a number of ways you can increase your chances of aging with a healthy cardiovascular system.

## LO 1 | CURRENT TRENDS: SOCIAL AND ECONOMIC IMPACT OF CVD

Discuss the social and economic burden of cardiovascular disease in the United States and the importance of ideal cardiovascular health.

In 2015–2016, the American Heart Association (AHA) reported that death rates from **cardiovascular disease (CVD)**—diseases associated with the heart and blood vessels, such as high blood pressure, coronary heart disease (CHD), heart failure, stroke, and congenital cardiovascular defects—had declined in the United States by nearly 33 percent in the last decade.[4] In spite of the promising decline, nearly 86 million Americans, more than 1 out of every 3 adults, suffer from one or more types of CVD.[5]

Much of the improvement in death rates is due to better diagnosis, early intervention and treatment, and a multibillion-dollar market in drugs designed to keep the heart and circulatory system ticking along. People are living longer with their underlying diseases. Although we've improved our understanding of risk factors, CVD continues to exact a heavy toll on individuals, families, the health care system, and the economy. Although we can't put a dollar value on *premature deaths, years of potential life lost,* or *disability* for millions of Americans, the measureable direct and indirect costs of CVD total nearly $1 billion per day.[6] This includes health care costs and lost productivity, and doesn't fully account for recent skyrocketing costs for essential drugs and procedures.[7] As Americans live longer with chronic diseases, costs will continue to increase. How much? Based on current trends, projections of total direct and indirect costs of CVD will surpass $918 billion, almost triple current costs, by 2030![8]

## History and Future Goals: Ideal Cardiovascular Health

Although these statistics may seem grim, the reality is that CVD has been the leading killer of both men and women in the United States every year since 1918, when a pandemic flu killed more people.[9] Recognizing that selected risk factors are key to changing the future course of CVD, the American Heart Association (AHA) has established goals designed to improve Americans' cardiovascular health by 20 percent and to reduce death from CVDs and stroke by 20 percent—all by the year 2020.[10]

As part of this strategy, the AHA is focusing on **ideal cardiovascular health (ICH)** and health promotion rather than morbidity and mortality rates. ICH is defined as the absence of CVD and indicators of CVD, the presence of *favorable health factors and behaviors*, and the simultaneous presence of the following seven behavioral and health factors.[11]

Behaviors:
- Not smoking
- Sufficient physical activity
- A healthy diet
- An appropriate energy balance and normal body weight

**cardiovascular disease (CVD)** Disease of the heat and blood vessels.

**ideal cardiovascular health (ICH)** The absence of clinical indicators of CVD and the presence of certain favorable behavioral and health factor metrics.

# $918 BILLION

in projected annual direct **MEDICAL COSTS** will be associated with cardiovascular diseases by 2030.

**Health Factors:**

- Optimal total cholesterol without medication
- Optimal blood pressure without medication
- Optimal fasting blood glucose without medication

So, how are we doing with respect to these *ideal CVD* measures today? One percent of adults don't meet any of the criteria; 16 percent meet only one; 63% meet two, three, or four of the ideal criteria; 13 percent meet five criteria; 5 percent meet six criteria; and fewer than 1 percent meet all seven behavioral criteria at ideal levels.[12] Meeting ideal cardiovascular health is both age and sex related, with younger adults and women more likely to meet more criteria overall.[13] While we clearly have a long way to go, understanding how the cardiovascular system works and how your actions can impact how it functions is an important first step.

## LO 2 | ESSENTIALS: UNDERSTANDING THE CARDIOVASCULAR SYSTEM

Describe the anatomy and physiology of the heart and circulatory system and the importance of healthy heart function.

The **cardiovascular system** is the network of organs and vessels through which blood flows as it carries oxygen and nutrients to all parts of the body. It includes the *heart, arteries, arterioles* (small arteries), *veins, venules* (small veins), and *capillaries* (minute blood vessels).

## The Heart: A Mighty Machine

The heart is a muscular pump, roughly the size of your fist. It is a highly efficient, extremely flexible organ that contracts 100,000 times each day and pumps the equivalent of 2,000 gallons of blood through the body. In a 70-year lifetime, an average human heart beats 2.5 billion times.

Under normal circumstances, the human body contains approximately 6 quarts of blood, which transports nutrients, oxygen, waste products, hormones, and enzymes throughout the body. Blood also helps regulate body temperature, cellular water levels, and acidity levels of body components, and it helps defend the body against toxins and harmful microorganisms.

The heart has four chambers that work together to circulate blood constantly throughout the body. The two upper chambers, called **atria**, are large collecting chambers that receive blood from the rest of the body. The two lower chambers, known as **ventricles**, pump the blood out again. Small valves both regulate the steady, rhythmic flow of blood and prevent leakage or backflow between chambers.

**Heart Function** Heart activity depends on a complex interaction of biochemical, physical, and neurological signals. There are four basic steps involved in heart function (see **FIGURE 16.1**).

> **cardiovascular system** Organ system, consisting of the heart and blood vessels, that transports nutrients, oxygen, hormones, metabolic wastes, and enzymes throughout the body.
>
> **atria (singular: atrium)** The heart's two upper chambers, which receive blood.
>
> **ventricles** The heart's two lower chambers, which pump blood through the blood vessels.

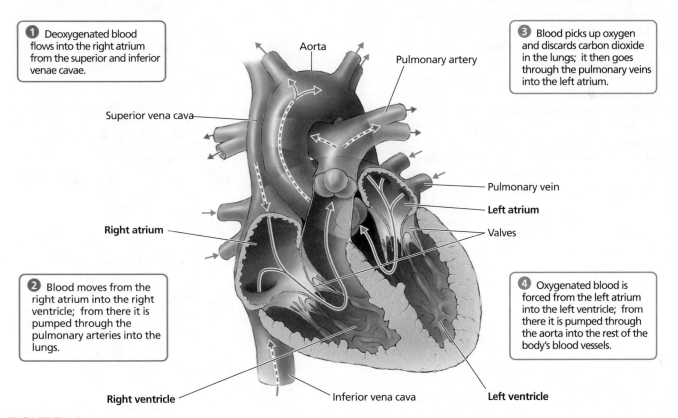

1. Deoxygenated blood flows into the right atrium from the superior and inferior venae cavae.

2. Blood moves from the right atrium into the right ventricle; from there it is pumped through the pulmonary arteries into the lungs.

3. Blood picks up oxygen and discards carbon dioxide in the lungs; it then goes through the pulmonary veins into the left atrium.

4. Oxygenated blood is forced from the left atrium into the left ventricle; from there it is pumped through the aorta into the rest of the body's blood vessels.

Aorta
Pulmonary artery
Superior vena cava
Pulmonary vein
Left atrium
Valves
Right atrium
Right ventricle
Inferior vena cava
Left ventricle

**FIGURE 16.1** Blood Flow within the Heart

1. Deoxygenated blood enters the right atrium after circulating through the body.
2. Blood moves to the right ventricle and is pumped through the pulmonary artery to the lungs, where it receives oxygen.
3. Oxygenated blood returns to the left atrium of the heart.
4. Blood from the left atrium moves into the left ventricle. The left ventricle pumps blood through the aorta to all body parts.

Various blood vessels perform different parts of this process. **Arteries** carry blood away from the heart; all arteries carry oxygenated blood, *except* for pulmonary arteries, which carry deoxygenated blood to the lungs where it picks up oxygen and gives off carbon dioxide. As the arteries branch off from the heart, they branch into smaller blood vessels called **arterioles**, and even smaller blood vessels known as **capillaries**. Capillaries have thin walls that permit exchange of oxygen, carbon dioxide, nutrients, and waste products with body cells. Carbon dioxide and other waste products are transported to the lungs and kidneys through **veins** and **venules** (small veins).

For the heart to function properly, its four chambers must beat in an organized manner. Your heartbeat is governed by an electrical impulse that travels across the heart and directs the heart muscle to move, resulting in sequential contraction of the four chambers. This signal starts in a small bundle of highly specialized cells, the **sinoatrial node (SA node)**, located in the right atrium. The SA node serves as a natural pacemaker. People with a damaged SA node must often have a mechanical pacemaker implanted to ensure the smooth passage of blood through the heartbeat's sequential phases.

At rest, the average adult heart beats 70 to 80 times per minute; a well-conditioned heart may beat only 50 to 60 times per minute to achieve the same results. If your resting heart rate is routinely in the high 80s or 90s, it may indicate that you are out of shape or suffering from an underlying illness. When overly stressed, a heart may beat more than 200 times per minute. A healthy heart functions more efficiently and is less likely to suffer damage from overwork.

# 750,000

Americans have a **HEART ATTACK** each year in the U.S.; 116,000 of whom die and 200,000 of whom will have another heart attack within 5 years.

## LO 3 | CARDIOVASCULAR DISEASE: AN EPIDEMIOLOGICAL OVERVIEW

Explain the incidence, prevalence, outcomes, and impacts of cardiovascular disease in the United States and globally.

Although rates have declined by over 30 percent in recent decades, it is important to recognize that over 2,200 people in the United States die from CVD *each day*—the equivalent of *ten 757* jetliners crashing each day.[14] For decades, cardiovascular diseases have surpassed cancer and other diseases as the leading cause of death; however, improvements in diagnosis and treatment have led to dramatic improvements in CVD death rates. It is important to note that there are vast differences in death rates by age, race, socioeconomic status, and gender (**FIGURE 16.2**).

### U.S. Disparities: Differences by Age, Sex, and Race

Many populations continue to be underinsured or uninsured and seek health care only in the later stages of their disease. When that happens, the disease ends up being more costly to treat, more disabling, and has poorer outcomes. Some CVD areas are

**arteries** Vessels that carry blood away from the heart to other regions of the body.
**arterioles** Branches of the arteries.
**capillaries** Minute blood vessels that branch out from the arterioles and venules; their thin walls permit exchange of oxygen, carbon dioxide, nutrients, and waste products among body cells.
**veins** Vessels that carry blood back to the heart from other regions of the body.
**venules** Branches of the veins.
**sinoatrial node (SA node)** Cluster of electric pulse–generating cells that serves as a natural pacemaker for the heart.

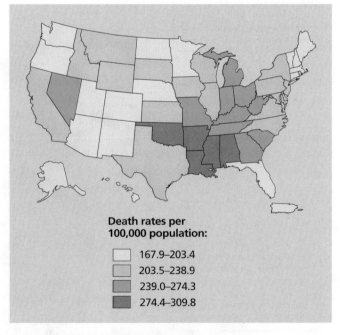

**Death rates per 100,000 population:**

- 167.9–203.4
- 203.5–238.9
- 239.0–274.3
- 274.4–309.8

**FIGURE 16.2** Major Cardiovascular Disease Age-Adjusted Death Rates by State

Source: D. Mozaffarian et al., "Heart Disease and Stroke Statistics—2016 Update: A Report From the American Heart Association," *Circulation* 133, no. 4 (2016): e200.

particularly devastating for different age, sex, and racial groups. Consider the following:

- Almost 50 percent of African American adults suffer from some form of CVD.[15]
- Many CVD-related fatalities are **sudden cardiac deaths (SCDs)**, an abrupt, profound loss of heart function (cardiac arrest) that causes death either instantly or shortly after symptoms occur. Technically different from a heart attack, where blockage occurs, SCD is typically not due to blockage. SCD strikes most often in those in their mid-30s and 40s, and affects men twice as often as women.[16]
- More men suffer from CVD at every age and stage of life until age 80, when women surpass men in prevalence rates (see **FIGURE 16.3**). Women also have a higher lifetime prevalence of stroke.[17]
- Heart disease is the leading killer of African American and white women in the United States. Among Hispanic women, heart disease causes as many deaths as cancer does. For American Indian or Alaska Native and Asian or Pacific Islander women, the second most common cause of death is heart disease.[18]
- Heart disease is the number one killer for men in most racial and ethnic groups in the United States, including African Americans, American Indians or Alaska Natives, Hispanics, and whites. For Asian American or Pacific Islander men, heart disease is the second greatest killer.[19]

## An Emerging Global Threat

Cardiovascular disease is not a uniquely American health problem. With an international trend toward obesity, more and more countries face epidemic CVD rates (see **TABLE 16.1**). In fact, according to the most recent World Health Organization (WHO) estimates, CVD accounts for over 31 percent of all deaths globally.[20] Over 75 percent percent of the world's CVD deaths occur in low- and middle-income countries, places where people have more risks and fewer options for prevention and treatment.[21] People with CVD in these countries die at younger ages, often during their most productive years.

## LO 4 | UNDERSTANDING THE MAJOR CARDIOVASCULAR DISEASES

Review major types of cardiovascular disease and their symptoms, as well as at-risk populations.

**sudden cardiac death (SCD)** an abrupt, profound loss of heart function (cardiac arrest) that causes death either instantly or shortly after symptoms occur.

Although there are several types of CVD, this chapter focuses on those with the greatest morbidity and mortality in U.S. populations: *hypertension, atherosclerosis,*

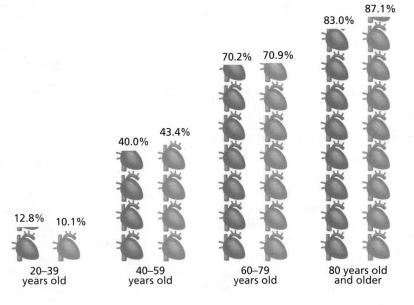

Men with CVD; each heart = 10% of the population

Women with CVD; each heart = 10% of the population

**FIGURE 16.3** Prevalence of Cardiovascular Diseases (CVDs) in Adults Aged 20 and Older by Age and Sex

Source: Data from D. Mozaffarian et al., "Heart Disease and Stroke Statistics—2016 Update: A Report From the American Heart Association," *Circulation* 133, no> 4 (2016): e192.

**TABLE 16.1** | Death Rates from CVD in Selected Countries

| Country | Rate* |
| --- | --- |
| Russian Federation | 1087.0 |
| Ukraine | 1067.0 |
| Romania | 595.0 |
| United States | 234.0 |
| Germany | 197.0 |
| United Kingdom | 178.5 |
| New Zealand | 164.8 |
| Sweden | 158.0 |
| Italy | 141.0 |
| Spain | 133.0 |
| Japan | 132.0 |
| France | 121.0 |
| Israel | 114.0 |

(*Rates per 100,000 people.)

Source: Data from D. Mozaffarian et al., "Heart Disease and Stroke Statistics—2016 Update: A Report From the American Heart Association, Table 13-3 Death Rates for Cardiovascular Diseases and All Causes in Selected Countries," *Circulation* 133, no. 4 (2016): e190–1.

# 31%

of all global deaths are attributable to **CVD**—making it the number one cause of death in the U.S. and globally. Over 80% of those deaths occur in low- and middle-income countries.

*peripheral arterial disease (PAD), coronary heart disease (CHD), angina pectoris, arrhythmia, congestive heart failure,* and *stroke.* **FIGURE 16.4** presents a breakdown of deaths by key cardiovascular diseases in the United States. Knowing more about your specific CVD risks, your limitations, and what you can do about them is key to taking healthy action.

## Hypertension

**hypertension** Sustained elevated blood pressure.

**resistant hypertension** A form of HBP that is difficult to control and may require three or more different classes of antihypertensive drugs to begin to control blood pressure.

**systolic blood pressure** The upper number in the fraction that measures blood pressure, indicating pressure on the walls of the arteries when the heart contracts.

**diastolic blood pressure** The lower number in the fraction that measures blood pressure, indicating pressure on the walls of the arteries during the relaxation phase of heart activity.

Blood pressure measures how hard blood pushes against vessel walls as your heart pumps. Sustained high blood pressure is called **hypertension**. Known as the "silent killer," it has few overt symptoms. Untreated hypertension damages blood vessels and increases your chance of a number of other CVDs. Hypertension can also cause kidney damage and contribute to vision loss, erectile dysfunction, and memory problems.[22]

Today, over 80 million adults—nearly 1 in 3 over the age of 20—in

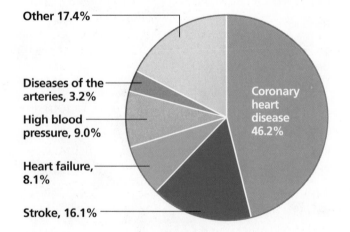

**FIGURE 16.4** Percentage Breakdown of Deaths Attributable to Cardiovascular Disease

**Source:** Data from D. Mozaffarian et al., "Heart Disease and Stroke Statistics—2016 Update: A Report From the American Heart Association," *Circulation* 133, no. 4 (2016): e193.

---

**TABLE 16.2** | Blood Pressure Classifications

| Blood Pressure Category | Systolic mm Hg (upper #) | | Diastolic mm Hg (lower #) |
|---|---|---|---|
| Normal | less than 120 | and | less than 80 |
| Prehypertension | 120 – 139 | or | 80 – 89 |
| High Blood Pressure (Hypertension) Stage 1 | 140 – 159 | or | 90 – 99 |
| High Blood Pressure (Hypertension) Stage 2 | 160 or higher | or | 100 or higher |
| Hypertensive Crisis (Emergency care needed) | Higher than 180 | or | Higher than 110 |

**Source:** American Heart Association, "Understanding Blood Pressure Readings," March 23, 2016, http://www.heart.org/HEARTORG/Conditions/HighBloodPressure/AboutHighBloodPressure/Understanding-Blood-Pressure-Readings_UCM_301764_Article.jsp#.VyVG1aT2aUk.

---

the United States have high blood pressure; based on current trends, rates may reach 41.4 percent by 2030.[23] There are large disparities in self-reported hypertension by race/ethnicity, age, sex, level of education, and state. At approximately 45 percent, African Americans have the highest rates of high blood pressure in the United States and globally.[24] Rates are also much higher among older adults, men, and those without a high school education.[25] Although awareness of hypertension has increased and most diagnosed individuals are using hypertension medications, only 53 percent of those on meds have their hypertension under control.[26] Many others have **resistant hypertension**, a difficult form of HBP that may require three or more classes of antihypertensive drugs to control.[27]

Blood pressure is measured by two numbers, for example, 110/80 mm Hg, stated as "110 over 80 millimeters of mercury." The top number, **systolic blood pressure**, refers to the pressure of blood in the arteries when the heart muscle contracts, sending blood to the rest of the body. The bottom number, **diastolic blood pressure**, refers to the pressure of blood on the arteries when the heart muscle relaxes as blood reenters the heart chambers. Normal blood pressure varies depending on age, weight, and physical condition, and high blood pressure is usually diagnosed when systolic pressure is 140 or above (see **TABLE 16.2**). When only systolic pressure is high, the condition is known as *isolated systolic hypertension* (*ISH*), the most common form of high blood pressure in older Americans. See the Health Headlines box for more on what it means to have "normal" blood pressure.

Systolic blood pressure tends to increase with age, whereas diastolic blood pressure typically increases until age 55 and then declines. Men under the age of 45 are at nearly twice the risk of becoming hypertensive as their female counterparts.[28] Men and women have nearly the same rates of HBP between the ages of 45 and 64.[29] Women have higher rates of hypertension after age 65.[30]

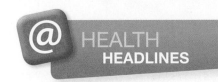
# NEW BLOOD PRESSURE GUIDELINES CAUSE CONTROVERSY

What does it really mean to have *normal* blood pressure? Should everyone, at every age, be treated to make sure they are at the ideal 120/80 mm Hg? Experts have debated whether individuals with high blood pressure need their levels to drop all the way to the ideal or whether somewhere below the high blood pressure limit would suffice. Should a 75-year-old woman in otherwise good health who has an elevated blood pressure of 140–150/90 mm Hg be put on a high-dose or multiple-drug regimen of antihypertensive medications to bring her blood pressure down to 120/80? Or are the potential risks from side effects from the drugs greater than the risks of a stroke or other CVD event? How low should blood pressure levels go, and do the benefits of using drugs to bring BP down always outweigh the risks? In 2014, a new study, *The Systolic Blood Pressure Intervention Trial (SPRINT)*, showed that if people cut their blood pressure below what was currently recommended they could slash their risk of heart failure and death. However,

questions arose about *how low is low enough* and if everyone needed the same low goal.

Based on new guidelines on blood pressure, most people in good health and without major CVD risks would use the current 120/80 mm Hg "healthy blood pressure" standard as their guide. However, the new recommendations say that those between the ages of 60 and 75 in otherwise good health should start medications at 150/90 mm Hg rather than 140/90 mm Hg. Those with CVD risks such as diabetes or chronic kidney disease should start medications at 140/90 mm Hg, but those under age 60 without other risks should be counseled about diet and exercise by their doctor. Critics argue that raising the BP treatment to 150 mm Hg is a mistake and that those with systolic BP between 140 and 149 face a 70 percent increased risk of stroke compared to those with lower BP readings. Proponents of raising the measures for treatment argue that the benefits of treatment at higher BP levels are outweighed by

fewer drug side effects. They point out that the recommendations consider the many studies that show that significant reductions in blood pressure may actually increase the risk of harm in some populations trying to achieve levels below 140/90 mm Hg with high doses of several BP-lowering drugs. Side effects such as persistent cough, erectile dysfunction, and frequent urination are among some of the typical side effects. Those considering these treatments should discuss risks and benefits with their doctor.

**Sources:** J. T. Wright et al., "A Randomized Trial of Intensive versus Standard Blood-Pressure Control," *New England Journal of Medicine* 373, no 22 (2015): 2103–2116; C. Rosendorf et al., "Treatment of Hypertension in Patients with Coronary Artery Disease: A Scientific Statement from the American Heart Association, American College of Cardiology, and American Society of Hypertension," *Journal of the American College of Cardiology* 65, no. 18 (2015): 1998–2038; X. Xie, et al. "Effects of Intensive Blood Pressure Lowering on Cardiovascular and Renal Outcomes: Updated Systematic Review and Meta Analysis," *The Lancet* 387 (2015): 435–43; R. Touyz and A Domiczak, "Hypertension Guidelines: Is it Time to Reappraise Blood Pressure Thresholds and Targets?" *Hypertension* (2016), doi: 10.1161. HypertensionAHA.116.07090.

## WHAT DO YOU THINK?

**Why are certain populations within the United States especially at risk for CVD?**

- Why are developing regions of the world experiencing major increases in CVD rates?
- With all of the media focus on reducing risks for CVD, why do you think we aren't seeing more dramatic reductions in CVD deaths?

## Atherosclerosis

**Arteriosclerosis**, thickening and hardening of the arteries, is a condition underlying many cardiovascular health problems. **Atherosclerosis** is a type of arteriosclerosis, where fatty substances, cholesterol, cellular waste products, calcium, and fibrin (a clotting material in the blood) accumulate in the inner lining of an artery. **Hyperlipidemia** (abnormally high

More and more people (over 30 percent of the population) are considered to be **prehypertensive**— blood pressure is above normal, but not yet in the hypertensive range. These individuals have a significantly greater risk of becoming hypertensive.[31] Importantly, over 17 percent of those with high blood pressure don't even know it.[32]

blood levels of *lipids*, which are non-water-soluble molecules, such as fats and cholesterol) is a key factor in this process, and the resulting buildup is referred to as **plaque**.

As plaque accumulates, it adheres to the inner lining of the blood vessels. Vessel walls become narrow and may eventually block blood flow or rupture. This is similar to putting your thumb over the end of a hose while water is running through it. Pressure builds within arteries just as pressure builds in the hose. If vessels are weakened and pressure persists, the artery may become weak and eventually burst. Fluctuation in blood pressure levels within arteries may actually damage their internal walls, making it even more likely that plaque will accumulate.

Atherosclerosis is the most common form of *coronary artery disease (CAD)*, which occurs as plaque builds in vessel walls and restricts blood flow and

**prehypertensive** Blood pressure is above normal, but not yet in the hypertensive range.

**arteriosclerosis** A general term for thickening and hardening of the arteries.

**atherosclerosis** Condition characterized by deposits of fatty substances (plaque) in the inner lining of an artery.

**hyperlipidemia** Abnormally high blood levels of *lipids*, which are non-water-soluble molecules, such as fats and cholesterol.

**plaque** Buildup of deposits in the arteries.

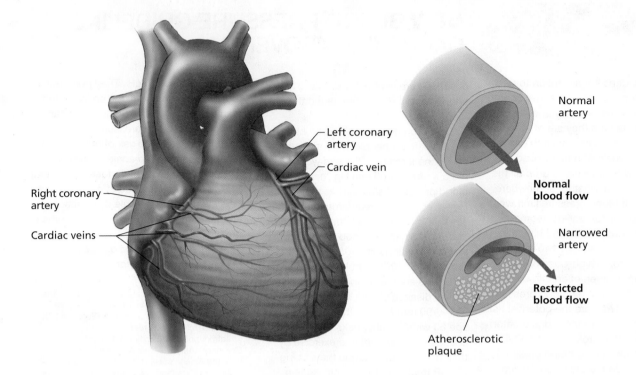

**FIGURE 16.5** **Atherosclerosis and Coronary Heart Disease** The coronary arteries are located on the exterior of the heart and supply blood and oxygen to the heart muscle itself. In atherosclerosis, arteries become clogged by a buildup of plaque. When atherosclerosis occurs in coronary arteries, blood flow to the heart muscle is restricted and a heart attack may occur.

**Source:** From Joan Salge Blake, *Nutrition & You*, and Michael D. Johnson, *Human: Biology: Concepts and Current Issues*, 7th ed. Both copyright © 2014 Pearson Education, Inc. Adapted by permission.

▶ **VIDEO TUTOR**
Atherosclerosis and Coronary Artery Disease

oxygen to the body's main coronary arteries, often eventually resulting in a heart attack (see **FIGURE 16.5**). When circulation is impaired and blood flow to the heart is limited, the heart may become starved for oxygen—a condition known as **ischemia**. Sometimes coronary artery disease is referred to as ischemic heart disease.

## Peripheral Artery Disease

When atherosclerosis occurs in the upper or lower extremities—such as in the arms, feet, calves, or legs—and causes narrowing or complete blockage of arteries, it is often called **peripheral artery disease (PAD)**. In the United States, over 8.5 million people—particularly people over age 65, non-Hispanic blacks, and women—have PAD; many receive no treatment because they are asymptomatic or don't recognize symptoms until they have a heart attack or stroke.[33] Others have pain, cramping, and aching in the legs, calves, or feet upon walking/exercising, relieved by rest (known as *intermittent claudication*); they may note that their feet feel colder than other areas.

Discussing symptoms with your doctor is a critical first step in intervention. A simple **ankle-brachial index (ABI)** test that measures blood pressure in your feet compared to your arm to determine blood flow might be warranted. The blood pressure in your feet is normally about 90 percent of that in your arm. If testing shows it much lower, and if you have PAD symptoms, a more sophisticated test may be required.

PAD is a leading cause of disability in people over age 50, and men develop it more frequently.[34] Risk factors include inflammation, smoking, high blood pressure, high cholesterol, and diabetes.[35] Sometimes PAD in the arms can be caused by trauma, certain diseases, radiation therapy or surgery, repetitive motion syndrome, or the combined risks of these factors and atherosclerosis.

## Coronary Heart Disease

Of all the major cardiovascular diseases, **coronary heart disease (CHD)** is the greatest killer, accounting for nearly 1 in 7 deaths in the United States.[36] Over 15 million Americans have CHD—7.6 percent of men and 5.0 percent of women.[37] Each year there are over 600,000 new coronary events and 305,000

**ischemia** Reduced oxygen supply to a body part or organ.

**peripheral artery disease (PAD)** Atherosclerosis occurring in the lower extremities, such as in the feet, calves, or legs, or in the arms.

**ankle-brachial index (ABI)** test in which a measure of blood pressure in your feet is compared to blood pressure in your arm to determine blood flow

**coronary heart disease (CHD)** A narrowing of the small blood vessels that supply blood

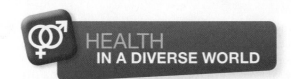
# WOMEN AND HEART ATTACKS
## *Different from Men?*

"Having a heart attack" usually brings to mind an older man gasping for breath, clutching his chest, toppling over in the middle of a workout. So, the story of comedian and former talk show host Rosie O'Donnell's heart attack doesn't seem to fit the mold: O'Donnell, 50, didn't immediately know she'd had one. At first, she wondered if she might have strained a muscle. Later she felt hot and clammy, and vomited. Fortunately, she took an aspirin and eventually went to the doctor, despite initially doubting a serious problem. It turned out O'Donnell had an almost complete blockage of an artery that required a stent.

Unfortunately, women's heart attack symptoms often don't "look" like what people have come to expect, sometimes ignored until it is too late. Women who suffer heart attacks under the age of 55 are not only less likely to have classic chest pain or pressure, but they also tend to delay going to the doctor. When they do seek medical attention, they often report atypical symptoms, such as shortness of breath, or pain in the neck, shoulder, arms, and stomach. Many women chalk up heart symptoms to stress, flu, or lack of exercise. Because of treatment delays, women are more likely to have heart damage and to die from a heart attack than are men of the same age. Here are some differences in the ways men and women experience heart attack symptoms:

| Sign or Symptom | Gender That Most Commonly Experiences It |
|---|---|
| Crushing or squeezing chest pain | More common in men |
| Pain radiating down arm, neck, or jaw | More common in men |
| Chest discomfort or pressure with shortness of breath, nausea/vomiting, or lightheadedness | Women more likely to feel pressure than pain. Shortness of breath and nausea and lightheadedness common in both women and men, but *more* common in women. |
| Shortness of breath without chest pain; discomfort in back, neck, or jaw or in one or both arms | More common in women |
| Unusual weakness | More common in women |
| Unusual fatigue | More common in women |
| Sleep disturbances | More common in women |
| Indigestion, flulike symptoms | More common in women |

If you or someone you know has any of these symptoms, don't delay. Crush or chew a full-strength aspirin and swallow it with water. Then have someone drive you to a health care facility for evaluation, or call 9-1-1 to get an ambulance.

**Sources:** American Heart Association, "Heart Attack Symptoms in Women," April 18, 2016, http://www.heart.org/HEARTORG/Conditions/HeartAttack/WarningSignsofaHeartAttack/Heart-Attack-Symptoms-in-Women_UCM_436448_Article.jsp#; National Coalition for Women with Heart Disease, "Am I Having a Heart Attack?" Accessed May 2016, http://www.womenheart.org/?page=Support_AmIHaving.

reoccurrences.[38] A **myocardial infarction (MI)**, or **heart attack**, involves an area of the heart that suffers permanent damage because its normal blood supply has been blocked—often brought on by a **coronary thrombosis** (formation of a clot) or an atherosclerotic narrowing that blocks a coronary artery. When a clot, or **thrombus**, becomes dislodged and moves through the circulatory system, it is called an **embolus**. Whenever blood does not flow readily, there is a corresponding decrease in oxygen flow to tissue below the blockage. If the blockage is extremely minor, an otherwise healthy heart will adapt over time by enlarging existing blood vessels and growing new ones to reroute needed blood through other areas. This system, called *collateral circulation*, is a form of self-preservation that allows an affected heart muscle to cope with damage.

When heart blockage is more severe, however, the body is unable to adapt on its own, and outside lifesaving support is critical. See the **Health in a Diverse World** box and the **Making Changes Today** box on page 432 for what to do in case of a heart attack.

## Arrhythmias

Over the course of a lifetime, most people experience some type of **arrhythmia**, an irregularity in heart rhythm that occurs when the electrical impulses that coordinate heartbeat don't work properly. Often described as a heart "fluttering" or racing, these irregularities send many people to the emergency room, only to find they are fine. A racing heart in the absence of exercise or anxiety may be *tachycardia*, the medical term for abnormally fast heartbeat. On the other end of the continuum is *bradycardia*, or abnormally slow heartbeat. When a heart goes into **fibrillation**, it beats in a sporadic,

**myocardial infarction (MI; heart attack)** A blockage of normal blood supply to an area in the heart.

**coronary thrombosis** A clot or an atherosclerotic narrowing that blocks a coronary artery.

**thrombus** A clot or blockage in the blood vessels.

**embolus** When a clot becomes dislodged and moves through the circulatory system.

**arrhythmia** An irregularity in heartbeat.

**fibrillation** A sporadic, quivering pattern of heartbeat that results in extreme inefficiency in moving blood through the cardiovascular system.

quivering pattern, resulting in extreme inefficiency in moving blood through the cardiovascular system. If untreated, fibrillation may be fatal.

Not all arrhythmias are life-threatening. In many instances, excessive caffeine or nicotine consumption can trigger an episode. However, severe cases may require drug therapy or external electrical stimulus to prevent serious complications. When in doubt, check with your doctor.

**angina pectoris** Chest pain occurring as a result of reduced oxygen flow to the heart.

**congestive heart failure (CHF)** An abnormal cardiovascular condition that reflects impaired cardiac pumping and blood flow; pooling blood leads to congestion in body tissues.

**cardiomyopathy** Damage to heart muscle.

**congenital cardiovascular defect** Cardiovascular problem that is present at birth.

## Angina Pectoris

**Angina pectoris** is a symptom of CHD that occurs when not enough oxygen supplies the heart muscle and is an indicator of underlying heart disease. Over 8 million people in the United States suffer from angina symptoms, ranging from heartburn-like symptoms to palpitations and crushing chest pain.[39] Mild cases may be treated with rest.

Drugs such as *nitroglycerin* can dilate veins and provide pain relief. Other medications such as *calcium channel blockers* can relieve cardiac spasms and arrhythmias, lower blood pressure, and slow heart rate. *Beta-blockers* can control potential overactivity of the heart muscle.

## Heart Failure

When the heart muscle is damaged or overworked and lacks the strength to circulate blood normally, blood and fluids begin to back up into the lungs and other body tissues, sometimes causing swelling of the feet, ankles, and legs, along with shortness of breath and tiredness. Known as heart failure or **congestive heart failure**, this condition is increasingly common, particularly among those with a history of CVD. Nearly 5.1 million adults have heart failure in the United States, with cases estimated to approach 10 million by 2030.[40]

Underlying causes of HF may include heart injury that results in damage to heart muscle (**cardiomyopathy**), affects heart valves, or causes problems with heart rhythms. Infectious diseases such as rheumatic fever can damage heart valves. Bacteria and viruses can inflame blood vessels, increasing atherosclerotic plaque formation. Uncontrolled high blood pressure, coronary artery disease, diabetes, and other chronic conditions can all lead to heart failure. Certain prescription drugs such as NSAIDS and diabetes medications also increase risks, as do chronic drug and alcohol abuse. In some cases, radiation or chemotherapy treatments for cancer cause damage.[41]

Untreated, HF can be fatal. However, most cases respond well to treatment that includes *diuretics* ("water pills") to relieve fluid accumulation; drugs, such as *digitalis*, that increase the heart's pumping action; and drugs called *vasodilators*, which expand blood vessels and decrease resistance, allowing blood to flow more freely and making the heart's work easier. Prevention of underlying CVD risks, such as reducing sodium intake and following a heart-smart diet, are the best ways to reduce your risks of HF.

## Congenital and Rheumatic Heart Disease

Approximately 40,000 infants are born in the United States each year with some form of **congenital cardiovascular defect** (*congenital* means the problem is present at birth).[42] Some are relatively minor, such as slight *murmurs* (low-pitched sounds caused by turbulent blood flow through the heart) caused by valve irregularities that some children outgrow. About 25 percent of those born with congenital heart defects must undergo invasive procedures to correct problems within the first year of life.[43] The underlying causes of these defects are unknown, but a variety of factors may contribute, such as heredity, maternal rubella during pregnancy, maternal drug use, smoking during the first trimester, and folate deficiency during pregnancy.[44] Paternal factors such as exposure to solvents, phthalates, and pesticides may increase fetal risks.[45] Because of advances in prenatal care, diagnosis, and pediatric cardiology, the prognosis for children with congenital heart defects is better than ever before.

**rheumatic heart disease** A heart disease caused by untreated streptococcal infection of the throat.

**stroke** A condition occurring when the brain is damaged by disrupted blood supply; also called *cerebrovascular accident.*

**aneurysm** A weakened blood vessel that may bulge under pressure and, in severe cases, burst.

**Rheumatic heart disease** is attributed to *rheumatic fever,* an inflammatory disease caused by an unresolved *streptococcal infection* of the throat (strep throat). Over time, this strep infection can affect many connective tissues of the body, especially those of the heart, joints, brain, or skin. In some cases, this infection can lead to an immune response in which antibodies attack the heart as well as the bacteria. Many of the thousands of operations on heart valves performed per year in the United States are related to rheumatic heart disease.

## Stroke

Like heart muscle, brain cells require a continuous supply of oxygen. A **stroke** (also called a *cerebrovascular accident*) occurs when blood supply to the brain is interrupted. Strokes may be either *ischemic* (caused by plaque formation that narrows blood flow or a clot that obstructs a blood vessel) or *hemorrhagic* (due to a bulging or rupturing blood vessel). **FIGURE 16.6** illustrates some of the blood vessel disorders that can lead to a stroke. An **aneurysm** (a widening or bulge in a blood vessel that may become hemorrhagic) is the most well-known hemorrhagic stroke. When any of these events occurs, oxygen deprivation kills brain cells.

Some strokes are mild and cause only temporary dizziness, slight weakness, or numbness. More serious blood flow interruptions may impair long-term speech, swallowing, memory, or motor control. Other strokes affect parts of the brain that

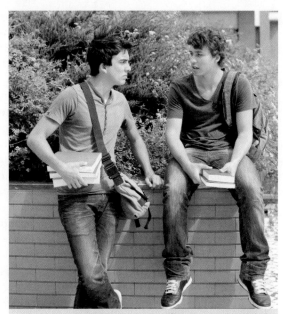

Young men, in particular, are at an elevated risk for stroke. What factors may contribute to this disparity in death rates?

regulate heart and lung function, killing within minutes. Fortunately, strokes have declined by nearly 20 percent since 2003, largely due to reductions in smoking, decreases in high-fat diets, improvements in diagnosis and treatment, and other factors. Despite overall decreases, stroke still affects nearly 6.5 million Americans every year, killing 129,000 people, making it the fifth leading cause of death in the United States.[46] Ten percent of all strokes occur in people aged 18 to 50. Strokes are on the increase among infants, youth, adolescents and younger adults.[47]

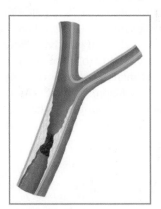 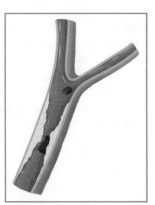 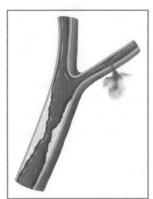 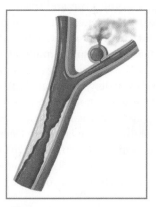

**a** A thrombus is a blood clot that forms inside a blood vessel and blocks the flow of blood at its origin. A thrombus in a cerebral artery can lead to an ischemic stroke.

**b** An embolus is a blood clot that breaks off from its point of formation and travels in the bloodstream until it lodges in a narrowed vessel and blocks blood flow. Emboli in brain blood vessels can cause ischemic strokes.

**c** A hemorrhage occurs when a blood vessel bursts, allowing blood to flow into the surrounding tissue or between tissues. There are two types of hemorrhagic strokes: subarachnoid, in which a vessel on the brain's surface bursts, and intracerebral, in which a vessel within the brain bursts.

**d** An aneurysm is the bulging of a weakened blood vessel wall. Aneurysms in the brain can cause hemorrhagic strokes if they burst.

**FIGURE 16.6** Blood Vessel Disorders That Can Lead to Stroke

**SEE IT!** VIDEOS

See how two young women have regained their lives after experiencing a stroke. Watch **Stroke in Young Adults**, available on **MasteringHealth.**

Many strokes are preceded days, weeks, or months by **transient ischemic attacks (TIAs)**, brief interruptions of the blood supply to the brain that cause only temporary impairment. Symptoms of TIAs include dizziness, particularly when first rising in the morning, weakness, temporary paralysis or numbness in the face or other regions, temporary memory loss, blurred vision, nausea, headache, slurred speech, or other unusual physiological reactions. While some may experience unexpected falls or have blackouts, others may have no obvious symptoms. TIAs often indicate an impending major stroke. The earlier a stroke is recognized, the more effective treatment will be (best results are seen if treatment begins within the first 1–2 hours). See the Making Changes Today box for tips on recognizing signs of a possible stroke.

Stroke survival rates have improved significantly in recent years, in part because of a greater recognition that *time is critical*. Greater awareness of stroke symptoms and faster medical attention, improvements in emergency medicine protocols and medicines, and a greater emphasis on fast rehabilitation and therapy have helped many survive. Newer treatments, including *tissue plasminogen activator* or *tPA*, the only FDA-approved treatment for ischemic stroke, dissolves clots and improves blood flow to affected areas, resulting in less damage and better chances of recovery. *Intra-arterial treatment (IAT)* is a technique in which a catheter delivers clot-dissolving drugs like tPA right to the site of injury, allowing for quick blood restoration and less long-term damage. Improvements in Emergency Medical Services protocols and treatments also significantly improve survival and recovery.[48] One promising new treatment, *stent retriever therapy*, involves inserting a catheter in the groin and snaking it through the body to the blocked artery. Once there, a wire mesh device opens and grabs the clot, often immediately restoring blood flow. Techniques like these often result in minimal or no disability in 91 percent of patients if used quickly after a stroke diagnosis.[49]

Unfortunately, stroke survivors do not always fully recover. Problems with speech, memory, swallowing, activities of daily living, and other consequences can persist, even with physical therapy and medications. Depression and anxiety are also issues for many poststroke survivors.[50] Preventing strokes and other cardiovascular diseases before they occur is clearly the best option. The earlier you start, the better!

## LO 5 | REDUCING YOUR CVD RISKS

Describe the modifiable and nonmodifiable risk factors for cardiovascular disease and methods of prevention.

**Cardiometabolic risks** are the combined risks that indicate physical and biochemical changes that can lead to both CVD and type 2 diabetes. Some of these risks result from choices and behaviors, and so are modifiable. Others are inherited

or intrinsic (such as your age and gender) and cannot be modified.

According to the *U.S. Burden of Disease Collaborators*, the greatest contributor to CVD is *suboptimal diet*, followed by tobacco smoking, high body mass index, high blood pressure, high fasting plasma glucose, and physical inactivity.[51] Newer research indicates that for people aged 12 to 39, smoking, high body fat, and high blood glucose increase the chances of dying from CVD-related complications before age 60.[52] As mentioned previously, hypertension doesn't just wreak havoc with your heart and circulatory system; it may also lead to inflammation in artery walls and the buildup of plaque—ultimately increasing risks for stroke, heart attack, and Alzheimer's disease.[53] Fortunately, you can take key steps to reduce your risk of CVD and complications.[54]

### Metabolic Syndrome: Quick Risk Profile

A cluster of combined cardiometabolic risks, variably labeled as *syndrome X*, *insulin resistance syndrome*, and, most recently, **metabolic syndrome (MetS)** are believed to increase the risk for atherosclerotic heart disease by as much as three times the normal rates.[55]

**transient ischemic attacks (TIAs)** Brief interruption of the blood supply to the brain that causes only temporary impairment; often an indicator of impending major stroke.

**cardiometabolic risks** Risk factors that impact both the cardiovascular system and the body's biochemical metabolic processes.

**metabolic syndrome (MetS)** A group of metabolic conditions occurring together that increases a person's risk of heart disease, stroke, and diabetes.

Women are more likely than men to have metabolic syndrome overall.[56] The highest prevalence occurs among Hispanics, followed by non-Hispanic whites and blacks.[57] As age increases, so does MetS, affecting over 18 percent of 20- to 39-year-olds to nearly 47 percent of those age 60.[58] Although different professional organizations have slightly different criteria for the syndrome, the National Cholesterol Education Program's Adult Treatment Panel (NCEP/ATP III) is most commonly used. A person with three or more of the following risks is diagnosed with metabolic syndrome (FIGURE 16.7):[59]

- Abdominal obesity (waist measurement of more than 40 inches in men or 35 inches in women).
- Elevated blood fat (triglycerides greater than 150) or on drug treatment for elevated triglycerides
- Low levels of HDL ("good") cholesterol (less than 40 in men and less than 50 in women) or on drug treatment for HDL reduction
- Elevated blood pressure greater than 130/85 or on drug treatment for BP reduction
- Elevated fasting glucose greater than 100 mg/dL (a sign of insulin resistance or glucose intolerance) or on drug treatment for elevated glucose

## Modifiable Risks for CVD

It may surprise you that CVD is not something you get as you hit middle age. In fact, you are a CVD work in progress right now. From the first moments of your life, you were genetically preprogrammed with some risks. How that genetic predisposition plays out is influenced significantly by your lifestyle. Your behaviors set the stage for risks in your 30s, 40s, and beyond. Making the following lifestyle modifications can have a significant effect on your future health profile.[60]

**Avoid Tobacco** Today, smoking rates in the United States are down dramatically—from 51 percent of men smoking in 1965 to 19 percent in 2014, and from 34 percent of women in 1965 to 15 percent in 2014. These declines are part of the reason heart disease rates are down, along with factors such as improved blood pressure, cholesterol control, and diet improvements.[61] Still, some populations continue to smoke despite overwhelming evidence of the consequences. For example, 27.1 percent of adults aged 18 to 20 years are current smokers.[62] In addition, racial disparities in smoking rates persist (see Chapter 12). Just how great a risk is smoking when it comes to CVD? Consider this:[63]

- Smokers are two to four times more likely to develop CHD than nonsmokers.
- Cigarette smoking doubles a person's stroke risk.
- Smokers are over 10 times more likely to develop peripheral vascular diseases than nonsmokers.

Smoking is thought to damage the heart in several ways. Nicotine increases heart rate, blood pressure, and oxygen use by heart muscles, which over time forces the organ to work harder. Additionally, chemicals in smoke may damage and inflame coronary arteries, increasing blood pressure and allowing plaque to accumulate more easily.

The sooner you quit, the better. People who stop smoking before they turned age 40 drastically cut their changes of dying early from smoking-related causes—by about 90 percent![64] Those who quit between the ages of 45 and 54 lower their chances of early death by about 66 percent.[65] Even those who develop cancer should quit immediately, as their prognosis is likely to improve.[66]

**Changing Fat and Cholesterol Recommendations** Cholesterol is a fatty, waxy substance found in the bloodstream and body cells. Cholesterol plays an important

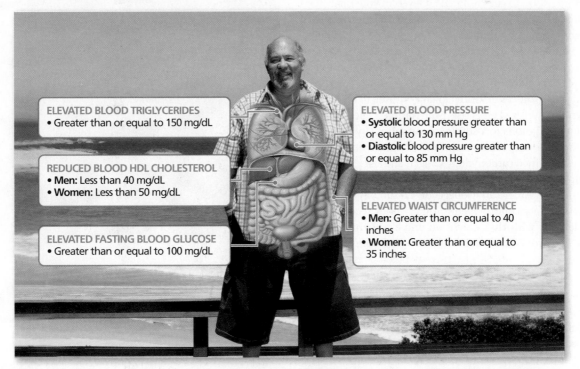

**FIGURE 16.7** Risk Factors Associated with Metabolic Syndrome

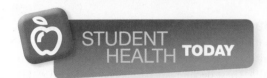
# EMERGING CONCERN
## *Gut Bacteria a Culprit in CVD Risk?*

While the high levels of saturated fat in red meat and high-fat dairy can lead to clogged arteries, new research suggests the way the bacteria in your gut process these substances might put you at risk for CVD rather than the fat level itself!

According to researchers, a chemical by-product created by digesting animal products actually may harm the linings of blood vessels, contributing to atherosclerosis. The by-product, known as *trimethylamine (TMA)*, changes into *trimethylamine-N-oxide (TMAO)* in the liver, apparently doubling the risk of heart attack, stroke, and death. While we need good bacteria in the gut, bacterial interactions with substances found in animal cells end up contributing to TMAO development and cholesterol accumulation on vessel walls.

If levels of TMAO are elevated according to a blood test, reductions in high-fat animal products may be warranted. It's just one more reason to cut the saturated fat levels in your diet to less than 10 percent of total calories.

**Source:** J. Brown and S. Hazen, "The Gut Microbial Endocrine Organ: Bacterially Derived Signals Driving Cardiometabolic Diseases," *Annual Review of Medicine* 66 (2015): 343.

---

role in the production of cell membranes and hormones (estrogen and testosterone), it protects nerves, is a good source of antioxidants, and it helps with digestion as well as processing vitamin D. For years, cholesterol has been seen as a key culprit in CVD risk, rather than an essential part of our diets. However, in early 2016, surprising reversals in the "cholesterol is bad" mantra emerged with the new *Dietary Guidelines*.[67]

As a result of years of study, the new *2015–2020 Dietary Guidelines for Americans, Eighth Edition*, out in early 2016, eased up on recommendations focused on cutting cholesterol. It turns out, with 75 percent of blood cholesterol produced by your liver and other cells—mostly out of your control as part of your genetic risk—much of your CVD risk has little to do with your dietary intake of cholesterol.[68] Eggs and other cholesterol-rich foods are now on the "eat" list, as experts put the emphasis on reducing saturated fat from high-fat meats and dairy to 10 percent of the daily diet.[69] See the **Student Health Today** box for one more reason to cut saturated fat levels in your diet.

Still, just because eggs are off the "bad" list doesn't mean you can gorge on bacon or high-fat steak or burgers on a regular basis. Many factors influence the other 25 percent of cholesterol in your bloodstream—most importantly, the amount of saturated fat and *trans* fat in the diet. High-fat dairy, red meat, and other sources of saturated fat continue to be sources of concern for increased CVD risk. Moderation is the key, with new recommendations focusing more on a healthy diet with leaner meats, poultry, nuts, fish, and shellfish and drastic reductions in refined carbohydrates, sugar, and salt.[70]

To help guide public behavior, the American Heart Association and the American College of Cardiology came up with new cardiovascular prevention guidelines recommending people work with their physician and assess their risk. A new "risk equation" assesses factors such as gender, race, age, current blood pressure control and medications, total cholesterol, HDL cholesterol, diabetes, smoking status, overall lifestyle, and genetic/family CVD risks. For certain risk factors, your doctor may prescribe *statins*—heart medicines designed to lower cholesterol and significantly reduce stroke and CVD risk. The *Guidelines* recommend statin therapy for the following groups:[71]

- People 40 to 75 years old, without CVD, who have a 7.5 percent or higher risk of stroke or heart attack within 10 years.
- People who have had a cardiovascular event (heart attack, stroke, angina, peripheral artery disease, transient ischemic attack, etc.) in the past.

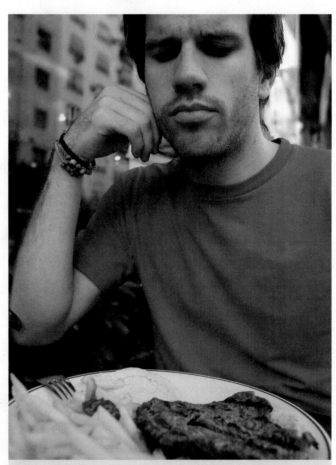

New guidelines indicate that reduction of saturated fat in the diet, particularly from meat and dairy, is more important than reducing cholesterol when it comes to CVD risks.

## SEE IT! VIDEOS

Can you find a way of eating to reduce your risk of heart disease? Watch **Diet Could Help Reduce Heart Disease**, available on **MasteringHealth.™**

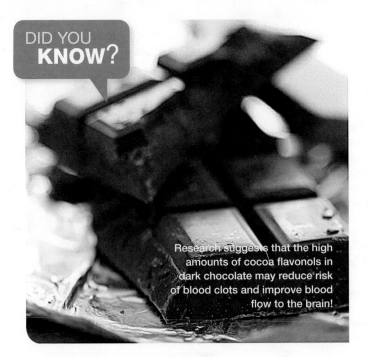

Research suggests that the high amounts of cocoa flavonols in dark chocolate may reduce risk of blood clots and improve blood flow to the brain!

- Adults age 21 and older with high levels of "bad" cholesterol (190 mg/dL or higher).
- People 40 to 75 years old who have diabetes.

Currently, about 45 percent of adults aged 20 and over have cholesterol levels at or above 200 mg/dL, and another 16 percent have levels in excess of 240 mg/dL.[72] Over 28 percent of Americans over the age of 40 in the United States are taking a cholesterol-lowering prescription; 93% of those are on statins.[73]

Historically, total cholesterol hasn't been the only level to be concerned with; the focus has been on two major types of blood cholesterol: *low-density lipoprotein (LDL)* and *high-density lipoprotein (HDL)*. Low-density lipoprotein, often referred to as "bad" cholesterol, is believed to build up on artery walls. In contrast, high-density lipoprotein, or "good" cholesterol, appeared to remove cholesterol from artery walls, thus serving as a protector. In theory, if LDL levels got too high or HDL levels too low, cholesterol would accumulate inside arteries and lead to cardiovascular problems. There is still controversy over whether this long-held theory is valid or not.

In general, LDL (or "bad" cholesterol) is more closely associated with cardiovascular risk than is total cholesterol. Until recently, most authorities agreed that looking only at LDL ignored the positive effects of "good" cholesterol (HDL) and that raising HDL was an important goal. There has been general agreement that the best method of evaluating risk is to examine the ratio of HDL to total cholesterol. If the level of HDL is lower than 35 mg/dL, cardiovascular risk increases dramatically. To reduce risk, the goal has been to manage the ratio of HDL to total cholesterol by lowering LDL levels, raising HDL, or both. New research indicates that trying to raise HDL as a means of preventing negative CVD outcomes may not be as beneficial as once thought.[74] However, many professional groups continue to believe that reducing LDL levels through aggressive drug therapy is the right goal for many at-risk

populations, along with increased exercise levels, weight control, healthy diet, and avoidance of tobacco.[75]

Today, *triglycerides* continue to be a focus of attention as a key factor in CVD risk. When you consume extra calories, the body converts them to triglycerides, which are stored in fat cells. Hormones release triglycerides throughout the day to provide energy. High levels of blood triglycerides are often found in people who have high cholesterol levels, heart problems, or diabetes or who are overweight. As people get older, heavier, or both, their triglyceride and cholesterol levels tend to rise. It has been recommended that a baseline cholesterol test (known as a lipid panel or lipid profile) be taken at age 20, with follow-ups every 5 years. This test, which measures triglyceride levels as well as HDL, LDL, and total cholesterol levels, requires that you fast for 12 hours prior to the test, are well hydrated, and avoid coffee and tea prior to testing. Men over the age of 35 and women over the age of 45 have been advised to have their lipid profile checked annually, with more frequent tests for those at high risk. Whether any or all of these recommendations will still be in force after the *Dietary Guidelines* are considered for their clinical implications remains unclear. See **TABLE 16.3** for current recommended levels of cholesterol and triglycerides and the **Health Headlines** box on page 438 for information about foods and dietary practices that can help maintain healthy cholesterol levels.

**Strive for a Heart-Healthy Diet** Research continues into other dietary modifications that may affect heart health. An overall approach, such as the DASH (Dietary Approaches to Stop Hypertension) eating plan from the

**TABLE 16.3** | Recommended Cholesterol Levels for Lower/Moderate-Risk Adults

| Total Cholesterol Level (lower numbers are better) | |
|---|---|
| Less than 200 mg/dL | Desirable |
| 200–239 mg/dL | Borderline high |
| 240 mg/dL and above | High |
| **HDL Cholesterol Level (higher numbers are better)** | |
| Less than 40 mg/dL (for men) | Low |
| 60 mg/dL and above | Desirable |
| **LDL Cholesterol Level (lower numbers are better)** | |
| Less than 100 mg/dL | Optimal |
| 100–129 mg/dL | Near or above optimal |
| 130–159 mg/dL | Borderline high |
| 160–189 mg/dL | High |
| 190 mg/dL and above | Very high |
| **Triglyceride Level (lower numbers are better)** | |
| Less than 150 mg/dL | Normal/desirable |

**Source:** National Heart Lung and Blood Institute, "What is Cholesterol?" April, 2016. http://www.nhlbi.nih.gov/health/health-topics/topics/hbc/diagnosis.

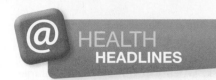

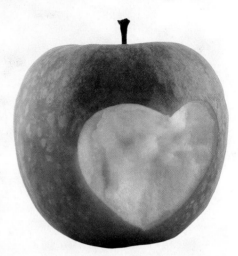

# HEALTH HEADLINES

# HEART-HEALTHY SUPER FOODS

The foods you eat play a major role in your CVD risk. While many foods can increase your risk, several have been shown to reduce the chances that cholesterol will be absorbed in the cells, reduce levels of LDL cholesterol, or enhance the protective effects of HDL cholesterol. To protect your heart, include the following in your diet:

- **Dark chocolate.** Dark chocolate contains 70 percent or more of flavonoid-rich cocoa, and much less sugar than milk chocolate. If you must indulge, buy the highest percent cocoa you can find, and savor the 1 to 2 ounces a bit at a time. Moderation is the key.
- **Fish high in omega-3 fatty acids.** Consumption of fish such as salmon, sardines, and herring may help reduce blood pressure and the inflammation that leads to plaque formation; however, new research is showing conflicting results about the benefits of omega-3s.
- **Olive oil.** Using monounsaturated fats in cooking, particularly extra virgin olive oil, helps lower total cholesterol and raise your HDL levels. Canola oil; margarine labeled *trans* fat–free; and cholesterol-lowering margarines such as Benecol, Promise Activ, or Smart Balance are also excellent choices.
- **Whole grains and fiber.** Getting enough fiber each day in the form of 100 percent whole wheat, steel-cut oats, oat bran, flaxseed, fruits, and vegetables helps lower LDL or bad cholesterol. Soluble fiber, in particular,

seems to keep cholesterol from being absorbed in the intestines.

- **Plant sterols and stanols.** These essential components of plant membranes are found naturally in vegetables, fruits, and legumes. In addition, many food products, including juices and yogurt, are now fortified with them. These compounds are believed to benefit your heart health by blocking cholesterol absorption in the bloodstream, thus reducing LDL levels.
- **Nuts.** Long maligned for being high in calories, walnuts, almonds, and other nuts are naturally high in omega-3 fatty acids, which are important in lowering cholesterol and good for the blood vessels themselves.
- **Green tea.** Several studies have indicated that green tea may reduce LDL cholesterol. The flavonoids in it act as powerful antioxidants that may protect the cells of the heart and blood vessels; however, other studies indicate that the FDA should *not* endorse health claims for green tea. Research in support is methodologically weak, and there are safety issues with the wide range of unfiltered tea available on the market.
- **Red wine.** In recent years, many observational studies have indicated that one glass of red wine may be protective and reduce your risk of CHD. Although the research is promising, the American Heart Association is slow to endorse drinking alcohol to reduce CVD risk and instead recommends dietary modification, exercise, and stress reduction, while supporting

additional research. While one drink of red wine might be protective, adding additional doses of wine doesn't appear to help.

**Sources:** A. Tresserra-Rimbau et al., "Moderate Red Wine Consumption is Associated with Lower Prevalence of the Metabolic Syndrome in the PREDIMED population," *British Journal of Nutrition* 113, no. S2 (2015): S121–S130; American Heart Association, "Alcoholic Beverages and Cardiovascular Disease," 2015, www.heart.org/HEARTORG/GettingHealthy/NutritionCenter/HealthyEating/Alcohol-and-Heart-Health_UCM_305173_Article.jsp; S. Kalesi, J. Sun, and N. Buys, "Green Tea Catechins and Blood Pressure: A Systematic Review and Meta Analysis of Randomized Controlled Trials," *European Journal of Nutrition* (2014), doi: 10.1007/s00394-014-0720-1; M. Murray, C. Walcuk, M. Suh, and P. J. Jones, "Green Tea Catechins and Cardiovascular Risk Factors. Should a Health Claim be Made by U.S. FDA?," *Trends in Food Science and Technology* 41, no. 2 (2015): 188–97; American Heart Association, "Fish and Omega 3 Fatty Acids," June 15, 2015, www.heart.org/HEARTORG/General/Fish-and-Omega-3-Fatty-Acids_UCM_303248_Article.jsp.

**plant sterols** Essential components of plant membranes that, when consumed in the diet, appear to help lower cholesterol levels.

National Heart, Lung, and Blood Institute (**FIGURE 16.8**), has strong evidence to back up its recommendations. DASH guidelines include:

- Reduce sodium intake.
- Consume 5 to 10 milligrams per day of soluble fiber from sources such as oat bran, fruits, vegetables, and seeds. This may result in a 5 percent drop in LDL levels.
- Consume about 2 grams per day of **plant sterols**, which are naturally present in many plant-based foods. Intake of plant sterols can reduce LDL by another 5 percent.

**Maintain a Healthy Weight** Researchers are not sure whether high-fat, high-sugar, high-calorie diets are a direct risk for CVD or whether they invite risk by causing obesity, which strains the heart, forcing it to push blood through the many miles of capillaries that supply each pound of fat. A heart that has to continuously move blood through an over-abundance of vessels may become damaged. Overweight people are more likely to develop heart disease and stroke even if they have no other risk factors. This is especially true if you're an "apple" (thicker around your upper body and waist) rather than a "pear" (thicker around your hips and thighs).

**Exercise Regularly** Even modest levels of low-intensity physical activity—walking, gardening, housework,

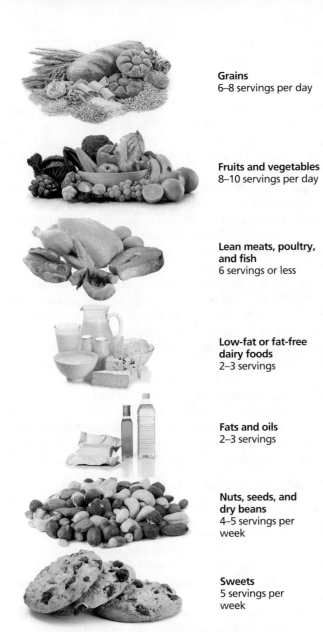

**Grains**
6–8 servings per day

**Fruits and vegetables**
8–10 servings per day

**Lean meats, poultry, and fish**
6 servings or less

**Low-fat or fat-free dairy foods**
2–3 servings

**Fats and oils**
2–3 servings

**Nuts, seeds, and dry beans**
4–5 servings per week

**Sweets**
5 servings per week

**FIGURE 16.8** **The DASH Eating Plan** Based on a 2,000-calorie/day diet. All serving suggestions are per day unless otherwise noted.

**Source:** National Heart, Lung, and Blood Institute, "Following the DASH Eating Plan," September 2015, www.nhlbi.nih.gov/health/health-topics/topics/dash/followdash.html.

dancing—are beneficial if done regularly and over the long term. Exercise can increase HDL, lower triglycerides, and reduce coronary risks in several ways.[76]

## Control Diabetes
Heart disease death rates among adults with diabetes are two to four times higher than the rates for adults without diabetes. At least 65 percent of people with diabetes die of some form of heart disease or stroke.[77] However, through a prescribed regimen of diet, exercise, and medication, they can control much of their increased risk for

CVD. (See **Focus On: Minimizing Your Risk for Diabetes** starting on page 446 for more on preventing and controlling diabetes.)

**Control Your Blood Pressure** In general, the higher your blood pressure, the greater your risk for CVD. Key factors in increasing blood pressure include obesity, lack of exercise, atherosclerosis, kidney damage from diabetes complications, and other factors.[78] Treatment of hypertension should involve dietary changes, particularly cutting sodium as it plays a key role in increasing blood pressure. The AHA recommends consuming less than 1500 mg (less than 3/4 teaspoon) of sodium per day to reduce risk of heart disease and stroke. Because our current levels are so high, getting sodium levels down to 2300 mg/day (less than 1 tsp) would also reduce risks.[79]

**Manage Stress** In recent years, scientists have shown compelling evidence that both acute and chronic stress may trigger acute cardiac events or even sudden cardiac death, as well as increase risks of hypertension, stroke, and elevated cholesterol levels.[80] Multiple life stressors can have tsunami-like effects on people young and old.[81] See Chapter 3 for more on effects of and coping with stress.

## Nonmodifiable Risks

Unfortunately, not all risk factors for CVD can be prevented or controlled. The most important are:

- **Race and ethnicity.** African Americans tend to have the highest overall rates of CVD and hypertension and the lowest rates of physical activity. Mexican Americans have the highest percentage of adults with cholesterol levels exceeding 200 mg/dL and the highest rates of obesity and overweight.[82]
- **Heredity.** A family history of heart disease increases risk of CVD significantly. The amount of cholesterol you produce, tendencies to form plaque, and other factors seem to have genetic links. The difficulty comes in sorting out genetic influences from the modifiable factors shared by family members, such as environment, stress, dietary habits, and so on. Newer research has focused on studying the interactions between nutrition and genes (*nutrigenetics*) and the role that diet may play in increasing or decreasing risks among certain genetic profiles.[83]
- **Age.** Advanced age and multiple risk factors increase the risk of CVD for all.[84]
- **Gender.** Men are at greater risk for CVD until about age 60, when women begin to catch up, taking the lead at age 80. Otherwise healthy women under age 35 have a fairly low risk, although oral contraceptive use and smoking increase risks. After menopause, or after estrogen levels are otherwise reduced (for example, because of hysterectomy), women's LDL levels tend to go up, which increases the chance for CVD. Women also have poorer health outcomes and higher death rates than men when they have a heart attack or stroke.[85]

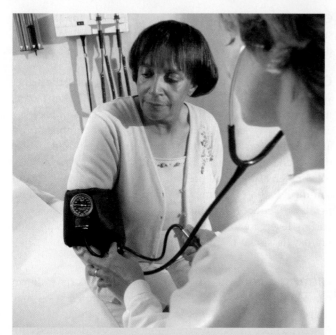

If there is a history of CVD in your family or your racial or ethnic background indicates a propensity for CVD, it is all the more important for you to have regular blood pressure and blood cholesterol screenings and for you to avoid lifestyle risks, including tobacco use, physical inactivity, and poor nutrition.

## Other Risk Factors Being Studied

Although risk factors for CVD are widely known, most people who die suddenly of a heart attack don't have obvious symptoms before it happens. New tests and emerging risk factors are being studied. Two fairly new CVD risks include high levels of inflammation in the vessels and homocysteine levels.

**Inflammation and C-Reactive Protein** Occurring when tissues are injured by bacteria, trauma, toxins, or heat, among other things, inflammation is increasingly being considered a culprit in atherosclerotic plaque formation. Injured vessel walls are more prone to plaque formation. To date, several factors, including cigarette smoke, high blood pressure, high LDL cholesterol, diabetes mellitus, certain forms of arthritis, gastrointestinal problems, and exposure to toxic substances have all been linked to increased risk of inflammation. However, the greatest risk appears to be from certain infectious disease pathogens, most notably *Chlamydia pneumoniae*, a common cause of respiratory infections; *Helicobacter pylori* (a bacterium that causes ulcers); herpes simplex virus (a virus that most of us have been exposed to); and *Cytomegalovirus* (another herpes virus infecting most Americans before the age of 40). During an inflammatory reaction, **C-reactive proteins** tend to be present at high levels. A recent meta-analysis of over 38 studies with nearly 170,000 subjects has shown a strong association between C-reactive proteins in the blood and increased risks for atherosclerosis and CVD.[86] Blood tests can test these proteins using a highly sensitive assay called *hs-CRP* (high-sensitivity C-reactive protein); if levels are high, action could be taken to reduce inflammation.

**C-reactive protein (CRP)** A protein whose blood levels rise in response to inflammation.

**homocysteine** An amino acid normally present in the blood that, when found at high levels, may be related to higher risk of cardiovascular disease.

**SEE IT! VIDEOS**
What habits can you change now to improve your heart health? Watch **Importance of Heart Health in Your Youth**, available on MasteringHealth.™

The FDA recently approved a new, nonfasting blood test that predicts heart attack in people with no history of heart disease. Known as *PLAC*, the test measures activity of inflammatory enzymes in the blood, which cause plaque to form. More inflammatory enzymes mean more plaque in vessels—and greater risk. The PLAC test could increase our ability to spot and treat potential heart attacks early in the process.[87]

Fish oil, flax, and other foods high in omega-3 have been recommended by the AHA and other groups for their anti-inflammatory properties, but questions have arisen about the role of omega-3 in reducing CVD.[88] In spite of conflicting reports, major professional organizations continue to recommend dietary omega-3 supplementation for risk reduction, particularly in reducing abnormal heartbeats that can lead to sudden death and in decreasing triglycerides and plaque formation.[89] More research is necessary to determine the actual role that inflammation plays in increased risk of CVD or if there is something unique about inflammation that omega-3 may work to counter.[90]

**Homocysteine** In the last decade, an increasing amount of attention has been given to the role of **homocysteine**—an amino acid normally present in the blood—in increased risk for CVD. When present at high levels, homocysteine may be related to higher risk of coronary heart disease, stroke, and peripheral artery disease. Although more research is needed, scientists hypothesize that homocysteine works like C-reactive proteins—inflaming the inner lining of the arterial walls, promoting fat deposits on the damaged walls, and encouraging blood clot development.[91] When early studies indicated that folic acid and other B vitamins may help break down homocysteine in the body, food manufacturers responded by adding folic acid to a number of foods and touting the CVD benefits. With conflicting research, the jury is still out on the role of folic acid in CVD risk reduction. In fact, professional groups such as the American Heart Association do not currently recommend taking folic acid supplements to lower homocysteine levels and prevent CVD.[92] For now, a healthy diet is the best preventive action.

## LO 6 | DIAGNOSING AND TREATING CARDIOVASCULAR DISEASE

Examine current strategies for diagnosis and treatment of cardiovascular disease.

Today, CVD patients have many diagnostic, treatment, prevention, and rehabilitation options that were not available a generation ago. Medications can strengthen heartbeat, control arrhythmias, remove fluids, reduce blood pressure, improve heart function, and reduce pain. Beyond statins, some common groups of drugs include *ACE inhibitors*, which cause the muscles surrounding blood vessels to contract, thereby lowering blood pressure, and *beta-blockers*, which reduce blood pressure by blocking the effects of the hormone epinephrine. New treatment procedures and techniques are saving countless lives. Even long-standing methods of cardiopulmonary resuscitation (CPR) have been changed to focus primarily on chest compressions rather than mouth-to-mouth breathing, the rationale being that people will be more likely to do CPR if the risk for exchange of body fluids is reduced—and any effort to save a person in trouble is better than inaction.

## Techniques for Diagnosing Cardiovascular Disease

Several techniques are used to diagnose CVD, including electrocardiogram, angiography, and positron emission tomography scans. An **electrocardiogram (ECG)** is a record of the electrical activity of the heart. Patients may undergo a *stress test*—standard exercise on a stationary bike or treadmill with an electrocardiogram and no injections—or a *nuclear stress test*, which involves injecting a radioactive dye and taking images of the heart to reveal problems with blood flow. In **angiography** (often referred to as *cardiac catheterization*), a needle-thin tube called a *catheter* is threaded through heart arteries, a dye is injected, and an X-ray image is taken to discover which areas are blocked. *Positron emission tomography (PET)* produces three-dimensional images of the heart as blood flows through it. Other tests include:

- **Magnetic resonance imaging (MRI).** This test uses powerful magnets to look inside the body. Computer-generated pictures can help physicians identify damage from a heart attack and evaluate disease of larger blood vessels such as the aorta.
- **Ultrafast computed tomography (CT).** This is an especially fast form of X-ray imaging of the heart designed to evaluate bypass grafts, diagnose ventricular function, and measure calcium deposits.
- **Cardiac calcium score.** This test measures the amount of calcium-containing plaque in the coronary arteries, a marker for overall atherosclerotic buildup. The more calcium, the higher your calcium score and the greater your risk of heart attack. Concerns have been raised over higher-than-average exposure to radiation from these tests.

## Surgical Options: Bypass Surgery, Angioplasty, and Stents

**Coronary bypass surgery** has helped many patients who suffered coronary blockages or heart attacks. In a *coronary artery bypass graft (CABG)*, referred to as a "cabbage," a blood vessel is taken from another site in the patient's body (usually the saphenous vein in the leg or the internal thoracic artery in the chest) and implanted to bypass blocked coronary arteries

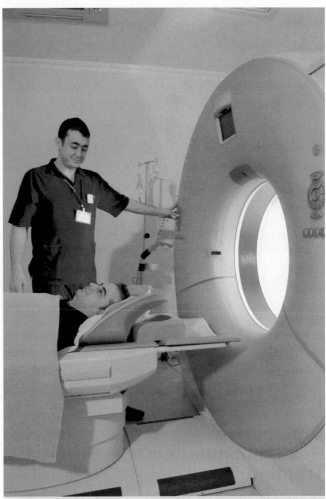

Magnetic resonance imaging is one of several methods used to detect heart damage, abnormalities, or defects.

and transport blood to heart tissue. Increasing numbers of heart surgeries are done using a minimally invasive bypass surgery in which the chest is not cut into; the surgeon enters the body through a series of ports and performs the surgery with cameras.

Another procedure, **angioplasty** (sometimes called *balloon angioplasty*), carries fewer risks. As in angiography, a thin catheter is threaded through blocked heart arteries. The catheter has a balloon at the tip, which is inflated to flatten fatty deposits against the artery walls, allowing blood to flow more freely. A stent (a mesh-like stainless steel tube) may be inserted to prop open the artery. Although highly effective, stents can result in inflammation and tissue growth in the area that can actually lead to more blockage and problems. In about 30 percent of patients, the

**electrocardiogram (ECG)** A record of the electrical activity of the heart; may be measured during a stress test.

**angiography** A technique for examining blockages in heart arteries.

**coronary bypass surgery** A surgical technique whereby a blood vessel taken from another part of the body is implanted to bypass a clogged coronary artery.

**angioplasty** A technique in which a catheter with a balloon at the tip is inserted into a clogged artery; the balloon is inflated to flatten fatty deposits against artery walls and a stent is typically inserted to keep the artery open.

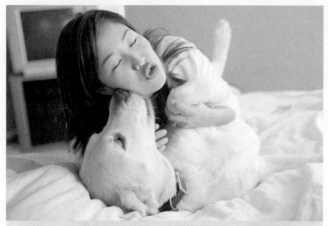

Depression, anxiety and insomnia are often part of the challenges facing those who have had a heart attack or stroke. Having a pet is a good way to help you focus on something positive besides your health.

treated arteries become clogged again within 6 months. Newer stents are usually medicated to reduce this risk. Nonetheless, some surgeons argue that, given this high rate of recurrence, bypass may be a more effective treatment. Newer forms of laser angioplasty and *atherectomy*, a procedure that removes plaque, are being done in several clinics.

## Changing Aspirin Recommendations and Other Treatments

Although aspirin has been touted for its blood-thinning qualities and possibly reducing risks for future heart attacks among those who already have had MI events, the benefits of an aspirin regimen for otherwise healthy adults has been controversial. New recommendations focus on those over the age of 50, as the

**thrombolysis** Injection of an agent to dissolve clots and restore some blood flow, thereby reducing the amount of tissue that dies from ischemia.

evidence for aspirin use in younger, low-risk adults is inconclusive. Those with a history of heart attack, or at risk for a heart attack or stroke, should consult with a doctor to discuss aspirin use. Those with risks of gastrointestinal bleeding or a history of stroke due to bleeding in the brain should discuss risks versus benefits before use. Ultimately, the FDA indicates it may be helpful to those who have had a heart attack or stroke in preventing a recurrence; however, it shouldn't be taken forever.[93] Furthermore, once a patient has taken aspirin regularly for possible protection against CHD, stopping this regimen may, in fact, increase his or her risk.[94]

Beyond aspirin, if a victim reaches an emergency room and is diagnosed fast enough, a form of clot-busting therapy called **thrombolysis** can be performed. Thrombolysis involves injecting an agent such as *tissue plasminogen activator* (*tPA*) to dissolve the clot and restore some blood flow to the heart (or brain), thereby reducing the amount of tissue that dies from ischemia.[95] These drugs must be administered within 1 to 3 hours after a cardiovascular event.

## Cardiac Rehabilitation and Recovery

Every year, millions survive heart attacks and utilize medical interventions to survive and thrive. In spite of our best diagnostic and treatment options, many cardiac patients find recovery difficult and live in fear of subsequent attacks. Others are disabled, have difficulty breathing and need supportive oxygen, retain fluid due to congestive heart failure, and have difficulties with activities of daily living. Those with friends and family for support and the financial ability to purchase necessary medication and travel for follow-up care can live out their lives with minimal dysfunction.

Perhaps the biggest deterrent is fear of having another attack due to exercise. The benefits of cardiac rehabilitation (including increased stamina and strength and faster recovery), however, far outweigh the risks when these programs are run by certified health professionals.

# STUDY **PLAN**

Customize your study plan—and master your health!—
in the Study Area of **MasteringHealth**.

## ASSESS YOURSELF

**What do your behaviors and family history tell you
about your CVD risk?** Want to find out? Take the **What's Your
Personal CVD Risk?** assessment available on

### MasteringHealth.™

## CHAPTER **REVIEW**

To hear an MP3 Tutor Session,
scan here or visit the Study
Area in **MasteringHealth**.

### LO 1 | Current Trends: Social and Economic Impact of CVD

- CVD exacts a heavy toll on individual health, families, communities, and the health care system, costing at least $1 billion per day, as well as being a huge burden in terms of years of potential life lost, disability, and other factors.
- Ideal cardiovascular health refers to the absence of CVD and the presence of seven favorable health factors and behaviors. Rather than focusing on mortality and morbidity, IDH focuses on healthy lifestyle.

### LO 2 | Essentials: Understanding the Cardiovascular System

- The cardiovascular system consists of the heart and circulatory system and is a carefully regulated, integrated network of vessels that supplies the body with the nutrients and oxygen necessary to perform daily functions.

### LO 3 | Cardiovascular Disease: An Epidemiological Overview

- Cardiovascular disease is the leading cause of death in the United States and globally. African Americans have the highest rates of CVD deaths out of any group in the United States.
- Although CVD used to be a problem of affluent, developed countries of the world, increasing prevalence in lower-income, developing countries is a cause for concern. Huge disparities in diagnosis, treatment, and outcomes continue to exist globally.

### LO 4 | Understanding the Major Cardiovascular Diseases

- Cardiovascular diseases include atherosclerosis, coronary artery disease, peripheral artery disease, coronary heart disease, stroke, hypertension, angina pectoris, arrhythmias, congestive heart failure, and congenital and rheumatic heart disease.

### LO 5 | Reducing Your CVD Risks

- *Cardiometabolic risks* refer to combined factors that increase a person's chances of CVD and diabetes. A person who possesses three or more cardiometabolic risk factors may have *metabolic syndrome*. Metabolic syndrome is increasing at all levels—among young and old, rich and poor, and in all races and ethnicities.
- Many risk factors for cardiovascular disease can be modified through your own lifestyle, such as cigarette smoking, high blood cholesterol and triglyceride levels, hypertension, lack of exercise, obesity, diabetes, emotional stress, and a diet high in saturated fat, sodium, and total calories. Some

risk factors, such as age, gender, and heredity, cannot be modified. The more risks you have, the greater your chances of developing CVD at an early age. Starting now to prevent CVD risks is key to future risk.

### LO 6 | Diagnosing and Treating Cardiovascular Disease

- Coronary bypass surgery is an established treatment for heart blockage; however, increasing numbers of angioplasty procedures and stents are being used with great success. Increasing numbers of pharmacological interventions such as statins are being used to reduce risk and prevent problems. Drug therapies can be used to prevent and treat CVD. Policies that improve the emergency medical response for victims, improve early diagnosis, and motivate people to take action can all reduce risks.

## POP **QUIZ**

Visit **MasteringHealth** to personalize your
study plan with Chapter Review Quizzes
and Dynamic Study Modules.

### LO 1 | Current Trends: Social and Economic Impact of CVD

1. Which of the following is *not* correct?
   a. CVD is a leading cause of death in the United States and globally
   b. Direct and indirect costs of CVD are more than $1 billion per day

c. Ideal cardiovascular health refers to having a perfect genetic, physiological, and health profile with zero cardiovascular risk throughout one's lifetime

d. Ideal cardiovascular health refers to a goal of no CVD disease and the presence of seven positive health and lifestyle behaviors

## Essentials: Understanding the Cardiovascular System
LO 2

2. The heart's upper chambers are called the
   a. valves.
   b. ventricles.
   c. atria.
   d. sinoatrial node.

3. Which type of blood vessels carry oxygenated blood away from the heart?
   a. Ventricles
   b. Arteries
   c. Pulmonary arteries
   d. Venules

## Cardiovascular Disease: An Epidemiological Overview
LO 3

4. Which of the following is true about CVD?
   a. It's only a problem in developed nations.
   b. It claims the lives of more men than women every year.
   c. Risk factors are only an issue starting at age 50.
   d. It's the leading cause of death in America.

## Understanding the Major Cardiovascular Diseases
LO 4

5. A stroke results
   a. when a heart stops beating.
   b. when cardiopulmonary resuscitation has failed to revive the stopped heart.
   c. when blood flow in the brain has been compromised, either due to blockage or hemorrhage.
   d. when blood pressure rises above 120/80 mm Hg.

6. An irregularity in the heartbeat is called a(n)
   a. fibrillation.
   b. bradycardia.
   c. tachycardia.
   d. arrhythmia.

7. Severe chest pain due to reduced oxygen flow to the heart is called
   a. angina pectoris.
   b. arrhythmias.
   c. myocardial infarction.
   d. congestive heart failure.

## Reducing Your CVD Risks
LO 5

8. What are the latest recommendations about cholesterol and fats in the diet as prevention for CVD?
   a. Cholesterol is a significant risk for atherosclerosis and dramatic reductions in cholesterol are recommended.
   b. Saturated fats are no longer on the "area of concern" list when it comes to CVD; hence you can eat all the bacon and burgers you want without worrying!
   c. Eggs are back "in" and cholesterol is no longer a major reason for concern in CVD risks.
   d. C-reactive proteins are part of the good element of cholesterol and having high levels of them in the blood are protective against CVD.

9. The "bad" type of cholesterol that we have been concerned about in recent years, which is found in the arteries, is known as
   a. high-density lipoprotein (HDL).
   b. low-density lipoprotein (LDL).
   c. total cholesterol.
   d. triglyceride.

## Diagnosing and Treating Cardiovascular Disease
LO 6

10. The surgery in which a blood vessel is taken from another site in the patient's body and implanted to bypass the blocked artery and transport blood to the heart is called
    a. atherosclerosis surgery.
    b. thrombolysis.

c. coronary bypass surgery.
d. angioplasty.

*Answers to the Pop Quiz can be found on page A-1. If you answered a question incorrectly, review the section identified by the Learning Outcome. For even more study tools, visit* **MasteringHealth**.

# THINK ABOUT IT!

## Current Trends: Social and Economic Impact of CVD
LO 1

1. What are the major social impacts of CVD on society today? What can individuals, communities, and health care systems do to reduce these impacts?

## Essentials: Understanding the Cardiovascular System
LO 2

2. What can your resting heart rate tell you about your overall health? What are some reasons a person's resting heart rate might be higher or lower than the median?

## Cardiovascular Disease: An Epidemiological Overview
LO 3

3. Why do you think hypertension rates are rising among today's college students? Do you know your own blood pressure levels? What factors are affecting your blood pressure right now?

## Understanding the Major Cardiovascular Diseases
LO 4

4. List the different types of CVD. Compare and contrast their symptoms, risk factors, prevention, and treatment. Which of these are you at greatest risk for? Explain.

## Reducing Your CVD Risks
LO 5

5. Discuss the role that exercise, stress management, dietary changes, medical checkups, sodium reduction, and other

factors can play in reducing risk for CVD. What role might infectious diseases play in CVD risk?

6. Discuss why age is an important factor in women's risk for CVD. Do men face the same age-related risks? Why or why not? What can be done to decrease women's risk in later life?

LO **6** **Diagnosing and Treating Cardiovascular Disease**

7. Describe some of the diagnostic, preventive, and treatment alternatives for CVD. If you had a heart attack today, which treatment would you prefer? Explain why.

## ACCESS YOUR HEALTH ON THE INTERNET

For links to the websites below, visit **MasteringHealth.**

Today, resources for those struggling with CVD risks abound. Quick links can open a world of CVD information.

**American Heart Association**. This is the home page of the leading private organization dedicated to heart health. This site provides information, statistics, and resources regarding cardiovascular care, including an opportunity to test your risk for CVD. **www.heart.org**

**National Heart, Lung, and Blood Institute**. This valuable resource provides information on all aspects of cardiovascular health and wellness. **www.nhlbi.nih.gov**

**Global Cardiovascular Infobase**. This site contains epidemiological data and statistics for cardiovascular diseases for countries throughout the world, with a focus on developing nations. **www.cvdinfobase.ca**

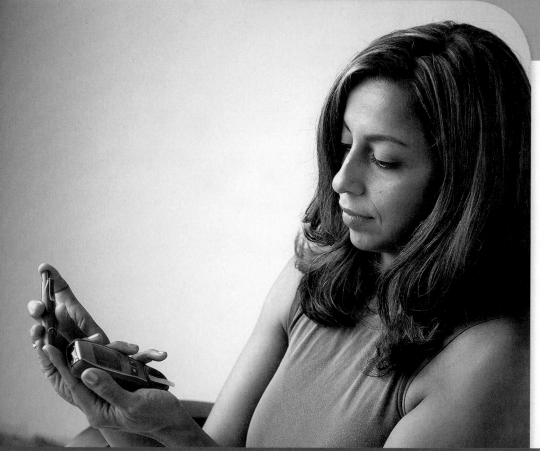

## LEARNING OUTCOMES

LO **1** Explain trends in diabetes in the United States and globally, describe the effect of diabetes on the body, and differentiate among types of diabetes and their risk factors.

LO **2** Describe the main tests for, symptoms of, and complications associated with diabetes.

LO **3** Explain how diabetes can be prevented and treated.

## WHY SHOULD I CARE?

Millennials, or Generation Y's—those 18- to 34-year-olds in the prime years of health—may also be among the fastest-growing segment of the obesity and type 2 diabetes epidemic in the United States. Over 1.2 percent of college students are reported diabetics, with an estimated 1.7 million new cases among young adults overall each year.[1] Millions more Millennials are believed to be prediabetic and the triple whammies of increasing hypertension, obesity, and progression to diabetes put more and more "under-45" adults at risk for serious problems, including stroke, kidney problems, vision problems, and other complications.[2] The mystique of "invincibility," vague early symptoms, and the perception that major health issues are the curse of older adults keep many from seeking early assistance aimed at prevention and treatment.

ia is overweight and out of shape. She used to figure it was no big deal and that she would diet and exercise more when she wasn't so busy with classes and trying to find a job. She was surprised to get a call from her mom, who seemed a bit distracted and down. It turned out that she had just been diagnosed with type 2 diabetes—at the age of 38. Her voice sounded shaky as she reminded Tia about her own mother's death from kidney failure—a complication of diabetes—at age 52. Although she had never brought up Tia's weight, she hinted that they *both* needed to try to lose weight and exercise more before she hung up. Later, Tia searched online for information about her risk for diabetes. Her Hispanic ethnicity, family history, high stress level and lack of sleep, excessive weight, and sedentary lifestyle made her a prime candidate.

Tia made an appointment for a diabetes screening. She was instructed to fast the night before. At her visit, the nurse practitioner took a blood sample. The next day, the NP called Tia to tell her that her blood glucose was elevated, and although she wasn't diabetic yet, she needed to make changes to her diet and lifestyle to reduce her risk for developing type 2 diabetes like her mom.

Diabetes is one of the fastest-growing health threats in the world today, with over 422 million people classified as diabetic in 2014. Over half of all adult diabetes cases occur in five countries: China, India, the United States, Brazil, and Indonesia. Those diagnosed with diabetes are expected to exceed 700 million by 2035.[3] While the number of people with diabetes has increased in virtually all countries of the world, with the fastest rates of growth occurring in low- and middle-income countries where access to prevention and treatment may be lacking.

Over the past two decades, diabetes rates in the United States have increased dramatically[4] (see **FIGURE 1**). The Centers for Disease Control and Prevention (CDC) estimates that nearly 30 million people—almost 10 percent of the U.S. population—have diabetes, and another 86 million have *prediabetes*.[5] Experts predict that at current rates, more than

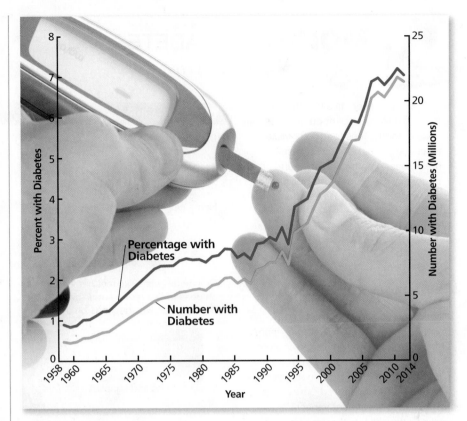

**FIGURE 1** Percentage and Number of U.S. Population with Diagnosed Diabetes, 1958–2014

Source: CDC, "Long-Term Trends in Diabetes," April 2016, https://www.cdc.gov/diabetes/statistics/slides/long_term_trends.pdf.

1 in 3 Americans will have diabetes by 2050. Diabetes kills more Americans each year than breast cancer and AIDS combined, and millions suffer the physical, emotional, and economic burdens of dealing with this difficult disease.[6]

Diabetes rates increase as age and weight increase. Among persons aged 18 to 44 years, approximately 2.4 percent have diabetes, compared to roughly 12.3 percent of those aged 45 to 64, 22.1 percent of those 65 to 74, and 19.8 percent of those 75 and over.[7] The economic burden of diagnosed diabetes, gestational diabetes, undiagnosed diabetes, and prediabetes was over $322 billion in 2012.[8] At current rates, this economic burden is projected to increase to over $512 billion by 2021.[9] Costs for diagnosed diabetics average nearly $11,400 per person per year, while undiagnosed diabetes averages just over $4,400.[10] For an explanation of the personal financial toll that comes with diabetes, read the **Money & Health** box on page 448.

## LO 1 | WHAT IS DIABETES?

Explain trends in diabetes in the United States and globally, describe the effect of diabetes on the body, and differentiate among types of diabetes and their risk factors.

**Diabetes mellitus** is a group of diseases, each with its own mechanism, all characterized by a persistently high level of glucose, a type of sugar, in the blood. One sign of diabetes is the production of an unusually high volume of glucose-laden urine, a fact reflected in its name: *Diabetes* derives from a Greek word meaning "to flow through," and *mellitus* is the Latin word for "sweet." The high blood glucose levels—or **hyperglycemia**—seen in diabetes can

---

**diabetes mellitus** A group of diseases characterized by elevated blood glucose levels.

**hyperglycemia** Elevated blood glucose level.

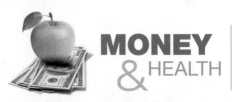

# DIABETES
## At What Cost?

One in every five health care dollars is spent on diabetes care today: fees for doctor visits, testing supplies, laboratory results, medicines to control glucose and others to control side effects, as well as the costs for other necessities often only partially covered, even for those with insurance. If you are underinsured or uninsured, the *diabetes drain* on your bank account could be major. Average medical costs for a person diagnosed with type 2 diabetes runs nearly $14,000 per year, with about $8,000 of that directly attributable to the disease. This is nearly two to three times more than someone without diabetes incurs each year. Complications from diabetes can quickly mount, with specialized treatment often required.

Costs of treatment varies tremendously; whether you have insurance, the nature of your deductibles and co-pays, proximity to pharmacies with a supply of generics, and the number and dosage of drugs necessary to control your blood glucose are all factors. As with most pharmaceuticals, prices for drugs have increased dramatically in the last few years. Newer drugs may not be more effective, yet they may cost significantly more. Often, after a person takes one drug for a period of time, the drug becomes less effective and additional drugs are necessary. This is especially true when people with diabetes ignore dietary guidelines and eat as they did prior to diagnosis, using their medications as the prevention strategy rather than making lifestyle changes. To give you an idea of what it might cost someone who is diagnosed with type 2 diabetes and who doesn't have insurance, consider these very conservative monthly estimates.

The American Diabetes Association estimates costs of between $350 and $1,000 per month for the typical type 2 diabetic without complications. However, those whose diabetes is difficult to control and those who must use insulin or use multiple drug therapy may have costs that are two to three times higher.

| Diabetic Health Care Need | Estimated Monthly Cost |
|---|---|
| Doctor visit for monitoring and testing | $200–1,000, depending on number of visits and specialists seen |
| Lab tests: Fasting blood glucose test, glucose tolerance, A1C tests | $50–250 for fasting blood glucose; $100–200 for A1C |
| Home glucose meter, test strips | Meter = $35–50<br>Test strips = roughly $2 each.<br>Average = $100/month |
| Lancets and lancing devices, alcohol wipes | $5–10/month |
| Oral medications like metformin (depends on dosage and type); Actos (depends on dosage); Januvia (depends on dosage) | *Metformin*: $13–15 at low end per month; less at big-box stores, more for different dosage<br>*Actos*: $220–370/month<br>*Januvia*: $265/month, newer drugs may not have generic version yet and insurance may not pay for newest |
| Insulin pumps and supplies | $7,000 or more without insurance; co-pays may run $2,000 or more |

**Sources:** American Diabetes Association. "The Costs of Diabetes," June 2015, http://www.diabetes.org/advocacy/news-events/cost-of-diabetes.htm; C. Iliades, M.D. "Budgeting for Diabetes Health Costs." Everyday Health. http://www.everydayhealth.com/hs/type-2-diabetes/budgeting-for-diabetes-health-costs; American Diabetes Association, "What Are My Options," March 2015, http://www.diabetes.org/living-with-diabetes/treatment-and-care/medication/oral-medications/what-are-my-options.html.

lead to many serious health problems and even premature death.

In a healthy person, the digestive system breaks down the carbohydrates we eat into glucose—one of our main energy sources—which it releases into the bloodstream for use by body cells. Our red blood cells can only use glucose to fuel functioning, and brain and other nerve cells prefer glucose over other fuels. When glucose levels drop below normal, you may feel unable to concentrate, and certain mental functions may be impaired. When more glucose is available than required to meet immediate needs, the excess is stored as glycogen in the liver and muscles for later use. The average adult has about 5 to 6 grams of glucose in the blood at any given time, enough to provide energy for about 15 minutes under normal activity levels. Once that circulating glucose is used, the body begins to draw upon its glycogen reserves.

Glucose can't simply cross cell membranes on its own. Instead, cells have structures that transport glucose across in response to a signal generated by the **pancreas**, an organ located just beneath the stomach. Whenever a surge of glucose enters the bloodstream, the pancreas secretes a hormone called **insulin**. Insulin stimulates cells to take up glucose from the bloodstream and carry it into the cell, where it's used for immediate energy. Conversion of glucose to glycogen for storage in the liver and muscles is also assisted by insulin. When levels of

**pancreas** Organ that secretes digestive enzymes into the small intestine and hormones, including insulin, into the bloodstream.

**insulin** Hormone secreted by the pancreas and required by body cells for the uptake and storage of glucose.

glucose fall, the pancreas stops secreting insulin—until the next influx of glucose arrives.

# Type 1 Diabetes

The more serious and less prevalent form of diabetes, called **type 1 diabetes** (or insulin-dependent diabetes), is an autoimmune disease in which the individual's immune system attacks and destroys the insulin-making cells in the pancreas. Destruction of these cells causes a dramatic reduction, or total cessation, of insulin production. Without insulin, cells cannot take up glucose, leaving blood glucose levels permanently elevated. Too much glucose in the bloodstream can wreak havoc with tissues and organs in the body, damaging the kidneys and the nerves in the hands and feet and causing a wide range of other serious health consequences. The higher and longer sustained the blood glucose level, the greater the risk.

Only about 5 percent of diabetic cases are type 1.[11] People inherit a predisposition to type 1 diabetes and something in the environment triggers it.[12] Type 1 diabetes is more common in predominantly white, European populations, those with a genetic predisposition, those living in cold climates, children who are not breastfed, and those with a history of certain viral infections.[13] People with type 1 diabetes require daily insulin injections or infusions and must carefully monitor their diet and exercise levels. Often they face unique challenges as the "lesser known" diabetic type, with fewer funds available for research and fewer options for treatment.

# Type 2 Diabetes

**Type 2 diabetes** (non-insulin-dependent diabetes) accounts for 90 to 95 percent of all cases, with genetics and lifestyle playing significant roles in its development.[14] (In type 2, either the pancreas does not make sufficient insulin, or body cells are resistant to its effects—a condition called **insulin resistance**—and don't use it efficiently (**FIGURE 2**).

## Development of Type 2 Diabetes

Type 2 diabetes usually develops slowly. In early stages, cells throughout the body begin to resist the effects of insulin over time, or the body may not produce enough insulin. An overabundance of free fatty acids concentrated in a person's fat cells (as may be the case in an obese individual) inhibit glucose uptake by body cells and suppress the liver's sensitivity to insulin. As a result, the liver's ability to self-regulate its conversion of glucose into glycogen begins to fail, and blood levels of glucose gradually rise.

The pancreas attempts to compensate by producing more insulin, but it cannot maintain hyperproduction indefinitely. More and more pancreatic

**type 1 diabetes** Form of diabetes mellitus in which the pancreas is not able to make insulin, and therefore blood glucose cannot enter the cells to be used for energy.

**type 2 diabetes** Form of diabetes mellitus in which the pancreas does not make enough insulin or the body is unable to use insulin correctly.

**insulin resistance** State in which body cells fail to respond to the effects of insulin; obesity increases the risk that cells will become insulin resistant.

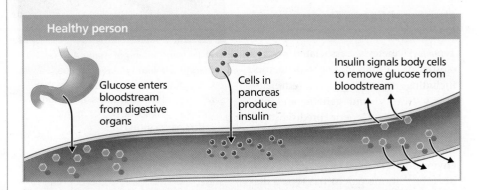

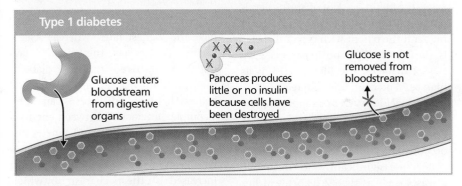

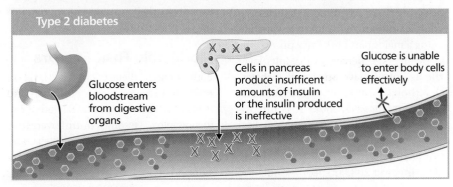

**FIGURE 2 Diabetes: What It Is and How It Develops** In a healthy person, a sufficient amount of insulin is produced and released by the pancreas and used efficiently by the cells. In type 1 diabetes, the pancreas makes little or no insulin. In type 2 diabetes, either the pancreas does not make sufficient insulin, or resistant to insulin and are not able to use it efficiently.

▶ VIDEO TUTOR
How Diabetes Develops

# 1 IN 2

Odds your child will develop type 2 **DIABETES** if both you and your partner have type 2 diabetes.

insulin-producing cells become non-functional, insulin output declines, and blood glucose levels rise high enough to warrant a diagnosis of type 2 diabetes.

## Nonmodifiable Risk Factors

Type 2 diabetes is associated with a cluster of nonmodifiable risk factors, including increasing age, ethnicity, family history, and genetic and biological factors. Genetic predisposition plays a stronger role in type 2 diabetes than in type 1 diabetes, even though environment is a key to triggering both diseases.[15] If one parent has type 2 diabetes, the lifetime risk of offspring development is up to 40 percent and slightly higher if the parent with type 2 diabetes is the mother.[16] If both parents have type 2 diabetes, the lifetime risk is as high as 70 percent.[17] Several recent studies have yielded evidence supporting the theory that, during pregnancy, aspects of a woman's health—such as obesity or consumption of a high-fat diet—contribute significantly to metabolic diseases such as type 2 diabetes in her offspring.[18] Clearly, type 2 diabetes is a complex disease, with lifestyle variables being a major part of the risk profile.

Nearly 26 percent of adults over the age of 65 have a form of diabetes.[19] Although it used to be referred to as *adult-onset diabetes*, today it is increasingly diagnosed among children and teens.[20] Currently diabetes is one of the leading chronic diseases in youth, affecting over 208,000 people under the age of 20, or 1 in every 400 youth.[21]

Non-Hispanic whites, Native Americans, and non-Hispanic black youth

**prediabetes** Condition in which blood glucose levels are higher than normal, but not high enough to be classified as diabetes.

Halle Berry is one of many Americans diagnosed with type 2 diabetes. Each day, over 3800 Americans are diagnosed with diabetes, and many more are undiagnosed or in the prediabetes stage.

**Source:** American Diabetes Association, "The Staggering Costs of Diabetes.," Accessed July 2016, http://www.diabetes.org/diabetes-basics/statistics/infographics/adv-staggering-cost-of-diabetes.html#sthash.Vay8Lmnq.dpuf.

have the highest rates, whereas Asian/Pacific Islanders have the lowest.[22] Having a close relative with type 2 diabetes is a significant risk factor. Most experts believe that type 2 diabetes is caused by a complex interaction between environmental factors, lifestyle, and genetic susceptibility. Although numerous genes have been identified as likely culprits in increased risk, the mechanisms by which inherited diabetes develops remains poorly understood.[23]

## Modifiable Risk Factors

Body weight, dietary choices, level of physical activity, sleep patterns, and stress level are all diabetes-related factors people have some control over. Type 2 diabetes is linked to overweight and obesity, particularly a genetic predisposition to central body obesity. In adults, a body mass index (BMI) of 25 or greater increases risks, with significantly higher risks for each 5 kg/m$^2$ increase.[24] In particular, excess weight carried around the waistline—a condition called *central adiposity*—and measured by waist circumference is a significant risk factor

for older women.[25] People with type 2 diabetes who lose weight and increase their physical activity can significantly improve their blood glucose levels.

Inadequate sleep may contribute to the development of both obesity and type 2 diabetes, possibly due to the fact that sleep-deprived people tend to eat more and engage in food-finding activities more frequently and tend to expend less energy in physical activity.[26] People routinely sleep deprived are also at higher risk for *metabolic syndrome* (discussed shortly), a cluster of risk factors that include poor glucose metabolism.[27] A recent review of the accumulated research indicates that Type 2 Diabetes risk increases among those experiencing trauma or stressful working conditions; those with a history of depression; and those with personalities that often lead to conflict with others.[28] In addition, diabetes is more common among those who have experienced persistent low socioeconomic status (SES) in their lives and in racial and ethnic minorities, independent of current SES.[29]

### SEE IT! VIDEOS

Could fewer, larger meals be better for people with diabetes? Watch **Two Meals a Day Could Help Diabetics Control Blood Sugar**, available on **MasteringHealth.**™

## Prediabetes

An estimated 86 million Americans age 20 or older—37 percent of the population over age 20—and 51 percent of those over 65—have **prediabetes**, a condition involving higher-than-normal blood glucose levels, but not high enough to be classified as diabetes. Nine out of 10 people with prediabetes do not know they have it.[30] Current rates of prediabetes in college students are unknown; however, results from several smaller studies indicate that increased rates of obesity and "sitting behavior" or "sedentariness" increase rates of type 2 diabetes—not only in American college students, but in college populations in other countries.[31] Often, prediabetes is one of the risk factors linked to overweight and obesity that together constitute *metabolic syndrome (MetS).*

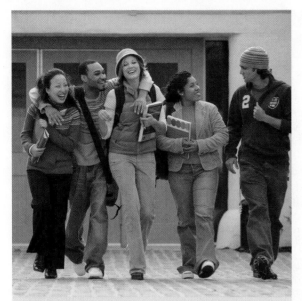

About 208,000 people younger than age 20 have type 1 or type 2 diabetes, with over 5,000 new cases each year. Thousands more are believed to have prediabetes.

**Source:** American Diabetes Association, "Fast Facts: Data and Statistics about Diabetes," December 2015, http://professional2.diabetes.org/admin/UserFiles/0%20-%20Sean/Documents/Fast_Facts_12-2015a.pdf.

Currently, MetS affects about 35 percent of U.S. adults and increases their risks of cardiovascular disease, stroke, and diabetes, as well as accumulation of fatty deposits in blood vessel walls.[32] Overweight, obesity, sedentary lifestyle, and genetics are all key risks for MetS. [33] A person who has metabolic syndrome is five times more likely to develop type 2 diabetes than is a person without it.[34] Overall, Mexican Americans have the highest rates of metabolic syndrome, with white Americans and African Americans not far behind.[35] Women

### WHAT DO YOU THINK?

**Why do you think prediabetes and type 2 diabetes are increasing in the United States?**

- Why is it increasing so quickly among young people?
- Why do you think that so many people are prediabetic or are undiagnosed diabetics and don't have a clue that they have it? What do you think should be done to increase awareness, particularly among high-risk minority populations?

with uterine fibroids or ovarian cysts are also at increased risk.[36] See Chapter 6 and Chapter 16 for more on MetS.

Without weight loss and increases in moderate physical activity, 15 to 30 percent of those with prediabetes will develop type 2 diabetes within 5 years.[37] Lack of knowledge—less than 14 percent of the population knows what prediabetes is—poses a major challenge to slowing increasing diabetes rates.[38] A prediabetes diagnosis represents an opportunity to adjust your lifestyle. Increasing physical activity can have a significant positive effect on type 2 diabetes as well as reducing risks of blood lipids, hypertension, and other diabetic complications.[39] See tips for halting or slowing the progression of diabetes in the Making Changes Today box on page 452.

## Gestational Diabetes

**Gestational diabetes (GD)** is a state of high blood glucose levels during pregnancy, posing risks for both mother and child. Thought to be associated with metabolic stresses that occur in response to changing hormonal levels, as many as 18 percent of pregnancies have been affected by gestational diabetes.[40] Although there has been significant variability, most reports have indicated that between 40 and 50 percent—and as many as 60 percent—of women with a history of GD will progress to type 2 diabetes within a decade of initial diagnosis if they don't lose weight, improve their diet, and exercise. If excess weight is never lost, higher "normal" weight increases risk of progression to type 2 diabetes with subsequent births.[41] New research indicates that there is tremendous variability in progression rates and that recent changes in diagnostic criteria for GD will mean that many more women will be diagnosed; recommended aggressive treatment may

signal a decline in progression to type 2 diabetes in the future.[42]

Improved diagnosis, as well as increased emphasis on prevention and follow-up, are important to the overall health of the mother and her baby. Women with GD also have increased risk of high blood pressure, high blood acidity, increased infections, and death.[43] A result of the excess fat accumulation that is a hallmark sign of gestational diabetes, women can give birth to large babies—increasing the risk of birth injuries and the need for caesarean sections. High blood sugar and excess weight in a pregnant woman can trigger high insulin levels and blood sugar fluctuations in the newborn. Babies born to women with gestational diabetes are also at risk for malformations of the heart, nervous system, and bones; respiratory distress; and fetal death.[44]

## LO 2 | WHAT ARE THE SYMPTOMS OF DIABETES?

Describe the main tests for, symptoms of, and complications associated with diabetes.

The symptoms of diabetes are similar for both type 1 and type 2, including:

- **Thirst.** Kidneys filter excessive glucose by diluting it with water. This can pull too much water from the body and result in dehydration.
- **Excessive urination.** For the same reason, increased need to urinate occurs.
- **Weight loss.** Because so many calories are lost in the glucose that passes into urine, a person with diabetes often feels hungry. Despite eating more, he or she typically loses weight.
- **Fatigue.** When glucose cannot enter cells, fatigue and weakness occur.

**gestational diabetes** Form of diabetes mellitus in which women who have never had diabetes have high blood sugar (glucose) levels during pregnancy.

# MAKING CHANGES TODAY

## What Can You Do to Reduce Your Risks?

If you are wondering if you might be showing symptoms of prediabetes or diabetes, set up an appointment with your doctor either at home or on campus (check your insurance policy first to determine if you are covered for selected blood tests). Tell the doctor about your potential genetic risks; your weight, diet, and exercise behaviors; and your concerns. Be honest, be assertive, and ask for these tests: blood chemistry and lipid profile, fasting blood glucose test, and an A1C test.

Since weight loss, healthy diet, exercise, stress management, and sound sleep are all parts of the formula for risk reduction, take your risks seriously. Even if your blood tests all are normal, you need to pay attention to genetic risks like parents, siblings, or other relatives with a history of diabetes. It gets harder to lose weight and get in shape as you age. Starting now on a lifelong behavior change is key to your long-term health future.

The good news is that you can reduce your risks significantly and even if you have genetic risks for diabetes, you can increase the number of healthy years you live diabetes free or avoid developing it. Proven strategies include:

- **Careful with the carbs!** Remember that carbohydrates in any form will ramp up blood glucose. Even foods that are otherwise full of nutrients, such as refined grains with beans and squash, will raise your blood sugar rapidly. Balancing your carb intake with lean protein and healthy fats can help slow those spikes. Avoid high-sugar beverages, sweets, and hidden sugar found in foods. Focus on the veggies and complex carbohydrates. Watch portion control and stick to small!

- **Lose weight!** By losing just 7 percent of your body weight by improving your diet and increasing exercise, you can prevent diabetes and bring glucose levels back to normal.

- **Get moving!** Although you may not like it much at first, as you lose and feel better and see your glucose levels decrease and the "flab" start to fade, moving may become one of your most enjoyable parts of the day. Thirty minutes per day over 5 days a week is the minimum. Remember, those 30 minutes can be broken into three 10-minute bouts throughout the day.

- **Quit smoking.** In addition to cancer and heart disease, smoking increases blood glucose levels.

- **Reduce or eliminate alcohol consumption.** It's high in calories and can interfere with blood glucose regulation. If you drink, go for drinks with low sugar and carbohydrates, and decide ahead of time which healthy munchies you can have.

- **Get enough sleep.** Inadequate sleep may contribute to the development of type 2 diabetes.

- **Destress.** What you think is so important won't seem important to you in a few days or weeks. Keep things in perspective. Learn to take yourself less seriously, find time for fun, develop a strong support network, and use relaxation skills as part of a mindful life.

- **Get regular checkups.** If you have a family history, or several risk factors, get regular checkups with your doctor. If you need help with any of the above, talk to someone in the counseling or student health center.

- **Get support.** Check to see if there are any campus or community seminars or meetings focused on weight loss, prediabetes prevention, and/or starting an exercise program. Prioritize your time to get to one of these meetings. If you have a dietician working through your student health center, set up a meeting with him or her and ask for help in reducing your personal risk. Find a CDC-sponsored Lifestyle Change Program in your area. For details, go to: https://www.cdc.gov/diabetes/prevention/lifestyle-program/experience/index.html.

**Sources:** Centers for Disease Control and Prevention, "National Diabetes Prevention Program," 2015, www.cdc.gov/diabetes/prevention/recognition/curriculum.htm; ADA, "Living with Type 2 Diabetes Program Plan," https://donations.diabetes.org/site/SPageServer/?pagename=LWT2D_English&loc=dorg_diabetes-myths&s_src=dorg&s_subsrc=diabetes-myths.

---

- **Nerve damage.** A high glucose concentration damages the smallest blood vessels of the body, including those supplying nerves in the hands and feet. This can cause numbness and tingling.
- **Blurred vision.** Too much glucose causes body tissues to dry out—particularly damaging to the eyes.
- **Poor wound healing and increased infections.** High levels of glucose can affect the body's ability to ward off infections and may affect overall immune system functioning.

## Complications of Diabetes

The main complications of poorly controlled diabetes include:[45]

- **Diabetic coma.** A coma from high blood acidity known as *diabetic ketoacidosis* can occur when, in the absence of glucose, body cells break down stored fat for energy. The process produces acidic molecules called *ketones*. Too many ketones can raise blood acid level dangerously high.

The diabetic person slips into a coma and, without medical intervention, will die.
- **Cardiovascular disease.** Because many diabetics are also overweight or obese, hypertension is often present. Blood vessels become damaged and more prone to fatty plaque formation as glucose-laden blood flows sluggishly and essential nutrients and other substances are not transported as effectively.
- **Kidney disease.** Diabetes is the leading cause of kidney failure. The

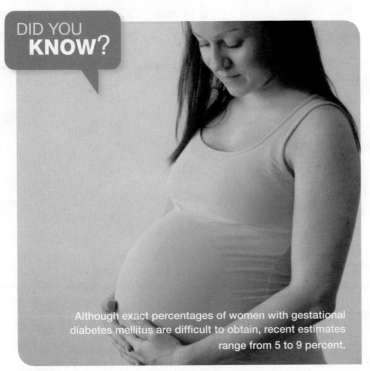
kidneys become scarred by overwork and the high blood pressure in their vessels. More than 247,000 Americans are currently living with kidney failure caused by diabetes.[46] In fact, 35 percent of those age 20 or older with diabetes have kidney failure.[47] Many of these people are on dialysis or are waiting for a kidney transplant that may never come.

■ **Amputations.** An impaired immune response combined with damaged blood vessels and neuropathy in hands and feet makes it easier for people with diabetes not to notice injury until damage is extensive. Lack of circulation to the area increases risk of infection and difficulty of treatment, leading to tissue death and amputation. More than 60 percent of nontraumatic amputations of legs, feet, and toes are due to diabetes[48] (see **FIGURE 3A**). In fact, each year nearly 73,000 nontraumatic lower-limb amputations are performed on people with diabetes (180 per day).[49]

■ **Eye disease and blindness.** High blood glucose levels damage microvessels in the eye, leading to vision loss. Nearly 7.7 million people over the age of 40 have early-stage retinopathy, swelling of capillaries in the eye, which could lead to blindness without treatment (**FIGURE 3B**).[50]

■ **Infectious diseases.** Persons with diabetes have increased risk of poor wound healing and greater susceptibility to infectious diseases, particularly influenza and pneumonia. Once infection occurs, it may be more difficult to treat.

■ **Tooth and gum diseases.** Research indicates that persons with diabetes are more susceptible to bacterial infections of the mouth that can lead to *gingivitis* (an early stage of gum disease) and *periodontitis*—a more serious inflammation of the gums that can lead to decay, tooth loss, and a variety of other health risks.[51] Emerging research suggests that the relationship between diabetes and gum disease may be a two-way street, with those who have gum disease being more susceptible to problems with blood glucose control, increasing the risk of progression to diabetes.[52]

■ **Other complications.** Diabetics may have foot neuropathy and chronic pain that makes walking, driving, and simple tasks more difficult. Persons with diabetes are more likely to suffer from depression, making intervention and treatment more difficult. Depressed individuals are 60 percent more likely to develop type 2 diabetes.

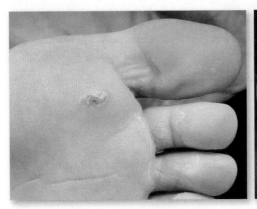

ⓐ Diabetics are prone to wounds that don't heal on the feet as nerves may be damaged, healing impaired and sensation diminished. Blisters, infections and other irritants can easily progress to more serious problems.

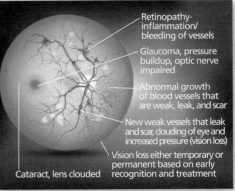

Retinopathy-inflammation/bleeding of vessels

Glaucoma, pressure buildup, optic nerve impaired

Abnormal growth of blood vessels that are weak, leak, and scar

New weak vessels that leak and scar, clouding of eye and increased pressure (vision loss)

Vision loss either temporary or permanent based on early recognition and treatment

Cataract, lens clouded

ⓑ Uncontrolled diabetes can damage the eye, causing swelling, rupture of blood vessels.

**FIGURE 3** Complications of Uncontrolled Diabetes: Amputation and Eye Disease

## Diagnosing Diabetes

Diabetes and prediabetes are diagnosed when a blood test reveals elevated blood glucose levels. Generally, a physician orders one of the following blood tests:

- The *fasting plasma glucose (FPG) test* requires a patient to fast for 8 to 10 hours. Then, a small sample of blood is tested for glucose concentration. An FPG level greater than or equal to 100 mg/dL indicates prediabetes, and a level greater than or equal to 126 mg/dL indicates diabetes (**FIGURE 4**).

- The *oral glucose tolerance test (OGTT)* requires the patient to drink concentrated glucose. A sample of blood is drawn for testing 2 hours after drinking. A reading greater than or equal to 140 mg/dL indicates prediabetes; a reading greater than or equal to 200 mg/dL indicates diabetes.

- A third test, *A1C* or *glycosylated hemoglobin test (HbA1C)*, doesn't require fasting and gives the average value of a patient's blood glucose over the past 2 to 3 months, instead of at one moment in time. In general, an A1C of 5.7 to 6.4 means high risk for diabetes or being prediabetic. If the A1C is 6.5 or higher, then diabetes may be diagnosed.[53] **Estimated average glucose (eAG)** shows how A1C numbers correspond to blood glucose numbers. For example, someone with an A1C value of 6.1 would be able to look at a chart and see that his or her average blood glucose was around 128—a high level that should encourage healthy lifestyle modifications.

People with diabetes need to check blood glucose levels several times each day to ensure they stay within their target range. To check blood glucose, diabetics must prick their finger to obtain a drop of blood. A handheld glucose meter can then evaluate the blood sample.

**estimated average glucose (eAG)** A method for reporting A1C test results that gives the average blood glucose levels for the testing period using the same units (milligrams per deciliter [mg/dL]) that patients are used to seeing in self-administered glucose tests.

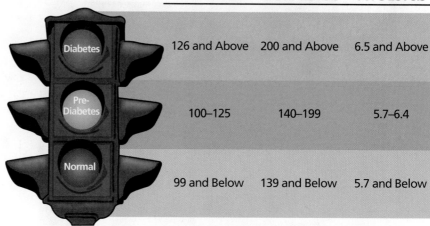

| | FPG Levels | OGTT Levels | A1C Levels |
|---|---|---|---|
| Diabetes | 126 and Above | 200 and Above | 6.5 and Above |
| Pre-Diabetes | 100–125 | 140–199 | 5.7–6.4 |
| Normal | 99 and Below | 139 and Below | 5.7 and Below |

**FIGURE 4** **Blood Glucose Levels in Prediabetes and Untreated Diabetes** The fasting plasma glucose (FPG) test measures levels of blood glucose after a person fasts overnight. The oral glucose tolerance test (OGTT) measures levels of blood glucose after a person consumes a concentrated amount of glucose. The A1C test is a blood test that measures average glucose levels over a 3-month period.

**Source:** American Diabetes Association, "Diagnosing Diabetes and Learning about Prediabetes," June 9, 2015, www.diabetes.org/diabetes-basics/diagnosis.

## LO 3 | TREATING DIABETES

Explain how diabetes can be prevented and treated.

Treatment options for people with prediabetes and diabetes vary according to type and progression of the disease.

### Lifestyle Changes

Studies have shown that lifestyle changes can prevent or delay the development of type 2 diabetes by up to 58 percent.[54] Even for people with type 2 diabetes, lifestyle changes can sometimes prevent or delay the need for medication or insulin injections.

### Losing Weight

A landmark clinical trial, the *Diabetes Prevention Program (DPP)* study, showed that a loss of as little as 5 to 7 percent of current body weight and regular physical activity significantly lowered the risk of progressing to diabetes.[55] If you have diabetes, weight loss and exercise can improve your blood glucose and other health indicators.

### Adopting a Healthy Diet

To prevent surges in blood sugar, people with diabetes must pay attention

# 30%

The reduced risk of diabetes among those in a major research trial who were on a Mediterranean diet.

to the glycemic index and glycemic load of the foods they eat. Glycemic index compares the potential of foods containing the same amount of carbohydrate to raise blood glucose. The concept of glycemic load was developed by scientists to simultaneously describe the quality (glycemic index) and quantity of carbohydrate in a meal.[56] By learning to combine high—and low—glycemic index foods to avoid surges in blood glucose, diabetics can help control average blood glucose levels throughout the day.

Researchers have studied a variety of specific foods for their effect on blood glucose levels. Here is a brief summary of their findings:

- **Whole grains.** A diet high in whole grains may reduce a person's risk of developing type 2 diabetes.[57]

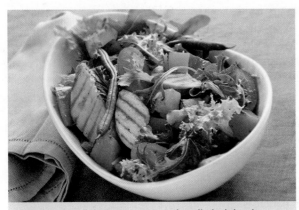

People with diabetes can occasionally indulge in sweets in moderation, particularly if they balance carbohydrates with lean protein and healthy fat. However, meals low in saturated and *trans* fats and high in fiber, like this salad of salmon and fresh vegetables, are recommended for helping to control blood glucose and body weight.

- **High-fiber foods.** Recent research indicates that eating high-fiber foods may reduce diabetes risk.[58]
- **Fatty fish.** An impressive body of evidence has linked the consumption of fish high in omega-3 fatty acids with decreased progression of insulin resistance. However, more research has called this high fish intake and risk reduction for diabetes into question.[59] Likewise, studies linking fatty fish consumption with reduced risk of MetS, a diabetes risk factor, have indicated only a weak association at best.[60] More research is necessary to determine the role fatty acids play in diabetes risk reduction.[61]

## Increasing Physical Fitness

The DPP and other organizations recommend at least 30 minutes of moderate-intensity physical activity 5 days a week to reduce your risk of type 2 diabetes.[62] Exercise increases sensitivity to insulin. The more muscle mass you have and the more you use your muscles, the more efficiently cells use glucose for fuel, meaning there will be less glucose circulating in the bloodstream. For most people, activity of moderate intensity can help keep blood glucose levels under control.

## Medical Interventions

Lifestyle changes are not always sufficient to control diabetes. Sometimes medication is necessary. In cases where medications are less effective, bariatric surgery may be an option for slowing or halting the progression of prediabetes and type 2 diabetes.

## Oral Medications

When lifestyle changes fail to control type 2 diabetes, oral medications may be prescribed. Some medications reduce glucose production by the liver, whereas others slow the absorption of carbohydrates from the small intestine. Other medications increase insulin production by the pancreas, whereas still others work to increase the insulin sensitivity of cells. The newest class of diabetes drugs is known as SGLT2 inhibitors. These drugs cause the kidneys to excrete more glucose, lowering levels of glucose circulating in the body. Some people use diabetes medications without altering lifestyle, thinking the drugs are taking care of the problem. With time, medications become less effective and treatment options increasingly scarce. It is best to follow American Diabetes Association recommendations on diet, exercise, and lifestyle, in general. All diabetic drugs have side effects and contraindications; however, each person must balance risks of medications with risks of elevated blood glucose.

Currently, there is much discussion about whether using another drug, metformin, along with lifestyle intervention and counseling, is effective for those with significant risk factors and who show evidence of prediabetes. Although sources indicate potential benefits, metformin is not without side effects and risks, particularly for those with cardiovascular risks and those who have a history of gastrointestinal problems. If you or a loved one has prediabetes or diabetes, talk with your doctor about the best drug regimen, weight loss program, and exercise program for you.[63]

## Weight Loss Surgery

People who undergo any of several options for bariatric surgery (including gastric bypass, biliopancreatic diversion/duodenal switch, and sleeve gastrectomy) for weight loss have shown significant greater reductions in blood glucose and diabetes symptomatology than those engaged in lifestyle interventions more than 2 years postsurgery.[64] Those who combined gastric bypass or sleeve gastrectomy with intensive medical therapy had similar outcomes.[65] In many cases, former diabetics can stop taking medications for some of their cardiovascular risks, and stop diabetes symptoms altogether. Many professional groups are pushing for wider

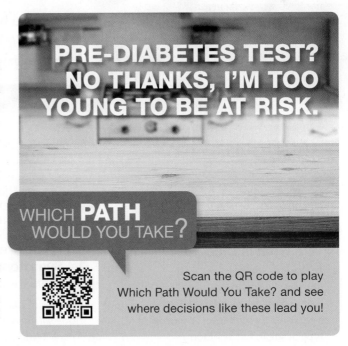

PRE-DIABETES TEST? NO THANKS, I'M TOO YOUNG TO BE AT RISK.

WHICH **PATH** WOULD YOU TAKE?

Scan the QR code to play Which Path Would You Take? and see where decisions like these lead you!

use of these more drastic weight loss methods, particularly for those who are severely obese and who have health risks and complications.[66] Gastric bypass surgeries are not without risks, however, and can include serious complications and even death. (See Chapter 6 for more on gastric bypass surgeries.)

## Insulin Injections

For people with type 1 diabetes, insulin injections or infusions are absolutely essential for daily functioning because their pancreases can no longer produce adequate amounts of insulin. In addition, people with type 2 diabetes whose blood glucose levels cannot be adequately controlled with other treatment options require insulin injections. Because insulin is a protein and would be digested in the gastrointestinal tract, it cannot be taken orally and must be injected into the fat layer under the skin; from there, it is absorbed into the bloodstream.

People with diabetes used to need two or more daily insulin injections.

Now, many use an *insulin infusion pump* to deliver minute amounts of insulin throughout the day. The external portion is only about the size of an MP3 player and can easily be hidden by clothes, while a thin tube and catheter is inserted under the patient's skin. Infusion over time is less painful and more effective than a few larger doses of insulin.

To overcome current insulin therapy limitations, researchers are working to link glucose monitoring and insulin delivery by developing an artificial pancreas. An artificial pancreas would mimic, as closely as possible, the way a healthy pancreas detects changes in blood glucose levels, responding automatically to secrete appropriate amounts of insulin. Although the first prototype devices received FDA approval, they cannot yet do the job of a fully functional pancreas.[67] Promising results from a recent clinical trial indicate that artificial pancreases appear to perform better than the current version of insulin pumps in regulating glucose.[68] Stay tuned. These may be available in the near future.

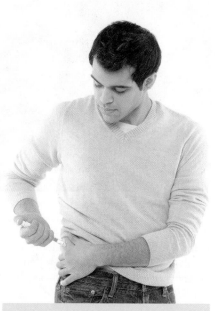

Some type 2 diabetics can control their condition with changes in diet and lifestyle habits or with oral medications. However, some type 2 diabetics and all type 1 diabetics require insulin injections or infusions.

# STUDY **PLAN**

Customize your study plan—and master your health!— in the Study Area of **MasteringHealth**.

## **ASSESS** YOURSELF

**Could you have diabetes?** Want to find out what behaviors and symptoms to look out for? Take the **Are You at Risk for Diabetes?** assessment available on **MasteringHealth.**™

## CHAPTER **REVIEW**

To hear an MP3 Tutor Session, scan here or visit the Study Area in **MasteringHealth**.

### LO **1** | What Is Diabetes?

- *Diabetes mellitus* is a group of diseases, each with its own mechanics. All are characterized by a persistently high level of glucose, a type of sugar, in the blood.

- Complications can range from cardiovascular disease to visual and gum problems, neuropathy, poor wound healing, and a host of other health problems.

### LO **2** | What Are the Symptoms of Diabetes?

- Symptoms of diabetes vary, but may include *polydypsia* (increased thirst), *polyphagia* (increased hunger), *polyuria* (increased urination), fatigue, blurred vision, nausea and light-headedness, slow wound healing, numbness or tingling in hands and feet, frequent infections of the skin, and tendency to bruise easily, among others.

- Key tests for diabetes include a fasting plasma glucose test taken after an 8- to 10-hour fast; an oral glucose tolerance test, taken 2 hours after consuming a concentrated glucose drink; and an estimated average glucose test.

## LO 3 | Treating Diabetes

- Prevention of diabetes include life-style changes such as a healthy/balanced diet, healthy weight, regular exercise, sufficient sleep, and stress reduction.

- Treatment of diabetes may include oral or injectable medications such as insulin, use of infusion pumps and other technologies, appropriate visits to the doctor, monitoring of glucose levels, and possible weight loss surgery.

## POP QUIZ

Visit **MasteringHealth** to personalize your study plan with Chapter Review Quizzes and Dynamic Study Modules.

## LO 1 | What Is Diabetes?

1. Which of the following is *not* correct?
   a. Type 1 diabetes is an autoimmune disease in which the body does not produce insulin.
   b. Type 2 diabetes is a disease in which the body may not produce sufficient amounts of insulin, or it may not be utilized properly.
   c. Gestational diabetes is only a problem for the mother while she is pregnant.
   d. Increased weight gain, high stress, lack of sleep, and sedentary lifestyle are key contributors to risks for type 2 diabetes.

## LO 2 | What Are the Symptoms of Diabetes?

2. Which of the following is *not* an accurate match between blood glucose level and diabetes-related problems in adults?
   a. A fasting plasma glucose of 100–126 mg/dL indicates prediabetes.
   b. An A1C test of 6.8 is normal.
   c. A fasting blood glucose level of 130 mg/dl indicates diabetes.
   d. An A1C test of <5.7 % is normal.

## LO 3 | Treating Diabetes

3. Which of the following statements is *correct*?
   a. People with type 2 diabetes must totally eliminate sweets or high-sugar foods from their diets.
   b. Skipping meals and eating two high-protein meals/no-carbohydrate meals per day is the best way to control blood sugar.
   c. Regular exercise, weight control, a balanced diet, adequate sleep, and stress management are key factors in blood glucose prevention and control.
   d. Most people with prediabetes know they have it.

*Answers to the Pop Quiz questions can be found on page A-1. If you answered a question incorrectly, review the section identified by the Learning Outcome. For even more study tools, visit **MasteringHealth**.*

# 17 Reducing Your Cancer Risk

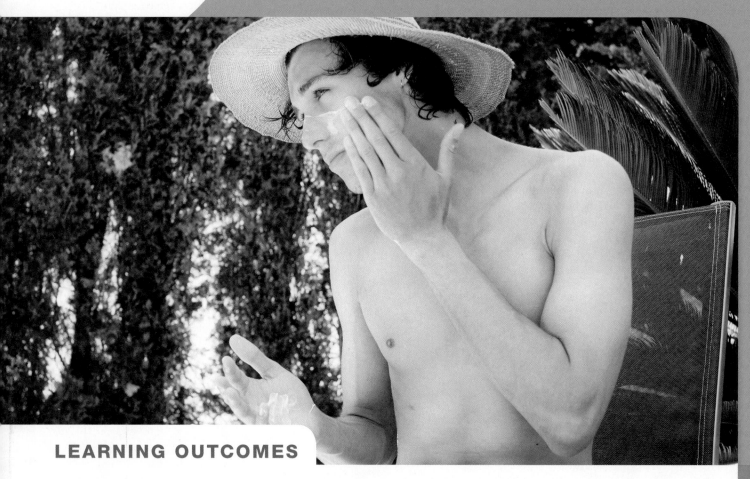

## LEARNING OUTCOMES

LO **1** Describe cancer's impact on people in the United States as compared to other major health problems in terms of morbidity/mortality, costs, and overall effectiveness of prevention and control.

LO **2** Describe cancer and how it develops, as well as key risk factors.

LO **3** Explain the suspected causes of cancer, and describe your own risks based on genetics and your lifestyle.

LO **4** Describe the different types of cancer and the risks they pose to people at different ages and stages of life, as well as key actions to prevent cancer development.

LO **5** Discuss the most current and effective methods of cancer detection and treatment, including areas of significant progress and future challenges.

LO **6** Discuss what it really means to be a "cancer survivor" and how it means more than living cancer free for 5 years after diagnosis.

As recently as 50 years ago, a cancer diagnosis was typically a death sentence. Health professionals could only guess at the cause, and treatments were often as deadly as the disease itself. Because we didn't understand the disease process, fears about "catching cancer" from those who had it led to ostracism and bigotry. Fortunately, we've come a long way in our understanding of cancer, our willingness to talk about the disease openly, and our ability to prevent certain forms of cancer and treat it.

Knowledge of risks and symptoms, early detection, and significant developments in technology and treatment have dramatically improved the prognosis for most cancer patients, particularly those diagnosed in early stages. There are also many actions individuals and society can take to prevent cancer. Understanding the facts, recognizing your own risk, and taking action to reduce risks are important steps in the battle.

## LO 1 | AN OVERVIEW OF CANCER

Describe cancer's impact on people in the United States as compared to other major health problems in terms of morbidity/mortality, costs, and overall effectiveness of prevention and control.

Cancer is the second most common cause of death in the United States, exceeded only by heart disease.[2] There were nearly 1.7 million *new* cancer diagnoses—not including **carcinoma *in situ*** (noninvasive) or basal and squamous skin cancers (which are not reported to cancer registries)—in 2016, and nearly 600,000 deaths (over 1,630 people per day!).[3] While those numbers may sound bleak, we've made remarkable progress in cancer death rates in recent decades. Cancer deaths were on an epidemic rise through much of the twentieth century, peaking at an all-time high in 1991; yet today, more people are surviving cancer than ever before. Why? Increased emphasis on education and awareness and on prevention and early intervention, advancements in diagnosis and treatment, and policies and programs designed to decrease disparities in early access and treatment, as well as decreased environmental risks all contribute to declining cancer rates and increasing survival rates.[4]

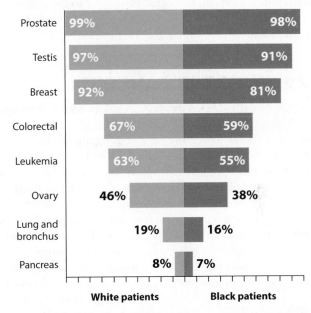

**FIGURE 17.1 Five-Year Survival Cancer Rates by Site and Race** Since the 1970s, survival rates have increased steadily for nearly all types of cancer. The exception to this trend has been lung cancer survivorship. Its survival rates remain both relatively steady and low, most likely due to the late stage at which most lung cancer cases are detected.

**Source:** N. Howlader et al., "SEER Cancer Statistics Review, 1975–2013" (Bethesda, MD: National Cancer Institute, April 2016), Available at http://seer.cancer.gov/csr/1975_2013/.

The **5-year relative survival rates** (the percent of people alive 5 years after diagnosis divided by the percentage expected to be alive and cancer-free based on normal life expectancy) have increased greatly from the 50 percent of past generations (**FIGURE 17.1**). Today, about 69 percent of people diagnosed with cancer each year will be alive 5 years after diagnosis.[5] But 5-year survival rates should be viewed with caution. Relative survival rates don't distinguish between people who are truly cancer-free, those in **remission** (responding to treatment with cancer under control), those who have relapsed, and those still

**Carcinoma *in situ*** Localized, noninvasive carcinoma

**5-year relative survival rates** The percent of people alive (usually 5 years) after diagnosis divided by the percentage expected to survive with the absence of cancer based on normal life expectancy.

**remission** Meaning the cancer is responding to treatment and under control.

in treatment whose cancer is not controlled.[6] Survival rates for people with many cancers caught in their earliest stages approach 90 to 99 percent.[7] While survival rates provide a good indicator of progress, they may not reflect outcomes from the most recent advances in treatment since they are calculated based on patients diagnosed years earlier. Also, they don't account for individual differences in age, overall health status, and **comorbidities** (the presence of other illnesses and conditions that might affect treatment outcomes).[8] It's important to remember that, although treatments and survival statistics have improved dramatically, there continue to be huge disparities based on socioeconomic status, race, geographical location, and other variables.[9] In the following sections, we provide an overview of factors that increase risk of cancer and discuss ways to reduce those risks.

## LO 2 | **WHAT** IS CANCER?

Describe cancer and how it develops, as well as key risk factors.

**Cancer** is the general term for a large group of diseases in which abnormal cells divide uncontrollably and invade tissues and organs. These cancer cells spread, or **metastasize**, via the blood and lymphatic system. It might be helpful to think of them as traitorous cells that overpower our body's defenses and ultimately deplete our reserves. If we are already weakened by virtue of age, other comorbidities, immune system breakdown, chronic stress, exposure to toxins, lack of sleep, or other health risks, cancers have a better chance of successfully invading and spreading. When cancer cells invade and ramp up their growth, they interrupt normal cell programming and develop into a **neoplasm**, a new growth of tissue serving no physiological function. This neoplasmic mass often forms a clump of cells known as a **tumor**. Tumors can grow rapidly or take months or years to cause noticeable symptoms.

Not all tumors are **malignant** (cancerous). In fact, most are **benign** (noncancerous). Benign tumors are generally harmless unless they grow to obstruct or crowd out normal tissues. A benign tumor of the brain, for instance, becomes life-threatening when it grows enough to restrict blood flow and cause a stroke. The only way to determine whether a tumor is malignant is through **biopsy**, the removal and microscopic examination of a cell sample.

Benign tumors generally consist of ordinary-looking cells enclosed in a fibrous shell or capsule that prevents their spreading. Malignant tumors are usually not enclosed in a protective capsule and can therefore spread to other organs or tissue more readily (**FIGURE 17.2**). This *metastatic* spread makes some forms of cancer particularly aggressive. By the time they are diagnosed, some malignant tumors have already metastasized throughout the body, making treatment extremely difficult. Malignant cells invade surrounding tissue, emitting clawlike protrusions that disturb the RNA and DNA within normal cells. Disrupting these substances, which control cellular metabolism and reproduction, produces **mutant cells** that differ in form, quality, and function from normal cells.

*Cancer staging* is a classification system that describes how much a cancer has spread at the time it is diagnosed; it helps doctors and patients decide on appropriate treatments

**comorbidities** The presence of other illnesses at the same time and other conditions that might affect treatment outcomes.

**cancer** A large group of diseases characterized by the uncontrolled growth and spread of abnormal cells.

**metastasize** To spread from one area to different areas of the body.

**neoplasm** A new growth of tissue that results from uncontrolled, abnormal cellular development and serves no physiological function.

**tumor** A neoplasmic mass that grows more rapidly than surrounding tissue.

**malignant** Very dangerous or harmful; refers to a cancerous tumor.

**benign** Harmless; refers to a noncancerous tumor.

**biopsy** Removal and examination of a tissue sample to determine if a cancer is present.

**mutant cells** Cells that differ in form, quality, or function from normal cells.

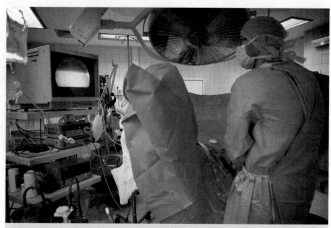

Physicians usually order biopsies of tumors to determine whether they are cancerous. Newer techniques, such as the minimally invasive "optical biopsy" shown here, allow microscopic examination of tissue without doing a physical biopsy.

NOT ME! I'M A SOCIAL SMOKER, I'LL NEVER BECOME ADDICTED.

WHICH **PATH** WOULD YOU TAKE?

Scan the QR code to play Which Path Would You Take? and see where decisions like these lead you!

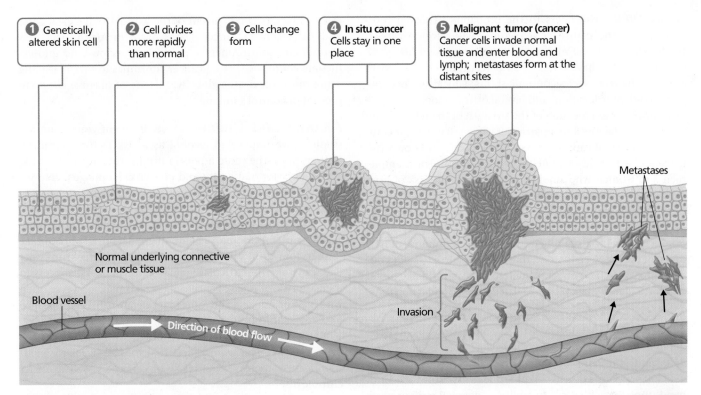

| ① Genetically altered skin cell | ② Cell divides more rapidly than normal | ③ Cells change form | ④ In situ cancer Cells stay in one place | ⑤ Malignant tumor (cancer) Cancer cells invade normal tissue and enter blood and lymph; metastases form at the distant sites |

Metastases

Normal underlying connective or muscle tissue

Blood vessel

Direction of blood flow

Invasion

**FIGURE 17.2 Metastasis** A mutation to the genetic material of a skin cell triggers abnormal cell division and changes cell formation, resulting in a cancerous tumor. If the tumor remains localized, it is considered *in situ* cancer. If the tumor spreads, it is considered a malignant cancer.

→ **VIDEO TUTOR** Metastasis

and estimate a person's life expectancy. Cancers are typically staged based on the size of a tumor, how deeply it has penetrated, the number of affected lymph nodes, and the degree of metastasis or spread, known as the *TNM* (for *tumor, node,* **and** *metastasis*) **staging system**. The most commonly known staging system assigns a number from 0 to IV to the disease, with IV being most advanced (**TABLE 17.1**). In addition to staging, many tumors are assigned a grade based on the degree of cell abnormality. Typically, the lower the stage and grade, the better the prognosis.[10]

## TABLE **17.1** | Cancer Stages

| Stage | Definition |
|-------|------------|
| 0 | Early cancer, when abnormal cells remain only in the place they originated. |
| I–III | Higher numbers indicate more extensive disease: Larger tumor size and/or spread of the cancer beyond the organ in which it first developed to nearby lymph nodes and/or organs adjacent to the location of the primary tumor. |
| IV | Cancer has spread to other organs |

**Source:** National Cancer Institute, National Institutes of Health, "Fact Sheet, Cancer Staging, 2015," January 6, 2015, www.cancer .gov/cancertopics/diagnosis-staging/staging/staging-fact-sheet.

## LO **3** | **WHAT** CAUSES CANCER?

Explain the suspected causes of cancer, and describe your own risks based on genetics and lifestyle.

Causes are generally divided into two categories of risk factors: *hereditary* and *acquired* (environmental). Where heredity factors cannot be changed, we have control over some infectious agents, certain medical treatments, drug and alcohol consumption, amount of sun exposure, and exposure to **carcinogens** (cancer-causing agents) in food. Hereditary and environmental factors may interact to make cancer more likely, accelerate cancer progression, or increase susceptibility during certain periods of life. The mechanisms underlying cancer development are not fully understood. Two people with seemingly identical risk factors may end up with very different experiences when it comes to developing cancer, and the reasons for these differences remain a mystery.

## Lifestyle Risks for Cancer

Cancer occurs in all age groups, but the older you are, the greater your risk. In fact, 78 percent of all cancers are diagnosed in adults over age 55.[11] Cancer researchers refer to one's cancer risk when they assess risk

**TNM staging system** A system for classifying cancer staging by assessing tumor size, nodal involvement, and degree of metastasis.

**carcinogens** Cancer-causing agents.

factors. *Lifetime risk* refers to the probability that an individual, over the course of a lifetime, will develop cancer. In the United States, men have a lifetime risk of about 42 percent; women have a risk of 33 percent, or 1 in 3.[12] Risks also vary by race, socioeconomic status, education, occupation, geographic location, and several other factors.

*Relative risk* is a measure of the strength of the relationship between risk factors and a particular cancer. Basically, it compares your risk of cancer if you engage in certain known risk behaviors with that of someone who does not. For example, men and women who smoke have 25 times the risk of lung cancer of a nonsmoker—a relative risk of 25.[13]

Over the years, researchers have found that diet, a sedentary lifestyle, overconsumption of alcohol, tobacco use, stress, and other factors play a key role in the incidence (number of new cases) of cancer. Keep in mind that a high relative risk does not guarantee cause and effect. It merely indicates the likelihood of a particular risk factor being related to a particular outcome.

## Tobacco Use

In the United States, smoking has the dubious distinction of being the *leading cause of preventable death* and is responsible for nearly 1 in 5 deaths, or about 480,000 premature deaths—42,000 due to exposure to secondhand smoke—each year.[14] In addition, nearly 9 million more people suffer from smoking-related diseases, such as chronic bronchitis, emphysema, and cardiovascular disease (CVD).[15]

In the 1960s, over 42 percent of Americans smoked. The good news is that today, only about 17 percent of Americans smoke—a higher percentage than we'd like, yet a vast improvement.[16] Continued declines in smoking rates, improvements in smoking policies, and better environmental controls provide a promising outlook for the future.

Smoking is associated with increased risk of at least 15 different cancers. According to the 2014 *Surgeon General Report on the Health Consequences of Smoking*, several compelling associations between smoking and cancer were reported, including causal relationships between smoking and liver cancer, colorectal polyps, oral cancer, and colorectal cancer.[17]

Cigar smokers, users of smokeless tobacco, e-cigarette smokers, and those exposed to tobacco smoke via secondhand smoke all run increased risks for various illnesses, including cancer. Quitting smoking can significantly reduce risks of cancer and other illnesses (see Chapter 12 for more information on the benefits of quitting).[18]

Over the years, cigarette smoking has declined in many regions of the world, largely due to efforts aimed at prevention and control through education, policy development programs that mandate plain packaging and less glamorous appeal, media campaigns, advertising bans, and taxation. Still, developing countries continue to be disproportionately affected by increasing numbers of cancer cases and high smoking

Of the several lifestyle risk factors for cancer, tobacco use is the most significant—and the most preventable.

rates. In fact, over 60 percent of the world's total cancer cases and 70 percent of cancer deaths occur in Africa, Asia, and Central and South America, particularly in low- and middle-income countries.[19] Lung cancer continues to be the leading cause of cancer deaths globally, in spite of massive efforts to prevent or control smoking.[20]

## Alcohol and Cancer Risk

In recent years, countless studies have implicated alcohol as a risk factor for cancer. Bottom line—the more a person drinks, the greater the risk, particularly for oral cavity and pharynx, esophagus, colorectal, liver, larynx, and female breast cancer. There is increasing evidence that moderate to high levels of drinking are associated with some other cancers such as pancreas and prostate cancer and melanoma.[21] Light to moderate alcohol intake (one to four drinks per day for men; one to three drinks per day for women), particularly among nonsmokers, appears to increase risk of breast cancer among women; however, men who are nonsmokers and light to moderate drinkers appear to have no significant increased risk.[22]

Both men and women who binge-drink (more than 8 drinks per week for women and 15 drinks per week for men) significantly increase their risks of cancer as well as other chronic diseases.[23]

## Poor Nutrition, Physical Inactivity, and Obesity

Mounting evidence suggests nearly one-third of annual cancer deaths in the United States may be due to lifestyle factors such as overweight or obesity, physical inactivity, and poor nutrition and that obesity may be a key contributor in 1 out of 5 cancer deaths.[24] Aside from choosing not to use tobacco, dietary choices and physical activity are the most important modifiable determinants of cancer risk. Several studies indicate a relationship between a high body mass index (BMI) and death rates from cancers of the esophagus, colon, rectum, liver, stomach, kidney, pancreas, and others, as well as high risk of endometrial cancer among younger women aged 18 to 25 with higher BMIs and rapid weight gain.[25] Overall, risk of breast cancer appears to increase with BMI and age, and is a significant risk for postmenopausal women. Furthermore, women with higher BMI have a significantly greater risk of dying from endometrial and breast cancer.[26] Men also increase their risk of cancers with BMI and waist circumference increases. A new study following 150,000 men in Europe for 14 years showed that for every 4-inch increase in waistline, the risk of developing aggressive prostate cancer goes up by 18 percent![27] Having a high BMI increases the risk of dying from prostate cancer significantly.[28]

The relative risk of colon cancer in men is 40 percent higher for obese men than it is for nonobese men.[29] The relative risk of gallbladder cancer is five times higher in obese individuals than in individuals of healthy weight.[30] Numerous other studies support the link between various forms of cancer and obesity.[31] The higher the BMI, the greater the cancer risk.[32]

**Stress and Psychosocial Risks** Although stress has been implicated in increased susceptibility to several types of cancers, most reports of cancer being caused by stress are observational in nature, and many of these studies lack scientific rigor or are simply too small to show definitive results. A recent large meta-analytic study found no relationship between job strain and risk for colorectal, lung, breast, or prostate cancer.[33] That said, people who are under chronic, severe stress or who suffer from depression or other persistent emotional problems show higher rates of cancer than their healthy counterparts. Sleep disturbances, unhealthy diet, and emotional or physical trauma may weaken the body's immune system, increasing susceptibility to cancer. Other possible contributors to cancer are poverty and the health disparities associated with low socioeconomic status.

## Genetic and Physiological Risks

If one of your close family members develops cancer, does it mean that you have a genetic predisposition for it? Scientists believe that between 5 and 10 percent of all cancers are strongly hereditary.[34] It seems that some people may be more predisposed to the malfunctioning of genes that ultimately cause cancer.[35]

Suspected cancer-causing genes are called **oncogenes**. Although these genes are typically dormant, certain conditions such as age, stress, and exposure to carcinogens, viruses, and radiation may activate them. Once activated, oncogenes cause cells to grow and reproduce uncontrollably. Scientists are uncertain whether only people who develop cancer have oncogenes or whether we all have genes that can become oncogenes under certain conditions.

Certain cancers—particularly those of the breast, stomach, colon, prostate, uterus, ovaries, and lungs—appear to run in families. For example, a woman runs a much higher risk of breast cancer if her mother or sisters have had the disease (particularly at a young age), or if she inherits the breast cancer susceptibility genes (*BRCA1* or *BRCA2*). Hodgkin disease and certain leukemias show similar familial patterns. Can we attribute these familial patterns to genetic susceptibility or to the fact that people in the same families experience similar environmental risks? Research in this area is inconclusive. It is possible that we can inherit a tendency toward a cancer-prone, weak immune system or, conversely, that we

can inherit a cancer-fighting potential. But the complex interaction of heredity, lifestyle, and environment on the development of cancer makes it a challenge to determine a single cause. Even among those predisposed to mutations, avoiding risks may decrease chances of cancer development.

**Reproductive and Hormonal Factors** The effects of reproductive factors on breast and cervical cancers have been well documented. Increased numbers of fertile or menstrual cycle years (early menarche, late menopause), not having children or having them later in life, recent use of birth control pills or hormone replacement therapy, and opting not to breast-feed all appear to increase risks of breast cancer.[36] While the above factors appear to play a significant role in increased risk for non-Hispanic white women, they do not appear to have as strong an influence on Hispanic women, who may have more protective reproductive patterns (an overall lower age at first birth and greater number of births). They also use less hormone replacement therapy and have a lower utilization rate for mammograms, making comparisons difficult.[37]

## Inflammation and Cancer Risks

An emerging theory in cancer research is that inflammatory processes in the body play a significant role in the development of cancer—from initiation and promoting cancer cells to paving the way for them to invade, spread, and weaken the immune response.[38] Others have found an association between childhood trauma and an increased risk of psychological distress in adulthood that may weaken the immune system.[39] According to some researchers, the vast majority of cancers (90%) are caused by cellular mutations and environmental factors that occur as a result of inflammation.[40] These same researchers believe that up to 20 percent of cancers are the result of chronic infections, 30 percent are the result of tobacco smoking and inhaled particulates such as asbestos, and 35 percent are due to dietary factors.[41]

The common denominator in these threats is inflammation that primes the system for cancer to gain a foothold and spread. Inflammation appears to be a key factor in colorectal cancer, with inflammatory bowel disease, Crohn's disease, colitis, and other gastrointestinal (GI) tract inflammatory problems having a higher risk of cancer development.[42] If

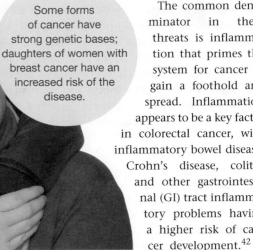

Some forms of cancer have strong genetic bases; daughters of women with breast cancer have an increased risk of the disease.

inflammation is indeed a key factor, reducing inflammation via stress reduction, sleep, dietary supplements, low-dose aspirin, and other behaviors may prove beneficial in reducing cancer risks.

## Occupational and Environmental Risks

Workplace hazards account for only a small percentage of all cancers, but various substances are known to cause cancer when exposure levels are high or prolonged. Asbestos—a fibrous material once widely used in the construction, insulation, and automobile industries—nickel, chromate, and chemicals such as benzene, arsenic, and vinyl chloride have been shown to be carcinogens. Also, people who routinely work with certain dyes and radioactive substances may have increased risks for cancer. Working with coal tars, as in the mining profession, or with inhalants, as in the auto-painting business, is hazardous. So is working with herbicides and pesticides, although evidence is inconclusive for low-dose exposures. Several federal and state agencies are responsible for monitoring such exposures and ensuring that businesses comply with standards designed to protect workers.

**Radiation** Ionizing radiation (IR)—radiation from X-rays, radon, cosmic rays, and ultraviolet radiation (primarily UVB radiation)—is the only form of radiation proven to cause human cancer. Evidence that high-dose IR causes cancer comes from studies of atomic bomb survivors, patients receiving radiotherapy, and certain occupational groups, such as uranium miners. Virtually any part of the body can be affected by IR, but bone marrow and the thyroid are particularly susceptible. Radon exposure in homes can increase lung cancer risk, especially in cigarette smokers. To reduce the risk of harmful effects, diagnostic medical and dental X-rays are set at the lowest dose levels possible.

Nonionizing radiation produced by radio waves, cell phones, microwaves, computer screens, televisions, electric blankets, and other products has been a topic of great concern in recent years, but research has not proven excess risk to date. Although a wide range of studies have been conducted, none have shown a consistent link between cell phone use and cancers of the brain, nerves, or other tissues of the head or neck. Additionally, most of the key policymaking and health organizations have indicated that existing research does not support a cell phone–cancer link. In the meantime, simple strategies can help ensure that even if future studies identify prolonged cell usage as a risk factor for cancer, you will have reduced your risk. First and foremost, use a hands-free device, and try to keep as much space as possible between your head and your phone. When hands free isn't available, limit your talk time, keep the phone away from your bed, and use the speaker function on your phone to get it as far from your head/body as possible.[43] (See Chapter 21 for more on the potential hazards of both ionizing and nonionizing radiation.)

**Chemicals in Foods** Much of the concern about chemicals in food centers on the possible harm caused by

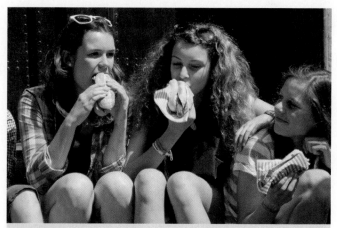

Concern about the carcinogenic properties of nitrates, which are often used to preserve hot dogs, hams, and luncheon meats, has led to the introduction of meats that are nitrate-free or contain reduced levels of the substance.

pesticide and herbicide residues. Whereas some of these chemicals cause cancer at high doses in experimental animals, the government considers the very low concentrations found in some foods to be safe. Continued research regarding pesticide and herbicide use is essential, and scientists and consumer groups stress the importance of a balance between chemical use and the production of high-quality food products.

## Infectious Diseases and Cancer Risks

Over 10 percent of all cancers in the United States are caused by infectious agents such as viruses, bacteria, or parasites.[44] Worldwide, approximately 15 to 20 percent of human cancers have been traced to infectious agents.[45] Infections are thought to influence cancer development in several ways, most commonly through chronic inflammation, suppression of the immune system, or chronic stimulation.

### Hepatitis B, Hepatitis C, and Liver Cancer

Viruses that cause chronic forms of hepatitis B (HBV) and C (HCV) are believed to stimulate growth of cancer cells in the liver because they chronically inflame liver tissue. This may prime the liver for cancer or make it more hospitable for cancer development. Global increases in hepatitis B and C rates and concurrent rises in liver cancer rates seem to provide evidence of such an association. Vaccines that prevent hepatitis B may reduce the risk of liver damage as well as cancer.

### Human Papillomavirus and Cervical Cancer

Every year in the United States, nearly 18,000 women and 9,300 men get cancer linked to *human papillomavirus (HPV)* infection, which is believed to be a major cause of cervical cancer, as well as cancers of the back of the throat, tongue, and tonsils.[46] HPV can also cause cancers of the vulva and vagina in women, cancer of the penis in men, and cancer of the anus in women and men. The good news is that vaccines are available to help protect men and women from being infected with HPV and increased cancer susceptibility. While vaccines don't completely prevent all of these cancers, they seem to be effective in reducing risks of cervical and penile cancer.[47] (For more information on the HPV vaccine, and usage among college students, see the discussion in Chapter 15.)

### *Helicobacter pylori* and Stomach Cancer

*Helicobacter pylori* is a potent bacterium found in the stomach lining of approximately 30 percent of Americans.[48] It causes inflammation, scarring, and ulcers, damaging the lining of the stomach and leading to cellular changes that may lead to cancer. More than half of all cases of stomach cancer are thought to be linked to *H. pylori* infection, even though most infected people don't develop cancer.[49] Treatment with antibiotics often cures the ulcers, which appears to reduce risk of new stomach cancer.[50]

## Medical Factors

Some medical treatments can increase a person's risk for cancer. For example, estrogen use for relieving menopausal symptoms is now recognized to contribute to multiple cancer risks and provides fewer benefits than originally believed. Prescriptions for estrogen therapy have declined dramatically, and many women are trying to reduce or eliminate use of the hormone.

Ironically, medicines used to treat cancers, such as selected chemotherapy drugs, have been shown to increase risks for other cancers. Weighing the benefits versus harms of these treatments is always necessary.

## LO 4 | TYPES OF CANCERS

Describe the different types of cancer and the risks they pose to people at different ages and stages of life, as well as key actions to prevent cancer development.

Cancers are grouped into four broad categories based on the type of tissue from which each arises:

- **Carcinomas.** Epithelial tissues (tissues covering body surfaces and lining most body cavities) are the most common sites for cancers; cancers occurring in epithelial tissue are called *carcinomas*. These cancers affect the outer layer of the skin and mouth as well as mucous membranes. They metastasize through the circulatory or lymphatic system initially and form solid tumors.
- **Sarcomas.** Sarcomas occur in the mesodermal, or middle, layers of tissue—for example, in bones, muscles, and general connective tissue. In early stages, they metastasize primarily via the blood. Sarcomas are less common but generally more virulent than carcinomas. They also form solid tumors.
- **Lymphomas.** Lymphomas develop in the lymphatic system—the infection-fighting regions of the body—and metastasize through the lymphatic system. Hodgkin disease is an example. Lymphomas also form solid tumors.
- **Leukemias.** Cancer of the blood-forming parts of the body, particularly the bone marrow and spleen, is called leukemia. A nonsolid tumor, leukemia is characterized by an abnormal increase in the number of white blood cells that the body produces.

**FIGURE 17.3** shows the most common sites of cancer and the number of new cases and deaths from each type that were estimated to have occurred in 2016. A comprehensive discussion of the many different forms of cancer is beyond the scope of this book, but we discuss the most common types in the next sections.

## Lung Cancer

Lung cancer is the leading cause of cancer deaths for both men and women in the United States. It killed an estimated 224,390 Americans in 2015, accounting for nearly 14 percent of all cancer deaths.[51] The lifetime risks for males and females getting lung cancer is 1 in 14 and 1 in 17, respectively. Risks begin to rise around age 40 and continue to climb through all age groups thereafter.[52]

Since 1987, more women have died each year from lung cancer than breast cancer, which had been the leading cause of cancer deaths in women for 40 years prior.[53] Although past reductions in smoking rates bode well for cancer statistics, there is growing concern about the number of young people, particularly young women and persons of low income and low educational levels, who continue to pick up the habit.

# 32%

of all U.S. **CANCER DEATHS** are attributable to smoking.

There is also growing concern about the increase in lung cancers among lifelong *never smokers*—a group of people who, as the name suggests, have never smoked or used tobacco products, but still make up 20% of those who die from lung cancer.[54] Never smokers' lung cancer is believed to be related

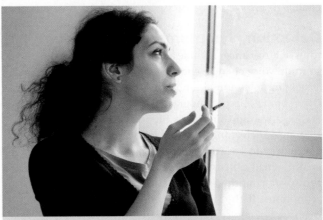

Stopping smoking at any time will reduce your risk of lung cancer. Studies show that within 5 years of quitting, women's risk of death from lung cancer decreases by 21 percent, compared to people who continue smoking.

| Estimated New Cases of Cancer * | | Estimated Deaths from Cancer * | |
|---|---|---|---|
| **Female** | **Male** | **Female** | **Male** |
| **Breast**<br>246,660 (29%) | **Prostate**<br>180,890 (21%) | **Lung & bronchus**<br>72,160 (26%) | **Lung & bronchus**<br>85,920 (27%) |
| **Lung & bronchus**<br>106,470 (13%) | **Lung & bronchus**<br>117,920 (14%) | **Breast**<br>40,450 (14%) | **Prostate**<br>26,120 (8%) |
| **Colon & rectum**<br>63,670 (8%) | **Colon & rectum**<br>70,820 (8%) | **Colon & rectum**<br>23,170 (8%) | **Colon & rectum**<br>26,020 (8%) |
| **Uterine corpus**<br>60,050 (7%) | **Urinary bladder**<br>58,950 (7%) | **Pancreas**<br>20,330 (7%) | **Pancreas**<br>21,450 (7%) |
| **Thyroid**<br>49,350 (6%) | **Melanoma of the skin**<br>46,870 (6%) | **Ovary**<br>14,240 (5%) | **Liver & intrahepatic bile duct**<br>18,280 (6%) |
| **Non-Hodgkin lymphoma**<br>32,410 (4%) | **Non-Hodgkin lymphoma**<br>40,170 (5%) | **Uterine corpus**<br>10,470 (4%) | **Leukemia**<br>14,130 (4%) |
| **Melanoma of the skin**<br>29,510 (3%) | **Kidney & renal pelvis**<br>39,650 (5%) | **Leukemia**<br>10,270 (4%) | **Esophagus**<br>12,720 (4%) |
| **Leukemia**<br>26,050 (3%) | **Oral cavity & pharynx**<br>34,780 (4%) | **Liver & intrahepatic bile duct**<br>8,890 (3%) | **Urinary bladder**<br>11,820 (4%) |
| **Kidney & renal pelvis**<br>23,050 (3%) | **Leukemia**<br>34,780 (4%) | **Non-Hodgkin lymphoma**<br>8,630 (3%) | **Non-Hodgkin lymphoma**<br>11,520 (4%) |
| **All Sites**<br>843,820 (100%) | **Liver & intrahepatic bile duct**<br>28,410 (3%) | **Brain & other nervous system**<br>6,610 (2%) | **Brain & other nervous system**<br>9,440 (3%) |
| | **All Sites**<br>841,390 (100%) | **All Sites**<br>281,400 (100%) | **All Sites**<br>314,290 (100%) |

*Excludes basal and squamous cell skin cancers and in situ carcinoma except urinary bladder. Percentages may not total 100% due to rounding.

**FIGURE 17.3** Leading Sites of New Cancer Cases and Deaths, 2016 Estimates

**Source:** Data from American Cancer Society, *Cancer Facts & Figures 2016*, Table (Atlanta, GA: American Cancer Society; 2016), 10. Note that percentages do not add up to 100 due to omissions of certain rare cancers as well as rounding of statistics.

to genetic mutations that increase risk, exposure to second-hand smoke, radon gas, asbestos, indoor wood-burning stoves, exposure to environmental agents that increase risk, and aerosolized oils caused by cooking with oil and deep fat frying.[55] Unfortunately, because doctors often don't think of lung cancer when a never smoker presents with a cough, patients are often put on antibiotics or cough suppressants as therapy. By the time they recognize that it's really lung cancer, their cancer is likely to be more advanced and treatment is more challenging.

### Detection, Symptoms, and Treatment Symptoms of lung cancer include a persistent cough, blood-streaked sputum, voice change, chest pain or back pain, and recurrent attacks of pneumonia or bronchitis. Newer tests, such as low-dose computerized tomography (CT) scans, molecular markers in saliva, and improved biopsy techniques, have helped to improve screening accuracy for lung cancer, but they have a long way to go. Treatment depends on the type (small cell or non–small cell) and stage of the cancer. Surgery, radiation therapy, chemotherapy, and targeted biological therapies are all options. If the cancer is localized, surgery is usually the treatment of choice. If it has spread, surgery is combined with radiation, chemotherapy, and other targeted drug treatments. Fewer than 15 percent of lung cancer cases are diagnosed at the early, localized stages.[56] Despite advances in medical technology, survival rates 1 year after diagnosis are only 44 percent

overall.[57] The 5-year survival rate for all stages combined is only 17 percent.[58]

### Risk Factors and Prevention Risks for cancer increase dramatically based on the quantity of cigarettes smoked and the number of years smoked, often referred to as *pack years*. The greater the number of pack years smoked, the greater the risk of developing cancer. Quitting smoking does substantially reduce the risk of developing lung cancer.[59] Exposure to industrial substances or radiation also highly increases the risk for lung cancer.

## Breast Cancer

Breast cancer is a group of diseases that cause uncontrolled cell growth in breast tissue, particularly in the glands that produce milk and the ducts that connect those glands to the nipple. Cancers can also form in the connective and lymphatic tissues of the breast. In 2016, approximately 246,660 women and 2,600 men in the United States were diagnosed with invasive breast cancer for the first time.[60] In addition, 61,000 new cases of *in situ* breast cancer, a more localized cancer, were diagnosed.[61] About 41,000 women (and 440 men) died, making breast cancer the second leading cause of cancer death for women.[62] Women have a 1 in 8 lifetime risk of being diagnosed with breast cancer.[63] For women from birth to age 49, the chance is about a 1 in 53, with significantly higher rates after menopause.[64] This is why most health groups have advocated screening for breast cancer more thoroughly after age 40.

## Detection

The earliest signs of breast cancer are usually observable on mammograms, often before lumps can be felt. However, mammograms are not foolproof, and there is debate regarding the optimal age at which women should start regularly receiving them. Although mammograms detect between 80 and 90 percent of breast cancers in women without symptoms, a newer form of *magnetic resonance imaging* (*MRI*) appears to be even more accurate, particularly in women with genetic risks for tumors or those who have suspicious areas of the breast or surrounding tissue that warrant a clearer image.[65] If you are referred for a breast MRI, be sure to check with your insurance company as these are costly and may not be covered unless you are considered high risk. Also, go to a facility where they can perform a breast biopsy if there are any areas that need further investigation.[66]

## Breast Awareness and Self-Exam

Breast self-exam (BSE) has been recommended by major health organizations as a form of early breast cancer screening for the last two decades (**FIGURE 17.4**). However, a 2009 "study of studies" done by the U.S. Preventive Services Task Force determined that breast self-exams did not decrease suffering and death and, in fact, often lead to unnecessary worry, unnecessary tests, and increased health care costs.[67] As a result of this research, several groups have downgraded the recommendation about BSE from "do them and do them regularly" to "learn how to do them, and if you desire, do them to know your body and be able to recognize changes."

To do a breast self-exam, begin by standing in front of a mirror to inspect the breasts, looking for their usual symmetry. Some breasts are not symmetrical, and if this is not a change, it is okay. Raise and lower both arms while checking that the breasts move evenly and freely. Next, inspect the skin, looking for areas of redness, thickening, or dimpling, which might have the appearance of an orange peel. Look for any scaling on the nipple.

To feel for lumps, raise one arm above your head while either standing or lying. This will flatten out the breast, making it easier to feel the tissue. Using the index, middle, and fourth fingers of your opposite hand, gently push down on the breast tissue and move the fingers in small circular motions, varying pressure from light to more firm. Start at one edge of the breast and move upward and then downward, working your way across the breast until all of the breast tissue has been covered. Often breast tissue will feel dense and irregular, and this is usually normal. It helps to do regular self-exams to become familiar with what your breast tissue feels like; then, if there is a change, you will notice. Cancers usually feel like a dense or firm little rock and are very different from the normal breast tissue.

Next, lower the arm and reach into the top of the underarm and pull downward with gentle pressure feeling for any enlarged lymph nodes. To complete the exam, squeeze the tissue around the nipple. If you notice discharge from the nipple and you have not recently been breast-feeding, consult your doctor. Likewise, if you notice any asymmetry, skin changes, scaling on the nipple, or new lumps in the breast, you should see your doctor for evaluation.

## Symptoms and Treatment

If breast cancer grows large enough, it can produce the following symptoms: a lump in the breast or surrounding lymph nodes, thickening, dimpling, skin irritation, distortion, retraction or scaliness of the nipple, nipple discharge, or tenderness.

Treatments range from a lumpectomy to radical mastectomy to various combinations of radiation or chemotherapy. Among nonsurgical options, promising results have been noted among women using *selective estrogen-receptor modulators* (*SERMs*) such as tamoxifen and raloxifene, particularly among women whose cancers appear to grow in response to estrogen. These drugs, as well as new *aromatase inhibitors*, work by blocking estrogen. The 5-year survival rate for people with localized breast cancer has risen from 80 percent in the 1950s to 99 percent today.[68] However, these statistics vary dramatically, based on the stage of the cancer when it

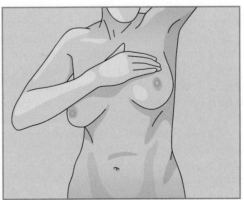

❶ Face a mirror and check for changes in symmetry.

❷ Either standing or lying down, use the pads of the three middle fingers to check for lumps. Follow an up-and-down pattern on the breast to ensure all tissue gets inspected.

**FIGURE 17.4** Breast Awareness and Self-Exam

**Source:** Adapted from Breast Self-Exam Illustration Series, National Cancer Institute Visuals Online Collection, U.S. National Institutes of Health, https://visualsonline.cancer.gov.

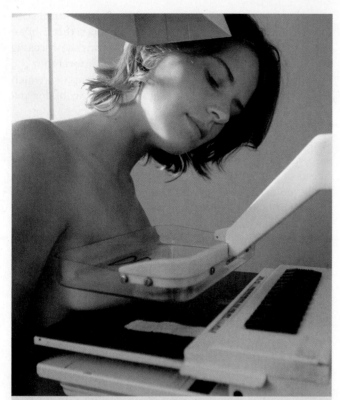

Early detection through mammography and other techniques greatly increases a woman's chance of surviving breast cancer. New 3D machines are available.

is first detected and whether it has spread.[69] Having access to early diagnosis and treatment is key to survival.

### Risk Factors and Prevention
The incidence of breast cancer increases with age. Although there are many possible risk factors, those that are well supported by research include family history of breast cancer, menstrual periods that started early and ended late in life, weight gain after the age of 18, obesity after menopause, recent use of oral contraceptives or postmenopausal hormone therapy, never bearing children or bearing a first child after age 30, consuming two or more alcoholic drinks per day, and physical inactivity. In addition, there is new evidence that heavy smoking, particularly among women who started smoking before their first pregnancy, increases risk. Other factors that increase risk include having dense breasts, type 2 diabetes, high bone mineral density, and exposure to high-dose radiation.[70] Although the *BRCA1* and *BRCA2* gene mutations are rare and occur in less than 1 percent of the population, they account for approximately 5 to 10 percent of all cases of breast cancer.[71] Cancers are also more likely to occur in both breasts in women with the genes as compared to women without these genes. Because these genes are rare, routine screening for them is not recommended unless there is a strong family history (particularly among younger primary relatives) of breast cancer.[72]

International differences in breast cancer incidence correlate with variations in diet, especially fat intake, although a causal role for these dietary factors has not been firmly

established. Sudden weight gain has also been implicated. Research also shows that regular exercise can reduce risk.[73] In particular, two large meta-analyses of studies focused on the role of dietary fiber indicate strong inverse relationships between dietary fiber and breast cancer. In short, if you eat more fiber, breast cancer rates seem to go down, and if you eat less, rates seem to increase.[74]

## Colon and Rectal Cancers

Colorectal cancers (cancers of the colon and rectum) continue to be the third most commonly diagnosed cancer in both men and women and the third leading cause of cancer deaths, even though death rates are declining.[75] In 2016 there were 95,270 cases of colon cancer and 39,220 cases of rectal cancer diagnosed in the United States, as well as 49,190 deaths attributed to colon or rectal cancer.[76] While rates of colon cancer appear to be declining in those over age 50, they are increasing among people under age 50.[77] Younger men and women have approximately a 1 in 300 risk of developing colon and rectal cancer from birth to age 49, increasing to about 1 in 21–22.[78]

### Detection, Symptoms, and Treatment
Because colorectal cancer tends to spread slowly over a period of 10 to 20 years, the prognosis is quite good for those who receive recommended screenings and are diagnosed in early stages; in fact, when caught at an early, localized stage, 5-year survival rates are over 90 percent; however, if caught in the later stage, survival rates are only 13 percent.[79] Through education, screening tests, and timely treatment, we've made remarkable progress in reducing the incidence and death rates of this cancer. The bad news is that, in its early stages, colorectal cancer typically has no clear symptoms and only 39 percent of cases are caught in the earliest stage.[80] Because early symptoms may be vague, far too many colorectal cancer diagnoses occur at later stages when 5-year survival rates are much lower. Men, who as a group are more reluctant to seek medical care early, tend to have a 30 to 40 percent higher rate of colorectal cancer incidence and mortality.[81] As the disease progresses, stool changes, bleeding, cramping or pain in the lower abdomen, unusual urges to have a bowel movement, unusual weight loss, decreased appetite, and unusual fatigue are the major warning signals.

Colonoscopies and other screening tests should begin at age 50 for most people. Virtual colonoscopies and fecal DNA testing are newer diagnostic techniques that have shown

## 59%
of people over the age of 50 actually get the recommended SCREENING TESTS for colorectal cancer.

promise. However, only 10 percent of all Americans over age 50 have had the most basic screening test—the at-home *fecal occult blood* test (FOBT)—in the past year, and slightly over 50 percent have had an colonoscopy test.[82] Rates are even lower in those who are nonwhite, have fewer years of education, lack health insurance, and are recent immigrants.[83]

Treatment often consists of radiation or surgery. Chemotherapy, although not used extensively in the past, is today a possibility.

## Risk Factors and Prevention

The older you are, the greater your chances of colorectal cancer. Although anyone can develop it, people who are over age 50, who are obese, who have a family history of colon and rectal cancer, who have a personal or family history of polyps (benign growths) in the colon or rectum, or who have inflammatory bowel problems such as colitis run an increased risk. A history of diabetes also seems to increase risk. Other possible risk factors include diets high in fat or low in fiber, high consumption of red and processed meats, smoking, sedentary lifestyle, high alcohol consumption, and low intake of fruits and vegetables.

Following recommended screenings and paying attention to your own bowel activity are key factors in early diagnosis. If you have a history of inflammatory bowel problems such as irritable bowel syndrome (IBS), colitis, or Crohn's disease and/or a history of type 2 diabetes, talk with your doctor about whether or not you should begin colorectal screening before age 50. Regular exercise, a diet with lots of fruits and other plant foods, maintaining a healthy weight, avoiding tobacco products, and moderation in alcohol consumption appear to be among the most promising prevention strategies. Consumption of milk and calcium and having higher blood levels of vitamin D decrease risks. However, other factors, such as use of nonsteroidal anti-inflammatory drugs (NSAIDS), diet, vitamins, and calcium have shown conflicting results in studies.[84]

## Skin Cancer

Skin cancer is the most common form of cancer in the United States today, although exact numbers of cases remain in question because skin cancer is not reported to cancer registries.[85] Although millions of people are diagnosed each year, and millions of dollars are spent on sun protection, rates of the two most common forms—basal cell and squamous cell carcinomas—continue to increase. The good news is that most cases are highly treatable, and not life-threatening, even though they can cause pain and be disfiguring if they are in advanced stages. Most skin cancer deaths—nearly 13,500 in 2016—are from a much more serious form of skin cancer known as melanoma.[86] Melanoma affects over 76,000 people in the United States each year.[87] The majority of these deaths are in white men over the age of 50, with only rare cases among African Americans. With improved knowledge about risks, as well as greater awareness of symptoms and improved preventive behaviors, diagnosis, and treatments, death rates are declining in whites under the age of 50. Death rates have increased slightly among those over 50, reflecting past work exposure and too much "sun time." Between 65 and 90 percent of melanomas are caused by exposure to ultraviolet (UV) light or sunlight.[88]

## Detection, Symptoms, and Treatment

Basal and squamous cell carcinomas show up most commonly on the face, ears, neck, arms, hands, and legs as warty bumps, colored spots, or scaly patches. Bleeding, itching, pain, or oozing are other symptoms that warrant attention. Surgery may be necessary to remove them, but they are seldom life threatening.

Although malignant melanoma may appear to be a harmless form of cancer initially, its size, shape, and color often undergo distinctive changes over time. Unless one takes note of these changes, it can invade body organs and tissues with devastating consequences. Like other cancers, survival is largely dependent on how advanced the cancer is when diagnosed. If melanoma has not yet penetrated the underlying layers of skin, chances of survival are over 90 percent. However, if it is diagnosed after deeper layers of skin are penetrated and it has spread to other organs, the survival rate falls to 17 percent.[89] **FIGURE 17.5** compares melanoma with basal cell and squamous cell carcinomas.

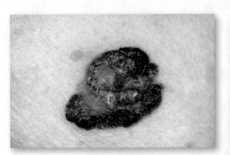 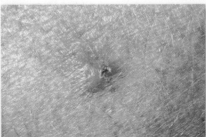 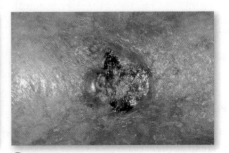

**ⓐ** Malignant melanoma    **ⓑ** Basal cell carcinoma    **ⓒ** Squamous cell carcinoma

**FIGURE 17.5 Types of Skin Cancers** Preventing skin cancer includes keeping a careful watch for any new pigmented growths and for changes to any moles. The ABCDE warning signs of melanoma (a) include *asymmetrical* shapes, irregular *borders*, *color* variation, an increase in *diameter*, and the characteristics have *evolved* over time. Basal cell carcinoma (b) and squamous cell carcinoma (c) should be brought to your physician's attention, but they are not as deadly as melanoma.

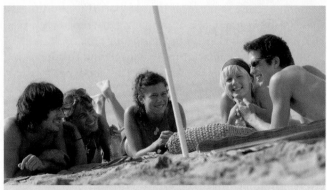

There is no such thing as a "safe" tan because a tan is visible evidence of UV-induced skin damage. According to the American Cancer Society, tanned skin provides only the equivalent of sun protection factor (SPF) 4 sunscreen—much too weak to be protective.

The *ABCDE* rule can help you remember the warning signs of melanoma:[90]

- **Asymmetry.** One half of the mole or lesion does not match the other half.
- **Border irregularity.** The edges are uneven, notched, or scalloped.
- **Color.** Pigmentation is not uniform. Melanomas may vary in color from tan to deeper brown, reddish black, black, or deep bluish black.
- **Diameter.** Diameter is greater than 6 millimeters (about the size of a pea).
- **Evolving.** The symmetry, size, shape, color, border, or other characteristics have changed over time.

Treatment of skin cancer depends on the type of cancer, its stage, and its location. Surgery, laser treatments, topical chemical agents, *electrodesiccation* (tissue destruction by heat), and *cryosurgery* (tissue destruction by freezing) are all common forms of treatment. Melanoma treatments have advanced significantly in recent years, with targeted therapies showing much promise in addition to newer surgical, radiation, and chemotherapy regimens.

**SEE IT! VIDEOS**

Is there such a thing as a "safe" tan? Watch **Extreme Tanning**, available on **MasteringHealth.**

**Risk Factors and Prevention** Anyone who overexposes him- or herself to ultraviolet (UV) radiation without adequate protection is at risk for skin cancer. The risk is greatest for people who:

- Have fair skin; blonde, red, or light brown hair; blue, green, or gray eyes
- Always burn before tanning or burn easily and peel readily
- Don't tan easily but spend lots of time outdoors
- Use no or low sun protection factor (SPF) sunscreens or expired suntan lotions

- Have had skin cancer or a family history of skin cancer
- Experienced severe sunburns during childhood. Contrary to popular thinking, there is no such thing as getting a base tan that protects against damage. The greater the exposure dose and the longer the time periods of exposure, the greater the risk.

Preventing skin cancer is a matter of limiting exposure to harmful UV rays and applying broad-spectrum suntan lotions liberally and often when exposed. What happens when you expose yourself to sunlight? The skin responds to *photodamage* by increasing its thickness and the number of pigment cells (melanocytes), which produce the "tan" look. (A tan is actually the body's way of trying to protect itself or defend against UV attack.

**WHAT DO YOU THINK?**

How should we determine whether a behavior or substance is a risk factor for a disease and whether programs should be enacted to reduce the risk or stop a behavior?

- Do you think that there should be federal legislation banning the use of tanning booths/beds in all 50 states? Why or why not? Would you favor such bans for minors only? Adults?

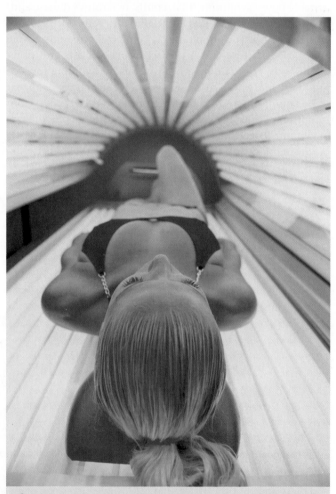

Gaining that "savage tan" in a tanning booth can significantly increase risks of melanoma.

## MAKING CHANGES TODAY

### Tips for Protecting Your Skin in the Sun

◉ Seek shade from 10:00 A.M. to 4:00 P.M., when the sun's rays are strongest. Even on a cloudy day, up to 80 percent of the sun's rays can get through.

◎ Apply a sunscreen with SPF 15 or higher evenly to all uncovered skin before going outside. Look for a broad-spectrum sunscreen that protects against both UVA and UVB radiation. If the sunscreen label does not specify otherwise, assume you need to apply it 15 minutes before going outside.

◎ Know your SPFs. You may think that a 15 SPF is only half as good as a 30 SPF and that a 100 SPF is going to block 100 percent of the damaging sun rays. Not so! An SPF 15 product typically blocks about 94 percent of UVB rays while an SPF 30 may block 97 percent. If you pay for a 70 to 100 SPF product, you are probably just wasting your money. New regulations are in play designed to simply say 50+ SPF so that consumers are not led on a merry chase, paying more for no more benefit.

◎ Check the expiration date on your sunscreen. Sunscreens lose effectiveness over time. Ditch that suntan lotion in your medicine cabinet from 3 to 5 years ago when you went to Florida for spring break. If it doesn't *have* an expiration date, it is probably so old that they weren't required. Don't waste your time with expired products!

◎ Put sunscreen on your lips, nose, ears, neck, hands, and feet. If you don't have much hair, apply sunscreen to the top of your head, too. Most people do not apply sunscreen liberally enough! Did you know that you should probably apply half a typical tube of lotion at each sun outing? One to 2 ounces are suggested, applied liberally and often.

◎ Reapply sunscreen at least every 2 hours. It is recommended that you apply at least 15 minutes before getting into water or before lying out on the beach so that it is absorbed and likely to protect you. The label will tell you how often you need to do this. If it isn't waterproof, reapply after swimming or if you are sweating.

◎ Wear loose-fitting, light-colored clothing. For extra protection, in most sporting goods stores you can now purchase clothing that has SPF protection. A wide-brimmed hat will protect your head and face.

◎ Buy good-quality sunglasses from reputable companies rather than the $5 to $10 versions available at beach-side stands. Make sure they cover your entire eye and don't allow sunlight in the corners and edges of your eye. Use sunglasses with 99 to 100 percent UV protection to protect your eyes. Look for polarized lenses.

◎ Tanning booths are *not* safer than the sun. Avoid them.

◎ Check your skin for cancer, keeping an eye out for changes in birthmarks, moles, or sunspots.

**Sources:** U.S. Food and Drug Administration, "FDA Sheds Light on Sunscreens," 2013, www.fda.gov/ForConsumers/ConsumerUpdates/ucm258416.htm; NCSL, "Indoor Tanning Restrictions for Minors—A State-by-State Comparison," March 31, 2016, www.ncsl.org/research/health/indoor-tanning-restrictions.aspx; American College of Dermatology, "Dangers of Indoor Tanning," May 17, 2016, https://www.aad.org/public/spot-skin-cancer/learn-about-skin-cancer/dangers-of-indoor-tanning.

It can fight the onslaught only for a short time before damage begins to accrue.) Ultraviolet light damages the skin's immune cells, lowering the normal immune protection of the skin and priming it for cancer. Photodamage also causes wrinkling by impairing the elastic substances (collagens) that keep skin soft and pliable. See the Making Changes Today box for tips on staying safe in the sun.

In spite of the risks, many Americans are still "working on a tan," either outdoors or in tanning salons, prompting some psychologists to speculate that there might be a form of compulsion to tan termed *tanorexia*. Tanning is thought to be addictive due to some form of brain response to UVR light, prompting physiological or psychological responses. Recent studies of young adults exposed to indoor tanning suggest a possible link to tanning dependence and activation of the reward system.[91] However, critics argue that this research is preliminary and that significant, large-scale clinical trials are necessary to confirm an association.

## Prostate Cancer

After skin cancer, prostate cancer is the most frequently diagnosed cancer in American males today.[92] It is the second leading cause of cancer deaths in men after lung cancer.[93] In 2016, about 181,000 new cases of prostate cancer were diagnosed in the United States, with 26,120 estimated deaths.[94] Although the reasons are unclear, African American rates of prostate cancer are about 70 percent higher than in non-Hispanic whites.[95] About 1 in 6 men will be diagnosed with prostate cancer during his lifetime.[96] However, with improved screening and early diagnosis, 5-year survival rates are nearly 99 percent for all but the most advanced cases, which have a much more bleak outcome, with only 13 percent surviving.[97] Men who are obese and smoke have an increased risk of dying from prostate cancer.[98]

**Detection, Symptoms, and Treatment** The prostate is a muscular, walnut-sized gland that surrounds part

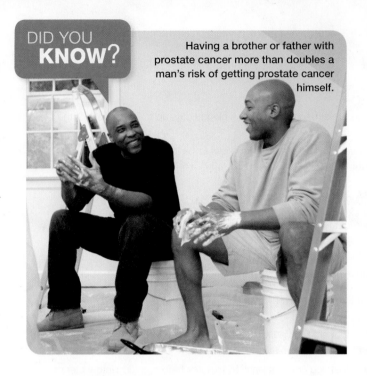

of a man's urethra, the tube that transports urine and sperm out of the body. A part of the reproductive system, its primary function is to produce seminal fluid. Often, early stages of prostate cancer have no symptoms. As the disease progresses, symptoms may include weak or interrupted urine flow; difficulty starting or stopping urination; feeling the urge to urinate frequently, particularly at night; pain on urination; and blood in the urine. Prostate cancer often spreads to the bones if not treated early; unexplained pain in the hips, low back, ribs, or other areas may indicate the cancer has spread.

Men over age 40 should have an annual digital rectal prostate examination. Another screening method for prostate cancer is the **prostate-specific antigen (PSA)** test, a blood test that screens for an indicator of prostate cancer. However, the United States Preventive Services Task Force recommends that otherwise asymptomatic men no longer receive the routine PSA test because, overall, it does not save lives and may in fact lead to painful, unnecessary cancer treatments. If you have a family history or other symptoms, consult with your physician.

**Risk Factors and Prevention** Increasing age is one of the biggest risks for prostate cancer, as is African ancestry or a family history of prostate cancer. In fact, more than 60 percent of prostate cancers are diagnosed in men over the age of 65, and over 97 percent of all cases occur in men over the age of 50.[99]

Black men in the United States and Caribbean men of African descent have the highest documented prostate cancer incidence rates in the world. Genetics may account for between 5 and 10 percent of prostate cancers overall.[100] They are also more likely to be diagnosed at more advanced stages than other racial groups.[101]

Having a father or brother with prostate cancer more than doubles a man's risk of getting prostate cancer. Men who have had several relatives with prostate cancer, especially those with relatives who developed prostate cancer at younger ages, are also at higher risk.[102]

Eating more fruits and vegetables, particularly those containing *lycopene*, a pigment found in tomatoes and other red fruits, may lower the risk of prostate cancer death; however, more research is necessary to determine the validity of these claims.[103] Diets high in processed meats or dairy and obesity also appear to increase risks.[104] The best advice is to follow the dietary recommendations of the U.S. Department of Agriculture, discussed in Chapter 5, and maintain a healthy weight.

## Ovarian Cancer

Ovarian cancer is the fifth leading cause of cancer deaths for women, with nearly 23,000 diagnoses in 2016 and just over 14,000 deaths.[105] Ovarian cancer causes more deaths than any other cancer of the reproductive system because women tend not to discover it until the cancer is at an advanced stage, when 5-year survival is only 27 percent.[106] Younger women (under the age of 65) are much more likely to survive 5 years compared to those 65 or older. For all stages, the 5-year survival is 46 percent.[107]

**Detection, Symptoms, and Treatment** Ovarian cancer symptoms are often not obvious, and it is common for women to have no early symptoms and be diagnosed at later, more difficult to treat stages. A woman may complain of feeling bloated, having pain in the pelvic area, feeling full quickly, or feeling the need to urinate more frequently. Some may experience persistent digestive disturbances, while other symptoms include fatigue, pain during intercourse, unexplained weight loss, unexplained changes in bowel or bladder habits, and incontinence. If these vague symptoms persist for more than a week or two, prompt medical evaluation is a must.

Treatment for early-stage ovarian cancer typically includes surgery, chemotherapy, and occasionally radiation therapy. Depending on the patient's age and her desire to bear children in the future, one or both ovaries, fallopian tubes, and the uterus may be removed.

**Risk Factors and Prevention** Primary relatives (mother, daughter, sister) of a woman who has had breast or ovarian cancer are at increased risk, as are those with a family or personal history of breast or colon cancer (particularly those with positive *BRCA1* or *BRCA2* tests). Women who have never been pregnant are more likely to develop ovarian cancer than those who have given birth, and the more children a woman has had, the less risk she faces. The use of estrogen alone as postmenopausal therapy may increase a woman's risk, as will smoking and obesity.[108]

Research shows that long-term use of oral contraceptives, adhering to a low-fat diet, having multiple children, breastfeeding, and tubal ligation may reduce your risk of ovarian cancer.[109] So, should you get pregnant or start taking birth control pills to reduce risk? No. General prevention strategies such as focusing on diet, exercise, sleep, stress management, and weight control are good ideas for combating cancer risk.

**prostate-specific antigen (PSA)** An antigen found in prostate cancer patients.

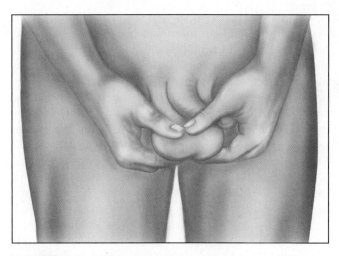

**SEE IT! VIDEOS**

How can you prevent cervical cancer? Watch **Preventing Cervical Cancer**, available on **MasteringHealth.™**

To protect yourself, get a complete annual pelvic examination. Women over age 40 should have a cancer-related checkup every year. Uterine ultrasound or a blood test is recommended for those with risk factors or unexplained symptoms.

## Cervical and Endometrial (Uterine) Cancer

Most uterine cancers develop in the body of the uterus, usually in the endometrium. The rest develop in the cervix, located at the base of the uterus. In 2015, nearly 13,000 new cases of cervical cancer and over 60,000 cases of endometrial cancer were diagnosed in the United States, with nearly 10,500 deaths.[110] As more women have regular **Pap test** screenings—a procedure in which cells taken from the cervical region are examined for abnormal activity—rates should decline even further in the future. As of 2016, it is recommended women get a Pap test every 2 years beginning at age 21. Between ages 30 and 65, women should have an HPV and Pap test every 5 years and a Pap test alone every 3 years. Those with parents and/or siblings with breast cancer should talk with their doctor about having tests more frequently.

Although Pap tests are very effective for detecting early-stage cervical cancer, they are less effective for detecting cancers of the uterine lining. Women have a lifetime risk of 1 in 157 for being diagnosed with cervical cancer and a 1 in 36 risk of being diagnosed with uterine corpus cancer.[111] Early warning signs of uterine cancer include bleeding outside the normal menstrual period or after menopause, or persistent unusual vaginal discharge.

Risk factors for cervical cancer include early age at first intercourse, multiple sex partners, cigarette smoking, and a history of infection with HPV (the cause of genital warts). Today, both young men and women have the option of getting vaccinated with either *Gardasil* or *Cervarix*, designed to protect against the two types of HPV that cause most cervical cancers. For endometrial cancer, age is a risk factor; however, estrogen and obesity (particularly abdominal obesity) are also strong risk factors. In addition, risks are increased by treatment with tamoxifen for breast cancer, metabolic syndrome, late menopause, never bearing children, a history of polyps in the uterus or ovaries, a history of other cancers, and race (white women are at higher risk).[112]

## Testicular Cancer

Testicular cancer is one of the most common types of solid tumors found in young adult men, affecting nearly 8,720 young men in 2016.[113] Over one-half of all cases occur between the ages of 20 and 34, with steady increases in this group over the last few years.[114] However, with a 95.4 percent 5-year survival rate, it is one of the most curable forms of cancer, particularly if caught in localized stages.[115] Although the cause of testicular cancer is unknown, several risk factors have been identified.

**FIGURE 17.6** Testicular Self-Exam

**Source:** From Michael Johnson, *Human Biology: Concepts and Current Issues*, 3rd ed. Copyright © 2006. Reprinted with permission of Pearson Education, Inc.

Men with undescended testicles appear to be at greatest risk, and some studies indicate a genetic influence. Risk is also higher if you are white, have HIV or AIDS, or if a primary relative (father or brother, in particular) has had testicular cancer.[116]

> **Pap test** A procedure in which cells taken from the cervical region are examined for abnormal cellular activity.

**Testicular Self-Exam** In general, testicular tumors first appear as an enlargement of the testis or thickening in testicular tissue. Some men report a heavy feeling, dull ache, or pain that extends to the lower abdomen or groin area. Testicular self-exams have long been recommended for teen boys and young men to perform monthly as a means of detecting testicular cancer (**FIGURE 17.6**). However, recent studies discovered that findings from monthly self-exams result in testing for noncancerous conditions and thus are not cost-effective. For this reason, the U.S. Preventive Services Task Force has dropped their recommendation for monthly testicular exams. Regardless, most cases of testicular cancer are discovered through self-exam, and there is currently no other screening test for the disease.

The testicular self-exam is best done after a hot shower, which will relax the scrotum and make the exam easier. Standing in front of a mirror, hold the testicle with one hand while gently rolling its surface between the thumb and fingers of your other hand. Feel underneath the scrotum for the tubes of the epididymis and blood vessels that sit close to the body. Repeat with the other testicle. Look for any lump, thickening, or pea-like nodules, paying attention to any areas that may be painful over the entire surface of the scrotum. When done, wash your hands with soap and water. Doing regular self-exams will help you to know what is normal for you and to note any irregularity. Consult a doctor if you notice anything that is unusual.

## Leukemia

Leukemia is a cancer of the bone and blood-forming tissues that leads to proliferation of millions of immature white blood cells. These abnormal cells crowd out normal white blood cells (which fight infection), platelets (which control hemorrhaging), and red blood cells (which carry oxygen to body cells). Resulting symptoms include fatigue, paleness, weight loss, bone and joint pain, easy bruising, repeated infections, and nosebleeds. Leukemia can be *acute* and come on rather suddenly or *chronic* and progress over months or years with vague symptoms. It is classified into four types based on cell type and growth rate: *acute lymphocytic (ALL), chronic lymphocytic (CLL), acute myeloid (AML),* and *chronic myeloid (CML)*. Of particular relevance for young adults is the fact that the majority of leukemia cases (91 percent) occur in adults aged 20 and older.[117] Among adults, the most common types are CLL (37%) and AML (31%), while ALL is more common among youth.[118] Over 60,000 new cases will be diagnosed in 2016 in the United States.[119] Risk factors include exposure to ionizing radiation often used in treatment for cancers, working in the rubber industry, and having Down syndrome and other genetic factors.[120] Depending on type of leukemia and stage at diagnosis, a variety of treatments, including chemotherapy, radiation, bone marrow and stem cell transplants, and other strategies, are among the most effective.

## Lymphoma

Just a few short years ago, not many people had heard much about lymphomas, a group of cancers of the lymphatic system that include Hodgkin disease and non-Hodgkin lymphoma. Today, however, lymphomas are among the fastest-growing cancers, with over 81,000 cases and over 21,000 deaths in 2016.[121] Much of this increase has occurred in women and, like many cancers, risk increases with age. The cause is unknown; however, a weakened immune system is suspected— particularly one that has been exposed to viruses such as HIV, hepatitis C, Epstein-Barr virus (EBV), and others. Treatment and prognosis for lymphoma varies by type and stage; however, chemotherapy and radiotherapy are commonly used. If detected early, survival rates are high.

## Pancreatic Cancer

In 2016, nearly 53,070 will be diagnosed with pancreatic cancer, and 41,780 will die from it, making it one of the deadliest forms of cancer.[122] In spite of advances in diagnosis and treatment, only 27 percent of patients survive 1 year after diagnosis, and only 7 percent survive 5 years.[123] Although most cases occur after age 50, there are increasing numbers of cases at earlier ages. Overall, rates are higher in African Americans and in populations with lower socioeconomic status and education levels. They are also about 30 percent higher in men than in women.[124]

**magnetic resonance imaging (MRI)** A device that uses magnetic fields, radio waves, and computers to generate an image of internal tissues of the body for diagnostic purposes without the use of radiation.

**computerized axial tomography (CAT) scan** A scan by a machine that uses radiation to view internal organs not normally visible in X-rays.

**stereotactic radiosurgery** A type of radiation therapy that can be used to zap tumors; also known as gamma knife surgery.

**gamma knife surgery** *See* stereotactic radiosurgery.

Key risk factors appear to be tobacco use, obesity, consuming high levels of red meat, and a high-fat diet. Family history, genetic links, and a history of chronic inflammation of the pancreas (*pancreatitis*) also seem to increase risk. There appears to be a greater risk among diabetics and those who have had infections with hepatitis B and C and the *Helicobacter* bacteria. Because pancreatic cancer has few early symptoms, there is no reliable test to detect it in its early stages. When symptoms begin, weight loss, stomach discomfort, and pain that may radiate to the back may occur. Often, by the time it is diagnosed via CAT or MRI examinations, it is too advanced to treat effectively.

## LO 5 | FACING CANCER

Discuss the most current and effective methods of cancer detection and treatment, including areas of significant progress and future challenges.

There is much you can do to reduce your own risk of cancer. Make a realistic assessment of your own risk factors, avoid behaviors that put you at risk, and increase healthy behaviors. Even if you have significant risks, those are factors you can control. Avoid known carcinogens and other environmental hazards, and follow the recommendations for self-exams and medical checkups in **TABLE 17.2**. The earlier cancer is diagnosed, the better the prognosis will be.

## Detecting Cancer

If you are at high risk for developing cancer, or if you notice potential cancer symptoms, your health care provider might use one or more tests to diagnose or rule out cancer. **Magnetic resonance imaging (MRI)** uses a huge electromagnet to detect tumors by mapping the vibrations of the atoms in the body on a computer screen. The **computerized axial tomography (CAT) scan** uses X-rays to examine parts of the body. In both of these painless, noninvasive procedures, cross-sectioned pictures can reveal a tumor's shape and location more accurately than can conventional X-rays. *Prostatic ultrasound* (a rectal probe using ultrasonic waves to produce an image of the prostate) is being investigated as a means to increase the early detection of prostate cancer. New three-dimensional mammogram machines offer significant improvements in imaging and breast cancer detection, but deliver nearly double the radiation risk of conventional mammograms.

## Cancer Treatments

Cancer treatments vary according to the type and stage of cancer. Surgery, in which the tumor and surrounding tissue are removed, is one common strategy. It may be performed alone or in combination with other treatments. The surgeon may operate using traditional surgical instruments such as a scalpel, or by using a laser, laparoscope, or other tools for less invasive results. Pain and infection are the most common problems after surgery.

**Stereotactic radiosurgery**, also known as **gamma knife surgery**, uses a targeted dose of gamma radiation to zap tumors

| Cancer Site | Screening Procedure | Age and Frequency of Test |
|---|---|---|
| Breast | Mammograms | The NCI recommends that women in their 40s and older have mammograms every 1 to 2 years. Women who are at higher-than-average risk of breast cancer should talk with their health care provider about whether to have mammograms before age 40 and how often to have them. |
| Cervix | Pap test (Pap smear) | Testing is generally recommended to begin at age 21 and to end at age 65, as long as recent results have been normal. Most women should have a Pap test at least once every 3 years. |
| Colon and rectum | ***Fecal occult blood test:*** Sometimes cancer or polyps bleed. This test can detect tiny amounts of blood in the stool. ***Sigmoidoscopy:*** Checks the rectum and lower part of the colon for polyps. ***Colonoscopy:*** Checks the rectum and entire colon for polyps and cancer. | People aged 50 and older should be screened. People who have a higher-than-average risk of cancer of the colon or rectum should talk with their doctor about whether to have screening tests before age 50 and how often to have them. |
| Prostate | Prostate-specific antigen (PSA) test | Some groups encourage yearly screening for men over age 50, and some advise men who are at a higher risk for prostate cancer to begin screening at age 40 or 45. Many expert groups no longer recommend routine PSA testing as studies have shown little or no effect on prostate cancer deaths. It also leads to overdiagnosis and overtreatment. Currently, Medicare provides coverage for an annual PSA test for all men age 50 and older. |

**Source:** National Cancer Institute, National Institutes of Health, "Screening Tests," March 24, 2015, http://www.cancer.gov/about-cancer/screening/screening-tests.

with pinpoint accuracy without any blood loss or ever using a scalpel. **Radiotherapy** (the use of radiation) or **chemotherapy** (the use of drugs) to kill cancerous cells are also used. Radiation destroys malignant cells or stops cell growth. It is most effective in treating localized cancer masses because it can be targeted to a particular area of the body. Over the course of several weeks, patients are treated by a machine that exposes the designated

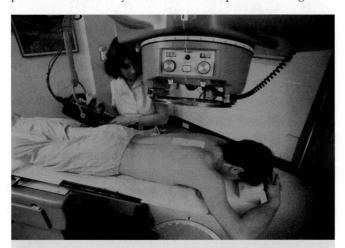

Radiation therapy is often used to target and destroy cancerous tumors. The machine in this photograph emits gamma rays, which are typically used to treat localized secondary cancers and also provide pain relief for otherwise untreatable cancers. Gamma rays are less powerful than the X-rays emitted from linear accelerators, another machine frequently used in radiation therapy.

part of the body to high-energy rays. Radiotherapy usually takes place on an outpatient basis. Side effects include fatigue, changes to the skin in the affected area, and a small increase in the chance of developing another type of cancer.

Chemotherapy may be used to shrink a tumor before surgery or radiation therapy, after surgery or radiation therapy to kill remaining cancer cells, or on its own. Powerful drugs, often targeted for specific tumors, are given, usually in on-and-off cycles so the body can recover from their effects. Side effects may include nausea, hair loss, fatigue, increased chance of bleeding, bruising, infection, and anemia, among others. These usually diminish as the drugs leave the body after treatment. Other possible effects include loss of fertility, damage to blood vessels, and memory loss. In the process of killing malignant cells, some healthy cells are also destroyed, and long-term damage to the cardiovascular system and other body systems can be significant.

Participation in clinical trials (people-based studies of new drugs or procedures) has provided a new source of hope for many patients undergoing cancer treatment. Because of the many unknown variables, deciding whether to participate in a clinical trial can be a difficult decision. Despite the risks, thousands of clinical trial participants have benefited from treatments that would otherwise be unavailable to them.

Several newer treatments described in the **Health Headlines** box on page 476 are either being used in clinical trials or have become available in selected cancer centers throughout the country. In addition,

**radiotherapy** The use of radiation to kill cancerous cells.

**chemotherapy** The use of drugs to kill cancerous cells.

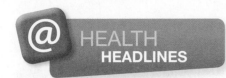
Surgery, chemotherapy, and radiation therapy remain the most common treatments for all types of cancer. However, newer techniques are constantly being investigated that may be more effective for certain cancers or certain patients:

- **Immunotherapy.** The goal of immunotherapy is to enhance the body's own disease-fighting systems. Biological response modifiers such as interferon and interleukin-2 are under study. Immunotherapies have been particularly effective against melanomas and certain kidney cancers.

- **Biological therapies.** One of the most exciting new approaches for spurring the immune system to ward off cancer is the use of *cancer-fighting vaccines*. These alert the body's immune defenses to good cells that have gone bad. Rather than preventing disease as other vaccines do, they help people who are already ill.

- **Gene therapies.** Research on the effectiveness of *gene therapy* has moved into early clinical trials.

Scientists have found signs of a virus carrying genetic information that makes the cells it infects (such as cancer cells) susceptible to an antiviral drug. Scientists are also looking at ways to transfer genes that increase the patient's immune response to the cancerous tumor or that confer drug resistance to the bone marrow to allow higher doses of chemotherapeutic drugs.

- **Angiogenesis inhibitors.** Researchers are testing compounds that may stop tumors from forming new blood vessels, a process called *angiogenesis*. Without adequate blood supply, tumors either die or grow very slowly, giving other chemotherapeutic agents a better chance to fight them.

- **Disrupting cancer pathways.** In recent years, scientists have identified various steps in what is termed the *cancer pathway*. These include oncogene actions, hormone receptors, growth factors, metastasis, and angiogenesis. Preliminary studies are under way to design compounds that inhibit actions at these various steps.

- **Smart "bullet" drugs.** Drugs such as T-DM1 (which combines chemotherapy and targeted antibodies), Herceptin, Gleevec, and Avastin are new forms of *targeted smart-drug therapies* that deliver chemotherapy to attack only the cancer cells and avoid healthy cells, which helps patients avoid severe sickness during aggressive treatments.

- **Enzyme inhibitors.** A powerful enzyme inhibitor, TIMP2, shows promise for slowing the metastasis of tumor cells. A metastasis suppressor gene, *NM23*, has also been identified. Both of these therapies are aimed at disrupting cancer pathways.

- **Neoadjuvant chemotherapy.** This method (which uses chemotherapy to shrink the tumor and then surgically remove it) has been tried against various types of cancers.

- **Stem cell research.** When a patient's bone marrow has been destroyed by disease, chemotherapy, or radiation, transplants of stem cells from donor bone marrow may successfully restore blood stem cells (the cells that divide to produce blood cells).

---

psychosocial and behavioral research has become increasingly important as health professionals learn more about lifestyle factors that influence risk and survivability. Health practitioners have begun to tailor treatment programs to meet the diverse psychological needs of patients and families.

Before beginning any form of cancer therapy, you need to be a vigilant and vocal consumer. Read and seek information from cancer support groups. Check the skills of your surgeon, your radiation therapist, and your doctor in terms of clinical experience and interpersonal interactions. Look at *Oncolink* and other websites supported by the National Cancer Institute and the American Cancer Society (ACS), and check out clinical trials, reports on effectiveness of various treatments, new experimental therapies, and other options. Although you may like and trust your family doctor, it is always a good idea to seek advice or consultation from large cancer facilities that see many patients and are well equipped to deal with all situations. Do not be afraid to question health care providers about options and their reasons for selecting one course of treatment over another. Check the credentials and specialty areas of your oncologist and try to find the best match for your type of cancer. See the **Student Health Today** box for more on being your own advocate or an advocate for someone you love.

## LO 6 | **CANCER** SURVIVORS

Discuss what it really means to be a "cancer survivor" and how it means more than living cancer free for 5 years after diagnosis.

Today, an increasing number of people in the United States and globally survive cancer with less disease burden and disability, better outcomes in terms of healthy years, and fewer problems than any previous generation. Although a diagnosis of cancer is never easy, living with cancer is less traumatic than ever before, largely due to heightened public awareness, less stigma, and a much greater level of support for cancer patients. Cancer patients are much less likely to face cancer alone or make decisions about treatment in isolation. Cancer support groups, cancer information workshops, and low-cost medical consultation are widely available via a wide range of information networks. Groups such as the Susan G. Komen for the Cure Foundation have provided support for survivors and their families and have helped people realize that cancer is not a death sentence or something to be hidden. Coping with cancer can be difficult, but there are ways to ease the burden and make surviving less challenging for all concerned.[125]

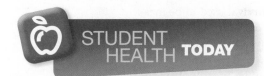

# BEING A HEALTH ADVOCATE FOR YOURSELF OR SOMEONE YOU LOVE

When cancer is diagnosed, people often react with anxiety, fear, and anger. Emotional distress is sometimes so intense that patients and their loved ones are unable to make critical health care decisions. Sometimes, they are unable to understand how a treatment will really work or what the risks versus benefits are. If you or a loved one is diagnosed with cancer, the following actions can help you remain calm as you check out available treatment options:

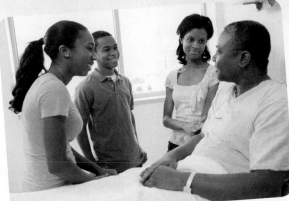

If you or someone you love is diagnosed with cancer, it is important to seek out all the help and information that you can find.

- **Pair up for doctor appointments.** Even suspecting cancer can cause fear and shock, and that can prevent a patient from asking important questions or from hearing key details. Bring a trusted friend or relative with you to the doctor, and talk together about what you heard later.
- **Find out as much as possible about the cancer.** Before you go to your appointment, *read widely* about your suspected cancer. There are numerous sources that can help you understand your treatment options, long-term prognosis, and overall options. Don't be afraid to ask questions. If your doctor acts too busy to answer or acts annoyed, find another doctor. Questions you might ask include an explanation of the type and stage of cancer, the recommended treatment plan, and the potential risks and benefits. Read about your cancer on reliable websites such as the American Cancer Society or the National Cancer Institute. If your doctor recommends that you participate in a clinical drug trial, request a copy of the documents outlining potential risks and benefits. Remember that not everyone in a clinical trial gets the experimental treatment right away. If you are in the control group (placebo)

group, when will you get the treatment? Can you afford to wait?
- **Get a second opinion.** Request a copy of the diagnostic test results and get an "out-of-group" physician (someone unaffiliated with your original doctor) to review them. Find an oncologist (cancer specialist) at a big teaching hospital where they see a large number of patients with your type of cancer. Don't worry about hurting the original doctor's feelings. This is a common practice. Remember, it's your life!
- **Check out the credentials of the hospital, surgeon, and treatment specialist.** If surgery is recommended, find out about the patient-to-caregiver ratio in the hospital and the plan for aftercare. Ask for recommendations from patients who've had the procedures that are planned for you. When you go in for scans, ask if they have the newest generation of CT scanners and other radiation-emitting equipment. Older-generation scanners can expose you to more radiation than newer scanners.
- **Find local resources and support groups.** It can be helpful to talk with someone who isn't emotionally

involved in your personal situation. Survivor support groups can provide information you can get only from people who have lived through cancer. Talking with a counselor is another good way to keep the focus on getting well.
- **Get your personal ducks in a row.** Write down financial information, where to find important papers, passwords for computer files, and key bits of information. It's always a good idea to have a file box with detailed documentation of the above, as well as your advanced directives and other medical wishes, even when you don't have an actual cancer diagnosis. Find someone to take care of your home and pets if you will be hospitalized and someone who can bring you home when you are released.
- **Know what insurance does and doesn't cover.** Call your insurer ahead of time and know what procedures require permission. Find out what percentage of the bill is the patient's responsibility and how this may change if you need to see specialists. If you do not have insurance, talk with social service agencies, your student health center financial director, or others who can help you come up with a plan for payment.
- **Mobilize family and friends to help.** If you or your loved one will be bedridden, ask friends to make and deliver dinners, do errands, take you for follow-up appointments, or help around the house. Don't be afraid to ask for the help you need. Friends and family usually want to have some concrete way to help in times of crisis. Let others "in." Encourage your loved ones to share thoughts and fears.

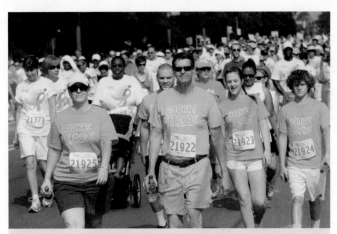

There may be physical and emotional issues as well as financial issues related to health insurance and cost of care to cope with for years after cancer diagnosis and treatment. Survivors also have to live with the possibility of a recurrence. However, cancer survivors can and do live active, productive lives despite these challenges. Many survivors and their relatives find it emotionally satisfying to participate in cancer research fundraiser walks and other events.

Although survival used to be measured almost exclusively by whether a person had gone 5 years without cancer symptoms, **survivorship** is now viewed much more broadly in terms of both years and the quality of life that a person experiences after diagnosis. Today, survivorship comprises the unique ways in which people survive and thrive after cancer has been diagnosed. The National Cancer Institute defines this term as the "physical, psychological, emotional, and economic issues of cancer from diagnosis until the end of life."[126]

Accumulating evidence makes it clear that breast cancer survivorship, for example, is influenced by a constellation of important factors, including age, socioeconomic status, availability of support services, education level, relationship status, social support, sexual identity, race, stress level, coping style, spirituality, and depression.

Rather than looking only at the number of years people survive, quality of the survival experience is becoming increasingly important. In fact, quality-of-life measures may influence whether a person actually reaches the 5-year survivor milestone.

**survivorship** Physical, psychological, emotional, and economic issues of cancer from diagnosis until the end of life.

# STUDY **PLAN**

Customize your study plan—and master your health!—in the Study Area of **MasteringHealth**.

## ASSESS YOURSELF

**Could you be at risk for cancer?** Want to find out? Take the **What's Your Personal Risk for Cancer?** assessment available on **MasteringHealth.**™

# CHAPTER **REVIEW**

To hear an MP3 Tutor Session, scan here or visit the Study Area in **MasteringHealth**.

## LO **1** | An Overview of Cancer

■ Cancer is the second most common cause of death in the United States. The current 5-year survival rates for cancer have greatly increased from those of previous generations.

## LO **2** | What Is Cancer?

■ Cancer is a group of diseases characterized by uncontrolled growth and spread of abnormal cells. These cells may create tumors. Benign (noncancerous) tumors grow in size but do not spread; malignant (cancerous) tumors spread to other parts of the body.

## LO **3** | What Causes Cancer?

■ Lifestyle factors for cancer include smoking and obesity as well as poor diet, lack of exercise, stress, and other factors. Biological factors include inherited genes, age, and gender. Potential environmental carcinogens include asbestos, radiation, preservatives, and pesticides. Infectious agents may increase your risks for cancer; those that appear most likely to cause cancer are chronic hepatitis B and C,

human papillomavirus, and genital herpes. Medical factors may elevate the chance of cancer.

## LO **4** | Types of Cancers

■ There are many different types of cancer, each of which poses different risks, depending on several factors. Common cancers include that of the lung, breast, colon and rectum, skin, prostate, testis, ovary, and uterus; leukemia; and lymphomas.

## LO **5** | Facing Cancer

■ The most common treatments for cancer are surgery, chemotherapy, and radiation; however, newer therapies, including biologicals, smart drugs, immunotherapy, and others, show promising results and should always be considered.

- Early diagnosis improves survival rate. Disparities exist based on race, geographical location, socioeconomic status, education, and other variables. Self-exams for breast, testicular, and skin cancer aid early diagnosis.

## LO 6 | Cancer Survivors

- The number of cancer survivors is at an all-time high for most cancer types. Surviving cancer is viewed in terms of both the years of life and the quality of life a person experiences from diagnosis to end of life.

# POP QUIZ

Visit **MasteringHealth** to personalize your study plan with Chapter Review Quizzes and Dynamic Study Modules.

## LO 1 | An Overview of Cancer

1. Overall, which cancer has the worst 5-year survival rate today?
   a. Prostate
   b. Pancreas
   c. Melanoma
   d. Breast

## LO 2 | What Is Cancer?

2. When cancer cells have *metastasized,*
   a. they have grown into a malignant tumor.
   b. they have spread to other parts of the body.
   c. the cancer is retreating and cancer cells are dying off.
   d. the tumor is localized and considered *in situ.*

3. A cancerous *neoplasm* is
   a. a type of biopsy.
   b. a form of benign tumor.
   c. a type of treatment for a tumor.
   d. a malignant group of cells or tumor.

## LO 3 | What Causes Cancer?

4. "If you are male and smoke, your chances of getting lung cancer are 23 times greater than those of a nonsmoker." This statement refers to a type of risk assessed statistically, known as

   a. relative risk.
   b. comparable risk.
   c. cancer risk.
   d. genetic predisposition.

5. One of the biggest factors in increased risk for cancer is
   a. increasing age.
   b. not having children.
   c. being of long-lived parents.
   d. increased consumption of fruits and vegetables.

## LO 4 | Types of Cancers

6. Who is at the highest risk for developing skin cancer?
   a. People who sunburned badly during childhood
   b. People who have dark skin
   c. People without a base tan
   d. People who wear sunscreen daily but tan easily

7. The cancer that causes the most deaths for men and women in the United States is:
   a. colorectal cancer.
   b. pancreatic cancer.
   c. lung cancer.
   d. stomach cancer.

8. Which of the following is *true* with respect to cancer?
   a. Black men in the United States and Caribbean men of African descent have the highest prostate cancer incidence in the world.
   b. Leukemia is primarily a childhood disease; few adults ever develop it.
   c. Number of skin cancer cases reported to cancer registries in the United States totalled 20 million in 2016.
   d. Colorectal cancer is the second most diagnosed cancer among men and women in the United States behind breast cancer in women and prostate cancer in men.

## LO 5 | Facing Cancer

9. Which of the following treatment methods uses drugs to kill cancerous cells?
   a. Radiotherapy
   b. Chemotherapy
   c. Stem cell therapy
   d. Stereotactic radiosurgery

## LO 6 | Cancer Survivors

10. What does the term cancer *survivorship* mean?
    a. The likeliness of surviving cancer during the treatment process and for 1 year following
    b. The emotional and physical states of relatives who have lost loved ones to cancer
    c. The likeliness of living with cancer past the 5-year survival rate
    d. The physical, psychological, emotional, and economic issues of surviving cancer

*Answers to the Pop Quiz can be found on page A-1. If you answered a question incorrectly, review the section identified by the Learning Outcome. For even more study tools, visit* **MasteringHealth***.*

# THINK ABOUT IT!

## LO 1 | An Overview of Cancer

1. What are some of the factors that account for the great increase in 5-year survival rates for people with cancer in recent years?

## LO 2 | What Is Cancer?

2. What is cancer? How does it spread? What is the difference between a benign tumor and a malignant tumor?

## LO 3 | What Causes Cancer?

3. List the likely causes of cancer. Which of these causes would be a risk for you, in particular? What can you do to reduce these risks? What risk factors do you share with family members? Friends?

## LO 4 | Types of Cancers

4. What are the symptoms of lung, breast, prostate, and testicular cancers? How can you reduce your risk of developing these cancers or increase your chances of surviving them?

5. What are the differences between carcinomas, sarcomas, lymphomas, and leukemia? Which is the most common? Least

common? Why is it important that you know the stage of your cancer?

LO **5** | **Facing Cancer**

6. Why are breast and testicular self-exams especially important for college students? What factors keep you from doing your own self-exams? What could you do to make sure you do regular self-exams?

LO **6** | **Cancer Survivors**

7. How has the idea of survivorship changed the way people think about the years after diagnosis? What are some ways people cope with and fight through a cancer diagnosis?

# ACCESS YOUR HEALTH ON THE INTERNET

Visit **MasteringHealth** for links to the websites and RSS feeds.

The following websites explore further topics and issues related to cancer.

**American Cancer Society.** This private organization is dedicated to cancer prevention. Here you'll find information, statistics, and resources regarding cancer. **www.cancer.org**

**National Cancer Institute.** On this site you will find valuable information on cancer facts, results of research, new and ongoing clinical trials, and the Physician Data Query (PDQ), a comprehensive database of cancer treatment information. **www.cancer.gov**

**National Women's Health Information Center (NWHIC).** A wealth of information about cancer in women is presented on this site, which is cosponsored by the National Cancer Institute. **http://womenshealth.gov**

**Oncolink.** Sponsored by the University of Pennsylvania Cancer Center, this site educates cancer patients and their families by offering information on support services, cancer causes, screening, prevention, and common questions. **www.oncolink.com**

**Susan G. Komen for the Cure.** Up-to-date information about breast cancer, issues in treatment, and support groups are presented here; there is also a wealth of videos and information. This site is especially useful for diagnosed patients looking for additional support and advice. **www.komen.org**

**National Coalition for Cancer Survivorship.** Cancer survivors share their experiences advocating for themselves during and after cancer treatment. **www.canceradvocacy.org**

# 18

# Reducing Risks and Coping with Chronic Conditions

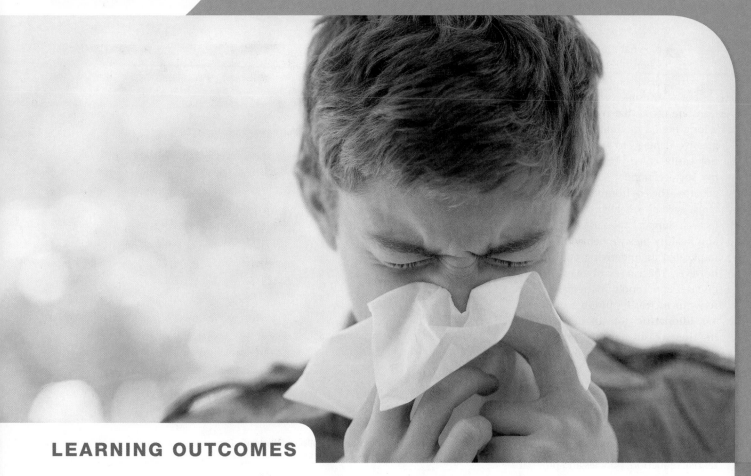

## LEARNING OUTCOMES

LO **1** Describe the prevalence and symptoms of key respiratory diseases such as bronchitis, emphysema, and asthma, including their risk factors and impact on society.

LO **2** Describe the allergic response and complications associated with allergies as well as who is susceptible to allergy development.

LO **3** Explain common neurological disorders, including headaches and seizure disorders, with emphasis on risk factors, possible causes, and what is being done to control them.

LO **4** Outline risk factors, symptoms, and strategies for preventing major digestive disorders affecting adults in the United States today.

LO **5** Explain the risk factors and symptoms of various musculoskeletal diseases, including arthritis and low back pain, and suggest strategies for prevention.

Chronic conditions represent the single greatest threat to health in the United States, responsible for 7 out of 10 deaths and over 86 percent of our nation's health care costs.[1] While cardiovascular disease, cancer, and diabetes get most of the media attention, respiratory diseases and allergies and musculoskeletal, neurological, and gastrointestinal problems, just to name a few, cause significant pain, suffering, emotional and mental distress, and disability for millions of Americans. They wreak havoc on the lives of youth, young adults, and older adults from all socioeconomic, racial, and ethnic groups across locations, and can cause much distress for today's college students. The good news is that many of them are preventable or their impact on your daily life can be greatly diminished.

So, what do we really mean when we talk about chronic diseases and conditions? Chronic diseases and conditions are those that often develop over a long period of time, that cause progressive damage to the body, and are not easily cured. They are influenced by socioeconomic status, education, genetics, the environment, support systems, access to health care, and other factors. Support for self-empowerment and healthy lifestyle behaviors are also implicated as underlying contributors; however, the causes of many chronic diseases and conditions remain a mystery. An increasing number of diseases are **idiopathic** (of unknown cause). In these cases, health professionals often use **palliative treatments**, those treatments designed to treat or ease symptoms but not cure the disease. In general, prevention or intervention for chronic diseases requires investment in education about risks where they are known, lifestyle changes, environmental risk reduction, policies and programs that support positive behavior change, and assistance via pharmaceuticals and other medical interventions. Public support in the form of targeted research is also key to increasing our understanding of risks and our ability to reduce illness and deaths.

Clearly, chronic diseases pose a major risk for Americans, even though people are living longer with cardiovascular disease, cancer, and diabetes today. Projections for the future point to dramatic increases in rates for many chronic ailments—meaning a staggering hit to our health care and economic expenses:[2]

Today, one out of every two adults in the United States suffer from one or more chronic ailments.[3] Because we have already discussed leading chronic diseases—cardiovascular disease, cancer, and diabetes—the focus of this chapter is on the "other," lesser known, but extremely important chronic conditions that affect young and old alike. (The **Health in a Diverse World** box discusses maladies specific to women.) Knowledge and action are key weapons in reducing risks, preventing disease, and controlling threats to health both now and in the future (**FIGURE 18.1**). The sooner people take action to prevent chronic illness—and policymakers and community agencies act to enable behavior changes for all—the greater the chance of real progress.

**idiopathic** Of unknown cause.
**palliative treatment** Those treatments designed to treat or ease symptoms but not cure the disease.

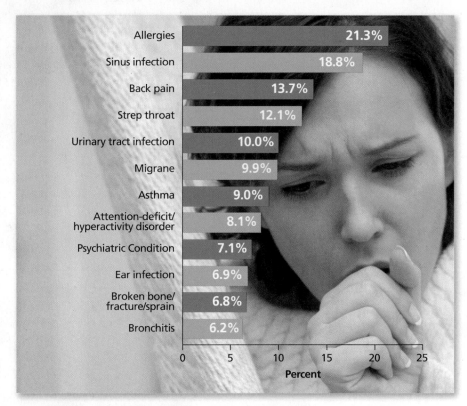

**FIGURE 18.1** Proportion of College Students Diagnosed with or Treated for Chronic Conditions in the Past 12 Months

**Source:** Data are from American College Health Association, *American College Health Association— National College Health Assessment II (ACHA-NCHA II): Reference Group Data Report, Fall 2015* (Baltimore: American College Health Association, 2016).

Chart data:
- Allergies 21.3%
- Sinus infection 18.8%
- Back pain 13.7%
- Strep throat 12.1%
- Urinary tract infection 10.0%
- Migrane 9.9%
- Asthma 9.0%
- Attention-deficit/ hyperactivity disorder 8.1%
- Psychiatric Condition 7.1%
- Ear infection 6.9%
- Broken bone/ fracture/sprain 6.8%
- Bronchitis 6.2%

Percent

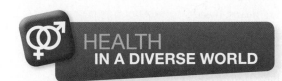
# MALADIES SPECIFIC TO WOMEN

Men and women frequently experience different rates of chronic conditions. In addition, there are some conditions that are specific to one gender or the other because they affect body structures and organs associated with reproductive functions.

## Fibrocystic Breast Condition

Over 50 percent of all women in the United States, particularly those over the age of 30, have a noncancerous condition called *fibrocystic breast condition*. Indeed, it is so common that many experts have taken it out of the disease category and refer to it as *benign breast changes*.

Symptoms range from one small, palpable lump to large masses of irregular tissue found in both breasts. Although most cysts consist of fibrous tissue, some are filled with fluid. The underlying causes of the condition are unknown; it may relate to an imbalance between estrogen and progesterone or to hormonal changes that occur during the normal menstrual cycle. Some experts believe that caffeine raises hormone levels, which can increase susceptibility to fibrous tissue buildup. Women with certain types of fibrocystic tissue may have a slightly higher risk of breast cancer, but this may be because fibrous tissue makes it more difficult to notice an abnormal lump. Treatment, if needed, often involves removing fluid from the affected area or surgically removing the cyst.

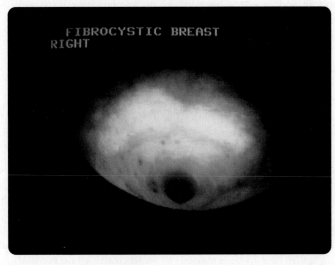

**This image, created by computerized analysis of the light absorption of tissues, shows a fibrocystic breast.**

FIBROCYSTIC BREAST
RIGHT

## Endometriosis

Endometriosis is a hormonal and immune system disease affecting at least 8.5 million women and girls in the United States and more than 176 million worldwide. Endometriosis is characterized by abnormal growth and development of endometrial tissue (the tissue lining the uterus) in regions of the body other than the uterus. One of the top three causes of female infertility, it is readily treatable if diagnosed; however, it is often misdiagnosed. The most widely used diagnostic strategy is a laparoscopic biopsy of uterine tissue, and the average age for first diagnosis is 27 years.

Symptoms of endometriosis include severe cramping during and between menstrual cycles, irregular periods, unusually heavy or light menstrual flow, abdominal bloating, fatigue, painful bowel movements with periods, painful intercourse, constipation, blood in the urine, pelvic pain, diarrhea, infertility, and low back pain. Among the most widely accepted theories concerning the causes of endometriosis are the transmission of endometrial tissue to other regions of the body during surgery or through the birthing process, the movement of menstrual fluid backward through the fallopian tubes during menstruation, and abnormal cell migration through body-fluid movement. Women with cycles shorter than 27 days or flows longer than a week are at increased risk. The more aerobic exercise a woman engages in and the earlier she starts it, the less likely she is to develop endometriosis.

Treatment for endometriosis ranges from bedrest and stress reduction to *hysterectomy* (surgical removal of the uterus) or surgical removal of one or both ovaries and the fallopian tubes. More conservative treatments involve dilation and curettage, surgically scraping endometrial tissue off the fallopian tubes and other reproductive organs. Combinations of hormone therapy have also become more acceptable.

**Sources:** Mayo Clinic, "Fibrocystic Breasts," March, 2016, http://www.mayoclinic.org/diseases-conditions/fibrocystic-breasts/home/ovc-20194898; The Endometriosis Foundation of America. "Endometriosis," Accessed June 2016, www.endofound.org/endometriosis; National Institutes of Health, Medline Plus, "Endometriosis," May 2016, www.nlm.nih.gov/medlineplus/endometriosis.html.

# $4.2 TRILLION

The economic burden of **CHRONIC DISEASES** projected by 2022, equal to 20% of GDP.

## LO 1 | COPING WITH RESPIRATORY PROBLEMS

Describe the prevalence and symptoms of key respiratory diseases such as bronchitis, emphysema, and asthma, including their risk factors and impact on society.

The normal adult takes 12 to 15 breaths per minute at rest—varying by age and overall cardiorespiratory health and fitness level.[4] Our respiratory systems move fresh air into the body

**chronic lower respiratory disease (CLRD)** Lung diseases such as emphysema, asthma, and some forms of bronchitis that are long term in nature.

**dyspnea** Shortness of breath, usually associated with disease of the heart or lungs.

**chronic obstructive pulmonary disease (COPD)** A collection of chronic lung diseases, including emphysema and chronic bronchitis, where some form of obstruction interferes with a person's ability to breathe.

**bronchitis** An inflammation and eventual scarring of the lining of the bronchial tubes.

**chronic bronchitis** Bronchitis type diagnosed when a person has bronchitis symptoms for at least 3 months of the year in 2 consecutive years and which is part of the COPD grouping.

and waste gases out. Breath really is *life*, but the respiratory system does much more than push air in and out. When healthy, the respiratory system is a finely tuned machine: It filters the air you breathe, and it protects you from invaders by trapping and expelling harmful particles that you inhale with a cough or a sneeze.

Unfortunately, several respiratory diseases are on the rise. **Chronic lower respiratory disease (CLRD)** (including *bronchitis*, *emphysema*, and *asthma*) is the third leading cause of death in the United States (right after heart disease and cancer), killing nearly 150,000 people in 2015.[5]

Virtually any disease or disorder that impairs lung function is considered a lung disease. The lungs can be damaged by a single exposure to a toxic chemical or severe heat or be impaired from years of inhaling the tar and chemicals in tobacco smoke. Exposure to toxic environmental substances such as asbestos, silica dust, paint fumes and lacquers, pesticides, or secondhand smoke in the home can cause lung deterioration. Cancers, infections, and degenerative changes can also wreak havoc with lung function. When the lungs are impaired, a condition known as **dyspnea**, a choking type of breathlessness, can occur, even with mild exertion. As the body is deprived of oxygen, the heart is forced to work harder and, over time, cardiovascular problems, suffocation, and death can occur. Symptoms of compromised lungs can lead to prolonged coughing, shortness of breath, excess mucus production, wheezing, pain, and coughing up phlegm or blood. Fatigue, increased heart rate, and a host of other problems may occur. Keeping your lungs healthy is an important part of overall health.

## Chronic Obstructive Pulmonary Disease (COPD)

**Chronic obstructive pulmonary disease (COPD)** is a progressive lung disease that slowly makes it more and more difficult for a person to breathe. COPD may begin with shortness of breath after little exertion, but may eventually leave patients gasping for air and needing onboard oxygen to perform even the simplest tasks. In the United States, the term *COPD* refers to two specific diseases, *chronic bronchitis* and *emphysema*, which often occur together and can lead to problems with inhalation and exhalation. Currently, nearly 15 million people aged 18 and over have impaired lung function caused by COPD; however, these numbers are believed to grossly underestimate the over 24 million people believed to have undiagnosed lung impairment.[6]

Women are nearly twice as likely to be diagnosed with chronic bronchitis as their male counterparts. While men have historically been more likely to be diagnosed with emphysema, women have now surpassed men in emphysema diagnoses and emphysema deaths.[7] The vast majority of people with COPD are either former or current smokers. Other risk factors include a history of asthma, heredity, respiratory infections, and many of the risk factors for CLRDs listed earlier.

There is no cure for COPD; however, there is much that can be done to prevent it, including quitting smoking, avoiding secondhand smoke, and maximizing lung function through exercise. While lifestyle changes are important, vaccines for the flu and pneumonia are also important preventive options to help reduce risk of infection-related lung damage. Some occupations continue to pose risks, but major improvements in air cleaning and ventilation systems have reduced exposures in recent years. Reading labels, wearing protective devices, and making sure areas where toxins accumulate are ventilated when spraying chemicals and cleaning products are important. If you have symptoms, such as a chronic cough, shortness of breath, rapid heart rate, or note your lips or nail beds are gray or blue, see a doctor as soon as possible. Early treatment and regular follow-up are important. There are many options for relieving symptoms, preventing further damage, and improving lung function. The **Health Headlines** box describes ways to minimize exposure to household chemicals.

**Bronchitis** **Bronchitis** involves inflammation and eventual scarring of the lining of the bronchial tubes (*bronchi*) that connect the windpipe to the lungs. When the bronchi become inflamed or infected with bacteria, less air is able to flow from the lungs and heavy mucus begins to form. Although some mucus is normal and necessary, bronchitis sufferers typically have numerous coughing spasms in a day as they try to rid their bodies of phlegm. Frequent clearing of the throat, a sensation of tightness in the chest, back pain, and shortness of breath are other bronchitis symptoms.

Inhaling certain chemicals such as tobacco, marijuana, or e-cigarette smoke can trigger bronchitis. Cosmetic sprays, perfumes, hairsprays, household cleaners, and air fresheners can also be triggers. The more common *acute bronchitis* is often caused by other infectious diseases. Symptoms often begin to go away in a week or two once the sources are removed and any inflammation and infections are treated.

When the symptoms of bronchitis last for at least 3 months of the year for 2 consecutive years, the condition is considered **chronic bronchitis**. In some cases, this chronic inflammation and irritation goes undiagnosed for years, particularly

**WHAT DO YOU THINK?**

Have you or any of your friends or family experienced any of the conditions discussed in this section?

- Why do you think the incidence of COPD is increasing?
- What actions can you or the people in your community take to reduce risks and problems from these diseases on campus? in your homes? in your communities?

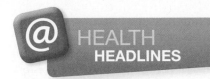

# BE ECO-CLEAN AND ALLERGEN FREE

Exposure to household chemicals, dust, and pet dander may exacerbate asthma, allergies, and other respiratory problems. Reduce exposure to noxious household chemicals and create a clean, comfortable home by using cleaning supplies and household products that are less toxic to the home environment. Read labels carefully, and look for independent certifications such as the Green Seal and the Environmental Protection Agency's (EPA's) Design for the Environment program.

- For a handy glass and surface cleaner, mix 1/2 cup of white vinegar with 4 cups of water. Pour the solution into a spray bottle, and keep the remainder for a quick and cheap refill. You can make another surface cleaner by combining 2 tablespoons of lemon juice with 4 cups of water.

**Making your own cleansers from natural products such as vinegar and water, ensures that they are not harmful to your health.**

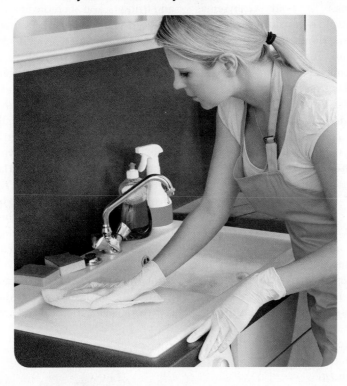

- Baking soda is a great deodorizer and cleaner. Use it to remove carpet odors and to scour sinks, toilets, and bathtubs.

- Because chlorine can damage lungs, skin, and eyes, and chlorine production adds toxic chemicals such as carcinogenic dioxins to our environment, use a chlorine bleach alternative. For example, use 1/2 cup of hydrogen peroxide in your laundry or try oxygen-based bleaches.
- An all-purpose cleaner can be made of 1/2 cup of Borax (found in the laundry aisle) and 1 gallon of hot water.
- For green air fresheners, use essential oils, such as lemon or lavender. Many store-bought air fresheners contain phthalates, often called "fragrance," that are related to respiratory problems and other noninfectious conditions. Place a few drops of essential oils on a piece of tissue paper, in a bowl of warm water, or in a store-bought diffuser.

As you transition to green cleaning, do not just throw old products in the trash, as these can wind up polluting landfills and leaching into water supplies. Instead, take them to a hazardous chemical recycling facility.

---

in smokers who feel it's a normal part of their lives (smoker's cough). By the time these individuals receive medical care, the damage to their lungs is severe and may lead to heart and respiratory failure or to a chronic need to carry oxygen to aid in breathing. Coal miners, grain handlers, metalworkers, autobody painters, hairstylists, and others exposed to fumes, dusts, and hazards are particularly susceptible. Nearly 9 million Americans, the majority of whom are women, suffer from chronic bronchitis; 33 percent are under age 45.[8] White Americans experience more chronic bronchitis than any other group.[9]

To help prevent the problems associated with bronchitis, stop smoking and avoid particulates that trigger bronchitis attacks. Avoid smoke-filled bars or other settings that make your situation worse. If the pollution index is high, stay indoors, make sure windows and doors are closed, and use air filtration systems. See a doctor promptly if you have recurrent symptoms. Prescription drugs can reduce inflammation, prevent mucus buildup, and stop secondary bacterial infections from setting in.

**Emphysema** Over 3.4 million Americans suffer from **emphysema**.[10] While emphysema was historically a "man's disease" (largely due to higher smoking rates and more occupational exposures), today, more women than men are diagnosed.[11] Emphysema involves the gradual, irreversible destruction of the **alveoli** (tiny air sacs through which gas exchange occurs) of the lungs. Destruction of the alveoli walls impairs the transfer of oxygen and carbon dioxide into and out of the blood and makes the lungs less elastic, which makes it harder to breathe. As the alveoli are destroyed, the affected person finds it more and more difficult to exhale. People with emphysema liken this experience to engaging in heavy exercise while breathing through a straw. What most of us take for granted—the easy, rhythmic flow of air in and out of the lungs—becomes a continuous, anxious, and life-threatening struggle.

> **emphysema** A respiratory disease in which the alveoli become distended or ruptured and are no longer functional.
> **alveoli** Tiny air sacs of the lungs where gas exchange occurs (oxygen enters the body and carbon dioxide is removed).

**asthma** A chronic
respiratory disease that
blocks airflow into and out
of the lungs, characterized
by attacks of wheezing,
shortness of breath, and
coughing spasms.

The cause of emphysema is uncertain. As with most respiratory ailments, there is a strong relationship between emphysema and long-term cigarette smoking and exposure to air pollution. (See Chapter 12 for more on the connection between smoking and emphysema.) To avoid emphysema, don't smoke. If you smoke, quit. Avoid occupational exposure that involves inhaling chemicals and fumes. If you must take a job that involves inhaling toxins, use appropriate protection.

A key to coping with emphysema is compliance with doctor's orders, both in terms of taking prescribed medications and healthy lifestyle, including diet, exercise, sleep, and stress management. Many persons tied to oxygen supplementation have difficulty coping and find counseling and help from social services and support groups helpful. Help for the caregiver in terms of respite care is also essential.

## Asthma

**Asthma** is a long-term, chronic inflammatory disorder that blocks airflow into and out of the lungs. Asthma causes tiny airways in the lung to overreact with spasms in response to certain triggers (**FIGURE 18.2**). Symptoms include wheezing, difficulty breathing, shortness of breath, and coughing spasms. Although most asthma attacks are mild, severe attacks can trigger *bronchospasms* (contractions of the bronchial tubes in the lungs) that are so severe that, without rapid treatment, death may occur. Between attacks, most people have few symptoms. Approximately 18 million adults and just over 6 million children in the United States have asthma.[12] It is the most common chronic disease of childhood, affecting nearly 9 percent of all children in the United States and nearly 7.5 percent of adults (**FIGURE 18.3**).[13]

Asthma falls into two distinctly different types. The more common form, *extrinsic* or *allergic asthma*, is typically associated with allergic triggers; it tends to run in families and develop in childhood. Often by adulthood, a person has few episodes, or the disorder completely goes away. The less common form of asthma, *intrinsic* or *nonallergic asthma*, may be triggered by anything except an allergy.

Several factors—including medical conditions, animal dander and saliva, mold, cockroach allergens, dust mites, perfumes, exercise, smoke, food allergies, weather changes, pollen, and air pollution—can trigger asthma flare-ups. In fact, even emotions such as anger, fear, or stress can trigger an asthma attack.[14] Genetics may play a role in asthma development. If your mom or dad has asthma, or if family members have a history of allergies, asthma is more likely. If you had respiratory infections when you were younger, such as colds, the flu, or sinus infections, or if you are exposed to environmental allergens and irritants, you are more likely to develop asthma.[15] Certain medications, particularly fever reducers or anti-inflammatory drugs such as NSAIDs, beta-blockers, and ACE inhibitors, used to treat cardiovascular problems may also be triggers.[16]

Asthma can occur at any age, but is most likely to appear in children between infancy and age 5, with a spike in prevalence between ages 15 and 34, and tapering off after age 35. In childhood, asthma strikes more boys than girls; in adulthood, it strikes more women than men. Even with advances in treatment, asthma deaths among young people have more than doubled, with over 3,600 deaths last year in the United States.[17]

Poverty, low education, and risky home and work environments as well as limited access to health care lead to clear disparities in asthma treatment and control. African Americans have the highest rates of asthma in the United States at 9.6 percent, followed by whites at 7.6 percent and Hispanics at 6.7 percent.[18]

The Making Changes Today box on page 488 suggests ways to reduce asthma attacks. In addition to avoiding triggers, finding the most effective medications can help asthmatics cope with their condition and avoid severe attacks.

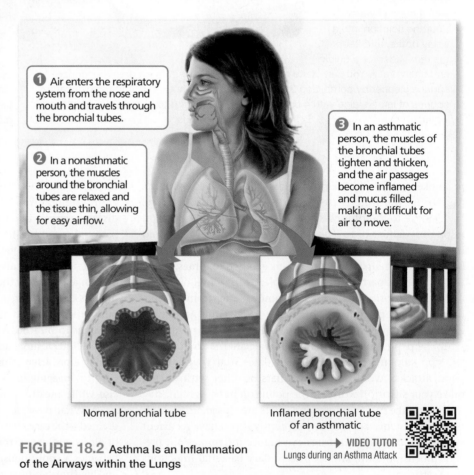

**①** Air enters the respiratory system from the nose and mouth and travels through the bronchial tubes.

**②** In a nonasthmatic person, the muscles around the bronchial tubes are relaxed and the tissue thin, allowing for easy airflow.

**③** In an asthmatic person, the muscles of the bronchial tubes tighten and thicken, and the air passages become inflamed and mucus filled, making it difficult for air to move.

Normal bronchial tube

Inflamed bronchial tube of an asthmatic

**FIGURE 18.2 Asthma Is an Inflammation of the Airways within the Lungs**

VIDEO TUTOR
Lungs during an Asthma Attack

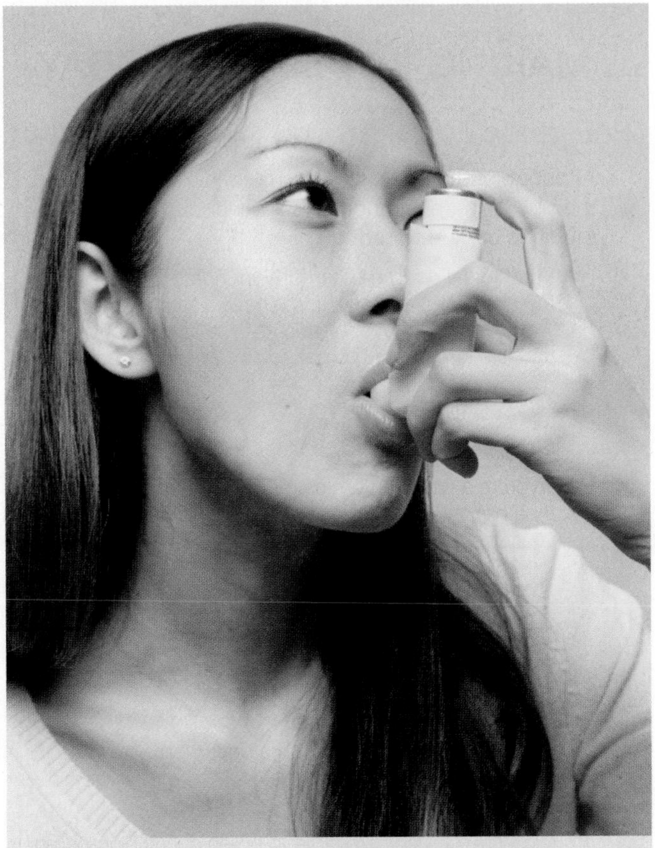

People with asthma can generally control their symptoms through the use of inhaled medications, and most asthmatics keep a "rescue" inhaler of bronchodilating medication on hand to use in case of a flare-up.

## LO 2 | COPING WITH ALLERGIES

Describe the allergic response and complications associated with allergies as well as who is susceptible to allergy development.

**Allergies** are diseases characterized by an overreaction of the immune system to a foreign protein substance (*allergen* or *antigen*) that is swallowed, breathed into the lungs, injected, or touched.[19] When foreign substances or pathogens such as bacteria or viruses enter the body, the body responds by producing *antibodies* to destroy these invaders. Normally, antibody production is a positive element in the body's defense system. However, for unknown reasons, sometimes the body develops an overly elaborate protective mechanism against relatively harmless substances. The resulting *hypersensitivity reaction* to specific allergens or antigens in the environment is fairly common, as anyone who has awakened with a runny nose or itchy eyes can attest. People with severe allergies can suffer much more extreme responses, including hives, vomiting, and **anaphylaxis**—a particularly severe sensitivity reaction to an allergic trigger such as a bee sting or drug that can begin a few minutes after exposure. Dizziness, breathing difficulties, blood pressure drops and racing heart rate, swelling of the tongue and throat, and unconsciousness can occur rapidly and lead to *anaphylactic shock*—a life-threatening combination of the above symptoms. Globally, up to 20 percent of anaphylaxis deaths are due to drug reactions.[20]

Allergies are grouped by the kind of trigger, time of year, or where symptoms appear on the body into *outdoor* or *indoor allergies, food and drug allergies, latex allergies, insect allergies, skin allergies,* and *eye allergies.*[21] Environmental triggers can include molds, animal dander, pollen, grasses, ragweed, particulate matter, air pollution, or dust that leads to spikes in the air quality index. Other triggers include foods such as peanuts, shellfish, or milk; insect bites; and medicines (both over-the-counter and prescription drugs). Once excessive antibodies to these antigens are produced, they, in turn, trigger the release of **histamine**, a chemical substance that dilates blood vessels, increases mucous secretions, swells tissues, and produces other allergy symptoms, particularly in the respiratory system (**FIGURE 18.4**). Many people have

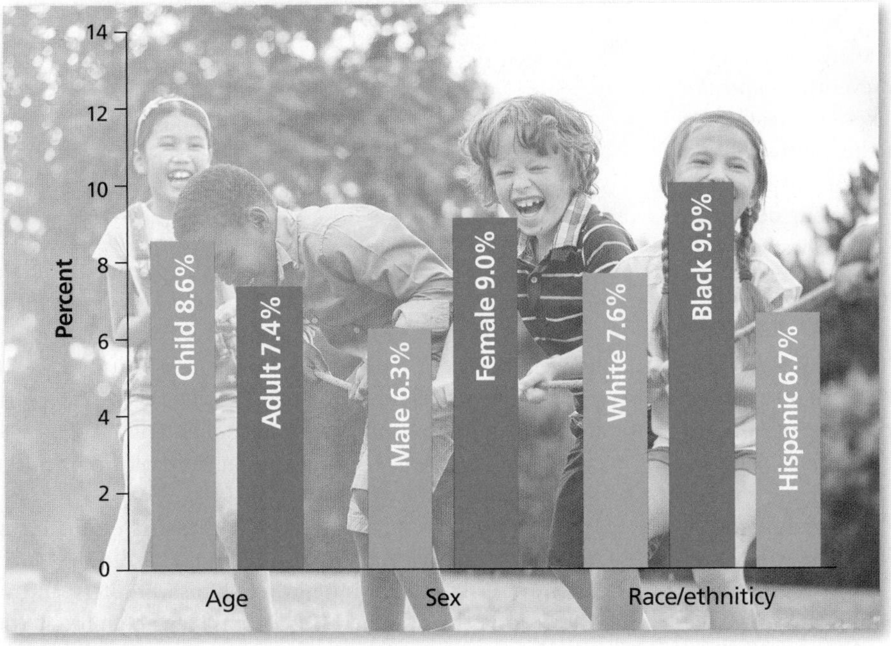

**allergies** Hypersensitivity reactions in which the body produces antibodies to a normally harmless substance in the environment.

**anaphylaxis** A severe sensitivity reaction to an allergic trigger such as a bee sting, or chemical reaction that can begin a few minutes after exposure.

**histamine** Chemical substance that dilates blood vessels, increases mucus secretions, and triggers other allergy symptoms.

**FIGURE 18.3** Asthma Prevalence by Age, Sex, and Race/Ethnicity, United States, 2014

**Source:** CDC, "Data, Statistics and Surveillance: Asthma Surveillance," March 2016, http://www.cdc.gov/asthma/asthmadata.htm.

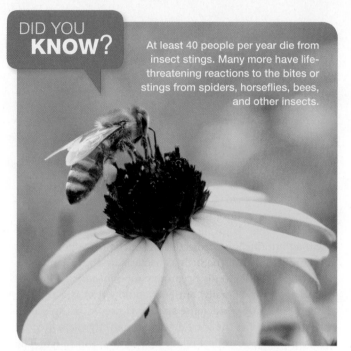

**Source:** American College of Allergy, Asthma, and Immunology, "Types of Allergies: Insect Sting Allergy," Accessed June 2016, http://acaai.org/allergies/types/insect-sting-allergies.

found that **immunotherapy** treatment, or "allergy shots," somewhat reduces the severity of their symptoms. In most cases, once the offending antigen is removed, allergy-prone people suffer few symptoms.

Globally, between 40 and 50 percent of all school-aged children are currently sensitized to one or more of the common allergens.[22] Allergies were the single greatest reason that college students (over 21 percent of them) sought professional help in 2015.[23] Asthma (discussed previously) is a unique disease in that it is typically considered to be both a key respiratory disease as well as one of the major allergic diseases.[24] Prevention of allergies usually focuses on preventing exposure to things that cause you to react. If you are exposed, treatments may be as simple as quickly washing off the substance you came in contact with, taking antihistamines or getting shots to avoid serious reactions, and working with your doctor to come up with a treatment regimen that will work best for you.

## Hay Fever

**Hay fever**, or *pollen allergy*, occurs throughout the world and is one of the most common chronic diseases in the United States, affecting over 19 million adults and 6 million children each year.[25] It is usually considered a seasonal disease because it is most prevalent when ragweed, grass pollen, and flowers are blooming; it can make going outside a miserable experience. Hay fever attacks are characterized by sneezing, itchy and watery eyes, runny nose, and sore throat. As with other

**immunotherapy** Treatment strategies based on the concept of regulating the immune system, as by administering antibodies or desensitization shots of allergens.

**hay fever** A chronic allergy-related respiratory disorder that is most prevalent when ragweed and flowers bloom, also known as *pollen allergy*.

**allergist** Medical doctor focusing on the diagnosis and treatment of allergies.

allergies, hay fever results from an overzealous immune system that is hypersensitive to certain substances. You are more likely to have hay fever if you have a family history of allergies, are male, were born during pollen season, are a firstborn child, were exposed to cigarette smoke during your first year of life, or are exposed to dust mites. As grass pollen and other pollen levels increase in the late spring and ragweed blossoms in the fall, outdoor allergy reports spike.

Typical over-the-counter treatment consists of antihistamines. These work well for mild cases, but may become less effective over time. Air-conditioning, whole-house air filters, and air purifiers can also help relieve symptoms. To determine if you have pollen allergy, the best bet is to get tested by an **allergist**—a doctor specializing in allergies. Typical treatments include prescription medications and/or allergy shots. While allergy shots are one of the most effective ways of treatment, side effects are possible and doctors recommend them for limited time periods.

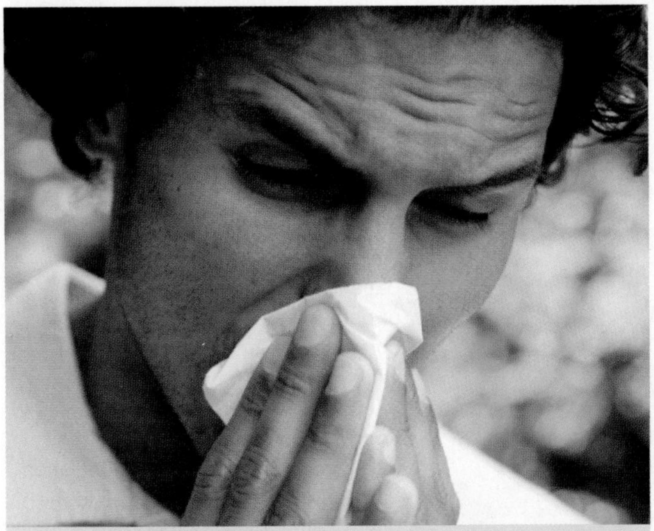

## Food Allergies

A **food allergy** is an exaggerated immune response to certain foods, such as milk, eggs, peanuts, tree nuts, shellfish, fish, wheat, and soy. Symptoms of a food allergy typically include hives or rash; hoarse voice; wheezing and trouble breathing; swelling of the tongue, lips, or face; abdominal pain; diarrhea or vomiting; difficulty swallowing; and itching.[26] The reaction can be so severe that the victim goes into anaphylactic shock. Each year, over 200,000 people end up in the emergency room due to food allergies.[27]

Food allergies should not be confused with **food intolerance**, which is the inability to properly digest a particular food due to problems with physical, hormonal, enzyme, or biochemical systems in your gastrointestinal (GI) tract. *Food intolerance* typically causes stomach or GI pain, gas, cramps, and/or diarrhea, but not true allergic reactions. Some estimate that 5 percent of children and 4 percent of adults may have food allergies.[28] There are increasing numbers of media reports and marketing around food allergies, even though actual diagnoses are not widely available. Sometimes, people may think they have an allergy when they are reacting to specific pathogens in the food and really have a food-borne illness.

Although some food allergies can be outgrown, there is no cure. If you have an allergy, you can avoid many reactions by reading labels, asking questions in restaurants, and knowing exactly what you are eating. Wear a medical alert bracelet or necklace that says you have food allergies, and let your friends, family members, and instructors know that you react to certain foods. Carry antihistamines or autoinjector devices containing epinephrine (adrenaline) so that you can quickly respond in the event of accidental exposure.

**food allergy** An immune response against a specific food that the majority of people can eat without problem.

**food intolerance** Difficulty or inability to digest certain foods due to problems with the physical, hormonal, or biochemical systems in your digestive tract.

## LO 3 | COPING WITH NEUROLOGICAL DISORDERS

Explain common neurological disorders, including headaches and seizure disorders, with emphasis on risk factors, possible causes, and what is being done to control them.

While stroke is the fourth leading cause of death (see Chapter 16) and *Alzheimer's disease* (AD) (see Chapter 22) is the sixth leading cause of death, with a rapid rise in prevalence in the last decade, there are more than 600 diseases and disorders that can affect the nervous systems of over 50 million Americans each year.[29] These diseases can

To minimize your exposure to hay fever, keep windows closed, stay indoors when pollen counts are highest (typically 10:00 A.M. to 4:00 P.M.), and change clothes or shower after spending time outdoors.

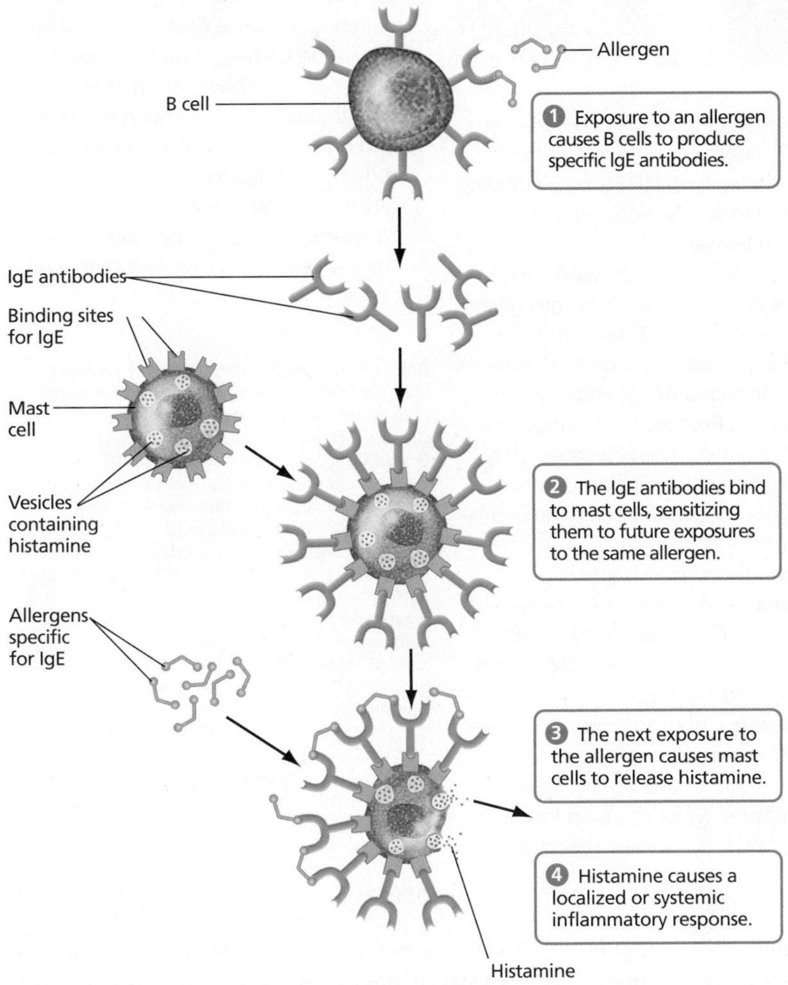

B cell

Allergen

**1** Exposure to an allergen causes B cells to produce specific IgE antibodies.

IgE antibodies

Binding sites for IgE

Mast cell

Vesicles containing histamine

**2** The IgE antibodies bind to mast cells, sensitizing them to future exposures to the same allergen.

Allergens specific for IgE

**3** The next exposure to the allergen causes mast cells to release histamine.

**4** Histamine causes a localized or systemic inflammatory response.

Histamine

**FIGURE 18.4** Steps of an Allergic Response

**Source:** Adapted from Johnson, Michael D., *Human Biology: Concepts and Current Issues*, 7th Ed., © 2014, p. 211. Printed and electronically reproduced by permission of Pearson Education, Inc., Upper Saddle River, New Jersey.

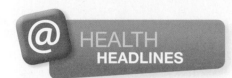
# TREATING CHRONIC PAIN

Chronic pain is pain that persists and keeps neurons firing for days, weeks, or even months. For those who have it, it is a nagging, often agonizing, threat to their mental and physical health and overall well-being. Over 100 million people in the United States suffer from chronic pain every day, exacting a heavy toll on individuals, families, businesses, and society. The collective direct and indirect costs of unresolved pain are estimated to be over $635 billion. Chronic pain affects more Americans than diabetes, heart disease, and cancer combined. Pain disrupts activities of daily living while contributing to mental health problems such as depression and anxiety. Even with pain medications, 50 to 75 percent of patients die in moderate to severe pain.

## Who Suffers Most from Pain?

- Women are more likely to suffer from pain.
- Adults aged 18 to 44 are more likely to experience migraines or severe headaches.
- Poor or near-poor families are more likely to experience pain from all causes.

Newer research suggests that two groups of people may be more likely to experience pain in their lifetimes: people with abnormalities in the structure of their brain and people who experienced chronic pain during childhood. Based on magnetic resonance imaging (MRI) scans, scientists have been able to predict with 85 percent accuracy who would experience chronic pain based on irregular markers on the axons, pathways for nerve transmission in white matter of the brain. Overall, pain from most conditions increases with age, particularly among those 65 and over.

Chronic pain sufferers have a variety of treatment options:

- **Over-the-counter (OTC) medications.** Available without prescription

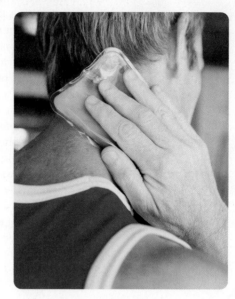

**Cold packs are one of many options for pain and inflammation treatment.**

are medications such as acetaminophen (Tylenol) and nonsteroidal anti-inflammatory drugs (NSAIDs), including ibuprofen (Advil, Motrin), aspirin, and naproxen (Aleve).
- **Prescription medications.** A variety of these are available. They may give faster results than OTC drugs, but they also present increased risks for patients in terms of addiction and drug interactions. Prescription painkillers are the second most abused category of drugs in the United States, contributing to over 14,000 unintentional deaths each year.
- **Cold and heat treatments.** Cold packs are used to numb areas, reduce swelling, and ease joint aches. Hot packs relax muscles, bring blood to an area, and aid healing.
- **Acupuncture, acupressure, and massage.** All are designed to reduce pain, relax the patient, and speed healing. (See Chapter 18 for more on these options and their rates of effectiveness.)

- **Physical therapy.** Physical therapists use a variety of modalities—heat and cold, electrical stimulation, stretching, and others—to work with patients experiencing a wide range of pain-related conditions, increasing core strength and range of motion, while retraining muscles to function effectively and reduce pain.
- **Local electrical stimulation.** Transcutaneous electrical nerve stimulation (TENS) blocks pain messages to the brain and modifies perceptions of pain. Brief electrical pulses to nerve endings provide pain relief.
- **Psychological treatment.** Among a small percentage of pain sufferers, pain appears to be precipitated by emotional or psychological trauma or suffering. In these cases, counseling, relaxation training, water therapy, meditation, biofeedback, aromatherapy, light therapy, dietary changes, yoga, and other mind–body techniques can reduce the severity of pain or eventually make it go away.
- **Surgery.** If someone has tried everything else and nothing seems to work, surgery may be a last option.

**Sources:** NINDS, "Chronic Pain Information Page," March 9, 2016, www.ninds.nih.gov/disorders/chronic_pain/chronic_pain.htm; Centers for Disease Control and Prevention. "Prescription Opioid Overdose Data," June 21, 2016, http://www.cdc.gov/drugoverdose/data/overdose.html American Medical Communication, "Disease State Report: Pain," October 2015, http://www.managedcaremag.com/sites/default/files/graphics/DiseaseStateReport-PAIN.pdf; American Academy of Pain Medicine, "AAPM Facts and Figures on Pain," Accessed June 2016, www.painmed.org/patientcenter/facts_on_pain.aspx; A. Mansour et al., "Brain White Matter Structural Properties Predict Transition to Chronic Pain," *PAIN* 154, no. 10 (2013): 2160, doi: 10.1016/j.pain.2013.06.044; American Pain Society, "Links of Childhood Pain to Adult Chronic Pain, Fibromyalgia," *ScienceDaily*, December 19, 2013, www.sciencedaily.com/releases/2013/12/131219162532.htm.

affect your movement, speech, swallowing, autonomic functions such as heart rate and breathing, ability to learn, memory, sensations, and emotions. At their worst, they can cause loss of life and/or major disability. They can cause you to lose "you" inside of a fleshy shell that no longer remembers or reacts. They are also responsible for a tremendous burden on family members, health care providers, social service workers, workplaces, and patients themselves. Some of these disorders, such as Alzheimer's disease, multiple sclerosis, migraine headaches, and epilepsy, are well known, but there are many lesser-known disorders and some that elude diagnosis. (See the **Health Headlines** box for pain treatment options.)

# Headaches

Headaches are one of the most common reasons for emergency room visits each year. Adults aged 18 to 44 are more likely to visit emergency rooms for headaches than other age groups.[30] Most of the time, headaches are not the sign of a serious disease and go away fairly quickly,

Generally, headaches can be broken down into two major categories. *Primary headaches*, including tension headaches, migraines, and cluster headaches, are not related to other medical conditions and make up the majority of all headaches. *Secondary headaches* are those that are the result of other medical conditions, including a sinus infection, medications, head injury, visual ailments, trauma, or a serious health threat such as stroke or brain tumor (**TABLE 18.1**).[31] More women than men get headaches; in fact, about 70 percent of headache sufferers are women.[32] To give you an idea of the scope of headache investigations, many things cause your head to "ache"; in fact, there are over 150 different types of headaches![33]

## TABLE 18.1 | Types of Headaches

| Type | Symptoms | Precipitating Factors | Treatment | Prevention |
|---|---|---|---|---|
| **Allergy** | Generalized headache; Nasal congestion, watery eyes | Seasonal allergens such as pollen, molds. Allergies to food are not usually a factor. | Antihistamine medication; topical, nasal cortisone-related sprays, or desensitization injections | None |
| **Caffeine-withdrawal** | Throbbing headache caused by rebound dilation of the blood vessels, occurring multiple days after consumption of large quantities of caffeine | Caffeine | In extreme cases, treat by terminating caffeine consumption | Avoid excess caffeine |
| **Exertion** | Generalized head pain of short duration (minutes to 1 hour) during or following physical exertion (running, jumping, or sexual intercourse) or passive exertion (sneezing, coughing, moving one's bowels, etc.) | For these headaches, 10% caused by organic diseases (aneurysms, tumors, or blood vessel malformation); 90% are related to migraine or cluster headaches | Cause must be accurately determined. Most commonly treated with aspirin, indomethacin, or propranolol. Extensive testing is necessary to determine the headache cause. Surgery to correct organic disease is occasionally indicated. | Alternative forms of exercise; avoid jarring exercises |
| **Eyestrain** | Usually frontal, bilateral pain, directly related to eyestrain; rare cause of headache | Muscle imbalance; uncorrected vision, astigmatism | Correction of vision | Same as treatment |
| **Hangover** | Migraine-like symptoms of throbbing pain and nausea not localized to one side | Alcohol, which causes dilation and irritation of the blood vessels of the brain and surrounding tissue | Liquids (including broth); consumption of fructose (honey, tomato juice are good sources) to help burn alcohol | Drink alcohol only in moderation |
| **Hunger** | Pain strikes just before mealtime. Caused by muscle tension, low blood sugar, rebound dilation of the blood vessels, oversleeping, or missing a meal. | Strenuous dieting or skipping meals | Regular, nourishing meals containing adequate protein and complex carbohydrates | Same as treatment |
| **Sinus** | Gnawing pain over nasal area, often increasing in severity throughout the day. Caused by acute infection, usually with fever, producing blockage of sinus ducts and preventing normal drainage. Sinus headaches are rare. Migraine and cluster headaches are often misdiagnosed as sinus in origin. | Infection, nasal polyps, anatomical deformities, such as a deviated septum, that block the sinus ducts | Treat with antibiotics, decongestants, surgical drainage if necessary | None |

**Source:** Adapted from "The Complete Headache Chart," 2010, www.headaches.org. Reprinted by permission of the National Headache Foundation.

**SEE IT! VIDEOS**

Plagued by serious headaches? Watch **Migraine Breakthrough**, available on MasteringHealth.™

## Tension-Type Headaches

Up to 80 percent of the population occasionally have the most common type of headache, *tension-type headache*, during their lives. Another 3 percent have a more chronic version of tension headache. Numbers of cases peak up to the age of 40; however, they can occur at any age.[34] Symptoms include dull, aching head pain on either or both sides of the head; a sensation of tightness or pressure across the forehead, sides, and back of your head; tenderness on the scalp, neck, and shoulder muscles; and, occasionally, loss of appetite.[35]

There is a wide range in the frequency and severity of symptoms, ranging from episodic to *chronic*, with varying pain and frequency. While the cause(s) of tension headaches remain unknown, possible triggers include stress, depression and anxiety, jaw clenching, poor posture, or working in an awkward position. Red wine, lack of sleep, extreme fasting, hormonal changes, and certain food additives or preservatives have also been implicated.[36]

Tension-type headaches are most often prevented by reducing triggers. If stress is a trigger, try to relax with a hot bath, relaxing music, hot compresses, massage, or other relaxation techniques. Aspirin, ibuprofen, acetaminophen, and naproxen sodium often are effective pain relievers. If headaches occur more frequently and are difficult to treat with OTC medications, they are probably *chronic tension headaches*—the result of physical or psychological problems or depression. These more difficult forms of tension headaches warrant a visit to the doctor to assess the underlying cause.

## Migraine Headaches

Over 36 million Americans, or nearly 12 percent of the population—three times more women than men—suffer from **migraines**, an inherited neurological disorder that is characterized by overexcitability of specific areas of the brain, particularly the vascular network.[37] Symptoms include moderate to severe pain on one or both sides of the head, head pain with a pulsating or throbbing quality, pain that worsens with physical activity or interferes with regular activity, nausea with or without vomiting, and sensitivity to light and sound. In fact, 1 out of 4 households has a migraine sufferer.[38] Usually, migraine incidence peaks in young adulthood (between ages 20 and 45). Migraines appear to run in families: If both your parents experience migraines, you have a 75 percent chance of experiencing them, too; if only one parent has them, you have a 50 percent chance.[39]

Whereas all headaches can be painful, migraines can be disabling. Symptoms vary greatly by individual, and attacks can last anywhere from 4 to 72 hours, with distinct phases of symptoms. In about one-third of cases, migraines are preceded by a sensory warning sign called an *aura*, which includes flashes of light, flickering vision, blind spots, tingling in arms or legs, or a sensation of odor or taste.[40] The triggers of a migraine vary widely from one person to the next and include stress, fatigue, too much or too little sleep, fasting or missing meals, food or drugs that change blood vessel diameter, caffeine, chocolate, alcohol (particularly red wine), menses, hormonal changes, changes in humidity, and altitude changes, as well as certain food additives such as MSG, nitrates, and nitrites.[41] Although vascular abnormalities in the brain have long been thought to be underlying causes, experts are beginning to believe that migraines may be triggered within the brain itself as a result of a complex biochemical and inflammatory process.[42]

Because triggers for migraine vary by individual, treatment varies. Keeping a careful diary and noting when migraine occurs is important in identifying your triggers and making appropriate changes in behavior where possible. Healthy lifestyle in the form of diet and exercise is important. When true migraines occur, relaxation is only minimally effective as a treatment. Often, prescription pain relievers are necessary. See your doctor for more information or go to the National Headache Foundation website (*www.headaches.org*) for the latest information on treatments.

**migraine** A type of headache characterized by debilitating symptoms that possibly results from alternating dilation and constriction of blood vessels.

Patients report that migraines can be triggered by emotional stress, fatigue, too much or not enough sleep, fasting, caffeine, chocolate, alcohol, menses, hormone changes, altitude, weather, and certain foods. What triggers a migraine in one person may relieve it in another.

### WHAT DO YOU THINK?

Have you ever experienced a migraine or tension-type headache? How did you alleviate the pain?

- What actions can you take to reduce your risks of severe headaches in the future?

**Cluster Headaches** The severe pain of a cluster headache has been described as "killer" or "suicidal." Usually, these headaches cause excruciating, stabbing pain on one side of the head, behind the eye, or in one defined spot. Fortunately, cluster headaches are relatively rare, affecting men at twice the rate of women.[43] Young adults between the ages of 20 and 40 tend to be particularly susceptible.[44]

Cluster headaches can last for weeks and disappear quickly. More commonly, they last for 40 to 90 minutes and often occur in the middle of the night, usually during rapid eye movement (REM) sleep. Oxygen therapy, drugs, and even surgery have been used to treat severe cases.[45]

## Seizure Disorders

The word **epilepsy** derives from the Greek *epilepsia*, meaning "seizure." Approximately 5.1 million people in the United States suffer from epilepsy or some other seizure-related disorder, including about 460,000 children.[46]

Seizure disorders are generally caused by abnormal electrical activity in the brain and are characterized by loss of control of muscular activity and unconsciousness. Risk factors include taking certain drugs, withdrawing from drugs, having a high fever and abnormal blood levels of sodium or glucose, or experiencing physical, chemical, or temperature trauma. Symptoms vary widely and can range from temporary confusion to major seizure activity.

Although causes of nearly half of seizure disorders are unknown, likely contributors include stroke, congenital abnormalities, injury or illness resulting in inflammation of the brain or spinal column, high fever, drug reactions, tumors, nutritional deficiency, and heredity. (See the appendix at the end of this book for information on providing first aid to someone experiencing a seizure.)

Public ignorance and stigma associated with seizure disorders can have a significant impact on sufferers and their families as they cope with the challenges of treatment and daily living. In most cases, people with these disorders can lead normal, seizure-free lives as a result of advancements in diagnosis and treatment.

## LO 4 | COPING WITH DIGESTION-RELATED DISORDERS AND DISEASES

Outline risk factors, symptoms, and strategies for preventing major digestive disorders affecting adults in the United States today.

The *gastrointestinal tract* (GI tract), otherwise known as the *digestive system*, is a remarkable and fine-tuned machine, responsible for the breakdown of food into smaller molecules for absorption, fueling the body, and eliminating waste products. Every inch of that system has a job to do in keeping you healthy and maintaining bodily function. When any of several key indicators of digestive problems shows up—severe abdominal pain and cramping, bloody stool, stool that changes dramatically in size or shape, diarrhea/constipation, weight loss, and changes in bowel habits—it should tell you something has run amuck and a visit to the doctor might be in order.

Today, digestive disorders are among the fastest growing and most costly problems that Americans of all ages and stages of life face. Each year, over 70 million people suffer from one or more digestive problems, with nearly 49 million visiting a doctor.[47] Unfortunately, the causes of digestive disorders are often complex, symptoms are often subtle, and there is great variability in type of treatment and effectiveness. Two of the most common reported disorders are *lactose intolerance* and *celiac disease*); disorders not related to a specific nutrient are described here. See **TABLE 18.2** for discussion of gallbladder disease, another common digestive disorder, as well as several other modern maladies.

## Inflammatory Bowel Disease

**Inflammatory bowel disease (IBD)** is an umbrella term for a group of disorders in which the intestines become inflamed. Causes are not known, but symptoms tend to come and go. Typically, they are severe, with stomach cramping, bloating, pain, and bloody bouts of diarrhea (as many as 20 bouts a day). The most common types of IBD are *ulcerative colitis* and *Crohn's disease*. About 25 percent of those with IBD develop it before age 20, with the majority of additional cases in the 15- to 35-year-old age range, especially among those who have a family history of the disease.[48] As many as 2 million people in the United States have been diagnosed, with the majority of cases being among whites, particularly persons of Jewish descent.[49] Numbers of cases in African Americans and Latinos are increasing without clear patterns by geographical region. Asian Americans tend to have lower rates than do whites and African Americans.[50]

**Ulcerative Colitis** **Ulcerative colitis** is a condition occurring when the lining of the large intestine, also known as the *colon*, becomes inflamed, or develops sores or ulcers that become pus filled and trigger cramping, pain, and frequent bloody diarrhea bouts. These symptoms happen when the immune system begins to misfire and signals "invader" when food, bacteria, and other pathogens are introduced. A full-fledged attack by your own protective cells leads to inflammation and ulcers. Affecting nearly 700,000 Americans and on the increase, it often first flares up in the teens, with most diagnoses in those in their 30s.[51] Men and women are equally likely to suffer from it, but men are more likely to develop it later in life.[52]

Why this happens is controversial, with environmental, pathogenic, stress, smoking, and genetics as possible factors, but with no clear explanation. Research indicates that up to 20 percent of people

**epilepsy** A neurological disorder caused by abnormal electrical brain activity; can be accompanied by altered consciousness or convulsions.

**inflammatory bowel disease (IBD)** A group of disorders in which the intestines become inflamed.

**ulcerative colitis** An inflammatory bowel disease that affects the mucous membranes of the large intestine and can lead to ulcers, erosion of the outer lining of the colon, and serious bleeding.

# TABLE 18.2 | Other Modern Maladies

| Disease | Who is Affected? | Causes and Risk Factors | Symptoms | Treatment | Prevention |
|---|---|---|---|---|---|
| **Fibromyalgia** Extreme fatigue; painful, aching joints and muscles | Affects 2% of the population; rates increase with age | Unknown; affects primarily women in their 30s and 40s | Numbness, tingling, pain, headache, dizziness | Pain medications, anti-inflammatories, rest, stress management | Rest, dietary adjustments; avoid extreme temperatures |
| **Gallbladder diseases** Most common are cholecystitis (inflammation) and cholelithiasis (gallstones) | Affects 10–15% of the population, twice as many women as men; highest in Mexican Americans and Native Americans | Chemical exposure, infections, traumatic injury, obesity, cirrhosis of liver, rapid weight loss, diabetes, cholesterol-lowering drugs | Acute pain in the upper right quadrant of abdomen, particularly after eating fatty food; nausea and vomiting; often asymptomatic | Medications to relieve inflammation or cause of inflammation; removal of gallstones through lithotripsy or surgery | Reduce dietary fat; avoid alcohol, fried foods, whole grains |
| **Multiple sclerosis** Degenerative, autoimmune neurological disease caused by breakdown of protective sheath around nerves | Over 400,000 cases, most between ages 20 and 40; over 10,000 new cases per year | Suspected causes include genetics, viruses, allergies, and environmental toxins; Caucasians are at greatest risk | From minor numbness, blurred vision, fatigue, balance issues to severe disability; intermittent course for some | No cure, but drug therapy, climate change, and lifestyle choices can reduce symptoms and increase healthy years | Flare-up prevention possible with healthy lifestyle, adequate sleep, healthy diet, stress management, and avoidance of temperature extremes |
| **Parkinson's disease** Chronic, progressive neurological disease that affects motor function | There are 50,000–60,000 new cases per year; nearly 2 million total, mostly over age 50 | Cause currently unknown | Tremors of limbs and head; rigidity, postural instability, slowness, balance issues, shuffling gait; speech difficulties | No cure, but medications can relieve symptoms; deep brain stimulation and gamma knife surgery may help | None obvious; healthy lifestyle may help slow progression |
| **Raynaud's syndrome** Exaggerated constriction of small arteries in the extremities | Affected are 5–10% of adults, primarily women | Unknown | Fingers and toes become numb, turn white or purple; throbbing pain | Topical medications to reduce symptoms | More common in those exposed to extreme cold repeatedly, so avoid frostbite or medications that affect blood flow |
| **Rosacea** Inflammatory skin condition causing redness and small red bumps or pustules on the face | Affects over 14 million Americans; more common in menopausal women and people with fair skin/sensitive skin | Still unknown, but many suspects, ranging from genetic predisposition to blushing, skin mites, bacteria; none conclusive | Can progress from flushing and spider veins on face to lumps and bumps; skin thickening, red itchy eyes, bulbous nose in later stages | No cure, but controls include prescription medications and lotions, less irritating soaps, surgery, laser treatments, freezing | Unknown |
| **Systemic lupus erythematosus** Autoimmune disease in which antibodies destroy or injure organs such as kidneys, brain, and heart | 1.5 million people with this disease, the majority of whom are women | Cause unknown; possible genetic predisposition combined with environment and hormones | Sensitivity to light, arthritis, swelling, tendency toward increased infections, butterfly-shaped rash across nose and cheeks | Medications such as steroids to reduce symptoms and complications | Healthy lifestyle; other possible preventive measures unknown |

**Sources:** NIH, Medline Plus, "Fibromyalgia," 2014, www.nlm.nih.gov/medlineplus/fibromyalgia.html; A. Mohamed and M. Solan, "Gallbladder Disease," *Healthline*, October 2015, http://www.healthline.com/health/gallbladder-disease#Overview1; C. Hersch, "Multiple Sclerosis," *Cleveland Clinic,* June 2014, http://www.clevelandclinicmeded.com/medicalpubs/diseasemanagement/neurology/multiple_sclerosis/; National MS Society, "Multiple Sclerosis FAQs," Accessed June 2016, http://www.nationalmssociety.org/What-is-MS/MS-FAQ-s; P. Sweeney, "Parkinson's Disease," Cleveland Clinic, Center for Continuing Education, May 2013, www.clevelandclinicmeded.com/medicalpubs/diseasemanagement/neurology/parkinsons-disease; The National Rosacea Society, "All about Rosacea," Accessed June 2016, https://www.rosacea.org/patients/allaboutrosacea.php; Centers for Disease Control and Prevention, "Systemic Lupus Erythematosus (SLE)" April 2015, http://www.cdc.gov/arthritis/basics/lupus.htm.

affected have close relatives who have it; it is most common in white populations of European descent and Jewish populations.[53] Determining the cause of colitis is difficult because the disease can go into remission and then recur without apparent reason. This pattern often continues over periods of years and may be related to increased risks for colorectal cancer.[54]

Because the cause is unknown, it is important to treat symptoms and avoid substances that may trigger attacks. Keeping a food diary and recording potential flare-ups of colitis is an important part of prevention. Treatment focuses on relieving the symptoms by decreasing foods that are hard to digest (raw vegetables, seeds, nuts, and high-fiber foods); taking probiotics; and taking anti-inflammatory drugs, steroids, and other medications to reduce inflammation and soothe irritated intestinal walls.

## Crohn's Disease

Although often confused with colitis, **Crohn's disease** can affect any area of the gastrointestinal tract from the mouth to the anus, particularly the small intestine. It causes major pain, inflammation, and bleeding and can lead to tears in the GI tract.[55] Genes, environmental exposures, and an autoimmune reaction are among the most likely culprits.[56] Crohn's disease tends to affect adolescents and young adults aged 15 to 35, although it can affect people of any age, with increased risk among those who smoke and those with a family history of Crohn's.[57] It is characterized by intense stomach pain, often in the lower right area, fever, weight loss, joint pain, mouth ulcers, and watery diarrhea. Intestinal bleeding may also occur and can be serious enough to cause anemia, fatigue, and immune system dysfunction. The most common complication is actually bowel obstruction due to swelling and scar tissue and ulcers that erode and form little infection-prone out-pouches known as fistula. Those diagnosed with this disease must carefully monitor their diet to ensure adequate nutrition, be "tuned in" to their body and changes that may occur, see their doctors if symptoms develop, and take medications to reduce inflammation and prevent infection.[58] Surgery to remove damaged or obstructed portions of the bowel may be necessary.

## Irritable Bowel Syndrome (IBS)

Inflammatory bowel disease (IBD) and **irritable bowel syndrome (IBS)** are not the same condition, although they may sound as if they were. Irritable bowel syndrome is a *functional bowel disorder* (affecting how the bowel, including the colon and rectum, works). The exact cause is unknown, but in individuals with IBS, the normal muscular contractions in the intestines don't work properly and food isn't processed or eliminated as it should be.[59] Irritable bowel syndrome affects an estimated 10 to 15 percent of adults in the United States—particularly women—and usually begins in adolescence or early adulthood, with those under age 35 being most susceptible.[60] It is also the second leading cause of work absenteeism after the common cold.[61]

Irritable bowel syndrome may begin after an infection, a stressful life event, or onset of maturity, without any other

# 20%

of adults in the U.S., most of whom are women, suffer from IRRITABLE BOWEL SYNDROME.

medical indicators. Characterized by nausea, pain, gas, diarrhea, bloating, or cramps after eating certain foods or during unusual stress, IBS can be uncomfortable, but usually does not permanently harm the intestines unless symptoms are severe. Symptoms may vary from week to week and can fade for long periods of time. Researchers suspect that people with IBS have digestive systems that are overly sensitive to what they eat and drink, to stress, and to certain hormonal changes. Often, because symptoms are so similar to other gastrointestinal tract diseases, IBS is only diagnosed after all the other gastrointestinal diseases have been ruled out.

Although there is no cure for IBS, treatments attempt to relieve symptoms; stress management, relaxation techniques, regular activity, and diet changes (including gradual increases in fiber and fluids and reductions in fat to help control cramps, diarrhea, and constipation) can help control symptoms for many.

# Gastroesophageal Reflux Disease

**Gastroesophageal reflux disease (GERD)**, commonly referred to as *heartburn* or *acid reflux*, affects millions of people throughout the world. Risk factors include age, diet, alcohol use, obesity, pregnancy, and smoking. At any given time, people of all ages and stages of life suffer from a sensation of heartburn, or backflow of stomach acid into the esophagus, characterized by discomfort or a burning sensation behind the breastbone. Symptoms usually occur after a meal and can include coughing, choking, or vomiting. When these symptoms are severe and occur more than two to three times per week, GERD is often the diagnosis.

Prevention of GERD focuses on determining which foods or beverages trigger symptoms (coffee, sodas, high-acid food and juices, and alcohol are the big culprits) and avoiding spicy or fried foods. Dietary control is often a key in reducing heartburn symptoms. Also, it is important to find out whether there are mechanical causes of reflux, such as sleeping or sitting in positions that exacerbate symptoms. For persistent problems, see your doctor.

**Crohn's disease** An autoimmune inflammatory bowel disease that can affect several parts of the gastrointestinal tract as well as other body organs and systems.

**irritable bowel syndrome (IBS)** A functional bowel disorder caused by certain foods or stress that is characterized by nausea, pain, gas, or diarrhea.

**gastroesophageal reflux disease (GERD)** Chronic condition in which stomach acid backflows into the esophagus, causing heartburn and potential damage to the esophagus.

# LO 5 | COPING WITH MUSCULOSKELETAL DISEASES

Explain the risk factors and symptoms of various musculoskeletal diseases, including arthritis and low back pain, and suggest strategies for prevention.

Musculoskeletal diseases—including back pain, arthritis, bodily injuries, and osteoporosis—are more common than any other health condition in the United States and exact a tremendous toll in disability, pain, and suffering. Every year, a large proportion of all days of work missed due to a major medical condition result from musculoskeletal problems such as joint pain, arthritis, and back/neck pain (FIGURE 18.5). As the population ages and becomes increasingly overweight and sedentary, the musculoskeletal system has seen epidemic increases in problems.

## Arthritis and Related Conditions

Nearly 23 percent of Americans, or 53 million people, have one of the doctor-diagnosed forms of **arthritis**.[62] With the aging of the baby boomers, these numbers are projected to exceed 78 million, over 25 percent of the population, by 2040.[63] Arthritis consists of more than 100 conditions that wreak havoc on joints, bones, muscles, cartilage, and connective tissues, leading to disability and pain. Osteoarthritis and rheumatoid arthritis are the most common types, with symptoms that range from minor aches and pains to crippling disability. Arthritis is not just a disease of old age; in fact, nearly two-thirds of those with arthritis are under the age of 65, with nearly 300,000 children affected.[64]

**Osteoarthritis** Also called *degenerative joint disease*, **osteoarthritis (OA)** is the most common form of arthritis, affecting nearly 31 million adults in the United States.[65] If you notice that your parents or grandparents are slow to get up or walk stiffly after getting out of bed, they may be showing early signs of OA. Before age 45, more men than women have osteoarthritis; after age 45, more women have it.[66] This progressive deterioration of cartilage, bones, and joints has been associated with the "wear-and-tear" theory of aging.

Although age and injury are undoubtedly factors in osteoarthritis, heredity, abnormal joint use, diet and excess weight,

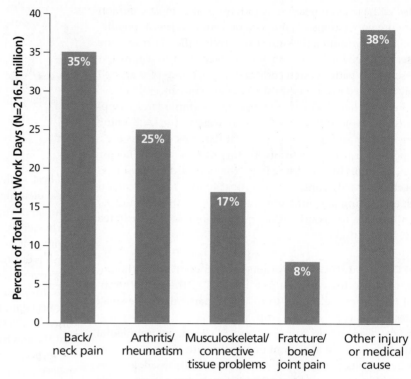

**FIGURE 18.5** Proportion of Lost Work Days for Persons Aged 18 and Older by Medical Cause

**Sources:** Adapted from The Burden of Musculoskeletal Diseases in the United States, "Bed and Lost Work Days Due to Musculoskeletal Injuries," Source of data: CDC National Center for Health Statistics, "National Health Interview Survey (NHIS) Adult Sample, 2012," July 2, 2013, www.cdc.gov/nchs/nhis/nhis_2012_data_release.htm.

abnormalities in joint structure, and impaired blood supply to the joint may also contribute. For most people, anti-inflammatory drugs and pain relievers such as aspirin and cortisone-related agents ease discomfort. In some sufferers, applications of heat, mild exercise, and massage also relieve the pain. When joints become so distorted that they impair activity, surgical intervention is often necessary.

**Rheumatoid Arthritis** The most crippling form of arthritis, **rheumatoid arthritis (RA)** is an autoimmune disease involving chronic inflammation. Over 1.5 million people have RA, with nearly three times as many women as men.[67] It typically affects women at younger ages than men. Increasing numbers of cases are occurring in people in their 20s.[68] Symptoms include stiffness, pain, redness, and swelling of

---

**arthritis** Painful inflammatory disease of the joints.

**osteoarthritis (OA)** Progressive deterioration of bones and joints that has been associated with the wear-and-tear theory of aging; also called *degenerative joint disease*.

**rheumatoid arthritis (RA)** An autoimmune inflammatory joint disease.

---

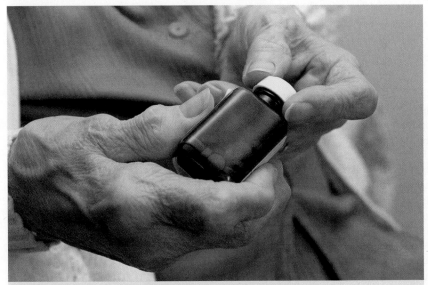

Arthritis can make even a simple task painful and difficult.

and vitamin D, and regular weight-bearing exercise and strength training—are among key recommendations to reduce risks of developing osteoporosis.

## Low Back Pain

If you're like 85 percent of the population, at some point you will experience **low back pain (LBP)**, the number one cause of activity limitation and work absence worldwide.[72] The resulting pain may be mild, involving short-lived muscle spasms, or it may be more severe, involving damage to discs, dislocation, a fracture, or another form of spinal trauma. In about 23 percent of LBP cases, pain is chronic and comes and goes with activities as varied as sneezing, bending over, and lifting heavy objects.[73] About 12 percent of those with LBP become permanently disabled.[74]

> **osteoporosis** A disease in which bones become brittle and break easily.
>
> **low back pain (LBP)** Pain or discomfort in the lumbosacral region (lowest vertebrae) of the back.

multiple joints, particularly those of the hands and wrists, and can be gradually progressive or sporadic, with occasional unexplained remissions. Although the cause of rheumatoid arthritis is unknown, some believe that invading microorganisms take over the joint and cause the immune system to begin attacking the body's own tissues. Exposure to toxic chemicals and stress are also possible triggers, as are hormonal influences.[69] Genetic markers that seem to increase risk have also been identified.

Treatment of rheumatoid arthritis emphasizes pain relief and improved functional mobility. In some instances, immunosuppressant drugs can reduce the inflammatory response, and in advanced cases, surgery may be necessary. Advanced rheumatoid arthritis often involves destruction of the bony ends of joints. The remedy for this condition is typically bone fusion, which leaves the joint immobile. In some instances, joint replacement may be a viable alternative.

## Osteoporosis

**Osteoporosis** is a disease in which bones become brittle and weak and break easily. Most commonly, bones in the spine fracture, which results in back pain, loss of height over time, and a stooped posture. Ultimately, bones in other parts of the body fracture easily too, including the hands, wrists, and hip.

Osteoporosis affects men and women of all races. But white and Asian women—especially those who are past menopause—are at highest risk.

The good news is that recent research has shown significant decreases in osteoporosis in persons age 50 and over in recent years, due to improved early diagnosis, medications, and lifestyle changes. Nevertheless, an estimated 200 million people globally have osteoporosis.[70] Nearly 40 percent of women with osteoporosis and 15 to 30 percent of men will have one or more fragility fractures in their lifetimes.[71] Prevention strategies—including regular exams, adequate amounts of calcium

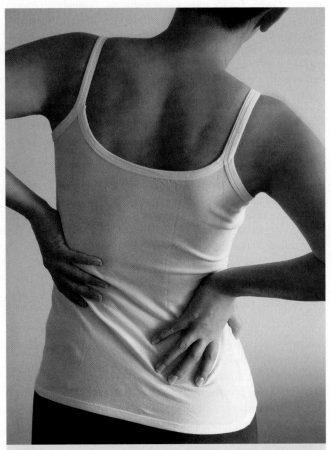

In the United States, low back pain is the major cause of disability for people aged 20 to 45, who suffer more frequently and severely from this problem than older people do. It is one of the most common chronic ailments among college students.

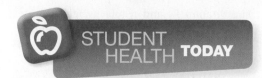
# COLLEGE STUDENTS AND LOW BACK PAIN *Oh, My Aching Backpack?*

Did you know that more than half of your college peers suffer from back problems? Why are there so many issues with the back? Although athletics, exercise regimens, sitting for hours while studying, and other normal activities can cause problems, modern conveniences may also be a huge factor. Not surprisingly, lugging heavy backpacks over one shoulder or messenger bags jammed with books and devices, water bottles, and quick changes of clothes can really bog you down, inflame muscles, and cause back strain and pain. It's no surprise that back pain is one of the top conditions that college students end up at the doctor's office each year.

Whereas hikers have long recognized the importance of internal frames and heavy-duty hip straps to displace the weight of heavy packs, most college students carry less supportive (and cheaper) daypacks that contain as much as 30 to 40 pounds of stuff, supported with only one shoulder strap. Over time, this weight can wreak havoc on even the most fit and healthy backs and shoulders. Increasing numbers of students are experiencing knee and foot problems related to backpack overload. Neuromas, flat feet, plantar foot pressure injuries, and other problems are on the increase among those who add unnecessary weight to their packs.

College students are not alone; even elementary school–age children are toting heavy backpacks—sometimes carrying amounts that are 10 to 15 percent of their total body weight. Because such repetitive strain on the back can result in

a lifetime of pain and disability, prevention is imperative. If you must carry a pack all day, protect your back by following this advice:

- Opt for the lightest pack available and make sure that it has a heavy-duty hip strap so that you are not carrying the bulk of the weight around your back and shoulders. Adjust the strap so the weight is primarily on your hips in the center of your back instead of a huge purse or messenger bag.
- If you can afford a small internal-frame pack, buy one. There are many excellent packs available from outdoor recreation supply companies, or consider a rolling computer case.
- If your pack has two straps, use them both, rather than putting additional strain on one side of your body.
- Use and carry the lightest computer possible. If you have to carry larger devices, don't let your ego get in the way. Let a roller bag take the weight rather than your back! Don't bring your books to class unless your instructor asks you to. Plan ahead and bring only those study materials to campus that you can complete while you're there; carry a smaller notepad; store files on a jump drive and upload to a campus computer to do work.
- Limit the amount of personal items you carry each day. Wallets, makeup, hair products, and so on should be kept to a minimum.
- When lifting your pack to put it on your back, stand with both feet on the

**Overstuffed backpacks can lead to a lifetime of back pain.**

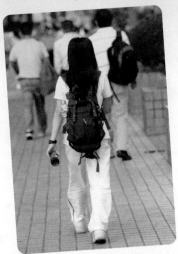

ground, knees slightly flexed, and your back straight. Twisting the back while swinging up the load can cause back injuries.

- Pack heavy items on the bottom and as close to your back as possible.
- Once you're ready to go, weigh the pack. If it's over 15 pounds, reassess what is necessary and ditch the rest.

**Sources:** H. Son, "The Effect of Backpack Load on Muscle Activities of the Trunk and Lower Extremities and Plantar Foot Pressure in Flatfoot," *Journal of Physical Therapy Science* 25, no. 11 (2013): 1383–6; American College Health Association, *American College Health Association–National College Health Assessment II: Reference Group Executive Summary Fall 2015* (Hanover, MD: American College Health Association, 2016).

---

Treatment may involve medication, rehabilitation, injections, and surgery, with varying results. A comprehensive analysis of recent research indicates that strength and resistance exercise, particularly for acute low back pain, and exercises focusing on coordination and stabilization are among the most effective strategies for long-term low back pain relief, particularly under the guidance of a physical therapist.[75]

Low back pain is increasingly common, especially among young adults (see the **Student Health Today** box for one possible cause).[76] These injuries tend to be shorter lived initially, but over time they progress toward more recurrent and long-term disability and costs.[77]

The following factors contribute to LBP:

- **Age.** People between the ages of 20 and 45 run the greatest risk of LBP. At age 50, the condition becomes less common. After age 65, the incidence again rises, apparently because of bone and joint deterioration. For college students, heavy purses or backpacks can be major precipitators of back problems, particularly among those who are primarily sedentary or who have weak core muscles.
- **Body type.** Many studies indicate that people who are very tall, have a high body mass index (BMI), or have a lanky body type run an increased risk of LBP. Other sources say

that being slightly overweight helps reduce the risk of LBP, as the weight helps strengthen core muscles. However, much of this research is controversial.

- **Posture.** Poor posture may be one of the greatest contributors to LBP. If you routinely slouch, particularly over a computer or workstation, you run an increased risk of LBP.
- **Strength and fitness.** People with LBP tend to have less overall core strength than other people. The total level of fitness and conditioning is also a factor—the fitter you are, the better. Sedentary people who suddenly decide to "get fit" often are among those most at risk for LBP, as they engage in strenuous activity without first strengthening supporting muscles.
- **Psychological factors.** Numerous psychological factors appear to increase risk for LBP. Depression, apathy, inattentiveness, boredom, emotional upsets, drug abuse, and family and financial problems all heighten risk.
- **Occupational risk.** The type of work you do and the conditions you do it in greatly affect risk. For example, truck drivers, who must endure the bumps and jolts of the road while in a sitting position, frequently suffer from back pain.

## Repetitive Motion Disorders

It's the end of the term, and you have finished the last of several papers. After hours of nonstop typing, your hands are numb and you feel an intense, burning pain that makes the thought of typing one more word almost unbearable. If this happens, you may be suffering from a *repetitive motion disorder* (RMD). Repetitive motion disorders include carpal tunnel syndrome, bursitis, tendonitis, ganglion cysts, and others.[78] Twisting of the arm or wrist, overexertion, and incorrect posture or position are usually contributors, particularly among those spending hours texting or on gaming or other devices. One of the most common RMDs is **carpal tunnel syndrome** with resultant numbness, tingling and pain in the fingers, wrist and hands. (See **Focus On: Reducing Your Risk of Unintentional Injury** on page 549, for a more complete description of this painful chronic condition.)

> **carpal tunnel syndrome** An occupational injury in which the median nerve in the wrist becomes irritated, causing numbness, tingling, and pain in the fingers and hands.

# STUDY **PLAN**

Customize your study plan—and master your health!— in the Study Area of **MasteringHealth**.

## ASSESS YOURSELF

**Could you be at risk for chronic illness?** Want to find out? Take the **Are You at Risk for Chronic Illness?** assessment available on

## MasteringHealth.™

# CHAPTER **REVIEW**

To hear an MP3 Tutor Session, scan here or visit the Study Area in **MasteringHealth**.

### LO **1** Coping with Respiratory Problems

- Chronic lower respiratory disease (CLRD) (including bronchitis, emphysema, and asthma) is the third leading cause of death in the United States (right after heart disease and cancer).

### LO **2** Coping with Allergies

- Allergies occur as the immune system responds to allergens. They can be triggered by pollens, foods, or other substances.

### LO **3** Coping with Neurological Disorders

- Neurological conditions include headaches and seizure disorders such as epilepsy. The most

common types of headache are tension, migraine, and cluster headaches.

### LO **4** Coping with Digestion-Related Disorders and Diseases

- Inflammatory bowel disease includes ulcerative colitis and Crohn's disease. Irritable bowel syndrome (IBS) and other digestive problems affect increasing numbers of adults.

## LO 5 | Coping with Musculoskeletal Diseases

■ Musculoskeletal problems such as arthritis, repetitive motion disorders, low back pain, and osteoporosis cause significant pain and disability in millions of people. Many of these problems are preventable.

# POP **QUIZ**

Visit **MasteringHealth** to personalize your study plan with Chapter Review Quizzes and Dynamic Study Modules.

## LO 1 | Coping with Respiratory Problems

1. The gradual destruction of the alveoli in a smoker's lung usually causes which COPD characterized by difficulty in exhaling?
   a. Dyspnea
   b. Bronchitis
   c. Emphysema
   d. Asthma

2. Margaret experiences occasional wheezing, shortness of breath, and coughing spasms. What chronic respiratory disorder is she likely suffering from?
   a. Sleep apnea
   b. Bronchitis
   c. Asthma
   d. COPD

3. The leading chronic disease in school-aged children today is
   a. bronchitis.
   b. common cold.
   c. attention-deficit disorder.
   d. asthma.

## LO 2 | Coping with Allergies

4. Julie has found that she cannot eat nuts without suffering from itching and nausea. What condition is she likely to be suffering from?
   a. Irritable bowel syndrome
   b. Ulcerative colitis
   c. Food allergy
   d. Diabetes mellitus

5. Which of the following statements is correct?
   a. Lactose intolerance is an example of a food allergy.
   b. Children are more likely than adults to outgrow allergies to foods.
   c. Food allergies and food intolerance are the same thing.
   d. Food allergies appear to be decreasing in the United States.

## LO 3 | Coping with Neurological Disorders

6. If you experience an aura, a sensory warning sign that may include flickering vision or blind spots, you are likely to
   a. have an asthma attack.
   b. have a migraine headache.
   c. have a tension-type headache.
   d. be showing symptoms of glaucoma.

7. Which of the following is correct?
   a. Migraine incidence usually peaks in older adulthood (between ages 60 and 80).
   b. Men have more cluster headaches than women.
   c. Tension-type headaches are often preceded by an aura.
   d. If untreated, migraines can progress into epilepsy or another seizure-related disorder.

## LO 4 | Coping with Digestion-Related Disorders and Diseases

8. Which of the following is correct?
   a. Irritable bowel syndrome often occurs before age 35.
   b. Irritable bowel disease and irritable bowel syndrome are the same thing.
   c. Consuming fruit juices lessens heartburn associated with gastroesophageal reflux disease.
   d. Smokers have a lower risk of ulcerative colitis.

## LO 5 | Coping with Musculoskeletal Diseases

9. Which of the following conditions is the leading cause of employee sick time and lost productivity in the United States?
   a. Low back pain
   b. Upper respiratory infections
   c. Asthma
   d. On-the-job injuries

10. After Dylan spent days on his computer finishing all of his final papers, he noticed numbness, tingling, and pain in his left wrist. Dylan is most likely experiencing
    a. rheumatoid arthritis.
    b. osteoporosis.
    c. osteoarthritis.
    d. carpal tunnel syndrome.

*Answers to the Pop Quiz can be found on page A-1. If you answered a question incorrectly, review the section identified by the Learning Outcome. For even more study tools, visit **MasteringHealth**.*

# THINK ABOUT IT!

## LO 1 | Coping with Respiratory Problems

1. List common respiratory diseases affecting Americans. Which of these has
   a. a genetic basis?
   b. an environmental basis?
   c. an individual basis?
   d. What are the combined risks?

## LO 2 | Coping with Allergies

2. Why do you think allergies are the top medical conditions that college students seek medical care for each year? What can you do to reduce your risks for allergies?

## LO 3 | Coping with Neurological Disorders

3. Compare and contrast the different types of headaches. What are some of the major factors that put people at risk for migraines?

## LO 4 | Coping with Digestion-Related Disorders and Diseases

4. Compare the symptoms of ulcerative colitis, gastroesophageal reflux disease, and Crohn's disease. How can you tell whether your stomach is reacting to final exams or telling you that you have a serious medical condition?

## LO 5 | Coping with Musculoskeletal Diseases

5. What are the major disorders of the musculoskeletal system? Which, if any, have you or your family members experienced in the last year? Were they preventable? If so, what actions might have prevented them?

# ACCESS YOUR HEALTH ON THE INTERNET

Visit **MasteringHealth** for links to the websites and RSS feeds.

The following websites explore further topics and issues related to chronic conditions.

**American Academy of Allergy, Asthma, and Immunology.** This site presents an overview of asthma and allergy information, particularly as it applies to children with allergies. It also offers interactive quizzes to test your knowledge and an ask-the-expert section. **www.aaaai.org**

**American Lung Association.** The latest news on asthma and lung disease is available here. **www.lungusa.org**

**National Center for Chronic Disease Prevention and Health Promotion.** A wide range of information is available from this organization, which is dedicated to chronic diseases and health promotion. The organization is linked to the Centers for Disease Control and Prevention. **www.cdc.gov/chronicdisease**

**National Institute of Neurological Disorders and Stroke.** This site contains up-to-date information to help individuals cope with pain-related difficulties. **www.ninds.nih.gov**

**National Institute for Diabetes and Digestive and Kidney Diseases (NIDDK).** This valuable resource provides key information about diabetes and the major digestive and kidney diseases, as well as resources for prevention and treatment options. **www2.niddk.nih.gov**

# 19 Making Smart Health Care Choices

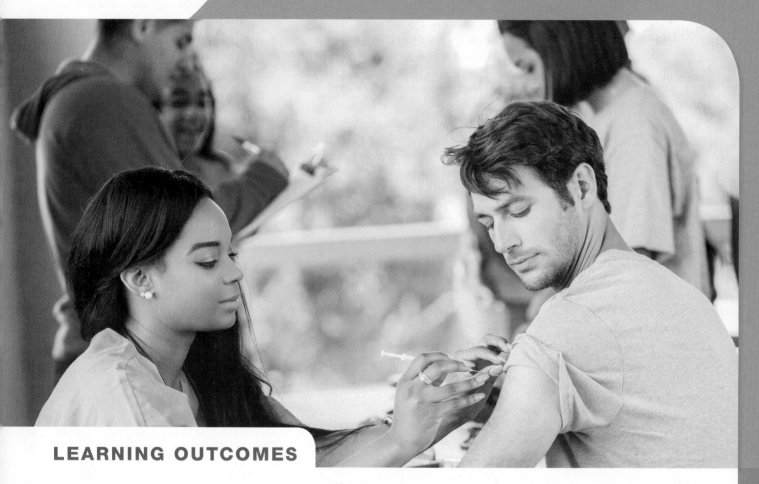

## LEARNING OUTCOMES

**LO 1** Explain why it is important to be a responsible health care consumer, and identify several factors to consider when making health care decisions.

**LO 2** Discuss conventional health care, including types of practitioners and the health care products and treatments available.

**LO 3** Discuss complementary and integrative health care, identifying three basic categories and the most commonly used approaches within each.

**LO 4** Describe the U.S. health care system in terms of types of insurance; the changing structure of the systems; and issues concerning cost, quality, and access to services.

**LO 5** Explain key issues facing our health care system today and possible actions that could improve the system.

Have you ever wondered whether you were sick enough to go to your campus health clinic? Have you left visits with your health care provider feeling that he or she didn't give a thorough exam or that you had more questions than you did when you arrived? Do you understand health insurance provisions and what your options are in terms of health care systems and services? If you were suddenly injured or became very ill, would you know where to go for help? Have you ever had to help a loved one make health care decisions? Are you among the nearly 15 percent of young adults aged 18 to 24 in the United States who do not have health insurance?[1]

If you answered yes or are unsure about any of these questions, then you will find the information in this chapter valuable for becoming a better health care consumer. Learning how to navigate the health care system is an important part of taking charge of your health.

## LO 1 | TAKING RESPONSIBILITY FOR YOUR HEALTH CARE

Explain why it is important to be a responsible health care consumer, and identify several factors to consider when making health care decisions.

Acting responsibly in times of illness can be difficult. If you are not feeling well, you must first decide whether you really need to seek medical advice. For ailments like colds or minor injuries, self-care may be the best course of action. In more serious cases, not seeking treatment—whether because of high costs or limited coverage—or trying to medicate yourself when a professional diagnosis and treatment are needed, is potentially dangerous. It's important to know the benefits and limits of self-care.

### Self-Care

Individuals can practice behaviors that promote health and reduce the risk of disease as well as treat minor afflictions without seeking professional help. Self-care consists of knowing your body, paying attention to its signals, and taking appropriate action to stop the progression of illness or injury. Common forms of self-care include:

- Diagnosing symptoms or conditions that occur frequently but may not require physician visits (e.g., the common cold, minor abrasions)
- Using over-the-counter remedies to treat mild, infrequent, and unambiguous pain and other symptoms
- Performing first aid for common, uncomplicated injuries and conditions
- Having periodic checks for blood pressure, blood glucose, blood lipids, or other levels as prescribed by a physician
- Learning from reliable self-help books, websites, and videos
- Performing meditation or other relaxation techniques
- Maintaining a healthful diet, getting adequate rest, and exercising

In addition, a vast array of at-home diagnostic kits are now available to test for pregnancy, allergies, HIV, prediabetes, genetic disorders, and many other conditions. Caution is in order here: Diagnoses from these devices are not always accurate, or you may need professional interpretation to explain the ramifications of test results. Moreover, home health tests are not substitutes for regular, complete examinations by a trained practitioner.

Taking prescription drugs used for a previous illness to treat your current illness, using unproven self-treatment, or using other people's medications are examples of inappropriate self-care. Using self-care methods appropriately takes effort, education, and the ability to make informed decisions based on scientific evidence.

**HEAR IT! PODCASTS**

Want a study podcast for this chapter? Download the podcast **Consumerism: Selecting Health Care Products and Services**, available on MasteringHealth.™

### When to Seek Help

Effective self-care also means understanding when to seek medical attention and how to access the most cost-effective and appropriate level of care. Generally, you should consult a physician if you experience *any* of the following:

- Serious accident or injury
- Sudden or severe chest pains, especially if they cause breathing difficulties
- Trauma to the head or spine accompanied by persistent headache, blurred vision, loss of consciousness, vomiting, convulsions, or paralysis
- Sudden high fever or recurring high temperature (over 102°F for children and 103°F for adults) and/or sweats

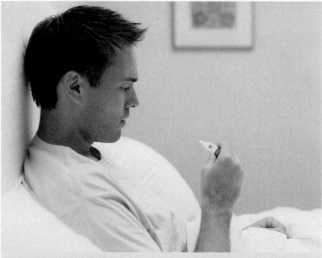

Deciding when to contact a physician can be difficult. Most people first try to diagnose and treat a minor condition themselves.

- Tingling sensation in the arm accompanied by slurred speech or impaired thought processes
- Adverse reactions to a drug or insect bite (shortness of breath, severe swelling, or dizziness)
- Sudden unexplained weight loss
- Persistent or recurrent diarrhea or vomiting
- Blue-tinted lips, eyelids, or nail beds
- Any lump, swelling, thickness, or sore that does not subside or that grows for over a month
- Any blood in the stool or urine, or significant pain, or marked, persistent change in bowel or bladder habits
- Yellowing of the skin or the whites of the eyes
- Sudden severe pain that has no apparent cause
- Any symptom that is unusual, persists, or recurs over time
- Pregnancy

See the Making Changes Today box for pointers on taking an active role in your own health care.

# 35.1 MILLION

Americans are admitted to a **HOSPITAL** each year.

## Assessing Health Professionals

Suppose you decide that you do need medical help. How should you go about assessing the qualifications of a health care provider? Numerous studies show that the most satisfied patients are those who feel their health care provider takes

## MAKING **CHANGES** TODAY

### Be Proactive in Your Health Care

The following points help you communicate well with health care providers:

- Research your personal and family medical history. Visit https://familyhistory.hhs.gov/FHH/html/index.html to create a family health portrait you can share with your health care providers.

- Research your condition—causes, physiological effects, possible treatments, and prognosis. Don't rely solely on the health care provider.

- Write out your questions in advance. Asking questions is your right as a patient.

- Bring someone with you to appointments to listen, take notes, and ask for clarification if necessary. If you go alone, take notes.

- Ask the practitioner to explain the problem and possible tests, treatments, and medications. If you don't understand something, ask for clarification.

- If the health care provider prescribes any medications, ask whether you can take generic equivalents that cost less.

- Ask for a written summary of the results of your visit and any lab tests.

- Seek a second opinion about important tests or treatment recommendations.

- After an appointment, write down an account of what happened and what was said. Include the names of the provider and all other people involved in your care, the date, and the place.

- When filling prescriptions, read the pharmacist-provided drug information sheet that lists medical considerations and details about potential drug and food interactions.

time to listen, explains diagnosis and treatment options thoroughly, and demonstrates competency, respect, and genuine concern.[2]

When evaluating health care providers, consider the following questions:

- Do they listen to you, respect you as an individual, and give you time to ask questions? Do you feel that they are in a rush to finish and move on to the next patient or are they "tuned in" to you? Do they return your calls, and are they available to answer questions between visits? How quickly could you get in to see them in an emergency? Does your insurance cover their care?
- What professional education and training have they had and what are their credentials? What license or board certification(s) do they hold? Note an important difference: *Board certified* indicates that the physician has passed

the national board examination for his or her specialty (e.g., pediatrics) and has been certified as competent in that specialty. In contrast, *board eligible* merely means that the physician is eligible to take the exam, but not that he or she has passed it. Do they have a record of any malpractice claims?

- Are they affiliated with an accredited medical facility or institution? *The Joint Commission* is an independent non-profit organization that evaluates and accredits more than 20,500 health care organizations and programs in the United States. Accreditation requires institutions to verify all education, licensing, and training claims of their affiliated practitioners.[3]
- Are they open to complementary or integrative strategies (discussed shortly)? Would they refer you for different treatment modalities if appropriate?
- Do they clearly identify possible treatment options, the pros and cons of each, and the effectiveness of a given treatment in the short and long terms? What might be the side effects of a treatment and what possible symptoms might you expect?
- Who will be responsible for your care when your physician is on vacation or off call? Are they part of a practice group with colleagues who can help you when they are not available? Will they refer you out of their group if you would like to see another specialist or do they try to keep your business in-house?
- Are there professional reviews and information on any lawsuits against them available online?

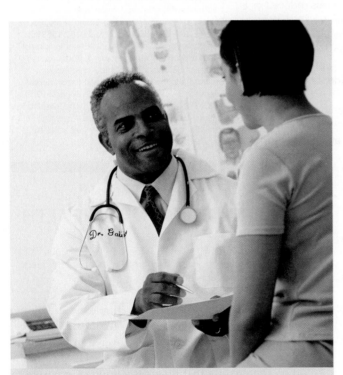

It's important to understand recommendations that your health care provider makes. Questions to ask include how often the practitioner has performed a procedure and risks, the proportion of successful outcomes for the treatment or procedure, and why a test has been ordered.

Be prepared for appointments. Do some background investigation about your symptoms and ask the right questions. Work in partnership with your health care provider. Many patients find that writing questions down before an appointment helps them get the answers they need. Don't accept a defensive or hostile response; if you are not satisfied with how a practitioner communicates, go elsewhere. It is also important that you provide honest answers to the provider's questions about your symptoms, condition, lifestyle, and medical history.

Active participation in your treatment is the only sensible course in a health care environment that encourages *defensive medicine*, in which providers take certain actions primarily to avoid a **malpractice** claim. Today, the third leading cause of death in America is preventable medical error: hospital errors, errors in diagnosis, injuries from medications, and other health care errors.[4] In a complex, often overtaxed health care system, mistakes can happen. Being a savvy health care consumer is the best way to reduce your risks.

## Your Rights as a Patient

More than asking questions, being proactive in your health care also means being aware of your rights as a patient, as follows:[5]

1. The right of **informed consent** means that before receiving care, you should be fully informed of what is planned; risks and potential benefits; and possible alternative forms of treatment, including the option of no treatment. Your consent must be voluntary and without coercion. It is critical to read consent forms carefully and amend them as necessary before signing.
2. You are entitled to know whether the treatment you are receiving is standard or experimental. In experimental conditions, you have the legal and ethical right to know if any drug is being used as part of a research project for a purpose not approved by the U.S. Food and Drug Administration (FDA) and if the study is one in which some people receive treatment while others receive a **placebo**. (See the **Student Health Today** box on page 506 for more on placebos and the placebo effect.)
3. You have the right to make decisions regarding the health care that is recommended by the physician.
4. You have the right to confidentiality, which

**malpractice** Improper or negligent treatment by a health practitioner that results in loss, injury, or harm to the patient.

**informed consent** Acknowledgment that you have been told of the potential risks and benefits of a recommended test or treatment, understand what you have been told, and agree to the care.

**placebo** Inactive substance used as a control in a clinical test to determine the effectiveness of a particular drug; the *placebo effect* occurs when patients given a placebo drug or treatment experience an improved state of health owing to the belief that they are receiving something that will be of benefit.

**SEE IT! VIDEOS**

Knowing your medical history can keep you informed of health risks. Watch **Your Medical History**, available on **MasteringHealth.™**

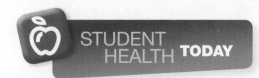

# STUDENT HEALTH TODAY

# THE PLACEBO EFFECT
*Mind over Matter?*

The *placebo effect* is an apparent cure or improved state of health brought about by a substance, product, or procedure that has no generally recognized therapeutic value. Patients often report improvements in a condition based on what they expect, desire, or were told would happen after receiving a treatment, even though the treatment was, for example, simple sugar pills instead of powerful drugs. Placebo-controlled studies are often used to determine the effectiveness of medications. Patients with a particular condition are given either the drug that is being tested or a placebo. If a significantly greater number of patients receiving the drug have a significantly better outcome than the patients receiving the placebo, the treatment can be considered effective. Most such studies are double-blind; that is, neither the patients nor the doctors involved are told until the study ends who had the real treatment.

There is also a *nocebo effect*, in which a practitioner's negative assessment of a patient's symptoms leads to a worsening of the condition, such as increased anxiety and pain. Similarly, a negative assessment of a treatment's potential efficacy induces a failure to respond to that treatment.

Researchers are investigating how and why expectation appears to change physiology. Evidence from pain studies suggests that use of a placebo for pain

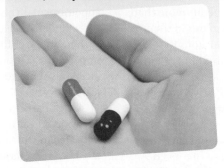

**Is it real medicine or a placebo? In some cases, it may not make a difference.**

control causes the brain to release the same endogenous (natural) opioids it releases when the study participant uses a pain medication with an active ingredient. But pain is not the only factor to respond to expectation.

■ A study of resting tremor (such as involuntary finger tapping) in patients with Parkinson's disease found that positive or negative expectations of a treatment's effectiveness reduced or increased patient tremor when they were given the same valid medication or the same placebo.

■ A recent review study of thousands of clinical trials of antidepressants concluded that their therapeutic benefits reflect a combination of effects, including those induced pharmacologically as well as placebo effects.

■ Several studies have found a significant placebo effect in trials of medications to treat alcohol dependency; alcohol-dependent patients consume fewer alcoholic drinks and report less alcohol dependence and cravings, regardless of whether they are receiving the drug or a placebo.

If you're curious to learn more about the scientific evidence behind a drug prescribed for you, get online. A quick search using the exact name of the medication and the words "drug studies" should provide links to the information you're looking for.

**Sources:** L. Colloca and C. Grillon, "Understanding Placebo and Nocebo Responses for Pain Management," *Current Pain and Headache Reports* 18, no. 6 (2014): 419, doi: 10.1007/s11916-014-0419-2; A. Keitel et al., "Expectation Modulates the Effect of Deep Brain Stimulation on Motor and Cognitive Function in Tremor-Dominant Parkinson's Disease," *PLoS One* 8, no. 12 (2013): e81878, doi: 10.1371/journal.pone.0081878; T. Bschor and L.L. Kilarski, "Are Antidepressants Effective?: A Debate on Their Efficacy for the Treatment of Major Depression in Adults," *Expert Review of Neurotherapeutics* 16, no. 4 (2016): 367–74, doi 10.1586/14737175.2016.1155985; R. A. Litten et al., "The Placebo Effect in Clinical Trials for Alcohol Dependence: An Exploratory Analysis of 51 Naltrexone and Acamprosate Studies," *Alcoholism, Clinical and Experimental Research* 37, no. 12 (2013): 2128–37, doi: 10.1111/acer.12197; G. L. Petersen et al., "The Magnitude of Nocebo Effects in Pain: A Meta-Analysis," *Pain* 155, no. 8 (2014), 1426–34, doi: 10.1016/j.pain.2014.04.016.

---

**allopathic medicine** Conventional, Western medical practice; in theory, based on scientifically validated methods and procedures.

includes the source of payment for treatment and care. It also means you have the right to make personal decisions concerning all reproductive matters.

5. You have the right to receive adequate health care, as well as to refuse treatment and to cease treatment at any time.
6. You are entitled to have access to all of your medical records and to have those records remain confidential.
7. You have the right to continuity of health care.
8. You have the right to seek the opinions of other health care professionals regarding your condition.
9. You have the right to courtesy, respect, dignity, responsiveness, and timely attention to health needs.

## LO 2 | CONVENTIONAL HEALTH CARE

Discuss conventional health care, including types of practitioners and the health care products and treatments available.

- - - - - - - - - - - - - - - - - - - - - - - - - - - - - - - - - - - -

Conventional health care, also called **allopathic medicine**, mainstream medicine, or traditional Western medical practice, is the dominant type of health care delivered in the United States, Canada, Europe, and much of the developed world. It is based on the premise that illness is a result of exposure to harmful environmental agents, or organic changes in the body. The prevention of disease and the restoration of health involve vaccines, drugs, surgery, and other treatments.

Be aware, however, that not all allopathic treatments have had the benefit of extensive, long-term, unbiased clinical trials that would conclusively prove effectiveness in various populations. Even when studies appear to support the benefits of a particular treatment or product, their findings can be subject to bias. A comprehensive review of drug studies found, for example, that those funded by the pharmaceutical industry are far more likely to report positive response to the drug and fail to report negative effects as compared to studies of the same drug funded by outside sources.[6] This is one reason that later studies without sponsorship bias often refute earlier claims. Also, recommended treatments may change dramatically as new technologies and medical advances replace older practices. Like other professionals, medical doctors must keep up with new research and changing practices in their field(s) of specialty.

One of the ways health care providers maintain the quality of care they provide is by practicing **evidence-based medicine**. Decisions regarding patient care are based on clinical expertise, patient values, and current best scientific evidence. Clinical expertise refers to the clinician's cumulative experience, education, and clinical skills. The patient brings his or her own personal and unique concerns, expectations, and values. The best evidence is usually found in clinically relevant research conducted using sound methodology.

# Conventional Health Care Practitioners

Selecting a **primary care practitioner (PCP)**—a medical practitioner whom you can visit for routine ailments, preventive care, general medical advice, and appropriate referrals—is not an easy task. The PCP for most people is a family practitioner, an internist, or, for women, an obstetrician-gynecologist (ob-gyn). Many people routinely see nurse practitioners or physician assistants who work for an individual doctor or a medical group, and others use nontraditional providers as their primary source of care. As a college student, you may opt to visit a PCP at your campus health center.

Doctors undergo rigorous training before they can begin practicing. After 4 years of undergraduate work, students typically spend 4 additional years studying for their doctor of medicine degree (MD). After this general training, some students choose a specialty, such as pediatrics, cardiology, oncology, radiology, or surgery, and spend another year in an internship and several years doing a residency. Some doctors receive additional training in order to specialize in certain elective surgeries (see the Student Health Today box on page 508). Some specialties also require a fellowship, so additional training after receiving a medical degree can take up to 8 years.

**Osteopaths** are general practitioners who receive training similar to that of a medical doctor but who place special emphasis on the skeletal and muscular systems. Their treatments may involve manipulation of the muscles and joints. Osteopaths receive the degree of doctor of osteopathy (DO) rather than an MD.

Eye care specialists can be either ophthalmologists or optometrists. An **ophthalmologist** holds a medical degree and can perform surgery and prescribe medications. An **optometrist** typically evaluates visual problems and fits glasses but is not a trained physician. If you have an eye condition requiring diagnosis and treatment, see an ophthalmologist.

**Dentists** diagnose and treat diseases of the teeth, gums, and oral cavity. They attend dental school for 4 years and receive the title of doctor of dental surgery (DDS) or doctor of medical dentistry (DMD). They must also pass both state and national board examinations before receiving their licenses to practice. The field of dentistry includes specialties; for example, *orthodontists* specialize in the alignment of teeth, *periodontists* treat diseases of the gums and other tissues surrounding the teeth, and *oral surgeons* perform surgical procedures to correct problems of the mouth, face, and jaw.

**Nurses** are trained health care professionals who provide a wide range of services for patients and their families, including patient education, counseling, community health and disease prevention information, and administration of medications. Registered nurses (RNs) in the United States complete either a 4-year program leading to a bachelor of science in nursing (BSN) degree or a 2-year associate degree program, and must also pass a national certification exam. Lower-level licensed practical or vocational nurses (LPN or LVN) complete a 1- to 2-year training program, which may be based in either a community college or hospital, and take a licensing exam.

**Nurse practitioners (NPs)** are nurses with advanced training obtained through either a master's degree program or a specialized nurse practitioner program. Nurse practitioners have the training and authority to conduct diagnostic tests and prescribe medications (in some states). They work in a variety of settings, including clinics and student health centers, and can specialize in areas such as pediatrics or acute care. Nurses and nurse practitioners may also earn the clinical doctor of nursing degree (ND), doctor of nursing science (DNS and DNSc degrees), or a research-based PhD in nursing.

**Physician assistants (PAs)** are licensed to examine and diagnose patients, offer treatment, and write prescriptions under a physician's supervision. An important difference between a PA and an NP is that the PA must practice under a physician's supervision. Like other health care providers, PAs are licensed by state boards of medicine.

You can locate licensing information about a physician or

**evidence-based medicine** Decisions regarding patient care based on clinical expertise, patient values, and current best scientific evidence.

**primary care practitioner (PCP)** Medical practitioner who provides preventive care and treats routine ailments, gives general medical advice, and makes appropriate referrals when necessary.

**osteopath** General practitioner who receives training similar to a medical doctor's but with an emphasis on the skeletal and muscular systems; may use spinal manipulation as part of treatment.

**ophthalmologist** Physician who specializes in the medical and surgical care of the eyes, including prescriptions for lenses.

**optometrist** Eye specialist whose practice is limited to prescribing and fitting lenses to correct vision problems.

**dentist** Physician who diagnoses and treats diseases of the teeth, gums, and oral cavity.

**nurse** Health professional who provides patient care in a variety of settings.

**nurse practitioner (NP)** Nurse with advanced training obtained through either a master's degree program or a specialized nurse practitioner program.

**physician assistant (PA)** Health care practitioner trained to handle most routine care under the supervision of a physician.

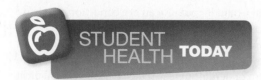

# CHOOSING SURGERY
## *Elective Procedures*

Elective medical procedures are surgeries and other treatments that are planned; that is, they are not performed on an emergency basis. Although not considered medically necessary, many types of elective procedures, from musculoskeletal to weight loss surgeries, greatly improve people's health and functioning, and some can reduce the patient's risk for chronic disease. Even purely cosmetic surgeries can enhance the patient's self-esteem.

If a procedure is considered not medically necessary, it may not be covered by insurance. In some cases, insurance companies may require a second opinion before approving payment on elective surgical procedures. If you are considering elective surgery, review your coverage requirements with your health insurance carrier before scheduling the procedure.

An elective surgical procedure is typically performed by a surgeon or qualified physician in either a hospital or an ambulatory center. Some simple, minimally invasive procedures may even be performed in a doctor's office. The type of surgery will mandate the qualifications and background of the surgeon or physician who performs it. The following are some of the more common elective surgeries.

## LASIK

Millions of Americans have had surgery to reduce their dependence on contact lenses or glasses. The most common technique is called LASIK (laser-assisted in situ keratomileusis), in which a surgeon uses a razor-like instrument or laser to cut a flap in the cornea, the clear covering on the front of the eye, and then reshapes the exposed area using a laser. The surgery alters the way the eye focuses light, correcting nearsightedness, farsightedness, and some astigmatism. However, LASIK is not effective at treating close-up vision problems in middle-aged or older adults.

The procedure usually takes less than 30 minutes, uses numbing drops to eliminate pain, and the patient is awake the

entire time. For a few days after surgery, the eye may itch, burn, or feel gritty. Postoperative complications can include infection or night glare—starbursts or halos that appear when viewing lights at night. It may take 3 to 6 months for vision to stabilize.

## Cosmetic Surgery

Cosmetic surgery is performed to enhance appearance. Over the past two decades, the number of cosmetic surgeries performed in the United States has nearly doubled. In 2015, over 1.9 million were performed. The five most common are:

- *Liposuction*, the removal of pockets of fatty tissue with a vacuum-like device, to slim the hips, thighs, abdomen, or other areas
- *Breast augmentation*, the surgical placement of an implant behind each breast to increase breast volume and enhance shape
- *Breast lift*, removal of excess skin and tightening, reshaping, and supporting remaining breast tissue
- *Abdominoplasty*, commonly called a "tummy tuck," to remove excess abdominal skin and fat and restore weakened or separated muscles
- *Blepharoplasty*, to improve the appearance of the eyelids
- *Rhinoplasty*, correction and reconstruction of the nose, and rhytidectomy, commonly called a facelift, are other common procedures.

Risks and complications of cosmetic surgery include infection, bruising, numbness, bleeding, and poor healing.

## Nonsurgical Cosmetic Procedures

Nonsurgical cosmetic procedures are more than five times as common as cosmetic surgeries, with nearly 10.9 million performed in 2015. And their rate has increased more than fivefold over the past 15 years. The most common nonsurgical procedure is injection of botulinum toxin to reduce facial wrinkles; in 2015, more than 4 million were performed. A similar procedure uses hyaluronic acid to fill

**If you have a vision problem, you have a wide range of options, including corrective lenses and surgery, for correcting them. Make sure you investigate the procedure and the care provider thoroughly before deciding on any elective surgery.**

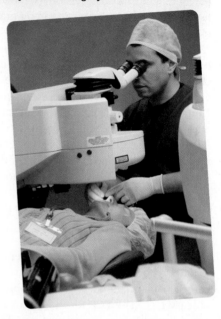

wrinkles and plump lips. Other common procedures include microdermabrasion, a surgical scraping of the top layers of the skin to remove fine wrinkles, acne scars, and skin growths; hair removal; and chemical peels.

Although women account for more than 90 percent of all surgical and nonsurgical cosmetic procedures, nearly 10 percent are performed on men. Liposuction, facelifts, and breast reduction are all top procedures among men. During the last two decades, the number of men choosing such procedures has more than tripled.

**Sources:** U.S. Food and Drug Administration, "LASIK," June 9, 2014, www.fda.gov/MedicalDevices/ProductsandMedicalProcedures/SurgeryandLifeSupport/LASIK/default.htm; American Society for Aesthetic Plastic Surgery, "Quick Facts, Highlights of the ASAPS 2015 Statistics on Cosmetic Surgery," 2015, http://www.surgery.org/sites/default/files/2015-quick-facts.pdf.

other medical provider you're considering by searching the DocFinder database from the Administrators in Medicine (AIM) at *www.administratorsinmedicine.org*. The database also provides physician profiles, including information about any disciplinary action that may have been taken in relation to the provider.

What about nonmedical providers you might be considering, such as nutritionists, therapists, counselors, coaches, and trainers? These terms are not regulated; thus, there are no guarantees that individuals using them have any formal education, training, certification, license, or experience in any health care field. Individuals qualified to provide nutrition counseling are registered dietitians. Qualified mental health professionals are identified in Table 2.1 on page 25. Before working with a "life coach," "fitness counselor," "healer," or any other unlicensed individual, investigate their education, training, and certification.

## Conventional Medication

Prescription drugs can be obtained only with a written prescription from a physician, while over-the-counter drugs can be purchased without a prescription. Both types are approved and regulated by the FDA. Making wise decisions about medication is an important aspect of responsible health care.

### Prescription Drugs
In almost three-fourths of doctor visits, the physician administers or prescribes at least one medication.[7] In fact, prescription drug use has increased steadily over the past decade: over 48 percent of Americans report having used one or more prescription drugs in the previous 30 days, and more than 10 percent of Americans have used five or more.[8] Even though these drugs are administered under medical supervision, the wise consumer still takes precautions. Adverse effects and complications arising from the use of prescription drugs are common, as is failure to respond to a medication.

Consumers have a variety of resources available to help them make educated decisions about whether to take a certain drug. One of the best resources is the FDA's Center for Drug Evaluation and Research website (*www.fda.gov/drugs*), which provides current information for consumers on the risks and benefits of prescription drugs.

Common types of prescription drugs discussed in this text include antidepressants and antianxiety drugs (Chapter 2); hormonal contraceptives (Chapter 10); weight-loss aids (Chapter 6); smoking-cessation aids (Chapter 12); stimulants, sedatives, and narcotic analgesics (Chapter 13); antibiotics (Chapter 14); and statins and other cholesterol-lowering drugs (Chapter 16).

**Generic drugs**, prescription medications sold under a chemical name rather than a brand name, contain the same active ingredients as brand-name drugs but are usually much less expensive. Not all drugs are available as generics. If your doctor prescribes medication, ask if a generic equivalent exists and if it would be safe and effective for you to try.

Although generic medications behave very similarly to brand-name versions and show a similar efficacy, there is some concern that substitutions made in minor ingredients

might reduce a patient's response to the drug or cause side effects.[9] Always tell your doctor about any reactions you have to medications.

### Over-the-Counter Drugs
Medications available without a prescription are referred to as *over-the-counter (OTC)* drugs. American consumers spend billions of dollars yearly on OTC preparations for relief of everything from runny noses to ingrown toenails. Those most commonly used are pain relievers; cold, cough, and allergy medications; stimulants; sleeping aids and relaxants; and dieting aids.

Despite a common belief that OTC products are safe and effective, indiscriminate use and abuse can occur with these drugs as with all others. For example, people who frequently use eye drops to "get the red out" or pop antacids after every meal are likely to become dependent. Many people also experience adverse side effects because they ignore warnings on drug interactions and other cautions printed on labels. The FDA has developed a standard label that appears on most OTC products (see **FIGURE 19.1**). It includes directions for use, active and inactive ingredients, warnings, and other useful information. Bear in mind that, as discussed in Chapter 6 (page 169), the FDA does not classify dietary supplements—including vitamins and minerals, amino acids, herbs, diet aids, and similar preparations—as drugs, and therefore does not evaluate their safety or effectiveness.

## LO 3 | COMPLEMENTARY AND INTEGRATIVE HEALTH CARE

Discuss complementary and integrative health care, identifying three basic categories and the most commonly used approaches within each.

Complementary health approaches are practices and products commonly used together with conventional medicine.[10] A patient with chronic back pain, for example, may combine massage therapy with prescription medication. In contrast, alternative health approaches are used in place of conventional medicine, such as following a special diet or herbal remedy to treat cancer instead of using surgery, radiation, or other conventional treatments. The *National Center for Complementary and Integrative Health (NCCIH)* reports that, in the United States, true alternative medicine is rare; most people who use nonmainstream approaches use them alongside conventional treatments.[11]

Doctors of medicine (MDs), doctors of osteopathy (DOs), nurses, and various allied health professionals practice conventional medicine. These practitioners may recommend massage therapy, specific vitamin or mineral supplements, or other complementary therapies for individual patients. However, some practitioners incorporate complementary therapies into their conventional

**generic drugs** Medications marketed by chemical names rather than brand names.

**complementary health approaches** Health care practices and products commonly used together with conventional medicine.

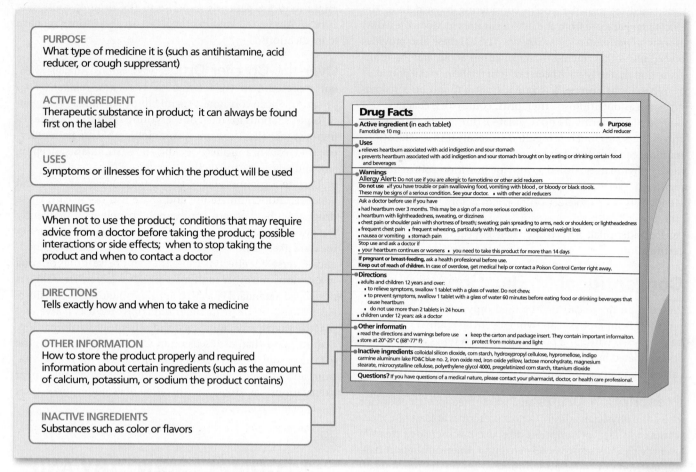

**FIGURE 19.1** The Over-the-Counter Medicine Label

**Source:** Consumer Healthcare Products Association, OTC Label. Courtesy of CHPA Educational Foundation, www.otcsafety.org.

→ **VIDEO TUTOR**
Being a Good Health Care Consumer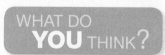

health care, often working closely with alternative specialists in a coordinated, purposeful way. This approach is known as **integrative medicine.**[12]

A survey conducted by the NCCIH revealed that 33 percent of U.S. adults use one or more complementary therapies.[13] **FIGURE 19.2** identifies those most commonly used. Why do so many people find complementary approaches appealing? Many people turn to these therapies to promote their general wellness or to relieve symptoms associated with a chronic disease or the side effects of conventional medicine.[14] They may also be seeking a *holistic* approach; that is, care that focuses on the mind and the whole body, rather than just an isolated symptom or body part. They may also desire a less invasive, gentler approach to healing, one that allows them a greater measure of control over their treatment.

Although practitioners of most complementary health approaches spend many years in training, each approach has a different set of training standards, guidelines for practice, and licensure procedures. Also, states may differ in their requirements and regulations.

Before you consider using any complementary therapy, visit the website of the NCCIH, a division of the National Institutes of Health (NIH). Its mission is to study complementary health approaches using rigorous scientific methods, and build an evidence base regarding their safety and effectiveness. The organization serves as an information clearinghouse and conducts research, education, and outreach programs.

The NCCIH groups the complementary health approaches (**FIGURE 19.3**) into three general categories of practice: natural products, mind and body practices, and other complementary health approaches—what we'll call complementary medical systems.

**integrative medicine** The integration of complementary health approaches into conventional health care in a purposeful way.

**WHAT DO YOU THINK?**

Do you believe that patients should have access to information about practitioners' and facilities' malpractice records?

■ What about information on success and failure rates or outcomes of various procedures?

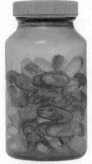
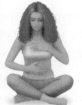

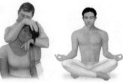

| 17.7% | 10.9% | 10.1% | 8.4% | 8.0% | 6.9% | 3.0% | 2.2% | 2.1% | 1.7% |
| Natural products | Deep breathing | Yoga, tai chi, or qi gong | Chiropractic & osteopathic | Meditation | Massage | Special diets | Homeopathic treatment | Progressive relaxation | Guided imagery |

**FIGURE 19.2** The Ten Most Common Complementary Therapies among U.S. Adults

Source: Data are from T. C. Clarke, et al., "Trends in the Use of Complementary Health Approachs among Adults: United States, 2002–2012," *National Health Statistics Reports*, no. 79 (2015), February 2015, www.cdc.gov/nchs/data/nhsr/nhs079.pdf.

 **VIDEO TUTOR**
CAM: Risks vs. Benefits

## Complementary Medical Systems

**Complementary medical systems** reflect specific theories of physiology, health, and disease that have developed outside the influence of conventional medicine. Many have been practiced throughout the world for centuries. For example, Native American, Aboriginal, African, Middle Eastern, South American, and Asian cultures have their own unique healing systems. Here, we discuss those most commonly available in the United States.

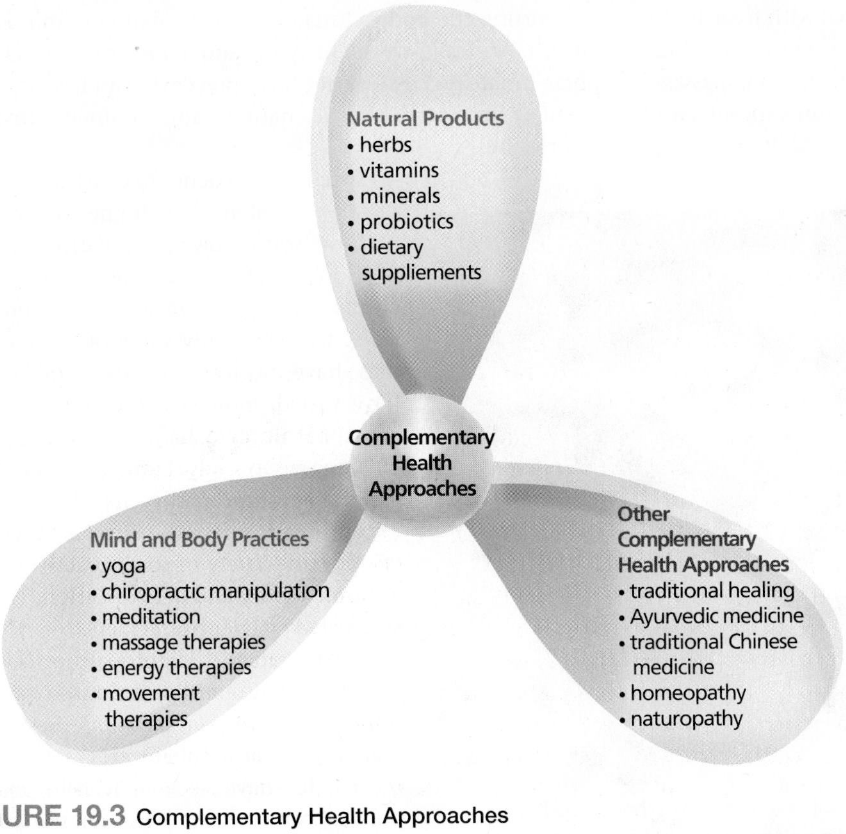

**Traditional Chinese Medicine** The concept of *qi* (pronounced "chee"), or vital energy, is foundational to **traditional Chinese medicine (TCM)**. When *qi* is in balance, the person is in a state of health; imbalance of *qi* results in disease. Diagnosis is based on personal history, observation of the body (especially the tongue), palpation, and pulse diagnosis, a detailed procedure requiring considerable skill. Techniques such as acupuncture, herbal medicine, massage, and *qigong* (a form of energy therapy) are among the TCM approaches to health and healing. TCM is complex, and research into its effectiveness is limited.[15] Analysis of Chinese herbal medicines have found some of them to be contaminated by toxic heavy metals, drugs not listed on the label, and other potentially harmful ingredients.[16]

Traditional Chinese medicine practitioners within the United States must have completed a graduate program in a college or university approved by the Accreditation Commission for

**Natural Products**
- herbs
- vitamins
- minerals
- probiotics
- dietary supplements

**Complementary Health Approaches**

**Mind and Body Practices**
- yoga
- chiropractic manipulation
- meditation
- massage therapies
- energy therapies
- movement therapies

**Other Complementary Health Approaches**
- traditional healing
- Ayurvedic medicine
- traditional Chinese medicine
- homeopathy
- naturopathy

**FIGURE 19.3** Complementary Health Approaches

Source: Based on National Center for Complementary and Integrative Health, "Complementary, Alternative, or Integrative Health: What's In a Name?" April 12, 2016, https://nccih.nih.gov/health/integrative-health#types.

**complementary medical systems** Broad approaches to health care that reflect specific theories of physiology, health, and disease that have developed outside the influence of conventional medicine.

**traditional Chinese medicine (TCM)** Ancient comprehensive system of healing that uses herbs, acupuncture, massage, and qigong to bring vital energy, *qi*, into balance and to remove blockages of *qi* that lead to disease.

**Ayurveda (Ayurvedic medicine)** A comprehensive system of medicine, originating in ancient India, that places equal emphasis on the body, mind, and spirit and strives to restore the body's innate harmony through diet, exercise, meditation, herbs, massage, sun exposure, and controlled breathing.

**homeopathy (homeopathic medicine)** Unconventional Western system of medicine based on the principle that "like cures like" and the "law of minimum dose."

**naturopathy (naturopathic medicine)** System of medicine in which practitioners work to support the body's innate healing mechanisms and use treatment approaches such as diet, exercise, and massage that are minimally invasive.

Acupuncture and Oriental Medicine (ACAOM). Graduate programs usually involve an extensive 3- or 4-year clinical internship. In addition, the student must pass a certification and licensing examination by the National Commission for the Certification of Acupuncture and Oriental Medicine.

### Ayurveda

The "science of life," **Ayurveda** (**Ayurvedic medicine**) is one of the world's oldest medical systems, evolving over 3,000 years ago in India. Ayurveda seeks to integrate and balance the body, mind, and spirit to restore harmony in the individual.[17] Practitioners use techniques including questioning, observation, and pulse palpation to determine which of three vital energies, or *doshas*, is dominant in the patient. Treatment plans aim to bring the doshas into balance, thereby reducing symptoms. Dietary modification and herbal remedies drawn from the botanical wealth of the Indian subcontinent are common. Research into Ayurveda is limited, but studies have shown some of its herbal remedies to be effective for certain joint and digestive disorders.[18] However, like some TCMs, some Ayurvedic remedies sold online have been found tainted with toxic heavy metals, including lead, mercury, or arsenic.[19] Other Ayurvedic treatments include certain yoga postures, meditation, massage, steam baths, changes in sleep patterns and sun exposure, and controlled breathing.

Training of Ayurvedic practitioners varies. There is no national standard for certification, although professional groups are working toward creating licensing guidelines.

### Homeopathy

**Homeopathy (homeopathic medicine)** is an unconventional Western system of medicine based on the principle that "like cures like." In other words, the same substance that in a large dose produces the symptoms of an illness—and may even be fatal—will in a small dose prompt the body's own defenses to cure the illness. Developed in the late 1700s by Samuel Hahnemann, a German physician, homeopathy follows the "law of minimum dose," which asserts that the lower the dose of a remedy, the greater its effectiveness. Thus, homeopathic remedies, which are derived from a wide range of natural, sometimes toxic, substances such as arsenic and belladonna, may be so diluted that no molecules of the original substance remain.[20] The NCCIH reports that certain foundational concepts in homeopathy are at odds with foundational concepts of physics and chemistry, and that little evidence supports homeopathy for treatment of any specific condition.[21]

Homeopathic training varies considerably, from diploma programs to correspondence courses. Only Arizona, Connecticut, and Nevada have homeopathic licensing boards. Requirements to practice vary from state to state.

### Naturopathy

**Naturopathy (naturopathic medicine)** is a system of medicine that emphasizes the power of nature to restore health. Naturopathic physicians view their role as supporting the body's innate ability to maintain and restore health, typically by identifying and removing obstacles to these innate processes. They favor prevention and, when treatment is necessary, holistic, natural, and minimally invasive approaches.[22]

Specific approaches to care include diet; dietary supplements; homeopathy; spinal and soft-tissue manipulation; detoxification using fasting, juice diets, colon cleansing, or other means; and therapeutic counseling. Only some of these therapies have been researched, and results have varied; moreover, the complexity of naturopathic care has made this system challenging to study. Limited research suggests that naturopathy may be effective for chronic lower-back pain. However, the efficacy and safety of some practices, such as homeopathy and detoxification, are not supported by scientific evidence.[23]

Several major naturopathic schools in the United States and Canada provide training. *Naturopathic physicians* have completed a 4-year graduate program and, in most states, have passed a licensing examination. Naturopaths who are not physicians may have received varied training and typically are unlicensed.

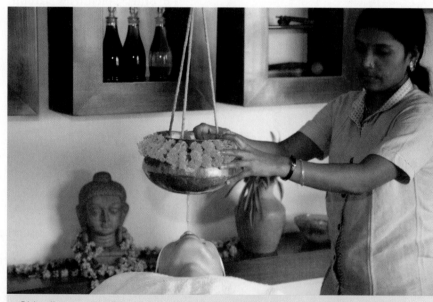

*Shirodhara*—a traditional Ayurvedic treatment in which warm, herbalized oil is poured over the forehead in guided rhythmic patterns—is said to relieve stress and anxiety, treat insomnia and chronic headaches, and improve memory.

# 32%

of 18- to 44-year-olds in the U.S. report having used some form of COMPLEMENTARY HEALTH APPROACH.

## Mind and Body Practices

Mind and body practices are a large and diverse group of complementary health approaches that a trained practitioner or teacher often teaches or administers.[24] They include movement reeducation therapies, as well as modalities in which the practitioner directly manipulates body tissues, attempts to shift the flow of body energy, or teaches the client techniques to promote relaxation or manage stress. As shown in FIGURE 19.2, several relaxation techniques for stress management—including yoga, deep breathing, meditation, and progressive relaxation—are among the ten most commonly used complementary therapies in the United States (see Chapter 3). **Manipulative therapies** are approaches based on manipulation or movement of body tissues and structures.

### Chiropractic Medicine
**Chiropractic medicine** has been practiced for more than 100 years and focuses on disorders of the muscular and skeletal system and the use of various modalities to reduce health effects from these disorders.[25] Over the decades, allopathic medicine and chiropractic medicine have been in direct competition. Today, many health care providers work closely with chiropractors, and many insurance companies pay for chiropractic treatment, particularly if it is recommended by a medical doctor.

Chiropractic medicine is based on the principle that energy flows through the nervous system, including the spinal cord. If the spine is partly misaligned or dislocated, that force is disrupted. Chiropractors use a variety of techniques to manipulate the spine into proper alignment so energy can flow unimpeded. Typically chiropractors treat low-back pain; neck pain; and pain in the arms, legs, and feet, as well as headaches. Spinal manipulation, a common technique in chiropractic care, appears to be as beneficial in relieving low-back pain as pain-relief medications and other common remedies.[26]

Chiropractic training typically begins with a premedical undergraduate degree followed by entrance into a 4-year chiropractic program involving intensive coursework similar to that of medical school programs, combined with hands-on clinical training. Graduates must also pass a licensing examination given by the National Board of Chiropractic Examiners. Chiropractic practice is licensed and regulated in all 50 states.[27]

### Massage Therapy
References to massage exist in numerous ancient texts, including those of Greece, Rome, Japan, China, Egypt, and India.[28] **Massage therapy** is soft tissue manipulation by trained therapists for relaxation and healing. Therapists manipulate the patient's muscles and connective tissues to loosen the fibers and break up adhesions, improve the body's circulation, and remove waste products. The NCCIH reports that research evidence supports the effectiveness of massage therapy to temporarily relieve musculoskeletal pain such as low-back and neck pain, and it may help to promote relaxation and relieve depression.[29]

The course of study in massage schools varies greatly by state, but typically covers sciences such as anatomy and physiology as well as massage techniques, and business, ethical, and legal considerations.[30] For licensing, many states require a minimum of 500 hours of training and a passing grade on a national certification exam. Massage therapists work in private studios and health spas and in medical and chiropractic offices, nursing homes, hotels, and fitness centers.[31]

### Movement Therapies
A broad range of Eastern and Western complementary health approaches use movement,

**manipulative therapies** Treatments involving manipulation or movement of one or more body structures or the whole body.

**chiropractic medicine** System of treatment that involves manipulation of the spine and neuromuscular structures to promote proper energy flow.

**massage therapy** Soft tissue manipulation by trained therapists for relaxation and healing.

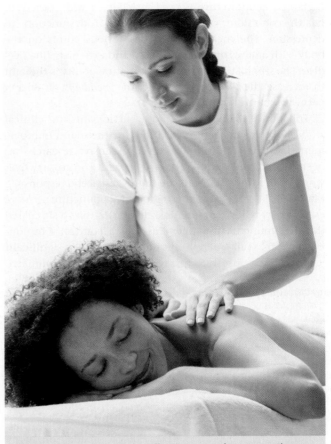

Many studies support the effectiveness of massage therapy for musculoskeletal pain.

including postural realignment, to increase physical, mental, and emotional well-being and reduce limitations in body functioning. Two commonly available approaches include:

- The *Alexander technique*, a movement education method designed to release harmful tension in the body to improve ease of movement, balance, and coordination.
- The *Feldenkrais method*, a system of gentle movements and exercises designed to improve movement, flexibility, coordination, and overall functioning through techniques that enhance the client's awareness and retrain the nervous system.

## Energy Therapies

**Energy therapies** focus either on energy fields thought to originate within the body (biofields) or from other sources (electromagnetic fields). The existence of these fields has not been experimentally proven. Popular examples of energy therapy include acupuncture, acupressure, qigong, Reiki, and therapeutic touch.

## Acupuncture

One of the oldest and most popular TCM therapies, **acupuncture** is used to relieve a wide variety of health conditions, from musculoskeletal dysfunction to depression. The therapist stimulates various points on the body with a series of precisely placed and extremely fine needles. The stimulation of these acupuncture points is thought to increase the flow of *qi* through the *meridians*, or energy pathways, in the body (**FIGURE 19.4**).

Following acupuncture, most participants in clinical studies report satisfaction with the treatment and improvement in their condition; however, extensive research has been inconclusive, and there is significant controversy over whether or not such results are simply a placebo response.[32] Many studies, for example, have found acupuncture no more effective for relieving musculoskeletal pain than a simulated (fake) acupuncture treatment used as a control.[33] In contrast, a 2014 meta-analysis did find a statistically significant increased response rate for acupuncture over a simulated treatment for back pain, neck pain, and chronic headaches.[34]

Most U.S. states require a license, certification, or registration to practice acupuncture. Licensing requirements vary by state; however, most states require a diploma from the National Certification Commission for Acupuncture and Oriental Medicine. In addition, many conventional physicians and dentists practice acupuncture.[35]

**energy therapies** Therapies using energy fields, such as electromagnetic fields or biofields.

**acupuncture** Technique of traditional Chinese medicine that involves the placement of long, thin needles to affect flow of energy (*qi*) along energy pathways (meridians) within the body.

**acupressure** Technique of traditional Chinese medicine that uses application of pressure to selected points along meridians to balance energy.

**Acupressure** Like acupuncture, **acupressure** is based on the principles of energy flow as *qi*. Instead of inserting needles, however, the therapist applies pressure. The goal of the therapy is for *qi* to be evenly distributed and flow freely throughout the body. Practitioners typically have the same basic training and understanding of meridians and acupuncture points as do acupuncturists.

**Other Forms of Energy Therapy** *Qigong*, a technique of TCM, brings together movement, meditation, and regulation of breathing to increase the flow of *qi*, enhance blood circulation, and improve immune function. A 2015

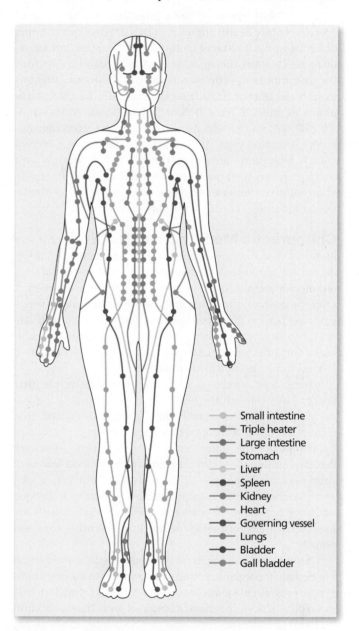

| | Small intestine |
| | Triple heater |
| | Large intestine |
| | Stomach |
| | Liver |
| | Spleen |
| | Kidney |
| | Heart |
| | Governing vessel |
| | Lungs |
| | Bladder |
| | Gall bladder |

**FIGURE 19.4 The Main Meridian Channels** Acupuncture and acupressure are two therapies within traditional Chinese medicine based on the belief that vital energy flows through meridian channels in the body.

**Source:** Courtesy of the Association for Energy and Meridian Therapies (The AMT), East Sussex, UK, http://theamt.com.

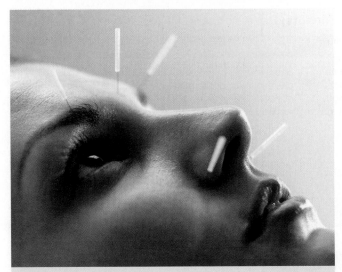

In acupuncture, long, thin needles are inserted into specific points along the body. This is theorized to increase the flow of a vital energy known as *qi*, providing many physical and mental benefits.

systematic review of meta-analyses found that the practice of qigong and other meditative movement therapies was associated with statistically significant improvements in pain management and other aspects of health-related quality of life for people recovering from breast cancer, as well as people with low-back pain, heart failure, and other conditions.[36]

*Reiki* is a nontouch form of energy therapy that originated in Japan. The name is derived from the Japanese words representing "universal" and "vital energy," or *ki*. Reiki is based on the belief that by channeling *ki* to the patient, the practitioner facilitates healing. In two related nontouch energy therapies, *therapeutic touch* and *healing touch*, the therapist attempts to perceive, through his or her hands held just above the patient's body, imbalances in the patient's energy. The therapist promotes healing by increasing the flow of the body's energies and bringing them into balance. Although a 2014 systematic review found at least a partial therapeutic response from nontouch energy therapies, the variety of experimental designs and small size of the studies prevented the researchers from drawing conclusions about their effectiveness.[37]

## Natural Products

Natural products include functional foods and dietary supplements (for definitions and basic descriptions, see Chapter 7). They are the most commonly used and perhaps the most controversial of complementary health approaches because of the sheer number of options available, the many claims that are made about their effects, and their less stringent regulation.

First, although it's tempting to assume that natural products are safe because they are labeled "natural," the FDA has not developed a definition for the term *natural*, and cautions consumers to avoid assuming that any food or dietary supplement claiming to be "natural" is safe.[38] For example, in recent years, dietary supplements have caused a variety of health problems, such as liver damage, heart problems, and miscarriage, and some have been found to be contaminated with bacteria, toxic metals, and hidden drug ingredients, as well as grass, gluten, or other potential allergens. When seeking out supplements, choose those labeled with the U.S. Pharmacopoeia Verified Mark (FIGURE 19.5)—a label that means what it says on the bottle is in the bottle, that the labeled supplement doesn't contain unsafe levels of contaminants, and that the product was created with well-controlled, sanitary processes.[39]

The NCCIH "Alerts and Advisories" web page continually releases notifications of natural products that are contaminated or contain hidden drug ingredients. A 2016 FDA recall, for example, involved two weight-loss products containing ingredients that had been withdrawn from the market by the FDA because of their association with potentially fatal heart attacks, strokes, serious gastrointestinal disturbances, and cancer.[40] Moreover, the NCCIH has reported that some natural products can be dangerous when combined with prescription or over-the-counter drugs, can disrupt the normal action of the drugs, or can cause unusual side effects.[41]

In recent years, there have been increasing media claims about the health benefits of various hormones, enzymes, and other biological and synthetic compounds. Although a few products, such as melatonin (a hormone) or zinc lozenges (a mineral), have been widely studied, there is little quality research to support the claims of many others. TABLE 19.1 gives an overview of some of the most common dietary supplements on the market.

Individuals must take an active role in their health care, which means staying educated. See the Making Changes Today box on page 517 for tips on how to make smart decisions about integrating complementary therapies into your health care.

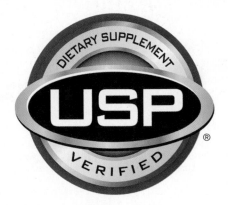

FIGURE 19.5 The USP Verified Mark is only given to those products that meet a set of testing criteria, including accurately labeling content, no unsafe levels of contaminants, and sanitary processes. Registered Trademark of U.S. Pharmacopeial Convention (USP). Used with Permission.

Source: U.S. Pharmacopoeial Convention, "USP Verified Dietary Supplements," Accessed May 2016, http://www.usp.org/usp-verification-services/usp-verified-dietary-supplements.

## TABLE 19.1 | Common Dietary Supplements: Benefits, Research, and Risks

| Herb | Claims of Benefits | Research Findings | Potential Risks |
|---|---|---|---|
| Echinacea (purple coneflower, *Echinacea purpurea, E. angustifolia, E. pallida*) | Stimulates the immune system and helps fight infection. Used to both prevent and treat colds and flu. | Some studies have provided preliminary evidence of its effectiveness in treating respiratory infections, but two recent studies found no benefit either for prevention or treatment. | Allergic reactions, including rashes, increased asthma, gastrointestinal problems, and anaphylaxis (a life-threatening allergic reaction). |
| Flaxseed (*Linum usitatissimum*) and flaxseed oil | Used as a laxative and for hot flashes and breast pain, as well as to reduce cholesterol levels and risk of heart disease and cancer. | Flaxseed contains soluble fiber and may have a laxative effect. Study results are mixed on whether flaxseed decreases hot flashes. Insufficient data are available on the effect of flaxseed on cholesterol levels, heart disease, or cancer risks. | Delays absorption of medicines, but otherwise has few side effects. Oil taken in excess could cause diarrhea. Should be taken with plenty of water. |
| Ginkgo (*Ginkgo biloba*) | Popularly used to prevent cognitive decline, dementia, and Alzheimer's disease, and general vascular disease. | Although some small studies have had promising results, the large Ginkgo Evaluation of Memory study found ginkgo did not reduce Alzheimer's disease or dementia, slow cognitive decline, or reduce blood pressure. | Gastric irritation, headache, nausea, dizziness, difficulty thinking, memory loss, and allergic reactions. Ginkgo seeds are highly toxic; only products made from leaf extracts should be used. |
| Ginseng (*Panax ginseng*) | Claimed to increase resistance to stress, boost the immune system, lower blood glucose and blood pressure, and improve stamina and sex drive. | Some studies suggest that ginseng may improve immune function and lower blood glucose; however, research overall is inconclusive. | Headaches, insomnia, and gastrointestinal problems are the most commonly reported adverse effects. |
| Green tea (*Camellia sinensis*) | Useful for lowering cholesterol and risk of some cancers, protecting the skin from sun damage, bolstering mental alertness, and boosting heart health. | Although some studies have shown promising links between green and white tea consumption and cancer prevention, recent research questions the ability of tea to significantly reduce the risk of breast, lung, or prostate cancer. | Insomnia, liver problems, anxiety, irritability, upset stomach, nausea, diarrhea, or frequent urination. |
| Zinc (mineral) | Supports immune system; lozenges used to lessen duration and severity of cold symptoms. | Some research suggests that zinc lozenges can reduce the severity and duration of a cold if taken within 24 hours of onset of symptoms. | Use of zinc lozenges can cause nausea. Excessive use can reduce immune function. |

**Sources:** National Center for Complementary and Alternative Medicine, "Herbs at a Glance," January 2014, http://nccih.nih.gov/health/herbsataglance.htm; American Cancer Society, "Green Tea," May 2012, www.cancer.org; Office of Dietary Supplements, National Institutes of Health, "Dietary Supplement Fact Sheets." April 2014, http://ods.od.nih.gob/Health_Informaion_About_Individual_Dietary_Supplements.aspx

## LO 4 | **HEALTH** INSURANCE

Describe the U.S. health care system in terms of types of insurance; the changing structure of the systems; and issues concerning cost, quality, and access to services.

No matter how you access health care, chances are you'll use some form of health insurance to pay for your care. Insurance typically allows you to pay into a pool of funds and then bill the insurance carrier for covered charges you incur. The fundamental principle of insurance underwriting is that the cost of health care can be predicted for large populations. This is how health care **premiums** are determined. Policyholders pay

**premium** Payment made to an insurance carrier, usually in monthly installments, that covers the cost of an insurance policy.

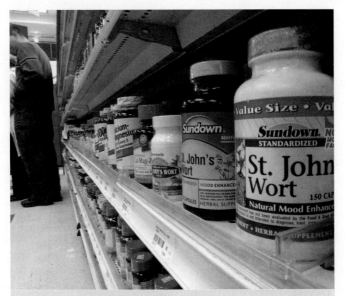

To prevent potentially serious adverse effects, avoid combining herbs with prescription or over-the-counter medications without approval from your primary care practitioner. St. John's wort, for example, has potentially dangerous interactions with some prescription antidepressants and should never be taken with them.

premiums into a pool from which insurance companies pay claims. When you are sick or injured, the insurance company pays your care provider out of the pool regardless of your total contribution. If you require a great deal of medical care, you may never pay anything close to the actual cost of that care. Or, if you are basically healthy, you may pay more in insurance premiums than the total cost of your medical bills. Health insurance is based on the idea that policyholders pay affordable premiums so they never have to face catastrophic bills. In profit-oriented systems, insurers prefer to have healthy people in their plans who pour money into risk pools without taking money out.

In 2010, Congress passed the Patient Protection *and* Affordable Care Act (ACA), (commonly referred to as "*Obamacare*"). Among other provisions, it mandates that all Americans have at least minimal essential health insurance coverage or pay a penalty known as the *individual insurance shared responsibility payment*. The amount is paid when the individual or couple files their tax return. The precise payment changes annually and can be calculated in a variety of ways. For example, in 2016, the per-person calculation was $695 for one adult.[42] The mandate—along with other provisions of the ACA that increase affordability of health insurance for Americans—have increased enrollment in private plans, managed care, and government-funded programs. We discuss each of these types here.

## Private Health Insurance

Originally, health insurance consisted solely of coverage for hospital costs (it was called *major medical*), but was gradually extended to cover routine physicians' treatment and other services, such as dental, vision care, and pharmaceuticals. These payment mechanisms laid the groundwork for today's steadily rising health care costs as hospitals were reimbursed for the costs of providing care plus an amount for profit. This system provided no incentive to contain costs, limit the number of procedures, or curtail capital investment in redundant equipment and facilities. Physicians were reimbursed on a fee-for-service (indemnity) basis determined by "usual, customary, and reasonable" fees. This system encouraged physicians to charge high fees, raise them often, and perform as many procedures as possible. Until the mid- to late twentieth century, most insurance did not cover routine or preventive services, and consumers generally waited until illness developed to see a doctor instead of seeking preventive care. Consumers were also free to choose any provider or service they wished, including even inappropriate—and often expensive—levels of care.

To limit potential losses, private insurance companies began increasingly

### WHAT DO YOU THINK?

**Why is it important that private insurance cover preventive or lower-level care as well as hospitalization and high-tech interventions?**

- ▪ What kinds of incentives would cause you to seek care early rather than delay care?

employing the following cost-sharing mechanisms and coverage limits:

- *Deductibles* are payments (which can range from about $500 to $5,000 annually) you make for health care before insurance coverage kicks in to pay for eligible services.
- *Co-payments* are set amounts that you pay per service or product received, regardless of the total cost (e.g., $20 per doctor visit or per prescription filled).
- *Coinsurance* is the percentage of costs that you must pay based on the terms of the policy (e.g., 20% of the total bill).
- Some group plans specify a *waiting period* that cannot exceed 90 days before they will provide coverage. Waiting periods do not apply to plans purchased by individuals.
- All insurers set some limits on the types of *covered services* (e.g., most exclude cosmetic surgery, private rooms, and experimental procedures).
- *Preexisting condition clauses* once limited the insurance company's liability for medical conditions that a consumer had before obtaining coverage. Under the ACA, no one can be discriminated against due to a preexisting condition.
- Some plans imposed an *annual upper limit* or *lifetime limit*, after which coverage would end. The ACA makes this practice illegal.

During the past few decades, private health insurance has become increasingly unaffordable for many Americans. To address this concern, the ACA authorized the U.S. Centers for Medicare and Medicaid Services to sponsor an online health insurance "marketplace" (at *www.healthcare.gov*) where Americans can compare the benefits and costs of plans available in their region. As they choose a plan, those with qualifying incomes are notified of their eligibility for federal subsidies to reduce their premiums. The marketplace and its federal subsidies have boosted enrollments not only in private health insurance plans, but also in managed care plans and government-funded programs.

## Managed Care

**Managed care** describes a health care delivery system consisting of the following:

- A network of physicians, hospitals, and other providers and facilities linked contractually to deliver comprehensive health benefits within a predetermined budget and sharing economic risk for any budget deficit or surplus
- A budget based on an estimate of the annual cost of delivering health care for a given population
- An established set of administrative rules regarding how services are to be obtained from participating health care providers under the terms of the health plan

Many managed care plans pay their contracted health care providers through **capitation**, a fixed monthly amount paid

**managed care** Type of health insurance plan based on coordination of care and cost-reduction strategies; emphasizes health education and preventive care.

**capitation** Prepayment of a fixed monthly amount for each patient without regard to the type or number of services provided.

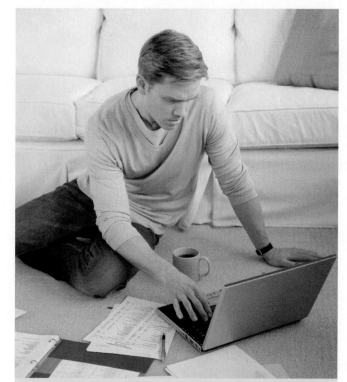

Choosing a health insurance plan can be confusing. Some things to think about include how comprehensive your coverage needs to be, how much you are willing to spend on premiums and co-payments, and whether the services of the plan meet your needs.

for each enrolled patient regardless of services provided. Some plans pay health care providers a salary, and some are still fee-for-service plans. Doctors participating in managed care networks are motivated (and sometimes incentivized) to keep their patient pool healthy and avoid preventable catastrophic illnesses. Prevention and early intervention are often capstone components of such plans.

The three most common types of managed care available in the United States are *health maintenance organizations* (HMOs), *preferred provider organizations* (PPOs), and *point of service* (POS).[43]

**Health Maintenance Organizations** The most common type of managed care plan is the *health maintenance organization* (HMO). More than 90 million Americans were enrolled in HMOs in 2015.[44] HMOs provide a wide range of covered health benefits (e.g., physician visits, lab tests, surgery) for a fixed amount prepaid by the patient, the employer, Medicaid, or Medicare. Usually, HMO premiums are the least expensive form of managed care, but they are also the most restrictive (offering more limited choices of staff and health care facilities). Premiums are 8 to 10 percent lower than for traditional plans, there are low or no deductibles or coinsurance payments, and co-payments are small.

The downside of HMOs is that patients are required to use the plan's doctors and hospitals. Within an HMO, the PCP serves as a *gatekeeper*, coordinating the patient's care and providing referrals to specialists and other services. As more and more people enroll in HMOs, concerns have arisen about care allocation and access to services, profit-motivated medical decision making, and the degree of focus on prevention and intervention.

## Preferred Provider Organization

A *preferred provider organization* (PPO) is a network of independent doctors and hospitals that contracts to provide care at discounted rates. Although PPOs often offer a broader choice of providers than HMOs do, they are less likely to coordinate a patient's care. Members may choose to see doctors who are not on the preferred list at a higher percentage of out-of-pocket costs.

## Point of Service

A hybrid of HMO and PPO plans are *point of service* (POS) plans. They provide a more familiar form of managed care for people used to traditional indemnity insurance in which services are directly reimbursed, a factor that may explain why POS plans are among the fastest-growing of managed care plans. Under POS plans, members select an in-network PCP, but they can go to nonnetwork providers for care without a referral and must pay the extra cost.

## Other Types of Managed Care

*Independent practice associations* (IPAs) comprise independent physicians who maintain their own offices, but who also agree to enroll members of an organization for a negotiated fee for each assigned patient, or a negotiated fee-for-service basis. IPAs can help eliminate isolation, risks, and expenses associated with independent private practice. *Exclusive provider organizations* (EPOs) are a type of managed care in which no coverage is typically provided for services received outside the EPO. Treatment or care received outside of the approved network must be paid by the patient.

## Elite Plans: "Concierge" Options

For those frustrated with long waits to see a doctor and impersonal care, concierge medicine allows you to get to know your doctor very well—for a price. Concierge patients select a doctor or specialist and for a fee—as much as $5,000 to $10,000 in some cities—a person receives unlimited access to their doctor, usually within a day. Patients maintain their regular health insurance as these plans normally don't pay for lab tests, diagnostic tests, hospital, or specialized treatments. They are designed for people who feel like just another number in a long list of patients, to be seen quickly, have individualized interactions and the peace of mind that someone is watching over them—as long as they have money. Critics argue that such care for those with means creates yet another tier system for care. Proponents argue that if you've worked hard and can pay for extra care, you should be able to do so.

No matter what type of plan you have, a variety of strategies can help you maximize your care while minimizing your costs. See the **Money & Health** box on page 520 to find out how.

# Government-Funded Programs

The federal government, through programs such as Medicare and Medicaid, currently funds about 45 percent of the total U.S. health care spending.[45]

## Medicare

A federal insurance program that employees and employers pay into over the course of a person's working life, **Medicare** is a form of long-term savings plan for health insurance and health care, rather than an "entitlement" program. The funds are used to cover a broad range of services, excluding long-term care. Medicare covers citizens or permanent residents of the United States who are 65 or older, have any of certain disabilities, or have permanent end-stage kidney damage. Currently, 53.8 million people receive Medicare (44.9 million aged 65 or older, and 8.9 million disabled persons).[46] As the costs of medical care have continued to increase (over $600 billion in 2014), Medicare has placed limits on the amount of reimbursement to providers.[47] As a result, some providers no longer accept Medicare patients or those new to their practice.

Currently Medicare is divided into two major parts. Part A is the hospital insurance portion and helps pay for care while in hospitals, skilled nursing facilities, hospice care, and limited home health care. Part B covers outpatient services, medical equipment, and supplies and certain preventive services and tests. Part B requires monthly payments (typically deducted from the individual's Social Security check). Those with a higher income pay more than lower-income individuals. Typically, Part B covers most of your care as long as your provider or facility "*accepts assignment*"—meaning that they agree to charge only what Medicare reimburses.

To control hospital costs, the federal government set up a prospective payment system based on *diagnosis-related groups (DRGs)* for Medicare as well as other insurance plans. Nearly 500 groupings establish how much a hospital would be reimbursed for caring for a patient diagnosed with particular conditions. DRGs are based on the assumption that patients with similar health status and conditions require a similar level of care. If the costs of treating a patient are less than the predetermined amount, the hospital can keep the difference. However, if a patient's care costs more than the set amount, the hospital typically must absorb the difference. This system motivates hospitals to discharge patients quickly, to hold them in observation rooms (which are often curtained areas rather than admitting them to more expensive traditional rooms where Medicare may only pay part of their charges), to provide more ambulatory care, and to admit patients classified into the most favorable (profitable) DRGs. Many private health insurance companies have also adopted reimbursement rates based on DRGs.

The Centers for Medicare and Medicaid Services (CMS) has encouraged the growth of HMO plans for Medicare-eligible persons. Under this system, commercial managed care insurance plans receive a fixed per capita premium from CMS and then offer more preventive services with lower out-of-pocket co-payments. These managed care plans encourage providers and patients to utilize health care resources under administrative rules similar to commercial HMO plans.

## Medicare Supplemental Plans

If providers charge more than Medicare allows, either the individual or a so-called *Medigap* plan must make

**Medicare** A federal health insurance program that covers people over the age of 65, permanently disabled people, and people with end-stage kidney failure.

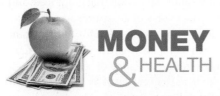

# MONEY & HEALTH | MAXIMIZING CARE WHILE MINIMIZING COSTS

**M**aybe you're like the 3.2 percent of college students who reported in a 2015 survey that they had no health insurance. Or maybe you're on your parents' plan or one sponsored by your college or university, but there's a hefty deductible or co-payment. Or the test or medication you need isn't covered. Whatever your situation, following a few strategies will help you get the best care for the lowest cost.

- **If you have health insurance read the summary plan description (SPD).** This explains what types of care providers, tests, and treatments are covered. The SPD also outlines any co-payments, annual deductibles, and in- and out-of-network rules for seeing specialists. When you know the answers to these questions, you're less likely to make decisions resulting in large bills.
- **Make sure you need health care, not self-care.** The number one reason behind doctor visits is the common cold—for which there's no treatment. For many conditions, rest, nutritious fluids, and the passage of time are the only healers. So think before you spend money on health care you don't need.
- **Try the least expensive health care options first.** For instance, your student health center may be able to provide exactly the level of care you need for little or no cost. Or call the nurse hotline available on your insurance plan. Use the hospital emergency department (ED) only for emergencies. Care in an ED can cost

If you are uninsured or underinsured, ask your doctor for generic prescriptions to save on your costs.

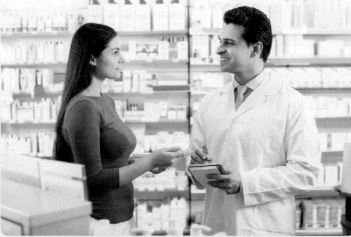

10 times as much as the same care in a walk-in clinic.

- **Ask your doctor to help you get the lowest cost care.** For instance, generic versions of most prescription medications are available, at a cost that may be 50 to 75 percent lower than that of the brand-name drug. Ask the doctor for the generic version of the drug, when possible. If you're still concerned that you can't afford a prescription drug, find out if you qualify for assistance by visiting the website of the Partnership for Prescription Assistance at www.pparx.org. Also talk to your pharmacist, who may be able to direct you to a prescription discount program or online coupon for commonly prescribed drugs.
- **Check bills and benefits statements for accuracy.** Medical bill errors are common, especially duplicated charges and simple typos. Also review the explanation of benefits from your plan to determine whether or not you received the reimbursements you'd expected.

- If your plan denies coverage for a test or treatment that your physician says is necessary, appeal the decision. Check your SPD for your plan's appeals process.
- **Consider opening up a health care spending account.** As long as you're not claimed as a dependent on someone else's tax return, you can open either a Flexible Spending Account through your employer or a Health Savings Account through your bank. These plans give you the opportunity to save money tax free to be used toward qualified health care expenses. If you currently pay out of pocket for more than one or two health care visits a year, for a few prescriptions, contact lenses, etc., and the money you use for these expenses comes from taxable income, then a health care savings plan might be worth a closer look. Contact your employee benefits specialist, your tax preparer, or a customer service provider at your bank.

**Sources:** American College Health Association, *American College Health Association–National College Health Assessment II: Reference Group Executive Summary, Spring 2015* (Baltimore: American College Health Association, 2015); U.S. Department of Labor; Top 10 Ways to Make Your Health Benefits Work for You, www.dol.gov/ebsa/publications/10working4you.html, accessed April 26, 2016; Aetna, Six Ways to Save Money with Your Aetna Student Health Benefits, Aetnastudenthealth.com, www.aetnastudenthealth.com/schools/SavingMoneyFlyer.pdf, accessed April 26, 2016.

up the difference. Medigap plans cover such "gaps" in charges, as well as certain services that Medicare doesn't cover—such as emergency international travel or additional stays in the hospital.

Medicare Advantage plans (often called Medicare Part C) are private plans that contract with Medicare, which funds their coverage of Medicare Part A and B; however, the plans also typically cover other services and operate like an HMO or PPO—forming a sort of hybrid Medicare plan. Some Advantage plans offer dental, vision, or prescription drug coverage. It is important to note that states differ in types of Advantage plans and coverage and that some health care organizations do not accept Medicare Advantage plans.

In an era of rapidly increasing drug costs, prescription drug coverage is an essential part of any Medicare plan. Part A and B Medicare typically covers only minimal drugs, making the purchase of an additional drug plan, known as Medicare Part D, sensible for many individuals. People who opt for Advantage plans must check to find out whether or not their prescriptions are covered.

**Medicaid** A federal–state matching funds program, **Medicaid** provides health insurance for approximately 70 million low-income Americans, including 33 million children.[48] Because each state determines income eligibility, covered services, and payments to providers, there are vast differences in the way Medicaid operates from state to state. The ACA provides generous federal subsidies to states that expand Medicaid coverage to all Americans with incomes up to 133 percent (and, in some states, 138 percent) of the federal poverty threshold (in 2016 the poverty threshold was $24,300 for a four-person household).[49] Although states are not responsible for the costs to expand Medicaid until 2020, at which time states will be required to fund just 10 percent of the costs, some have refused; however, state compliance with the Medicaid expansion brought insurance coverage to 12.3 million previously uninsured low-income Americans between 2013 and 2015.[50]

The Children's Health Insurance Program (CHIP) provides health insurance coverage to more than 8 million uninsured children whose family income is too high to qualify for Medicaid.[51] Like Medicaid, it is jointly funded by federal and state funds and is administered by state governments. Americans seeking health insurance can find out whether or not they qualify for Medicaid or CHIP at *www.healthcare.gov*.

## Insurance Coverage by the Numbers

For 2016, the average family's annual health insurance premium was estimated to exceed $17,500.[52] For workers employed in organizations that offer health care insurance, most of this cost is hidden: The worker pays 15 to 25 percent of the full premium, usually as a deduction from his or her paycheck, and earns lower wages in return for the remaining cost of the coverage.

However, people who are self-employed or work in companies that do not provide group health insurance must pay their premiums independently, often at extremely high rates. Despite the implementation of the ACA, 28.8 million uninsured Americans (over 9 percent of Americans) do not find health insurance affordable.[53] The vast majority of uninsured Americans work or are dependents of workers.

Lack of health insurance has been associated with delayed health care and increased mortality. *Underinsurance* (i.e., the inability to pay out-of-pocket expenses despite having insurance) also may result in adverse health consequences. We noted earlier that, among Americans aged 18 to 24, nearly 15 percent lack health insurance coverage; among those aged 25 to 34, nearly 18 percent lack coverage.[54] College students as a group fare better than noncollege adults when it comes to insurance. In a 2015 national survey of college students, 3.2 percent of respondents said they did not have health insurance.[55] (Hanover, MD: American College Health Association, 2015). People without adequate health care coverage are less likely than other Americans to have their children immunized, seek early prenatal care, obtain annual blood pressure checks and other screenings, and seek attention for symptoms of health problems. Forgoing preventative care because of cost, they tend to rely on emergency care at later stages of illness. Because emergency care is far more expensive than other types of care, uninsured and underinsured patients are often unable to pay, and the cost is absorbed by "the system" in the form of higher hospital costs, insurance premiums, and taxes for all.

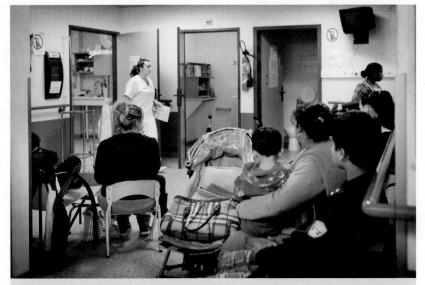

People without insurance can't gain access to preventive care, so they seek care only in an emergency. Because emergency care is extraordinarily expensive, they often are unable to pay, and the cost is shifted to others in the form of increased health care costs, increased insurance rates, and taxes.

Explain key issues facing our health care system today and possible actions that could improve the system.

As mentioned earlier, in 2010, Congress passed the Patient Protection and Affordable Care Act (ACA) to provide a means for all Americans to obtain affordable health care. In addition to increasing access to care, the ACA is addressing the high cost of care and improving the overall quality of care.

## Access

The most significant factors in determining access to health care are the supply and proximity of providers and facilities and availability of insurance coverage.

### Access to Providers, Facilities, and Treatments
In 2014, there were more than 708,000 physicians in the United States.[56] However, there is an oversupply of higher-paid specialists and a shortage of lower-paid primary care physicians (family practitioners, internists, pediatricians, etc.). Moreover, the majority of nongovernment hospitals in the United States are located in urban areas, leaving many rural communities with a lack of facilities.[57]

Managed care health plans determine access on the basis of participating providers, health plan benefits, and administrative rules, which means that consumers have little say in who treats them or what facility they can use.

The ACA and other government investments have increased training for many new health care providers, as well as encouraged primary care providers to set up their practices in high-need areas. Some of these efforts have included:

- Investing in new primary care training programs like the National Health Service Corps and the Graduate Medical Education program.
- Training new primary care providers through increased funding of medical training programs.
- Supporting mental and behavioral health training to boost numbers of those practicing in mental and behavioral health.

### Access to Quality Health Insurance
Because not everyone has the same insurance (or any at all), not everyone gets the same level of care.[58] Key provisions in the ACA aim to increase access to quality health insurance among Americans. These include the following:

- Insurers are now required to cover 15 preventive services (22 for women), such as health screenings for breast, cervical, and colorectal cancer; blood glucose and cholesterol screenings for patients of certain ages or with certain health risks; immunizations; contraception; and counseling on topics such as losing weight, quitting smoking, treating depression, and reducing alcohol use.
- Insurers are required to cover young adults on a parent's plan through age 26.

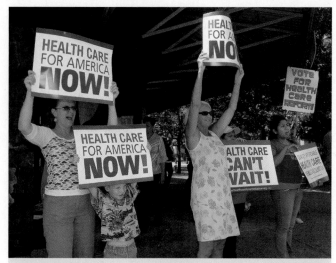

Access to healthcare continues to be a contentious issue in America. Some advocate a taxpayer-financed single-payer system for all, whereas others oppose even the modest provisions of the Affordable Care Act. Meanwhile, millions of Americans remain uninsured.

- Coverage is in place for prescription medications, including psychotropic medications.
- Americans with preexisting conditions cannot be denied coverage.
- No annual and lifetime limits on benefits are allowed.
- An online insurance "marketplace" helps consumers shop for and enroll in plans as well as apply for federal subsidies that lower the cost of premiums for many Americans.
- Small businesses, which typically paid as much as 18 percent more than large businesses, now qualify for special tax credits to help fund insurance plans.

Even before passage of the ACA, Congress provided assistance with insurance coverage for employees who change jobs. Under the Consolidated Omnibus Budget Reconciliation Act (COBRA), former employees, retirees, spouses, and dependents have the option to continue their insurance for up to 18 months at group rates. People who enroll in COBRA do pay a higher amount than they did when they were employed because they are covering both the personal premium and the amount previously covered by the employer.

## Cost

Both per capita and as a percentage of gross domestic product (GDP), the United States spends more on health care than any other nation. In 2014, our national health expenditures were estimated to exceed $3 trillion, about $9,523 for every man, woman, and child.[59] Health care expenditures are projected to grow by 5.8 percent each year, and climb to over 20 percent of our projected GDP by 2025.[60]

Why are U.S. health care costs so high? Many factors are involved: duplication of services; an aging population; growing rates of obesity, inactivity, and related health problems; demand for new diagnostic and treatment technologies; an

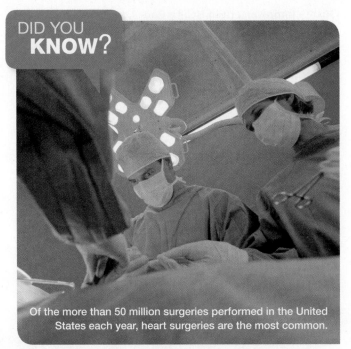

**DID YOU KNOW?**

Of the more than 50 million surgeries performed in the United States each year, heart surgeries are the most common.

**Source:** U.S. Centers for Disease Control and Prevention, "Inpatient Surgery," April, 2016, http://www.cdc.gov/nchs/fastats/inpatient-surgery.htm.

emphasis on crisis-oriented care instead of prevention; physician overtreatment; and inappropriate use of services.

Our insurance system is also to blame. Currently, more than 2,000 companies provide health insurance in the United States, each with different coverage structures and administrative requirements. This lack of uniformity prevents our system from achieving the *economies of scale* (bulk purchasing at a reduced cost) and administrative efficiency realized in countries with a single-payer delivery system. On average, America's commercial insurance companies commonly spend about 16 percent of their total premiums on administrative costs.[61] These expenses contribute to the high cost of health care. See **FIGURE 19.6** for a breakdown of how health care dollars are spent.

The ACA's 80/20 rule mandates that insurance companies that spend less than 80 percent of premium dollars on medical care in a given year now must send enrollees a rebate. Also, insurance companies now have to publicly justify their actions if they plan to raise rates by 10 percent or more.

Another way our insurance system contributes to America's high health care costs is through increasing consolidation. Excluding HMOs and other forms of managed care, just four companies dominate 83 percent of the private health insurance market, a market share that expanded from 74 percent a decade ago.[62] Since

**AN ESTIMATED**

# 440,000

people die each year from **PREVENTABLE MEDICAL ERRORS** in hospitals.

affordable insurance depends on rivalry within the market, reduced competition promotes higher premiums. Moreover, despite the fact that these large companies serve more patients within a geographic area and thus have been able to negotiate lower charges from hospitals and physicians, they have not passed this savings along to their policyholders in the form of lower premiums.[63]

## Quality

The United States has several mechanisms for ensuring quality services: Providers are assessed according to education, licensure, certification/registration, accreditation, peer review, and the legal system of malpractice litigation. Over-the-counter and prescription medications, as well as medical devices, must be approved by the FDA. Insurance companies and the U.S. Centers for Medicare and Medicaid Services may also require a higher level of quality by linking payment to whether a practitioner is board certified, a facility is accredited, or a treatment is an approved therapy. In addition, most insurance plans now

**2013 total expenditures = $2.5 trillion**

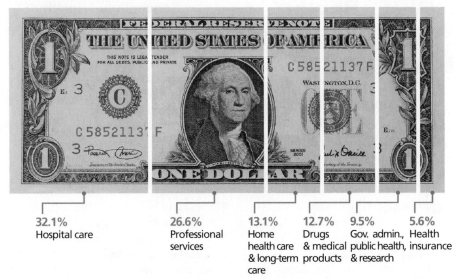

| 32.1% | 26.6% | 13.1% | 12.7% | 9.5% | 5.6% |
|---|---|---|---|---|---|
| Hospital care | Professional services | Home health care & long-term care | Drugs & medical products | Gov. admin., public health, & research | Health insurance |

**FIGURE 19.6** Where Do We Spend Our Health Care Dollars?

**Source:** U.S. Department of Health and Human Services, "Health, United States, 2014," National Center for Health Statistics, May 2015, www.cdc.gov/nchs/data/hus/hus14.pdf.

require prior authorization and/or second opinions, not only to reduce costs, but also to improve quality of care.

Although our health care spending far exceeds that of any other nation, we rank far below many other nations in key indicators of quality such as infant mortality, years of health-related quality of life, and others. For example, in 2016, the Central Intelligence Agency ranked the United States 43rd in life expectancy among 224 nations ranked.[64] At a projected 79.7 years, U.S. life expectancy was a decade below that of the top-ranked country, Monaco.[65] And our *infant mortality rate*, at 5.9 deaths per every 1,000 live births, is higher than that of 57 other nations.[66] The ACA is intended to improve the quality of health care in the United States. As a first step, in 2011 the Department of Health and Human Services released to Congress a National Strategy for

Quality Improvement in Health Care. Updated annually, the National Quality Strategy emphasizes promoting the safest, most preventive, and most effective care; making care affordable for individuals, families, employers, and governments; increasing communication and coordination among providers; and ensuring that patients and families are engaged as partners in their care.[67]

Although many public health experts and citizens feel that the ACA does not go far enough in addressing the unequal access, high cost, and poor quality of our health care system, others believe that it is a step in the right direction. They contend that gradual improvements in technology and implementation and increased state acceptance of federal funding will help the ACA achieve its overall goals of improved cost, quality, and access to care for all Americans.

# STUDY PLAN

Customize your study plan—and master your health!—in the Study Area of **MasteringHealth.**

## ASSESS YOURSELF

**What could you do to become a better health care consumer?** Want to find out? Take the **Are You a Smart Health Care Consumer?** assessment available on **MasteringHealth.™**

## CHAPTER REVIEW

To hear an MP3 Tutor Session, scan here or visit the Study Area in **MasteringHealth.**

### LO 1 Taking Responsibility for Your Health Care

- Knowing when to take care of yourself and when to seek professional help will save you money and improve your health status. Advance planning can help you navigate health care treatment in unfamiliar situations or emergencies. Assess health professionals by considering their qualifications, their record of treating similar problems, and their ability to work with you. Know and advocate for your rights as a patient.

### LO 2 Conventional Health Care

- In theory, conventional Western (allopathic) medicine is based on scientifically validated methods and procedures. Medical doctors, specialists of various kinds, nurses, physician assistants, and other health care professionals practice allopathic medicine.
- Prescription drugs are obtained through a written prescription from a physician, whereas over-the-counter-drugs can be purchased without a prescription. Both are approved and regulated by the U.S. Food and Drug Administration.

### LO 3 Complementary and Integrative Health Care

- Throughout the world, people are using complementary and integrative health care in increasing numbers. Complementary medical systems include traditional Chinese medicine (TCM), ayurveda, homeopathy, and naturopathy. Mind and body practices include chiropractic medicine, massage therapy, movement therapies, and energy therapies. The most commonly used complementary health approach is the broad group of natural products, including functional foods and dietary supplements.

- Consumers need to understand that the FDA does not approve dietary supplements before they are brought to market. Thus, there is no guarantee of their safety or effectiveness. However, they can be removed from the market if they are found to make fraudulent claims or cause harm to consumers.

## LO 4 | Health Insurance

- Health insurance is based on the concept of spreading risk. Insurance is provided by private insurance companies (which charge premiums) and the government Medicare and Medicaid programs (which are funded by taxes). Managed care (in the form of HMOs, PPOs, and POS plans) attempts to control costs by streamlining administrative procedures and promoting preventive care, among other initiatives. Despite implementation of the Affordable Care Act (ACA), more than 9 percent of Americans (28.8 million) are uninsured and millions more are underinsured.[68]

## LO 5 | Issues Facing Today's Health Care System

- Concerns about the U.S. health care system include access, cost, and quality. Lack of uniformity in our health insurance system and increasing consolidation of insurance companies contribute to high costs, as do our aging population, high levels of obesity, physician overtreatment, and many other factors. The Patient Protection and Affordable Care Act, passed by Congress in 2010, has increased access to insurance for millions of Americans, and has mandated quality improvements such as full coverage for certain types of preventive care and coverage for Americans with preexisting conditions. However, many public health experts feel that it does not go far enough.

# POP QUIZ

Visit **MasteringHealth** to personalize your study plan with Chapter Review Quizzes and Dynamic Study Modules.

## LO 1 | Taking Responsibility for Your Health Care

1. Of the following conditions, which would be appropriately managed by self-care?
   a. A persistent temperature of 104°F or higher
   b. Sudden weight loss of more than a few pounds without changes in diet or exercise patterns
   c. A sore throat, runny nose, and cough that persist for several days
   d. Yellowing of the skin or the whites of the eyes

2. A component of your rights as a patient includes *informed consent*. Informed consent means that before you receive any care you:
   a. should be fully informed of what is being planned.
   b. should know the risks and potential benefits.
   c. have the option to refuse treatment.
   d. all of the above.

## LO 2 | Conventional Health Care

3. Which medical system is based on treating the patient's symptoms using scientifically validated methods?
   a. Allopathic medicine
   b. Nonallopathic medicine
   c. Ayurvedic medicine
   d. Alternative medicine

4. Which is a common type of over-the-counter drug?
   a. Antibiotics
   b. Hormonal contraceptives
   c. Antidepressants
   d. Antacids

## LO 3 | Complementary and Integrative Health Care

5. Complementary health approaches focus on treating the mind and the whole body, which makes them part of a
   a. natural approach.
   b. psychological approach.
   c. holistic approach.
   d. gentle approach.

6. What type of medicine addresses imbalances of *qi*?
   a. Chiropractic medicine
   b. Ayurvedic medicine
   c. Traditional Chinese medicine
   d. Homeopathic medicine

## LO 4 | Health Insurance

7. What is the term for an amount paid directly to a provider by a patient before his or her insurance carrier will begin paying for services?
   a. Coinsurance
   b. Cost sharing
   c. Co-payment
   d. Deductible

8. Of the following, the type of managed care that most greatly restricts choice of physicians and services is
   a. fee-for-service plans.
   b. health maintenance organizations.
   c. point of service plans.
   d. preferred provider organizations.

9. Deborah, 28, is a single parent of two children who works full time as a cashier. Her income is 130% of the federal poverty threshold. Which of the following statements about her health insurance coverage is true?
   a. Deborah and her two children are eligible for insurance coverage through the CHIP.
   b. Deborah and her two children qualify for insurance coverage through Medicaid, presuming their state has accepted federal Medicaid expansion funding.

c. Deborah is most likely receiving insurance coverage through Medicare, whereas her two children are most likely covered through the CHIP.

d. Deborah makes too high an income to qualify for a federal health insurance program; however, she can purchase a "marketplace" plan, for which she may qualify for premium subsidies.

### LO 5 | Issues Facing Today's Health Care System

10. Which of the following is a key provision of the ACA?
   a. Insurers are required to cover only major medical emergencies.
   b. Lifetime limits on benefits are allowed if costs exceed a set amount.
   c. Insurers are required to cover young adults on a parent's plan through age 21.
   d. Americans with preexisting conditions can't be denied coverage.

*Answers to the Pop Quiz can be found on page A-1. If you answered a question incorrectly, review the section identified by the Learning Outcome. For even more study tools, visit MasteringHealth.*

## THINK ABOUT IT!

### LO 1 | Taking Responsibility for Your Health Care

1. List several conditions for which you wouldn't need to seek medical help. When would you consider each condition to be bad enough to require medical attention? How would you decide where to go for treatment?

### LO 2 | Conventional Health Care

2. Describe your rights as a patient. Have you ever received treatment that violated these rights? If so, what action, if any, did you take?

### LO 3 | Complementary and Integrative Health Care

3. What are some of the potential benefits and risks of complementary health approaches? Why do you think these practices and products are so popular?

### LO 4 | Health Insurance

4. What are the inherent benefits and risks of managed care health insurance plans?

5. Explain the differences between traditional private health insurance plans and managed health care. Should insurance companies dictate reimbursement rates for various medical tests and procedures in an attempt to keep prices down? Why or why not?

### LO 5 | Issues Facing Today's Health Care System

6. Discuss how the Affordable Care Act (ACA) has increased access to health care for Americans. What are the key provisions of the ACA?

## ACCESS YOUR HEALTH ON THE INTERNET

Visit **MasteringHealth** for links to the websites and RSS feeds.

The following websites explore further topics and issues related to health care.

**Agency for Healthcare Research and Quality (AHRQ).** This provides links to sites that can address health care concerns and information on what questions to ask, what to look for, and what you should know when making critical decisions about personal care.
**www.ahrq.gov**

**Food and Drug Administration (FDA).** This website provides news on the latest government-approved home health tests and other health-related products.
**www.fda.gov**

**PubMed.** Find research abstracts—and increasingly entire studies—on health care topics of interest to you. This site is a service of the National Library of Medicine at the National Institutes of Health.
**www.ncbi.nlm.nih.gov/pubmed**

**HealthGrades.** This company provides quality reports on physicians as well as hospitals, nursing homes, and other health care facilities.
**www.healthgrades.com**

**National Committee for Quality Assurance (NCQA).** The NCQA assesses and reports on the quality of managed care plans, including HMOs.
**www.ncqa.org**

**Healthcare.gov.** Visit this website for information regarding health care reform in the United States and to access the online health insurance "marketplace" where Americans can enroll in plans and learn about their eligibility for federal subsidies, Medicaid, or CHIP.
**www.healthcare.gov**

**Physician Compare.** The Affordable Care Act mandated this website be established to provide basic information on physicians for consumers to use to assist them in finding a doctor.
**https://www.medicare.gov/physiciancompare/search.html**

**National Center for Complementary and Integrative Health.** A division of the National Institutes of Health, the NCCIH is dedicated to providing the latest information and research on complementary health approaches.
**http://nccih.nih.gov**

**National Institutes of Health, Office of Dietary Supplements.** This excellent resource includes access to a database of federally funded research projects pertaining to dietary supplements.
**http://ods.od.nih.gov**

# 20 Preventing Violence and Abuse

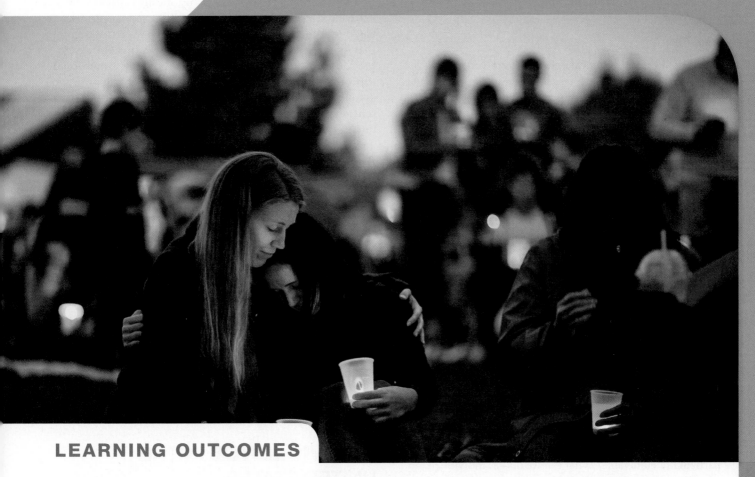

## LEARNING OUTCOMES

LO **1** Differentiate between intentional and unintentional injuries and discuss societal and personal factors that contribute to violence in American society and on college campuses.

LO **2** List and explain factors that contribute to homicide, domestic violence, intimate partner violence, sexual victimization, and other intentional acts of violence.

LO **3** Explain the prevalence and common causes of homicide, hate crimes, domestic violence, child abuse, sexual victimization, and other forms of interpersonal violence.

LO **4** Describe factors that contribute to gang violence and to terrorist activities.

LO **5** Articulate personal strategies for minimizing the risk of violence.

LO **6** Explain potential strategies that campus leaders, law enforcement officials, and individuals can develop to prevent students from becoming victims.

LO **7** Describe community-wide strategies for preventing violence.

Violence threatens us on many levels. While deaths and injuries make the headlines, the repercussions of violence can permeate our physical, social/interpersonal, and psychological lives, leading to a broad range of problems. We are victimized regardless of whether we experience, see, or merely fear violence. Fear changes us in subtle ways. We live our lives differently and relate to others differently; we view the world differently.

*Fear follows crime, and is its punishment.*
—*Voltaire, 1694–1778*[1]

Wars, political upheaval, terrorism, mass shootings, hate crimes, increases in homicides, rapes, bullying, domestic violence, child abuse, and fears over unknown threats seem to permeate our media and our thoughts. Increasingly, violence seems to be the expected norm that we are helpless to counteract. Is global violence an inevitable part of our future?

It may surprise you to know that violence is not a new phenomenon. Throughout history, violence has played a major role in human lives as people sought to dominate others or react to real or perceived threats. However, at no other time in history have we been able to view hate and carnage within minutes of its happening. We see it displayed over and over, seemingly 24/7. In this environment, many live in fear, increasingly frustrated by what seems to be a mean-spirited and violent world. We worry about being victimized at home, at work, at school, at athletic events, while traveling, or going to the movies. No place seems entirely safe. Are these fears justified? Is violence in the United States worse than ever? And to which kinds of violence are college students particularly vulnerable? What can we do—as individuals, and as a society—to reduce our risks?

First, it's important to understand what the word *violence* means. The World Health Organization (WHO) defines **violence** as "the intentional use of physical force or power, threatened or actual, against oneself, another person, or a group or community that results in or has a high likelihood of resulting in injury, death, psychological harm, maldevelopment or deprivation."[2] Today, most experts realize that emotional and psychological violence can be as devastating as physical violence.

**HEAR IT! PODCASTS**

Want a study podcast for this chapter? Download the podcast **Violence and Abuse: Creating Healthy Environments**, available on MasteringHealth.™

**violence** Aggressive behaviors that produce injuries and can result in death.

**intentional injuries** Injury, death, or psychological harm inflicted with the intent to harm.

**unintentional injuries** Injury, death, or psychological harm caused unintentionally or without premeditation.

The U.S. Public Health Service historically categorized violence resulting in injuries as either *intentional* or *unintentional*, based on the intent to cause harm. Today, experts recognize that intent is not always completely clear and that distinguishing cause and intent can be difficult. Typically, **intentional injuries**—those committed with intent to harm—include assaults, homicides, self-inflicted injuries, and suicides. **Unintentional injuries** are those committed without apparent intent to harm, such as motor vehicle crashes and other accidents. (See **Focus On: Reducing Your Risk of Unintentional Injury** on page 549.)

Intentional injury can be categorized into three major types: *interpersonal violence, collective violence,* and *self-directed violence,* with some degree of overlap among these groups.[3] Interpersonal violence and collective violence are discussed later in the chapter. (Self-directed violence is discussed in Chapter 2.)

Why focus on violence in an introductory health text? Because young adults are disproportionately affected by violence and injury. In fact, suicide and homicide are the second and third leading causes of death among individuals aged 15 to 34 in the United States.[4] Globally, violence is the fourth leading cause of death for people aged 10 to 29.[5] Add statistics from intimate partner violence, bullying, assaults, harassment, and other forms of physical and mental abuse, and the actual global toll is staggering.

## LO 1 | VIOLENCE IN THE UNITED STATES

Differentiate between intentional and unintentional injuries and discuss societal and personal factors that contribute to violence in American society and on college campuses.

Although violence has been part of the American landscape since colonial times, it wasn't until the 1980s that the U.S. Public Health Service gave violence *chronic disease status*, indicating that it was a pervasive threat to society. Violent crimes involve force or threat of force, and include four offenses: *murder and non-negligent manslaughter, forcible rape, robbery,* and *aggravated assault.* Statistics from the Federal Bureau of Investigation (FBI) have shown that, after steadily increasing from 1973 to 2006, the rates of overall crime and certain types of violent crime began a slow decline, falling by more than

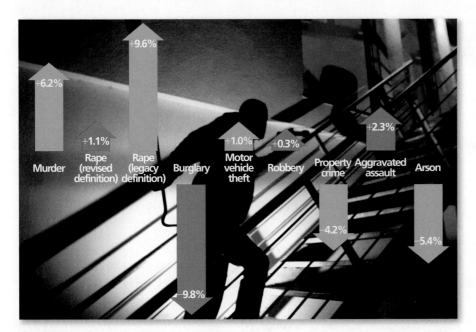

**FIGURE 20.1** **Changing Crime Rates** FBI statistics show reported violent crimes increased early in 2015 after declines in previous years. Rates of crimes vary by type of crime, location, sex, and other variables, with the most violent crimes on the increase overall.

**Source:** FBI Crime in the United States, 2015, "Preliminary Semiannual Uniform Crime Report, January–June 2015," Accessed July 2016, www.fbi.gov.

10 percent between 2012 and 2014.[6] In contrast, the Bureau of Justice Statistics reported little change in violent crime during 2014.[7]

Which report was right? Actually, both! Historically, we use two measures for violence in the United States: the FBI's *Uniform Crime Reporting (UCR) Program* and the Bureau of Justice Statistics' *National Crime Victimization Survey (NCVS)*. While the FBI's UCR collects data on violent crimes involving force or threat reported to law enforcement agencies, the Bureau of Justice Statistics collects detailed information on the frequency and nature of certain crimes twice a year through surveys of nearly 160,000 people in 90,000 homes.[8] In addition to using different methods, the Bureau of Justice Statistics does not track homicides or crimes against businesses.

Where are we today? Based on data from the first 6 months of 2015, violent crime, particularly homicide and rape, are on the increase, with some areas of the United States reporting dramatic increases. Other areas seem to be showing declines.[9] See **FIGURE 20.1** for the percent change of violent crimes reported in 2015 and **FIGURE 20.2** for the frequency of different types of crimes.

Violence trends are difficult to assess, but whether total crime rates are up or down, huge disparities in crime rates based on race, sex, age, socioeconomic status, location, crime type, and other factors exist. Importantly, it is believed that current numbers may not reflect actual offenses, as over 54 percent of violent victimizations are not reported to the police.[10] Rates of nonreporting are even higher for some offenses such as rape. If those nonreports suddenly become reported, we might have a dramatically different profile. The good news is that, even

though crime rates ebb and flow over the years, overall rates are considerably lower (nearly one-third less) than they were in the early 1990s.[11]

Even if we have never physically been victims ourselves, we all are victimized by violent acts that cause us to be fearful; impinge on our liberty; and damage the reputation of our campus, city, or nation. If you don't go out for a walk or run at night, have to keep your doors and windows locked at all times; if the thought of going to a concert or sitting in a large stadium for an athletic event makes you nervous, or you avoid an international vacation because you are worried about being attacked, you are a victim of societal violence.

## Violence on U.S. Campuses

Violence on campuses seems to be increasingly covered in the media, with gun violence making headline news far too many times in recent years. Whether at Virginia Tech University, where 32 people died in the deadliest campus shooting in U.S. history, or at Umpqua Community College in Roseburg, Oregon, where 10 people were gunned down and many more injured in 2016, or dozens of others in the last two decades, campus shootings are on the rise. Tragedies like these have sparked dialogue and action across the nation, prompting increases in campus security and safety measures. Today, it would be hard to find a campus without some form of safety plan in place to prevent and respond to violent attacks.

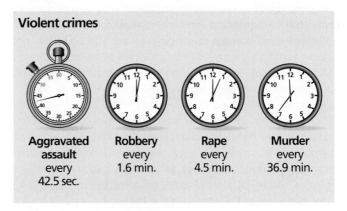

**Violent crimes**

**Aggravated assault** every 42.5 sec.

**Robbery** every 1.6 min.

**Rape** every 4.5 min.

**Murder** every 36.9 min.

**FIGURE 20.2** **Crime Clock** The crime clock represents the annual ratio of crime to fixed time intervals. The crime clock should not be taken to imply a regularity in the commission of crime.

**Source:** Adapted from Federal Bureau of Investigation, "Crime in the United States, 2014," Accessed July 2016, https://ucr.fbi.gov/crime-in-the-u.s/2014/crime-in-the-u.s.-2014/figs/crime-clock.jpg.

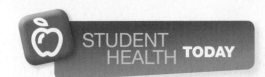
# HAZING
*Over the Top and Dangerous for Many*

Many people don't fully understand just what hazing is, or the legal ramifications of hazing or being hazed. So, what is **hazing**? Essentially it is *"any activity expected of someone joining or participating in a group that humiliates, degrades, abuses, or endangers them regardless of a person's willingness to participate."* Typically, it involves forcing students to consume excessive alcohol; dress in humiliating garb; undergo forced sleep deprivation; or endure verbal abuse from group members or physical abuse in the form of beatings, heat or cold exposure, or forced sexual acts. For those who are victimized and don't find their forced hazing humorous, psychological and physical damage can be serious.

More common than expected, even in today's campus settings where it is explicitly outlawed, details about the nature and extent of hazing are scarce. We only tune in when there are hazing deaths on the national media; yet, over 250,000 college students are hazed each year and as many as 50 percent of those on athletic teams receive some form of hazing. However, unconfirmed reports of hazing by "newbies" on athletic teams, in sororities and fraternities, and in other social groups are common on campus. According to a recent national study, 55 percent of college students involved in clubs, teams, and organizations experience hazing, and 47 percent of students come to college already having experienced hazing. Yet many students are unaware of its dangers or legal implications, and 9 out of 10 students who experience hazing in college do not realize they've been hazed.

Most hazing cases are never reported or prosecuted. In part, this may be due to fear of retribution or fear of falling out of group favour. Also, many regard hazing as a "rite of passage" and as long as no one is physically harmed, it may foster a sense of belonging. Students also report that school administrators do little to prevent hazing beyond maintaining a "hazing is not tolerated" stance. If schools are to have an impact on the prevalence of hazing on their campuses, they need to implement broader prevention and intervention efforts and work to educate their campus community on the physical and legal perils of hazing.

**Source:** J. Waldron, "Predictors of Mild Hazing, Severe Hazing, and Positive Initiation Rituals in Sport," *International Journal of Sport Science and Coaching* 10, no. 6 (2015): 1089–1101; "Am I My Brother's Keeper?: Reforming Criminal Hazing Laws Based on Assumption of Care," *Emory Law Journal* (2014), www.law.emory.edu/fileadmin/journals/elj/63/63.4/Chamberlin.pdf.

Knowing what actions will be taken in the event of a school shooting can help save lives, and help avoid the inevitable anxiety and fear that occurs when lives are threatened.

While shootings make national news, many forms of campus violence continue to be hidden behind a veil of secrecy, with many victims reluctant to report assaults.

Relationship violence is one of the most prevalent problems on campus. In the most recent American College Health Association survey, 10.3 percent of women and 5.8 percent of men reported being emotionally abused in the past 12 months by a significant other.[12] Over 6 percent of women and 2.5 percent of men reported being stalked, and 2.2 percent of women and 1.2 percent of men reported being involved in a physically abusive relationship.[13] Nearly 1 percent of men and 2.4 percent of women reported being in a sexually abusive relationship.[14]

The statistics on reported campus violence represent only a glimpse of the big picture. It is believed that fewer than 25 percent of campus crimes in general are reported to *any* authority.[15] Even though as many as 20 to 25 percent of college women will be raped or sexually assaulted before they graduate, 95 percent of them never report these crimes.[16]

Why do so few report these assaults? Typical reasons include privacy concerns, fear of retaliation, embarrassment, lack of support, perception that the crime was too minor or they were at fault, or uncertainty it was a crime. This is particularly true in situations where a victim knew her rapist, or where drinking was involved and crime details were fuzzy, as well as instances of stalking and hazing. See the **Student Health Today** box for more on hazing.

## LO **2** | **FACTORS** CONTRIBUTING TO VIOLENCE

**List and explain factors that contribute to homicide, domestic violence, intimate partner violence, sexual victimization, and other intentional acts of violence.**

While no single criterion can explain what causes people to become violent offenders, key risk factors include:[17]

- **Community contexts.** Environments where interactions with unsafe neighborhoods, schools, and workplaces predominate increase risks of exposure to drugs, guns, and gangs. Inadequately staffed police and social services add to the risks.[18]
- **Societal factors.** Policies and programs that seek to remove inequality/disparity and discourage discrimination decrease risks; social and cultural norms that support male dominance over women and violence as a means of settling problems increase risks.[19]
- **Religious beliefs and differences.** Extreme religious beliefs can lead people to think that violence against others is justified.

**hazing** Any activity expected of someone joining or participating in a group that humiliates, degrades, abuses, or endangers them regardless of a person's willingness to participate.

- **Political differences.** Civil unrest and differences in political party affiliations and beliefs have historically been triggers for violent acts.
- **Breakdowns in the criminal justice system.** Overcrowded prisons and inadequate availability of mental health services can encourage repeat offenses and future violence.
- **Stress, depression, or other mental health issues.** People who are in crisis, depressed, feel threatened, or are under stress are more apt to be highly reactive, striking out at others, displaying anger, or acting irrationally.[20]

## What Makes Some Individuals Prone to Violence?

Personal factors can also increase risks for violence. Emerging evidence suggests that the family and home environment may be the greatest contributor to eventual violent behavior among family members.[21] The following are among key predictors of aggressive behavior, including anger and irrational beliefs, genetic predispositions toward anger, and influences of coercive and contagious peers.[22]

**Anger** Anger is a well-known catalyst for violence. Anger typically occurs when there is a *triggering event* or a person has learned that acting out in angry ways can get him or her what he or she wants. Anger tends to be an active, attack-oriented emotion in which people feel powerful and in control for a short period.[23] Learning to assess the underlying "self-talk" or beliefs that lead to anger is an important part of prevention. (For more suggestions on anger management, see Chapter 3.)

People who anger quickly may have physiological and genetic factors influencing this short fuse. Increasing evidence suggests those who act violently and unemotionally may be most likely to have a genetic basis for increased anger and aggression; however, researchers acknowledge that there are several pathways by which a person may act violently.[24] Typically, anger-prone people also come from families that are disruptive, chaotic, and unskilled in emotional expression and where anger, domestic violence, and abuse occur regularly.[25] Those who have been bullied in school may also be prone to react with violence in future situations and suffer from PTSD as adults.[26]

*Aggressive* behavior is often a key aspect of violent interactions. **Primary aggression** is goal-directed, hostile, and destructive self-assertion. **Reactive aggression** is more often emotional and brought about by frustrating life experiences. Whether reactive or primary, aggression is most likely to flare up in times of acute stress.

**Substance Abuse** Alcohol and drug abuse are often catalysts for violence at all levels of society, both nationally and internationally.[27]

- Forty percent of all violent crimes today include alcohol as a factor; the Department of Justice reports that 37 percent of nearly 2 million convicted offenders in jail at present report imbibing in alcohol when they were arrested.[28]
- An estimated 80 percent of American offenses leading to prison, such as domestic violence, property offenses, and public-order offenses, include the involvement of alcohol and drugs.[29]
- Research indicates higher rates of alcohol use and violence in some athlete populations when compared to nonathlete populations. Masculinity, antisocial norms, and violent social identity connected to certain sports may contribute to violence among athletes.[30]
- Numbers of suicide attempts and completions are highly correlated to drug and alcohol intake.[31]

## How Much Impact Do the Media Have?

After countless shootings and episodes of terrorism in the United States and globally, people invariably ask *why* such things happen to innocent people. The media focus their attention squarely on what are widely perceived to be causes of violence: (1) too many high-capacity assault rifles and handguns, as well as easy access to guns; (2) inadequate mental health resources; and (3) a daily dose of media violence. Does a regular diet of violence from video games, TV, and movies make people more likely to engage in murder and mayhem? Is there such a thing as becoming so desensitized or "numbed" to violence that life and death scenarios feel commonplace?

Although the media are blamed for having a major role in the escalation of violence, this association has been challenged continuously. While early studies seemed to support a link between excessive exposure to violent

Most adults learn to control outbursts of anger in a rational manner. However, some people act out their aggressive tendencies in much the same way they did as children—with anger and violence that are a form of self-assertion or a response to frustration.

**primary aggression** Goal-directed, hostile self-assertion that is destructive in nature.

**reactive aggression** Hostile emotional reaction brought about by frustrating life experiences.

media and subsequent violent behavior, much of this research has now been criticized for methodological problems such as poor/inconsistent measures of violence, biased subject selection, and sample size issues.[32] More recent studies of a possible relationship between media violence and violent acts seem to point a weak finger toward a connection between media violence and short-term aggression; however, the link to homicides and assaults is much less clear.[33] Other researchers continue to point out that exposure to violent videos has neither long- nor short-term effects of either positive or negative behaviors.[34]

Despite evidence to the contrary, some still believe that viewing violent media numbs people to humanity, allows people to commit violence without empathy or regret, or even triggers violent events.[35] Several potential restrictions have been proposed to ban violent media for youth. The Supreme Court has steadfastly rejected them, echoing the claims that a relationship between violent acts and the consumption of violent media has not been proven through consistent, rigorous research. During his term in office, President Barack Obama and several professional groups called for more research to better understand the complex factors that prompt violence and what might be done to reduce risks.

Critics of previous studies point out that today's young people are exposed to more media violence than any previous generation, yet rates of

**homicide** Death that results from intent to injure or kill.

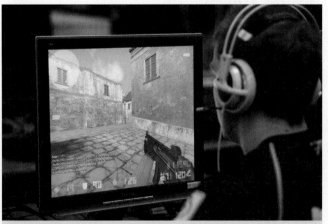

Arguably, Americans today—especially children—are exposed to more depictions of violence than ever before, but research has not shown a clear link between a person's exposure to violent media and his or her propensity to engage in violent acts.

violent crime among youth have fallen to 40-year lows.[36] Still, concerns have been raised about those who spend a disproportionate amount of time online instead of interacting in real-time, face-to-face communication. Will they miss the important lessons that come from talking with people in person and learning to get along with others? What will be the result of a generation that opts out of significant "live" interactions with their peers? When problems arise in face-to-face interactions and we can't click delete, will we know how to respond?

## LO 3 | INTERPERSONAL VIOLENCE

Explain the prevalence and common causes of homicide, hate crimes, domestic violence, child abuse, sexual victimization, and other forms of interpersonal violence.

Interpersonal violence includes intentionally using "physical force or power, threatened or actual," to inflict violence against an individual that results in injury, death, or psychological harm.[37] Homicide, hate crimes, domestic violence, child abuse, elder abuse, and sexual victimization all fit into this category.

## Homicide

**Homicide**, defined as murder or nonnegligent manslaughter (killing another human), is the 13th leading cause of death in the United States, the second leading cause of death for persons aged 15 to 24, and the fourth leading cause of death for those 25 to 44. Overall, it is among the top five leading causes of death for those aged 1 to 44.[38] Nearly half of all homicides occur among people who know one another.[39] In two-thirds of these cases, the perpetrator and the victim are friends or acquaintances; in one-third, they are family members.[40]

Homicide rates reveal clear disparities across race, gender, and age. Homicides are the fifth leading cause of death for African American males, the sixth leading cause of death for Native Americans, and the ninth leading cause of death in Latino populations; however, homicide is not a leading cause of death for females, or for white and Asian/Pacific Islander males.[41] See the **Health Headlines** box for a discussion of guns and violence.

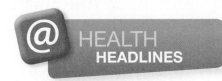

# BRINGING THE GUN DEBATE TO CAMPUS

On average, each year in the United States 100,000 people are shot. Over 31,000 of them die, and of those who survive, many experience significant physical and emotional repercussions. Some facts about guns and gun violence include:

- Handguns are consistently responsible for more murders than any other type of weapon.
- Today, 35 percent of American homes have a gun on the premises, with nearly 300 million privately owned guns registered—and millions more that are unregistered and/or illegal.
- Firearms are the weapons most often used in attacks on American campuses. The most common reason for an incident is "related to an intimate relationship," followed by "retaliation for a specific action."
- The presence of a gun in the home triples the risk of a homicide in that location and increases suicide risk more than five times.

What factors contribute to gun deaths in the United States? Currently, this country has somewhere between 270 million and 350 million guns—meaning that, by some counts, there may be more guns than there are people. No other country on the planet even comes close in terms of civilian gun ownership. Advocates of background checks for weapons purchases and more strict gun control legislation argue that the uniquely large numbers of guns—particularly semi-automatic assault weapons with high-capacity magazines—in the United States as well as relatively easy access to powerful weapons are the main culprits. However, gun-rights advocates say that the problem lies not with guns themselves, but with the people who own them.

High-profile shootings at schools and other public places have brought the gun debate to campuses. Over the last decade, numerous states have allowed concealed weapon carry, some of which allow them on campus. Critics argue that this is a dangerous situation where

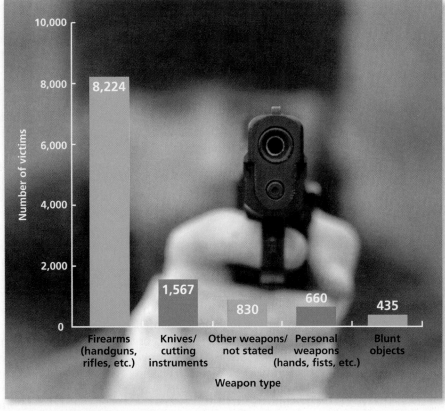

**Homicide in the United States by Weapon Type, 2014**
The vast majority of murders in the United States are committed using firearms, far outweighing all other weapons combined.

Source: Data from U.S. Department of Justice, Federal Bureau of Investigation, "Crime in the United States, 2014, Expanded Homicide Data Table 8—Murder Victims by Weapon—2010–2014," 2015, https://www.fbi.gov/about-us/cjis/ucr/crime-in-the-u.s/2014/crime-in-the-u.s.-2014/tables/expanded-homicide-data/expanded_homicide_data_table_8_murder_victims_by_weapon_2010-2014.xls.

alcohol and anger may converge to increase risks for faculty and students alike. Gun advocates argue that if people in mass-shooting situations had weapons, deaths and assaults would be prevented. What do you think?

- How would you feel about students in your classes having guns? Would it make you feel more or less safe? What about bringing a gun to a sporting event, party on campus, or other venue? Should instructors carry weapons?
- Do you think making guns illegal on campus would prevent students from bringing guns to school? Why or why not?
- What factors should be taken into consideration as states vote on guns on campus?

Sources: C. Ingraham, "There are Now More Guns than People in the United States," *The Washington Post,* October 5, 2015, https://www.washingtonpost.com/news/wonk/wp/2015/10/05/guns-in-the-united-states-one-for-every-man-woman-and-child-and-then-some/; J. Davidson and H. Jones, "The Orlando Shooting is a Haunting Reminder of Just How Many Guns are in America," *Time,* June 14, 2016, http://time.com/4188456/orlando-shooting-mass-shootings-gun-control/; D. Drysdale, W. Modzeleski, and A. Simons, *Campus Attacks: Targeted Violence Affecting Institutions of Higher Learning* (Washington, DC: United States Secret Service, United States Department of Education, and the Federal Bureau of Investigation, 2010); National Conference of State Legislatures, "Guns on Campus: Overview," 2015, http://www.ncsl.org/research/education/guns-on-campus-overview.aspx.

## Hate and Bias-Motivated Crimes

A **hate crime** is a crime committed against a person, property, or group of people motivated by bias based on race, gender or gender identity, religion, disability, sexual orientation, or ethnicity.[42] As a result of national efforts to promote understanding and appreciation of diversity, reports of hate crimes have declined to 5,479 reported incidents in 2014, according to the FBI[43] (**FIGURE 20.3**). Of these hate crimes, over 47 percent were a result of bias toward a particular race; nearly 19 percent were motivated by bias based on sexual orientation, nearly 19 percent toward religion, 11.9 percent by ethnicity/national origin bias; 1.5 percent reflected bias toward disabilities; 1.8 were based on gender identity; and 0.6% were based on gender.[44]

Although newer data are not yet available, when a representative sample of Americans completed the anonymous National Crime Victimization Survey, an estimated 294,000 violent and property hate crimes occurred in 2012![45] Clearly, based on reported increases in violence by agencies such as the FBI, and shootings like the 2016 mass murders in a gay nightclub in Orlando, hate crimes are on the increase. As with many crimes, fear of retaliation keeps many hate crimes hidden. While over 60 percent of hate crimes may never be reported, only about one-fourth of those reported are reported by victims themselves.[46]

*Bias-related crime*, sometimes referred to as **ethnoviolence**, describes violence based on prejudice and discrimination among ethnic groups in the larger society. **Prejudice** is an irrational attitude of hostility directed against an individual, group, or race or the supposed characteristics of an individual, group, or race. **Discrimination** constitutes actions that deny equal treatment or opportunities to a group of people, often based on prejudice. Often prejudice and discrimination stem from fear and a desire to blame others when forces such as the economy and crime seem out of control. Teaching tolerance, understanding, and respect for people from different backgrounds can reduce bias-related crimes.

Common reasons given to explain bias-related and hate crimes include (1) *thrill seeking* by multiple offenders through a group attack; (2) *feeling threatened* that others will take their jobs or property or harass them in some way; (3) *retaliating* for some real or perceived insult or slight; and (4) *fearing the unknown or differences*. For other people, hate crimes are a part of their mission in life, either due to religious zeal, lack of understanding, or distorted moral beliefs.

Unfortunately, accurate and current statistics on bias and hate crimes in the general public and on campus are difficult to come by. However, increasing media attention focused on actions on campuses and in communities has put these issues in the national spotlight. Campuses have responded to reports of hate crimes by offering courses that emphasize diversity, having zero tolerance for violations, training faculty appropriately, and developing policies that enforce punishment for hate crimes.

## Domestic Violence

**Domestic violence** refers to the use of force to control and maintain power over another person in the home environment. It can occur between parents and children, between spouses or intimate partners, or between siblings or other family members. The violence may involve emotional abuse, verbal abuse, threats of physical harm, and physical violence ranging from slapping and shoving to beatings, rape, and homicide.

### Intimate Partner Violence and Women

**Intimate partner violence (IPV)** describes physical, sexual, or psychological harm done by a current or former partner or spouse. It is a growing problem. How bad is it? On average, each

---

**hate crime** Crime targeted against a particular societal group and motivated by bias against that group.

**ethnoviolence** Violence directed at persons affiliated with a particular ethnic group.

**prejudice** A negative evaluation of an entire group of people that is typically based on unfavorable and often wrong ideas about the group.

**discrimination** Actions that deny equal treatment or opportunities to a group, often based on prejudice.

**domestic violence** The use of force to control and maintain power over another person in the home environment, including both actual harm and the threat of harm.

**intimate partner violence (IPV)** Describes physical, sexual, or psychological harm by a current or former partner or spouse.

---

**SEE IT! VIDEOS**

Murder over a parking spot or something more? Watch **Was North Carolina Killing a Hate Crime?**, available on MasteringHealth.™

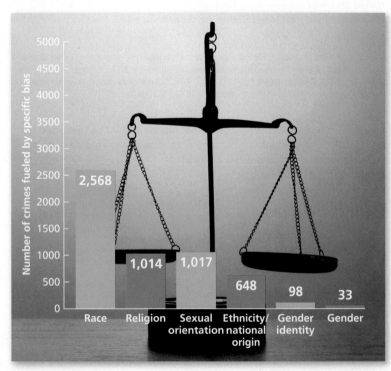

**FIGURE 20.3** Bias-Motivated Crimes, Single-Bias Incidence, 2014

**Source:** Data from Federal Bureau of Investigation, "Hate Crime Statistics, 2014," Table 1, www.fbi.gov. November, 2015.

*Y-axis: Number of crimes fueled by specific bias*

- Race: 2,568
- Religion: 1,014
- Sexual orientation: 1,017
- Ethnicity/national origin: 648
- Gender identity: 98
- Gender: 33

minute, there are 20 new victims of physical violence at the hands of an intimate partner in the United States.[47] This type of violence can occur among all types of couples and does not require sexual intimacy. Although we often think of violence as something perpetrated by a stranger, in truth, Americans are more likely to be victims of physical and psychological abuse, stalking, and other offenses by an intimate partner—often someone they know or who is living with them. Nearly 75 percent of all murder-suicides were perpetrated by an intimate partner.[48] Homicide committed by a current or former intimate partner is the leading cause of death and injury of pregnant women in the United States.[49]

Nearly half of all women and men in the United States have experienced psychological aggression by an intimate partner in their lifetime.[50] Women who are poor, less educated, live in high-poverty areas, socially isolated, and dependent on drugs and alcohol are at greatest risk of IPV.[51] This abuse can take the form of constant criticism, verbal attacks, displays of explosive anger meant to intimidate, and controlling behavior. Those who have experienced this violence are three times more likely to report mental health problems, such as depression, anxiety, high stress, insomnia, and other issues.[52]

### The Cycle of IPV and Battered Woman Syndrome

Have you ever heard of a woman who is repeatedly beaten by her partner and wondered, "Why doesn't she just leave him?" There are many reasons some women find it difficult to break their ties with abusers. Some women, particularly those with small children, are financially dependent on their partners. Others fear retaliation. Some hope the situation will change with time, and others stay because cultural or religious beliefs forbid divorce. Others are socially isolated from family and friends due to the abuser's control and manipulation. (Ironically, technology meant to connect people, like social media and smartphones, can allow perpetrators to stalk their victim and monitor their activities, cutting them off from support systems and services.) Finally, some women still love the abusive partner and are concerned about what will happen to him if they leave.

In the 1970s, psychologist Lenore Walker developed a theory called the *cycle of violence* that explained predictable, repetitive patterns of psychological and/or physical abuse that seemed to occur in abusive relationships. The cycle consisted of three major phases:[53]

1. **Tension building.** Prior to the overtly abusive act, tension building includes breakdowns in communication, anger, psychological aggression, growing tension, and fear.
2. **Incident of acute battering.** When the acute attack is over, he may respond with shock and denial about his own behavior or blame her for making him do it.
3. **Remorse/reconciliation.** During a "honeymoon" period, the batterer may be kind, loving, and apologetic, swearing that he will work to change his behavior.

After refining her work with the insights of other researchers, Walker's research has been expanded to focus on *battered woman syndrome*.[54] Today, battered woman syndrome is considered to be a subgroup of posttraumatic stress disorder (PTSD) and is often used to describe someone who has gone through the above cycle at least twice.

## Causes of Domestic Violence and IPV

There is no single reason that explains abuse in relationships. Alcohol abuse is often associated with such violence, as are having a history of family violence and marital dissatisfaction. Poor communication patterns within abusive relationships are often common. Stress, mental health issues, economic uncertainty/frustration, jealousy, issues of power/control and gender roles, and issues with self-esteem are among common reasons given for IPV.[55]

## Intimate Partner Violence: Men as Victims

We may think that intimate partner violence happens only to women, but 1 in 7 men in the United States experience assaults by an intimate partner or spouse, male or female.[56] In fact, gay men appear to be just as susceptible to male-perpetrated violence as are women in heterosexual relationships, and abuse of heterosexual men by their female partners is likely more common than statistics show.[57] Although men are sexually assaulted, men's assaults tended to be less severe and less likely to end in fatality.[58]

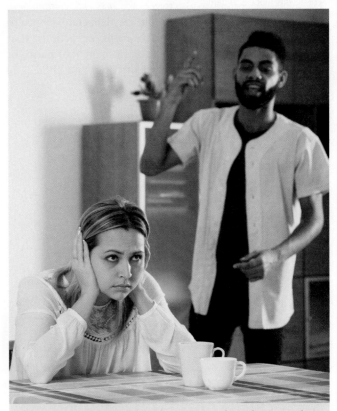

People who stay with their abusers may do so because they are dependent on the abuser, because they fear the abuser, or even because they love the abuser. In some cultures, women may not be free to leave an abusive relationship because of restrictive laws, religious beliefs, or social mores.

Why don't men report abuse? Reasons include:

- A sense of humiliation and/or fear that no one will believe them
- Abuse that has reached the point that they believe they deserve bad treatment
- Belief that not hitting back is a sign of honor, strength, or masculinity
- Lack of awareness and support services for men in abusive relationships

Recognizing that a problem exists, communities across the nation are responding with education and awareness programs and resources, such as support groups and counseling, to help male victims protect themselves and make positive changes in their lives.

## Child Abuse and Neglect

Children living in families in which domestic violence or sexual abuse occurs are at great risk for damage to personal health and well-being. **Child maltreatment** is defined as any act or series of acts of commission or omission by a parent or caregiver that results in harm, potential for harm, or threat of harm to a child.[59] **Child abuse** refers to *acts of commission*, which are deliberate or intentional words or actions that cause harm, potential harm, or threat of harm to a child. The abuse may be sexual, psychological, physical, or any combination of these. **Neglect** is an *act of omission*, meaning a failure to provide for a child's basic physical, emotional, or education needs or to protect a child from harm or potential harm. Failure to provide food, shelter, clothing, medical care, or supervision or exposing a child to unnecessary environmental violence or threat are examples of ne-glect. Although reported cases may only represent a fraction of actual causes, **FIGURE 20.4** provides an overview of the most recent reported cases, representing over 3 million.[60]

There is no single profile of a child abuser. Frequently, the perpetrator is a young adult in his or her mid-20s without a high school diploma, living at or below the poverty level, depressed, socially isolated, with a poor self-image, and having difficulty coping with stressful situations. In many instances, the perpetrator has experienced violence and is frustrated by life.

Child abuse occurs at every socioeconomic level, across ethnic and cultural lines, within all religions, and at all levels of education. Not all violence against children is physical. Mental health can be severely affected by psychological violence—assaults on personality, character, competence, independence, or general dignity as a human being. Victims of child abuse have a higher risk of depression, unintended pregnancy, sexually transmitted diseases (STIs), suicide, drug and alcohol abuse, and an overall lowered life expectancy, particularly among those repeatedly victimized.[61]

**child maltreatment** Any act or series of acts of commission or omission by a parent or caregiver that results in harm, potential for harm, or threat of harm to a child.

**child abuse** Deliberate, intentional words or actions that cause harm, potential for harm, or threat of harm to a child.

**neglect** Failure to provide a child's basic needs such as food, clothing, shelter, and medical care.

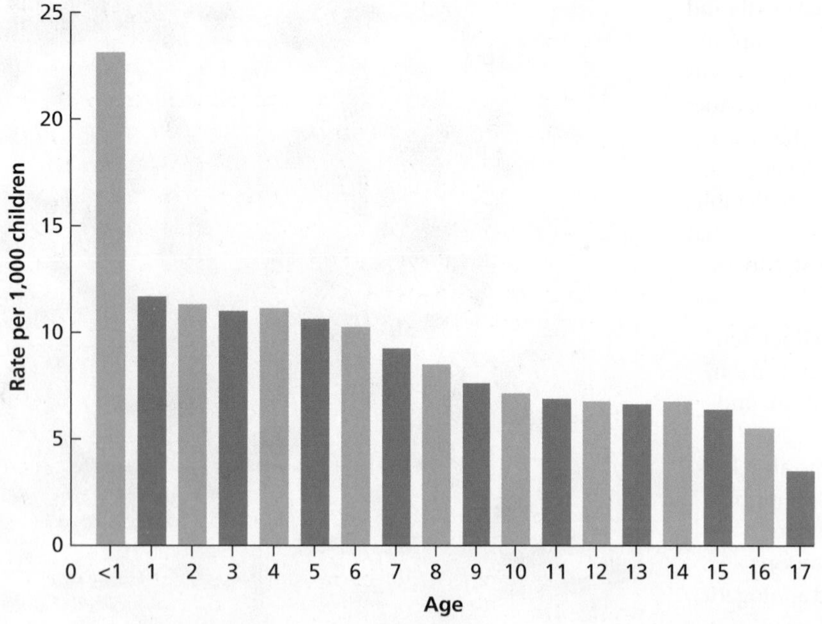

## Elder Abuse

By 2030, the number of people in the United States over the age of 65 will exceed 71 million—nearly double their number in 2000. Each year, hundreds of thousands of adults over the age of 60 are abused, neglected, or financially exploited as they enter the later years of life, and these statistics are likely an underestimate.[62] Many victims fail to report abuse because they are embarrassed or because they don't want the abuser to get in trouble or retaliate by putting them in a nursing home or escalating the abuse. A variety of social services focus on protecting our seniors, just as we endeavor to protect other vulnerable populations.

## Sexual Victimization

The term *sexual victimization* refers to any situation in which an individual is coerced or forced to comply with or endure another's sexual acts or overtures. It can run the gamut from harassment to stalking to assault and rape by perpetrators known or unknown to the victim. It can even include sexual coercion and rape by spouses within the confines of marriage. Sexual victimization and violence can have devastating and far-reaching effects on people of any age. Fear, sexual avoidance, sleeplessness, anxiety, and depression are

**FIGURE 20.4** Child Abuse and Neglect Victims by Age, 2013

**Source:** U.S. Department of Health and Human Services, Administration for Children and Families, Administration on Children, Youth and Families, Children's Bureau, 2015, Child Maltreatment 2013, Table 3-5, www.acf.hhs.gov/programs/cb/research-data-technology/statistics-research/child-maltreatment.

just a few of the long-term consequences for victims of sexual victimization.[63]

**Sexual Assault and Rape** **Sexual assault** is any act in which one person is sexually intimate with another person without that person's consent. This may range from simple touching to forceful penetration and may include, for example, ignoring indications that intimacy is not wanted, threatening force or other negative consequences, and actually using force.

Considered the most extreme form of sexual assault, **rape** is typically thought of as forcible penetration without the victim's consent. However, a new, clarified definition of rape includes: "Penetration, no matter how slight, of the vagina or anus with any body part or object, or oral penetration by a sex organ of another person, without the consent of the victim. This includes the offenses of rape, sodomy, and sexual assault with an object."[64]

Incidents of rape generally fall into one of two types—simple or aggravated. A **simple rape** is a rape perpetrated by one person, whom the victim knows, and does not involve a physical beating or use of a weapon. An **aggravated rape** is any rape involving one or multiple attackers, strangers, weapons, or physical beatings. Most rapes are classified as simple rape, but that terminology should not be taken to mean that a simple rape is any less violent or criminal.

Nearly 1 in 5 women and 1 in 59 men in the United States have been raped at some time in their lives, with nearly 80 percent of female rape victims experiencing their first rape before the age of 25.[65] More than one-fourth of male rape victims were raped before they were 10 years old.[66]

By most indicators, reported cases of rape appear to have declined in the United States since the early 1990s, even as reports of other forms of sexual assault have increased. This decline is thought to be due to shifts in public awareness and attitudes about rape, combined with tougher crime policies, major educational campaigns, and media attention. These changes enforce the idea that rape is a violent crime and should be treated as such. However, numerous sources indicate that rape is among one of the most underreported crimes, particularly on college campuses.[67]

**Acquaintance Rape** The terms *date rape* and *acquaintance rape* have been used interchangeably in the past. However, most experts now believe that the term *date rape* is inappropriate because it implies a consensual interaction in an

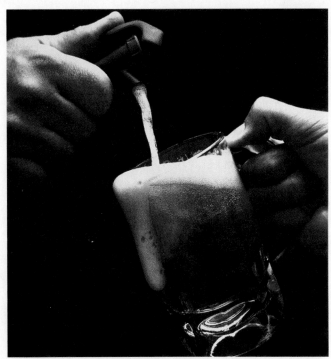

# A lot of campus rapes start here.

Whenever there's drinking or drugs, things can get out of hand. So it's no surprise that many campus rapes involve alcohol.

But you should know that under any circumstances, sex without the other person's consent is considered rape. A felony, punishable by prison. And drinking is no excuse.

That's why, when you party, it's good to know what your limits are. You see, a little sobering thought now can save you from a big problem later.

Acquaintance rape is particularly common on college campuses, where alcohol and drug use can impair young people's judgment and self-control.

➜ **VIDEO TUTOR**
Acquaintance Rape on Campus

arranged setting and may, in fact, minimize the crime of rape when it occurs. Today, **acquaintance rape** refers to any rape in which the rapist is known to the victim. Acquaintance rape is more common when drugs or alcohol have been consumed by the offender or victim, making the campus party environment a high-risk venue. Alcohol is frequently involved in rape, as are a growing number of rape-facilitating drugs such as Rohypnol, ketamine, and gamma-hydroxy-butyrate (GHB).

**Rape on U.S. Campuses** In 1986, Jeanne Clery, a freshman at Lehigh University, was brutally raped and murdered. After finding out that campus security and reported violence cases were lacking, Jeanne's parents pushed for some of the first major changes in campus security and reporting

**sexual assault** Any act in which one person is sexually intimate with another without that person's consent.

**rape** Sexual penetration without the victim's consent.

**simple rape** Rape by one person, usually known to the victim, that does not involve physical beating or use of a weapon.

**aggravated rape** Rape that involves one or multiple attackers, strangers, weapons, or physical beating.

**acquaintance rape** Any rape in which the rapist is known to the victim (replaces the formerly used term *date rape*).

# 1 IN 5

College women were victims of **RAPE OR ATTEMPTED RAPE** during their freshmen year, with the most falling prey during their first 3 months on campus. These numbers increased during subsequent years.

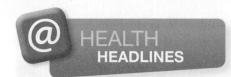
# SEXUAL ASSAULT
## Changing the Culture of Silence?

Responding to increased evidence of major issues and increased pressure to take action, President Obama formed a National Task Force to study sexual assault and make recommendations for change. Its report notes that over 20 percent of college students are sexually assaulted as undergraduates. As part of its recommendations, colleges are being asked to do the following:

■ Identify the problem. Consider using mandatory anonymous surveys where experiences with unwanted sexual contact, sexual assault, rape, and sexual harassment are reported.

■ Teach the definition of consent and the legal ramifications of any actions that are undertaken without clear consent.

■ Effectively respond when there is a report.

■ Increase transparency and improve enforcement.

■ Teach "bystander education" to show students how to intervene in potentially harmful situations.

As part of the *Campus Sexual Violence Elimination Act*, passed by Congress in 2014, rape, domestic violence, dating violence, sexual assault, and stalking

The reluctance to report sexual assault on campus and the difficulty of pursuing criminal proceedings in the campus environment can create turmoil in victims' lives while too rarely leading to punishment of offenders.

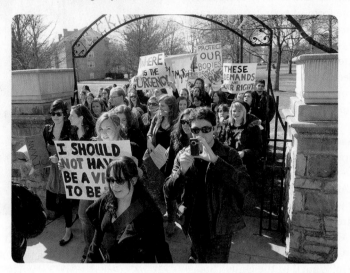

cases must be reported on annual campus crime reports. The White House is asking for measures that would levy harsh penalties for not taking strong action to prevent assaults.

In 2014, the State of California became the first in the nation to implement a *"yes means yes"* law, changing the definition of sexual consent to require "an affirmative, conscious, and voluntary agreement to engage in sexual activity." If one party is unable to give consent due to intoxication or other factors, the perpetrator could be prosecuted for sexual assault. Beyond changing definitions, the law also

requires schools who receive funding from the state to develop policies around numerous situations related to sexual assault.

Ironically, as campuses improve education/awareness, increase reporting, and call for zero tolerance, as well as a clarification of the definition of rape, the number of reported forcible rapes and assaults increased. These increases are believed to be due to a greater willingness of victims to come forward as well as a better understanding of the actions that constitute rape or sexual assault. Efforts are underway to change campus culture by educating students about their options, informing counselors and support staff of their legal responsibilities, and improving reporting protocols. However, the process is slow. Schools fear negative publicity and image tarnishing from reports of rape and sexual assault, which could affect enrollment and fundraising.

**Sources:** White House Task Force to Protect Students from Sexual Assault, *Not Alone: First Report of White House Task Force to Protect Students from Sexual Assault*, April 2014, www.whitehouse.gov/sites/default/files/docs/report_0.pdf; B. Chappell, "California Enacts 'Yes means Yes' Law, Defining Sexual Consent," September 29, 2014, www.npr.org/blogs/thetwo-way/2014/09/29/352482932/california-enacts-yes-means-yes-law-defining-sexual-consent.

via the *Clery Act*, which later become the *Violence Against Women Act*.[68] In 1992, President George H. W. Bush and Congress passed the Campus Sexual Assault Victim's Bill of Rights, known as the *Ramstad Act*. The act gave victims the right to call in off-campus authorities to investigate serious campus crimes and required universities to develop educational programs and notify students of available counseling. More recent provisions of the act specify notification procedures and options for victims, rights of victims and accused perpetrators, and consequences, including possible loss of federal support, if schools do not comply. It also asks campuses to conduct climate surveys, report rapes, and provide assessments of prevention activities to the U.S. Department of Education.[69] Despite these changes, in 2014, many campuses who were not receiving

Federal funds did not report campus violence. In fact, as many as 500 of them reported no rapes or sexual assaults at all, prompting considerable national concern in the media.[70] As a result, several sources published rankings of those campuses with the highest rape occurrences—a scathing indictment of campus safety.

With a flurry of national media exposure, President Obama has raised the issue of rape on campus to the level of a national crisis with his "You are Not Alone" program.[71] For more information, see the **Health Headlines** box on sexual assault on campus.

**Marital Rape** Although its legal definition varies within the United States, *marital rape* can be any unwanted intercourse

# 78%

of **SEXUAL VIOLENCE** involves an offender who is a family member, intimate partner, friend, or acquaintance of the victim.

or penetration (vaginal, anal, or oral) obtained by force, threat of force, or when the spouse is unable to consent. This problem has undoubtedly existed since the origin of marriage as a social institution, and it is noteworthy that marital rape did not become a crime in all 50 states until 1993. Unfortunately, as many as 13 states still allow "marital exemptions" from prosecution, meaning that the judicial system may treat it as a lesser crime.[72]

Decades of research have indicated that marital rape is not that uncommon, but exact percentages are difficult to assess due to differences in marital rape laws and perceptions of whether rape within the confines of marriage is the same as rape by an acquaintance or a stranger. Does "no" mean "no" regardless of the setting? If a spouse doesn't want to have sex and yet feels that she or he must succumb to perform her or his spousal marital duty, is that rape? What if power/control issues make resistance futile and she or he is unable to physically resist? Internationally, women raised in cultures where male dominance is the norm and women are treated as property tend to have higher rates of forced sex within the confines of marriage. Women who are pregnant, ill, separated, or divorced have higher rates, as do women from homes where other forms of domestic violence are common and where there is a high rate of alcoholism or substance abuse.

**Child Sexual Abuse** Sexual abuse of children by adults or older children includes sexually suggestive conversations; inappropriate kissing; touching; petting; oral, anal, or vaginal intercourse; and other kinds of sexual interaction. In 2015, there were 315,000 reported cases of child sexual abuse in the United States.[73] Recent studies indicate that the rates of sexual abuse in children range from 1 to 35 percent of all children, with 1 in 4 girls and 1 in 6 boys being sexually abused before the age of 18.[74]

The shroud of secrecy surrounding this problem makes it likely that the number of actual cases is grossly underestimated both in the United States and globally. Unfortunately, the programs taught in schools today, often with an emphasis on "stranger danger," may give children the false impression that they are more likely to be assaulted by a stranger. In reality, 90 percent of child sexual abuse victims know their perpetrator, with nearly 70 percent of children abused by family members, usually an adult male.[75]

People who were abused as children bear spiritual, psychological, and/or physical scars. Studies have shown that child sexual abuse has an impact on later life: Children who experience sexual abuse are at increased risk for anxiety disorders, depression, eating disorders, PTSD, and suicide attempts.[76]

Youth who have been sexually abused are 25 percent more likely to experience teen pregnancy, 30 percent more likely to abuse their own children, and are much more likely to have problems with alcohol abuse or drug addiction.[77]

**Sexual Harassment** **Sexual harassment** is defined as unwelcome sexual conduct that is related to any condition of employment or evaluation of student performance. Unwelcome sexual advances, requests for sexual favors, and other verbal or physical conduct of a sexual nature constitute sexual harassment when:

- Submission to such conduct is made either explicitly or implicitly a term or condition of an individual's employment or education;
- Submission to or rejection of such conduct by an individual is used as the basis for employment or education-related decisions affecting such an individual; or
- Such conduct is sufficiently severe or pervasive that it has the effect, intended or unintended, of unreasonably interfering with an individual's work or academic performance because it has created an intimidating, hostile, or offensive environment and would have such an effect on a reasonable person of that individual's status.[78]

Commonly, people think of harassment as involving only faculty members or persons in power, where sex is used to exhibit control of a situation. However, peers can harass one another too. Sexual harassment may include unwanted touching; unwarranted sex-related comments or subtle pressure for sexual favors; deliberate or repeated humiliation or intimidation based on sex; and gratuitous comments, jokes, questions, or remarks about clothing or body, sexuality, or past sexual relationships.

Most schools and companies have sexual harassment policies in place, as well as procedures for dealing with harassment problems. Faculty, students, and employees on U.S. campuses are protected from sexual harassment and other sexual offenses under *Title IX of the Education Amendment of 1972*, which prohibits discrimination based on sex in all education programs or activities that receive federal funds.

**SEE IT! VIDEOS**

Are college administrations liable for sexual assaults on campus? Watch **95 Colleges Under Federal Investigation**, available on **MasteringHealth.**

**WHAT DO YOU THINK?**

What policies does your school have regarding consensual relationships between faculty members and students?

- Should consenting adults have the right to become intimate or interact socially, regardless of their positions within a school system or workplace?
- What are the potential dangers of such interactions? Are such interactions ever okay?

**sexual harassment** Any form of unwanted sexual attention related to any condition of employment, education, or performance evaluation.

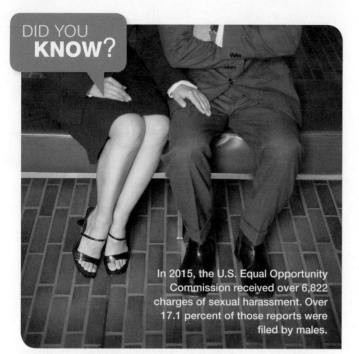

In 2015, the U.S. Equal Opportunity Commission received over 6,822 charges of sexual harassment. Over 17.1 percent of those reports were filed by males.

**Source:** Data are from U.S. Equal Employment Opportunity Commission, "Charges Alleging Sexual Harrassment, FY2010–FY2015," Accessed July 2016, https://www.eeoc.gov/eeoc/statistics/enforcement/sexual_harassment_new.cfm.

If you feel you are being harassed, the most important thing you can do is be assertive:

- **Tell the harasser to stop.** Be clear and direct. Tell the person if it continues that you will report it. If the harassing is via phone or Internet, block the person.
- **Document the harassment.** Make a record of each incident. If the harassment becomes intolerable, a record of exactly what occurred (and when and where) will help make your case. Save copies of all communication from the harasser.
- **Try to make sure you aren't alone in the harasser's presence.** Witnesses to harassment can ensure appropriate validation of the event.
- **Complain to a higher authority.** Talk to legal authorities or your instructor, adviser, or counseling center psychologist about what happened.
- **Remember that you have not done anything wrong.** You will likely feel awful after being harassed (especially if you have to complain to superiors). However, feel proud that you are not keeping silent.

**stalking** Willful, repeated, and malicious following, harassing, or threatening of another person.

**cyberstalking** Stalking that occurs online or via smart technology/tracking devices.

**bullying** Unwanted aggressive behavior, real or perceived power imbalances, and repeating behaviors designed to demean others

### Stalking and Cyberstalking

Stalking can be defined as a course of conduct directed at a specific person that would cause a reasonable person to feel fear. This may include repeated visual or physical proximity, nonconsensual written or verbal communication, and implied or explicit threats.[79]

Stalking that occurs online is referred to as **cyberstalking**; more than 1 in 4 victims report being stalked through the use of some form of technology.[80] (See the **Tech & Health** box for information on staying safe when using social networking sites.)

The most common stalking behaviors included unwanted phone calls and messages, spreading rumors, spying on the victim, and showing up at the same places as the victim without having a reason to be there.[81] Over 15 percent of women and nearly 6 percent of men have been a victim of stalking during their lifetimes.[82] The vast majority of stalkers are persons involved in relationship breakups or are other dating acquaintances; fewer than 10 percent of stalkers are strangers to their victims.[83] Adults between the ages of 18 and 24 experience the highest rates of stalking. Like sexual harassment, stalking is an underreported crime. Often students do not think a stalking incident is serious enough to report, or they worry that the police will not take it seriously.

**Social Contributors to Sexual Violence** Sexual violence and intimate partner violence share common factors that increase the likelihood of their occurrence. Certain societal assumptions and traditions can promote sexual violence, including:

- **Trivialization.** Many people think that rape committed by a husband or intimate partner doesn't count as rape.
- **Blaming the victim.** In spite of efforts to combat this type of thinking, there is still the belief that a scantily clad woman "asks" for sexual advances.
- **Pressure to be macho.** Males are taught from a young age that showing emotions is a sign of weakness. This portrayal often depicts men as aggressive and predatory, and females as passive targets.
- **Male socialization.** Many still believe ideas like "sowing wild oats" and "boys will be boys" are merely a normal part of male development. Women are often *objectified* (treated as sexual objects) in the media, which contributes to the idea that it's natural for men to be predatory.
- **Male misperceptions.** With media implying that sex is the focus of life, it's not surprising that some men believe that when a woman says no, she is really asking to be seduced. Later, these same men may be surprised when the woman says she was raped.
- **Situational factors.** Dates in which the male makes all the decisions, pays for everything, and generally controls the entire situation are more likely to end in an aggressive sexual scenario. Alcohol and other drugs increase the risk and severity of assaults.

## Bullying

When we think of "bullies," think elementary students physically and emotionally beating on the weaker and less popular. Typically, **bullying** is defined as unwanted aggressive behavior, real or perceived power imbalances, and repeating behaviors designed to demean others.[84] There are several major types of bullying:

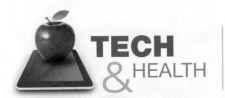

# TECH & HEALTH | SOCIAL NETWORKING SAFETY

Nearly 18 million Americans became victims of identity fraud in 2014, the majority of which involved the fraudulent use of existing credit cards or the unauthorized use or attempted use of personal information to open a new account under a different identity.

Very real threats to health, reputation, financial security, and future employment lie in wait for those who post indiscriminately and unwisely to the Web or who fail to do regular checks of their accounts and credit ratings. The following tips will help you remain safe and protect your identity when you express yourself online:

- Don't post compromising pictures, videos, or other things that you wouldn't want your mother or coworkers to see.
- Never agree to meet a stranger whom you've met only online without bringing a trusted friend, or at the very least, notifying a close friend or family member of where you will be and when you will return. Choose a well-established, public place and only meet during daylight hours. Don't give your address or traceable phone numbers to the person you are meeting.
- Change your passwords and security questions often, and don't write them all down where someone can find them.
- Avoid banking or accessing sensitive personal financial documents when

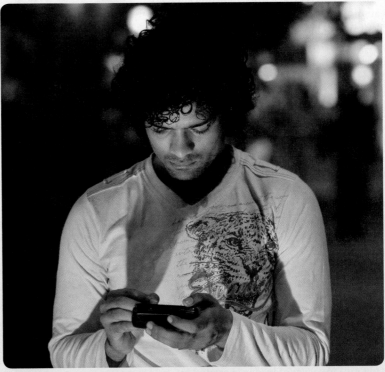

Cybercrime in the form of identity theft and hacking. Staying safe requires vigilence and use of the best available security on all your devices.

using public WiFi servers. Make sure your cell phone is not posting your location publically.
- Check for software updates for your devices and run full scans often.
- When you get rid of phones or other devices, make sure you wipe them of your data and close all accounts.
- Never give credit card information or personal information over the phone.

- Invest in a high quality micro shredder.
- Only use locking mailboxes
- Only leave small amounts of money in an overdraft fund. If you have a larger savings account, don't let it be a source of overdraft funds.

**Sources:** 2016 NCVRW Resource Guide, "Financial Crime," April 2016, Available at www. ncjrs.gov. Bureau of Justice Statistics. "Victims of Identity theft." 2015. http://www.bjs.gov/content/pub/pdf/vit14_sum.pdf

---

1. *Verbal bullying* includes saying or writing mean things, teasing people, taunting them, name-calling, and threats, either directly or indirectly.
2. *Social bullying*, also known as relational bullying, involves hurting someone's reputation, trying to demean them and turn others against them, or leaving them out of social interactions.
3. *Physical bullying* involves hitting, spitting on, or injuring someone or their possessions.
4. *Cyberbullying* is bullying usually carried out online, via social media or otherwise.

Unfortunately, elementary school bullies don't suddenly stop bullying when they go to college. They carry the same

insecurities and learned behaviors with them, using more insidious and subtle forms of bullying to torment their peers. Typically, college bullying includes gossip and rumors, shaming for purported sexual exploits, and sexual bullying. The period after a nasty breakup is often a high-risk time. Twenty to 25 percent of students report noncyberbullying victimization during college and 10 to 15 percent report cyberbullying victimization. Another 20 percent reported cyberbullying others, with no significant differences based on race or gender.[85]

More colleges and universities are increasing awareness on campus about bullying, adopting zero-tolerance programs for those found guilty of physical, social, or emotional threats to others. Unfortunately, unless stopped, bullies continue to bully in the workplace, using harassment, verbal assaults, and the same strategies that worked for them earlier in life. If you are threatened or victimized by a bully, consider the following actions:

- **Ignore and report.** Because they want a response, don't give them one. Walk away. If it is a threatening contact, report it to campus security.
- **Cut communication.** Block their numbers and e-mails. Unfriend them from Facebook or change your social media accounts. Change your routines.
- **Document.** Keep a log of bullying occurrences, noting specific times and dates and witnesses. Ask your friends to keep copies of any attacks.
- **Be proactive.** If a written antibullying policy doesn't exist on your campus, petition school administrators to implement one.
- **Stay positive.** Most importantly, don't doubt yourself, your character, or your work ethic. Don't blame yourself if you are a target. It's the bully who has a problem, not you.

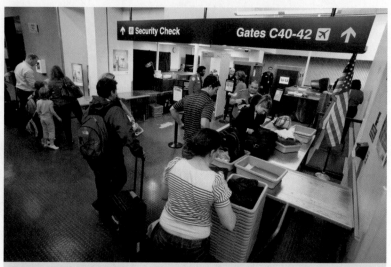
The threat of terrorism has affected many aspects of our daily lives.

## LO 4 | COLLECTIVE VIOLENCE

Describe factors that contribute to gang violence and to terrorist activities.

**Collective violence** is violence perpetrated by groups against other groups and includes violent acts related to political, governmental, religious, cultural, or social clashes. Gang violence and terrorism are two forms of collective violence that have become major threats in recent years.

## Gang Violence

Gang violence is increasing in many regions of the world; U.S. communities face escalating threats from gang networks engaged in drug trafficking, sex trafficking, shootings, beatings, thefts, carjackings, and the killing of innocent victims caught in the crossfire. Currently, there are over 33,000 gangs in the United States, with membership in excess of 1.4 million.[86] Gangs are believed to be responsible for 48 percent of U.S. violent crime overall, and in some locations, as much as 90 percent.[87]

Why do young people join gangs? Often, gangs give members a sense of self-worth, companionship, security, and excitement. In other cases, gangs provide economic security through drug sales, prostitution, and other types of criminal activity. Friendships with delinquent peers, lack of parental monitoring, negative life events, and alcohol and drug use appear to increase risks for gang affiliation. Other risk factors include low self-esteem, academic problems, low socioeconomic status, alienation from family and society, a history of family violence, and living in gang-controlled neighborhoods.[88] It becomes difficult to leave gangs once youth become involved, but prevention strategies appear to offer promise.

## Terrorism

Numerous terrorist attacks around the world reveal the vulnerability of all nations to domestic and international threats. Effects on our economy, travel restrictions, additional security measures, and military buildups are but a few of the examples of how terrorist threats have affected our lives. As defined in the U.S. Code of Federal Regulations, **terrorism** is the "unlawful use of force or violence against persons or property to intimidate or coerce a government, the civilian population, or any segment thereof in furtherance of political or social objectives."[89]

Over the past decade, the Centers for Disease Control and Prevention (CDC) established the *Emergency Preparedness and Response Division*. This group monitors potential public health problems, such as bioterrorism, chemical emergencies, radiation emergencies, mass casualties, national disaster, and severe weather; develops plans for mobilizing communities in case of emergency; and provides information about terrorist threats. In addition, the Department of Homeland Security works to prevent future attacks, and the FBI and other government agencies work to ensure citizens' health and safety.

## LO 5 | MINIMIZE YOUR RISK OF BECOMING A VICTIM OF VIOLENCE

Articulate personal strategies for minimizing the risk of violence.

It is far better to prevent a violent act than to recover from it. Both individuals and communities can play important roles in preventing violence and intentional injuries.

**collective violence** Violence perpetrated by groups against other groups.

**terrorism** Unlawful use of force or violence against persons or property to intimidate or coerce a government, civilian population, or any segment thereof in furtherance of political or social objectives.

## Self-Defense against Personal Assault and Rape

Assault can occur no matter what preventive actions you take, but common-sense self-defense tactics can lower the risk. Self-defense is a process that includes increasing your awareness, developing self-protective skills, taking reasonable precautions, and having the judgment necessary to respond quickly to changing situations. It is important to know ways to avoid and extract yourself from potentially dangerous situations.

Most attacks by unknown assailants are planned in advance. Many rapists use certain ploys to initiate their attacks. Examples include asking for help, offering help, staging a deliberate "accident" such as bumping into you, or posing as a police officer or other authority figure. Sexual assault frequently begins with a casual, friendly conversation.

Trust your intuition. Be assertive and direct with someone who is getting out of line or becoming threatening—this may convince a would-be attacker to back off. Don't try to be nice, and don't fear making a scene. Use the following tips to let a potential assailant know that you are prepared to defend yourself:

- **Speak in a strong voice.** State, "Leave me alone!" rather than, "Will you please leave me alone?" Sound like you mean it.

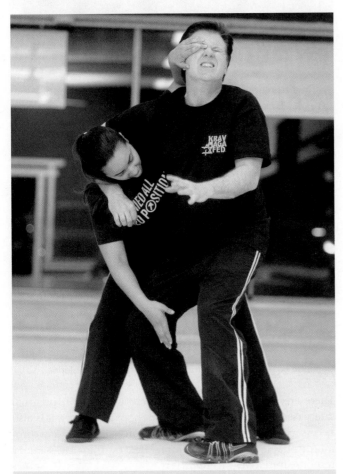

College campuses often offer safety workshops and self-defense classes to arm students with the physical and mental skills that may help them repel or deter an assailant.

- **Maintain eye contact.** This keeps you aware of the person's movements and conveys an aura of strength and confidence.
- **Stand up straight, act confident, and remain alert.** Walk as though you own the sidewalk.

If you are attacked, act immediately. Draw attention to yourself and your assailant. Scream "Fire!" as loudly as you can. Research has shown that passersby are much more likely to help if they hear the word *fire* rather than just a scream.

## What to Do if Rape Occurs

If you are a rape victim, report the attack. This gives you a sense of control. Follow these steps:

- Call 9-1-1.
- Do not bathe, shower, douche, clean up, or touch anything the attacker may have touched.
- Save the clothes you were wearing, and do not launder them. They will be needed as evidence. Bring a clean change of clothes to the clinic or hospital.
- Contact the rape assistance hotline in your area, and ask for advice on counseling if you need additional help.

If a friend is raped, here's how you can help:

- Believe the rape victim. Don't ask questions that may appear to imply that she or he is at fault in any way for the assault.
- Recognize that rape is a violent act and that the victim was not looking for this to happen.
- Encourage your friend to see a doctor immediately because she may have medical needs but feel too embarrassed to seek help on her own. Offer to go with her.
- Encourage her to report the crime.
- Be understanding, and let her know you will be there for her.
- Recognize that this is an emotional recovery, and it may take time for her to bounce back.
- Encourage your friend to seek counseling.

## LO 6 | CAMPUS-WIDE RESPONSES TO VIOLENCE

**Explain potential strategies that campus leaders, law enforcement officials, and individuals can develop to prevent students from becoming victims.**

Increasingly, campuses have become microcosms of the greater society, complete with the risks, hazards, and dangers that people face in the world. Many college administrators have been proactive in establishing violence-prevention policies, programs, and services. Campuses have begun to take a careful look at the aspects of campus culture that promote and tolerate violent acts.

## Prevention and Early Response Efforts

Campuses are conducting emergency response drills and reviewing the effectiveness of emergency messaging systems, including mobile phone alert systems. The REVERSE 9-1-1 system uses database and geographic information system (GIS) mapping technologies to notify campus police and community members in the event of problems, and other systems allow administrators to send out alerts in text, voice, e-mail, or instant message format. Some schools program the phone numbers, photographs, and basic student information for all incoming first-year students into a university security system so that in the event of a threat, students need only hit a button on their phones, whereupon campus police will be notified and tracking devices will pinpoint their location.

## Changes in the Campus Environment

There are many changes that can be made to the campus environment to improve safety. Campus lighting, parking lot security, emergency call boxes, removal of overgrown shrubbery, and stepped-up security are increasingly on the radar of campus safety personnel. Buildings can be designed with better lighting and enhanced security features, and security cameras can be installed in hallways, classrooms, and public places. Safe rides can be provided for students who have consumed too much alcohol, and health promotion programs can step up their violence prevention efforts through seminars on acquaintance rape, sexual assault, harassment, and other topics.

## Changes in Campus Policies

In response to increasing reports of rape and IPV, harassment, bullying, and other violence on campus, colleges and universities in the United States have begun to change policies and redefine violations as well as the rights of victims and offenders. However, we have a long way to go. Check with your own campus to see which policies are in affect, how policies are reported and enforced, and what actions you should take in the event of witnessing or experiencing a violent crime on campus.

## Campus Law Enforcement

Campus law enforcement has changed over the years by increasing both its numbers and its authority to prosecute student offenders. Attitudes of law enforcement have also changed so that more possible offenses and offenders are treated impartially and fairly. In fact, many campuses now hire state troopers or local law enforcement officers to deal with campus issues rather than maintain a separate police staff.

## Coping in the Event of Campus Violence

Although schools have worked tirelessly to prevent violence, it can and does still occur. In its aftermath, some may find it

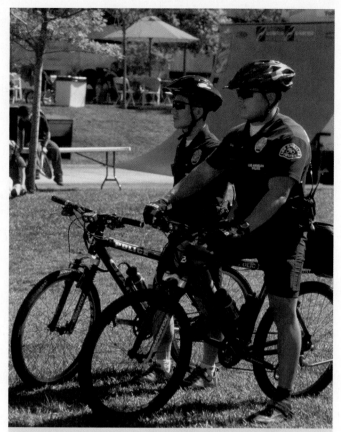

Presence and visibility of campus law enforcement have increased recently.

difficult to remain on campus, as it represents a place of violation and lack of safety; others may experience problems with concentration, studying, and other daily activities. Although there is no "fix" for these traumatic events, several strategies can be helpful. First, members of the campus community should be allowed to mourn. Memorial services and acknowledgment of grief, fear, anger, and other emotions are critical to healing. Second, students, faculty, and staff should be involved in planning to prevent future problems—it can help to impart a feeling of control. Third, students should seek out support groups, therapists who specialize in treating PTSD, and trusted family members or friends if they need to talk and work through their feelings. Journaling or writing about feelings can also help.

## LO 7 | COMMUNITY STRATEGIES FOR PREVENTING VIOLENCE

Describe community-wide strategies for preventing violence.

There are many steps you can take to ensure your personal safety (see the Making Changes Today box); however, it is also necessary to address the issues of violence and safety at a community level. Strategies recommended by the CDC's injury response initiatives include:

- Inoculate children against violence in the home. Teaching youth principles of respect and responsibility are fundamental to the health and well-being of future generations.

# MAKING **CHANGES** TODAY

## Stay Safe on All Fronts

Follow these tips to protect yourself from assault.

### OUTSIDE ALONE

- ◉ Carry a cell phone and keep it turned on, but stay off it. Be aware of what is happening around you. Don't walk to your car in a dark parking lot while chatting to others. Stay alert.
- ◎ If you are being followed, don't go home. Head for a location where there are other people. If you decide to run, run fast and scream loudly to attract attention.
- ◎ Vary your routes. Stay close to other people.
- ◎ Park in lighted areas; avoid dark areas where someone could hide.
- ◎ Carry pepper spray or other deterrents. Consider using your campus escort service.
- ◎ Tell others where you are going and when you expect to be back.

### IN YOUR CAR

- ◉ Lock your doors. Do not open your doors or windows to strangers.
- ◎ If someone hits your car, drive to the nearest gas station or other public place if you are able. Call the police or road service for help, and stay in your car until help arrives.
- ◎ If a car appears to be following you, do not drive home. Drive to the nearest police station.

### IN YOUR HOME

- ◉ Install dead bolts on all doors and locks on all windows. Make sure the locks work, and don't leave a spare key outside.
- ◎ Lock doors when at home, even during the day. Close blinds and drapes whenever you are away and in the evening when you are home.
- ◎ Rent apartments that require a security code or clearance to gain entry, and avoid easily accessible apartments, such as first-floor units. When you move into a new residence, pay a locksmith to change the keys and locks.
- ◎ Don't let repair people in without asking for identification, and have someone else with you when repairs are being made.
- ◎ Keep a cell phone near your bed and call 9-1-1 in emergencies. Buy phones that have E911 locators so that emergency personnel can find you even when you can't respond or don't know where you are.
- ◎ If you return home to find your residence has been broken into, don't enter. Call the police. If you encounter an intruder, it is better to give up money or valuables than to resist.

- Develop policies and laws that prevent violence. Enforce laws so offenders know you mean business in your settings.
- Develop skills-based educational programs that teach the basics of interpersonal communication, elements of healthy relationships, anger management, conflict resolution, appropriate assertiveness, stress management, and other health-based behaviors.
- Involve families, schools, community programs, athletics, music, faith-based organizations, and other community groups in providing experiences that help young people to develop self-esteem and self-efficacy.

- Promote tolerance and acceptance and establish and enforce policies that forbid discrimination. Offer diversity training and mandate involvement.
- Improve community services focused on family planning, mental health services, day care and respite care, and alcohol and substance abuse prevention.
- Make sure walking trails, parking lots, and other public areas are well lit, unobstructed, and patrolled regularly to reduce threats.
- Improve community-based support and treatment for victims and ensure that individuals have choices available when trying to stop violence in their lives.

# STUDY **PLAN**

Customize your study plan—and master your health!— in the Study Area of **MasteringHealth**.

## ASSESS YOURSELF

**How often are you at risk of being a victim of violence?** Want to find out? Take the **Are You at Risk for Violence?** assessment available on **MasteringHealth.™**

---

## CHAPTER **REVIEW**

To hear an MP3 Tutor Session, scan here or visit the Study Area in **MasteringHealth**.

### LO **1** | Violence in the United States

- Violence affects everyone in society—from the direct victims, to children and families who witness it, to those who modify their behaviors because they are fearful.

### LO **2** | Factors Contributing to Violence

- Factors that lead to violence include poverty or economic difficulties, unemployment, parental and family influences, cultural beliefs, discrimination or oppression, religious or political differences, breakdowns in the criminal justice system, and stress. Mental health problems, anger, and substance abuse can contribute to violence and aggression.

### LO **3** | Interpersonal Violence

- Interpersonal violence includes homicide, domestic violence, child abuse, elder abuse, and sexual victimization. Each of these causes significant emotional, social, and physical risks to health.

### LO **4** | Collective Violence

- Forms of collective violence, including gang violence and terrorism, result in fear, anxiety, and issues of discrimination.

### LO **5** | Minimize Your Risk of Becoming a Victim of Violence

- Individual strategies to reduce the risk of becoming a victim of violence include: recognize how to protect yourself and your friends; know where to turn for help; and have honest, straightforward dialogue about sexual matters in dating situations. Alcohol moderation is another key factor in reducing your risks.

### LO **6** | Campus-wide Responses to Violence

- With increasing reports of violence on campus, national attention has sharply focused what we can do to change a culture of violence. New recommendations by the White House are designed to encourage campuses to report, respond, engage, and support victims of violence and prevent violent assaults.

### LO **7** | Community Strategies for Preventing Violence

- Preventing violence is a public health priority that involves community activism, prioritizing mental and emotional health, and providing skills training in anger management, stress management, conflict resolution, and other key coping skills. Policies and procedures designed to increase security and enforce penalties are key to success.

---

## POP **QUIZ**

Visit **MasteringHealth** to personalize your study plan with Chapter Review Quizzes and Dynamic Study Modules.

### LO **1** | Violence in the United States

1. ___ is an example of an *intentional injury*.
   a. A car accident
   b. Murder
   c. Accidental drowning
   d. Road rage

### LO **2** | Factors Contributing to Violence

2. An emotional reaction brought about by a frustrating life experience is called
   a. reactive aggression.
   b. primary aggression.
   c. secondary aggression.
   d. tertiary aggression.

### LO **3** | Interpersonal Violence

3. When Jane began a new job with all male coworkers, her supervisor told her that he enjoyed having an attractive woman in the workplace, and he winked at her. His comment constitutes
   a. poor judgment, but not a problem if Jane likes compliments.
   b. sexual assault.
   c. sexual harassment.
   d. sexual battering.

4. In a sociology class, some students were discussing sexual assault. One student commented that some women dress too provocatively. The assumption this student made is
   a. minimization.
   b. trivialization.
   c. blaming the victim.
   d. "boys will be boys."

5. Which of the following statements is *correct*?
   a. In 8 out of 10 homicides, the victim is female.
   b. The majority of all sexual assaults against women are by men who the women know.
   c. "Date rape" is the appropriate ("politically correct") label for a rape by a person the woman knows well.
   d. Homicide is the leading cause of death for Hispanic women.

6. Jack beats his wife Melissa "to teach her a lesson." Afterward, he apologizes profusely and swears he'll never hurt her again. This illustrates which phase of the cycle of violence?
   a. Acute battering
   b. Fear/depression
   c. Remorse/reconciliation
   d. Tension building

## LO 4 | Collective Violence

7. Which of the following is an example of collective violence?
   a. Sexual assault
   b. Homicide
   c. Domestic violence
   d. Terrorism

## LO 5 | Minimize Your Risk of Becoming a Victim of Violence

8. Which of the following is recommended in the case of rape?
   a. Wait 24 hours before seeing a doctor.
   b. Call 9-1-1 immediately.
   c. Wash clothes the attacker touched.
   d. Shower immediately.

## LO 6 | Campus-wide Responses to Violence

9. Which of the following is *true* regarding responses to violence on campus?
   a. "Bystander" education is one of the new strategies for helping prevent a sexual assault.
   b. Most sexual assault programs should focus their money/effort on women only because they are the ones most likely to be victims.
   c. E-mail alerts and campus lockdowns are not effective ways of preventing a possible violent attack on campus.
   d. In the aftermath of media attention and White House reports designed to curb sexual violence, campus reports of violence have dropped dramatically.

## LO 7 | Community Strategies for Preventing Violence

10. Which of the following is a tip to protect yourself from assault?
    a. If a car is following you, drive home, go in, and lock your doors.
    b. If you get home and find your residence has been broken into, go inside, assess damages, and call the police.
    c. Talk or text on your phone when you're outside alone to look busy.
    d. If you're going somewhere alone, tell others where you are going and when you expect to be back.

*Answers to the Pop Quiz can be found on page A-1. If you answered a question incorrectly, review the section identified by the Learning Outcome. For even more study tools, visit* **MasteringHealth**.

# THINK ABOUT IT!

## LO 1 | Violence in the United States

1. What forms of violence do you think are most significant or prevalent in the United States today? Which ones are you most concerned about right now? Why? What programs/policies are in effect on your campus to prevent violent attacks? Would you know what to do if a campus lockdown occurred?

## LO 2 | Factors Contributing to Violence

2. Some people have said we have an "epidemic of meanness" in society today. Why do some people develop into violent or abusive adults and others become pacifists or peaceful adults? What key factors influence violent offenders to be violent? What three key things could we do to reduce violence in the United States? Globally?

## LO 3 | Interpersonal Violence

3. Have you known anyone personally who has been sexually assaulted on campus? What actions were taken to help him or her cope with the assault? What campus services, if any, were used?

## LO 4 | Collective Violence

4. Have you been affected by acts of terrorism or gang violence? What strategies can you take to discourage collective violence, as an individual and as a community?

## LO 5 | Minimize Your Risk of Becoming a Victim of Violence

5. What are some everyday decisions you can make to minimize your risk of becoming a victim of violence? How can you be a good friend to someone who has become a victim of violence?

## LO 6 | Campus-wide Responses to Violence

6. Is your campus safe? What steps has your campus administration and community taken to reduce levels of campus-wide violence?

## Community Strategies for Preventing Violence

7. What actions need to be taken to stem the tide of violence in the United States at the individual level? At the community level? In schools? On college campuses? Nationally?

# ACCESS YOUR HEALTH ON THE INTERNET

Visit **MasteringHealth** for links to the websites and RSS feeds.

The following websites explore further topics and issues related to violence and abuse.

**Not Alone.** This site houses the report of the White House Task Force to Protect Students from Sexual Assault and recommendations for reporting, responding, and preventing future assaults. Detailed recommendations and action plans.
www.whitehouse.gov/sites/default/files/docs/report_0.pdf

**Men Can Stop Rape.** Practical suggestions for men interested in helping to protect women from sexual predators and assault are provided on this site.
www.mencanstoprape.org

**Department of Homeland Security Active Shooter Preparedness.** The DHS website includes a lot of information on disaster preparation. In terms of violence preparation, there is a specific page, complete with a self-guided course, on what to do in the instance of an active shooter. In light of the ever growing number of shootings in the United States, it helps to be prepared.
https://www.dhs.gov/active-shooter-preparedness

**National Center for Injury Prevention and Control.** The Web-based Injury Statistics Query and Reporting System (WISQARS) database of this CDC section provides statistics and information on fatal and nonfatal injuries, both intentional and unintentional.
www.cdc.gov/injury

**National Sexual Violence Resource Center.** This is an excellent resource for victims of sexual violence.
www.nsvrc.org

# FOCUS ON

# Reducing Your Risk of Unintentional Injury

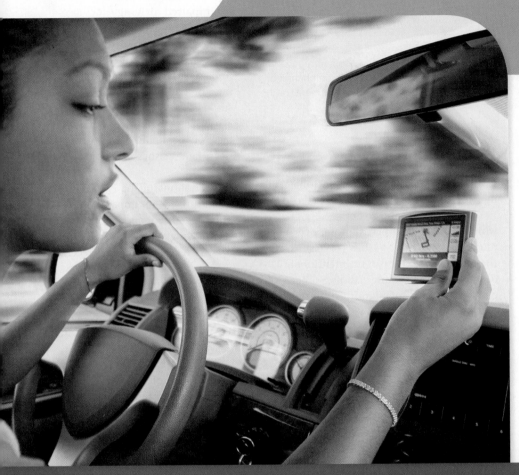

## LEARNING OUTCOMES

**LO 1** Discuss factors that contribute to motor vehicle crashes and how to reduce their occurrence.

**LO 2** Explain safety guidelines for recreational activities that are particularly prone to cause injury.

**LO 3** Discuss injuries that occur in the home and what you can do to prevent them.

**LO 4** Describe work-related injuries and what you can do to prevent them.

**LO 5** Explain how to prepare for and respond to natural disasters and severe weather events.

## WHY SHOULD I CARE?

Unintentional injuries are the leading causes of death for those aged 1 to 44 in the United States, killing more young people in the prime of their lives than any other cause each year.[1] Because the great majority of unintentional injuries occur as a result of people's poor choices, including use of alcohol and other risky behaviors, there are several actions you can take to reduce your risk. Strategies include changing your behavior or aspects of your environment that put you in harm's way.

When Matt planned his birthday trip for spring break, he never thought he'd be spending part of the day in a hospital room. After drinking for several hours at the cantina on the beach, he and his friends made their way back to their hotel to continue the party by the swimming pool. They were in a celebratory mood when two of Matt's friends picked him up and threw him into the water, shouting, "Happy Birthday!" When he hit the water, Matt started thrashing, but was too drunk to understand what was happening. All he knew was an all-consuming panic as he inhaled the water. Then he passed out. Fortunately, another hotel patron

**549**

sitting by the pool recognized what his friends were too intoxicated to realize: Matt was drowning. She jumped into the water and pulled Matt's limp body to the edge, screaming to his friends, "Dial 9-1-1!" Then she started cardiopulmonary resuscitation (CPR). As the ambulance arrived, Matt regained consciousness, but even hours later, in his hospital room, he had no memory of what had really happened to him.

Drowning is just one of many unintentional injuries in which substance abuse commonly plays a role. Other factors—such as drowsiness, distraction, and failing to take sensible precautions—also increase your risk of injury. In fact, although the term **unintentional injury** might sound academic, most health professionals shy away from the more familiar term *accidental injury* because it implies that these injuries occur without individuals having any control over their situation. As we saw with Matt's near-drowning, "accidents" often occur as a consequence of people's poor choices.

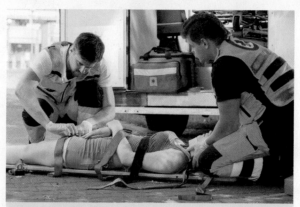

Unintentional injuries killed over 127,792 Americans in 2012. That's 350 people a day. Most strategies for preventing unintentional injuries focus on changing something about the person, the environment, or the circumstances that put people in harm's way.

# 47,500

Americans died in 2014 of a drug overdose, over 1.5 times the number killed in car accidents. Most involved a **PRESCRIPTION OPIOID** or heroin.

How big a problem is unintentional injury? In 2014, unintentional injury was the leading cause of death for Americans age 1 through 44, and it is

now the fourth leading cause of death overall.[2] More than 130,000 Americans of all ages were killed by unintentional injuries in 2014.[3] Recently, unintentional poisonings, the great majority of which are due to drug overdose, overtook motor vehicle crashes (MVCs) as the number one cause of unintentional death.[4] Among young adults, other common causes of significant unintentional mortalities each year include falls, drownings, and fires.

LO 1 | **MOTOR VEHICLE INJURIES**

Discuss factors that contribute to motor vehicle crashes and how to reduce their occurrence.

In 2014, 33,736 Americans of all ages died of injuries sustained in MVCs.[5] That's an average of 92 people every day, and makes motor vehicle crashes the second-leading cause of all unintentional injury deaths. What factors contribute to motor vehicle crashes? And how can you reduce your risk?

## Your Choices Affect Motor Vehicle Safety

Factors within your control—impaired driving because of intoxication or drowsiness, distracted driving via phone and text, speeding and other forms of aggressive driving, and vehicle safety issues

such as failure to wear a helmet or your seat belt—contribute to the great majority of motor vehicle crash fatalities.[6]

### Impaired Driving

In 2014, nearly one-third of all motor vehicle fatalities involved an alcohol-impaired driver, making alcohol the primary cause of **impaired driving**.[7] Of alcohol-impaired drivers involved in fatalities, 7 percent had a previous conviction for driving while impaired (DWI) and another 24 percent had a history of license suspension or revocation.[8] The age group with the highest percentage of alcohol-impaired drivers involved in fatal crashes is people aged 21 to 24.[9]

After alcohol, marijuana is the drug most often linked to impaired driving.[10] Marijuana use reduces attention, increases weaving in and out of traffic, and slows reaction time.[11] A recent study of fatal crashes in Colorado shows increases in the number of fatal crashes since the legalization of marijuana.[12] Prescription drugs, mainly opioids and sedatives, are also common factors in MVC fatalities.[13]

Drowsiness is a form of impairment that plays a major role in fatal crashes. Many researchers contend that driving while sleep-deprived is as dangerous as driving drunk. Drowsy driving is estimated to cause up to 6,000 fatal MVCs each year.[14]

Both public health and law enforcement agencies are cooperating on several measures to keep impaired drivers off the road. These include:

- Promotion of community-based designated driver programs, including measures such as public funding of "safe rides" for people who have been drinking, and training restaurant and bar staff to enforce drink

### SEE IT! VIDEOS

Are you at risk of falling asleep at the wheel? Watch **Dozing and Driving: 1 in 24 Asleep at Wheel**, available on MasteringHealth.™

---

**unintentional injury** Any injury committed or sustained without intent of harm.

**impaired driving** Driving under the influence of alcohol or other drugs.

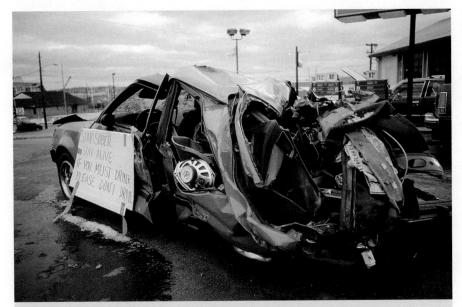

Driving under the influence of alcohol greatly increases the risk of being responsible for a fatal motor vehicle crash. In 2014, 31 percent of all fatal crashes involved an alcohol-impaired driver.

Source: NHTSA, "Traffic Safety Facts 2014 Data: Alcohol-Impaired Driving," DOT HS 812 231, December 2015, www-nrd.nhtsa.dot.gov/Pubs/812231.pdf.

limits and recognize and deny alcohol to impaired customers.

- Strict enforcement of existing laws defining impaired driving and the legal drinking age.
- Implementation of measures to prevent repeat offenses by anyone previously convicted of driving while impaired, whether due to alcohol or other drugs or to drowsiness: mandatory alcohol or other drug abuse treatment; installation of ignition interlock systems that prevent vehicle operation by anyone with a blood alcohol concentration above a specified safe level; revoking the driver's license.

## Distracted Driving

Three types of activities constitute **distracted driving**: taking your eyes off the road, taking your hands off the steering wheel, and taking your mind off driving.[15] Every day in the United States, more than 1,000 people are injured and 8 die in motor vehicle crashes involving distracted driving.[16]

Although there's no conclusive evidence identifying the forms of distraction most likely to contribute to MVCs, the behavior of greatest concern is texting. Overall, 31 percent of U.S. drivers aged 18 to 64 report texting while driving.[17] Highway safety experts estimate that the average text takes the driver's eyes off the road for long enough, traveling 55 miles per hour, to cross a football field.[18] Currently, 46 states ban texting while driving, and 14 states ban all handheld cell phone use of any kind while driving.[19]

## Aggressive Driving

The National Highway Traffic Safety Administration (NHTSA) describes **aggressive driving** as occurring "when an individual commits a combination of moving traffic offenses so as to endanger other persons or property."[20] Speeding is typically involved. Driver surveys suggest that many people speed because they don't perceive it as dangerous; they believe that traffic laws are overly restrictive and don't apply to them; they feel under time pressure, such as to arrive on time to work; or they simply enjoy the experience of speeding.[21] Although younger males in general are the population group most likely to speed, younger females are more likely to speed than older adults of either sex.[22] Every day, about 25 Americans die in speed-related car crashes; in 2014, speeding was a factor in

28 percent of all MVC fatalities, resulting in over 9,200 deaths.[23]

Speeding is not the only form of aggressive driving. Passing where prohibited, running red lights, weaving in and out of traffic, and tailgating are other forms, and all are linked to an increased MVC risk.

## Vehicle Safety Issues

Wearing a safety belt cuts your risk of death or serious injury in a crash by almost half.[24] Although about 87 percent of Americans report wearing a safety belt, 49 percent of all people killed in MVCs in 2014 were not wearing one at the time of the crash.[25] Each year, safety belt use is estimated to save more than 12,000 lives.[26] So buckle up, and insist any passengers do the same. If you're

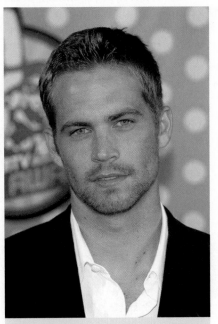

In November 2013 actor Paul Walker was killed when the Porsche driven by his friend Roger Rodas hit an electricity pole and a tree. Both men died within seconds of impact. Office police reports estimated that Rodas had been driving at a speed of more than 90 mph in a 45 mph zone.

**distracted driving** Driving while performing any nondriving activity that has the potential to distract someone from the primary task of driving and increase the risk of crashing.

**aggressive driving** Driving involving a combination of moving traffic offenses that endanger other persons or property.

transporting an infant or child in your vehicle, follow state laws governing use and location of age-appropriate safety seats.

In addition, buying vehicles with the highest crash safety ratings, side and knee airbags, antilock brakes, traction and stability controls, impact-absorbing crumple zones, strong compartment and roof supports, as well as automatic braking for impending frontal crashes and blind spot assistance, all make good sense if you are trying to keep yourself and loved ones safe on the road. Unfortunately, people who don't have the financial resources to drive vehicles with all of these safety features—and that group often includes college students—are at increased risk during MVCs.

Another factor in MVC safety is the size of the vehicles involved. All cars sold in the United States must meet U.S. Department of Transportation standards for crashworthiness, no matter their size. However, in 2014 there were nearly three times as many deaths per vehicle among minicars as compared to very large cars, and all of the 19 cars with the lowest rates of driver deaths were midsize or larger.[27] However, both size and weight matter, and hybrid electric vehicles, which are heavy because of their battery packs, are estimated to be about 25 percent safer than the same model of car with a traditional combustion engine.[28] Many college students drive small cars because they are more affordable and use less gas. If you're among them, consider a hybrid.

## Motorcyclists Face Unique Risks

Motorcycles are less visible to other drivers and less stable when turning, swerving, and braking quickly. Of

# 95%

of college students surveyed reported that they mostly or always wear a **SAFETY BELT** when driving or riding in a car.

---

# MAKING **CHANGES** TODAY

## Minimizing the Chance of Injury During a Motor Vehicle Crash

If a car crash is unavoidable, you can still behave in a way that lessens the chance of serious injury. Some tips include:

- Generally, it's safer to veer right rather than left. Drive onto the shoulder of the road if possible.

- Steer, don't skid, off the road to avoid rolling your vehicle.

- If you hear brakes screeching from a vehicle behind you and a rear-end collision seems unavoidable, put your foot on your brake pedal. This will help prevent your car from being propelled into the vehicle in front of you. Also, lean the back of your head against the headrest. This will help keep your head from being thrown back against the headrest and then forward again.

- If you are in a middle lane of a multilane road, and a vehicle in the oncoming lane veers into your lane and approaches you head-on, it's safer to sideswipe another vehicle traveling in your direction than to collide with the one in front of you.

- Avoid hitting pedestrians, motorcyclists, and bicyclists at all costs.

---

course, motorcyclists have less injury protection as well. As a result of these factors, per vehicle mile traveled, motorcyclists are about 26 times more likely than passenger car occupants to die in an MVC.[29] In 2014, this translated into over 4,500 motorcyclist deaths,[30] and 92,000 more were injured.[31]

The NHTSA reports that, in 2014, 39 percent of fatally injured motorcyclists were not wearing a helmet.[32] Moreover, the NHTSA estimates that helmets saved the lives of 1,669 motorcyclists in 2014.[33] Although the benefits of helmets and protective clothing are well established, only 19 states have full helmet requirements for anyone riding a motorcycle.[34] To find out what your state requirements are, go to *www.iihs. org/iihs/topics/laws/helmetuse*.

## Improve Your Driving Skills

Although you can't control what other drivers are doing, you can reduce your risk of injury in an MVC by practicing the following driving techniques:

- Don't use electronic devices while driving. Avoid talking on a cell phone while driving, even if the phone is hands free.

- Don't drink and drive—take a taxi or arrange for someone to be the designated driver.

- Keep your eyes on the road. Scan the road ahead of you and to both sides.

- Keep your mind on the road. Don't drive when tired, highly stressed, worried, or emotional.

- Avoid aggressive driving. This includes speeding, unnecessary lane changes, passing where prohibited, running red lights, and failing to yield the right of way. It also includes tailgating: The rear bumper of the car ahead of you should be at least 3 seconds' worth of distance away, making stopping safely possible. Increase the distance when visibility is reduced, speed is increased, or roads are slick.

- Drive with your low-beam headlights on, *day and night*, to make your car more visible to other drivers.

- Drive defensively. Be on the alert for unsignaled lane changes, sudden braking, or other unexpected maneuvers.

- Obey all traffic laws.

- Always wear a seat belt, whether you're the driver or the passenger.

Even the most careful drivers may find themselves having to avoid a crash at some time in their lives. See the **Making Changes Today** box for tips on how to reduce your risk of injury in a crash.

## LO 2 | RECREATIONAL INJURIES

Explain safety guidelines for recreational activities that are particularly prone to cause injury.

Recreational activities that commonly involve injury include biking, skateboarding, snow sports, swimming and boating, and using fireworks. The following basic guidelines can help you stay safe.

### Follow Bike Safety Rules

The National Highway and Traffic Safety Administration (NHTSA) reports that, in 2014, 726 bicyclists died in traffic collisions, and 50,000 were injured.[35] Most fatal collisions occur at nonintersections (60 percent) between the hours of 4:00 P.M. and midnight. Alcohol also plays a significant role in bicycle deaths and injuries: In about one-third of all fatal crashes between motor vehicles and bicycles, either the driver or the cyclist was drunk.[36]

Wearing a properly fitted bicycle helmet has been estimated to reduce the risk of head injury by half.[37] All cyclists should wear a properly fitted bicycle helmet every time they ride (**FIGURE 1**). In addition to wearing a helmet approved by the American National Standards Institute (ANSI) or the Snell Memorial Foundation, cyclists should consider the following suggestions:

- Watch the road and listen for traffic sounds! Never listen to an MP3 player or talk on a cell phone while cycling.
- Don't drink and ride.
- Follow all traffic laws, signs, and signals.
- Ride with the flow of traffic.
- Wear light or brightly colored reflective clothing that is easily seen at dawn, dusk, and during full daylight.
- Avoid riding after dark. If you must ride at night, use a front light and a red reflector or flashing rear light, as well as reflective tape or other markings on your bike and clothing.
- Use proper hand signals.
- Keep your bicycle in good condition.
- Use bike paths whenever possible.
- Stop at stop signs and traffic lights.

### Stay Safe on Your Board or Skis

According to the U.S. Consumer Product Safety Commission (CPSC), skateboard-related injuries are commonly due to riding in traffic, trick riding, excessive speed, and consumption of alcohol. Lack of protective equipment, poor board maintenance, riding on irregular road surfaces, inexperience,

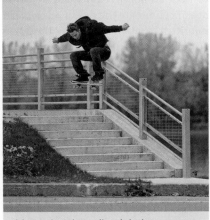

Many skateboarding injuries occur among people who have been practicing the sport for more than a year, often when they attempt a stunt beyond their level of skill. Wearing a helmet will help protect you in case of a fall.

and overconfidence also play a role.[38] A national skateboarding safety organization that tracks skateboard fatalities estimates an average of 29 deaths annually, the great majority of which occur when a skateboarder collides with a vehicle.[39] Skateboard safety tips from the CPSC include:[40]

- Wear an approved helmet designed for skateboarding, as well as gloves, wrist guards, knee and elbow pads, and flat-soled shoes.
- Maintain your board. Between uses, check it for loose, broken, sharp, or cracked parts.
- Examine the surface where you'll be riding for holes, bumps, and debris.
- Never skateboard in the street, and never hitch a ride from another vehicle.
- Don't speed.
- Don't ride alone.
- Don't drink and ride.

Snowboarding has a lower fatality rate than skateboarding. During the 2014–2015 ski season, there were six snowboarding fatalities in the United States.[41] Skiers don't fare as well: In the same year, there were 29 deaths of U.S. skiers.[42] Severe nonfatal injuries, such as head trauma and spinal cord injury, also occur.

Although one of the most important ways to protect yourself on the slopes is

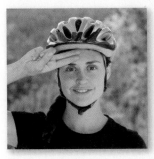

**1** The helmet should sit level on your head and low on your forehead—one or two finger-widths above your eyebrows.

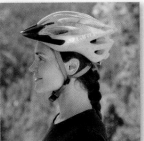

**2** The sliders on the side straps should be adjusted to form a "V" shape under, and slightly in front of, your ears. Lock the sliders if possible.

**3** The chin strap buckle should be centered under your chin. Tighten the strap until it is snug, so that no more than two fingers fit under the strap.

**FIGURE 1** **Fitting a Bicycle Helmet** Proper fit for helmets is an essential part of staying safe. Invest in a high-quality helmet and make sure it is fit properly.

 **VIDEO TUTOR** Biking Safety

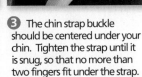

to wear an approved helmet, doing so doesn't eliminate the risk of severe head injuries and fatalities. During the 2014–2015 ski season, 26 of the 35 people who died were wearing helmets; therefore, skiers are warned against assuming that it's safe to take risks on the slopes because they're wearing a helmet.[43] It's also important to keep skis and snowboards in good condition, ski according to your ability, stay alert, and if you stop, move to the side of the trail.

The sun's ultraviolet (UV) rays can be up to eight times stronger on ski slopes than elsewhere.[44] When skiing in bright sunlight, wear sunscreen on exposed skin, as well as glasses or goggles designed for winter sports.

## Stay Safe in the Water

In 2014, 3406 Americans died by drowning, making it the fifth leading cause of unintentional injury death among Americans of all ages.[45] Children aged 1 to 4 have the highest rate of drowning, but young Americans aged 15 to 24 experience the most drownings—507 in 2014.[46] People who survive near-drownings may experience severe brain damage.[47]

### Drowning Risk Factors

Lack of swimming ability, lack of barriers around unsupervised swimming areas, lack of skilled supervision around water locations, failure to wear a **personal flotation device** (a life jacket), temperature extremes that cause hypothermia, riptides and other hazardous conditions, seizure disorders, and excess alcohol use all increase drowning risk. In fact, the vast majority of adults who drown are not wearing a personal flotation device (88 percent) and are under the influence of alcohol (70 percent).[48]

Most drownings occur during water recreation—either in backyard pools or natural water locations where people congregate to have fun. Often parents or lifeguards are not present. Many victims

**personal flotation device** A device worn to provide buoyancy and keep the wearer, conscious or unconscious, afloat with the nose and mouth out of the water; also known as a life jacket.

are strong swimmers, but can't get out of dangerous waters quickly enough. To be safe, take the following precautions around water:

- Learn how to swim. It is never too late.
- Learn CPR. When seconds can mean the difference between life and death, you want to be ready and able to save a loved one's life.
- Don't drink alcohol or take other drugs before or while swimming.
- Never swim alone, even if you are a skilled swimmer. Tell others where you are going.
- Pay attention to water temperature. Hypothermia can cause you to become disoriented and weak very quickly.
- Never leave a child unattended, even in extremely shallow water. Keep gates and barriers to backyard pools locked at all times.
- Before entering the water, check the depth. Most neck and back injuries result from diving into water that is too shallow.
- Never swim in a river with currents too swift for easy, relaxed swimming.
- Watch riptide warnings and beach conditions. If you are caught in a rip current, swim parallel to the shore. Once you are free of the current, swim toward the shore.

## Boating

In 2014, the U.S. Coast Guard received reports of 2,678 injured boaters and 610 deaths.[49] About 78 percent of these boating fatalities were drownings, and among those who drowned, 84 percent were not wearing a personal flotation device.[50]

Although operator inattention, inexperience, excessive speed, and mechanical failure also contributed to these deaths, alcohol consumption was the leading factor.[51] The U.S. Coast Guard and every state have "Boating under the Influence" (BUI) laws that carry stringent penalties for violation, including fines, license revocation, and even jail time.[52]

To stay safe when boating, the American Boating Association recommends sharing your plans for your outing, checking the weather ahead of time, making sure your boat is in good condition and has the proper safety equipment, and carrying an emergency radio and cell phone.[53] In addition, make sure you have enough life jackets for all who are on board, put on your life jacket before setting out, and wear it at all times while on the water.

If going on a snorkeling, diving, sailing, or other venture, check the qualifications and safety record of the company you are using. Also, don't

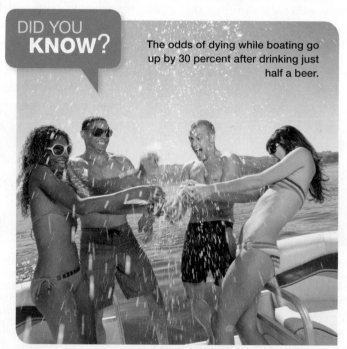

DID YOU **KNOW**?

The odds of dying while boating go up by 30 percent after drinking just half a beer.

**Source:** Data are from American Bating Association, "Alcohol Sharply Raises Death Risk for Boaters," 2016, www.americanboating.org/alcohol_in_deadly_accidents.asp.

sign up for trips where boat operators "party" with their passengers.

Like the snow, water re-flects UV rays. Wear sun-protective clothing, sunscreen on exposed skin, a hat, and sunglasses with UV protection.

## Have Fun with Fireworks—Safely

It's the Fourth of July, and you plan to celebrate with friends. If you bring along some fireworks, play it safe: In 2014, improper use of fireworks killed at least 11 Americans and caused 10,500 injuries treated in hospital emergency departments, often the loss of fingers or hands.[54] Here are some safety tips from the National Council on Fireworks Safety:[55]

- Only use fireworks outdoors in an open area, at least 50 feet from spectators, buildings, dry grasses, etc.
- Have plenty of water handy—either a hose or a bucket.
- When lighting fireworks, crouch down and reach out. Never bend over them, hold onto them, or throw them. Light the fuse and step away.
- Use only commercial fireworks. Homemade fireworks can kill you.
- Never tamper with fireworks. Use them only as packaged.
- Never try to relight a "dud" firework. It could explode in your hand. Set it aside for 20 minutes, then soak it in a bucket of water and discard.
- Alcohol and fireworks don't mix. Anyone who has been drinking should keep away from fireworks.

Before using any type of fireworks, check your state laws. You can find a state-by-state directory of fireworks-related laws at *www.fireworksafety.com*.

## LO 3 | INJURIES AT HOME

Discuss injuries that occur in the home and what you can do to prevent them.

Common unintentional injuries within the home include poisonings, falls, and burns. Although older adults are particularly vulnerable, thousands of young adults, teens, and children are brought to emergency rooms for treatment of such injuries.

## Prevent Poisoning

A **poison** is any substance that is harmful to your body when ingested, inhaled, injected, or absorbed through the skin. Unintentional poisoning is now the leading cause of unintentional injury deaths. In 2014, there were 42,032 poisoning deaths, and 28,000 of these were due to opioid overdose, including both prescription opioids and heroin.[56] Over-the-counter (OTC) drugs are also commonly implicated in overdose incidents. These include cough syrup and sleep medications, as well as aspirin and other pain relievers.

In 2014, 56 poison control centers in the United States logged more than 2.8 million calls for assistance with a poisoning.[57] The safety tips below were adapted from the American Association of Poison Control Centers:[58]

- Read and follow all usage and warning labels before taking medications or working with chemicals, including household products.
- Never share or sell your prescription drugs. Don't take prescriptions meant for others.
- Never take more than one medication at the same time without the approval of your health care provider. Also follow medication guidelines for alcohol consumption.
- When using household products, never mix them, as combinations of products can give off toxic fumes.
- When working with chemicals, wear a protective mask and make sure the area in which you are working is well ventilated. Wear gloves and other protective clothing if there is any possibility of skin contact and eyeglasses or an eye guard if splashing could occur.
- Program the national poison control number, 1-800-222-1222, into your cell phone. The line is open 24 hours a day, 7 days a week.

If you're with someone who is unconscious and you suspect the cause is a drug overdose or other poisoning, call 9-1-1. If you're trained in CPR (discussed shortly), provide CPR until paramedics arrive.

## Avoid Falls

Falls are the third most common cause of death from unintentional injury in the United States, causing 31,959 deaths in 2014.[59] About 20 percent of people who fall suffer serious injury, such as a hip fracture or a head injury. In fact, falls are the most common cause of both of these injuries.[60] Observe the following measures to reduce your risk of falls:

- Keep the floor and the stairs clear from all objects.
- Avoid using small scatter rugs and mats, which can slide out from under your feet. Use rubberized liners or strips to secure large rugs to the floor.
- Train your pets to stay away from your feet.
- Install slip-proof mats, treads, or decals in showers and tubs and on the stairs.
- Indoors or outdoors, if you need to access something beyond your reach, use an appropriate step stool or short ladder. Make sure it's stable before climbing.

## Reduce Your Risk of Fire

In 2013 more than 3,468 Americans died in a fire.[61] Although fire-related deaths are not common on college campuses in the United States, a total of 85 fatal campus fires occurred between January 2000 and May 2015, claiming 118 lives.[62]

Smoke alarms were missing or disconnected in 58 percent of these fatal fires. Alcohol was a factor in 76 percent; specifically, at least one of the students involved was legally drunk.[63] Intoxication increases the risk for not only a fire, but also for injury and death once a fire begins, in part because of less effective responses and evacuations. The primary causes of fires in campus housing are cooking, use of candles, smoking, faulty wiring, and arson.[64]

**poison** Any substance harmful to the body when ingested, inhaled, injected, or absorbed through the skin.

## Fire Prevention

Tips to prevent fires include:

- Extinguish all cigarettes in ashtrays before bed, and never smoke in bed!
- Set lamps and candles away from curtains, linens, paper, and other combustibles. Never leave candles unattended or burning while you sleep.
- In the kitchen, keep hot pads and kitchen cloths away from stove burners; avoid reaching over hot pans. Use caution when lighting barbecue grills.
- Avoid overloading electrical circuits with appliances and cords.
- Have the proper fire extinguishers ready in case of fire, and replace batteries in smoke alarms and test them periodically.

## What to Do in a Fire

If a fire breaks out in your dorm or apartment, your priority is to get out. Don't take time to phone before leaving. Don't gather up your stuff. First, feel the door handle: If it's hot, don't open the door!

**cardiopulmonary resuscitation (CPR)** Emergency technique to provide lifesaving chest compression and mouth-to-mouth resuscitation when an individual has stopped breathing and has no pulse. Use of an automated external defibrillator to reset the heart rhythm may be required.

Go to a window, open it as fully as possible, and call for help. Hang a sheet or piece of clothing from the window to let rescuers know where you are. If no one is outside, call 9-1-1. If smoke is entering the room, seal the cracks in the door with blankets, towels, or clothes. Then stay low until you're rescued—there is less smoke close to the floor.

If the door handle is not hot, open the door cautiously. If the hallway is clear to the exit, get out, yelling, "Fire!" and knocking on doors as you leave. If you encounter smoke, stay low to the floor—crawl if necessary—to make your way out. If you pass a fire alarm on your way out, pull it. Always use the stairs, never an elevator. Once you're outside, dial 9-1-1.

The same tips apply when you're staying in a hotel or motel. Always bring a flashlight with you when traveling, and study the evacuation plan posted in your room. Before going to bed, locate the two exits nearest your room and the fire alarms on your floor.

## Learn First Aid and CPR

If you were to encounter someone who is injured, would you offer assistance? Many bystanders don't because they lack training and are afraid their efforts will do more harm than good. However, one simple action can help any injury victim: Dial 9-1-1. As soon as your call is answered, describe the situation, then follow the advice you're given. (First aid measures are provided in Appendix B, "Providing Emergency Care.")

If you witness someone who has collapsed and you cannot detect a pulse, the American Heart Association advises that you call 9-1-1 and then begin chest compressions.[65] This technique simply requires you to push down in the middle of the victim's chest hard and fast (about 100 compressions per minute).

Traditional **cardiopulmonary resuscitation (CPR)** may involve chest compressions, mouth-to-mouth resuscitation, and use of an automated external defibrillator, a device that, in a person experiencing a cardiac arrest, shocks the heart to restore normal, rhythmic beating. Everyone is encouraged to get training in CPR, and the course is offered on most college campuses.

## Limit Your Exposure to Loud Noise

Our modern society is too often filled with excessive noise. Take a look at **FIGURE 2**, which shows the decibel (dB) levels of various common sounds. In general, chronic exposure to noise levels above 85 dB (about as loud as a diesel truck) can result in hearing loss. When you consider the many such noises people are exposed to every day, it should be no surprise that hearing loss is becoming increasingly common. In fact, an estimated 38 million Americans aged 18 and older have some degree of hearing loss.[66] This represents about 15 percent of this age group. Hearing loss becomes more common with each decade we age: 2 percent of adults aged 45 to 54 disabling hearing loss, but prevalence increases to 50 percent among those aged 75 and older.[67] The prevalence of disabling hearing loss in the United States is therefore expected to rise as the population ages overall.

Noise-induced hearing loss results when exposure to high-decibel noise, usually over extended periods of time, damages sensory receptors in the

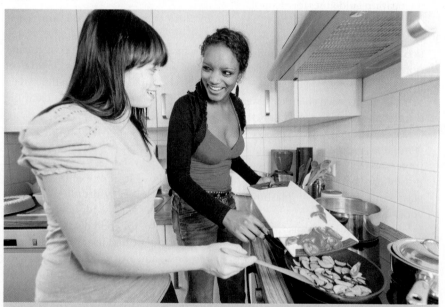

Cooking is the number one cause of residential fires, including those that result in injuries. Keep a fire extinguisher in your kitchen, and make sure you know how to use it.

**Source:** U.S Fire Administration, "U.S. Fire Statistics," April 27, 2016, https://www.usfa.fema.gov/data/statistics/index.html.

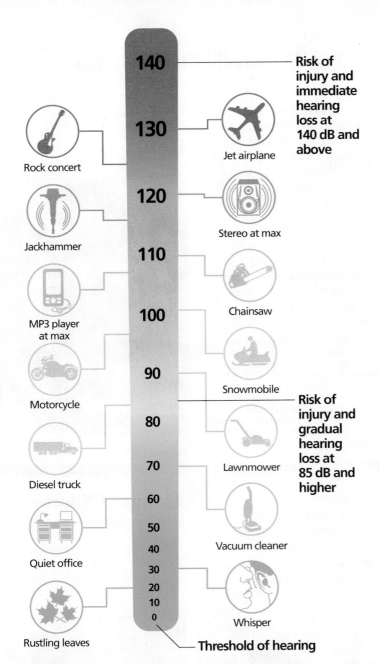

**FIGURE 2** Noise Levels of Various Sounds (dB) Decibels increase logarithmically, so each increase of 10 dB represents a tenfold increase in loudness.

**Source:** Adapted from National Institute on Deafness and Other Communication Disorders, "How Loud Is Too Loud? Bookmark," Updated July 2011, www.nidcd.nih. gov/health/hearing/rules.asp.

cochlea, or inner ear. Hearing loss can be temporary or permanent, and one of the highest rates of sudden noise-induced hearing loss is among adults aged 20 to 29. A recent survey of college students found that 39.6 percent had at least one noise-related hearing symptom such as ear pain, ringing in the ears, and so on, and 8 percent reported hearing loss.[68] The study authors identified playing in a band, using noisy tools, using firearms, and frequent attendance at sporting or music events as factors associated with an increased risk for hearing loss. Other studies have linked hearing loss in young adults to the use of personal music players. However, the precise decibel level, frequency, and duration of exposure that might correlate with hearing loss are currently under investigation.[69] Check out the **Student Health Today** box on

page 558 for more details and tips for protecting your hearing while enjoying your tunes.

## LO 4 | INJURIES AT WORK

Describe work-related injuries and what you can do to prevent them.

American adults spend most of their waking hours on the job. Although most job situations are safe, some pose hazards. Over 4,800 fatal work injuries occurred in the United States in 2014.[70] Transportation incidents made up the largest number of fatal work injuries (more than 40%). Contact with equipment, animals, and people accounted for another 31 percent.[71] In addition, workers in material moving, construction, and the service industry are at higher risk of fatal injuries.[72]

Although on-the-job deaths capture media attention, workers may also be seriously injured or disabled at their jobs. Common work injuries include cuts and lacerations, chemical burns, fractures, sprains and strains (often of the back), and repetitive motion disorders. Work injuries due to overexertion, poor body mechanics, or repetitive motion are largely preventable. We discuss these problems and share some prevention strategies here.

### Protect Your Back

Low back pain (LBP), usually as a result of injury, is epidemic throughout the United States. At some point, nearly 80 percent of American adults deal with low back pain, and it is the main cause of job-related disability.[73] In a recent survey, 12 percent of college students reported having seen their doctor in the previous year because of back pain.[74]

Frequently, sports injuries, occupational injuries, stress on spinal bones and tissues, or the sudden jolt of a car crash are the culprits in low back pain. Other times, sitting too long in the same position or hunching over your computer while you're pulling an all-nighter can prompt LBP. Carrying heavy backpacks between classes is another common source.

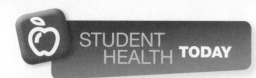
# TURNING DOWN THE TUNES

Increasingly, children and young adults experience hearing loss due to use of portable music devices such as MP3 players. High frequency, duration of use, and high volume all make hearing loss a high-risk side effect when using earphones. Long or repeated exposure to any sound above 75 decibels (dB) can cause hearing loss, and many people listen to music at volumes higher than this for several hours a day, every day. Most noise-induced hearing loss is caused by damage to delicate sensory cells (called hair cells) of the inner ear. These cells cannot regenerate: Once they're lost, they're gone for good.

What can you do to avoid hearing loss while still enjoying your music? A personal music player at full volume averages 105 dB. Listening at or close to this volume can quickly damage your hearing. So keep the volume below 75 dB—or at a level at which you can still comfortably carry on a conversation. If you do that, you won't need to limit the amount of time you spend listening to music. Another way to tell if your volume is set too loud is to ask people nearby if they can hear your music. If they can, it's definitely too loud. Finally, debate continues over the relative safety of over-the-ear earphones versus in-the-ear ear buds. Research indicates, however, that earphones are probably safer because, while delivering the music, they also muffle environmental noise. Therefore, people using earphones in noisy environments tend to set their MP3 players at a lower volume.

**Sources:** National Institute on Deafness and Other Communication Disorders, "Noise-Induced Hearing Loss," May 15, 2015, www.nidcd.nih.gov/health/noise-induced-hearing-loss#4; A.H. Sulaiman, R. Husain, and K. Seluakumaran, "Hearing risk among young personal listening device users: effects at high-frequency and extended high-frequency audiogram thresholds," *Journal of International Advanced Otology* 11, no. 2 (2015): 104–9.

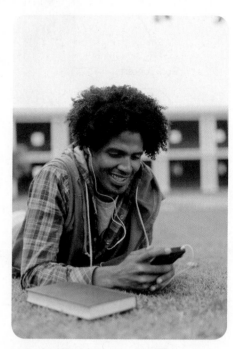

Because most injuries are in the lumbar spine area (the region above the tailbone), strengthening core abdominal muscles and stretching to avoid cramping and spasms are key prevention strategies. You can also reduce your risk by using the following common-sense strategies:

- Invest in a high-quality, supportive mattress.
- Avoid high-heeled shoes, which tilt the pelvis forward.
- Control your weight. Extra weight puts increased strain on your knees, hips, and back.
- Warm up and stretch before exercising or lifting heavy objects.
- When lifting something heavy, let your leg muscles take the weight (**FIGURE 3**). Do not bend from the waist or take the weight load on your back.
- Buy a desk chair with good lumbar support, and maintain an upright posture while using it.
- When driving, keep your car seat forward enough so that your knees are elevated slightly.

- Engage in exercise regularly, particularly in core exercises that strengthen the abdominal muscles and stretch the back muscles.
- Downsize your backpack.

## Maintain Alignment while Sitting

How many hours have you spent today glued to a laptop, tablet, smartphone, or book? Were you slouching, hunched

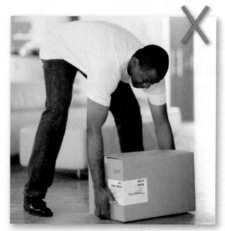

**ⓐ** Attempting to lift a heavy object by bending at your waist is a common cause of back injury.

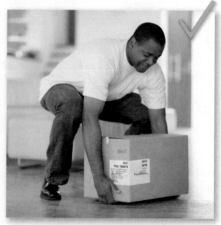

**ⓑ** Start as close to the object as possible, with it positioned between your knees as you squat down. Keep your feet parallel, or stagger one foot in front of the other. Keep the object close to your body as you stand, using your legs, not your back, to lift.

**FIGURE 3 Lifting a Heavy Object** Learning how to lift properly is key to reducing your risk of injury.

over, or sitting up straight? Your answers are probably reflected in the degree of aching and stiffness you may be feeling right now. Try these strategies to maintain a healthy alignment while you sit and work:

1. Sit comfortably with your feet flat on the floor or on a footrest, and your knees level with your hips. Raise or lower your chair, or move to a different chair, to achieve this position.

2. Your middle back should be firmly against the back of the chair. The small of your back should be supported, too. If you can't feel the chair back supporting your lumbar region, try placing a small cushion or even a rolled towel behind the curve of your lower back.

3. Keep your shoulders relaxed and straight, not rolled or hunched forward.

4. The angle of your elbows should be 90 degrees between your forearms and your upper arms. Change the height of your chair or desk or the position of your device to achieve this angle.

5. Ideally, you should be looking straight ahead, not peering down at a screen or book.

## Avoid Repetitive Motion Disorders

It's the end of the term, and you have finished the last of several papers. After hours of typing, your hands are numb and you feel an intense pain that makes the thought of typing one more word almost unbearable. If this happens, you may be suffering from one of several **repetitive motion disorders (RMDs)**, sometimes called *overuse syndrome*, *cumulative trauma disorders*, or *repetitive stress injuries*. These refer to a family of painful soft tissue injuries that begin with inflammation and gradually become disabling.

Repetitive motion disorders include carpal tunnel syndrome, bursitis, tendonitis, and ganglion cysts, among others. Twisting of the arm or wrist, overexertion, and incorrect posture or position are usually contributors. The areas most likely to be affected are the hands, wrists, elbows, and shoulders. Over time, RMDs can cause permanent damage to nerves, soft tissue, and joints.

Usually, RMDs are associated with repeating the same task in an occupational setting and gradually irritating the area in question. However, certain sports (tennis, golf, and others), gripping the wheel while driving, keyboarding or texting, and a number of newer technology-driven activities can also result in RMDs. Because many of these injuries occur during everyday activities, they are often not reported to national agencies that keep track of injury statistics.

One of the most common RMDs is **carpal tunnel syndrome (CTS)**, an inflammation of the tendons or other soft tissues within the "tunnel" through the carpal bones of the wrist (**FIGURE 4**). This puts pressure on the median nerve, which runs down the forearm through the tunnel to innervate the hand. Symptoms include numbness, tingling, and pain in the fingers and hands. Carpal tunnel syndrome typically results from spending hours typing, flipping groceries through computerized scanners, or manipulating other objects in jobs "made simpler" by technology. The risk for CTS can be reduced by proper design of workstations, protective wrist pads, and worker training. Physical and occupational therapy is an important part of treatment and recovery.

## LO 5 | PREPARING FOR NATURAL DISASTERS AND SEVERE WEATHER EVENTS

Explain how to prepare for and respond to natural disasters and severe weather events.

A **natural disaster** is any extreme environmental event that causes widespread destruction of land and/or property, injuries, and sometimes deaths. Some, such as hurricanes and volcanic eruptions, may be predictable, whereas others, like earthquakes and many tornadoes, can occur without warning. If a natural disaster were to strike without warning in your region, would you be prepared?

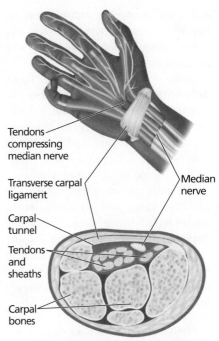

**Tendons compressing median nerve**

**Transverse carpal ligament**

**Median nerve**

**Carpal tunnel**

**Tendons and sheaths**

**Carpal bones**

Cross-section through wrist

**FIGURE 4 Carpal Tunnel Syndrome** The carpal tunnel is a space beneath the transverse carpal ligament and above the carpal bones of the wrist. The median nerve and the tendons that allow you to flex your fingers run through this tunnel. Carpal tunnel syndrome occurs when repetitive use prompts inflammation of the tissues and fluids of the tunnel. This in turn compresses the median nerve.

More common weather-related events, such as blizzards, dense fog, flash floods, high winds, and even hurricanes are typically forecast in advance. You can find advisories and preparedness information about such events in your area by visiting the National Weather Service website at *www.weather.gov*. Additionally, to learn more about specific types of disasters, log on to the Centers for Disease Control and Prevention (CDC) website at *www.cdc.gov* and search the event name. For instance, the CDC's hurricane page provides key facts; basic steps to prepare yourself, your residence,

---

**repetitive motion disorders (RMDs)** Injuries to soft tissue, tendons, muscles, nerves, or joints due to the physical stress of repeated motions.

**carpal tunnel syndrome (CTS)** A common occupational injury in which the median nerve in the wrist becomes irritated, causing numbness, tingling, and pain in the fingers and hands.

**natural disaster** Any extreme environmental event that causes widespread destruction of land and/or property, injuries, and sometimes deaths.

and even your pets; information on how to evacuate safely; and steps to take to get through the storm safely if you're ordered not to evacuate.

Some disasters, on the other hand, strike without warning. The first step in preparedness is to learn what types of natural disasters typically affect the area where you live. If you've relocated from New England to the Midwest to attend school, for example, you may want to learn about tornado preparedness. On the West Coast and elsewhere, earthquakes have a history of leaving people displaced. The best thing you can do, once familiar with common disasters in your area, is prepare yourself and your family in advance. Here are a few ways:[75]

- Choose a meeting place. In the instance that your house or home is impacted, or disaster strikes while you're separated from loved ones, choose a meeting place in advance.
- Build a disaster kit. Stockpile water (one gallon per person, per day, for at least 3 days). Fill a backpack or other bag with things like nonperishable food, emergency medical supplies, copies of important documents, and extra cash. Don't forget pet supplies if you have pets. It also doesn't hurt to include games and comfort items like a favorite (nonperishable) snack. If this is a bit much for your budget all at once, consider buying a few items for your kit each week until it's complete.
- Choose an out-of-state emergency contact. Sometimes, in large disasters like earthquakes, communication grids can become damaged or congested. Contacting someone out of state may be easier than calling someone down the block.

For more complete disaster planning info, visit *Ready.gov*. For more on the kinds of natural disasters common to your region, as well as an exhaustive emergency kit checklist, see the CDC's site on emergency preparedness and response at *https://emergency.cdc.gov*.

# STUDY **PLAN**

Customize your study plan—and master your health!—in the Study Area of **MasteringHealth**.

## ASSESS YOURSELF

**What could you do to be safer on the road?** Want to find out? Take the **Are You at Risk for a Motor Vehicle Crash?** assessment on **MasteringHealth.**™

## CHAPTER **REVIEW**

To head an MP3 Tutor Session, scan here or visit the Study Area in **MasteringHealth**.

### LO **1** | Motor Vehicle Injuries

- Unintentional motor vehicle injuries are the second leading cause of unintentional injury death for Americans. Impaired driving, distracted driving, and speeding and other forms of aggressive driving are key contributors to vehicular deaths and injuries. Motorcyclists are 26 times more likely than drivers in passenger cars to die on the road. To reduce your risk, use your safety belt and (for motocyclists) helmet, stay alert, and improve your driving skills.

### LO **2** | Recreational Injuries

- In the United States each year, thousands of cyclists sustain head injuries or other injuries and hundreds die. About one-third of these casualties involve alcohol. Wearing a helmet reduces the risk of head injury by about half. Other strategies are to stay alert and visible, ride with the flow of traffic, and obey all traffic signs and lights. Skateboarding, snowboarding, and skiing can also result in head injuries and fatalities, though not as commonly. In the United States, drowning is the fifth leading cause of unintentional injury death. As with many unintentional injuries, alcohol increases the risk of death, as does failure to wear a life jacket.

### LO **3** | Injuries at Home

- Unintentional poisoning is the number-one cause of unintentional injury death in the United States, and a majority of these deaths involve prescription opioids or heroin. Falls are the third leading cause of unintentional injury death, and are the most common cause of hip fractures and head injuries. Each year, thousands of

Americans die in fires. On campus, alcohol contributes to 76 percent of fatal fires. When someone is injured, the most important steps you can take are to call 9-1-1 and offer CPR or other first aid until help arrives. Noise-induced hearing loss occurs when high-decibel noise damages sensory receptors in the inner ear.

## LO 4 | Injuries at Work

- Over 4,800 workplace fatalities occurred in the United States in 2014. Transportation and construction are the leading industries affected. The most common cause of job-related disability is low back pain. Using proper body mechanics when lifting, driving, and sitting at a desk is essential to reduce your risk. Repetitive motion disorders are a family of soft tissue injuries that develop when repeated movements prompt inflammation. One of the most common is carpal tunnel syndrome.

## LO 5 | Weather Events

- Natural disasters are extreme environmental events that cause widespread destruction, injuries, and sometimes deaths. Preparedness is important for the types of natural disasters and severe weather events common in your geographic region. Both the U.S. Centers for Disease Control and Prevention and the National Weather Service are excellent resources.

# POP QUIZ

Visit **MasteringHealth** to personalize your study plan with Chapter Review Quizzes and Dynamic Study Modules.

## LO 1 | Motor Vehicle Injuries

1. The three types of activities that constitute distracted driving are
   a. driving while intoxicated, driving while using prescription or over-the-counter medications, and drowsy driving.
   b. speeding, tailgating, and running red lights.
   c. taking your eyes off the road, taking your hands off the steering wheel, and taking your mind off driving.
   d. texting, talking on a hand-held cellphone, or fiddling with the radio while driving.

## LO 2 | Recreational Injuries

2. Alcohol consumption greatly increases the risk of
   a. injuries and deaths involving cyclists.
   b. skateboarding injuries and deaths.
   c. drowning.
   d. all of the above.

## LO 3 | Injuries at Home

3. You wake in your dorm room to people shouting "Fire!" You jump out of bed. What is the first thing you should do?
   a. Feel the door handle.
   b. Call 9-1-1.
   c. Open a window and call for help.
   d. Gather your wallet, cell phone, and other valuable belongings.

## LO 4 | Injuries at Work

4. The primary cause of job-related disability is
   a. head injury.
   b. whiplash.
   c. low back pain.
   d. carpal tunnel syndrome.

## LO 5 | Weather Events

5. What United States agency provides information on preparing for the types of natural disasters common in your region of the country?
   a. the Centers for Disease Control and Prevention.
   b. the Environmental Protection Agency.
   c. the National Library of Medicine.
   d. the National Oceanic and Atmospheric Administration.

*Answers to the Pop Quiz can be found on page A-1. If you answered a question incorrectly, review the section identified by the Learning Outcome. For even more study tools, visit* **MasteringHealth**.

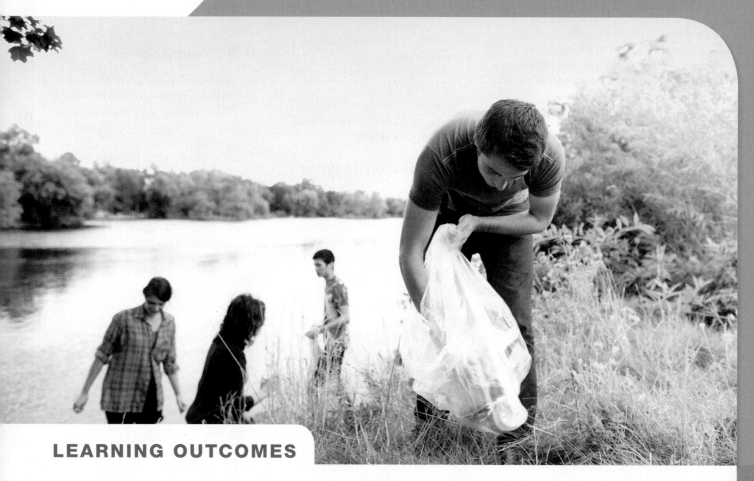

# 21 Preserving and Protecting Your Environment

## LEARNING OUTCOMES

LO **1** Explain the environmental impact associated with global population growth.

LO **2** Describe major causes of air pollution and the consequences of greenhouse gas accumulation and ozone depletion.

LO **3** Explain climate change and global warming, the underlying causes of each, impacts on health, and how alternative energy options and individual actions can reduce risks.

LO **4** Identify sources of pollution and chemical contaminants often found in water.

LO **5** Distinguish between municipal solid waste and hazardous waste and list strategies for reducing land pollution.

LO **6** List and explain key health concerns associated with ionizing and nonionizing radiation.

*. . . 2014 was the planet's warmest year on record. Now, one year doesn't make a trend, but this does—14 of the 15 warmest years on record have all fallen in the first 15 years of this century.*

—President Barack Obama, Excerpt from the 2015 State of the Union Address

The global population has grown more in the past 50 years than at any other time in human history. More people pose a potentially devastating threat to our water, air, food, and capacity to survive. Polar ice caps and glaciers are melting at rates that surpass even the most dire predictions of a decade ago, and threats of rising sea levels loom large. According to one report, we have lost half of the wild animals of the world in the last 40 years.[1] Drought, fires, floods, and a host of other natural calamities are daily news. Clean water is becoming scarce, fossil fuels are being depleted, and the amount of solid and hazardous waste is growing. In short, our collective disregard for the planet's life-sustaining resources may ultimately put all living things in peril unless we take action now.

This chapter provides an overview of the factors contributing to the global environmental crisis. It also provides a blueprint for action—by individuals, communities, policymakers, and governments. Staying informed, making important behavioral changes, and becoming an advocate for a healthy environment are key things you can do to help.

### HEAR IT! PODCASTS

Want a study podcast for this chapter? Download the podcast **Environmental Health**, available on **MasteringHealth.**™

## LO 1 | OVERPOPULATION: THE PLANET'S GREATEST THREAT

**Explain the environmental impact associated with global population growth.**

As anthropologist Margaret Mead put it, *"Every human society is faced not with one population problem, but two: how to beget and rear enough children and how not to beget and rear too many."*[2]

The United Nations projects that the world population will grow from its current level of 7 billion to between 9.3 and 10.5 billion by 2050, given recent jumps in **fertility rates**—the average number of births per woman in a specific country or region.[3] Current population projections have assumed a low, declining, or constant fertility rate. However, recent data indicate that rates have increased significantly, particularly in developing regions, meaning population projections may grossly underestimate the reality of our global population in the next decades. Add increasing fertility rates to increases in overall survival and increases in life expectancy at birth and other variables, and there's a perfect storm whereby future populations may exceed all previous projections, swelling to between 11 and 12.3 billion by 2100 (**FIGURE 21.1**).[4] Tomorrow's population will be significantly larger, younger, more industrialized, consume more resources, and produce even more waste than previous generations unless actions are taken to control population growth.[5]

**fertility rate** Average number of births a female in a certain population has during her reproductive years.

# 97%

of **GLOBAL POPULATION GROWTH** in the next four decades will happen in Asia, Africa, Latin America, and the Caribbean.

## Global Population Growth

A number of factors have led to the world population's increase. Key among them are changes in fertility and mortality rates. U.S. fertility rates have steadily declined from the high of 3.7 births per woman in the 1950s to 1.9 births in 2015.[6] While

### WHAT DO YOU THINK?

**Should individuals get tax breaks for having fewer children?**

- How would such policies compare to our current policies?
- Can you think of other policies that might be effective in encouraging population control and resource conservation in the United States?

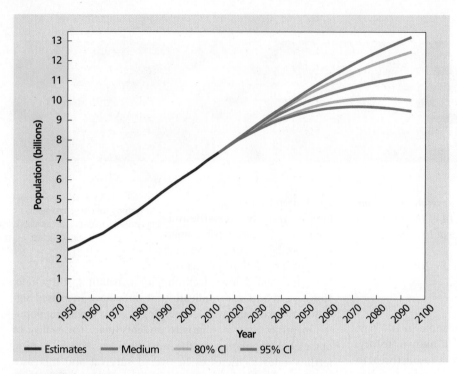

**FIGURE 21.1** Estimated Population of the World, 1950–2100, Medium-Variant Projection and 80 and 95 Percent Confidence Intervals

**Source:** United Nations, Department of Economic and Social Affairs, Population Division, *World Population Prospects: The 2015 Revision* (New York: United Nations, 2015).

consumption and add to the overall human footprint on the environment.

**Differing Growth Rates** The country projected to have the largest increase in population in coming decades is India, adding another 600 million people by 2050, surpassing China as the most populous nation on earth.[8]

With a current population of over 324 million and a net gain of one person every 11 seconds, the United States is among the fastest-growing industrialized nations.[9] It also has one of the largest *ecological footprints*—a measure of the biologically productive land and water area an individual or a population occupies and uses—exerting a greater impact on many of the planet's resources than do most other nations.[10]

## Measuring the Impact of People

Today, experts are analyzing the **carrying capacity of the Earth**—the largest population that can be supported indefinitely, given the resources available in the environment. At what point will we be unable to restore the balance between humans and nature? Since 1996, the global demand for natural resources has doubled. It now takes 1.5 years to regenerate the renewable resources humans use in 1 year. A significant report indicates that by 2030 it will take the equivalent of two planets to meet the demand for resources, and by 2100, we may need more than four planets to support human needs. Simply put, we are running out of the natural resources necessary to sustain us, and the problem is growing at an unprecedented rate.[11] Vast differences exist between countries that have the *biocapacity* to sustain their growth and those that are draining the global capacity to sustain life. When essential resources become unavailable, the likelihood of human conflict to ensure survival will increase, along with increased pressure on all living things.

Evidence of the effects of unchecked human population growth is everywhere:

■ **Impact on other species.** Changes in the **ecosystem** are resulting in mass destruction of many species and their habitats.[12] Over 477 vertebrate species have gone extinct since 1900—declining at rates over 100 times faster than normal rates of extinction, prompting some scientists to predict the *sixth mass extinction of living creatures*, similar to the fifth extinction that occurred with the demise of the dinosaurs.[13] According to a recent report by the International Union for the Conservation of Nature (IUCN), nearly 25 percent of all mammals on Earth are threatened with extinction.[14] African elephants, black rhinos, and

many developed countries have shown consistent declines in fertility rates in recent years, other countries, particularly those in the most impoverished areas, continue to have high rates. While some argue that lower fertility rates means slowing population growth, sheer population size, such as in India and China, can cause major increases, even if fertility rates remain constant or decline (**TABLE 21.1**).[7]

Historically, in countries where women have little education and little control over reproductive choices and where birth control is either not available or frowned upon, pregnancy rates continue to rise. As women become more educated, obtain higher socioeconomic status, work more outside of the home, and have more control over reproduction—as birth control becomes more accessible—fertility rates decline. Recognizing that population control will be essential in the decades ahead, many countries have enacted strict population control measures or have encouraged their citizens to limit the size of their families. Proponents of *zero population growth* believe that each couple should produce only two offspring, allowing the population to stabilize.

Mortality rates from chronic and infectious diseases have declined as a result of improved public health infrastructure, increased availability of drugs and vaccines, better disaster preparedness, and other factors. As people live longer, they add more years of resource

**carrying capacity of the Earth** The largest population that can be supported indefinitely given the resources available in the environment.

**ecosystem** Collection of physical (nonliving) and biological (living) components of an environment and the relationships between them.

## TABLE 21.1 | Selected Total Fertility Rates Worldwide, 2015

| Country | Number of Children Born per Woman* |
|---|---|
| Niger | 7.6 |
| Chad | 7.0 |
| Somalia | 6.9 ↑ |
| South Sudan | 6.9 ↑ |
| India | 2.3 ↑ |
| Mexico | 2.3 ↓ |
| United States | 1.9 |
| Australia | 1.9 |
| Canada | 1.6 |
| China | 1.7 ↑ |
| Russia | 1.8 ↑ |
| Germany | 1.5 ↑ |
| Japan | 1.4 |
| Afghanistan | 4.9 |
| Italy | 1.4 ↓ |

*Indicates average number of children that would be born per woman if all women lived to the end of their childbearing years and bore children according to a given fertility rate at each age.

↓↑ Denotes a change up or down from 2013 fertility rates.

**Source:** Data from Population Reference Bureau, "World Population Data Sheet," 2015, http://www.prb.org/pdf15/2015-world-population-data-sheet_eng.pdf.

by over 50 percent in the last 27 years, with virtual dead zones stretching for miles on ocean floors.[20] Massive storms, earthquakes, radiation, invasive species, and other threats hasten the demise of natural sea life and lead to increased aquaculture and fish farms rather than wild fish catches. In addition, fish farming can disrupt fragile ecosystems and waterways and increase disease in native species.[21]

- **Impact on the food supply.** We are currently fishing the oceans at rates that are 250 percent more than they can regenerate; scientists project a global collapse of all fish species by 2050.[22] Today, our global quest for food means increasing amounts of the earth's surface are used for agriculture. Because agriculture accounts for over 90 percent of our global water footprint, groundwater withdrawals have tripled in the last 50 years, putting increased pressure on dwindling water reserves.[23] Drought and erosion and natural disasters make growing food increasingly difficult, and food shortages and famine occur in many regions of the world with increasing frequency.

- **Land degradation and contamination of drinking water.** The per capita availability of freshwater is declining rapidly, and contaminated water remains the greatest single environmental cause of human illness. Unsustainable land use and climate change are increasing land degradation, including erosion, toxic chemical infiltration, nutrient depletion, deforestation, and other problems.

- **Energy consumption.** "Use it *and* lose it" is an apt saying for our use of nonrenewable energy sources in the form of **fossil fuels** (oil, coal, natural gas). Although there is a shift

> **fossil fuels** Carbon-based material used for energy; includes oil, coal, and natural gas.

walruses are among those being ruthlessly killed for high-priced horns and tusks.[15] In spite of major efforts to stop poaching of elephants for ivory, nearly 35,000 African elephants are slaughtered each year, outpacing births and ensuring extinction in the wild unless drastic measures are taken.[16] About a third of amphibians are threatened or extinct, and many of those that survive have chemically induced ailments or genetic mutations that will hasten their demise.[17] Along with mammals, rapid declines in plant species are reasons for concern.[18]

- **Impact on ecosystems.** Aquatic ecosystems continue to be heavily contaminated by chemical and human waste. Our oceans are 30 percent more acidic now than they were just 200 years ago, largely due to human-caused pollutants.[19] Living coral reefs that support aquatic life have declined

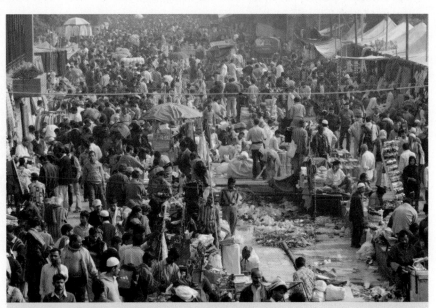

Every year the global population grows by 115 million, but Earth's resources are not expanding. Population increases are believed to be a key factor in our escalating pressure on increasingly scarce natural resources and climate change.

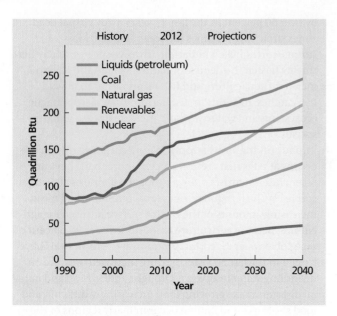

**FIGURE 21.2** World Energy Consumption by Fuel Type, 1990–2040 (Quadrillion Btu) Liquid fuels include petroleum. The last year with real data is 2012; years thereafter are projected estimates.

Source: U.S. Energy Information Administration, "International Energy Outlook 2016, Executive Summary," May 2016, Available at http://www.eia.gov/forecasts/ieo/exec_summ.cfm.

toward renewable energy sources, such as hydropower, solar and wind power, and biomass power, the predominant energy sources are still fossil fuels. China is the largest overall consumer of energy.[24] The United States is the largest consumer of petroleum/liquid fossil fuels and is the second largest consumer of coal and electricity.[25] In many developing regions of the world, greater industrialization and affluence has resulted in skyrocketing demand for limited fossil fuels (**FIGURE 21.2**).

## LO 2 | **AIR** POLLUTION

Describe major causes of air pollution and the consequences of greenhouse gas accumulation and ozone depletion.

The term *air pollution* refers to the presence, in varying degrees, of substances (suspended particles and vapors) not found in clean air. From the beginning of time, natural events, living creatures, and toxic by-products have polluted the environment. Air pollution is not new, but the array of **pollutants** that exist today and their potential effects are.

Air pollutants are either *naturally occurring* or *anthropogenic* (caused by humans). Naturally occurring air pollutants include *particulate matter*, such as ash from volcanic eruptions, soil, and dust. Anthropogenic sources include those caused by

*stationary sources* (e.g., power plants, factories, and refineries) and *mobile sources*, such as vehicles. Mobile sources are *on-road* vehicles (cars, trucks, and buses) or *off-road* sources (such as construction equipment). Planes, trains, and watercraft are considered *nonroad* sources.[26] Today, nearly 81 percent of all greenhouse gases are from carbon dioxide ($CO_2$)[27] In the United States, fossil fuels used to generate electricity contribute 37 percent of greenhouse gases, followed by transportation at 31 percent and industry at 15 percent.[28]

A new study focused on commuting polluters may surprise urbanites who think that gas-sipping mopeds are their way of helping save the planet. Those humming little two-stroke engines are at the top of the list of air polluters in much of Asia, Africa, and southern Europe. Scientists report that, whether idling or at full throttle, scooters/mopeds emit more than their share of fine-particle aromatic hydrocarbons (arenes) and other chemicals. Several countries have or are considering bans on two-stroke engines or establishment of lowered emission limits.[29]

**pollutant** Substance that contaminates some aspect of the environment and causes potential harm to living organisms.

## Components of Air Pollution

Concern about air quality prompted Congress to pass the *Clean Air Act* in 1970 and to amend it several times since then. The act established standards for six of the most widespread air pollutants that seriously affect health: sulfur dioxide, particulates, carbon monoxide, nitrogen dioxide, ground-level ozone, and lead. There have been major decreases in these six criteria pollutants, even as populations have increased in the United States. However, ozone and particulate matter continue to be present at significant levels, with over half of all Americans—166 million people—living

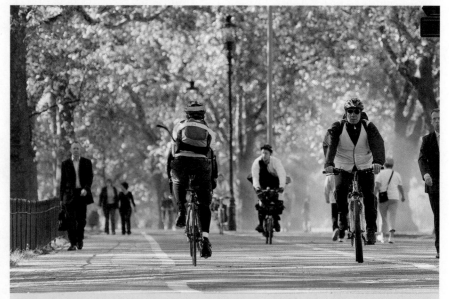

Making small changes such as driving less, riding your bike more, taking public transportation or carpooling, turning off lights, recycling, and composting can all help to reduce your carbon footprint.

## TABLE 21.2 | Sources, Health Effects, and Environmental Impacts of Other Major Air Pollutants

| Pollutant | Description | Sources | Health Effects | Welfare Effects |
|---|---|---|---|---|
| Carbon monoxide (CO) | Colorless, odorless gas | Motor vehicle exhaust; indoor sources include kerosene and wood-burning stoves | Headaches, reduced mental alertness, heart attack, cardiovascular diseases, impaired fetal development, death | Contributes to the formation of smog |
| Sulfur dioxide (SO$_2$) | Colorless gas that dissolves in water vapor to form acid and interacts with other gases and particles in the air | Coal-fired power plants, petroleum refineries, manufacture of sulfuric acid, and smelting of ores containing sulfur | Eye irritation, wheezing, chest tightness, shortness of breath, lung damage | Contributes to the formation of acid rain, visibility impairment, plant and water damage, aesthetic damage |
| Nitrogen dioxide (NO$_2$) | Reddish-brown, highly reactive gas | Motor vehicles, electric utilities, and other industrial, commercial, and residential sources that burn fuels | Susceptibility to respiratory infections, irritation of the lungs and respiratory symptoms (e.g., cough, chest pain, difficulty breathing) | Contributes to the formation of smog, acid rain, water quality deterioration, global warming, and visibility impairment |
| Particulate matter (PM) | Very small particles of soot, dust, or other matter, including tiny droplets of liquids | Diesel engines, power plants, industries, windblown dust, wood stoves | Eye irritation, asthma, bronchitis, lung damage, cancer, heavy metal poisoning, cardiovascular effects | Visibility impairment, atmospheric deposition, aesthetic damage |

**Source:** U.S. Environmental Protection Agency, "Air and Radiation: Air Pollutants," July 2016, www.epa.gov.

in counties with unhealthy levels of ozone and particulates.[30] See **TABLE 21.2** for an overview of the sources and effects of these pollutants.

## Photochemical Smog

**Smog** is a brownish haze produced by the photochemical reaction of sunlight with hydrocarbons, nitrogen compounds, and other gases in vehicle exhaust. It is sometimes called *ozone pollution* because ozone is a main component of smog. Smog tends to form in areas that experience a **temperature inversion**, in which a cool layer of air is trapped under a layer of warmer air, preventing the air from circulating. Smog is more likely to occur in valley areas surrounded by hills or mountains, such as Los Angeles or Mexico City. The most noticeable adverse effects of smog are difficulty breathing, burning eyes, headaches, and nausea. Long-term exposure poses serious health risks, particularly for children, older adults, pregnant women, and people with chronic respiratory disorders.

## Air Quality Index

The *Air Quality Index* (AQI) is a measure of how clean or polluted the air is on a given day and if there are any health concerns related to air quality. The AQI focuses on health effects that can happen within a few hours or days after breathing polluted air.

The AQI scale is from 0 to 500: The higher the AQI value, the greater the level of air pollution and associated health risks. An AQI value of 100 generally corresponds to the national air quality standard for the pollutant, which is the level the Environmental Protection Agency (EPA) has set to protect public health. AQI values below 100 are generally considered satisfactory. When AQI values rise above

| When the AQI is in this range: | ... air quality conditions are | ... as symbolized by this color: |
|---|---|---|
| 0 to 50 | Good | Green |
| 51 to 100 | Moderate | Yellow |
| 101 to 150 | Unhealthy for sensitive groups | Orange |
| 151 to 200 | Unhealthy | Red |
| 201 to 300 | Very unhealthy | Purple |
| 301 to 500 | Hazardous | Maroon |

**FIGURE 21.3 Air Quality Index** The EPA provides individual air quality indexes (AQIs) for ground-level ozone, particle pollution, carbon monoxide, sulfur dioxide, and nitrogen dioxide. All of the AQIs are presented using the general values, categories, and colors of this figure.

**Source:** U.S. Environmental Protection Agency, "Air Quality Index: A Guide to Air Quality and Your Health," Updated May 2014, www.airnow.gov/index.cfm?action=aqibasics.aqi.

100, air quality is considered unhealthy at certain levels for specific groups of people and at higher levels for everyone. As shown in **FIGURE 21.3**, the EPA has divided the AQI scale into six categories with corresponding color codes. National and local weather reports generally include information on the day's AQI.

**smog** Brownish haze that is a form of pollution produced by the photochemical reaction of sunlight with hydrocarbons, nitrogen compounds, and other gases in vehicle exhaust.

**temperature inversion** Weather condition that occurs when a layer of cool air is trapped under a layer of warmer air, preventing the air from circulating.

## Acid Deposition and Acid Rain

**Acid deposition** is replacing the term *acid rain* in scientific circles; it refers to the deposition of *wet* (rain, snow, sleet, fog, cloud water, and dew) and *dry* (acidifying particles and gases) acidic components that fall to the earth in dust or smoke.[31] Sulfur dioxide ($SO_2$) and nitrogen oxide ($NO_x$) cause damage to plants, aquatic animals, forests, and humans over time. In the United States, roughly two-thirds of all sulfur dioxides and one-fourth of all nitrogen oxides come from electric power generation that relies on burning fossil fuels such as coal.[32] When coal-powered plants, oil refineries, and other facilities burn these fuels, sulfur and nitrogen in the emissions combine with oxygen and sunlight to become sulfur dioxide and nitrogen oxide. Small acid particles are carried by the wind and combine with moisture to produce acidic rain or snow.[33]

Acid deposition gradually acidifies ponds, lakes, and other bodies of water. Once the acid content of the water reaches a certain level, plant and animal life cannot survive. Ironically, acidified lakes and ponds become a crystal-clear deep blue, giving the illusion of beauty and health even as they wreak destruction. Every year, acid deposition destroys millions of trees in Europe and North America. Sugar maples and other trees in the northeastern United States appear to be the newest victims of acid deposition, as they are having difficulty regenerating seedlings destroyed by these deposits. Scientists have concluded that much of the world's forestlands are now experiencing damaging levels of acid deposition.[34]

Acid deposition aggravates and may even cause bronchitis, asthma, and other respiratory problems, and people with emphysema or heart disease may suffer from exposure.[35] It may also be hazardous to fetuses. Acid deposition can cause metals such as aluminium, cadmium, lead, and mercury to **leach** out of the soil. If these metals make their way into water or food supplies, they can cause cancer in humans.

Although there have been substantial reductions in $SO_2$ and $NO_x$ emissions from power plants that use the fossil fuels coal, gas, and oil in the last decade, full recovery is still years away. Global pressure to reduce use and invest in technology to dramatically reduce emissions from coal production and burning has been a key focus of recent global environmental meetings in Rio de Janeiro and Paris. Although coal is "cleaner" than it was a decade ago from a production standpoint, the idea of "clean coal" is far from reality.

**acid deposition** Acidification process that occurs when pollutants are deposited by precipitation, clouds, or directly on the land.

**leach** To dissolve and filter through soil.

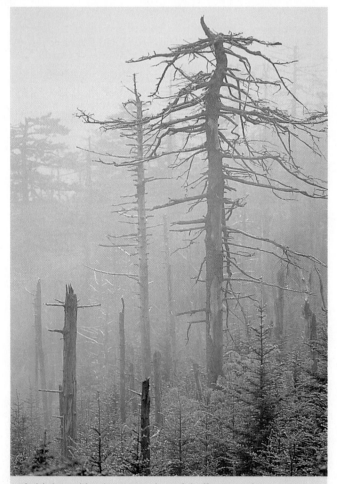

Acid deposition has many harmful effects on the environment. Because its toxins seep into groundwater and enter the food chain, it also poses health hazards to humans.

## Indoor Air Pollution

Mounting evidence indicates that air pollution levels within homes and other buildings, where we spend 90 percent of our time, may be two to five times higher than outdoor pollution levels.[36] Potentially dangerous chemical compounds can increase risks of cancer, contribute to respiratory problems, reduce the immune system's ability to fight disease, and increase problems with allergies and allergic reactions.

Indoor air pollution comes primarily from cooking stoves and furnaces, woodstoves and space heaters, household cleaners and solvents, mold, pesticides, asbestos, formaldehyde, radon, and lead. Today, more and more manufacturers are offering green building products and furnishings, such as natural fiber fabrics, untreated wood for furniture and floors, low-VOC (volatile organic compound) paints, and many other products. See the Making Changes Today box for ideas on how to become a more environmentally conscious consumer.

Multiple factors, including age, individual sensitivity, preexisting medical

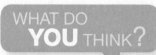

WHAT DO **YOU** THINK?

Think of the products you use each day. **How many of these could you do without?**

- What options do you have for cleaning products or personal care products that won't pollute the air in your home or contaminate the water supply?

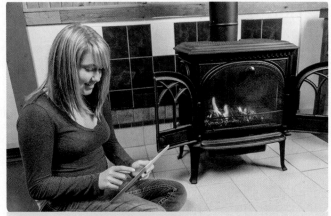

Inside air can be 10 to 40 times more hazardous than outside air. Indoor air pollution comes from woodstoves, furnaces, tobacco smoke, asbestos, formaldehyde, radon, lead, mold, and household chemicals.

conditions, liver function, and the condition of the immune and respiratory systems contribute to a person's risk for being affected by indoor air pollution.[37] Those with allergies may be particularly vulnerable, as may those living in newer, airtight, energy-efficient homes. Health effects may develop over years of exposure or may occur in response to toxic levels of pollutants. Room temperature and humidity also play a role. **TABLE 21.3** on page 570 lists major sources of indoor air pollution and possible health effects.

Preventing indoor air pollution should focus on three main areas: *source control* (eliminating or reducing individual contaminants), *ventilation improvements* (increasing the amount of outdoor air coming indoors), and *air cleaners* (removing particulates from the air).[38]

**Environmental Tobacco Smoke** Perhaps the greatest source of indoor air pollution is *environmental tobacco smoke (ETS)*, also known as secondhand smoke, which contains carbon monoxide and cancer-causing particulates. Today, a majority of all states have 100 percent smoking bans in restaurants and bars, municipal buildings, and in the workplace. Some cities have banned smoking in public places, including parks and beaches, and bans on smoking in automobiles while children are present are increasing.[39] For more on environmental tobacco smoke, see Chapter 12.

**Home Heating** Woodstoves emit significant levels of particulates and carbon monoxide in addition to other pollutants,

such as sulfur dioxide. If you rely on wood for heating, make sure that your stove is properly installed, vented, and maintained. Burning properly seasoned wood reduces particulates. Oil- or gas-fired furnaces also need to be properly installed, ventilated, and maintained. Inexpensive monitors are available to detect high carbon monoxide levels in the home.

**Asbestos** The mineral compound **asbestos** was once commonly used in insulating materials, vinyl flooring, shingles/roofing materials, heating pipe coverings, and many other products in buildings constructed before 1970. When bonded to other materials, asbestos is relatively harmless, but if its tiny fibers become loosened and airborne, they can embed themselves in the lungs. Their presence leads to cancer of the lungs, stomach, and chest lining and life-threatening lung diseases called *mesothelioma* and *asbestosis*. If asbestos is detected in the home, it must be removed or sealed off by a professional.

**Formaldehyde** **Formaldehyde** is a colorless, strong-smelling gas present in some carpets, draperies, furniture, particleboard, plywood, wood paneling, countertops, and many adhesives. It is released into the air in a process called *outgassing*. Outgassing is highest in new products, but can continue for many years. Exposure to formaldehyde can cause respiratory problems, dizziness, fatigue, nausea, and rashes. Long-term exposure can lead to central nervous system disorders and cancer. Ask about the formaldehyde content of products you are considering for your home, and avoid those that contain it.

**Radon** **Radon** is an odorless, colorless gas that penetrates homes through cracks, pipes, or sump pits, and other openings in the basement or foundation. The U.S. Surgeon General warns that radon is the second leading cause of lung cancer, after smoking, each year.[40] The EPA estimates that as many as 21,000

**asbestos** Mineral compound that separates into stringy fibers and lodges in the lungs, where it can cause disease.

**formaldehyde** Colorless, strong-smelling gas released through outgassing; causes respiratory and other health problems.

**radon** Naturally occurring radioactive gas resulting from the decay of certain radioactive elements.

## TABLE 21.3 | Health Effects of Selected Indoor Air Pollution

| Pollutant | Sources | Health Effects |
|---|---|---|
| Asbestos | Deteriorating or damaged insulation; fireproofing, acoustical materials, and floor tiles | Long-term risk of chest and abdominal cancers and lung diseases. Smokers are at higher risk of developing asbestos-induced lung cancer. |
| Biological contaminants (molds, mildew, viruses, animal dander, cat saliva, dust mites, cockroaches, and pollen) | Improper ventilation and moisture buildup, lack of cleanliness/sanitation, contaminated heating systems, faulty construction, household pets, rodents, insects, damp carpets | Allergic reactions, including hypersensitivity, rhinitis, asthma, infectious illnesses, sneezing, watery eyes, coughing, shortness of breath, dizziness, lethargy, fever, digestive problems |
| Combustion products | Unvented kerosene heaters, woodstoves, fireplaces, gas stoves | Carbon monoxide causes headaches, dizziness, weakness, nausea, confusion and disorientation, chest pain, death. Nitrogen dioxide causes irritation of nose and eyes, respiratory distress. Particles cause lung damage and irritation. |
| Benzene | Paint, new carpet, new drapes, upholstery, fast-drying glues, caulks | Headaches, eye/skin irritation, fatigue, cancer |
| Formaldehyde | Tobacco smoke, plywood, cabinets, furniture, particleboard, new carpet and drapes, wallpaper, ceiling tile, paneling | Headaches, eye/skin irritation, drowsiness, fatigue, respiratory problems, memory loss, depression, gynecological problems, cancer |
| Chloroform | Paint, new drapes, new carpet, upholstery | Headaches, asthma attacks, dizziness, eye/skin irritations |
| Toluene | All paper products, most finished wood products | Headaches, eye/skin irritation, sinus problems, dizziness, cancer |
| Hydrocarbons | Tobacco smoke, gas burners and furnaces | Headaches, fatigue, nausea, dizziness, breathing difficulty |
| Ammonia | Tobacco smoke, cleaning supplies, animal urine | Eye/skin irritation, headaches, nosebleeds, sinus problems |
| Trichloroethylene | Paints, glues, caulking, vinyl coatings, wallpaper | Headaches, eye/skin irritation, upper respiratory irritation |

Source: U.S. Environmental Protection Agency, "The Inside Story: A Guide to Indoor Air Quality," April, 2016, https://www.epa.gov/indoor-air-quality-iaq/publications-about-indoor-air-quality.

lung cancer deaths per year are attributable to excess radon in the home.[41] Since 1988, the EPA and the Office of the Surgeon General have recommended that homes be tested for radon below the third floor and that Americans test their homes every 2 years or when they move into a new home. Low-cost radon test kits are available online, in hardware stores, and through other retail outlets.

**Lead** Lead is a highly toxic metal common in paints used in many American homes before its banning in 1978. By some estimates, as many as 25 percent of U.S. homes still have lead-based paint hazards, and nearly 535,000 children aged 1 to 5 years old in the United States have blood lead levels above the 5 micrograms per deciliter (µg/dL) limit where the CDC recommends taking action for public health.[42] It is also found in batteries, soils, drinking water, older pipes, dishes, and other items. In recent years, toys produced in China and other regions of the world have been recalled owing to unsafe levels of lead. Low-income individuals living in older homes that may not be in compliance with newer recommended levels

**lead** Highly toxic metal found in emissions from lead smelters and processing plants; also sometimes found in pipes or paint in older buildings.

of lead exposure are at higher risk. Risk appears to be greatest during home remodeling and for persons with occupations in fields such as construction, e-waste/recycling, and demolition.[43]

Lead affects the circulatory, reproductive, urinary, and nervous systems, as well as the kidneys, and it can accumulate in bone and other tissues. It is particularly detrimental to children and fetuses, and can cause birth defects, learning problems, behavioral abnormalities, and other health problems. To reduce unsafe exposure at home, use water filters, keep areas where children play clean and dust free, regularly wash children's hands and toys, leave lead-based paint undisturbed if it is in good condition, or hire a professional contractor to remove it.

**Mold** Molds are fungi that live both indoors and outdoors in most regions of the country. Their tiny reproductive spores waft through the air. When they land on a damp spot indoors, they may begin growing and digesting whatever they are on, including wood, paper, carpet, and food. In general, molds are harmless; however, some people are sensitive or allergic to them. In such people, exposure to molds may lead to nasal stuffiness, eye irritation, wheezing, or skin irritation. For the very sensitive, molds may cause fever or shortness of breath.[44] Before purchasing a home, have a mold inspection. A history of mold can wreak havoc on home values as well as your health. For ways to reduce your exposure to mold, see the Making Changes Today box.

**Sick Building Syndrome** Sick building syndrome (SBS) occurs when people occupying a building experience severe health effects correlated to spending time in the building, but no specific source of the effects can be identified.[45] Poor ventilation is a primary cause, along with faulty furnaces, pet dander, mold, and dust. Volatile compounds from products such as hair spray, cleaners, and adhesives can cause problems, as can heavy metals such as lead, particularly in older buildings. Symptoms include eye irritation, sore throat, queasiness, and worsening of asthma.

Indoor air pollution and SBS are increasing concerns in the classroom and workplace. Studies show that significant numbers of U.S. schools have unsatisfactory indoor air quality, often due to poor ventilation, construction techniques that block outside air, and the use of synthetic materials.[46] Long-term exposure to poor air quality can affect student learning as well as trigger allergies, asthma, and other health problems among students.[47]

## Ozone Layer Depletion

The *ozone layer* forms a protective stratum in the stratosphere— the highest level of Earth's atmosphere, located 12 to 30 miles above the surface. The ozone layer protects our planet and its inhabitants from ultraviolet B (UVB) radiation, a primary cause of skin cancer. Such radiation damages DNA and weakens immune systems.

In the 1970s, scientists began to warn of a breakdown in the ozone layer. Instruments developed to test atmospheric contents indicated that certain chemicals, especially **chlorofluorocarbons (CFCs)**, were contributing to the ozone layer's rapid depletion. The U.S. government banned the use of aerosol sprays containing CFCs in the 1970s. The discovery of an ozone "hole" over Antarctica led to treaties whereby the United States and other nations agreed to further reduce the use of CFCs and other ozone-depleting chemicals. Today, more than 197 United Nations countries have agreed to basic protocols designed to preserve and protect the ozone layer.[48] Although the ban on CFCs is believed to be responsible for slowing the depletion of the ozone layer, some CFC replacements may also be damaging because they contribute to the **enhanced greenhouse effect**.

## LO 3 | CLIMATE CHANGE

Explain climate change and global warming, the underlying causes of each, impacts on health, and how alternative energy options and individual actions can reduce risks.

**Climate change** refers to a shift in typical weather patterns across the world. These changes can include fluctuations in seasonal temperatures, rain or snowfall amounts, and the occurrence of catastrophic storms. **Global warming** is a type of climate change in which average temperatures increase. Over 97 percent of scientists now agree the planet is warming, and over the last 50 years, this warming has been driven largely by the burning of fossil fuels.[49] Over the last 100 years, the average temperature of the earth has increased by 1.5°F, with the hottest year on record in 2014 and projections of another 2° to 11.5°F rise in the next 100 years.[50] The American Association for the Advancement of Science (AAAS) and other highly respected groups warn that our climate is being pushed toward abrupt, unpredictable, and irreversible change that could be extremely damaging to all living things.[51] According to the National Aeronautics and Space Administration (NASA), the National Oceanic and Atmospheric Administration (NOAA), and the National Research Council, climate change poses major risks to lives, and excess **greenhouse gases** are a key culprit.[52] The *greenhouse effect* is a natural phenomenon in

**sick building syndrome (SBS)** Describes a situation in which occupants of a building experience acute health effects linked to time spent there, but no specific illness or cause can be identified.

**chlorofluorocarbons (CFCs)** Chemicals that contribute to the depletion of the atmospheric ozone layer.

**enhanced greenhouse effect** Warming of the earth's surface due to increases in greenhouse gas concentration in the atmosphere, which traps more of the sun's radiation than is normal.

**climate change** A shift in typical weather patterns that includes fluctuations in seasonal temperatures, rain or snowfall amounts, and the occurrence of catastrophic storms.

**global warming** A type of climate change in which average temperatures increase.

**greenhouse gases** Gases that accumulate in the atmosphere, where they contribute to global warming by trapping heat near the earth's surface.

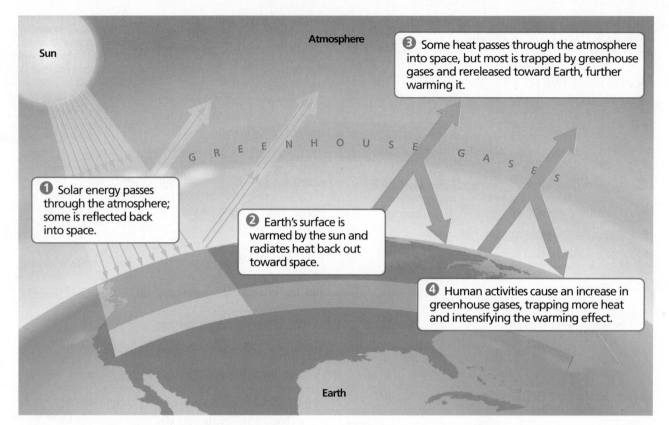

**Sun**

**Atmosphere**

G R E E N H O U S E    G A S E S

**① Solar energy passes through the atmosphere; some is reflected back into space.**

**② Earth's surface is warmed by the sun and radiates heat back out toward space.**

**③ Some heat passes through the atmosphere into space, but most is trapped by greenhouse gases and rereleased toward Earth, further warming it.**

**④ Human activities cause an increase in greenhouse gases, trapping more heat and intensifying the warming effect.**

**Earth**

**FIGURE 21.4 The Enhanced Greenhouse Effect** The natural greenhouse effect is responsible for making Earth habitable; it keeps the planet 33°C (60°F) warmer than it would otherwise be. An increase in greenhouse gases resulting from human activity is creating the *enhanced greenhouse effect*, trapping more heat and causing dangerous global climate change.

**Source:** OzCoasts (Geoscience Australia), "The enhanced greenhouse effect (Global warming)," 2013, http://www.ozcoasts.gov.au/indicators/greenhouse_effect.jsp.

→ **VIDEO TUTOR** Enhanced Greenhouse Effect

which greenhouse gases such as carbon dioxide, nitrous oxide, methane, CFCs, and hydrocarbons form a layer in the atmosphere, allowing solar heat to pass through and trapping some of the heat close to the surface, where it warms the planet (**FIGURE 21.4**). Excess carbon dioxide accounts for 82 percent of greenhouse gases emitted through human activity in the United States.[53]

## Scientific Evidence of Climate Change and Human-Caused Global Warming

According to data from U.S. and international sources, climate responds to changes in naturally occurring greenhouse gases as well as solar output and Earth's orbit; however, recent evidence points to unusual changes in climate that go beyond predictable natural causes. So, what evidence do we have? Consider the following:[54]

- Global sea levels rose 6.7 inches in the last 100 years, mostly in the last decade. With accelerated glacial and ice sheet melts, this rise is likely to increase dramatically.

- Since 1981, 20 of the warmest years ever have occurred, and 14 of the warmest years have been during the last 15 years.
- Greenland is losing 36 to 60 cubic miles of ice per year; Antarctica is losing 36 cubic miles of ice per year.
- Glaciers are receding at unprecedented and rapid rates. The arctic may have its first ice-free summer by 2040, driving arctic creatures to extinction and resulting in dramatic increases in sea level.

Multiple reconstructions of the earth's climate history show that the amounts of greenhouse gases in the atmosphere went up dramatically around the time of the industrial revolution—when humans began burning fossil fuels on a large scale—and correlates very closely with temperature increases.[55] Studies also indicate that large changes in climate can occur in decades rather than centuries or thousands of years.[56] Efforts to reduce the size and scope of our **carbon footprint**—the amount of $CO_2$ emissions created by society—are a huge part of reducing environmental destruction.

## Reducing the Threat of Global Warming

Climate change problems are largely rooted in our energy, transportation, and industrial practices.[57] However, the problem isn't just one of increased $CO_2$ production. Rapid

**carbon footprint** Amount of greenhouse gases produced, usually expressed in equivalent tons of carbon dioxide emissions

deforestation contributes to the rise in greenhouse gases. Trees take in carbon dioxide, transform it, store carbon for food, and release oxygen into the air. As we lose forests at the rate of hundreds of acres per hour, we lose the capacity to store and dissipate carbon dioxide.[58] Population increases and human destruction of natural resources pose additional threats.

## Toward Sustainable Development

To slow climate change, most experts agree that reducing consumption of fossil fuels and using mass transportation are all crucial, but clean energy, green factories, improved energy efficiency, and governmental regulation are also key. The *United Nations Conference on Sustainable Development (known as RIO+20)* took place in 2012 in Rio de Janeiro and outlined a plan for protecting the environment (called "The World We Want") through **sustainable development**—development that meets the needs of the present without compromising the needs of future generations.[59] A number of key nations (including the United States, France, Germany, and the United Kingdom) opted not to attend, and the plan lacked the "teeth" necessary for real change.

Late in 2015, nearly 190 nations, representing over 95 percent of the world's greenhouse gas emissions (including the United States this time) met in Paris to work toward slowing emissions and spurring alternative energy development. The Paris Agreement allowed countries to come up with their own **intended nationally determined contributions (INDCs)**. The United States goal for INDC is to reduce net greenhouse gas emissions 26 to 28 percent below 2005 levels by 2025.[60] Much of this reduction would come from obtaining compliance with existing policies, along with additional technological advances and improvements by individuals, communities, and industry.[61] Although promising, progress to date has been slow. Politics often get in the way, and other issues become priorities. Educating consumers about actions they can take can help.

**Promising Trends** Although getting all nations to form a plan that everyone can work toward may seem a bit like "herding cats," some glimmers of progress by individual nations may be occurring. Currently, the top three $CO_2$ producers (China, 29%; United States, 15%; and the European Union, 11%) contribute 55 percent of all emissions.[62] While China increased its emissions by 4.2 percent and the United States increased emissions by 2.5 percent, the European Union actually decreased emissions by 1.4 percent in 2013.[63] The good news is that the rate of emission increases has begun to slow, with overall global emissions increasing by only 2 percent in 2014 compared to years of double-digit increases.[64]

More wind, solar, and bioenergy use, reductions in natural gas prices, more strict emission standards, and public concerns about smog and pollution are likely reasons for these improvements in many regions.[65] Although stricter laws on

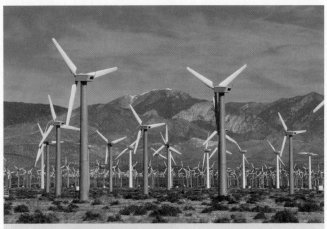

By reducing your use of fossil fuels, using high-efficiency vehicles, and supporting increased use of renewable resources such as solar, wind, and water power, you can help combat global warming.

vehicular carbon emissions and the development of cars that operate on electricity, hydrogen, biodiesel, ethanol, or other alternative energy sources are promising, we have a long way to go to reduce fossil fuel consumption. While hybrid cars often use much less gasoline, in areas where coal is the major source of electricity, issues arise as to whether using coal for electricity rather than gas really makes a car "green."

## Alternative Energy: Promising Future

Alternative energy refers to energy sources that don't utilize fossil fuels. Solar, wind, geothermal, hydroelectric, biomass, ocean, and hydrogen are the most common sources of alternative energy today (**FIGURE 21.5**).

**Solar Power** Solar power is one of the most promising methods of generating electricity, particularly in perpetually sunny places like Arizona and California. In 2016, solar accounted for about 2 percent of global electricity and is estimated to increase to about 16 percent by 2030.[66] Numbers of solar installations are soaring, with a compound annual growth rate of 60 percent in the last decade; up 20 percent in just the last 2 years.[67] It continues to power homes, businesses, city and highway lights, and more, with decreasing costs each year.[68]

**Wind Energy** After solar, wind is our next most used and most viable source of alternative power generation right now. As the wind blows, large turbines turn, harnessing its energy and capturing it in huge power stations. Energy is then fed to power grids, which power cities,

**sustainable development** Development that meets the needs of the present without compromising the ability of future generations to meet their own needs.

**intended nationally determined contributions (INDCs)** Goals that individual countries said they would achieve in order to do their part in the Paris Agreement and reduce global emissions.

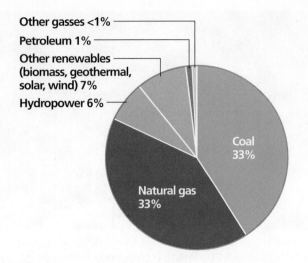

Other gasses <1%
Petroleum 1%
Other renewables
(biomass, geothermal,
solar, wind) 7%
Hydropower 6%

Coal 33%

Natural gas 33%

**FIGURE 21.5** Major Energy Sources and Percent Share of Total U.S. Electricity Generation, 2015

**Source:** U.S. Energy Information Administration, "What is the U.S. Energy Generation by Source?" April 2016, https://www.eia.gov/tools/faqs/faq.cfm?id=427&t=3.

industry, irrigation, wells, and a host of electrical options. Like solar, wind is a green alternative to fossil fuels. Although best suited to open areas with high winds, wind farms are growing in the United States, making up an ever increasing percentage of electric power generation. Concerns over noise and impact on wildlife, particularly birds, are currently being addressed.

### Geothermal Energy: Heating Up

Geothermal energy is another form of renewable, clean energy that works as an alternative to fossil fuels. Geothermal energy comes from heat found in molten rock deep beneath the earth's surface. Combine that superheated molten rock with water and steam is produced, which is captured by geothermal heat pumps. These pumps turn turbines, which in turn power generators. The United States has abundant hot-water geothermal reserves in several western states, providing an energy source that does use fossil fuels to get to produce steam and thus is fairly green as an energy source.[69]

### Hydroelectric Energy

One of the largest sources of energy production after coal, natural gas, and nuclear power is hydropower, produced by fast-moving water that turns great turbines, which in turn power generators. Although clean and renewable, hydroelectric energy has some downside in that it can change waterways through dams, damage fragile ecosystems and aquatic life, and divert water away from irrigation necessary for agriculture. Dams are also very expensive to build.

### Biomass and Other Alternative Energy Sources

Biomass, ocean, and hydrogen are a few more alternative energy sources. *Biomass* involves the conversion of biological materials (woods, crops, plants, landfill,

municipal and industrial wastes, trees, and agricultural products) into an energy source.[70] Experiments are currently underway to produce electricity as a result of wave and wind action in our oceans. Although in their infancy, these power options have huge potential for generating power; however, concerns over damage to fragile ocean ecosystems may be of concern in future years. Much research and huge investments of resources will be necessary for these to have widespread use.

## The Carbon Tax and Cap and Trade Policies: Options for Slowing Emissions

Many U.S. cities and states have begun to consider a **carbon tax** similar to those in Ireland, Sweden, Australia, Great Britain, Quebec, and British Columbia to help slow emissions. A carbon tax is the price a government charges for the carbon content in fuels. Diesel, gas, natural gas, jet fuel, and coal-fired electricity all emit percentages of carbon per unit of fuel. If you use more, you will pay more carbon tax. If your power is fueled by solar, wind, or hydro power, there is no $CO_2$ emission and no tax, incentivizing individuals to invest in noncarbon power generation—as well as drive less, turn down the heat, fly less, and reduce carbon footprints. The city of Boulder, Colorado, was the first to implement a carbon tax, and other states and cities are considering doing so.

**Cap and trade** policies are designed to set limits, or caps, on how much carbon large industrial polluters can emit. Large emitters would be issued permits for allowable levels of pollutants and then taxed on overages, unless they were able to acquire/trade/pay for more allowances from companies that produced lower carbon emissions. Although controversial among those who are antitax and antigovernment, carbon taxes and cap and trade policies are mechanisms for incentivizing green behaviors and motivating those with large carbon footprints to reduce emissions.[71]

## Campus-Wide Actions to Spur Sustainability: Going Green

Many communities and campuses have established plans to reduce their carbon footprint. Creating user-friendly bicycle lanes and monitored bike garages to prevent theft/vandalism and holding "bike to work" days motivate students to leave cars at home. Some campuses have raised fees for parking permits in the hopes of discouraging students from bringing cars to campus.

Many campuses in the United States have also taken steps to "green" their campuses. For example, Oregon State University has made great strides in sustainability through programs focused on recycling and reusing furniture and other items that are tossed out as students leave school in the spring. Its housing and dining services have initiated policies and procedures to help reduce waste and reliance on fossil fuels in products and make it easier for faculty, staff, and students to become more engaged. Its *"Eco2Go"* reusable containers allow people who buy take-out foods to simply rinse

**carbon tax** The price a government charges for the carbon content in fuels.

**cap and trade** Policies designed to set limits, or caps, on how much carbon large industrial polluters can emit.

them out and return them to centrally located spots on campus, where they will be picked up, sanitized, and reused, saving over 400,000 containers dumped in landfills each year.[72] Its priorities for using *locally produced and organic foods* in menus throughout campus reduces fossil fuels in transportation and also helps control exposure to preservatives and other chemicals used in packaging and in growing conventional produce. Other initiatives on campus are focused on waste management and conservation of energy. Is your campus doing it's part?

## LO 4 | WATER POLLUTION AND SHORTAGES

Identify sources of pollution and chemical contaminants often found in water.

Seventy-five percent of Earth is covered with water, but only 2.5 percent of all Earth's water is drinkable freshwater.[73] Approximately 1.2 percent of freshwater is surface water that comes from lakes, ground ice, swamps, marshes, rivers, and soil moisture.[74] Another 30.1 percent is groundwater from underwater wells and aquifers, and the rest of the freshwater (68.7 percent) is locked in glaciers and ice caps.[75] We draw our drinking water from groundwater and surface water; however, much of this water is too polluted or too difficult to reach and concerns over water shortages are on the increase.[76] Recent severe drought in many regions of the country and unseasonably hot weather have forced rationing, voluntary water reduction, and community efforts to conserve water by

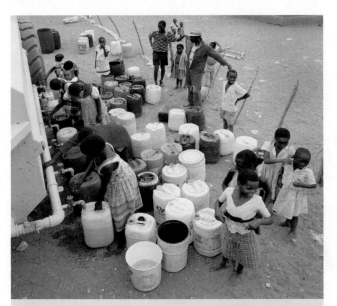

The lack of clean water and sanitation is a major global problem. *Closed basins* are regions where existing water cannot meet the agricultural, industrial, municipal, and environmental needs. The Stockholm International Water Institute estimates that 1.4 billion people live in a closed basin, and the problem is worsening.

individuals, industry, agriculture, and power generation in recent decades.

Although we have seen improvements in *gallons per capita per day* (*GPCD*) water usage from agriculture, thermoelectric power, municipal, and industrial sources in the United States—declining from 1,900 GPCD in 1900 to 1,100 GPCD in 2010—we continue to exceed most nations of the world in water consumption.[77] Residential use has also declined from nearly 120 GPCD in the 1980s to between 80 and 100 GPCD in 2015.[78] Water-saving toilets, faucets, showerheads, washers, and dishwashers and drip irrigation options are responsible for much of this decline.[79] While these changes are laudable, note that the GPCD residential consumption in parts of Africa is closer to 5 gallons![80]

We cannot take the safety of our water supply for granted. Over half the global population faces a shortage of clean water. More than 2.6 billion people, about 40 percent of the planet's population, have no access to basic sanitation or adequate toilet facilities. More than 1 billion have no access to clean water, and more than 4,500 children die every day from illnesses caused by lack of safe water and sanitation.[81] The U.N. estimates that by 2025, two-thirds of the world's population will live in water-stressed areas, increasing competition for scarce reserves and posing a major risk to global food supplies, energy supplies, and survival of all living things.[82] Some areas of the world will be at high risk due to extended drought, population increases, and dwindling supply. Poor sanitation, consumer waste, agricultural enterprises and development in areas that are historically arid, and public apathy all add to the burden.[83] The Making Changes Today box presents simple conservation measures that you can adopt to save water where you live.

# Water Contamination

Any substance that gets into the soil can potentially enter the water supply. Industrial pollutants and pesticides eventually work their way into the soil, then into groundwater. Underground storage tanks for gasoline may leak. U.S. Geological Survey researchers discovered the presence of low levels of many chemical compounds in a network of 139 targeted streams across the United States. Steroids, pharmaceuticals, personal care products, hormones, insect repellent, and wastewater compounds were all detected.[84]

Tap water in the United States is among the safest in the world. The Safe Drinking Water Act (SDWA) is the main federal law that ensures the quality of Americans' drinking water. Under the SDWA, the EPA sets standards for drinking water quality and oversees the states, localities, and water suppliers who implement those standards. Cities and municipalities have strict policies and procedures governing water treatment, filtration, and disinfection to screen out pathogens and microorganisms. However, their ability to filter out increasing amounts of chemical by-products and other substances is in question. According to a 2014 study of over 50 large wastewater sites in the United States, over half of the samples tested positive for at least 25 of the 56 prescription and over-the-counter drugs monitored[85] A more recent study of the drinking water of Americans estimates that the drinking water of over 41 million Americans is contaminated with pharmaceuticals.[86] These levels of drugs have been shown to have significant effects on aquatic life; however, more research needs to be done to examine human risks, particularly for more vulnerable populations.[87] Beyond pharmaceuticals, our aging infrastructure and poor water source choices can also lead to contamination (see the **Health Headlines** box for more on the Flint lead crisis).

Congress has coined two terms that describe general sources of water pollution. **Point source pollutants** enter a waterway at a specific location through a pipe, ditch, culvert, or other conduit. The major sources of point source pollution are sewage treatment plants and industrial facilities. **Nonpoint source pollutants**—commonly known as *runoff* and *sedimentation*—drain or seep into waterways from broad areas of land. Nonpoint source pollution results from a variety of land-use practices, including soil erosion and sedimentation, construction and engineering project wastes, pesticide and fertilizer runoff, urban street runoff, acid mine drainage, septic tank leakage, and sewage sludge (FIGURE 21.6).

Pollutants causing the greatest potential harm are:

- **Gasoline and petroleum products.** When the underground storage tank (UST) assessment program began, there were over 2 million underground tanks in the United States, containing a variety of petroleum products and other hazardous substances. Most of these tanks were located at filling stations and were made of steel, which rusted over time, posing major threats to groundwater and soil.[88] Today, there are only 560,000 tanks in operation, with over 70 percent compliance and much lower risk of contamination.[89]

- **Chemical contaminants.** *Organic solvents* are chemicals designed to dissolve grease and oil. These extremely toxic substances are used to clean clothing, painting equipment, plastics, and metal parts. Consumers often dump leftover products into the toilet or into street drains. Industries pour leftovers into barrels, which are then buried. Eventually, the chemicals eat through the barrels and leach into groundwater.

One potential threat to underwater aquifers and surface water is *hydraulic fracturing*, more commonly known as *fracking*. Fracking is a method of extracting natural gas from shale formations deep within the earth. Pressurized liquids containing chemicals are forced into shale rock formations, allowing oil and gas to flow to the surface. Proponents of fracking point to shale as a resource to help us avoid dependency on foreign oil, aiding in national security, and providing an economic boost. Critics point out that chemicals used in fracking pose the risk of contaminating underground wells, surface waters, and aquifers (see FIGURE 21.7 on page 578).[90] There are also noteworthy upticks in the frequency and intensity of earthquakes

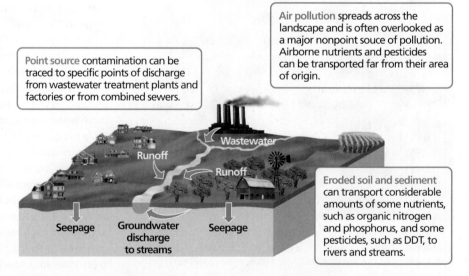

Point source contamination can be traced to specific points of discharge from wastewater treatment plants and factories or from combined sewers.

Air pollution spreads across the landscape and is often overlooked as a major nonpoint souce of pollution. Airborne nutrients and pesticides can be transported far from their area of origin.

Eroded soil and sediment can transport considerable amounts of some nutrients, such as organic nitrogen and phosphorus, and some pesticides, such as DDT, to rivers and streams.

Wastewater
Runoff
Runoff
Seepage
Groundwater discharge to streams
Seepage

**FIGURE 21.6** Potential Sources of Groundwater Contamination

**Source:** Adapted from U.S. Geological Survey, Wisconsin Water Science Center, "Learn More about Groundwater," 2008, http://wi.water.usgs.gov/gwcomp/learn.

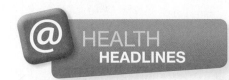
# THE FLINT LEAD CRISIS
## Are You at Risk From Lead Exposure?

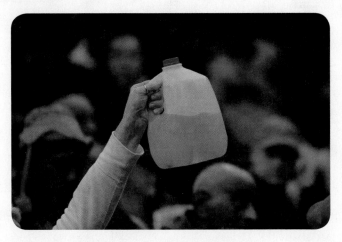

In 2011, facing financial crisis, Flint, Michigan, switched to a cheaper, closer water source than Lake Huron, their existing source about 70 miles away. Switching to the Flint River turned out to be a costly mistake, subjecting an entire city to a toxic brew of lead and a long list of dangerous chemicals and pathogens. While many of the threats could be controlled, some of the worst—including lead—infiltrated water lines in homes and businesses. When water turned smelly, foul-tasting, and rust-colored, people complained. However, since over 40 percent of the populace lives in poverty, complaints went "unheard" for months. In the meantime, children and adults were exposed to high levels of lead.

No level of lead exposure is safe. Children, in particular, face a wide range of health issues—from learning disabilities, to liver and kidney problems, to long-term neurological damage. While efforts to clean up Flint's disastrous lead situation continue, many fear that lead exposure may be more common in other regions of the country. Portland, Oregon, schools were forced to switch to bottled water after high levels of lead were found in the drinking water of several buildings in the spring of 2016. The Flint crisis has spurred increased testing and tuned people in to potential threats in other regions of the country.

How does lead get in the water? Old service lines were often made of lead-containing pipes in cities throughout the United States. Our infrastructure needs major updating, yet cities have been unable to invest in these major projects. Houses built before the 1930s often had lead pipes leading from service lines into homes, many of which have not been replaced. Even when replaced with copper pipes, the solder used to connect them contained high levels of lead, which can leech into water. Of course, lead may originate from primary water sources too, particularly in areas where there has been heavy industry near water supplies. Lead exposure can come from contaminated soils and other sources, too.

How can you find out if there is lead in your water? In some instances, you can just look and see if you have dull, gray older pipes in your home. If you stick a magnet on that metal-looking pipe, it will not stick. You can also look for copper piping where you see soldering joints. Check with your city water department to see if they publish an annual water report to see what is in city water. Have your home water tested by a reputable, certified lab. If you are living in student housing, see if your local community has water testing available and bring in a sample. Remember that hot water is more likely to pick up lead than cold water. Use cold whenever you can.

**Sources:** M. Kennedy, "Lead-Laced Water in Flint: A Step-By-Step Look at the Makings of a Crisis," *NPR,* April 20, 2016, http://www.npr.org/sections/thetwo-way/2016/04/20/465545378/lead-laced-water-in-flint-a-step-by-step-look-at-the-makings-of-a-crisis; EPA, "Flint Drinking Water Response," June 16, 2016, https://www.epa.gov/flint; National Institute of Environmental Health Sciences, "Lead," July 15, 2016, http://www.niehs.nih.gov/health/topics/agents/lead/.

---

in high fracking regions. The EPA and other groups are working to clarify and enforce regulations on discharge and disposal of waste and other potential threats.[91]

- **Polychlorinated biphenyls.** Fire resistant and stable at high temperatures, **polychlorinated biphenyls (PCBs)** were used for many years as insulating materials in high-voltage electrical equipment, such as transformers and older fluorescent lights. The human body does not excrete ingested PCBs but rather stores them in the liver and fatty tissues. PCB exposure is associated with birth defects, cancer, and skin problems. As of 1977, PCBs are no longer manufactured in the United States, but approximately 500 million pounds have been dumped into landfills and waterways, where they continue to pose an environmental threat.[92]

- **Dioxins. Dioxins** are found in herbicides (chemicals used to kill vegetation) and are produced during certain industrial processes. Dioxins have the ability to accumulate in the body and are much more toxic than PCBs. Long-term effects include possible immune system damage and increased risk of infections and cancer. Exposure to high concentrations of PCBs or dioxins for a short period of time can also have severe consequences, including nausea, vomiting, diarrhea, painful rashes and sores, and chloracne, an ailment in which the skin develops hard, black, painful pimples that may never heal.

- **Pesticides. Pesticides** are chemicals designed to kill insects, rodents, plants, and fungi. Americans use more than a billion pounds of pesticides each year, the

> **polychlorinated biphenyls (PCBs)** Toxic chemicals that were once used as insulating materials in high-voltage electrical equipment.
>
> **dioxins** Highly toxic chlorinated hydrocarbons contained in herbicides and produced during certain industrial processes.
>
> **pesticides** Chemicals that kill pests such as insects or rodents.

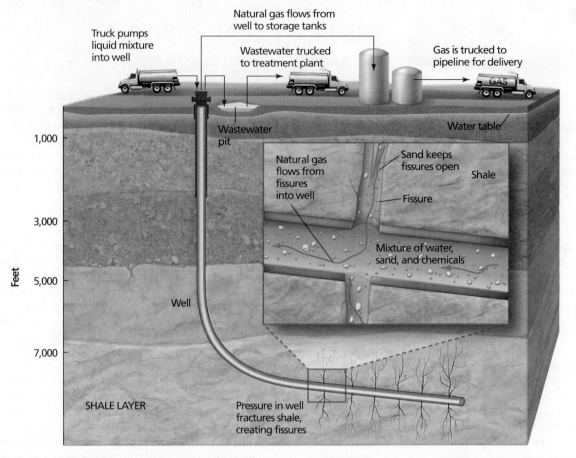

**FIGURE 21.7 Hydraulic Fracturing (Fracking)** Fracking has come under increasing fire for its potential contamination of vital aquifers, as well as increased earthquakes in high fracking areas.

**Source:** Adapted from schematic found in "Potential Relationships Between Hydraulic Fracturing and Drinking Water Resources," U.S. Environmental Protection Agency, 2010, http://www.epa.gov/ogwdw/uic/pdfs/presentations_hf_public_meetings_presentation.pdf.

**municipal solid waste (MSW)** Solid waste such as durable and nondurable goods, containers and packaging, food waste, yard waste, and miscellaneous waste from residential, commercial, institutional, and industrial sources.

majority of which settle on the land and in our air and water.[93] Pesticides evaporate readily and are often dispersed by winds over a large area or carried out to sea. In tropical regions, many farmers use pesticides heavily, and the climate promotes their rapid release into the atmosphere. Pesticide residues cling to fruits and vegetables and can accumulate in the body. Potential hazards associated with exposure to pesticides include birth defects, liver and kidney damage, and nervous system disorders.

of which is nonbiodegradable and some of which is directly harmful to living organisms.

## Solid Waste

Each day, every person in the United States generates nearly 4.4 pounds of **municipal solid waste (MSW)**, more commonly known as trash or garbage, totaling about 251 million tons of trash each year, with organic materials making up the largest share. Paperboard accounts for just over 27 percent, and yard trimmings and food scraps account for another 28 percent (**FIGURE 21.8**).[94]

Although we recycle only slightly over one-third of the waste we generate, experts believe we could recycle up to

## LO 5 | LAND POLLUTION

Distinguish between municipal solid waste and hazardous waste and list strategies for reducing land pollution.

Much of the waste that ends up polluting water starts out polluting the land. Growing population creates more pressure on the land to accommodate increasing amounts of refuse, much

# 254 MILLION

tons of **TRASH** is generated each day in the United States.

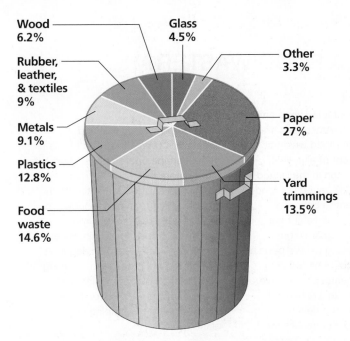

Wood
6.2%

Glass
4.5%

Other
3.3%

Rubber,
leather,
& textiles
9%

Metals
9.1%

Plastics
12.8%

Food
waste
14.6%

Paper
27%

Yard
trimmings
13.5%

**FIGURE 21.8 What's in Our Trash?** Americans throw out many items that could be recycled. Paper and food scraps are the biggest throwaways.

Source: Data are from U.S. Environmental Protection Agency, "Advancing Sustainable Materials Management, 2013 Fact Sheet," June 2015, Available at https://www.epa.gov/sites/production/files/2015-09/documents/2013_advncng_smm_fs.pdf.

90 percent of trash (**FIGURE 21.9**).[95] Currently, 34.3 percent of all MSW in the United States is recycled or composted, 12.9 percent is burned at combustion facilities, and the remaining 52.8 percent is disposed of in landfills.[96]

The number of U.S. landfills has actually decreased in the past decade, but their sheer mass has increased. Many people worry that we are rapidly losing our ability to dispose of all of the waste we create. As communities run out of landfill space, it is becoming common to haul garbage to other states or to dump it illegally in woods, waterways, or oceans, where it contaminates ecosystems, or to ship it to landfills in developing countries, where it becomes someone else's problem. In today's throwaway society, we need to become aware of the amount of waste we generate and to look for ways to recycle, reuse, and—most desirable of all—reduce what we consume.

Communities, businesses, and individuals can adopt several strategies to reduce MSW:

- *Source reduction (waste prevention)* involves altering the design, manufacture, or use of products and materials to reduce the amount and toxicity of waste. The most effective waste-reducing strategy is preventing waste from being generated in the first place. Do we really need to buy products that have three outer shells of plastic? Consumers can help by boycotting such packaging strategies.

- *Recycling* involves sorting, collecting, and processing materials to be reused in manufacturing new products. This process diverts items such as paper, cardboard, glass, plastic, and metals from the waste stream. Be responsible and recycle everything that is recyclable, particularly e-waste and paper.

- *Composting* involves collecting organic waste, such as food scraps and yard trimmings, and allowing it to decompose with the help of microorganisms (mainly bacteria and fungi). This process produces a nutrient-rich substance used to fertilize gardens and for soil enhancement. Many communities now have yard carts that allow you to mix your food scraps in with yard trimmings. Find out what options are available in your area. Not all organic waste is composted; see the **Money & Health** box on page 580 for more on the cost and prevalence of food waste.

- *Combustion with energy recovery* typically involves the use of boilers and industrial furnaces to incinerate waste and use the burning process to generate energy.

**WHAT DO YOU THINK?**

Do you know people who throw away recyclable items rather than recycling them?

- What do you think motivates their behavior?
- How might you encourage them to recycle more than they do now?

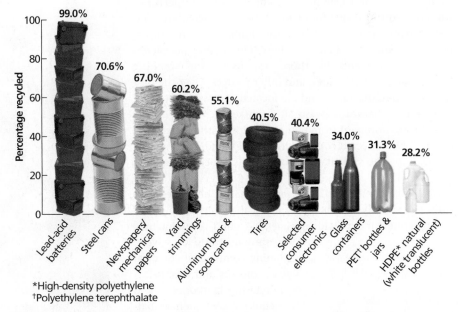

*High-density polyethylene
†Polyethylene terephthalate

99.0% Lead-acid batteries
70.6% Steel cans
67.0% Newspapers/mechanical papers
60.2% Yard trimmings
55.1% Aluminum beer & soda cans
40.5% Tires
40.4% Selected consumer electronics
34.0% Glass containers
31.3% PET† bottles & jars
28.2% HDPE* natural (white translucent) bottles

Percentage recycled

**FIGURE 21.9 How Much Do We Recycle?**

Source: EPA, "Advancing Sustainable Materials Management: 2013 Fact Sheet," June 2015, www.epa.gov/epawaste/nonhaz/municipal/pubs/2013_advncng_smm_fs.pdf.

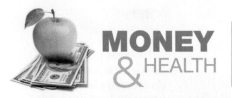

# MONEY & HEALTH | ARE YOU A FOOD WASTER?

At a time when starvation, hunger, and food insecurity plague people throughout the world, a new study by Britain's Institute of Mechanical Engineers indicates that *up to half of the food produced worldwide never makes it into consumer's mouths.* Over 2 billion tons of food could feed millions, but never reaches them.

Global consumer behaviors in more affluent nations are responsible for much of the waste. Big-box stores that promote "bigger size is cheaper" entice people to buy more than they can eat before it spoils. Freezers in homes encourage waste as food dries up before it is eaten, while other food sits on shelves until past its expiration date.

It isn't just our behaviors that contribute to the waste, however. When fresh produce is in surplus and demand is low, crops languish in fields. If weather or insects cause produce to be blemished, we reject it in stores and it is tossed in the trash. Americans are among the worst of the food wasters, wasting over 40 percent of all edible food. The average person in the United States dumps about 20 pounds of food each month, equivalent to between $28 and $43 per month. If we cut our food waste by just 15 percent, some estimate 26 million food-insecure people in the United States could be fed.

From an environmental perspective, when we waste food, we waste all of the time, effort, and resources that went into production and put unnecessary stress on the environment. By wasting less, we put less pressure on our vulnerable habitat.

What can you do?

- Be a better food planner. Make a list when shopping, and only buy what you will use.
- Buy locally.
- Don't be picky. Buy fruit and vegetables even if they don't have a perfect shape or are bruised, and eat them before they rot.
- Eat leftovers. Make a rule that you can't buy fast food or eat out when there is good food in your fridge.
- Eat lower on the food chain. By eating more vegetables, nuts, legumes, and other food crops, and reducing consumption of meat, dairy, and other animal products, you have a smaller footprint stomping on the planet.

**Sources:** B. Jensen, "America's Food Waste Problem Is Bigger Than You Think," *Johns Hopkins Magazine,* Fall 2015, http://hub.jhu.edu/magazine/2015/fall/america-food-waste/; Feeding America, "Food Waste in America," Accessed July 2016, http://www.feedingamerica.org/about-us/how-we-work/securing-meals/reducing-food-waste.html.

## Hazardous Waste

**Hazardous waste** is defined as waste with properties that make it capable of harming human health or the environment. In 1980, the Comprehensive Environmental Response, Compensation and Liability Act, known as the **Superfund**, was enacted to provide funds for cleaning up what are typically "abandoned" hazardous waste dump sites. This Superfund is financed by taxes on the chemical and petroleum industries, payments by those responsible for dumping waste, federal tax revenues, and other sources. Over the past three decades, the Superfund has located and assessed tens of thousands of hazardous waste sites, worked to protect people and the environment from contamination at the worst sites, and involved affected communities, states, and other groups in cleanup. The vast majority of sites have been cleared or "recovered."[97]

The large number of U.S. hazardous waste dump sites indicates the severity of our toxic chemical problem. American manufacturers and individuals generate around 40 million tons of hazardous waste each year, including commercial chemical refuse, solvents and oils, petroleum-refining by-products, and household wastes such as batteries, cleaning products, and paints.[98] Many wastes are now banned from land disposal or are being treated to reduce their toxicity before they become part of land disposal sites. The EPA has developed protective requirements for land disposal facilities, such as double liners, detection systems for substances that may leach into groundwater, and groundwater-monitoring systems.

**hazardous waste** Toxic waste that poses a hazard to humans or to the environment.

**Superfund** Fund established under the Comprehensive Environmental Response, Compensation, and Liability Act to be used for cleaning up toxic waste dumps.

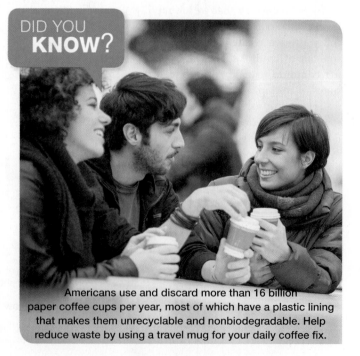

DID YOU **KNOW**?

Americans use and discard more than 16 billion paper coffee cups per year, most of which have a plastic lining that makes them unrecyclable and nonbiodegradable. Help reduce waste by using a travel mug for your daily coffee fix.

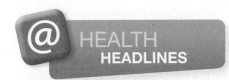

# E-CONCERNS
## Devices and Health Risks?

Given that mobile phone use has skyrocketed, only the most apathetic wouldn't be concerned about *radio (RF) frequency*. But what is the real risk? In theory, RF energy has the potential to penetrate the skull, neck, and upper torso. For the very young, whose skulls have not yet sufficiently hardened, the risk might be even greater. However, after more than a decade of research, epidemiological evidence indicates that radio frequency electromagnetic radiation exposure does not show an increased risk of brain tumors or other cancers of the head and neck. Nevertheless, experts in the field call for more research examining the heat-producing aspects of these waves, possible effects on glucose metabolism, and potential increased risks of exposure in youth and long-term super-users. Questions about increased exposure from wearable devices and larger screens with larger batteries also raise concerns. In the interim, it makes good sense to use caution. Go hands free. Check out the specific absorption rate (SAR) charts online or from your phone company before buying.

### Set-Top Box Power Guzzlers

While you are in class, out to dinner, or in bed sound asleep, your cable box is using more electricity than almost any appliance in your house! A recent report indicates that a set-top cable or satellite box can consume as much as 35 watts of power and cost about $8.00 a month in certain regions of the country. The nearly quarter of a million boxes currently in U.S. homes use as much electricity together as four nuclear power plants generate. Even when turned off, hard drives keep running, downloading, and updating. Unplugging can help, but can require a long reboot when you want to use the system. The answer might be to use fewer boxes in your home or do more streaming on lower-energy-use devices.

### E-Waste: Not in Your Backyard?

The global burden of e-waste (trashed computers, televisions, and tons of other electronic devices) has skyrocketed in recent years. Unfortanately, although many of these products can be reused or recycled through sustainable means, many end up in landfills. Others end up as part of a growing "trafficking in exports" of electronic parts and precious metals, as well as potential toxic components. In spite of calls for bans on these exports, they often end up in the poorest countries, exposing vulnerable populations to health-compromising conditions. What can you do to reduce this waste? Very simply, hang on to your devices for as long as possible. "Use it and *don't* lose it," so to speak. When you

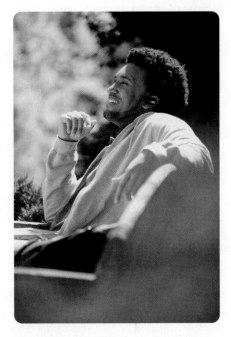

are thinking about *e-recycling*, check out www.ecyclingcentral.com for a state-by-state listing of e-recyclers in your area.

**Sources:** EPA, "Basic Information about Electronics Stewardship." April 26, 2016, https://www.epa.gov/smm-electronics/basic-information-about-electronics-stewardship#01; National Cancer Institute, Factsheet, "Cell Phones and Cancer Risk," May 27, 2016, www.cancer.gov/cancertopics/factsheet/Risk/cellphones; R. Vartabedian, "Cable TV Boxes Become 2nd Biggest Energy Users in Many Homes," *LA Times*, June 19, 2014, www.latimes.com/nation/la-na-power-hog-20140617-story.html#page=1.

---

## LO 6 | RADIATION

List and explain key health concerns associated with ionizing and nonionizing radiation.

Radiation is energy that travels in waves or particles. There are many different types of radiation, ranging from radio waves to gamma rays, all making up the electromagnetic spectrum. Exposure to radiation is an inescapable part of life on this planet, but only some of it poses a threat to human health.

## Nonionizing Radiation

**Nonionizing radiation** is radiation at the lower end of the electromagnetic spectrum, which moves in relatively long wavelengths. Examples of nonionizing radiation are radio waves, TV signals, microwaves, infrared waves, and visible light. Unlike ionizing radiation, which can disrupt molecular bonds and affect cells and health, nonionizing radiation doesn't have sufficient energy to break molecular bonds or cause significant damage to cells.[99] However, concerns have been raised about the safety of radio frequency waves generated by cell phones (see the **Health Headlines** box).

## Ionizing Radiation

**Ionizing radiation** is caused by the release of particles and electromagnetic rays from atomic nuclei during the normal process of disintegration. This type of radiation has enough energy to remove electrons from the atoms it passes through. Some naturally

**nonionizing radiation** Electromagnetic waves having relatively long wavelengths and enough energy to move atoms around or cause them to vibrate.

**ionizing radiation** Electromagnetic waves and particles having short wavelengths and energy high enough to ionize atoms.

occurring elements, such as uranium, emit ionizing radiation. The sun is another source of ionizing radiation, in the form of high-frequency ultraviolet rays—those against which the ozone layer protects us.

Radiation exposure is measured in **radiation-absorbed doses** or **rads** (also called *roentgens*). Radiation can cause damage at dosages as low as 100 to 200 rads. At this level, signs of radiation sickness include nausea, diarrhea, fatigue, anemia, sore throat, and hair loss. At 350 to 500 rads, these symptoms become more severe, and death may result because the radiation hinders bone marrow production of the white blood cells we need to protect us from disease. Dosages above 600 to 700 rads are fatal.

Recommended maximum "safe" exposure ranges from 0.5 to 5 rads per year.[100] Approximately 50 percent of the radiation to which we are exposed comes from background sources, including natural and human-made sources. Natural sources include radon gas in the air and cosmic radiation. Human-made sources include certain building materials. Another 45 percent comes from medical and dental X-rays. The remaining 5 percent is nonionizing radiation that comes from such sources as computer monitors, microwave ovens, televisions, and radar screens.[101] Most of us are exposed to far less radiation than the safe maximum dosage per year. The effects of long-term exposure to relatively low levels of radiation are unknown. Some scientists believe that such exposure can cause lung cancer, leukemia, skin cancer, bone cancer, and skeletal deformities.

## Nuclear Power Plants

Currently, nuclear power plants account for less than 1 percent of the total radiation to which we are exposed; however, the number of U.S. plants may increase in the next decade, so that percentage of exposure may increase. In addition, the use of nuclear power worldwide is expected to double in the next 35 years, particularly in China and other parts of Asia.[102] Proponents of nuclear energy believe that it is a safe and efficient way to generate electricity.

**radiation-absorbed dose (rad)** Unit of measure of radiation exposure.

**nuclear meltdown** Accident that results when the temperature in the core of a nuclear reactor increases enough to melt the nuclear fuel and breach the containment vessel.

Initial costs of building nuclear power plants are high, but actual power generation is relatively inexpensive. A 1,000-megawatt reactor produces enough energy for 650,000 homes and saves 420 million gallons of fossil fuels each year. In some areas where nuclear power plants were decommissioned, electricity bills tripled when power companies turned to hydroelectric or fossil fuel sources to generate electricity. Nuclear reactors discharge fewer carbon oxides into the air than do fossil fuel–powered generators. Advocates believe that converting to nuclear power could help slow global warming.

The advantages of nuclear energy must be weighed against the disadvantages. Disposal of nuclear waste is extremely problematic. In addition, a reactor core meltdown could pose serious threats to the immediate environment and to the world in general. A **nuclear meltdown** occurs when the temperature in the core of a nuclear reactor increases enough to melt the nuclear fuel and breach the containment vessel. Most modern facilities seal the reactors and containment vessels in concrete buildings with pools of cold water on the bottom. If a meltdown occurs, the building and the pool are supposed to prevent radiation from escaping.

The International Atomic Energy Agency ranks nuclear and radiological accidents and incidents by severity on a scale of 1 to 7. To date, we have had two major nuclear disasters that resulted in a 7, the highest severity rating, meaning that there was a major release of radioactive material with widespread health and environmental consequences. The first was the 1986 reactor core fire and explosion at the Chernobyl nuclear power plant in Russia, which has led to conservative estimates of from 2,000 to as many as 724,000 deaths. Many regions surrounding the area may be uninhabitable for decades.[103] The damage to the Fukushima Daiichi Nuclear Power Station in northern Japan caused by the March 2011 earthquake and tsunami was also listed as a level 7 nuclear disaster and has awakened worldwide fears about nuclear power. Some research suggests that there may be as many as 400,000 additional cancer patients and over 40,000 deaths from thyroid cancer alone among those within 200 kilometers of the Fukushima Daiichi plant; however, exact information is difficult to obtain. Effects of the Fukushima may be felt in waterways for decades.[104]

# STUDY **PLAN**

Customize your study plan—and master your health!—in the Study Area of **MasteringHealth**.

## ASSESS YOURSELF

**What measures can you take to preserve your environment?**
Want to find out? Take the **Are You Doing All You Can Do to Protect the Environment?** assessment available on

**MasteringHealth.™**

## CHAPTER **REVIEW**

To hear an MP3 Tutor Session, scan here or visit the Study Area in **MasteringHealth**.

### LO 1 | Overpopulation: The World's Greatest Threat

■ Population growth is the single largest factor affecting the environment. Demand for more food, water, and energy—as well as places to dispose of waste—puts unsustainable strain on Earth's resources.

### LO 2 | Air Pollution

■ The primary constituents of air pollution are sulfur dioxide, particulate matter, carbon monoxide, nitrogen dioxide, ozone, lead, carbon dioxide, and hydrocarbons. Indoor air pollution is caused primarily by tobacco smoke, woodstove smoke, furnace emissions, asbestos, formaldehyde, radon, lead, and mold.

### LO 3 | Climate Change

■ Air pollution is depleting Earth's protective ozone layer and contributing to global warming, a type of climate change, by enhancing the greenhouse effect. Alternative energy sources such as wind, solar, hydroelectric, biomass, geothermal, and other options are key to reducing climate

change and our dependence on fossil fuels.

### LO 4 | Water Pollution and Shortages

■ Water pollution can be caused by either point sources (direct entry) or nonpoint sources (runoff or seepage). Major contributors to water pollution include petroleum products, organic solvents, polychlorinated biphenyls (PCBs), dioxins, pesticides, and lead.

### LO 5 | Land Pollution

■ Municipal solid waste (MSW) includes household trash, plastics, glass, metals, and paper. Many of these items can be recycled. Limited landfill space creates problems in dealing with growing volumes of MSW. Hazardous waste is toxic; improper disposal creates health hazards for people in surrounding communities.

### LO 6 | Radiation

■ Nonionizing radiation comes from electromagnetic fields, such as those around power lines. Ionizing radiation results from the erosion of atomic nuclei. The disposal and storage of radioactive waste from nuclear power plants pose potential public health problems.

## POP **QUIZ**

Visit **MasteringHealth** to personalize your study plan with Chapter Review Quizzes and Dynamic Study Modules.

### LO 1 | Overpopulation: The World's Greatest Threat

1. The largest population that can be supported indefinitely given the resources available is known as Earth's
   a. maximum fertility rate.
   b. fertility capacity.
   c. maximum population growth.
   d. carrying capacity.

### LO 2 | Air Pollution

2. One source of indoor air pollution is a gas present in some carpets and home furnishings known as
   a. lead.
   b. asbestos.
   c. radon.
   d. formaldehyde.

3. Which substance separates into stringy fibers that can become embedded in the lungs and cause disease?
   a. Asbestos
   b. Particulate matter
   c. Radon
   d. Formaldehyde

4. The air pollutant that originates primarily from motor vehicle emissions is
   a. particulates.
   b. nitrogen dioxide.
   c. sulfur dioxide.
   d. carbon monoxide.

5. Which gas can potentially become cancer causing when it seeps into a home?
   a. Carbon monoxide
   b. Radon
   c. Hydrogen sulfide
   d. Ozone

## LO 3 | Climate Change

6. What is it called when gases such as carbon dioxide, nitrous oxide, methane, CFCs, and hydrocarbons form a layer in the atmosphere, allowing solar heat to pass through and trapping some of the heat close to the surface to warm the planet?
   a. Photochemical smog
   b. Ozone layer
   c. Gray air smog
   d. Greenhouse effect

## LO 4 | Water Pollution and Shortages

7. The terms *point source* and *nonpoint source* are used to describe the two general sources of
   a. water pollution.
   b. air pollution.
   c. noise pollution.
   d. ozone depletion.

8. Some herbicides contain toxic substances known as
   a. THMs.
   b. PCPs.
   c. dioxins.
   d. PCBs.

## LO 5 | Land Pollution

9. A DVD you recently purchased had less packaging than those you had bought previously. This change in packaging design is an example of reducing municipal solid waste by

   a. source reduction.
   b. recycling.
   c. composting.
   d. incineration.

## LO 6 | Radiation

10. What is the recommended safe level of rads exposure per year?
    a. 0.5 to 5 rads
    b. 5 to 100 rads
    c. 100 to 200 rads
    d. 200 to 350 rads

*Answers to the Pop Quiz can be found on page A-1. If you answered a question incorrectly, review the section identified by the Learning Outcome. For even more study tools, visit* **MasteringHealth**.

# THINK ABOUT IT!

## LO 1 | Overpopulation: The World's Greatest Threat

1. How are the rapid increases in global population and consumption of resources related to climate change? What are options for controlling population and less consumption of resources? Is population control the best solution? Why or why not?

## LO 2 | Air Pollution

2. What are the primary sources of air pollution? What actions can you take that will reduce air pollution? Which air pollution strategies seem to help reduce current threats and how can we best build upon those strategies?

## LO 3 | Climate Change

3. What are the causes and consequences of global warming? What can individuals do to reduce the threat of global warming? How do you feel about

a carbon tax? What policies do you think communities can take to reduce the threat of climate change and global warming?

## LO 4 | Water Pollution and Shortages

4. What are point and nonpoint sources of water pollution? What policies can communities enact that would help reduce or prevent water pollution? Policies on pesticide use and herbicides that pollute our water supply? What can you do to reduce your daily water consumption? To prevent toxic contamination of water in your home and environment?

## LO 5 | Land Pollution

5. How do you think communities and governments could encourage recycling efforts? Or should industry be forced to reduce packaging and waste? What are the pros and cons of a tax on the garbage individuals/families create weekly based on weight/volume? What would influence you to use less/recycle more?

## LO 6 | Radiation

6. What can you do to reduce your potential radiation exposure? Radiation in the community? National level radiation?

# ACCESS YOUR HEALTH ON THE INTERNET

Visit **MasteringHealth** for links to the websites and RSS feeds.

The following websites explore further topics and issues related to protecting the environment.

**Environmental Literacy Council.** This website is an excellent source of information about environmental issues in general. Topics range from how

the ozone layer works to why the rain forests are important ecosystems.
www.enviroliteracy.org

**Environmental Protection Agency (EPA).** The EPA is the U.S. government agency responsible for overseeing environmental regulation and protection issues.
www.epa.gov

**National Center for Environmental Health (NCEH).** This site provides information on a wide variety

of environmental health issues and includes a series of helpful fact sheets.
www.cdc.gov/nceh

**National Environmental Health Association (NEHA).** This organization provides educational resources and opportunities for environmental health professionals.
www.neha.org

**Environmental Working Group (EWG).** This organization provides

resources for consumers, such as a guide to fruits and vegetables that ranks the best to worst in terms of pesticide contaminants. It also works for national policy change.
www.ewg.org

**Global Footprint Network Footprint Calculator.** Use this tool to calculate your ecological footprint based on your current lifestyle.
www.footprintnetwork.org/en/index.php/GFN/page/calculators/

# 22 Preparing for Aging, Death, and Dying

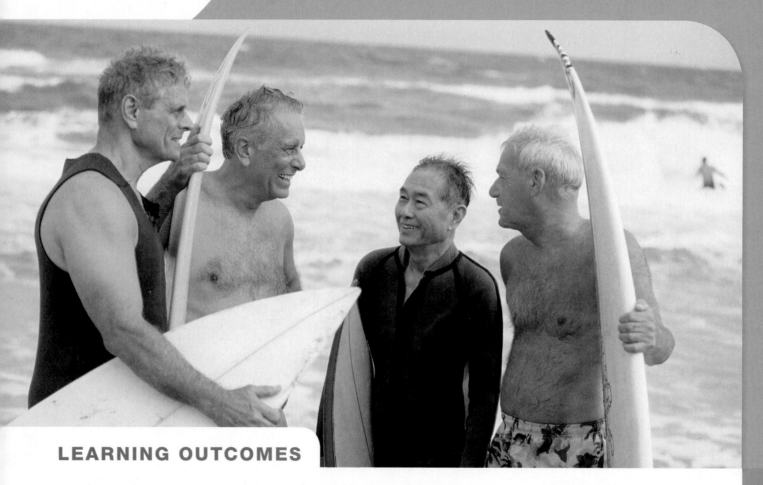

## LEARNING OUTCOMES

LO **1** Define *aging*, as well as the concepts of biological, psychological, social, legal, and functional age, and list the characteristics of successful aging.

LO **2** Explain how the growing population of older adults will affect society, including considerations of economics, health care, living arrangements, and ethical and moral issues.

LO **3** Explain the biological and psychosocial theories of aging and summarize major physiological changes that occur as a result of the normal aging process.

LO **4** Describe unique health challenges faced by older adults.

LO **5** List strategies for successful and healthy aging.

LO **6** Define death and discuss strategies for coping with death.

LO **7** Describe typical grief symptoms and the grieving process.

LO **8** Explain the ethical concerns that arise from the concepts of the right to die and rational suicide.

LO **9** Review the decisions that need to be made when someone is dying or has died, including hospice care, funeral arrangements, wills, and organ donation.

Aging isn't a process somewhere in the future—it's happening to every one of us every day. The way you live your life now has a direct impact on how you will live it in the future. Learning to cope with challenges and changes early in life develops attitudes and skills that contribute to a full and satisfying old age.

In a society that seems to worship youth, researchers have begun to offer good—even revolutionary—news about the aging process. Health promotion, disease prevention, and wellness-oriented activities can prolong vigor and productivity in older people, even among those who haven't always made healthful habits a priority. Numerous studies show that people who make even modest lifestyle changes can reap significant health benefits. In fact, getting older can mean getting better in many ways—particularly socially, psychologically, spiritually, and intellectually.

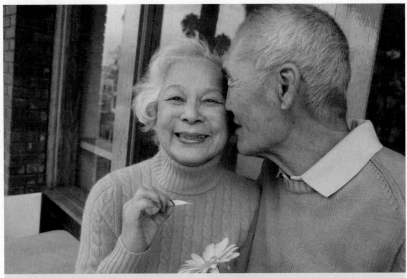

Grow old along with me! The best is yet to be, The last of life, for which the first was made . . .
—Robert Browning, *Rabbi Ben Ezra*

## LO 1 | AGING

Define *aging* as well as the concepts of biological, psychological, social, legal, and functional age, and list the characteristics of successful aging.

**Aging** has traditionally been described as the patterns of life changes that occur in members of all species as they grow older. Some believe that aging begins at the moment of conception. Others contend that it starts at birth. Still others believe that true aging does not begin until we reach our 40s. The study of individual and collective aging processes, known as **gerontology**, explores the reasons for aging and the ways in which people cope with and adapt to this process. Chronological age has traditionally been used to assign people to particular stages of life. However, definitions of aging that consider only years lived rather than quality of life warrant reexamination.

### HEAR IT! PODCASTS

Want a study podcast for this chapter? Download **Life's Transitions: The Aging Process**, available on

MasteringHealth.™

### Redefining Aging

Gerontologists have identified several age-related characteristics that define where a person is in terms of biological, psychological, social, legal, and functional life-stage development:[1]

- *Biological age* refers to the relative age or condition of a person's organs and body systems. Research shows that healthy lifestyle behaviors such as being active, eating a healthy diet, and not smoking are the most influential factors for how your body ages.[2]

- *Psychological age* refers to a person's adaptive capacities, such as coping abilities and intelligence, resilience and awareness of individual capabilities and self-efficacy, and general ability to adapt to new situations or adversity. Research demonstrates that many older adults maintain a positive attitude and successfully cope with the physical and cognitive changes associated with aging.[3]

- *Social age* refers to a person's habits and roles relative to society's expectations.

- *Legal age* is probably the most common definition of age. Based on chronological years lived, legal age is used as a factor in determining voting rights, driving privileges, eligibility for Social Security payments, and other rights and obligations.

- *Functional age* refers to a person's status in terms of physical and mental performance.

**What is Successful Aging?** Many older Americans lead active, productive lives. The majority of adults over age 65 continue to work, care for and help others, engage in social activities, and remain otherwise active. Ultimately, the question is not so much how many years someone has lived, but how much life the person has packed

> **aging** The patterns of life changes that occur in members of all species as they grow older.
>
> **gerontology** The study of individual and collective aging processes.

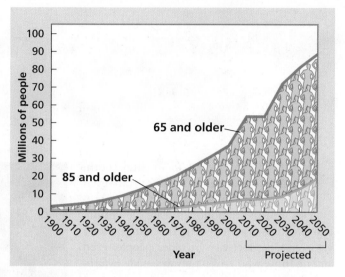

**FIGURE 22.1** Number of Americans 65 and Older (in millions), Years 1900–2008, and Projected 2010–2050

**Note:** Data for 2020–2050 are projections of the population.

**Source:** U.S. Department of Health and Human Services, "Projected Future Growth of the Older Population," Administration on Aging, (2014). http://www.aoa.acl.gov/Aging_Statistics/future_growth/future_growth.aspx.

into those years. This *quality-of-life index*, combined with the chronological process, appears to be the best indicator of "aging gracefully." Most experts agree that the best way to experience a productive, full, and satisfying old age is to lead a productive, full, and satisfying life prior to old age. See the Making Changes Today box for more specific characteristics of people who have aged well.

## LO 2 | OLDER ADULTS: A GROWING POPULATION

Explain how the growing population of older adults will affect society, including considerations of economics, health care, living arrangements, and ethical and moral issues.

The United States and much of the developed world are on the brink of a *longevity revolution*. Medical care breakthroughs and improved understanding of fitness and nutrition have steadily increased lifespan. According to the latest statistics, life expectancy for a child born in 2014 is 79.5 years—more than 30 years longer than for a child born in 1900.[4] In 2014 there were 46.2 million people age 65 or older in the United States, making up over 14 percent of the total population.[5] In comparison, the number of people age 65 and older has more than tripled since 1900 (see **FIGURE 22.1**).[6] Similar trends are true throughout the world, with the percentage of people over age 60 expected to hit 22 percent by 2050—a doubling or tripling since 2010![7]

Within the United States, the over-65 population will increase substantially over the next two decades due to the aging of the "baby boomer" generation, an especially large segment of the population who were born during the period of economic prosperity that began in the late 1940s and continued through the early 1960s. The oldest of the baby boomers are just beginning to retire, and their impact on the economy, housing market, health care system, and Social Security will be profound in the coming decades. For more on aging in the United States, particularly how we stack up against other countries, see the **Health in a Diverse World** box.

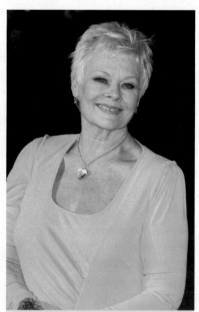

The people we often think of as aging gracefully—such as actress Dame Judi Dench—are those who continue to be active and productive; who are not frightened or ashamed of growing older; who adapt to the changing circumstances of their lives; and who strive to be emotionally and physically healthy, vibrant, and alive at any age.

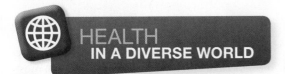

# AGING IN AMERICA
*How Do We Stack Up?*

By midcentury, the global population of people over the age of 65 is expected to triple to 1.5 billion. In the United States alone, the population of people age 65 and older is anticipated to exceed 84 million by 2050. In the United States, the nation that spends more money on health care than any other country, one would expect our length of life to exceed that of comparable countries. Furthermore, one would think the quality of life for our elderly would be vastly better in the United States than for the elderly in other countries. However, a report from the National Research Council documented that life expectancy at age 50 had been increasing at a slower rate than other high-income countries. Some of the reasons for this slower rate include:

■ The U.S. has the highest rates of infant mortality among high-income countries.*

■ Obesity and heart disease are at the highest rates among high income-nations.

■ The U.S. has one of the highest rates of people with physical limitations amongst our peer countries.

■ More American lives are lost to alcohol and drugs than any other nation. One of the most significant reasons why women in the United States do not reach 50 years of age is accidental poisonings linked to prescription opioid and heroin use.

Experts suggest that one approach to improving outcomes is to increase the amount of money spent on nonmedical social services such as education, daycare, job training, nutritional assistance, etc. Currently, the U.S. spends the most per person for health care and the least per person on nonmedical social services. It is this kind of approach that may significantly increase the likelihood of many more Americans living long, healthy lives.

**Sources:** J. McDonough, "Shorter Lives and Poorer Health on the Campaign Trail," *American Journal of Public Health* 106, no. 3, (2016): 395–7; S.H. Woolf and L. Aron, eds., *US Health in International Perspective: Shorter Lives, Poorer Health* (Washington, DC: National Academies Press, 2013), Available at http://www.nap.edu/catalog/13497/us-health-in-international-perspective-shorter-lives-poorer-health; L. Aron et al., "To Understand Climbing Death Rates Among Whites, Look to Women of Childbearing Age." *Health Affairs* blog, November 10, 2015, http://healthaffairs.org/blog/2015/11/10/to-understand-climbing-death-rates-among-whites-look-to-women-of-childbearing-age.

*Comparison countries: Australia, Austria, Canada, Denmark, Finland, France, Germany, Italy, Japan, Norway, Portugal, Spain, Switzerland, the Netherlands, and the United Kingdom

## Health Issues for an Aging Society

Advancing age is often associated with increasing vulnerability to a unique set of stressors that can have profound effects on health. Retirement, failing health, loss of loved ones, financial insecurity, problems with access to quality health care, and loss of independence and "change" are just a few of these issues. Meeting an older population's physical and emotional health needs, providing essential housing, health care, and support services, as well as addressing end-of-life ethical considerations are all of concern in an aging society. Many fear that the combination of fewer younger workers paying into the Social Security system and more older people drawing benefits for longer than ever before will result in tremendous government budget shortfalls. Enhancing health and reducing risks before health deteriorates are key to a healthy future health care system.

### Health Care Costs
Older Americans averaged $5,849 in out-of-pocket medical expenses in 2014, an increase of 50 percent since 2004.[8] About 68 percent of those costs, on average, went to pay for health insurance itself, whereas drugs or medical services not covered by insurance premiums accounted for roughly one-third of the costs.[9] As people live longer, the chances of developing a costly chronic disease increase, and as technology improves, chronic illnesses that once were quickly fatal may now be treated successfully for years. Most older adults have at least one chronic condition:

About 71 percent have hypertension or are taking antihypertensive medication, 49 percent have been diagnosed with arthritis, 30 percent have heart disease, 24 percent have cancer, and 21 percent have diabetes.[10]

### Housing and Living Arrangements
Most older adults never live in a nursing home. Many live with a spouse, partner, or alone; others live with family or friends or pay for home health services. An increasing number opt for assisted living in apartments, foster homes, or individual homes with supportive services like meals, help with housekeeping and medication, or other options that help seniors live independently (**FIGURE 22.2** on page 590). Other communities and facilities include 24/7 monitoring of unique needs, such as Alzheimer's cases or other disabilities. Newer, technologically advanced housing includes physiological monitoring that records heart rate and other life indicators to ensure prompt emergency services in case of problems. With increasing age comes an increased likelihood of some form of institutional

## 43%

Approximate number of Americans aged 65 to 74 that engage in regular **LEISURE-TIME ACTIVITY**. For people over age 75, it's 27%.

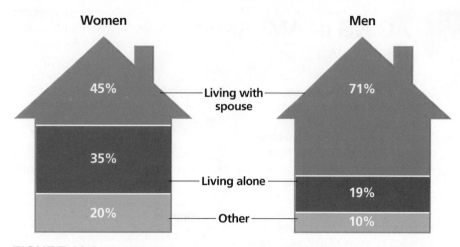

**Women** **Men**

45% — Living with spouse — 71%

35% — Living alone — 19%

20% — Other — 10%

**FIGURE 22.2** **Living Arrangements of Americans Age 65 and Older** Percentages may not total 100% due to rounding.

**Source:** Administration on Aging, U.S. Dept. of Health and Human Services, "A Profile of Older Americans: Living Arrangements, 2014," 2015, www.aoa.acl.gov/Aging_Statistics/Profile/2014/docs/2014-Profile.pdf.

setting, with just over 1 percent of those aged 65 to 74 years, 3 percent of those 75 to 85 years, and 10 percent of those over 85 years living in nursing homes.[11]

The average cost for institutional care varies tremendously by state and level of care, starting at more than $90,000 per year for a private room in a nursing home to $40,000 to $50,000 for an assisted living facility room.[12] Tremendous income-based disparities exist in caring for older adults, and even with significant savings, many elderly budgets will be stretched to the limit. Many American seniors live on small fixed incomes, and in 2014 the *supplemental poverty measure* calculated by the

**DID YOU KNOW?** The average cost for a private room in a nursing home is $250 per day, or nearly $7,700 per month. Could you or your parents afford a payment of this size?

**Source:** Genworth, "Compare Long-Term Care Costs across the United States," June, 2016, www.genworth.com/corporate/about-genworth/industry-expertise/cost-of-care.html.

government estimated that 10 percent of seniors lived in poverty in the United States.[13] Those without means are more likely to be shut out of all but the most meager health care and living situations. Those without friend and family supports will be in an even more precarious situation.

**Ethical and Moral Considerations** Difficult ethical questions arise when we consider the implications of an already overburdened health care system. The cost of care versus the quality and length of life it buys, particularly for terminally ill older people, is something each society must weigh. Is the prolonging of life at all costs a moral imperative, or will future generations devise a set of criteria for deciding who will be helped and who will not? Such debates leave much room for careful thought and discussion.

## LO 3 | THEORIES OF AGING

Explain the biological and psychosocial theories of aging and summarize major physiological changes that occur as a result of the normal aging process.

Social gerontologists, behaviorists, biologists, geneticists, and physiologists continue to explore various potential explanations for why the body breaks down over time. One explanation for the biological cause of aging is the *wear-and-tear theory*, which states that, like everything else, the human body wears out. Inherent in this theory is the idea that the more you abuse your body, the faster it will wear out.[14]

Another theory, the *cellular theory*, proposes that at birth we have only a certain number of usable cells, which are genetically programmed to reproduce a limited number of times. Once cells reach the end of their reproductive cycle, they die, and the organs they build begin to deteriorate, ultimately leading to body system failures and death.[15]

According to the *genetic mutation theory*, the number of body cells exhibiting unusual or different characteristics increases with age. Proponents of this theory believe that aging is related to the amount of mutational damage within the genes. The more mutation there is, the greater the chance that cells will not function properly.[16]

Finally, the *autoimmune theory* attributes aging to the decline of the body's immunological system. Studies indicate that as we age, the ability to produce necessary antibodies declines, and our immune systems become less effective in fighting disease. At the same time, the white blood cells active in the immune response become less able to recognize foreign invaders and more likely to mistakenly attack the body's own proteins.[17]

## LO 4 | **PHYSICAL** AND MENTAL CHANGES OF AGING

Describe unique health challenges faced by older adults.

Although the physiological consequences of aging can differ in severity and timing, certain standard changes occur as a result of the aging process. Many of these changes are physical (see **FIGURE 22.3**), whereas others are mental or psychosocial. Genetics, environment, and your behaviors can greatly influence the speed of age-related changes and how well an individual ages over time. Fortunately, there is much that you can do to remain strong and healthy and ensure that you age successfully. But first, let's explore some of the normal physical changes that are already starting to occur.

### The Skin

As a normal part of aging, the skin becomes thinner and loses elasticity, particularly in the outer surfaces. Fat deposits, which add to the soft lines and shape of the skin, diminish. Starting at about age 30, lines develop on the forehead as a result of smiling, squinting, and other facial expressions. During the 40s, these lines become more pronounced, with added "crow's feet" around the eyes. In the 50s and 60s, skin begins to sag and lose color, leading to pallor in the 70s. Body fat in underlying skin layers continues to be redistributed away from the limbs and extremities into the body's trunk region. Age spots increase because of excessive pigment accumulation under the skin, particularly in areas exposed to heavy sun.

### Bones and Joints

Throughout the lifespan, bones are continually changing because of the accumulation and loss of minerals. By the third or fourth decade of life, mineral loss from bones becomes more prevalent than mineral accumulation, which results in a weakening and porosity (diminishing density) of bony tissue. **Osteoporosis** is a disease characterized by low bone density and structural deterioration of bone tissue. These porous, fragile bones are susceptible to fracture and may lead to crippling malformation of the spine characteristic of the dowager's hump seen in stooped individuals.

Many people think osteoporosis is a disease affecting only older women, but it can occur at any age and affects men as well. More than 54 million Americans have low bone density or

**osteoporosis** A degenerative bone disorder characterized by increasingly porous bones.

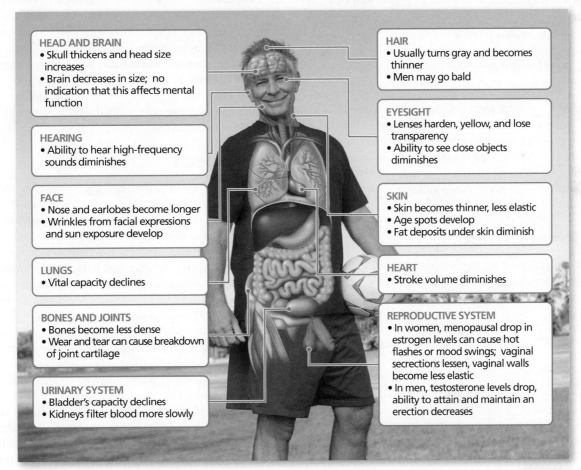

**HEAD AND BRAIN**
• Skull thickens and head size increases
• Brain decreases in size; no indication that this affects mental function

**HEARING**
• Ability to hear high-frequency sounds diminishes

**FACE**
• Nose and earlobes become longer
• Wrinkles from facial expressions and sun exposure develop

**LUNGS**
• Vital capacity declines

**BONES AND JOINTS**
• Bones become less dense
• Wear and tear can cause breakdown of joint cartilage

**URINARY SYSTEM**
• Bladder's capacity declines
• Kidneys filter blood more slowly

**HAIR**
• Usually turns gray and becomes thinner
• Men may go bald

**EYESIGHT**
• Lenses harden, yellow, and lose transparency
• Ability to see close objects diminishes

**SKIN**
• Skin becomes thinner, less elastic
• Age spots develop
• Fat deposits under skin diminish

**HEART**
• Stroke volume diminishes

**REPRODUCTIVE SYSTEM**
• In women, menopausal drop in estrogen levels can cause hot flashes or mood swings; vaginal secretions lessen, vaginal walls become less elastic
• In men, testosterone levels drop, ability to attain and maintain an erection decreases

**FIGURE 22.3** Normal Effects of Aging on the Body

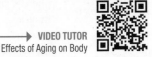

→ VIDEO TUTOR
Effects of Aging on Body

osteoporosis.[18] In fact, about 40 percent of women and 15 to 30 percent of men over 50 years of age will break a bone because of osteoporosis.[19] Bone density scans using dual-energy X-ray absorptiometry can screen for osteoporosis. With early detection, steps can be taken to reverse bone loss and prevent fractures.

Some of the factors that predispose a person to developing osteoporosis are intrinsic and cannot be controlled, including gender, age, body size, ethnicity, and family history. But there *are* some things you can do to prevent the disease. During your lifetime, bone is constantly being added (formation) and being broken down and removed (reabsorption). At around age 30, a person reaches *peak bone mass*. After this point, a slow and steady decline occurs. Individuals who develop strong, dense, healthy bones through proper diet and exercise can minimize this decline and reduce their risk for osteoporosis.

Adequate calcium intake is important, as is vitamin D, which helps the body absorb and use calcium more efficiently. Bone is a living tissue that grows stronger with exercise and weight-bearing activity; therefore, bone loss can be slowed or prevented with regular weight-bearing exercise, such as walking, jogging, and dancing, as well as through strength training. Unhealthy behaviors that contribute to bone loss include smoking, excessive alcohol consumption, and anorexia nervosa.

Another bone condition that afflicts almost 27 million Americans is *osteoarthritis*, a progressive breakdown of joint cartilage that becomes more common with age and is a major cause of disability in the United States.[20]

## Head and Face

With age, features of the head enlarge and become more prominent. Increased cartilage and a decrease of fatty tissue can give the face a sagging or drooping appearance. Earlobes may grow longer as a result of cartilage growth. Fat in the eyelid area settles more as we age, giving the appearance of sunken eyes. The muscle that supports the upper eyelid weakens as aging occurs, causing the eyelids to droop and skin around the eyes may wrinkle and sag.[21]

## The Urinary Tract

For about two-thirds of us, the 30s and 40s bring a gradual decrease in the size and weight of the kidneys, effectively reducing blood filtering and other functions. In addition, shrinkage/thinning of the bladder and urinary tract affect urination.[22] While age is a key factor in these changes, the fact that one-third of the aging population doesn't experience these declines supports the idea that other factors such as high blood pressure, lead exposure, smoking, inflammation, obesity, and plaque formation may also be important in kidney and urinary risks. If so, like many other things, urinary and kidney problems may not be inevitable.[23] Some changes, such as hormonal decreases in women, may increase bladder and urinary tract changes, leading to **urinary incontinence**, which ranges from passing a few drops of urine while laughing or sneezing to having no control over urination.

Incontinence can pose major social, physical, and emotional problems. Embarrassment and fear of wetting oneself may cause an older person to become isolated socially or increase frustrations for caregivers. Prolonged wetness and the inability to properly care for oneself can lead to tissue irritation, infections, and other problems.

However, incontinence is not inevitable. Causes range from persistent infections, to certain medications, to neurological problems that affect the central nervous system, weakness in the pelvic wall, and so on.[24] With exercises to strengthen the pelvic wall or a variety of other treatments, the incontinence is usually resolved.[25]

## Heart and Lungs

As people age, the size of the heart increases slightly, the walls of the heart become thicker, and the heart's chambers enlarge slightly. At rest, the heart rate is about the same as a younger heart, but during exercise the aging heart cannot pump out the same amount of blood as a younger heart.[26] Vital capacity, or the amount of air that moves when you inhale and exhale at maximum effort, also declines with age. Reduction in vital capacity results from changes in the body's lung tissue (air sacs can lose their elasticity and become slack), bones, and muscles in the chest and spine (i.e., weakened diaphragm). Exercise can do a great deal to preserve heart and lung function. Not smoking and avoiding smoke-filled environments are important ways of reducing risks.[27]

## The Senses

With aging, the senses (vision, hearing, touch, taste, and smell) become less acute. By the time a person reaches age 30, the lens of the eye begins to harden, which can cause problems by the early 40s. The lens also begins to yellow and lose transparency, and the pupil shrinks, allowing less light to penetrate. By age 60, depth perception declines and farsightedness often develops. **Cataracts** (clouding of the lens) and **glaucoma** (elevated pressure within the eyeball) become more likely. Eventually, a tendency toward color blindness may develop, especially for shades of blue and green. **Macular degeneration** is the breakdown of the light-sensitive area of the retina responsible for the sharp, direct vision needed to read or drive. Its effects can be devastating to independent older adults and causes are still being investigated.

*Presbycusis*, or age-related hearing loss, is one of the most common chronic conditions of the elderly—affecting 25 to 30 percent of people between the ages of 65 to 74 and between 40 and 50 percent of people over 75 years of age.[28] It appears that hearing loss may play a much greater role in maintaining health in older adults than was thought.

With age, the ear structure also experiences changes and often deteriorates. The eardrum thickens and the inner ear

**urinary incontinence** Inability to control urination.

**cataracts** Clouding of the lens that interrupts the focusing of light on the retina, resulting in blurred vision or eventual blindness.

**glaucoma** Elevation of pressure within the eyeball, leading to hardening of the eyeball, impaired vision, and possible blindness.

**macular degeneration** Breakdown of the macula, the light-sensitive part of the retina responsible for sharp, direct vision.

bones are affected. The inner ear controls balance (equilibrium). As a result, it often becomes difficult for a person to maintain balance. Studies have shown that exercises including resistance/strength training, yoga, and tai chi can improve balance in older adults.[29] The ability to hear high-frequency consonants (e.g., *s*, *t*, and *z*) also diminishes with age. Much of the actual hearing loss lies in the inability to distinguish extreme ranges of sound rather than in the inability to distinguish normal conversational tones.

Many studies have indicated that with age, there is a reduced or changed sensation of pain, vibration, cold, heat, pressure, and touch. Some of these changes may be caused by decreased blood flow to touch receptors or to the brain and spinal cord.[30] It may become difficult, for example, to tell the difference between cool and cold. Decreased temperature sensitivity increases the risk of injuries such as hypothermia and frostbite.

The senses of taste and smell are closely connected. The number of taste buds you have decreases, and taste buds themselves get smaller as you age. By the age of 60, sensitivity to the five tastes begin to diminish.[31] The sense of smell may diminish, especially after age 70. This may be related to loss of nerve endings in the nose. Studies on the cause of decreased sense of taste and smell have conflicting results. Some studies have indicated that normal aging produces very little change in taste and smell.[32] Therefore, changes may be related to chronic diseases, smoking, and environmental exposures over a lifetime. Medications may also have a significant effect on taste and smell.

## Sexual Function

As men age, they experience noticeable alterations in sexual function. Although the degree and rate of change vary greatly from man to man, several changes generally occur, including a slowed ability to obtain an erection, diminished ability to maintain an erection, and a decline in the angle of the erection. Men may also experience a longer refractory period between orgasms and shortened duration of orgasm.

Women also experience several changes in sexual function as they age. Menopause usually occurs between the ages of 45 and 55. Women may experience hot flashes, mood swings, weight gain, development of facial hair, or other hormone-related symptoms. The walls of the vagina become less elastic, and the epithelium thins, possibly making intercourse painful. Vaginal secretions, particularly during sexual activity, diminish. The breasts become less firm, and loss of fat in various areas leads to fewer curves, with a decrease in the soft lines of body contours.

Although these physiological changes may sound discouraging, sex is still an essential component in the lives of those in their mid-50s and older, and many people remain sexually active throughout their entire adult lives. According to a recent study, the majority of those 50 to 80 years old are still very engaged about sex and intimacy.[33] With the advent of drugs such as Viagra and medical interventions designed to treat sexual dysfunction, many older adults are able to be sexually active. However, older adults also report low percentages of condom use and rates of sexually transmitted infections (STIs) in older adults are rising. Nearly 25 percent of persons who have HIV/AIDS are over age 50, and growing faster than in people under the age of 40, signifying a need for education regarding the spread of STIs.[34]

## Mental Function and Memory

It's not true that you "can't teach an old dog new tricks." It may take a bit longer to learn, but, given an appropriate length of time, older people learn and develop skills in a manner similar to that of younger people. Researchers have also determined that what many older adults lack in speed of learning they make up for in practical knowledge—that is, the "wisdom of age." Memory loss is not necessarily a normal part of aging; however, as a person ages, drug interactions, vascular deficiencies, hormonal or biochemical imbalances, and other physiological changes can make memory lapses occur more frequently. Although short-term memory may fluctuate on a daily basis, the ability to remember events from past decades seems to remain largely unchanged in the absence of disease.[35]

**Staying Sharp in the Later Years** Generally, those who maintain their memory in old age have exercised and kept their cardiovascular system and mind healthy over the years. Researchers have found older adults who walk or jog perform better on memory tasks than those who are more sedentary.[36] Another key to maintaining memory is keeping your mind active as well. People who foster their creative side and engage their minds by reading books, solving mental puzzles, playing musical instruments, volunteering, and doing other brain-sharpening activities seem to fare much better in the memory department.[37] As with physical aspects of the body, "use it or lose it" applies to your brain acuity.

## Dementias and Alzheimer's Disease

Memory failure, errors in judgment, disorientation, or erratic behavior can occur at any age and for various reasons, including nutrient deficiency (such as vitamin B deficiency), alcohol

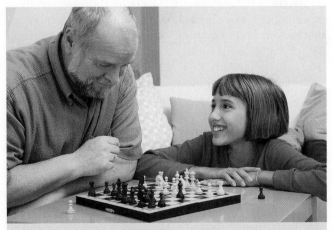

Certain physiological conditions or diseases may cause older people to experience memory loss, but in general the knowledge and memories gained through a lifetime remain intact.

**dementia** Progressive brain impairment that interferes with memory and normal intellectual functioning.

**dementia** Progressive brain impairment that interferes with memory and normal intellectual functioning.

**Alzheimer's disease (AD)** A chronic condition involving changes in nerve fibers of the brain that results in mental deterioration.

abuse, medication interactions, vascular problems, tumors, hormonal or metabolic imbalances, or any number of problems. Often, when the underlying issues are corrected, the memory loss and disorientation also improve. The terms *dementing diseases*, or **dementia**, are used to describe either reversible symptoms or progressive forms of brain malfunctioning.

Although there are many types of dementia, one of the most common forms is **Alzheimer's disease (AD)**. Affecting an estimated 1 in 9 Americans over the age of 65 (5.4 million), this disease is one of the most painful and devastating conditions that families can endure.[38] Alzheimer's disease is a degenerative illness in which areas of the brain develop "tangles" that impair the way nerve cells communicate with one another, eventually causing them to die. This disease characteristically progresses in stages, each of which is marked by increasingly impaired memory and judgment. In later stages of the disease, these symptoms can be accompanied by agitation and restlessness (especially at night), loss of sensory perceptions, muscle twitching, and repetitive actions. Many patients become depressed, combative, and aggressive.[39]

The final stage often includes complete disorientation, with patients becoming entirely dependent on the help of others to dress, eat, and perform other daily activities. Identity loss and speech problems are common. Eventually, control of bodily functions may be lost. Patients with AD live for an average of 4 to 6 years after diagnosis, although the disease can last for up to 20 years.[40]

Because of the growing number of people over age 65 in the United States, the annual number of new cases of Alzheimer's and other dementias is projected to almost triple by 2050.[41] An estimated 16 million family members and friends cared for a person with Alzheimer's disease or another dementia in 2015.[42] Caring for a person with AD can be a heavy burden for families. Approximately two-thirds of caregivers are women; 34 percent of those are over the age of 65.[43] On average, those providing care lose over $15,000 in annual income from cutting back on work or quitting work to give care.[44] Additionally, 28 percent of care providers struggle to have enough money for nutritious meals.[45]

Researchers are investigating several possible causes of the disease, including genetic predisposition, immune system malfunction, a slow-acting virus, chromosomal or genetic defects, chronic inflammation, uncontrolled hypertension, and neurotransmitter imbalance. No current treatment can stop the progression of AD, but there are medications that can prevent some symptoms from progressing for a short period of time or relieve symptoms such as sleeplessness, anxiety, and depression. Some researchers are looking at anti-inflammatory drugs, theorizing that AD may develop in response to an inflammatory ailment. Others are focusing on studying deposits of protein called plaques and their role in damaging and killing nerve cells.

## Depression

Contrary to what many think, most older adults lead healthy, fulfilling lives. However, research indicates that depression is the most common psychological problem affecting this population. It is estimated that between 1 and 5 percent of older people experience depression, which increases in those that require home health care or are in hospital.[46] Regardless of age, people who have a poor perception of their health, have multiple chronic illnesses, take a lot of medications, abuse alcohol or other drugs, lack social support, and do not exercise face more challenges to their emotional resilience.

## LO 5 | STRATEGIES FOR HEALTHY AGING

List strategies for successful and healthy aging.

The key factors to living long and well include maintaining a healthy lifestyle. Maintaining a healthy lifestyle includes avoiding unhealthy habits such as smoking, excessive alcohol use, and obesity. In addition, a healthy diet, engaging in an active lifestyle, staying positive and optimistic, and cultivating a strong social support network while building "social capital" are all key to successful aging. Focusing on *living healthy* can help you "stay" healthy.

## OVER 72,000

people, most of whom were women, were 100 years or older in the United States in 2014.

## Improve Fitness

Just about any moderate-intensity exercise that gets your heart beating faster and increases strength and/or flexibility will maximize your physical health and functional years. One of the physical changes that the body undergoes is *sarcopenia*, age-associated loss of muscle mass. The less muscle you have, the less energy you will burn even while resting. The lower your metabolic rate, the more likely you will gain weight. With regular strength training, you can increase your muscle mass, boost your metabolism, strengthen your bones, reduce your risk for osteoporosis, and, in general, feel better and function more efficiently.

Both aerobic and muscle-strengthening activities are critical for healthy aging. **TABLE 22.1** lists the basic recommendations for aerobic and strength-training

**SEE IT! VIDEOS**

Why do some people live longer than others? Watch **Myth-Busting Longevity**, available on **MasteringHealth.**™

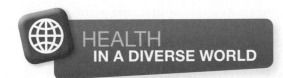
# KEEPING FIT AS WE AGE

Physical activity is the key for maintaining health and independence as people age, but regular physical activity is not widespread among older adults. According to the Administration on Aging, regular physical activity is reported by only 43 percent of those aged 65 to 74, and 27 percent of those aged 75 and older.

The Centers for Disease Control and Prevention identifies regular physical activity as one of the most important things that can be done to maintain your health as you age. The benefits include:

■ Maintenance and improvement of physical strength and fitness
■ Improvement of balance
■ Better management of diseases such as diabetes, heart disease, and osteoporosis
■ Reduction in feelings of depression and improved mood and overall well-being

**Adding variety to your fitness activities can make them fun and keep you motivated over time. Change it up!**

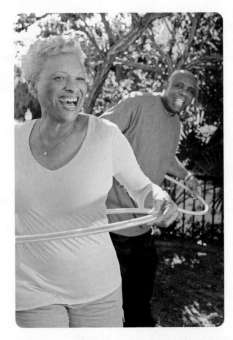

Recent studies have found that older adults who keep active may reduce their odds of losing their mental abilities. "If we want to become a healthy and fit nation, we need to increase the number of Americans who are healthy at every stage of life," former U.S. Surgeon General Dr. Regina Benjamin stated.

A new program called Go4Life (http://go4life.nia.nih.gov) is meant to encourage people age 50 and older to become and stay active to improve their health. Go4Life provides older adults with resources to be physically active, such as sample exercise programs and videos. Go4Life is based on studies demonstrating the benefits of exercise and physical activity for older people, including those with chronic health conditions.

**Source:** Administration on Aging, U.S. Department of Health and Human Services, "A Profile of Older Americans: 2015," 2016, http://www.aoa.acl.gov/Aging_Statistics/Profile/2015/14.aspx.

---

exercises in older adults. In addition to these, the Centers for Disease Control and Prevention recommends that people who are at risk of falling perform regular balance exercises.[47] It is also recommended that older adults or adults with chronic conditions develop an activity plan with a health professional to manage risks and take therapeutic needs into account. This will maximize the benefits of physical activity and ensure your safety. The **Health in a Diverse World** box describes more of the benefits of physical activity.

## Eat for Longevity

Although other chapters in this text provide detailed information about nutrition and weight control, certain nutrients are especially essential to healthy aging:

■ **Calcium.** Bone loss tends to increase in women, particularly in the hip region, shortly before menopause. During perimenopause and menopause, this bone loss accelerates rapidly, with an average of about 3 percent skeletal mass lost per year over a 5-year period. The result is an increased risk for fracture and disability. Adequate consumption of calcium throughout one's life can help prevent bone loss.

■ **Vitamin D.** Vitamin D is necessary for adequate calcium absorption, yet as people age, particularly in their 50s and 60s, they do not absorb vitamin D from foods as readily as they did in their younger years. If vitamin D is unavailable, calcium levels are also likely to be lower. However, new studies have emerged that indicate that too much vitamin D does not improve function in the lower body as it was once thought, but it actually may increase the risk for falls in older adults.[48]

**TABLE 22.1** | Exercise Recommendations for Adults over Age 65

| Option 1 | Option 2 | Option 3 |
|---|---|---|
| Moderate-intensity aerobic activity (e.g., brisk walking) at least 2 hours and 30 minutes every week | Vigorous-intensity aerobic activity (e.g., jogging or running) at least 1 hour and 15 minutes every week | An equal mix of moderate- and vigorous-intensity aerobic activity |
| *and* | *and* | *and* |
| muscle-strengthening activity, working all major muscle groups, 2 or more days a week | muscle-strengthening activity, working all major muscle groups, 2 or more days a week | muscle-strengthening activity 2 or more days a week |

**Source:** Centers for Disease Control, "How Much Physical Activity Do Older Adults Need?," 2015, www.cdc.gov.

- **Protein.** Recent research suggests that increased protein intake (slightly higher than the current RDA) has health benefits for older adults. So eating a diet high in protein helps reduce gradual loss of muscle mass (*sarcopenia*) that occurs most markedly after the age of 65.[49] Total calorie intake must be considered.

Other nutrients, including vitamin E, folic acid (folate), iron, potassium, and vitamin $B_{12}$ (cobalamin), are important to the aging process, and most of these are readily available in any diet that follows the U.S. Department of Agriculture's (USDA) MyPlate recommendations (www.choosemyplate.gov).

## Avoid Alcohol and Drug Use and Abuse

*Early in his life, Walter would have been called an "abstainer." With the exception of an occasional sip of wine on holidays or a beer with friends, Walter never drank. After his wife died, more of his friends began dying and his children moved away. Walter drank just in the evenings first, and then began drinking throughout the day as an escape and for companionship. Now in his mid-70s, Walter is an alcoholic.*

Alcoholism is a growing concern among older adults. Alcohol and drug abuse at any age is harmful, but for older adults there are a number of increased risks. The abuse of alcohol and drugs increases the risk of falls, interactions with medications, and as people age their sensitivity to alcohol and other drugs increases.[50] According to the National Council on Alcoholism and Drug Dependence, there are 2.5 million older adults with an alcohol or drug problem. Widowers over the age of 75 comprise those with the highest rates of alcoholism in the United States. Furthermore, older adults are hospitalized as often for alcohol-related problems as they are heart attacks.[51]

Those prone to alcoholism in their younger years are likely to continue drinking later in life. Alcohol abuse is more common among older men than it is among older women. Yet those age 65 and older have the lowest rates of drinking among any age group. Typically, those who do drink do so less than younger persons.[52]

If recent studies are accurate, the reason there aren't many heavy drinkers among older adults may be that very heavy drinkers tend to either die of complications with alcohol before they grow old or because they are afraid of combining alcohol with their prescription drugs. Most older adults who consume alcohol are not alcoholics but rather social drinkers.

Prescription medication misuse and abuse are growing problems among older adults.[53] Older adults are at a high risk for medication misuse because they tend to use a greater number of medications than other age groups.[54] Because of increased medication sensitivity, slower metabolism, and slower elimination, older adults are also likely to have problems with smaller quantities of medications.[55] Pain, sleep disorders, and anxiety are just some conditions that increase the likelihood of medication misuse or abuse.[56]

Currently, there is no one system that tracks all of a patient's prescriptions. To avoid drug interactions and other problems, older adults should use the same pharmacy consistently, ask questions about medicines, dosages, and possible drug interactions, and read directions carefully.

## Develop and Maintain Healthy Relationships

Social bonds and social support lend vigor and energy to life. Be willing to give to others and seek variety in your relationships rather than befriending only people who agree with you. By experiencing diverse people and points of view, we gain broader perspective. Positive relationships are important for well-being at any age, but as people age, support systems decrease, making it particularly important to remain socially active (see Chapter 8 for more information on healthy relationships).

## Enrich the Spiritual Side of Life

Cultivating a relationship with nature, the environment, a higher being, and yourself is a key factor in personal growth and development. Take time for thought and quiet contemplation, and enjoy the sunsets, sounds, and energy of life. Setting time aside for yourself will leave you invigorated and refreshed—better able to cope with the ups and downs of life.

## Financial Planning for Retirement

Financial planning for retirement should begin early in life. Consider reports that the average millennial will need to accumulate as much as $1.8 million by the time they reach retirement to be able to live comfortably.[57] Most millennials will have saved an average of only $10,000 at this point.[58] Aggressive saving is essential, particularly given that many jobs no longer come with retirement plans for workers.

Retirement generally means a change in finances. It may mean a stricter budget or even financial hardship if older adults have not been good financial planners. Starting early by putting aside small amounts of money in retirement savings accounts is one of the many ways to prepare for a comfortable retirement. Financial planning for retirement is especially important for women. Women are much less likely to be covered by pension plans. Women are also more likely to have worked at lower-paying jobs, or worked part time during childbearing years. Life expectancy for women is 81.2 years, and 76.4 years for men.[59] While the gap has been is narrowing, women still outlive men and are more likely to develop chronic disease later in life. To be sure they will be provided for as they age, women need to take a proactive role in both the day-to-day management of their finances and their retirement planning.

What you do today in terms of responsible saving and the support systems you put in place will have a tremendous influence on how you fare when you eventually reach retirement. Having a strong network of friends and family, having a plan for savings and health care insurance, and being knowledgeable in terms of options for living situations and access to health care are all key to how and where you live in your later years.

# LO 6 | UNDERSTANDING THE FINAL TRANSITIONS: DYING AND DEATH

Define death and discuss strategies for coping with death.

Throughout history, humans have attempted to determine the nature and meaning of death. Individuals' feelings about death vary widely, depending on many factors, including age, religious beliefs, family orientation, health, personal experience with death, and the circumstances of the death itself.

## Defining Death

According to the *Merriam-Webster Dictionary*, **death** can be defined as "a permanent cessation of all vital functions: the end of life."[60] This definition has become more significant as medical advances make it increasingly possible to postpone death. Legal and ethical issues led to the Uniform Determination of Death Act in 1981. This act, which several states have adopted, reads as follows: "An individual who has sustained either (1) irreversible cessation of circulatory and respiratory functions, or (2) irreversible cessation of all functions of the entire brain, including the brain stem, is dead. A determination of death must be made in accordance with accepted medical standards."[61]

The concept of **brain death**, defined as the irreversible cessation of all functions of the entire brainstem, has gained increasing credence. As defined by the Ad Hoc Committee of the Harvard Medical School, brain death occurs when the following criteria are met:[62]

- Unreceptivity and unresponsiveness—that is, no response even to painful stimuli
- No movement for a continuous hour after observation by a physician, and no breathing after 3 minutes off a respirator
- No reflexes, including brainstem reflexes; fixed and dilated pupils
- A "flat" electroencephalogram (EEG), which monitors electrical activity of the brain, for at least 10 minutes
- All of these tests repeated at least 24 hours later with no change
- Certainty that hypothermia (extreme loss of body heat) or depression of the central nervous system caused by use of drugs such as barbiturates are not responsible for these conditions

The Harvard report provides useful guidelines; however, the definition of death and all its ramifications continues to concern us.

## The Process of Dying

**Dying** is the process of decline in body functions that results in the death of an organism. It is a complex process that includes physical, intellectual, social, spiritual, and emotional dimensions. Now that we have examined the physical indicators of death, we must consider the emotional aspects of dying and "social death."

## Kübler-Ross and the Stages of Dying

Much of our knowledge about reactions to dying stems from the work of Elisabeth Kübler-Ross, a pioneer in **thanatology**, the study of death and dying. In 1969, Kübler-Ross published *On Death and Dying*, a sensitive analysis of the reactions of terminally ill patients. This pioneering work encouraged the development of death education as a discipline and prompted efforts to improve the care of dying patients. Kübler-Ross identified five psychological stages (**FIGURE 22.4**) that people coping with death often experience:[63]

1. **Denial** ("Not me, there must be a mistake"). A person intellectually accepts the impending death but rejects it emotionally and feels a sense of shock and disbelief. The patient is too confused and stunned to comprehend "not being" and thus rejects the idea.
2. **Anger** ("Why me?"). The person becomes angry at having to face death when others, including loved ones, are healthy and not threatened. The dying

**WHAT DO YOU THINK?**

Why is there so much concern over the definition of *death*?

- How does modern technology complicate the understanding of when death occurs?

> **death** The permanent ending of all vital functions.
>
> **brain death** The irreversible cessation of all functions of the entire brainstem.
>
> **dying** Process of decline in body functions that results in the death of an organism.
>
> **thanatology** The study of death and dying.

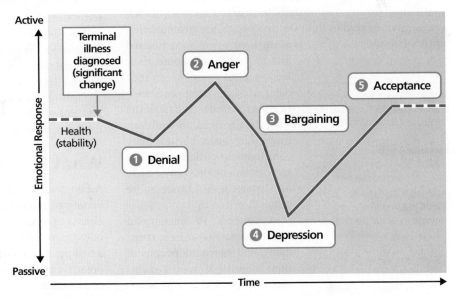

**FIGURE 22.4 Kübler-Ross's Stages of Dying** Kübler-Ross developed this model while working with terminally ill patients. She later expanded the model to apply to people experiencing grief or significant loss of any kind.

person perceives the situation as unfair or senseless and may be hostile to friends, family, physicians, or the world in general.

3. **Bargaining** ("If I'm allowed to live, I promise . . . "). The dying person may resolve to be a better person in return for an extension of life or may secretly pray for a short postponement of death in order to experience a special event, such as a family wedding or birth.

4. **Depression** ("It's really going to happen to me, and I can't do anything about it"). Depression eventually sets in as vitality diminishes and the person begins to experience symptoms with increasing frequency. The person's deteriorating condition becomes impossible for him or her to deny. Common feelings experienced during this stage include doom, loss, worthlessness, and guilt over the emotional suffering of loved ones and the arduous but seemingly futile efforts of caregivers.

5. **Acceptance** ("I'm ready"). This is often the final stage. The patient stops battling with emotions and becomes tired and weak. With acceptance, the person does not "give up" and become sullen or resentfully resigned to death, but rather becomes passive.

Some of Kübler-Ross's contemporaries consider her stage theory too neat and orderly. Subsequent research has indicated that the experiences of dying people do not fit easily into specific stages, and patterns vary from person to person. While some people might remain emotionally calm, others may pass back and forth between the stages. Even if it is not accurate in all its particulars, however, Kübler-Ross's theory offers valuable insights for those seeking to understand or deal with the process of dying.

## Social Death

The need for recognition and appreciation within a social group is nearly universal. Loss of being valued or appreciated by others can lead to **social death**, a situation in which a person is not treated like an active member of society. Numerous studies indicate that people are treated differently when they are dying, leading them to feel more isolated and unable to talk about their feelings: The dying person may be excluded from conversations or referred to as if he or she were already dead. In addition, inadequate pain control may contribute to patient suffering and anger or hostility, making caregiver assistance more difficult.

A decrease in meaningful social interaction often strips dying and bereaved people of their identity as valued members of society at a time when being able to talk, share, and make important decisions or say important things is critical.

**social death** A seemingly irreversible situation in which a person is not treated like an active member of society.

**bereavement** The loss or deprivation experienced by a survivor when a loved one dies.

**grief** An individual's reaction to significant loss, including one's own impending death, the death of a loved one, or a quasi-death experience; grief can involve mental, physical, social, or emotional responses.

**mourning** The culturally prescribed behavior patterns for the expression of grief.

LO **7** | ## COPING WITH LOSS

Describe typical grief symptoms and the grieving process.

Coping with the loss of a loved one is extremely difficult. The dying person, as well as close family and friends, frequently suffers emotionally and physically from the loss of critical relationships and roles.

**Bereavement** is generally defined as the loss or deprivation that a survivor experiences when a loved one dies. In the lives of the bereaved or of close survivors, the loss of loved ones leaves "holes" and inevitable changes. Understanding normal reactions, time, patience, and support from loved ones can do much to help the bereaved heal and move on.

**Grief** occurs in reaction to significant loss, including one's own impending death, the death of a loved one, or a *quasi-death* experience (a significant loss such as the end of a relationship or job, which involves separation, rejection, or a change in personal identity). Grief may be experienced as a mental, physical, social, or emotional reaction, and often includes changes in patterns of eating, sleeping, working, and even thinking.

When a person experiences a loss that cannot be openly acknowledged, publicly mourned, or socially supported, coping may be much more difficult. This type of grief is referred to as *disenfranchised grief*. It may occur among people who experience a miscarriage, who are developmentally disabled, or who are close friends rather than blood relatives of the deceased. It may also include relationships that are not socially approved, such as extramarital affairs or homosexual relationships.

Symptoms of grief vary in severity and duration, depending on the situation and the individual. However, the bereaved person can benefit from emotional and social support from family, friends, clergy, employers, and traditional support organizations. The larger and stronger the support system, the easier readjustment is likely to be. See the Making Changes Today box to learn about how you can best help a grieving friend.

The term *mourning* is often incorrectly equated with the term *grief*. As we have noted, *grief* refers to a wide variety of feelings and actions that occur in response to bereavement. **Mourning**, in contrast, refers to culturally prescribed and accepted time periods and behavior patterns for the expression of grief. In Judaism, for example, *sitting shivah* is a designated mourning period of 7 days that involves prescribed rituals and prayers. Depending on a person's relationship with the deceased, various other rituals may continue for up to a year.

## What is "Typical" Grief?

A bereaved person may suffer emotional pain and exhibit a variety of grief responses for many months after the death. Grief responses vary widely from person to person but frequently include periodic waves of prolonged physical distress, a feeling of tightness in the throat, choking and shortness of breath, a frequent need to sigh, feelings of emptiness and muscular weakness, or intense anxiety that is described as actually painful. Other common symptoms of grief include insomnia, memory lapses, loss of appetite, difficulty concentrating, a tendency to engage in repetitive or purposeless behavior, a

immediate aftermath of the event, some bereaved survivors feel numb or unable to accept the loss. Many feel shocked, lost, anxious, and depressed. For many, the pain from their loss can be intense and unrelenting. These emotional and bodily reactions may be very strong and can themselves be traumatizing, especially if they are unfamiliar and unexpected. This secondary reaction can further amplify the pain caused by the loss.

> **grief work** The process of accepting the reality of a person's death and coping with memories of the deceased.

It is important to realize that intense and unfamiliar emotionality is entirely normal and does not necessarily have implications for long-term emotional stability or health. However, if the symptoms linger and become increasingly debilitating, the condition turns into what is now being referred to as *unresolved*, *traumatic*, or *complicated grief*, which has features of both depression and posttraumatic stress disorder (PTSD). The most characteristic symptoms are intrusive thoughts and memories of the deceased person, a feeling of disbelief, intense images of the deceased person, or an inability to accept the loss and a painful yearning for his or her presence. Other complications are denial of the death, desperate loneliness and helplessness, anger and bitterness, and wanting to die. Complicated grief can occur after the loss of any close relationship. Complicated grief occurs about 10 to 20 percent of the time after the death of a romantic partner and more even more likely among parents who have experienced the loss of a child; it is more common when the death is sudden or violent as in a homicide, suicide, or an accident.[64] Treatment requires professional therapy and can include a promising new treatment called *traumatic grief therapy*, which uses cognitive-behavioral methods for traumatic symptoms and stress relief, along with interpersonal techniques to encourage reengagement with the world.

feeling of being removed from reality, difficulty making decisions, lack of organization, excessive talking, social withdrawal or hostility, guilty feelings, and preoccupation with the image of the deceased. Susceptibility to disease increases with grief and may even be life threatening in severe and enduring cases.

The rate of the healing process depends on the amount and quality of grief work that a person does. **Grief work** is the process of integrating the reality of the loss into everyday life and learning to feel better. Often, the bereaved person must deliberately and systematically work at reducing denial and coping with the pain that comes from remembering the deceased.

## Grief and Trauma

Disasters, war, and other events can leave many people suddenly bereaved of spouses, children, parents, close friends, and coworkers. In the

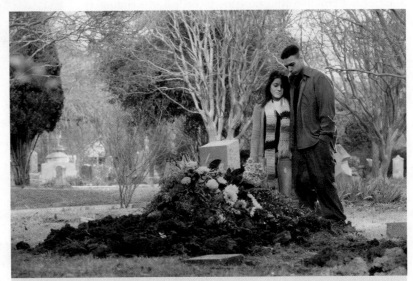

The most important thing you can do for a grieving friend is offer emotional support and a caring presence. Knowing what to say is less important than knowing how to listen.

## Worden's Model of Grieving Tasks

William Worden, a researcher into the death process, developed an active grieving model that suggests four developmental tasks that a grieving person must complete in the grief work process:[65]

1.  **Accept the reality of the loss.** This task requires acknowledging and realizing that the person is dead. Traditional rituals, such as the funeral, help many bereaved people move toward acceptance.

2.  **Work through the pain of grief.** It is necessary to acknowledge and work through the pain associated with loss, or it will manifest itself through other symptoms or behaviors.

3.  **Adjust to an environment in which the deceased is missing.** The bereaved may feel lonely and uncertain about a new identity without the person who has died. This loss confronts them with the challenge of adjusting their own sense of self.

4.  **Emotionally relocate the deceased and move on with life.** Individuals never lose memories of a significant relationship. They may need help in letting go of the emotional energy that used to be invested in the person who has died, and they may need help in finding an appropriate place for the deceased in their emotional lives.

## Children and Death

Children are highly valued in our society, and their deaths are considered major tragedies. No matter what the cause of death—miscarriage, fatal birth defects, childhood illness, accident, suicide, homicide, natural disaster, neglect, or war injuries—the grief experienced when a child dies may be overwhelming.

Siblings of a deceased child may have a particularly hard time with grief work and they may receive less social support and sympathy than their parents do. Feelings of guilt, relief, abandonment, anxiety, and confusion are not uncommon emotions of children who experience the loss of a sibling. If adults do not talk about this loss with their child, it is possible the child can feel isolated and withdraw from family and friends at a time they need their support and love the most.[66]

Bereaved children usually have limited experience with death and therefore have not yet learned how to deal with major loss. Often, when children suffer a loss, they will continue to behave "normally" to the adult observer. When it comes to complex emotional issues, children do not always show their feelings as openly as adults. They worry about whether they caused the death and whether they will die or will lose someone else they love, and they worry about what will happen to them and to the person who died. It can be helpful for family members to involve children in the dying process and to talk with them about the death while reassuring them of their safety.[67] A professional counselor may also be of help in assisting children who are coping with loss.

**living will** A type of advance directive.

**advance directive** A document that stipulates an individual's wishes about medical care; used to make treatment decisions when and if the individual becomes physically unable to voice his or her preferences.

# LIFE-AND-DEATH DECISION MAKING

Explain the ethical concerns that arise from the concepts of the right to die and rational suicide.

When a loved one is dying, many complex and emotional—and often expensive—life-and-death decisions must be made during a highly distressing period in people's lives.

## The Right to Die

Few people would object to the right to a dignified death. Going beyond that concept, however, many people today believe that they should be allowed to die if their condition is terminal and their existence depends on mechanical life-support devices or artificial feeding or hydration systems. Artificial life-support techniques that may be legally refused by competent patients include electrical or mechanical heart resuscitation, mechanical respiration by machine, nasogastric tube feedings, intravenous nutrition, gastrostomy (tube feeding directly into the stomach), and medications to treat life-threatening infections.

As long as a person is conscious and competent, he or she has the legal right to refuse treatment, even if this decision will hasten death. However, when a person is in a coma or otherwise incapable of speaking on his or her own behalf, medical personnel, family members, and administrative policy will dictate treatment. This issue has evolved into a battle involving personal freedom, legal rulings, health care administration policy, and physician responsibility. The **living will** and other **advance directives** were developed to assist in solving these

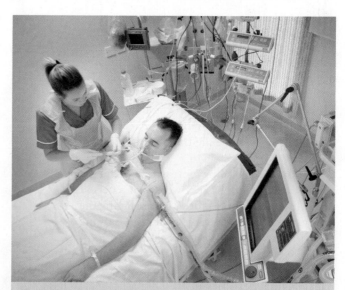

Today's sophisticated life-support technology can prolong a patient's life even in cases of terminal illness or mortal injury, yet not everyone would choose to have their life extended by such means. Living wills, advance directives, and health care proxies can protect your wishes and aid your loved ones should you become incapacitated.

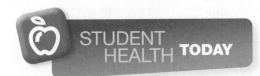

# PREPARING FOR ENDINGS

While college and those years immediately following graduation are not typically times we think about needing to prepare for death, we do know that life circumstances can change quickly for anyone. Here is a list of documents you should pull together in a central location, whether on a computer or in an old-fashioned file box.

**Source:** "25 Documents You Need before You Die," *The Wall Street Journal*, Accessed June 2014, http://online.wsj.com/news/interactive/DOC110702?ref=SB100014240527023036271 04576410234039258092.

**Marriage and Divorce**
• Marriage license
• Divorce papers

**Life Insurance/Retirement**
• Life insurance policies
• Individual retirement accounts
• 401(k) accounts

**Health Care**
• Personal and family medical history
• Authorization to release health-care information
• Durable power of attorney
• Living will
• Do-not-resuscitate order

**Bank Accounts**
• List of bank accounts
• List of all user names and passwords
• List of safe-deposit boxes and codes keys for access

**Proof of Ownership**
• Vehicle titles
• Proof of loans and debts owed
• Stock certificates and savings bonds

**The Essentials**
• Will
• Trust documents
• Last wishes for burial
• Executor of your estate

---

conflicts. See **Student Health Today** for a list of documents that you can put in order while you're in good health.

Even young, apparently healthy people need a living will. Consider Terri Schiavo, who collapsed at age 26 from heart failure that led to irreversible brain damage. Schiavo, unable to survive without life support, never left any written guidelines about her wishes should she become incapacitated. After a 15-year legal battle between her parents, who wanted her to be kept alive, and her husband, who felt she should be allowed to die, the courts sided with her husband, and she was removed from life support.

Many legal experts suggest that you take the following steps to ensure that your wishes are carried out:[68]

- **Complete an advance directive** that permits you to make very specific choices about a variety of procedures, including cardiopulmonary resuscitation (CPR); being placed on a ventilator; being given food, water, or medication through tubes; being given pain medication; and organ donation.
- **Name a health care proxy.** You may want to also appoint a family member or friend to act as your agent, or *proxy*, by completing a form known as either a *durable power of attorney for health care* or a *health care proxy*. This allows the person you designate to make medical decisions for you in the event you are incapacitated.
- **Discuss your wishes.** Discuss your preferences in detail with your proxy and your doctor. Once you have done this, fill out the legal forms detailing your wishes.
- **Deliver the directive.** Distribute several copies, not only to your doctor and your agent, but also to your lawyer and to immediate family members or a close friend. Make sure *someone* knows to bring a copy to the hospital in the event you are hospitalized.

One alternative to the traditional advance directive or living will is a document called "Five Wishes," which meets the legal requirements for advance directive statutes in most states. This document differs from most other living wills because it addresses personal, emotional, and spiritual needs, as well as medical needs.[69] It is available at low cost online at www.agingwithdignity.org.

## Rational Suicide and Euthanasia

It is estimated that thousands of terminally ill people every year decide to kill themselves rather than endure constant pain and slow decay. This alternative to the extended dying process is known as **rational suicide**. To these people, the prospect of an undignified death is unacceptable. This issue has been complicated by advances in death prevention techniques that allow terminally ill patients to exist in an irreversible disease state for extended periods of time.

Euthanasia is often referred to as "mercy killing." The term **active euthanasia** refers to ending the life of a person (or animal) who is suffering greatly and has no chance of recovery. An example might be a physician-prescribed lethal injection, as in physician-assisted suicide. **Passive euthanasia** refers to the intentional withholding of treatment that would prolong life. Deciding not to place a person with massive brain trauma on life support is an example of passive euthanasia. Advance directives, such as "do not resuscitate" orders, can provide legal justification for various forms of passive euthanasia.

**rational suicide** The decision to kill oneself rather than endure constant pain and slow decay.

**active euthanasia** "Mercy killing" in which a person or organization knowingly acts to end the life of a terminally ill person.

**passive euthanasia** The intentional withholding of treatment that would prolong life.

## LO 9 | **MAKING** FINAL ARRANGEMENTS

Review the decisions that need to be made when someone is dying or has died, including hospice care, funeral arrangements, wills, and organ donation.

Caring for a dying person and his or her bereaved loved ones involves a wide variety of psychological, legal, social, spiritual, economic, and interpersonal issues.

## Hospice Care: Positive Alternatives

Since the mid-1970s, **hospice** programs in the United States have grown from a mere handful to more than 5,800 and are available in nearly every community.[70] These programs are a form of **palliative care** that focuses on reducing pain and suffering while attending to the emotional and spiritual needs of dying individuals and their caregivers. Hospice may help survivors cope better with the death experience.

The primary goals of hospice programs are to relieve the dying person's pain; offer emotional support to the dying person and loved ones; and restore a sense of control to the dying person, family, and friends. Hospice programs also usually include the following characteristics:

- There is overall medical direction of the program, with all health care provided under the direction of a qualified physician. Emphasis is placed on symptom control, primarily the alleviation of pain.
- Services are provided by an interdisciplinary team.
- Coverage is provided 24 hours a day, 7 days a week, with emphasis on the availability of medical and nursing skills.
- Carefully selected and extensively trained volunteers who augment but do not replace staff service are an integral part of the health care team.
- Care of the family extends through the bereavement period.
- Patients are accepted on the basis of their health needs, not their ability to pay.

## Making Funeral Arrangements

Anthropological evidence indicates that all cultures throughout human history have developed some sort of funeral ritual. For this reason, social scientists agree that funerals assist survivors of the deceased in coping with their loss. In some faiths, the deceased may be displayed to formalize last respects and increase social support of the bereaved. This part of the funeral ritual is referred to as a *wake* or *viewing*. The funeral service may be held in a church, in a funeral chapel, or at the burial site. Some people choose to replace the funeral service with a simple memorial service held within a few days of the burial. Social interaction associated with funeral and memorial services is valuable in helping survivors cope with their losses.

In addition to details related to the type of funeral or memorial service and the method of burial or body disposition, loved ones must also consider the cost of funeral and memorial options. They usually have to contact friends and relatives, plan for the arrival of guests, choose markers, submit obituary information to newspapers, and deal with many other details. Even though funeral directors are available to facilitate decision making, the bereaved may experience undue stress, especially if the death is unexpected. People who make their own funeral arrangements ahead of time can save their loved ones the difficulty of having to make these decisions during a very stressful time.

## Wills

The issue of inheritance should be resolved before the person dies to reduce both conflict and needless expense. Unfortunately, many people are so intimidated by the thought of making a will that they never do so and die **intestate** (without a will). This is a mistake, especially because the procedure for establishing a legal will is relatively simple and inexpensive. If you don't make a will before you die, the courts (as directed by state laws) will make a will for you. Legal issues, rather than your wishes, will preside. Furthermore, settling an estate takes longer when a person dies without a will.

## Trusts

Trusts are estate-planning tools that can help you manage property during your life if you are disabled by accident or illness and ensure a smooth transition of affairs after your death. While a trust sounds appealing, there are some aspects to be aware of. A living trust is more expensive to set up than a typical will because it must be actively managed after it is created. Most importantly, however, a living trust is useless unless it is funded, and it can only control those assets that have been placed into it. If your assets have not been transferred or if you die without funding the trust, the trust will be of no benefit: Your estate will still be subject to probate, and there may be significant estate tax issues.

## Organ Donation

Organ donation takes healthy organs and tissues from one person for transplantation into another. Experts say that the organs from one donor can save or help as many as 50 people.[71] You can donate internal organs (kidneys, heart, liver, pancreas, intestines, lungs); skin; bone and bone marrow; and corneas. Most organ and tissue donations occur after the

**SEE IT! VIDEOS**

How might you lessen the sadness after a loved one passes? Watch **The Conversation: A Family's Private Decision**, available on **MasteringHealth.**™

**hospice** A concept of end-of-life care designed to maximize quality of life and help dying people have peace, comfort, and dignity.

**palliative care** Any form of medical care focused on relieving the pain, symptoms, and stress of serious illness in order to improve the quality of life for patients and their families.

**intestate** Dying without a will.

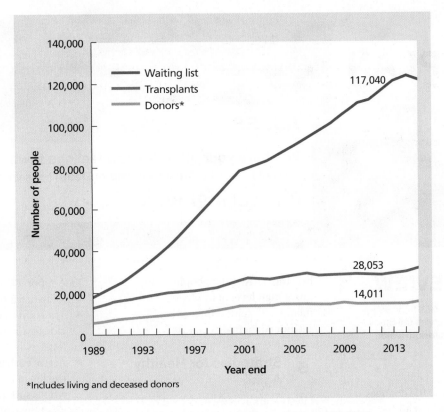

**FIGURE 22.5** Organ Donors and Patients Needing and Receiving Transplants, 1989–2015

**Source:** U.S Department of Health and Human Services, Organ Procurement and Transplantation Network, Accessed June 2016, http://optn.transplant.hrsa.gov.

donor has died, but some organs and tissues can be donated while the donor is alive.[72]

The number of patients waiting for organ donations greatly outnumbers available organs (**FIGURE 22.5**). Although some people are opposed to organ transplants and tissue donation, others experience personal fulfillment from knowing that their organs may extend and improve someone else's life after their own death. The most important step on the road to being an organ donor is to enroll in your state's donor registry. Go to www.organdonor.gov to sign up under your state. It is also a good idea to indicate your decision on your driver's license, tell your family and physician, and include the donation in your will and living will. Uniform donor cards are available through the U.S. Department of Health and Human Services and through many health care foundations and nonprofit organizations (**FIGURE 22.6**).

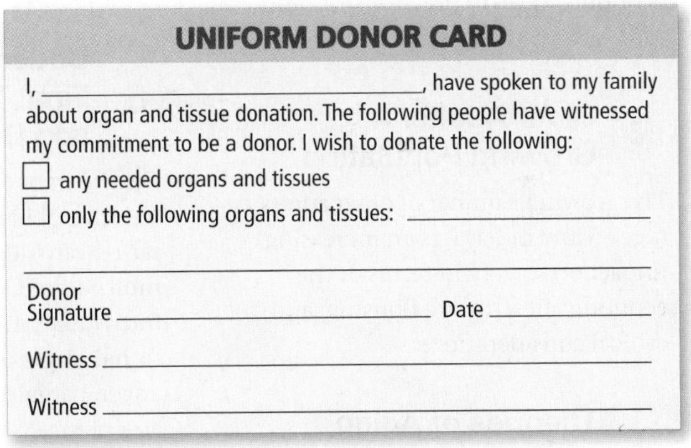

---

**UNIFORM DONOR CARD**

I, _____, have spoken to my family about organ and tissue donation. The following people have witnessed my commitment to be a donor. I wish to donate the following:

☐ any needed organs and tissues

☐ only the following organs and tissues: _____

_____

Donor
Signature _____ Date _____

Witness _____

Witness _____

**FIGURE 22.6 Organ Donor Card** Each organ and tissue donor can save or improve the lives of as many as 50 people.

# STUDY **PLAN**

Customize your study plan—and master your health!—in the Study Area of **MasteringHealth.**

## **ASSESS** YOURSELF

**What are your attitudes and feelings toward death?** Want to find out? Take the **Are You Afraid of Death?** assessment available on **MasteringHealth.**™

## CHAPTER **REVIEW**

To hear an MP3 Tutor Session, scan here or visit the Study Area in **MasteringHealth.**

### LO **1** | Aging

- Aging is the pattern of life changes that occur in members of all species as they grow older. The growing number of older adults (people aged 65 and older) has an increasing impact on society in terms of the economy, health care, housing, and ethical considerations.

### LO **2** | Older Adults: A Growing Population

- The growing number of older adults (age 65 and older) has an increasing impact on society in terms of the economy, health care housing, and ethical considerations.

### LO **3** | Theories of Aging

- Biological explanations of aging include the wear-and-tear theory, the cellular theory, the genetic mutation theory, and the autoimmune theory. Psychosocial theories center on adaptation and adjustments related to self-development.

### LO **4** | Physical and Mental Changes of Aging

- Aging changes the body and mind in many ways. Major physical concerns are osteoporosis, urinary incontinence, and changes in eyesight and

hearing. Most older people maintain a high level of intelligence and memory. Potential mental problems include Alzheimer's disease.

### LO **5** | Strategies for Healthy Aging

- Lifestyle choices we make today will affect health status later in life. Choosing to exercise, eat a healthy diet, foster lasting relationships, and enrich your spiritual side will contribute to healthy aging.

### LO **6** | Understanding the Final Transitions: Dying and Death

- *Death* can be defined biologically in terms of brain death or the cessation of vital functions. Dying is a multifaceted emotional process, and individuals may experience emotional stages of dying such as denial, anger, bargaining, depression, and acceptance. Social death results when a person is no longer treated as an active member of society.

### LO **7** | Coping with Loss

- Grief is the state of distress felt after loss. People differ in their responses to grief.

### LO **8** | Life-and-Death Decision Making

- Advanced directives assist people who believe they should be allowed to die if their condition is terminal and their existence depends on mechanical

life-support devices or artificial feeding or hydration systems.
- The right to die by rational suicide involves ethical, moral, and legal issues.
- Active euthanasia refers to ending the life of a person (or animal) who is suffering greatly and has no chance of recovery.

### LO **9** | Making Final Arrangements

- Hospice services are available to provide care for the terminally ill and their caregivers. After death, funeral arrangements must be made quickly and customs vary by family, region, religious affiliation, and cultural background. Decisions made in advance of illness and death, including wills and organ donation decisions, make the process easier for survivors.

## POP **QUIZ**

Visit **MasteringHealth** to personalize your study plan with Chapter Review Quizzes and Dynamic Study Modules.

### LO **1** | Aging

1. A person's adaptive capacities, such as coping abilities and intelligence, and the awareness of individual capabilities and self-efficacy is known as:
   a. biological age.
   b. psychological age.
   c. social age.
   d. legal age.

## LO 2 | Older Adults: A Growing Population

2. Within the United States, the over-65 population will increase substantially over the next two decades due to the aging of:
   a. generation X.
   b. millennials.
   c. the "baby boomer" generation.
   d. generation Y.

## LO 3 | Theories of Aging

3. Which biological theory of aging supports the concept that body cells are able to reproduce only so many times throughout life?
   a. Wear-and-tear theory
   b. Cellular theory
   c. Autoimmune theory
   d. Genetic mutation theory

## LO 4 | Physical and Mental Changes of Aging

4. The progressive breakdown of joint cartilage is known as
   a. osteoporosis.
   b. osteoarthritis.
   c. calcium loss.
   d. vitamin D deficiency.

5. Martha's ophthalmologist tells her that she has a condition that involves the breakdown of the light-sensitive area of the retina that is affecting her sharp, direct vision. What is this condition?
   a. Cataracts
   b. Glaucoma
   c. Macular degeneration
   d. Nearsightedness

## LO 5 | Strategies for Healthy Aging

6. The keys to successful aging include
   a. drinking red wine regularly.
   b. reducing protein intake.
   c. avoiding weight-bearing activities.
   d. eating sufficient calcium and vitamin D.

## LO 6 | Understanding the Final Transitions: Dying and Death

7. The Kübler-Ross stage of dying in which the individual rejects death emotionally and feels a sense of shock and disbelief is known as
   a. acceptance.
   b. bargaining.
   c. denial.
   d. anger.

## LO 7 | Coping with Loss

8. A culturally prescribed and accepted period of grief for someone who has died is known as
   a. bereavement.
   b. grief work.
   c. coping with loss.
   d. mourning.

## LO 8 | Life-and-Death Decision Making

9. Kerri's elderly grandmother is terminally ill and wants to die without medical intervention. Her family has agreed to withhold treatment that may prolong her life. This is called
   a. rational suicide.
   b. health care proxy.
   c. passive euthanasia.
   d. active euthanasia.

## LO 9 | Making Final Arrangements

10. Destiny's grandfather dies intestate. This means he
    a. had a health care proxy.
    b. did not have a will.
    c. received hospice care.
    d. did not have a trust.

*Answers to the Pop Quiz can be found on A-1. If you answered a question incorrectly, review the section identified by the Learning Outcome. For even more study tools, visit* **MasteringHealth**.

# THINK ABOUT IT!

## LO 1 | Aging

1. What are some of the different ways aging is defined? How are they different? How are they similar? How do you see it?

## LO 2 | Older Adults: A Growing Population

2. As the older population grows, how will it affect your life? Would you be willing to pay higher taxes to support government programs for older adults? Why or why not?

## LO 3 | Theories of Aging

3. What are the biological explanations of how and why we age? What do psychosocial theories focus on as important factors in aging?

## LO 4 | Physical and Mental Changes of Aging

4. List the major physical and mental changes that occur with aging. Which of these, if any, can you change?

## LO 5 | Strategies for Healthy Aging

5. How do the lifestyle choices we make now affect our health status later in life? What are some of the healthy choices and changes you could make today that will contribute to healthy aging later?

## LO 6 | Understanding the Final Transitions: Dying and Death

6. Discuss why so many of us deny death. How could death become a more acceptable topic to discuss?

# ACCESS YOUR HEALTH ON THE INTERNET

Visit **MasteringHealth** for links to the websites and RSS feeds.

The following websites explore further topics and issues related to aging.

**Administration on Aging.** This U.S. Department of Health and Human Services link is dedicated to addressing the health needs of older adults. **www.aoa.gov**

**Alzheimer's Association.** This site includes media releases, position statements, fact sheets, and research on Alzheimer's disease. **www.alz.org**

**Grieving.com.** This forum site addresses all aspects of grief and loss, including terminal illness, nondeath losses, and caregiving. **http://forums.grieving.com**

**National Hospice and Palliative Care Organization.** This site offers information on hospice care, including resources for finding a hospice, end-of-life issues, and advance directives. **www.nhpco.org**

**National Institute on Aging.** A site that provides information and research updates on aging related issues. **www.nia.nih.gov**

# APPENDIX A  ANSWERS TO POP QUIZ QUESTIONS

## Chapter 1
1. b; 2. d; 3. b; 4. a; 5. d; 6. b; 7. a; 8. a;
9. c; 10. b

## Chapter 2
1. b; 2. a; 3. d; 4. b; 5. c; 6. c; 7. c; 8. b;
9. b; 10. b; 11. a; 12. b; 13. b

## Chapter 2A Focus On
1. c; 2. b; 3. b

## Chapter 3
1. c; 2. b; 3. c; 4. a; 5. d; 6. c; 7. d; 8. b;
9. b; 10. c

## Chapter 3A Focus On
1. c; 2. a; 3. b

## Chapter 4
1. b; 2. c; 3. a; 4. d; 5. d

## Chapter 5
1. b; 2. b; 3. a; 4. c; 5. b; 6. a; 7. d; 8. c;
9. b; 10. d

## Chapter 6
1. b; 2. a; 3. c; 4. a; 5. c; 6. b; 7. c; 8. b;
9. d; 10. a

## Chapter 6A Focus On
1. a; 2. b; 3. d

## Chapter 7
1. d; 2. c; 3. c; 4. b; 5. b; 6. b; 7. a; 8. c;
9. b; 10. a

## Chapter 8
1. c; 2. d; 3. b; 4. c; 5. b; 6. a; 7. a; 8. d;
9. b; 10. d

## Chapter 9
1. c; 2. b; 3. c; 4. a; 5. b; 6. d; 7. a; 8. c;
9. c; 10. c

## Chapter 10
1. c; 2. a; 3. a; 4. c; 5. a; 6. b; 7. d; 8. b;
9. b; 10. a

## Chapter 10A Focus On
1. b; 2. d; 3. c; 4. b; 5. b.

## Chapter 11
1. c; 2. d; 3. c; 4. b; 5. d; 6. d; 7. b; 8. a;
9. a; 10. b

## Chapter 12
1. c; 2. b; 3. d; 4. c; 5. c; 6. d; 7. b; 8. b;
9. b; 10. a

## Chapter 13
1. b; 2. c; 3. c; 4. c; 5. b; 6. a; 7. d; 8. b;
9. d; 10. a

## Chapter 14
1. b; 2. c; 3. a; 4. a; 5. a; 6. c; 7. c; 8. b;
9. c; 10. b

## Chapter 15
1. d; 2. b; 3. c; 4. d; 5. b; 6. b

## Chapter 16
1. c; 2. c; 3. b; 4. d; 5. c; 6. d; 7. a; 8. c;
9. b; 10. c

## Chapter 16A Focus On
1. c; 2. b; 3. c

## Chapter 17
1. b; 2. b; 3. d; 4. a; 5. a; 6. a; 7. c; 8. a;
9. b; 10. d

## Chapter 18
1. c; 2. b; 3. d; 4. c; 5. b; 6. b; 7. b; 8. a;
9. a; 10. d

## Chapter 19
1. c; 2. d; 3. a; 4. d; 5. c; 6. c; 7. d; 8. b;
9. b; 10. d

## Chapter 20
1. b; 2. a; 3. c; 4. c; 5. b; 6. c; 7. d; 8. b;
9. a; 10. d

## Chapter 20A Focus On
1. c; 2. d; 3. a; 4. c; 5. a

## Chapter 21
1. d; 2. d; 3. a; 4. d; 5. b; 6. d; 7. a; 8. c;
9. a; 10. a

## Chapter 22
1. b; 2. c; 3. b; 4. b; 5. c; 6. d; 7. c; 8. d;
9. c; 10. b

deally, first-aid procedures should be performed only by someone who has received formal training from the American Red Cross or another reputable institution. (There are numerous classes and opportunities in most communities for updating your skills in these areas. Check for such classes at your university or local community college.) If you do not have such training, contact a physician or call your local emergency medical service (EMS) by dialing 9-1-1 or your local emergency number. In life-threatening situations, however, you may need to begin first aid immediately and continue until help arrives. This section contains basic information for various emergency situations. Simply reading these directions, however, may not prepare you fully to handle these situations. For this reason, you may want to enroll in a first-aid course.

## CALLING FOR EMERGENCY ASSISTANCE

When calling for emergency assistance, be prepared to give exact details. Be clear and thorough, and do not panic. Never hang up until the dispatcher has informed you that he or she has all the information needed. Be ready to answer the following questions:

- Where are you and the victim located? (This is the most important information that the EMS will need.)
- What is your phone number and name?
- What has happened? Was there an accident, or is the victim ill?
- How many people need help?
- What is the nature of the emergency? What is the victim's apparent condition?
- Are there any life-threatening situations that the EMS should know about (for example, fires, explosions, or fallen electrical lines)?
- Is the victim wearing a medic-alert tag (a tag indicating a specific medical condition such as diabetes)?

## ADMINISTERING FIRST AID

According to the laws in most states, you are not required to administer first aid unless you have a special obligation to the victim. For example, parents must provide first aid for their children, and a lifeguard must provide aid to a swimmer.

Before administering first aid, you should obtain the victim's consent. If the victim refuses aid, you must respect that person's rights. However, you should make every reasonable effort to persuade the victim to accept your help. In emergency situations, consent is *implied* if the victim is unconscious. Once you begin to administer first aid, you are required by law to continue. You must remain with the victim until someone of equal or greater competence takes over.

Can you be held liable if you fail to provide adequate care or if the victim is further injured? To protect people who render first aid, most states have Good Samaritan laws, which grant immunity (protection from civil liability) if you act in good faith to provide care to the best of your ability, according to your level of training. Because these laws vary, you should become familiar with the Good Samaritan laws in your state.

## First-Aid Supplies

Every home, car, and boat should be supplied with a basic first-aid kit, which should be stored in a convenient place but kept out of the reach of children. Following is a list of supplies that should be included:

- Bandages, including triangular bandages (36 inches by 6 inches), butterfly bandages, a roller bandage, rolled white gauze bandages (2- and 3-inch widths), adhesive bandages
- Sterile gauze pads and absorbent pads
- Adhesive tape (2- and 3-inch widths)
- Cotton-tip applicators
- Scissors
- Thermometer
- Antibiotic ointment
- Aspirin
- Calamine lotion
- Antiseptic cream or petroleum jelly
- Safety pins
- Tweezers
- Latex gloves
- Flashlight
- Paper cups
- Blanket

You cannot be prepared for every medical emergency, but these essential tools and a knowledge of basic first aid will help you cope with many emergency situations, including the ones discussed below.

## Cessation of Breathing

If someone has stopped breathing, you should perform mouth-to-mouth resuscitation. This involves the following steps:

1. Check for responsiveness by gently tapping or shaking the victim. Ask loudly, "Are you okay?"
2. Call the local EMS for help (usually 9-1-1).
3. Gently roll the victim onto his or her back.
4. Open the airway by tilting the victim's head back—place your hand nearest the victim's head on the victim's forehead, and apply backward pressure to tilt the head back and lift the chin.

5. Check for breathing (3 to 5 seconds): look, listen, and feel for breathing.
6. Give two slow breaths.
   - Keep the victim's head tilted back.
   - Pinch the victim's nose shut.
   - Seal your lips tightly around the victim's mouth.
   - Give two slow breaths, each lasting 1.5 to 2 seconds.
   - Watch for the chest to rise and fall.
7. Check for pulse at side of neck; feel for pulse for 5 to 10 seconds.
8. Begin rescue breathing.
   - Keep the victim's head tilted back.
   - Pinch the victim's nose shut.
   - Give one breath about every 5 seconds (12 breaths per minute).
   - Look, listen, and feel for breathing between breaths.
9. Recheck pulse every minute.
   - Keep the victim's head tilted back.
   - Feel for pulse for 5 to 10 seconds.
   - If the victim has a pulse but is not breathing, continue rescue breathing. If there is no pulse, begin CPR (see below).

There are some variations when performing this procedure on infants and children. For infants, at step 8, you should give one slow breath every 3 seconds. You should not pinch the nose. Instead, seal your lips tightly around the infant's nose and mouth. For children aged 1 to 8, at step 8, give one slow breath every 4 seconds.

## Sudden Collapse

If an adult has a sudden cardiac arrest, his or her survival depends largely on being given immediate cardiopulmonary resuscitation (CPR). People are often afraid to offer aid for fear of doing something wrong or making matters worse. In addition, some people are squeamish about performing the artificial respiration that is part of traditional CPR. However, studies have shown that simply providing hands-only CPR to an adult who has collapsed can double that person's chance of survival. The American Heart Association now recommends that anyone, trained or untrained, who witnesses an adult's sudden collapse should call 9-1-1 and then immediately begin hands-only CPR. That means uninterrupted chest compressions—pushing hard in the center of the victim's chest—at a rate of about 100 per minute until the EMS arrives.

Conventional CPR, a technique that involves a combination of artificial respiration and chest compressions, is still recommended for infants or children, drowning victims, drug overdose, or other respiratory problems, and on adult victims who are found already unconscious and not breathing normally. The American Red Cross, the American Heart Association, and other organizations offer courses in mouth-to-mouth resuscitation and CPR as well as general first aid. If you have taken a CPR course in the past, you should be aware that certain changes have been made in the procedure. Consider taking a refresher course.

## Choking

Choking occurs when an object obstructs the trachea (windpipe), thus preventing normal breathing. Failure to expel the object and restore breathing can lead to death within 6 minutes. The universal signal of distress related to choking is the clasping of the throat with one or both hands. Other signs of choking include not being able to talk and/or noisy and difficult breathing. If a victim can cough or speak, do not interfere. The most effective method for assisting choking victims is the Heimlich Maneuver (FIGURE 1), which involves the application of pressure to the victim's abdominal area to expel the foreign object, as described below.

### If the Choking Victim Is Standing or Seated

1. Recognize that the victim is choking. Without startling him or her, approach from behind.
2. Wrap your arms around the victim's waist, making a fist with one hand.
3. Place the thumb side of the fist on the middle of the victim's abdomen, just above the navel and well below the tip of the sternum.
4. Cover your fist with your other hand.
5. Press fist into victim's abdomen, with up to five quick upward thrusts.
6. After every five abdominal thrusts, check the victim and your technique.

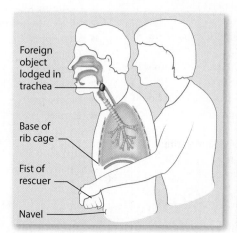

Foreign object lodged in trachea

Base of rib cage

Fist of rescuer

Navel

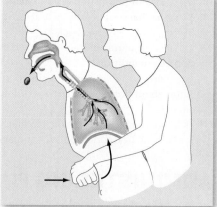

(a) Standing behind the victim, place a fist thumb-side in just above the victim's navel and cover it with your other hand.

(b) Press sharply upward and inward, using enough force to push the diaphragm and lungs up and create air pressure that will expel the object.

**FIGURE 1** Heimlich Maneuver
The Heimlich maneuver can be used to dislodge an object that is blocking a person's airway, causing him or her to choke. The technique shown here is appropriate for use on a person who is either sitting or standing.

**Source:** Adapted from Johnson, Michael D., *Human Biology: Concepts and Current Issues*, 5th, © 2010. Printed and Electronically reproduced by permission of Pearson Education, Inc., Upper Saddle River, New Jersey.

7. If the victim becomes unconscious, gently lower him or her to the ground.
8. Try to clear the airway by using your finger to sweep the object from the victim's mouth or throat.
9. Give two rescue breaths. If the passage is still blocked and air will not go in, repeat the Heimlich maneuver.

### If the Choking Victim Is Lying Down

1. Facing the person, kneel with your legs astride the victim's hips. Place the heel of one hand against the abdomen, slightly above the navel and well below the tip of the sternum. Put the other hand on top of the first hand.
2. Press inward and upward using both hands with up to five quick abdominal thrusts.
3. Repeat the following steps in this sequence until the airway becomes clear or the EMS arrives:
   - Finger sweep.
   - Give two rescue breaths.
   - Do up to five abdominal thrusts.

## Alcohol Poisoning

Alcohol overdose is considered a medical emergency when an irregular heartbeat or coma occurs. The two immediate causes of death in such cases are cardiac arrhythmia and respiratory depression. If a person is seriously uncoordinated and has possibly also taken a depressant, the risk of respiratory failure is serious enough that a physician should be contacted. When dealing with someone who is drunk, remember these points:

1. Stay calm. Assess the situation.
2. Keep your distance. Before approaching or touching the person, explain what you intend to do.
3. Speak in a clear, firm, reassuring manner.
4. Keep the person still and comfortable.
5. Stay with the person if she or he is vomiting. When helping him or her to lie down, turn the head to the side to prevent it from falling back. This helps to keep the person from choking on vomit.
6. Monitor the person's breathing.

## Seizures

If you are with someone experiencing a seizure, there are several steps you can take to help ensure his or her safety during and after the episode:

1. Note the length of the attack. Seizures in which a person remains unconscious for long periods of time should be monitored closely. If medical help arrives, be sure to tell them how long the person has been unconscious.
2. Remove obstacles that could harm the victim. Because seizure victims may lose motor control during a convulsion, they inadvertently thrash around. To reduce the chances of serious injury, clear away any objects that could pose a threat.
3. Loosen clothing, and turn the victim's head to the side. This will help ensure that the person can breathe freely and will allow fluids or vomit to drain from the mouth.
4. Do not force objects into the victim's mouth. Although seizure victims may bite their tongues, causing possible damage, they will not swallow them. If the victim's mouth is clamped

shut, forcing objects into the mouth may break teeth or cause more harm than doing nothing.
5. Get help. After you have completed steps 1 through 4, get help or send someone for help. This is particularly important if the victim does not regain consciousness within a few minutes.
6. Reassure the victim. Too often, the seizure victim regains consciousness only to face a crowd of staring people. When administering first aid, try to dissuade curious bystanders from hanging around. Calmly reassure the victim that everything is okay.
7. Allow the person to rest. After a seizure, many people will be exhausted. Allow them to sleep if possible.

## Bleeding

**External Bleeding** Control of external bleeding is an important part of emergency care. Survival is threatened by the loss of 1 quart of blood or more. There are three major procedures for the control of external bleeding:

- **Direct pressure.** The best method is to apply firm pressure by covering the wound with a sterile dressing, bandage, or clean cloth. Wearing disposable latex gloves or an equally protective barrier, apply pressure for 5 to 10 minutes to stop bleeding.
- **Elevation.** Elevate the wounded section of the body to slow the bleeding. For example, a wounded arm or leg should be raised above the level of the victim's heart.
- **Pressure points.** Pressure points are sites where an artery that is close to the body's surface lies directly over a bone (FIGURE 2). Pressing the artery against the bone can limit the flow of blood to the injury. This technique should be used only as a last resort when direct pressure and elevation have failed to stop bleeding.

For serious wounds, seek medical attention immediately.

**Internal Bleeding** Although internal bleeding may not be immediately obvious, you should be aware of the following signs and symptoms:

- Symptoms of shock (discussed below)
- Coughing up or vomiting blood
- Bruises or contusions of the skin
- Bruises on chest or fractured ribs
- Black, tarlike stools
- Abdominal discomfort or pain (rigidity or spasms)

In some cases, a person who has suffered an injury (such as a blow to the head, chest, or abdomen) that does not cause external bleeding may bleed internally. If you suspect internal bleeding, follow these steps:

1. Have the person lie on his or her back on a flat surface with knees bent.
2. Treat for shock. Keep the victim warm. Cover the person with a blanket, if possible.
3. Expect vomiting. If this occurs, keep the victim on his or her side for drainage, to prevent inhalation of vomit, and to prevent expulsion of vomit from the stomach.
4. Do *not* give the victim any medications or fluids.
5. Send someone to call for emergency medical help immediately.

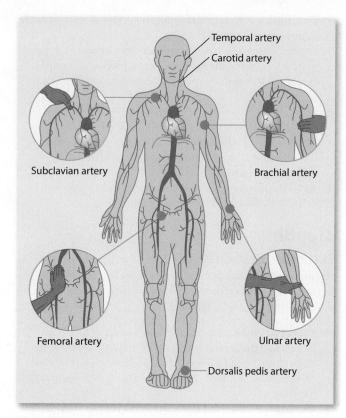

**FIGURE 2** Pressure Points

Pressure can be applied to these points to stop bleeding. However, unless absolutely necessary, avoid applying pressure to the carotid arteries, which supply blood to the brain. Never apply pressure to both carotid arteries at the same time.

## Nosebleeds

1. Have the victim sit down and lean slightly forward to prevent blood from running into the throat. If you do not suspect a fracture, pinch the person's nose firmly closed using the thumb and forefinger. Keep the nose pinched for at least 5 minutes.
2. While the nose is pinched, apply a cold compress to the surrounding area.
3. If pinching does not work, gently pack the nostril with gauze or a clean strip of cloth. Do not use absorbent cotton, which will stick. Be sure that the ends of the gauze or cloth hang out so that it can be easily removed later. Once the nose is packed with gauze, pinch it closed again for another 5 minutes.
4. If the bleeding persists, seek medical attention.

## Shock

Shock is a condition in which the cardiovascular system fails to provide sufficient blood circulation to all parts of the body. Victims of shock display some or all of the following symptoms:

- Dilated pupils
- Cool, moist skin
- Weak, rapid pulse
- Vomiting
- Delayed or unrelated responses to questions

All injuries result in some degree of shock. Therefore, treatment for shock should be given after every major injury. The following are basic steps for treating shock:

1. Have the victim lie flat with his or her feet elevated approximately 8 to 12 inches. (In the case of chest injuries, difficulty breathing, or severe pain, the victim's head should be slightly elevated if there is no sign of spinal injury.)
2. Keep the victim warm. If possible, wrap him or her in blankets or other material. Keep the victim calm and reassured.
3. Seek medical help.

## Treatment for Burns

**Minor Burns** For minor burns caused by fire or scalding water, apply running cold water or cold compresses for 20 to 30 minutes. Never put butter, grease, salt water, aloe vera, or topical burn ointments or sprays on burned skin. If the burned area is dirty, gently wash it with soap and water, and blot it dry with a sterile dressing.

**Major Burns** For major burn injuries, call for help immediately. Wrap the victim in a clean, dry sheet. Do not clean the burns or try to remove any clothing attached to burned skin. Remove jewelry near the burned skin immediately, if possible. Keep the victim lying down and calm.

**Chemical Burns** Remove clothing surrounding the burn. Wash skin that has been burned by chemicals by flushing with water for at least 20 minutes. Seek medical assistance as soon as possible.

## Electrical Shock

Do not touch a victim of electrical shock until the power source has been turned off. Approach the scene carefully, avoiding any live wires or electrical power lines. Pay attention to the following:

1. If the victim is holding onto the live electrical wire, do not remove it unless the power has been shut off at the plug, circuit breaker, or fuse box.
2. Check the victim's breathing and pulse. Electrical current can paralyze the nerves and muscles that control breathing and heartbeat. If necessary, give mouth-to-mouth resuscitation. If there is no pulse, CPR might be necessary. (Remember that only trained people should perform CPR.)
3. Keep the victim warm and treat for shock. Once the person is breathing and stable, seek medical help or send someone else for help.

## Poisoning

Among adults, almost all poisonings are caused by an overdose of a prescription drug, most commonly an opioid pain medication, or an illegal drug, such as cocaine or heroin. Among children, the majority of poisonings are caused by household products.

You should keep emergency telephone numbers for the poison control center and the local EMS close at hand. Many people keep these numbers on labels on their telephones. Check the front of your telephone book for these numbers. Be prepared to answer the following questions and to give the following information when calling for help:

- What was ingested? Have the container of the product and the remaining contents ready so you can describe it. Bring the container with you to the emergency room.
- When was the substance taken?
- How much was taken?
- Has vomiting occurred? If the person has vomited, save a sample to take to the hospital.
- Are there any other symptoms?
- How long will it take to get to the nearest emergency room?

When caring for a person who has ingested poison, keep these basic principles in mind:

1. Maintain an open airway. Make sure the person is breathing.
2. Call the local poison control center. Follow their advice for neutralizing the poison.
3. If the poison control center or another medical authority advises you to induce vomiting, then do so.
4. If a corrosive or caustic (that is, acid or alkali) substance was swallowed, immediately dilute it by having the victim drink at least one or two 8-ounce glasses of cold water or milk.
5. Place the victim on his or her left side. This position will delay advancement of the poison into the small intestine, where absorption into the victim's circulatory system is faster.

# Injuries of Joints, Muscles, and Bones

**Sprains** Sprains result when ligaments and other tissues around a joint are stretched or torn. The following steps should be taken to treat sprains:

1. Elevate the injured joint to a comfortable position.
2. Apply an ice pack or cold compress to reduce pain and swelling.
3. Wrap the joint firmly with a roller bandage.
4. Check the fingers or toes periodically to ensure that blood circulation has not been obstructed. If the bandage is too tight, loosen it.
5. Keep the injured area elevated, and continue ice treatment for 24 hours.
6. Apply heat to the injury after 48 hours if there is no further swelling.
7. If pain and swelling continue or if a fracture is suspected, seek medical attention.

**Fractures** Any deformity of an injured body part usually indicates a fracture. A fracture is any break in a bone, including chips, cracks, splinters, and complete breaks. Minor fractures (e.g., hairline cracks) might be difficult to detect and might be confused with sprains. If there is doubt, treat the injury as a fracture until X-rays have been taken.

Do not move the victim if a fracture of the neck or back is suspected, because this could result in a spinal cord injury. If the victim must be moved, splints should be applied to immobilize the fracture in order to prevent further damage and to decrease pain.

Following are some basic steps for treating fractures and applying splints to broken limbs:

1. If the person is bleeding, apply direct pressure above the site of the wound.
2. If a broken bone is exposed, do not try to move it back into the wound. This can cause contamination and further injury.
3. Do not try to straighten out a broken limb. Splint the limb as it lies.
4. The following materials are needed for splinting:
   - *Splint:* wooden board, pillow, or rolled up magazines and newspapers
   - *Padding:* towels, blankets, socks, or cloth
   - *Ties:* cloth, rope, or tape
5. Place splints and padding above and below the joint. Never put padding directly over the break. Padding should protect bony areas and the soft tissue of the limb.
6. Tie splints and padding into place.
7. Check the tightness of the splints periodically. Pay attention to the skin color, temperature, and pulse below the fracture to make sure the blood flow is adequate.
8. Elevate the fracture and apply ice packs to prevent swelling and reduce pain.

# Head Injuries

All head injuries can potentially lead to brain damage, which may result in a cessation of breathing and pulse.

## Minor Head Injuries

1. For a minor bump on the head resulting in a bruise without bleeding, apply ice to decrease the swelling.
2. If there is bleeding, apply even, moderate pressure. Do not use excessive pressure because the skull may be fractured.
3. Observe the victim for a change in consciousness.

Observe the size of pupils, including whether both pupils are dilated to the same degree, and note signs of inability to think clearly. Check for any signs of numbness or paralysis. Allow the victim to sleep, but wake him or her periodically to check for awareness.

## Severe Head Injuries

1. If the victim is unconscious, check the airway for breathing. If necessary, perform mouth-to-mouth resuscitation.
2. If the victim is breathing, check the pulse. If it is less than 55 or more than 125 beats per minute, the victim may be in danger.
3. Check for bleeding. If fluid is flowing from the ears or nose, do not stop it.
4. Do not remove any objects embedded in the victim's skull.
5. Cover the victim with blankets to maintain body temperature, but guard against overheating.
6. Seek medical help as soon as possible.

# Temperature-Related Emergencies

**Frostbite** Frostbite is damage to body tissues caused by intense cold, generally occurring at temperatures below 32°F. When skin is exposed to the cold, ice crystals form beneath the skin. Avoid rubbing frostbitten tissue, because the ice crystals can scrape and break blood vessels. The body parts most likely to suffer frostbite are the toes, ears, fingers, nose, and cheeks. To treat frostbite, follow these steps:

1. Bring the victim to a medical facility as soon as possible.
2. Cover and protect the frostbitten area. If possible, apply a steady source of external warmth, such as a warm compress. Avoid walking if the feet are frostbitten.
3. If the victim cannot be transported, warm the body part by immersing it in warm water (100°F to 105°F). Continue to warm until the frostbitten area is warm to the touch when removed from the bath. Do not allow the body part to touch the sides or bottom of the water container. After warming, dry gently and wrap the body part in bandages to protect from refreezing.

## Hypothermia
Hypothermia is a condition of generalized cooling of the body, resulting from exposure to cold temperatures or immersion in cold water. It can occur at any temperature below 65°F and can be made more severe by wind chill and moisture. The following are key symptoms of hypothermia:

- Shivering
- Vague, slow, slurred speech
- Poor judgment
- A cool abdomen
- Lethargy, or extreme exhaustion
- Slowed breathing and heartbeat
- Numbness and loss of feeling in extremities

After contacting the EMS, take the following steps:

1. Get the victim out of the cold.
2. Keep the victim in a flat position. Do not raise the legs.
3. Squeeze as much water as possible from wet clothing, and layer dry clothing over wet clothing. Removal of clothing may jostle the victim and lead to other problems.
4. Give the victim warm drinks only if he or she is able to swallow. Do not give the victim alcohol or caffeinated beverages, and do not allow the victim to smoke.
5. Do not allow the victim to exercise.

## Heatstroke
Heatstroke, the most serious heat-related disorder, results from the failure of the brain's heat-regulating mechanism (the hypothalamus) to cool the body. The following are signs and symptoms of heatstroke:

- Rapid pulse
- Hot, dry, flushed skin (absence of sweating)
- Disorientation leading to unconsciousness
- High body temperature

Body temperature should be reduced as quickly as possible. Immerse the victim in a cool bath, lake, or stream. If there is no water nearby, loosen clothing and use a fan to help lower the victim's body temperature.

## Heat Exhaustion
Heat exhaustion results from excessive loss of salt and water. The onset is gradual, with the following symptoms:

- Fatigue and weakness
- Anxiety
- Nausea
- Profuse sweating and clammy skin
- Normal body temperature

Move the victim to a cool place and have him or her lie down flat, with feet elevated 8 to 12 inches. Replace lost fluids slowly and steadily. Sponge or fan the victim.

## Heat Cramps
Heat cramps result from excessive sweating, resulting in an excessive loss of salt and water. Although heat cramps are the least serious heat-related emergency, they are the most painful. The symptoms include muscle cramps, usually starting in the arms and legs. To relieve symptoms, the victim should drink electrolyte-rich beverages or a light saltwater solution or eat salty foods.

# NUTRITIVE VALUE OF SELECTED FOODS AND FAST FOODS

This section presents nutritional information about a wide array of foods, including many fast foods. Values are given for calories, protein, carbohydrates, fiber, fat, saturated fat, and cholesterol for common foods and serving sizes. Use this information to assess your diet and make improvements. This is only a sampling of the most common foods. See the MyDietAnalysis database for a more extensive list of foods.

| MDA Code | Food Name | Amt | Wt (g) | Ener (kcal) | Prot (g) | Carb (g) | Fiber (g) | Fat (g) | Sat (g) | Chol (g) |
|---|---|---|---|---|---|---|---|---|---|---|
| **Beverages** | | | | | | | | | | |
| *Alcoholic Beverages* | | | | | | | | | | |
| 22831 | Beer | 12 fl. oz | 360 | 157 | 1 | 13 | | 0 | 0 | 0 |
| 34053 | Beer, light | 12 fl. oz | 353 | 105 | 1 | 5 | 0 | 0 | 0 | 0 |
| 22606 | Beer, nonalcoholic | 12 fl. oz | 353 | 73 | 1 | 14 | 0 | 0 | 0 | 0 |
| 22884 | Wine, red | 1 fl. oz | 29 | 24 | 0 | 1 | | 0 | 0 | |
| 22861 | Wine, white | 1 fl. oz | 29 | 24 | 0 | 1 | | 0 | 0 | |
| 22514 | Gin, 80 proof | 1 fl. oz | 28 | 64 | 0 | 0 | 0 | 0 | 0 | 0 |
| 22593 | Rum, 80 proof | 1 fl. oz | 28 | 64 | 0 | 0 | 0 | 0 | 0 | 0 |
| 22515 | Tequila, 80 proof | 1 fl. oz | 28 | 64 | 0 | 0 | 0 | 0 | 0 | 0 |
| 22594 | Vodka, 80 proof | 1 fl. oz | 28 | 64 | 0 | 0 | 0 | 0 | 0 | 0 |
| 22670 | Whiskey, 80 proof | 1 fl. oz | 28 | 64 | 0 | 0 | 0 | 0 | 0 | 0 |
| *Coffee, Tea, and Dairy Drink Mixes* | | | | | | | | | | |
| 20012 | Coffee, brewed | 1 cup | 237 | 2 | 0 | 0 | 0 | 0 | 0 | 0 |
| 20686 | Coffee, decaffeinated, brewed | 1 cup | 237 | 0 | 0 | 0 | 0 | 0 | 0 | 0 |
| 20439 | Coffee, espresso | 1 cup | 237 | 5 | 0 | 0 | 0 | 0 | 0.2 | 0 |
| 20402 | Coffee, from mix, French vanilla, sugar & fat free | 1 ea | 7 | 25 | 0 | 5 | 0 | 0 | 0.1 | 0 |
| 85 | Chocolate milk, prepared w/ syrup | 1 cup | 282 | 254 | 9 | 36 | 1 | 8 | 4.7 | 25 |
| 46 | Hot cocoa, w/ aspartame, sodium, vitamin A, prepared w/water | 1 cup | 256 | 74 | 3 | 14 | 2 | 1 | 0.4 | 0 |
| 48 | Hot cocoa, prep from dry mix w/ water | 1 cup | 275 | 151 | 3 | 32 | 1 | 2 | 0.9 | 0 |
| 166 | Hot cocoa, w/ marshmallows, from dry packet | 1 ea | 28 | 112 | 1 | 21 | 1 | 4 | 4.2 | 0 |
| 39 | Chocolate flavor, dry mix, prepared w/ milk | 1 cup | 266 | 226 | 9 | 32 | 1 | 9 | 4.9 | 24 |
| 41 | Strawberry flavor, dry mix, prepared w/ milk | 1 cup | 266 | 234 | 8 | 33 | 0 | 8 | 5.1 | 32 |
| 20014 | Tea, brewed | 1 cup | 237 | 2 | 0 | 1 | 0 | 0 | 0 | 0 |
| 20036 | Tea, herbal (not chamomile) brewed | 1 cup | 237 | 2 | 0 | 0 | 0 | 0 | 0 | 0 |
| *Fruit and Vegetable Beverages and Juices* | | | | | | | | | | |
| 71080 | Apple juice, canned or bottled, unsweetened | 1 ea | 262 | 121 | 0 | 30 | 1 | 0 | 0.1 | 0 |
| 20277 | Capri Sun All Natural Juice Drink, Fruit Punch | 1 ea | 210 | 99 | 0 | 26 | 0 | 0 | 0 | 0 |
| 5226 | Carrot juice, canned | 1 cup | 236 | 94 | 2 | 22 | 2 | 0 | 0.1 | 0 |
| 3042 | Cranberry juice cocktail | 1 cup | 253 | 137 | 0 | 34 | 0 | 0 | 0 | 0 |
| 20024 | Fruit punch, canned | 1 cup | 248 | 117 | 0 | 30 | 0 | 0 | 0 | 0 |
| 20035 | Fruit punch, from frozen concentrate | 1 cup | 247 | 114 | 0 | 29 | 0 | 0 | 0 | 0 |
| 20101 | Grape drink, canned | 1 cup | 250 | 152 | 0 | 39 | 0 | 0 | 0 | 0 |
| 3053 | Grapefruit juice, from frozen concentrate, unsweetened | 1 cup | 247 | 101 | 1 | 24 | 0 | 0 | 0 | 0 |
| 20045 | Lemonade flavor drink, from dry mix | 1 cup | 266 | 72 | 0 | 18 | 0 | 0 | 0 | 0 |
| 20047 | Lemonade w/ aspartame, low kcal, from dry mix | 1 cup | 237 | 7 | 0 | 2 | 0 | 0 | 0 | 0 |
| 20070 | Orange drink, canned | 1 cup | 248 | 122 | 0 | 31 | 0 | 0 | 0 | 0 |
| 20004 | Orange flavor drink, from dry mix | 1 cup | 248 | 122 | 0 | 31 | 0 | 0 | 0 | 0 |
| 71108 | Orange juice, canned, unsweetened | 1 ea | 263 | 124 | 2 | 29 | 1 | 0 | 0 | 0 |
| 3090 | Orange juice, fresh | 1 cup | 248 | 112 | 2 | 26 | 0 | 0 | 0.1 | 0 |
| 3091 | Orange juice, from frozen concentrate, unsweetened | 1 cup | 249 | 112 | 2 | 27 | 0 | 0 | 0 | 0 |
| 5397 | Tomato juice, canned w/o salt | 1 cup | 243 | 41 | 2 | 10 | 1 | 0 | 0 | 0 |
| 20849 | Vegetable and fruit, mixed juice drink | 4 oz | 113 | 33 | 0 | 8 | 0 | 0 | 0 | 0 |
| 20080 | Vegetable juice cocktail, canned | 1 cup | 242 | 46 | 2 | 11 | 2 | 0 | 0 | 0 |

**Ener** = energy (kilocalories); **Prot** = protein; **Carb** = carbohydrate; **Fiber** = dietary fiber; **Fat** = total fat; **Sat** = saturated fat; **Chol** = cholesterol.

| MDA Code | Food Name | Amt | Wt (g) | Ener (kcal) | Prot (g) | Carb (g) | Fiber (g) | Fat (g) | Sat (g) | Chol (g) |
|---|---|---|---|---|---|---|---|---|---|---|
| *Soft Drinks* | | | | | | | | | | |
| 20006 | Club soda | 1 cup | 237 | 0 | 0 | 0 | 0 | 0 | 0 | 0 |
| 20685 | Low-calorie cola, w/ aspartame, caffeine free | 12 fl. oz | 355 | 4 | 0 | 1 | 0 | 0 | 0 | 0 |
| 20843 | Cola, w/ higher caffeine | 12 fl. oz | 370 | 152 | 0 | 39 | 0 | 0 | 0 | 0 |
| 20008 | Ginger ale | 1 cup | 244 | 83 | 0 | 21 | 0 | 0 | 0 | 0 |
| 20032 | Lemon-lime soft drink | 1 cup | 246 | 98 | 0 | 25 | 0 | 0 | 0 | 0 |
| 20027 | Pepper-type soft drink | 1 cup | 246 | 101 | 0 | 26 | 0 | 0 | 0.2 | 0 |
| 20009 | Root beer | 1 cup | 246 | 101 | 0 | 26 | 0 | 0 | 0 | 0 |
| *Other* | | | | | | | | | | |
| 20033 | Soy milk | 1 cup | 245 | 132 | 8 | 15 | 1 | 4 | 0.5 | 0 |
| 20041 | Water, tap | 1 cup | 237 | 0 | 0 | 0 | 0 | 0 | 0 | 0 |
| **Breakfast Cereals** | | | | | | | | | | |
| 40095 | All-Bran/Kellogg | 0.5 cup | 30 | 78 | 4 | 22 | 9 | 1 | 0.2 | 0 |
| 40032 | Cap'n Crunch/Quaker | 0.75 cup | 27 | 109 | 1 | 23 | 1 | 2 | 1.1 | 0 |
| 40297 | Cheerios/Gen Mills | 1 cup | 30 | 110 | 3 | 22 | 3 | 2 | 0.3 | 0 |
| 40126 | Cinnamon Toast Crunch/Gen Mills | 0.75 cup | 30 | 130 | 2 | 24 | 1 | 3 | 0.4 | 0 |
| 40195 | Corn Flakes/Kellogg | 1 cup | 28 | 101 | 2 | 24 | 1 | 0 | 0 | 0 |
| 40089 | Corn Grits, instant, plain, prepared/Quaker | 1 pkg | 137 | 104 | 2 | 22 | 2 | 1 | 0.1 | |
| 40206 | Corn Pops/Kellogg | 1 cup | 31 | 117 | 1 | 28 | 0 | 0 | 0.1 | 0 |
| 40179 | Cream of Rice, prepared w/ salt | 1 cup | 244 | 127 | 2 | 28 | 0 | 0 | 0 | 0 |
| 40182 | Cream of Wheat, instant, prepared w/ salt | 1 cup | 241 | 149 | 4 | 32 | 1 | 1 | 0.1 | 0 |
| 40104 | Crispix/Kellogg | 1 cup | 29 | 109 | 2 | 25 | 0 | 0 | 0.1 | 0 |
| 40218 | Froot Loops/Kellogg | 1 cup | 30 | 112 | 2 | 26 | 3 | 1 | 0.6 | 0 |
| 40217 | Frosted Flakes/Kellogg | 0.75 cup | 31 | 114 | 1 | 28 | 1 | 0 | 0 | 0 |
| 11916 | Frosted Mini-Wheats, bite size/Kellogg | 1 cup | 55 | 189 | 6 | 45 | 6 | 1 | 0.2 | 0 |
| 40209 | Raisin Bran/Kellogg | 1 cup | 61 | 196 | 5 | 47 | 7 | 1 | 0.2 | 0 |
| 40210 | Rice Krispies/Kellogg | 1.25 cup | 33 | 128 | 2 | 28 | 0 | 0 | 0.1 | 0 |
| 60887 | Shredded wheat, large biscuit | 2 ea | 38 | 127 | 4 | 30 | 5 | 1 | 0.2 | 0 |
| 40211 | Special K/Kellogg | 1 cup | 31 | 117 | 7 | 22 | 1 | 0 | 0.1 | 0 |
| **Dairy and Cheese** | | | | | | | | | | |
| 500 | Cream, half & half | 2 Tbs | 30 | 39 | 1 | 1 | 0 | 3 | 2.1 | 11 |
| 11 | Milk, condensed, sweetened, canned | 2 Tbs | 38 | 123 | 3 | 21 | 0 | 3 | 2.1 | 13 |
| 19 | Milk, lowfat, 1% fat, chocolate | 1 cup | 250 | 158 | 8 | 26 | 1 | 2 | 1.5 | 8 |
| 218 | Milk, 2%, w/ added vitamins A & D | 1 cup | 245 | 130 | 8 | 13 | 0 | 5 | 3 | 20 |
| 6 | Milk, nonfat/skim, w/ added vitamin A | 1 cup | 245 | 83 | 8 | 12 | 0 | 0 | 0.1 | 5 |
| 1 | Milk, whole, 3.25% | 1 cup | 244 | 149 | 8 | 12 | 0 | 8 | 4.6 | 24 |
| 20 | Milk, whole, chocolate | 1 cup | 250 | 208 | 8 | 26 | 2 | 8 | 5.3 | 30 |
| 72088 | Yogurt, fruit variety, nonfat | 1 cup | 245 | 233 | 11 | 47 | 0 | 0 | 0.3 | 5 |
| 1287 | American cheese, nonfat slices | 1 pce | 21 | 32 | 5 | 2 | 0 | 0 | 0.1 | 3 |
| 13349 | Cheez Whiz cheese sauce/Kraft | 2 Tbs | 33 | 91 | 4 | 3 | 0 | 7 | 4.3 | 25 |
| 1014 | Cottage cheese, 2% fat | 0.5 cup | 113 | 97 | 13 | 4 | 0 | 3 | 1.1 | 11 |
| 1015 | Cream cheese | 2 Tbs | 29 | 99 | 2 | 1 | 0 | 10 | 5.6 | 32 |
| 1452 | Cream cheese, fat free | 2 Tbs | 29 | 30 | 5 | 2 | 0 | 0 | 0.2 | 3 |
| 1016 | Feta, crumbled | 0.25 cup | 38 | 99 | 5 | 2 | 0 | 8 | 5.6 | 33 |
| 47887 | Mozzarella, whole milk, slice | 1 ea | 34 | 102 | 8 | 1 | 0 | 8 | 4.5 | 27 |
| 1075 | Parmesan, grated | 1 Tbs | 5 | 22 | 2 | 0 | 0 | 1 | 0.9 | 4 |
| 1024 | Ricotta, part skim | 0.25 cup | 62 | 86 | 7 | 3 | 0 | 5 | 3.1 | 19 |
| 1064 | Ricotta, whole milk | 0.25 cup | 62 | 108 | 7 | 2 | 0 | 8 | 5.1 | 32 |
| **Eggs and Egg Substitutes** | | | | | | | | | | |
| 19525 | Egg substitute, liquid | 0.25 cup | 63 | 53 | 8 | 0 | 0 | 2 | 0.4 | 1 |
| 19506 | Egg, white, raw | 1 ea | 33 | 16 | 4 | 0 | 0 | 0 | 0 | 0 |
| 19509 | Egg, whole, fried | 1 ea | 46 | 90 | 6 | 0 | 0 | 7 | 2 | 210 |
| 19515 | Egg, whole, hard boiled | 1 ea | 37 | 57 | 5 | 0 | 0 | 4 | 1.2 | 157 |
| 19521 | Egg, whole, poached | 1 ea | 37 | 53 | 5 | 0 | 0 | 4 | 1.1 | 156 |
| 19516 | Egg, whole, scrambled | 1 ea | 61 | 102 | 7 | 1 | 0 | 7 | 2.2 | 215 |
| 19508 | Egg, yolk, raw, fresh | 1 ea | 17 | 53 | 3 | 1 | 0 | 4 | 1.6 | 205 |

| MDA Code | Food Name | Amt | Wt (g) | Ener (kcal) | Prot (g) | Carb (g) | Fiber (g) | Fat (g) | Sat (g) | Chol (g) |
|---|---|---|---|---|---|---|---|---|---|---|
| **Fruit** | | | | | | | | | | |
| 72101 | Apricots, canned, heavy syrup, drained | 1 cup | 182 | 151 | 1 | 39 | 5 | 0 | 0 | 0 |
| 3164 | Fruit cocktail canned in juice | 1 cup | 237 | 109 | 1 | 28 | 2 | 0 | 0 | 0 |
| 71079 | Apple w/ skin, raw | 1 cup | 125 | 65 | 0 | 17 | 3 | 0 | 0 | 0 |
| 3331 | Applesauce w/ added vitamin C | 0.5 cup | 128 | 97 | 0 | 25 | 2 | 0 | 0 | 0 |
| 3657 | Apricot, raw | 1 cup | 165 | 79 | 2 | 18 | 3 | 1 | 0 | 0 |
| 3210 | Avocado, California, peeled, raw | 1 ea | 173 | 289 | 3 | 15 | 12 | 27 | 3.7 | 0 |
| 71082 | Banana, peeled, raw | 1 ea | 81 | 72 | 1 | 19 | 2 | 0 | 0.1 | 0 |
| 71976 | Grapefruit, fresh | 0.5 ea | 154 | 60 | 1 | 16 | 6 | 0 | 0 | 0 |
| 3055 | Grapes, Thompson seedless, fresh | 0.5 cup | 80 | 55 | 1 | 14 | 1 | 0 | 0 | 0 |
| 3642 | Melon, fresh, wedge | 1 pce | 69 | 23 | 1 | 6 | 1 | 0 | 0 | 0 |
| 3168 | Mixed fruit (prune, apricot, & pear) dried | 1 oz | 28 | 69 | 1 | 18 | 2 | 0 | 0 | 0 |
| 3216 | Nectarine, raw | 1 cup | 138 | 61 | 1 | 15 | 2 | 0 | 0 | 0 |
| 3726 | Peach, peeled, raw | 1 ea | 79 | 31 | 1 | 8 | 1 | 0 | 0 | 0 |
| 3106 | Pear, raw | 1 ea | 209 | 121 | 1 | 32 | 6 | 0 | 0 | 0 |
| 3766 | Raisins, seedless | 50 ea | 26 | 78 | 1 | 21 | 1 | 0 | 0 | 0 |
| 72113 | Pineapple, fresh, slice | 1 pce | 84 | 38 | 0 | 10 | | 0 | | |
| 3085 | Orange, fresh | 1 ea | 184 | 86 | 2 | 22 | 4 | 0 | 0 | 0 |
| 3135 | Strawberries, halves/slices, raw | 1 cup | 166 | 53 | 1 | 13 | 3 | 0 | 0 | 0 |
| **Grain Products** | | | | | | | | | | |
| *Breads, Rolls, and Bread Crumbs* | | | | | | | | | | |
| 71170 | Bagel, cinnamon-raisin | 1 ea | 26 | 71 | 3 | 14 | 1 | 0 | 0.1 | 0 |
| 71167 | Bagel, egg | 1 ea | 26 | 72 | 3 | 14 | 1 | 1 | 0.1 | 6 |
| 71152 | Bagel, plain/onion/poppy/sesame, enriched | 1 ea | 26 | 67 | 3 | 13 | 1 | 0 | 0.1 | 0 |
| 42433 | Biscuit, w/ butter | 1 ea | 82 | 273 | 5 | 28 | 1 | 16 | 3.9 | 1 |
| 71192 | Biscuit, plain or buttermilk, refrig dough, baked, reduced fat | 1 ea | 21 | 63 | 2 | 12 | 0 | 1 | 0.3 | 0 |
| 42004 | Bread crumbs, dry, plain, grated | 1 Tbs | 7 | 27 | 1 | 5 | 0 | 0 | 0.1 | 0 |
| 49144 | Bread, crusty Italian w/ garlic | 1 pce | 50 | 186 | 4 | 21 | | 10 | 2.4 | 6 |
| 70964 | Bread, garlic, frozen/Campione | 1 pce | 28 | 101 | 2 | 12 | 1 | 5 | 0.8 | |
| 42069 | Bread, oat bran | 1 pce | 30 | 71 | 3 | 12 | 1 | 1 | 0.2 | 0 |
| 42095 | Bread, wheat, reduced kcal | 1 pce | 23 | 46 | 2 | 10 | 3 | 1 | 0.1 | 0 |
| 71247 | Bread, white, commercially prepared, crumbs/cubes/slices | 1 pce | 9 | 24 | 1 | 5 | 0 | 0 | 0.1 | 0 |
| 42084 | Bread, white, reduced kcal | 1 pce | 23 | 48 | 2 | 10 | 2 | 1 | 0.1 | 0 |
| 26561 | Buns, hamburger, Wonder | 1 ea | 43 | 117 | 3 | 22 | 1 | 2 | 0.4 | |
| 42021 | Hamburger/hot dog bun, plain | 1 ea | 43 | 120 | 4 | 21 | 1 | 2 | 0.5 | 0 |
| 42115 | Cornbread, prepared from dry mix | 1 pce | 60 | 188 | 4 | 29 | 1 | 6 | 1.6 | 37 |
| 71227 | Pita bread, white, enriched | 1 ea | 28 | 77 | 3 | 16 | 1 | 0 | 0 | 0 |
| 71228 | Pita bread, whole wheat | 1 ea | 28 | 74 | 3 | 15 | 2 | 1 | 0.1 | 0 |
| 71368 | Roll, dinner, plain, homemade w/ reduced fat (2%) milk | 1 ea | 43 | 136 | 4 | 23 | 1 | 3 | 0.8 | 15 |
| 42161 | Roll, French | 1 ea | 38 | 105 | 3 | 19 | 1 | 2 | 0.4 | 0 |
| 71056 | Roll, hard/kaiser | 1 ea | 57 | 167 | 6 | 30 | 1 | 2 | 0.3 | 0 |
| 42297 | Tortilla, corn, w/o salt, ready to cook | 1 ea | 26 | 58 | 1 | 12 | 1 | 1 | 0.1 | 0 |
| 90645 | Taco shell, baked | 1 ea | 5 | 23 | 0 | 3 | 0 | 1 | 0.3 | 0 |
| *Crackers* | | | | | | | | | | |
| 71451 | Cheez-its/Goldfish crackers, low sodium | 55 pce | 33 | 166 | 3 | 19 | 1 | 8 | 3.2 | 4 |
| 43507 | Oyster/soda/soup crackers | 1 cup | 45 | 189 | 4 | 33 | 1 | 4 | 0.9 | 0 |
| 70963 | Ritz crackers/Nabisco | 5 ea | 16 | 79 | 1 | 10 | 0 | 4 | 0.9 | |
| 43587 | Saltine crackers, original premium/Nabisco | 5 ea | 14 | 56 | 1 | 10 | 0 | 1 | 0 | 0 |
| 43545 | Sandwich crackers, cheese filled | 4 ea | 28 | 134 | 3 | 17 | 1 | 6 | 1.7 | 1 |
| 43546 | Sandwich crackers, peanut butter filled | 4 ea | 28 | 138 | 3 | 16 | 1 | 7 | 1.4 | 0 |
| 44677 | Snackwell Wheat Cracker/Nabisco | 1 ea | 15 | 62 | 1 | 12 | 1 | 2 | | |
| 43581 | Wheat Thins, baked/Nabisco | 16 ea | 29 | 140 | 3 | 20 | 1 | 6 | 0.9 | 0 |
| 43508 | Whole wheat cracker | 4 ea | 32 | 137 | 3 | 22 | 3 | 5 | 0.7 | 0 |
| *Muffins and Baked Goods* | | | | | | | | | | |
| 42723 | English muffin, plain | 1 ea | 57 | 132 | 5 | 26 | | 1 | 0.2 | |
| 62916 | Muffin, blueberry, commercially prepared | 1 ea | 11 | 43 | 1 | 5 | 0 | 2 | 0.4 | 4 |
| 44521 | Muffin, corn, commercially prepared | 1 ea | 57 | 174 | 3 | 29 | 2 | 5 | 0.8 | 15 |
| 44514 | Muffin, oatbran | 1 ea | 57 | 154 | 4 | 28 | 3 | 4 | 0.6 | 0 |
| 44518 | Toaster muffin, blueberry | 1 ea | 33 | 103 | 2 | 18 | 1 | 3 | 0.5 | 2 |

| MDA Code | Food Name | Amt | Wt (g) | Ener (kcal) | Prot (g) | Carb (g) | Fiber (g) | Fat (g) | Sat (g) | Chol (g) |
|---|---|---|---|---|---|---|---|---|---|---|
| *Noodles and Pasta* | | | | | | | | | | |
| 38048 | Chow mein noodles, dry | 1 cup | 45 | 237 | 4 | 26 | 2 | 14 | 2 | 0 |
| 38047 | Egg noodles, enriched, cooked | 0.5 cup | 80 | 110 | 4 | 20 | 1 | 2 | 0.3 | 23 |
| 38060 | Spaghetti, whole wheat, cooked | 1 cup | 140 | 174 | 7 | 37 | 6 | 1 | 0.1 | 0 |
| 38251 | Egg noodles, enriched, cooked w/ salt | 0.5 cup | 80 | 110 | 4 | 20 | 1 | 2 | | 23 |
| 38102 | Macaroni noodles, enriched, cooked | 1 cup | 140 | 221 | 8 | 43 | 3 | 1 | 0.2 | 0 |
| 38118 | Spaghetti noodles, enriched, cooked | 0.5 cup | 70 | 111 | 4 | 22 | 1 | 1 | 0.1 | 0 |
| *Grains* | | | | | | | | | | |
| 38076 | Couscous, cooked | 0.5 cup | 78 | 88 | 3 | 18 | 1 | 0 | 0 | 0 |
| 38080 | Oats | 0.25 cup | 39 | 152 | 7 | 26 | 4 | 3 | 0.5 | 0 |
| 38010 | Rice, brown, long grain, cooked | 1 cup | 195 | 216 | 5 | 45 | 4 | 2 | 0.4 | 0 |
| 38256 | Rice, white, long grain, enriched, cooked w/ salt | 1 cup | 158 | 205 | 4 | 45 | 1 | 0 | 0.1 | 0 |
| 38019 | Rice, white, long grain, instant, enriched, cooked | 1 cup | 165 | 193 | 4 | 41 | 1 | 1 | 0 | 0 |
| *Pancakes, French Toast, and Waffles* | | | | | | | | | | |
| 42156 | French toast, homemade, w/reduced fat (2%) milk | 1 pce | 65 | 149 | 5 | 16 | | 7 | 1.8 | 75 |
| 45192 | Pancake/waffle, buttermilk/Eggo/Kellogg | 1 ea | 42 | 99 | 3 | 16 | 0 | 3 | 0.6 | 5 |
| 45117 | Pancakes, plain, homemade | 1 ea | 77 | 175 | 5 | 22 | 1 | 7 | 1.6 | 45 |
| 45193 | Waffle, lowfat, homestyle, frozen | 1 ea | 35 | 83 | 2 | 15 | 0 | 1 | 0.3 | 9 |
| **Meat and Meat Substitutes** | | | | | | | | | | |
| *Beef* | | | | | | | | | | |
| 10093 | Beef, average of all cuts (1/4" trim), cooked | 3 oz | 85 | 260 | 22 | 0 | 0 | 18 | 7.3 | 75 |
| 10705 | Beef, average of all cuts, lean (1/4" trim), cooked | 3 oz | 85 | 184 | 25 | 0 | 0 | 8 | 3.2 | 73 |
| 10133 | Beef, whole rib, roasted, 1/4" trim | 3 oz | 85 | 305 | 19 | 0 | 0 | 25 | 10 | 71 |
| 58129 | Ground beef (hamburger), 25% fat, cooked, pan-browned | 3 oz | 85 | 236 | 22 | 0 | 0 | 15 | 6 | 76 |
| 58119 | Ground beef (hamburger), 15% fat, cooked, pan-browned | 3 oz | 85 | 218 | 24 | 0 | 0 | 13 | 5 | 77 |
| 58109 | Ground beef (hamburger), 5% fat, cooked, pan-browned | 3 oz | 85 | 164 | 25 | 0 | 0 | 6 | 2.9 | 76 |
| 10791 | Porterhouse steak, lean & fat (1/4" trim), broiled | 3 oz | 85 | 280 | 19 | 0 | 0 | 22 | 8.7 | 61 |
| 58257 | Rib eye steak, small end (ribs 10–12), 0" trim, broiled | 3 oz | 85 | 210 | 23 | 0 | 0 | 13 | 4.9 | 94 |
| 58094 | Skirt steak, trimmed to 0" fat, broiled | 3 oz | 85 | 187 | 22 | 0 | 0 | 10 | 4 | 51 |
| 58328 | Strip steak, top loin, 1/8" trim, broiled | 3 oz | 85 | 171 | 25 | 0 | 0 | 7 | 2.7 | 67 |
| 10805 | T-Bone steak, lean & fat (1/4" trim), broiled | 3 oz | 85 | 260 | 20 | 0 | 0 | 19 | 7.6 | 55 |
| 11531 | Veal, average of all cuts, cooked | 3 oz | 85 | 197 | 26 | 0 | 0 | 10 | 3.6 | 97 |
| *Chicken* | | | | | | | | | | |
| 15057 | Chicken breast, w/o skin, fried | 3 oz | 85 | 159 | 28 | 0 | 0 | 4 | 1.1 | 77 |
| 15080 | Chicken, dark meat, w/ skin, roasted | 3 oz | 85 | 215 | 22 | 0 | 0 | 13 | 3.7 | 77 |
| 15026 | Chicken, dark meat, w/o skin, fried | 3 oz | 85 | 203 | 25 | 2 | 0 | 10 | 2.7 | 82 |
| 15042 | Chicken drumstick, w/o skin, fried | 3 oz | 85 | 166 | 24 | 0 | 0 | 7 | 1.8 | 80 |
| 15048 | Chicken, wing, w/o skin, fried | 3 oz | 85 | 180 | 26 | 0 | 0 | 8 | 2.1 | 71 |
| 15059 | Chicken, wing, w/o skin, roasted | 3 oz | 85 | 173 | 26 | 0 | 0 | 7 | 1.9 | 72 |
| *Turkey* | | | | | | | | | | |
| 51151 | Turkey bacon, cooked | 1 oz | 28 | 108 | 8 | 1 | 0 | 8 | 2.4 | 28 |
| 51098 | Turkey patty, breaded, fried | 1 ea | 42 | 119 | 6 | 7 | 0 | 8 | 2 | 32 |
| 16110 | Turkey breast w/ skin, roasted | 3 oz | 85 | 130 | 25 | 0 | 0 | 3 | 0.7 | 77 |
| 16038 | Turkey breast, no skin, roasted | 3 oz | 85 | 115 | 26 | 0 | 0 | 1 | 0.2 | 71 |
| 16101 | Turkey, dark meat w/ skin, roasted | 3 oz | 85 | 155 | 24 | 0 | 0 | 6 | 1.8 | 100 |
| 16003 | Turkey, patty, ground, cooked | 1 ea | 82 | 193 | 22 | 0 | 0 | 11 | 2.8 | 84 |
| *Lamb* | | | | | | | | | | |
| 13604 | Lamb, average of all cuts (1/4" trim), cooked | 3 oz | 85 | 250 | 21 | 0 | 0 | 18 | 7.5 | 83 |
| 13616 | Lamb, average of all cuts, lean (1/4" trim), cooked | 3 oz | 85 | 175 | 24 | 0 | 0 | 8 | 2.9 | 78 |
| *Pork* | | | | | | | | | | |
| 12000 | Bacon, broiled, pan-fried, or roasted | 3 pcs | 19 | 103 | 7 | 0 | 0 | 8 | 2.6 | 21 |
| 28143 | Canadian bacon | 1 pce | 56 | 68 | 9 | 1 | | 3 | 1 | 27 |
| 12211 | Ham, cured, boneless, regular fat (11% fat), roasted | 1 cup | 140 | 249 | 32 | 0 | 0 | 13 | 4.4 | 83 |
| 12309 | Pork, average of retail cuts, cooked | 3 oz | 85 | 203 | 22 | 0 | 0 | 12 | 4.2 | 75 |
| 12097 | Pork, ribs, backribs, roasted | 3 oz | 85 | 315 | 21 | 0 | 0 | 25 | 9.4 | 100 |
| 12099 | Pork, ground, cooked | 3 oz | 85 | 253 | 22 | 0 | 0 | 18 | 6.6 | 80 |

| MDA Code | Food Name | Amt | Wt (g) | Ener (kcal) | Prot (g) | Carb (g) | Fiber (g) | Fat (g) | Sat (g) | Chol (g) |
|---|---|---|---|---|---|---|---|---|---|---|
| *Lunchmeats* | | | | | | | | | | |
| 13000 | Beef, thin slices | 1 oz | 28 | 33 | 5 | 1 | 0 | 1 | 0.3 | 14 |
| 58275 | Bologna, beef and pork, low fat | 1 ea | 14 | 32 | 2 | 0 | 0 | 3 | 1 | 5 |
| 13157 | Chicken breast, oven roasted deluxe | 1 oz | 28 | 29 | 5 | 1 | 0 | 1 | 0.2 | 14 |
| 13306 | Corned beef, cooked, chopped, pressed | 1 ea | 71 | 101 | 14 | 1 | 0 | 5 | 2 | 46 |
| 13264 | Ham, slices, regular (11% fat) | 1 cup | 135 | 220 | 22 | 5 | 2 | 12 | 4 | 77 |
| 13101 | Pastrami, beef, cured | 1 oz | 28 | 42 | 6 | 0 | 0 | 2 | 0.8 | 19 |
| 13215 | Salami, beef, cotto | 1 oz | 28 | 59 | 4 | 1 | 0 | 4 | 1.9 | 24 |
| 16160 | Turkey breast slice | 1 pce | 21 | 22 | 4 | 1 | 0 | 0 | 0.1 | 9 |
| 58279 | Turkey ham, sliced, extra lean, prepackaged or deli-sliced | 1 cup | 138 | 171 | 27 | 4 | 0 | 5 | 1.5 | 92 |
| *Sausage* | | | | | | | | | | |
| 13070 | Chorizo, pork & beef | 1 ea | 60 | 273 | 14 | 1 | 0 | 23 | 8.6 | 53 |
| 57877 | Frankfurter, beef | 1 ea | 45 | 148 | 5 | 2 | 0 | 13 | 5.3 | 24 |
| 13012 | Frankfurter, turkey | 1 ea | 45 | 100 | 6 | 2 | 0 | 8 | 1.8 | 35 |
| 57890 | Italian sausage, pork, cooked | 1 ea | 83 | 286 | 16 | 4 | 0 | 23 | 8 | 47 |
| 13021 | Pepperoni sausage | 1 pce | 6 | 27 | 1 | 0 | 0 | 2 | 0.8 | 6 |
| 13185 | Pork sausage links, cooked | 2 ea | 48 | 165 | 8 | 0 | 0 | 15 | 5.1 | 37 |
| 58227 | Sausage, pork, precooked | 3 oz | 85 | 321 | 12 | 0 | 0 | 30 | 9.9 | 63 |
| 58007 | Turkey sausage, breakfast links, mild | 2 ea | 56 | 132 | 9 | 1 | 0 | 10 | 2.1 | 90 |
| *Meat Substitutes* | | | | | | | | | | |
| 7509 | Bacon substitute, vegetarian, strips | 3 ea | 15 | 46 | 2 | 1 | 0 | 4 | 0.7 | 0 |
| 7722 | Garden patties, frozen/Worthington, Morningstar | 1 ea | 67 | 118 | 12 | 9 | 3 | 4 | 0.5 | 1 |
| 7674 | Harvest burger, original flavor, vegetable protein patty | 1 ea | 90 | 138 | 18 | 7 | 6 | 4 | 1 | 0 |
| 90626 | Sausage, vegetarian, meatless | 1 ea | 28 | 72 | 5 | 3 | 1 | 5 | 0.8 | 0 |
| 7726 | Spicy black bean burger/Worthington, Morningstar | 1 ea | 78 | 133 | 13 | 15 | 5 | 4 | 0.6 | 1 |
| Nuts | | | | | | | | | | |
| 4519 | Cashews, dry roasted w/ salt | 0.25 cup | 34 | 196 | 5 | 11 | 1 | 16 | 3.1 | 0 |
| 4728 | Macadamia nuts, dry roasted, unsalted | 1 cup | 134 | 962 | 10 | 18 | 11 | 102 | 16 | 0 |
| 4592 | Mixed nuts, w/ peanuts, dry roasted, salted | 0.25 cup | 34 | 203 | 6 | 9 | 3 | 18 | 2.4 | 0 |
| 4626 | Peanut butter, chunky w/ salt | 2 Tbs | 32 | 188 | 8 | 7 | 3 | 16 | 2.6 | 0 |
| 4756 | Peanuts, dry roasted w/o salt | 30 ea | 30 | 176 | 7 | 6 | 2 | 15 | 2.1 | 0 |
| 4696 | Peanuts, raw | 0.25 cup | 36 | 207 | 9 | 6 | 3 | 18 | 2.5 | 0 |
| 4540 | Pistachio nuts, dry roasted, salted | 0.25 cup | 32 | 182 | 7 | 9 | 3 | 15 | 1.8 | 0 |
| Seafood | | | | | | | | | | |
| 17029 | Bass, freshwater, cooked w/ dry heat | 3 oz | 85 | 124 | 21 | 0 | 0 | 4 | 0.9 | 74 |
| 17037 | Cod, Atlantic, baked/broiled (dry heat) | 3 oz | 85 | 89 | 19 | 0 | 0 | 1 | 0.1 | 47 |
| 19036 | Crab, Alaskan King, boiled/steamed | 3 oz | 85 | 83 | 16 | 0 | 0 | 1 | 0.1 | 45 |
| 17090 | Haddock, baked or broiled (dry heat) | 3 oz | 85 | 95 | 21 | 0 | 0 | 1 | 0.1 | 63 |
| 17291 | Halibut, Atlantic & Pacific, baked or broiled (dry heat) | 3 oz | 85 | 119 | 23 | 0 | 0 | 3 | 0.4 | 35 |
| 17181 | Salmon, Atlantic, farmed, cooked w/ dry heat | 3 oz | 85 | 175 | 19 | 0 | 0 | 11 | 2.1 | 54 |
| 17099 | Salmon, Sockeye, baked or broiled (dry heat) | 3 oz | 85 | 184 | 23 | 0 | 0 | 9 | 1.6 | 74 |
| 71707 | Squid, fried | 3 oz | 85 | 149 | 15 | 7 | 0 | 6 | 1.6 | 221 |
| 17066 | Swordfish, baked or broiled (dry heat) | 3 oz | 85 | 132 | 22 | 0 | 0 | 4 | 1.2 | 43 |
| 56007 | Tuna salad, lunchmeat spread | 2 Tbs | 26 | 48 | 4 | 2 | 0 | 2 | 0.4 | 3 |
| 17151 | White tuna, canned in water, drained | 3 oz | 85 | 109 | 20 | 0 | 0 | 3 | 0.7 | 36 |
| 17083 | White tuna, canned in oil, drained | 3 oz | 85 | 158 | 23 | 0 | 0 | 7 | 1.1 | 26 |
| **Vegetables and Legumes** | | | | | | | | | | |
| *Beans* | | | | | | | | | | |
| 7038 | Baked beans, plain or vegetarian, canned | 1 cup | 254 | 239 | 12 | 54 | 10 | 1 | 0.2 | 0 |
| 5197 | Bean sprouts, mung, canned, drained | 1 cup | 125 | 15 | 2 | 3 | 1 | 0 | 0 | 0 |
| 7012 | Black beans, boiled w/o salt | 1 cup | 172 | 227 | 15 | 41 | 15 | 1 | 0.2 | 0 |
| 5862 | Beets, boiled w/ salt, drained | 0.5 cup | 85 | 37 | 1 | 8 | 2 | 0 | 0 | 0 |
| 90018 | Cowpeas, cooked w/ salt | 1 cup | 171 | 198 | 13 | 35 | 11 | 1 | 0.2 | 0 |
| 7081 | Hummus, garbanzo or chickpea spread, homemade | 1 Tbs | 15 | 27 | 1 | 3 | 1 | 1 | 0.2 | 0 |
| 7087 | Kidney beans, canned | 1 cup | 256 | 215 | 13 | 37 | 14 | 2 | 0.3 | 0 |
| 7006 | Lentils, boiled w/o salt | 1 cup | 198 | 230 | 18 | 40 | 16 | 1 | 0.1 | 0 |
| 7051 | Pinto beans, canned | 1 cup | 240 | 206 | 12 | 37 | 11 | 2 | 0.4 | 0 |

| MDA Code | Food Name | Amt | Wt (g) | Ener (kcal) | Prot (g) | Carb (g) | Fiber (g) | Fat (g) | Sat (g) | Chol (g) |
|---|---|---|---|---|---|---|---|---|---|---|
| 6748 | Snap green beans, raw | 10 ea | 55 | 17 | 1 | 4 | 1 | 0 | 0 | 0 |
| 5320 | Snap yellow beans, raw | 0.5 cup | 55 | 17 | 1 | 4 | 2 | 0 | 0 | 0 |
| 90026 | Split peas, boiled w/ salt | 0.5 cup | 98 | 114 | 8 | 20 | 8 | 0 | 0.1 | 0 |
| 7054 | White beans, canned | 1 cup | 262 | 299 | 19 | 56 | 13 | 1 | 0.2 | 0 |

*Fresh Vegetables*

| MDA Code | Food Name | Amt | Wt (g) | Ener (kcal) | Prot (g) | Carb (g) | Fiber (g) | Fat (g) | Sat (g) | Chol (g) |
|---|---|---|---|---|---|---|---|---|---|---|
| 9577 | Artichokes (globe or French), boiled w/ salt, drained | 1 ea | 20 | 11 | 1 | 2 | 2 | 0 | 0 | 0 |
| 6033 | Arugula/roquette, raw | 1 cup | 20 | 5 | 1 | 1 | 0 | 0 | 0 | 0 |
| 90406 | Asparagus, raw | 10 ea | 35 | 7 | 1 | 1 | 1 | 0 | 0 | 0 |
| 5558 | Broccoli stalks, raw | 1 ea | 114 | 32 | 3 | 6 | 3 | 0 | 0.1 | 0 |
| 5036 | Cabbage, raw | 1 cup | 70 | 18 | 1 | 4 | 2 | 0 | 0 | 0 |
| 90605 | Carrots, baby, raw | 1 ea | 15 | 5 | 0 | 1 | 0 | 0 | 0 | 0 |
| 5049 | Cauliflower, raw | 0.5 cup | 50 | 12 | 1 | 2 | 1 | 0 | 0 | 0 |
| 90436 | Celery, raw | 1 ea | 17 | 3 | 0 | 1 | 0 | 0 | 0 | 0 |
| 7202 | Corn, white, sweet, ears, raw | 1 ea | 73 | 63 | 2 | 14 | 2 | 1 | 0.1 | 0 |
| 5900 | Corn, yellow, sweet, boiled w/ salt, drained | 0.5 cup | 82 | 79 | 3 | 17 | 2 | 1 | 0.2 | 0 |
| 5908 | Eggplant (brinjal), boiled w/ salt, drained | 1 cup | 99 | 33 | 1 | 8 | 2 | 0 | 0 | 0 |
| 5087 | Lettuce, looseleaf, raw | 2 pcs | 20 | 3 | 0 | 1 | 0 | 0 | 0 | 0 |
| 51069 | Mushrooms, brown, Italian, or crimini, raw | 2 ea | 28 | 6 | 1 | 1 | 0 | 0 | 0 | 0 |
| 90472 | Onions, chopped, raw | 1 ea | 70 | 28 | 1 | 7 | 1 | 0 | 0 | 0 |
| 5116 | Peas, green, raw | 1 cup | 145 | 117 | 8 | 21 | 7 | 1 | 0.1 | 0 |
| 7932 | Peppers, jalapeno, raw | 1 cup | 90 | 27 | 1 | 5 | 2 | 1 | 0.1 | 0 |
| 90493 | Peppers, sweet green, chopped/sliced, raw | 10 pcs | 27 | 5 | 0 | 1 | 0 | 0 | 0 | 0 |
| 6990 | Pepper, sweet red, raw | 1 ea | 10 | 3 | 0 | 1 | 0 | 0 | 0 | 0 |
| 9251 | Potatoes, red, flesh and skin, baked | 1 ea | 138 | 123 | 3 | 27 | 2 | 0 | 0 | 0 |
| 9245 | Potatoes, russet, flesh and skin, baked | 1 ea | 138 | 134 | 4 | 30 | 3 | 0 | 0 | 0 |
| 5146 | Spinach, raw | 1 cup | 30 | 7 | 1 | 1 | 1 | 0 | 0 | 0 |
| 90525 | Squash, zucchini w/ skin, slices, raw | 1 ea | 118 | 20 | 1 | 4 | 1 | 0 | 0.1 | 0 |
| 6924 | Sweet potato, baked in skin w/ salt | 0.5 cup | 100 | 92 | 2 | 21 | 3 | 0 | 0.1 | 0 |
| 5180 | Tomato sauce, canned | 0.5 cup | 123 | 30 | 2 | 7 | 2 | 0 | 0 | 0 |
| 90532 | Tomato, red, ripe, whole, raw | 1 pce | 15 | 3 | 0 | 1 | 0 | 0 | 0 | 0 |
| 5306 | Yam, peeled, raw | 0.5 cup | 75 | 88 | 1 | 21 | 3 | 0 | 0 | 0 |

*Soy and Soy Products*

| MDA Code | Food Name | Amt | Wt (g) | Ener (kcal) | Prot (g) | Carb (g) | Fiber (g) | Fat (g) | Sat (g) | Chol (g) |
|---|---|---|---|---|---|---|---|---|---|---|
| 7564 | Tempeh | 0.5 cup | 83 | 160 | 15 | 8 | | 9 | 1.8 | 0 |
| 7015 | Soybeans, cooked | 1 cup | 172 | 298 | 29 | 17 | 10 | 15 | 2.2 | 0 |
| 7542 | Tofu, firm, silken, 1" slice | 3 oz | 85 | 53 | 6 | 2 | 0 | 2 | 0.3 | 0 |

**Meals and Dishes**

| MDA Code | Food Name | Amt | Wt (g) | Ener (kcal) | Prot (g) | Carb (g) | Fiber (g) | Fat (g) | Sat (g) | Chol (g) |
|---|---|---|---|---|---|---|---|---|---|---|
| 92216 | Tortellini with cheese filling | 1 cup | 108 | 332 | 15 | 51 | 2 | 8 | 3.9 | 45 |
| 57658 | Chili con carne w/ beans, canned entree | 1 cup | 222 | 269 | 16 | 25 | 9 | 12 | 3.9 | 29 |
| 57703 | Chili, vegetarian chili w/ beans, canned entree/Hormel | 1 cup | 247 | 205 | 12 | 38 | 10 | 1 | 0.1 | 0 |
| 57068 | Macaroni and cheese, unprepared/Kraft | 1 ea | 70 | 260 | 9 | 48 | 1 | 4 | 2 | 15 |
| 70958 | Stir fry, rice & vegetables, w/ soy sauce/Hanover | 1 cup | 137 | 130 | 5 | 27 | 2 | 0 | | |
| 70943 | Beef & bean burrito/Las Campanas | 1 ea | 114 | 296 | 9 | 38 | 1 | 12 | 4.2 | 13 |
| 16195 | Chicken & vegetables/Lean Cuisine | 1 ea | 297 | 232 | 20 | 26 | 4 | 5 | 1.9 | 30 |
| 70917 | Hot Pockets, beef & cheddar, frozen | 1 ea | 142 | 403 | 16 | 39 | | 20 | 8.8 | 53 |
| 70918 | Hot Pockets, croissant pocket w/ chicken, broccoli, & cheddar, frozen | 1 ea | 128 | 301 | 11 | 39 | 1 | 11 | 3.4 | 37 |
| 56757 | Lasagna w/ meat sauce/Stouffer's | 1 ea | 215 | 249 | 17 | 27 | 2 | 8 | 4.1 | 28 |
| 11029 | Macaroni & beef in tomato sauce/Lean Cuisine | 1 ea | 283 | 326 | 21 | 40 | 3 | 9 | 3.7 | 32 |
| 5587 | Mashed potatoes, from granules w/ milk, prep w/ water & margarine | 0.5 cup | 105 | 122 | 2 | 17 | 1 | 5 | 1.2 | 2 |
| 70898 | Pizza, pepperoni, frozen | 1 ea | 146 | 432 | 16 | 42 | 3 | 22 | 7 | 22 |
| 56703 | Spaghetti w/ meat sauce/Lean Cuisine | 1 ea | 326 | 284 | 14 | 49 | 5 | 4 | 1.1 | 13 |

**Snack Foods**

| MDA Code | Food Name | Amt | Wt (g) | Ener (kcal) | Prot (g) | Carb (g) | Fiber (g) | Fat (g) | Sat (g) | Chol (g) |
|---|---|---|---|---|---|---|---|---|---|---|
| 10051 | Beef jerky | 1 pce | 20 | 81 | 7 | 2 | 0 | 5 | 2.1 | 10 |
| 63331 | Breakfast bars, oats, sugar, raisins, coconut | 1 ea | 43 | 200 | 4 | 29 | 1 | 8 | 5.5 | 0 |
| 61251 | Cheese puffs and twists, corn based, low fat | 1 oz | 28 | 123 | 2 | 21 | 3 | 3 | 0.6 | 0 |
| 44032 | Chex snack mix | 1 cup | 42 | 180 | 4 | 32 | 2 | 4 | 0.6 | |
| 23059 | Granola bar, hard, plain | 1 ea | 24 | 115 | 2 | 16 | 1 | 5 | 0.6 | 0 |
| 23104 | Granola bar, soft, plain | 1 ea | 28 | 126 | 2 | 19 | 1 | 5 | 2.1 | 0 |

| MDA Code | Food Name | Amt | Wt (g) | Ener (kcal) | Prot (g) | Carb (g) | Fiber (g) | Fat (g) | Sat (g) | Chol (g) |
|---|---|---|---|---|---|---|---|---|---|---|
| 44012 | Popcorn, air-popped | 1 cup | 8 | 31 | 1 | 6 | 1 | 0 | 0 | 0 |
| 44076 | Potato chips, plain, no salt | 1 oz | 28 | 152 | 2 | 15 | 1 | 10 | 3.1 | 0 |
| 5437 | Potato chips, sour cream & onion | 1 oz | 28 | 151 | 2 | 15 | 1 | 10 | 2.5 | 2 |
| 44015 | Pretzels, hard | 5 pcs | 30 | 114 | 3 | 24 | 1 | 1 | 0.1 | 0 |
| 44021 | Rice cake, brown rice, plain, salted | 1 ea | 9 | 35 | 1 | 7 | 0 | 0 | 0.1 | 0 |
| 44058 | Trail mix, regular | 0.25 cup | 38 | 173 | 5 | 17 | | 11 | 2.1 | 0 |

### Soups

| MDA Code | Food Name | Amt | Wt (g) | Ener (kcal) | Prot (g) | Carb (g) | Fiber (g) | Fat (g) | Sat (g) | Chol (g) |
|---|---|---|---|---|---|---|---|---|---|---|
| 50398 | Beef barley, canned/Progresso Healthy Classics | 1 cup | 241 | 142 | 11 | 20 | 3 | 2 | 0.7 | 19 |
| 50081 | Chicken noodle, chunky, canned | 1 cup | 240 | 89 | 8 | 10 | 1 | 2 | 1 | 12 |
| 50085 | Chicken rice, chunky, ready to eat, canned | 1 cup | 240 | 127 | 12 | 13 | 1 | 3 | 1 | 12 |
| 50088 | Chicken vegetable, chunky, canned | 1 cup | 240 | 166 | 12 | 19 | | 5 | 1.4 | 17 |
| 90238 | Chicken, chunky, canned | 1 cup | 240 | 170 | 12 | 17 | 1 | 6 | 1.9 | 29 |
| 50697 | Cup of Noodles, ramen, chicken flavor, dry/Nissin | 1 ea | 64 | 296 | 6 | 37 | | 14 | 6.3 | |
| 50009 | Minestrone, canned, made w/ water | 1 cup | 241 | 82 | 4 | 11 | 1 | 3 | 0.6 | 2 |
| 92163 | Ramen noodle, any flavor, dehydrated, dry | 0.5 cup | 38 | 166 | 4 | 24 | 1 | 6 | 2.9 | 0 |
| 50043 | Tomato vegetable, from dry mix, made w/ water | 1 cup | 253 | 56 | 2 | 10 | 1 | 1 | 0.4 | 0 |
| 50028 | Tomato, canned, made w/ water | 1 cup | 244 | 73 | 2 | 16 | 1 | 1 | 0.2 | 0 |
| 50014 | Vegetable beef, canned, made w/ water | 1 cup | 244 | 76 | 5 | 10 | 2 | 2 | 0.8 | 5 |
| 50013 | Vegetarian vegetable, canned, made w/ water | 1 cup | 241 | 67 | 2 | 12 | 1 | 2 | 0.3 | 0 |

### Desserts

| MDA Code | Food Name | Amt | Wt (g) | Ener (kcal) | Prot (g) | Carb (g) | Fiber (g) | Fat (g) | Sat (g) | Chol (g) |
|---|---|---|---|---|---|---|---|---|---|---|
| 62904 | Brownie, commercially prepared, square, lrg, 2-3/4" × 7/8" | 1 ea | 56 | 227 | 3 | 36 | 1 | 9 | 2.4 | 10 |
| 46062 | Cake, chocolate, homemade, w/o icing | 1 pce | 95 | 352 | 5 | 51 | 2 | 14 | 5.2 | 55 |
| 46091 | Cake, yellow, homemade, w/o icing | 1 pce | 68 | 245 | 4 | 36 | 0 | 10 | 2.7 | 37 |
| 71337 | Doughnut, cake, w/ chocolate icing, lrg, 3 1/2" | 1 ea | 57 | 258 | 3 | 29 | 1 | 14 | 7.7 | 11 |
| 45525 | Doughnut, cake, glazed/sugared, med, 3" | 1 ea | 45 | 192 | 2 | 23 | 1 | 10 | 2.7 | 14 |
| 47026 | Animal crackers/Arrowroot/Tea Biscuits | 10 ea | 12 | 56 | 1 | 9 | 0 | 2 | 0.4 | 0 |
| 90636 | Chocolate chip cookie, commercially prepared 3.5" to 4" | 1 ea | 40 | 190 | 2 | 26 | 1 | 9 | 4 | 0 |
| 47006 | Chocolate sandwich cookie, creme filled | 3 ea | 30 | 141 | 2 | 21 | 1 | 6 | 1.9 | 0 |
| 62905 | Fig bar, 2 oz | 1 ea | 57 | 197 | 2 | 40 | 3 | 4 | 0.6 | 0 |
| 90640 | Oatmeal cookie, commercially prepared, 3-1/2" to 4" | 1 ea | 25 | 112 | 2 | 17 | 1 | 5 | 1.1 | 0 |
| 47010 | Peanut butter cookie, homemade, 3" | 1 ea | 20 | 95 | 2 | 12 | | 5 | 0.9 | 6 |
| 62907 | Sugar cookie, refrigerated dough, baked | 1 ea | 23 | 111 | 1 | 15 | 0 | 5 | 1.4 | 7 |
| 57894 | Pudding, chocolate, ready to eat | 1 ea | 113 | 160 | 2 | 26 | 0 | 5 | 1.4 | 1 |
| 2612 | Pudding, vanilla, ready to eat | 1 ea | 113 | 147 | 2 | 26 | 0 | 4 | 1.1 | 1 |
| 2651 | Rice pudding, ready to eat | 1 ea | 142 | 168 | 5 | 28 | 1 | 4 | 2.5 | 26 |
| 57902 | Tapioca pudding, ready to eat | 1 ea | 113 | 147 | 2 | 25 | 0 | 4 | 1.1 | 1 |
| 71819 | Frozen yogurts, chocolate, nonfat | 1 cup | 186 | 199 | 8 | 37 | 4 | 1 | 0.9 | 7 |
| 72124 | Frozen yogurts, flavors other than chocolate | 1 cup | 174 | 221 | 5 | 38 | 0 | 6 | 4 | 23 |
| 2010 | Ice cream, light, vanilla, soft serve | 0.5 cup | 88 | 111 | 4 | 19 | 0 | 2 | 1.4 | 11 |
| 90723 | Ice popsicle | 1 ea | 59 | 47 | 0 | 11 | 0 | 0 | 0 | 0 |
| 42264 | Cinnamon rolls w/ icing, refrigerated dough/Pillsbury | 1 ea | 44 | 145 | 2 | 23 | 0 | 5 | 1.5 | 0 |
| 71299 | Croissant, butter | 1 ea | 67 | 272 | 5 | 31 | 2 | 14 | 7.8 | 45 |
| 45572 | Danish, cheese | 1 ea | 71 | 266 | 6 | 26 | 1 | 16 | 4.8 | 16 |
| 45593 | Toaster pastry, Pop Tart, apple-cinnamon/Kellogg | 1 ea | 52 | 205 | 2 | 37 | 1 | 5 | 0.9 | 0 |
| 23014 | Chocolate syrup, fudge-type | 2 Tbs | 38 | 133 | 2 | 24 | 1 | 3 | 1.5 | 0 |
| 510 | Whipped cream topping, pressurized | 2 Tbs | 8 | 19 | 0 | 1 | 0 | 2 | 1 | 6 |
| 54387 | Whipped topping, frozen, low fat | 2 Tbs | 9 | 21 | 0 | 2 | 0 | 1 | 1.1 | 0 |

### Fats, Oils, and Condiments

| MDA Code | Food Name | Amt | Wt (g) | Ener (kcal) | Prot (g) | Carb (g) | Fiber (g) | Fat (g) | Sat (g) | Chol (g) |
|---|---|---|---|---|---|---|---|---|---|---|
| 90210 | Butter, unsalted | 1 Tbs | 14 | 100 | 0 | 0 | 0 | 11 | 7.2 | 30 |
| 8084 | Oil, vegetable, canola | 1 Tbs | 14 | 124 | 0 | 0 | 0 | 14 | 1 | 0 |
| 8008 | Oil, olive, salad or cooking | 1 Tbs | 14 | 119 | 0 | 0 | 0 | 14 | 1.9 | 0 |
| 8111 | Oil, safflower, salad or cooking, greater than 70% oleic | 1 Tbs | 14 | 120 | 0 | 0 | 0 | 14 | 0.8 | 0 |
| 44483 | Shortening, household | 1 Tbs | 13 | 113 | 0 | 0 | 0 | 13 | 3.2 | 0 |
| 1708 | Barbecue sauce, original | 2 Tbs | 36 | 63 | 0 | 15 | | 0 | | |
| 27001 | Ketchup | 1 ea | 6 | 6 | 0 | 2 | 0 | 0 | 0 | 0 |
| 53523 | Cheese sauce, ready to eat | 0.25 cup | 63 | 110 | 4 | 4 | 0 | 8 | 3.8 | 18 |
| 54388 | Cream substitute, powdered, light | 1 Tbs | 6 | 25 | 0 | 4 | 0 | 1 | 0.2 | 0 |
| 50939 | Gravy, brown, homestyle, canned | 0.25 cup | 60 | 25 | 1 | 3 | | 1 | 0.3 | 2 |
| 23003 | Jelly | 1 Tbs | 19 | 51 | 0 | 13 | 0 | 0 | 0 | 0 |

| MDA Code | Food Name | Amt | Wt (g) | Ener (kcal) | Prot (g) | Carb (g) | Fiber (g) | Fat (g) | Sat (g) | Chol (g) |
|---|---|---|---|---|---|---|---|---|---|---|
| 25002 | Maple syrup | 1 Tbs | 20 | 52 | 0 | 13 | 0 | 0 | 0 | 0 |
| 44476 | Margarine, regular, 80% fat, with salt | 1 Tbs | 14 | 101 | 0 | 0 | 0 | 11 | 2 | 0 |
| 8145 | Mayonnaise, safflower/soybean oil | 1 Tbs | 14 | 99 | 0 | 0 | 0 | 11 | 1.2 | 8 |
| 8502 | Miracle Whip, light/Kraft | 1 Tbs | 16 | 37 | 0 | 2 | 0 | 3 | 0.5 | 4 |
| 435 | Mustard, yellow | 1 tsp | 5 | 3 | 0 | 0 | 0 | 0 | 0 | 0 |
| 23042 | Pancake syrup | 1 Tbs | 20 | 47 | 0 | 12 | 0 | 0 | 0 | 0 |
| 23172 | Pancake syrup, reduced kcal | 1 Tbs | 15 | 25 | 0 | 7 | 0 | 0 | 0 | 0 |
| 53524 | Pasta sauce, spaghetti/marinara | 0.5 cup | 125 | 109 | 2 | 17 | 3 | 3 | 0.9 | 2 |
| 53646 | Salsa picante, mild | 2 Tbs | 30 | 8 | 0 | 1 | 0 | 0 | | 0 |
| 504 | Sour cream, cultured | 2 Tbs | 29 | 56 | 1 | 1 | 0 | 6 | 3.3 | 15 |
| 53063 | Soy sauce | 1 Tbs | 18 | 11 | 2 | 1 | 0 | 0 | 0 | 0 |
| 53652 | Taco sauce, red, mild | 1 Tbs | 16 | 7 | 0 | 1 | 0 | 0 | | 0 |
| 53004 | Teriyaki sauce | 1 Tbs | 18 | 16 | 1 | 3 | 0 | 0 | 0 | 0 |
| 8024 | Thousand Island, regular | 1 Tbs | 16 | 58 | 0 | 2 | 0 | 5 | 0.8 | 4 |
| 8013 | Blue/Roquefort cheese, regular | 2 Tbs | 31 | 146 | 0 | 1 | 0 | 16 | 2.5 | 9 |
| 90232 | French, regular | 1 Tbs | 12 | 56 | 0 | 2 | 0 | 6 | 0.7 | 0 |
| 44498 | Italian, fat-free | 1 Tbs | 14 | 7 | 0 | 1 | 0 | 0 | 0 | 0 |
| 44696 | Ranch, reduced fat | 1 Tbs | 15 | 29 | 0 | 3 | 0 | 2 | 0.2 | 2 |
| 8035 | Vinegar & oil, homemade | 2 Tbs | 31 | 140 | 0 | 1 | 0 | 16 | 2.8 | 0 |
| **Fast Food** | | | | | | | | | | |
| 6177 | Baked potato, topped w/ cheese sauce | 1 ea | 296 | 474 | 15 | 47 | | 29 | 10.6 | 18 |
| 56629 | Burrito w/ beans & cheese | 1 ea | 93 | 189 | 8 | 27 | | 6 | 3.4 | 14 |
| 66023 | Burrito w/ beans, cheese, & beef | 1 ea | 102 | 166 | 7 | 20 | | 7 | 3.6 | 62 |
| 66024 | Burrito w/ beef | 1 ea | 110 | 262 | 13 | 29 | | 10 | 5.2 | 32 |
| 56600 | Biscuit w/ egg sandwich | 1 ea | 136 | 373 | 12 | 32 | 1 | 22 | 4.7 | 245 |
| 66029 | Biscuit w/ egg, cheese, & bacon sandwich | 1 ea | 144 | 433 | 17 | 35 | 0 | 25 | 8.5 | 239 |
| 66013 | Cheeseburger, double, condiments & vegetables | 1 ea | 166 | 417 | 21 | 35 | | 21 | 8.7 | 60 |
| 56649 | Cheeseburger, large, one meat patty w/ condiments & vegetables | 1 ea | 219 | 451 | 25 | 37 | 3 | 23 | 8.5 | 74 |
| 15063 | Chicken, breaded, fried, dark meat (drumstick or thigh) | 3 oz | 85 | 248 | 17 | 9 | | 15 | 4.1 | 95 |
| 15064 | Chicken, breaded, fried, light meat (breast or wing) | 3 oz | 85 | 258 | 19 | 10 | | 15 | 4.1 | 77 |
| 56000 | Chicken filet, plain | 1 ea | 182 | 515 | 24 | 39 | | 29 | 8.5 | 60 |
| 56635 | Chimichanga w/ beef & cheese | 1 ea | 183 | 443 | 20 | 39 | | 23 | 11.2 | 51 |
| 5461 | Cole slaw | 0.75 cup | 99 | 151 | 1 | 15 | 2 | 10 | 1.6 | 4 |
| 56606 | Croissant w/ egg & cheese sandwich | 1 ea | 127 | 368 | 13 | 24 | | 25 | 14.1 | 216 |
| 56607 | Croissant w/ egg, cheese, & bacon sandwich | 1 ea | 129 | 413 | 16 | 24 | | 28 | 15.4 | 215 |
| 66021 | Enchilada w/ cheese | 1 ea | 163 | 319 | 10 | 29 | | 19 | 10.6 | 44 |
| 66020 | Enchirito w/ cheese, beef, & beans | 1 ea | 193 | 344 | 18 | 34 | | 16 | 7.9 | 50 |
| 66031 | English muffin w/ cheese & sausage sandwich | 1 ea | 115 | 389 | 15 | 29 | 1 | 24 | 9.4 | 49 |
| 66010 | Fish sandwich w/ tartar sauce | 1 ea | 158 | 431 | 17 | 41 | | 23 | 5.2 | 55 |
| 90736 | French fries fried in vegetable oil, medium | 1 ea | 134 | 427 | 5 | 50 | 5 | 23 | 5.3 | 0 |
| 56638 | Frijoles (beans) w/ cheese | 0.5 cup | 84 | 113 | 6 | 14 | | 4 | 2 | 18 |
| 56664 | Ham & cheese sandwich | 1 ea | 146 | 352 | 21 | 33 | | 15 | 6.4 | 58 |
| 56662 | Hamburger, large, double, w/ condiments & vegetables | 1 ea | 226 | 540 | 34 | 40 | | 27 | 10.5 | 122 |
| 56659 | Hamburger, one patty w/ condiments & vegetables | 1 ea | 110 | 279 | 13 | 27 | | 13 | 4.1 | 26 |
| 66007 | Hamburger, plain | 1 ea | 90 | 266 | 13 | 30 | 1 | 10 | 3.2 | 30 |
| 5463 | Hash browns | 0.5 cup | 72 | 235 | 2 | 23 | 2 | 16 | 3.6 | 0 |
| 66004 | Hot dog, plain | 1 ea | 98 | 242 | 10 | 18 | | 15 | 5.1 | 44 |
| 2032 | Ice cream sundae, hot fudge | 1 ea | 158 | 284 | 6 | 48 | 0 | 9 | 5 | 21 |
| 6185 | Mashed potatoes | 0.5 cup | 121 | 100 | 3 | 20 | | 1 | 0.6 | 2 |
| 56639 | Nachos w/ cheese | 7 pcs | 113 | 346 | 9 | 36 | | 19 | 7.8 | 18 |
| 6176 | Onion rings, breaded, fried | 8 pcs | 78 | 259 | 3 | 29 | | 15 | 6.5 | 13 |
| 6173 | Potato salad | 0.33 cup | 95 | 108 | 1 | 13 | | 6 | 1 | 57 |
| 56619 | Pizza w/ pepperoni 12" | 1 pce | 108 | 275 | 15 | 30 | | 11 | 3.4 | 22 |
| 66003 | Roast beef sandwich, plain | 1 ea | 139 | 346 | 22 | 33 | | 14 | 3.6 | 51 |
| 56671 | Submarine sandwich, cold cuts | 1 ea | 228 | 456 | 22 | 51 | | 19 | 6.8 | 36 |
| 57531 | Taco | 1 ea | 171 | 371 | 21 | 27 | | 21 | 11.4 | 56 |
| 71129 | Shake, chocolate, 12 fl. oz | 1 ea | 250 | 318 | 8 | 51 | 5 | 9 | 5.8 | 32 |
| 71132 | Shake, vanilla, 12 fl. oz | 1 ea | 250 | 370 | 8 | 49 | 2 | 16 | 9.9 | 58 |

**Source:** This food composition table has been prepared for Pearson Education, Inc., and is copyrighted by ESHA Research in Salem, Oregon, the developer of the MyDietAnalysis software program.

# GLOSSARY

**% Daily Values (%DVs)** Percentages on food and supplement labels identifying how much of each listed nutrient or other substance a serving of food contributes to a 2,000 calorie/day diet.

**5-year relative survival rates** The percent of people alive (usually 5 years) after diagnosis divided by the percentage expected to survive with the absence of cancer based on normal life expectancy.

**abortion** Termination of a pregnancy by expulsion or removal of an embryo or fetus from the uterus.

**abstinence** Refraining from a behavior.

**accountability** Accepting responsibility for personal decisions, choices, and actions.

**acid deposition** Acidification process that occurs when pollutants are deposited by precipitation, clouds, or directly on the land.

**acquaintance rape** Any rape in which the rapist is known to the victim (replaces the formerly used term *date rape*).

**acquired immune deficiency syndrome (AIDS)** A disease caused by a retrovirus, the human immunodeficiency virus (HIV), that attacks the immune system, reducing the number of helper T cells and leaving the victim vulnerable to infections, malignancies, and neurological disorders.

**active euthanasia** "Mercy killing" in which a person or organization knowingly acts to end the life of a terminally ill person.

**acupressure** Technique of traditional Chinese medicine that uses application of pressure to selected points along meridians to balance energy.

**acupuncture** Technique of traditional Chinese medicine that involves the placement of long, thin needles to affect flow of energy (*qi*) along energy pathways (meridians) within the body.

**acute stress** The short-term physiological response to an immediate perceived threat.

**adaptive response** The physiological adjustments the body makes in an attempt to restore homeostasis.

**adaptive thermogenesis** Theoretical mechanism by which the brain regulates metabolic activity according to caloric intake.

**addiction** Persistent, compulsive dependence on a behavior or substance, including mood-altering behaviors or activities, despite ongoing negative consequences.

**advance directive** A document that stipulates an individual's wishes about medical care; used to make treatment decisions when and if the individual becomes physically unable to voice his or her preferences.

**aerobic capacity (power)** The functional status of the cardiorespiratory system; refers specifically to the volume of oxygen the muscles consume during exercise.

**aerobic exercise** Prolonged exercise that requires oxygen to make energy for activity.

**aggravated rape** Rape that involves one or multiple attackers, strangers, weapons, or physical beating.

**aggressive driving** Driving involving a combination of moving traffic offenses that endanger other persons or property.

**aging** The patterns of life changes that occur in members of all species as they grow older.

**alcohol abuse** Use of alcohol in a way that interferes with work, school, or personal relationships or that entails violations of the law.

**alcohol poisoning (acute alcohol intoxication)** Potentially lethal BAC that inhibits the brain's ability to control consciousness, respiration, and heart rate; usually occurs as a result of drinking a large amount of alcohol in a short period of time.

**alcohol use disorder** Refers to problem drinking so severe that at least two or more alcohol-related issues are present, such as engaging in risky behaviors, having problems at work or school, or issues with relationships.

**alcoholic hepatitis** Condition resulting from prolonged use of alcohol in which the liver is inflamed; can be fatal.

**Alcoholics Anonymous (AA)** Organization whose goal is to help alcoholics stop drinking; includes auxiliary branches such as Al-Anon and Alateen.

**alcoholism (alcohol dependence)** Condition in which personal and health problems related to alcohol use are severe, and stopping alcohol use results in withdrawal symptoms.

**allergies** Hypersensitivity reactions in which the body produces antibodies to a normally harmless substance in the environment.

**allergist** Medical doctor focusing on the diagnosis and treatment of allergies.

**allopathic medicine** Conventional, Western medical practice; in theory, based on scientifically validated methods and procedures.

**allostatic load** Wear and tear on the body caused by prolonged or excessive stress responses.

**alternative insemination** Fertilization procedure accomplished by depositing semen from a partner or donor into a woman's vagina via a thin tube.

**altruism** Giving of oneself out of genuine-concern for others.

**alveoli** Tiny air sacs of the lungs where gas exchange occurs (oxygen enters the body and carbon dioxide is removed).

**Alzheimer's disease (AD)** A chronic condition involving changes in nerve fibers of the brain that results in mental deterioration.

**amenorrhea** The absence of menstruation.

**amino acids** The nitrogen-containing building blocks of protein.

**amniocentesis** Medical test in which a small amount of fluid is drawn from the amniotic sac to test for Down syndrome and other genetic abnormalities.

**amniotic sac** Protective pouch surrounding the fetus.

**amphetamines** A large and varied group of synthetic agents that stimulate the central nervous system.

**anabolic steroids** Artificial forms of the hormone testosterone that promote muscle growth and strength.

**anal intercourse** Insertion of the penis into the anus.

**anaphylaxis** A severe sensitivity reaction to an allergic trigger such as a bee sting, or chemical reaction that can begin a few minutes after exposure.

**androgyny** Combination of traditional masculine and feminine traits in a single person.

**anemia** Condition that results from the body's inability to produce adequate hemoglobin.

**aneurysm** A weakened blood vessel that may bulge under pressure and, in severe cases, burst.

**angina pectoris** Chest pain occurring as a result of reduced oxygen flow to the heart.

**angiography** A technique for examining blockages in heart arteries.

**angioplasty** A technique in which a catheter with a balloon at the tip is inserted into a clogged artery; the balloon is inflated to flatten fatty deposits against artery walls and a stent is typically inserted to keep the artery open.

**ankle-brachial index (ABI)** Test in which a measure of blood pressure in your feet is compared to blood pressure in your arm to determine blood flow.

**annual percentage rate (APR)** The yearly cost of a credit card account, including interest and certain fees, expressed as a percentage.

**anorexia nervosa** Eating disorder characterized by deliberate food restriction, self–starvation, or extreme exercising to achieve weight loss, as well as an extremely distorted body image.

**antagonism** A type of interaction in which two or more drugs work at the same receptor site so that one blocks the action of the other.

**antibiotic/antimicrobial resistance** The ability of microbes to resist the effects of drugs, meaning the germs grow and proliferate.

**antibiotics** Medicines used to kill microorganisms, such as bacteria.

**antibodies** Substances produced by the body that are individually matched to specific antigens.

**antigen** Substance capable of triggering an immune response.

**antioxidants** Substances believed to protect against oxidative stress and resultant cell damage.

**anxiety disorders** Mental illness characterized by persistent feelings of threat and worry in coping with everyday problems.

**appetite** The learned desire to eat; normally accompanies hunger but is more psychological than physiological.

**appraisal** The interpretation and evaluation of information provided to the brain by the senses.

**arrhythmia** An irregularity in heartbeat.

**arteries** Vessels that carry blood away from the heart to other regions of the body.

**arterioles** Branches of the arteries.

**arteriosclerosis** A general term for thickening and hardening of the arteries.

**arthritis** Painful inflammatory disease of the joints.

**asbestos** Mineral compound that separates into stringy fibers and lodges in the lungs, where it can cause disease.

**asexual** A person who does not experience sexual attraction.

**Asperger syndrome** A form of high functioning autism.

**asthma** A chronic respiratory disease that blocks airflow into and out of the lungs, characterized by attacks of wheezing, shortness of breath, and coughing spasms.

**atherosclerosis** Condition characterized by deposits of fatty substances (plaque) in the inner lining of an artery.

**atria (singular: atrium)** The heart's two upper chambers, which receive blood.

**attention-deficit (hyperactivity) disorder (ADD/ADHD)** A learning disability usually associated with school-aged children, often involving difficulty concentrating, organizing things, listening to instructions, and remembering details.

**autism spectrum disorder (ASD)** A neurodevelopmental disorder (an impairment in brain development) where individuals learn and grow intellectually throughout their lives, but struggle to master communication and social behavior skills, impacting school and work performance.

**autoerotic behaviors** Sexual self-stimulation.

**autoimmune disease** Disease caused by an overactive immune response against the body's own cells.

**autoinoculate** Transmit a pathogen from one part of your body to another part.

**autonomic nervous system (ANS)** The portion of the central nervous system that regulates body functions that a person does not normally consciously control.

**avian influenza** An infectious disease of birds with some strains capable of crossing the species barrier and causing severe illness in humans that come in contact with bird droppings or fluids.

**Ayurveda (Ayurvedic medicine)** A comprehensive system of medicine, originating in ancient India, that places equal emphasis on the body, mind, and spirit and strives to restore the body's innate harmony through diet, exercise, meditation, herbs, massage, sun exposure, and controlled breathing.

**Babesiosis** A tick-borne disease whose parasite attacks and destroys red blood cells.

**background distressors** Environmental stressors of which people are often unaware.

**bacteria (singular: bacterium)** Simple, single-celled microscopic organisms; about 100 known species of bacteria cause disease in humans.

**barbiturates** Drugs that depress the central nervous system, have sedative and hypnotic effects, and are less safe than benzodiazepines.

**barrier methods** Contraceptive methods that block the meeting of egg and sperm by means of a physical barrier (such as a condom), a chemical barrier (such as a spermicide), or both.

**basal metabolic rate (BMR)** The rate of energy expenditure by a body at complete rest in a neutral environment.

**behavioral methods** Temporary or permanent abstinence or planning intercourse in accordance with fertility patterns.

**belief** Appraisal of the relationship between some object, action, or idea and some attribute of that object, action, or idea.

**benign** Harmless; refers to a noncancerous tumor.

**benzodiazepines** A class of central nervous system depressant drugs with sedative, hypnotic, and muscle relaxant effects; also called *tranquilizers*.

**bereavement** The loss or deprivation experienced by a survivor when a loved one dies.

**bidis** Hand-rolled flavored cigarettes.

**binge drinking** A pattern of drinking alcohol that brings BAC to 0.08 gram-percent or above; corresponds to consuming five or more drinks (adult male) or four or more drinks (adult female) in 2 hours.

**binge-eating disorder** A type of eating disorder characterized by gorging on food once a week or more, but not typically followed by a purge.

**biofeedback** A technique using a machine to self-monitor physical responses to stress.

**biopsy** Removal and examination of a tissue sample to determine if a cancer is present.

**biopsychosocial model of addiction** Theory of the relationship between an addict's biological (-genetic) nature and psychological and environmental influences.

**bipolar disorder** Form of mood disorder characterized by alternating mania and depression; also called *manic depressive illness*.

**birth control** Methods that reduce the likelihood of conception or childbirth.

**bisexual** Experiencing attraction to and preference for sexual activity with people of both sexes.

**blood alcohol concentration (BAC)** The ratio of alcohol to total blood volume; the factor used to measure the physiological and behavioral effects of alcohol.

**body composition** The relative proportions of fat and fat-free (muscle, bone, water, organs) tissues in the body.

**body dysmorphic disorder (BDD)** Psychological disorder characterized by an obsession with one's appearance and a distorted view of one's body or with a minor or imagined flaw in appearance.

**body image** How you see yourself in your mind, what you believe about your appearance, and how you feel about your body.

**body mass index (BMI)** A number calculated from a person's weight and height that is used to assess risk for possible present or future health problems.

**brain death** The irreversible cessation of all functions of the entire brainstem.

**bronchitis** An inflammation and eventual scarring of the lining of the bronchial tubes.

**budget** An estimate of spending and income over a set period of time.

**budget deficit** Spending more money than your income.

**budget surplus** Money left over for savings after expenses have been paid.

**bulimia nervosa** Eating disorder characterized by binge eating followed by inappropriate purging measures or compensatory behavior, such as vomiting or excessive exercise, to prevent weight gain.

**bullying** Unwanted aggressive behavior, real or perceived power imbalances, and repeating behaviors designed to demean others.

**burnout** A state of physical and mental exhaustion resulting from unrelenting stress.

**C-reactive protein (CRP)** A protein whose blood levels rise in response to inflammation.

**caffeine** A stimulant drug that is legal in the United States and found in coffee, tea, chocolate, energy drinks, and certain medications.

**calorie** A unit of measure that indicates the amount of energy obtained from a particular food.

**cancer** A large group of diseases characterized by the uncontrolled growth and spread of abnormal cells.

**candidiasis** Yeast-like fungal infection often transmitted sexually; also called *moniliasis* or *yeast infection*.

**cap and trade** Policies designed to set limits, or caps, on how much carbon large industrial polluters can emit.

**capillaries** Minute blood vessels that branch out from the arterioles and venules; their thin walls permit exchange of oxygen, carbon dioxide, nutrients, and waste products among body cells.

**capitation** Prepayment of a fixed monthly amount for each patient without regard to the type or number of services provided.

**carbohydrates** Basic nutrients that supply the body with glucose, the energy molecule most readily used by cells.

**carbon footprint** Amount of greenhouse gases produced, usually expressed in equivalent tons of carbon dioxide emissions.

**carbon monoxide** Gas found in cigarette smoke that reduces the ability of blood to carry oxygen.

**carbon tax** The price a government charges for the carbon content in fuels.

**carcinogens** Cancer-causing agents.

**Carcinoma** *in situ* Localized, non-invasive carcinoma

**cardiometabolic risks** Risk factors that impact both the cardiovascular system and the body's biochemical metabolic processes.

**cardiomyopathy** Damage to heart muscle.

**cardiopulmonary resuscitation (CPR)** Emergency technique to provide lifesaving chest compression and mouth-to-mouth resuscitation when an individual has stopped breathing and has no pulse. Use of an automated external defibrillator to reset the heart rhythm may be required.

**cardiorespiratory fitness** The ability of the heart, lungs, and blood vessels to supply oxygen to skeletal muscles during sustained physical activity.

**cardiovascular disease (CVD)** Disease of the heat and blood vessels.

**cardiovascular system** Organ system, consisting of the heart and blood vessels, that transports nutrients, oxygen, hormones, metabolic wastes, and enzymes throughout the body.

**carpal tunnel syndrome** An occupational injury in which the median nerve in the wrist becomes irritated, causing numbness, tingling, and pain in the fingers and hands.

**carrying capacity of the Earth** The largest population that can be supported indefinitely given the resources available in the environment.

**cataracts** Clouding of the lens that interrupts the focusing of light on the retina, resulting in blurred vision or eventual blindness.

**celiac disease** An inherited immune disorder causing malabsorption of nutrients from the small intestine and triggered by the consumption of gluten.

**celibacy** State of not engaging in sexual activity.

**cell-mediated immunity** Aspect of immunity that is mediated by specialized white blood cells that attack pathogens and antigens directly.

**cervical cap** Small cup made of silicone that is designed to fit snugly over the entire cervix; should always be used with spermicide.

**cervix** Lower end of the uterus that opens into the vagina.

**cesarean section (C-section)** Surgical birthing procedure in which a baby is removed through an incision made in the mother's abdominal wall and uterus.

**chancre** Sore often found at the site of syphilis infection.

**chemotherapy** The use of drugs to kill cancerous cells.

**chewing tobacco** Stringy form of tobacco that is placed in the mouth and then sucked or chewed.

**child abuse** Deliberate, intentional words or actions that cause harm, potential for harm, or threat of harm to a child.

**child maltreatment** Any act or series of acts of commission or omission by a parent or caregiver that results in harm, potential for harm, or threat of harm to a child.

**chiropractic medicine** System of treatment that involves manipulation of the spine and neuromuscular structures to promote proper energy flow.

**chlamydia** Bacterially caused STI of the urogenital tract.

**chlorofluorocarbons (CFCs)** Chemicals that contribute to the depletion of the atmospheric ozone layer.

**cholesterol** A type of lipid classified as a sterol and found in animal-based foods; it is also synthesized by the body.

**chorionic villus sampling (CVS)** Prenatal test that involves snipping tissue from the fetal sac to be analyzed for genetic defects.

**chronic bronchitis** Bronchitis type diagnosed when a person has bronchitis symptoms for at least 3 months of the year in 2 consecutive years and which is part of the COPD grouping.

**chronic disease** A disease that typically begins slowly, progresses, and persists, with a variety of signs and symptoms that can be treated but not cured by medication.

**chronic lower respiratory disease (CLRD)** Lung diseases such as emphysema, asthma, and some forms of bronchitis that are long term in nature.

**chronic mood disorder** Experience of persistent emotional states, such as sadness, despair, hopelessness, or euphoria.

**chronic obstructive pulmonary disease (COPD)** A collection of chronic lung diseases, including emphysema and chronic bronchitis, where some form of obstruction interferes with a person's ability to breathe.

**chronic stress** An ongoing state of physiological arousal in response to ongoing or numerous perceived threats.

**circadian rhythm** The 24-hour cycle by which you are accustomed to going to sleep, waking up, and performing habitual behaviors.

**cirrhosis** The last stage of liver disease associated with chronic heavy alcohol use, during which liver cells die and damage becomes permanent.

**cisgender** Having a gender identity that matches the biological sex an individual is assigned at birth.

**climate change** A shift in typical weather patterns that includes fluctuations in seasonal temperatures, rain or snowfall amounts, and the occurrence of catastrophic storms.

**clitoris** Pea-sized nodule of tissue located at the top of the labia minora; central to sexual arousal and pleasure in women.

**club drugs** Synthetic analogs that produce similar effects of existing drugs.

**codependence** A self-defeating relationship pattern in which a person is controlled by an addict's addictive behavior.

**cognitive restructuring** The modification of thoughts, ideas, and beliefs that contribute to stress.

**cognitive-behavioral therapy for chronic insomnia (CBTi)** A form of therapy that helps people better understand the thoughts and feelings that influence their behaviors and focus on changing habits that disrupt sleep.

**cohabitation** Intimate partners living together without being married.

**collective connectedness** Feeling that you are part of a community or group.

**collective violence** Violence perpetrated by groups against other groups.

**colonization** The process of bacteria or some other infectious organisms establishing themselves in a host without causing infection.

**common-law marriage** Cohabitation lasting a designated period of time (usually 7 years) that is considered legally binding in some states.

**comorbidities** The presence of other illnesses at the same time and other conditions that might affect treatment outcomes.

**complementary health approaches** Health care practices and products commonly used together with conventional medicine.

**complementary medical systems** Broad approaches to health care that reflect specific theories of physiology, health, and disease that have developed outside the influence of conventional medicine.

**complete proteins** Proteins that contain all nine of the essential amino acids.

**complex carbohydrates** Polysaccharides composed of long chains of glucose.

**compulsion** Preoccupation with a behavior and an overwhelming need to perform it.

**compulsive buying disorder** Compulsive shopping and spending disorder that cannot be controlled.

**compulsive exercise** Disorder characterized by a compulsion to engage in excessive amounts of exercise and feelings of guilt and anxiety if the level of exercise is perceived as inadequate.

**computerized axial tomography (CAT) scan** A scan by a machine that uses radiation to view internal organs not normally visible in X-rays.

**conception** Fertilization of an ovum by a sperm.

**conflict** Emotional state that arises when opinions differ or the behavior of one person interferes with the behavior of another.

**conflict resolution** Concerted effort by all parties to constructively resolve differences or points of contention.

**congeners** Forms of alcohol that are metabolized more slowly than ethanol and produce toxic by-products.

**congenital cardiovascular defect** Cardiovascular problem that is present at birth.

**congestive heart failure (CHF)** An abnormal cardiovascular condition that reflects impaired cardiac pumping and blood flow; pooling blood leads to congestion in body tissues.

**consummate love** A relationship that combines intimacy, compassion, and commitment.

**contemplation** Practice of concentrating the mind on a spiritual or ethical question or subject, a view of the natural world, or an icon or other image representative of divinity.

**contraception** Methods of preventing conception.

**contraceptive sponge** Contraceptive device containing nonoxynol-9 and made of polyurethane foam that fits over the cervix to create a barrier against sperm.

**coping** Managing events or conditions to lessen the physical or psychological effects of excess stress.

**coronary bypass surgery** A surgical technique whereby a blood vessel taken from another part of the body is implanted to bypass a clogged coronary artery.

**coronary heart disease (CHD)** A narrowing of the small blood vessels that supply blood

**coronary thrombosis** A clot or an atherosclerotic narrowing that blocks a coronary artery.

**corpus luteum** Cells that form from the remains of the graafian follicle following ovulation; it secretes estrogen and progesterone during the second half of the menstrual cycle.

**cortisol** Hormone released by the adrenal glands that makes stored nutrients more readily available to meet energy demands.

**countering** Substituting a desired behavior for an undesirable one.

**Cowper's glands** Glands that secrete a pre-ejaculate fluid that lubricates the urethra and neutralizes any acid remaining in the urethra after urination.

**credit** The ability to buy goods and services in advance of paying for them.

**credit limit** The maximum amount a person can charge on a credit card account.

**credit score** Numerical measure of an individual's creditworthiness.

**Crohn's disease** An autoimmune inflammatory bowel disease that can affect several parts of the gastrointestinal tract as well as other body organs and systems.

**cross-tolerance** Development of a tolerance to one drug that reduces the effects of another, similar drug.

**cunnilingus** Oral stimulation of a woman's genitals.

**cyberstalking** Stalking that occurs online or via smart technology/tracking devices.

**death** The permanent ending of all vital functions.

**debt** Money owed for goods and services that have been purchased.

**dehydration** Loss of water from body tissues.

**delayed ejaculation** Persistent difficulty in reaching orgasm despite normal desire and stimulation.

**delirium tremens (DTs)** State of confusion, delusions, and agitation brought on by withdrawal from alcohol.

**dementia** Progressive brain impairment that interferes with memory and normal intellectual functioning.

**denial** Inability to perceive or accurately interpret the self-destructive effects of the addictive behavior.

**dental dam** A square of latex used as a barrier between the mouth and a woman's genitals to protect from vaginal fluids.

**dentist** Physician who diagnoses and treats diseases of the teeth, gums, and oral cavity.

**Depo-Provera, Depo-subQ Provera** Injectable method of birth control that lasts for 3 months.

**depressants** Drugs that slow down the activity of the central nervous and muscular systems and cause sleepiness or calmness.

**determinants of health** The range of personal, social, economic, and environmental factors that influence health status.

**detoxification** The early abstinence period during which an addict adjusts physically and cognitively to being free from the influences of the addiction.

**diabetes mellitus** A group of diseases characterized by elevated blood glucose levels.

**diaphragm** Latex, cup-shaped device designed to cover the cervix and block access to the uterus; should always be used with spermicide.

**diastolic blood pressure** The lower number in the fraction that measures blood pressure, indicating pressure on the walls of the arteries during the relaxation phase of heart activity.

**Dietary Reference Intakes (DRIs)** Set of recommended intakes for each nutrient published by the Institute of Medicine.

**dietary supplements** Products taken by mouth and containing dietary ingredients such as vitamins and minerals that are intended to supplement existing diets.

**digestive process** The process by which the body breaks down foods into smaller components and either absorbs or excretes them.

**dilation and evacuation (D&E)** Abortion technique that uses a combination of instruments and vacuum aspiration.

**dioxins** Highly toxic chlorinated hydrocarbons contained in herbicides and produced during certain industrial processes.

**dipping** Placing a small amount of chewing tobacco between the lower lip and teeth for rapid nicotine absorption.

**disaccharides** Sugars combining two monosaccharides; include lactose, maltose, and sucrose.

**discretionary spending** Goods and services that are not life essentials.

**discrimination** Actions that deny equal treatment or opportunities to a group, often based on prejudice.

**disease prevention** Actions or behaviors designed to keep people from getting sick.

**disordered eating** A pattern of atypical eating behaviors that is used to achieve or maintain a lower body weight.

**distillation** Process in which alcohol vapors are condensed and mixed with water to make hard liquor.

**distracted driving** Driving while performing any nondriving activity that has the potential to distract someone from the primary task of driving and increase the risk of crashing.

**distress** Stress that can have a detrimental effect on health; negative stress.

**domestic violence** The use of force to control and maintain power over another person in the home environment, including both actual harm and the threat of harm.

**Down syndrome** A genetic disorder caused by the presence of an extra chromosome that results in mental disabilities and distinctive physical characteristics.

**downshifting** Taking a step back and simplifying a lifestyle that is hectic, packed with pressure and stress, and focused on trying to keep up; also known as *voluntary simplicity*.

**drug abuse** Excessive use of a drug.

**drug misuse** Use of a drug for a purpose for which it was not intended.

**drug resistance** The ability of pathogens to resist the effects of drugs, meaning the germs grow and proliferate.

**drugs** Nonfood, non-nutritional substances that are intended to affect the structure or function of the mind or body through chemical action.

**drunkorexia** A colloquial term to describe the combination of disordered eating, excessive physical activity, and heavy alcohol consumption.

**dying** Process of decline in body functions that results in the death of an organism.

**dyscalculia** A learning disability involving math.

**dysfunctional families** Families in which there is violence; physical, emotional, or sexual abuse; significant parental discord; or other negative family interactions.

**dysgraphia** A learning disability involving writing; individuals may have difficulty putting letters, numbers, and words on a page into order.

**dyslexia** Language-based learning disorder that can pose problems for reading, writing, and spelling.

**dysmenorrhea** Condition of pain or discomfort in the lower abdomen just before or during menstruation.

**dyspareunia** Pain experienced by women during intercourse.

**dyspnea** Shortness of breath, usually associated with disease of the heart or lungs.

**eating disorder** A psychiatric disorder characterized by severe disturbances in body image and eating behaviors.

**ecological or public health model** A view of health in which diseases and other negative health events are seen as a result of an individual's interaction with his or her social and physical environment.

**ecosystem** Collection of physical (nonliving) and biological (living) components of an environment and the relationships between them.

**ectopic pregnancy** Dangerous condition that results from the implantation of a fertilized egg outside the uterus, usually in a fallopian tube.

**ejaculation** Propulsion of semen from the penis.

**ejaculatory duct** Tube formed by the junction of the seminal vesicle and the vas deferens that carries semen to the urethra.

**electrocardiogram (ECG)** A record of the electrical activity of the heart; may be measured during a stress test.

**embolus** When a clot becomes dislodged and moves through the circulatory system.

**embryo** Fertilized egg from conception through the eighth week of development.

**emergency contraceptive pills (ECPs)** Drugs taken within 3 to 5 days after unprotected intercourse to prevent pregnancy.

**emotional health** The feeling part of psychological health; includes your emotional reactions to life.

**emotional intelligence (EI)** The ability to anticipate, identify, understand, and manage emotions in positive ways (yours and others'); to communicate effectively with others; and to empathize and avoid/diffuse potential conflicts.

**emotions** Intensified feelings or complex patterns of feelings.

**emphysema** A respiratory disease in which the alveoli become distended or ruptured and are no longer functional.

**enablers** People who knowingly or unknowingly protect addicts from the natural consequences of their behavior.

**endemic** Describing a disease that is always present to some degree.

**endometriosis** Disorder in which endometrial tissue establishes itself outside the uterus.

**endometrium** Soft, spongy matter that makes up the uterine lining.

**endorphins** Opioid-like hormones that are manufactured in the human body and contribute to natural feelings of well-being.

**energy therapies** Therapies using energy fields, such as electromagnetic fields or biofields.

**enhanced greenhouse effect** Warming of the earth's surface due to increases in greenhouse gas concentration in the atmosphere, which traps more of the sun's radiation than is normal.

**environmental tobacco smoke (ETS)** Smoke from tobacco products, including second-hand and mainstream smoke.

**epidemic** Disease outbreak that affects many people in a community or region at the same time.

**epidemiological triad of disease** The process explaining how a disease is likely to occur, including characteristics of the host (health of immune system, etc.), the agent (pathogen and its virulence), and the environment (whether conditions are conducive to spread)

**epididymis** Duct system atop the testis where sperm mature.

**epilepsy** A neurological disorder caused by abnormal electrical brain activity; can be accompanied by altered consciousness or convulsions.

**epinephrine** Also called *adrenaline*, a hormone that stimulates body systems in response to stress.

**episodic acute stress** The state of regularly reacting with wild, acute stress about one thing or another.

**erectile dysfunction (ED)** Difficulty in achieving or maintaining an erection sufficient for intercourse.

**ergogenic drugs** Substances believed to enhance athletic performance.

**erogenous zones** Areas of the body that, when touched, lead to sexual arousal.

**essential amino acids** The nine nitrogen-containing building blocks of human proteins that must be obtained from foods.

**estimated average glucose (eAG)** A method for reporting A1C test results that gives the average blood glucose levels for the testing period using the same units (milligrams per deciliter [mg/dL]) that patients are used to seeing in self-administered glucose tests.

**estrogen** Hormone secreted by the ovaries that controls the menstrual cycle and assists in the development of female secondary sex characteristics.

**ethnoviolence** Violence directed at persons affiliated with a particular ethnic group.

**ethyl alcohol (ethanol)** Addictive drug produced by fermentation that is the intoxicating substance in alcoholic beverages.

**eustress** Stress that presents opportunities for personal growth; positive stress.

**evidence-based medicine** Decisions regarding patient care based on clinical expertise, patient values, and current best scientific evidence.

**excessive daytime sleepiness** A disorder characterized by unusual patterns of falling asleep during normal waking hours.

**exercise** Planned, structured, and repetitive bodily movement done to improve or maintain one or more components of physical fitness.

**exercise addicts** People who exercise compulsively to try to meet needs of nurturance, intimacy, self-esteem, and self-competency.

**exercise metabolic rate (EMR)** The energy expenditure that occurs during exercise.

**extensively drug-resistant TB (XDR-TB)** Form of TB that is resistant to nearly all existing antibiotics.

**fallopian tubes** Tubes that extend from near the ovaries to the uterus; site of fertilization and passageway for fertilized eggs.

**family of origin** People present in the household during a child's first years of life—usually parents and siblings.

**fellatio** Oral stimulation of a man's genitals.

**female athlete triad** A syndrome of three interrelated health problems seen in some female athletes: disordered eating, amenorrhea, and poor bone density.

**female condom** Single-use nitrile sheath for internal use during vaginal intercourse to catch semen upon ejaculation.

**female orgasmic disorder** A woman's inability to achieve orgasm.

**fermentation** Process in which yeast organisms break down plant sugars to yield ethanol.

**fertility awareness methods (FAMs)** Several types of birth control that require alteration of sexual behavior rather than chemical or physical intervention in the reproductive process.

**fertility rate** Average number of births a female in a certain population has during her reproductive years.

**fertility** A person's ability to reproduce.

**fetal alcohol syndrome (FAS)** Pattern of birth defects, learning, and behavioral problems in a child caused by the mother's alcohol consumption during pregnancy.

**fetus** Developing human from the ninth week until birth.

**fiber** The indigestible portion of plant foods that helps move food through the digestive system and softens stools by absorbing water.

**fibrillation** A sporadic, quivering pattern of heartbeat that results in extreme inefficiency in moving blood through the cardiovascular system.

**fight-or-flight response** Physiological arousal response in which the body prepares to combat or escape a real or perceived threat.

**FITT** Acronym for frequency, intensity, time, and type; the terms that describe the essential components of a program or plan to improve a health-related component of physical fitness.

**flexibility** The range of motion, or the amount of movement possible, at a particular joint or series of joints.

**food allergy** An immune response against a specific food that the majority of people can eat without problem.

**food desert** Neighborhood or region where people lack access to affordable, nutritious food.

**food insecure** Lack of access to an adequate supply of nourishing food.

**food intolerance** Difficulty or inability to digest certain foods due to problems with the physical, hormonal, or biochemical systems in your digestive tract.

**formaldehyde** Colorless, strong-smelling gas released through outgassing; causes respiratory and other health problems.

**fossil fuels** Carbon-based material used for energy; includes oil, coal, and natural gas.

**frequency** As part of the FITT prescription, refers to how many days per week a person should exercise.

**functional foods** Foods believed to have specific health benefits beyond their basic nutrients.

**fungi** A group of multicellular and unicellular organisms that obtain their food by infiltrating the bodies of other organisms, both living and dead; several microscopic varieties are pathogenic.

**gambling disorder** Compulsive gambling that cannot be controlled.

**gamma knife surgery** *See* stereotactic radiosurgery.

**gastroesophageal reflux disease (GERD)** Chronic condition in which stomach acid backflows into the esophagus, causing heartburn and potential damage to the esophagus.

**gay** Sexual orientation involving primary attraction to people of the same sex.

**gender** Characteristics and actions associated with being feminine or masculine as defined by the society or culture in which one lives.

**gender identity** Personal sense or awareness of being masculine or feminine, a male or a female.

**gender roles** Expression of maleness or femaleness in everyday life that conforms to society's expectations.

**gender-role stereotypes** Generalizations concerning how men and women should express themselves and the characteristics each possess.

**general adaptation syndrome (GAS)** The pattern followed in the physiological response to stress, consisting of the alarm, resistance, and exhaustion phases.

**generalized anxiety disorder (GAD)** A constant sense of worry that may cause restlessness, difficulty in concentrating, tension, and other symptoms.

**generic drugs** Medications marketed by chemical names rather than brand names.

**genetically modified (GM) foods** Foods derived from organisms whose DNA has been altered using genetic engineering techniques.

**genital warts** Warts that appear in the genital area or the anus; caused by the human papillomavirus (HPV).

**gerontology** The study of individual and collective aging processes.

**gestational diabetes** Form of diabetes mellitus in which women who have never had diabetes have high blood sugar (glucose) levels during pregnancy.

**giardiasis** A common waterborne protozoan disease.

**glaucoma** Elevation of pressure within the eyeball, leading to hardening of the eyeball, impaired vision, and possible blindness.

**global warming** A type of climate change in which average temperatures increase.

**globesity** Global rates of obesity.

**glycogen** The polysaccharide form in which glucose is stored in the liver and, to a lesser extent, in muscles.

**gonads** Reproductive organs that produce germ cells and sex hormones; in males, the testes, and in females, the ovaries.

**gonorrhea** Second most common bacterial STI in the United States; if untreated, may cause sterility.

**graafian follicle** Mature ovarian follicle that contains a fully developed egg (ovum).

**greenhouse gases** Gases that accumulate in the atmosphere, where they contribute to global warming by trapping heat near the earth's surface.

**grief** An individual's reaction to significant loss, including one's own impending death, the death of a loved one, or a quasi-death experience; grief can involve mental, physical, social, or emotional responses.

**grief work** The process of accepting the reality of a person's death and coping with memories of the deceased.

**grit** A combination of passion and perseverance for a singularly important goal.

**hallucinogens** Substances capable of creating auditory or visual distortions and unusual changes in mood, thoughts, and feelings.

**hangover** Physiological reaction to excessive drinking, including headache, upset stomach, anxiety, depression, diarrhea, and thirst.

**happiness** A collective term for several positive states in which individuals actively embrace the world around them.

**hate crime** Crime targeted against a particular societal group and motivated by bias against that group.

**hay fever** A chronic allergy-related respiratory disorder that is most prevalent when ragweed and flowers bloom, also known as *pollen allergy*.

**hazardous waste** Toxic waste that poses a hazard to humans or to the environment.

**hazing** Any activity expected of someone joining or participating in a group that humiliates, degrades, abuses, or endangers them regardless of a person's willingness to participate.

**health** The ever-changing process of achieving individual potential in the physical, social, emotional, intellectual, spiritual, and environmental dimensions.

**health belief model (HBM)** Model for explaining how beliefs may influence behaviors.

**health care–associated infections (HAIs)** Infections that arise in patients while in treatment for other conditions.

**health disparities** Differences in the incidence, prevalence, mortality, and burden of diseases and other health conditions among specific population groups.

**health–income gradient** The relationship between the health of individuals or communities and income, where health outcomes increase as income increases.

**health promotion** The combined educational, organizational, procedural, environmental, social, and financial supports that help individuals and groups reduce negative health behaviors and promote positive change.

**health-related quality of life** Assessment of impact of health status—including elements of physical, mental, emotional, and social function—on overall quality of life.

**healthy life expectancy** Expected number of years of full health remaining at a given age, such as at birth.

**healthy weight** Those with BMIs of 18.5 to 24.9, the range of lowest statistical health risk.

**heat cramps** Involuntary and forcible muscle contractions that occur during or following exercise in hot and/or humid weather.

**heat exhaustion** A heat stress illness caused by significant dehydration resulting from exercise in hot and/or humid conditions.

**heatstroke** A deadly heat stress illness resulting from dehydration and overexertion in hot and/or humid conditions.

**hepatitis** A viral disease in which the liver becomes inflamed, producing symptoms such as fever, headache, and possibly jaundice.

**herpes simplex virus type 1 (HSV-1)** A family of infections characterized by sores or eruptions on the skin.

**herpes simplex virus type 2 (HSV-2)** (also called *genital herpes*) STI caused by the herpes simplex virus.

**heterosexual** Experiencing primary attraction to and preference for sexual activity with people of the opposite sex.

**high-density lipoproteins (HDLs)** Compounds that facilitate the transport of cholesterol in the blood to the liver for metabolism and elimination from the body.

**histamine** Chemical substance that dilates blood vessels, increases mucus secretions, and triggers other allergy symptoms.

**homeopathy (homeopathic medicine)** Unconventional Western system of medicine based on the principle that "like cures like" and the "law of minimum dose."

**homeostasis** A balanced physiological state in which all the body's systems function smoothly.

**homicide** Death that results from intent to injure or kill.

**homocysteine** An amino acid normally present in the blood that, when found at high levels, may be related to higher risk of cardiovascular disease.

**homosexual** Experiencing primary attraction to and preference for sexual activity with people of the same sex.

**hormonal methods** Contraceptive methods that introduce synthetic hormones into a woman's system to prevent ovulation, thicken cervical mucus, or prevent a fertilized egg from implanting.

**hormone replacement therapy (menopausal hormone therapy)** Use of synthetic estrogens and progesterone to compensate for hormonal changes in a woman's body during menopause.

**hospice** A concept of end-of-life care designed to maximize quality of life and help dying people have peace, comfort, and dignity.

**hostility** The cognitive, affective, and behavioral tendencies toward anger, distrust, and cynicism.

**human chorionic gonadotropin (HCG)** Hormone detectable in blood or urine samples of a mother within the first few weeks of pregnancy.

**human immunodeficiency virus (HIV)** The virus that causes AIDS by infecting helper T cells.

**human papillomavirus (HPV)** A group of viruses, many of which are transmitted sexually; some types of HPV can cause genital warts or cervical cancer.

**humoral immunity** Aspect of immunity that is mediated by antibodies secreted by white blood cells.

**hunger** The physiological impulse to seek food.

**hymen** In some women, a thin tissue covering the vaginal opening.

**hyperglycemia** Elevated blood glucose level.

**hyperlipidemia** Abnormally high blood levels of *lipids*, which are non-water-soluble molecules, such as fats and cholesterol.

**hyperplasia** A condition characterized by an excessive number of fat cells.

**hypertension** Sustained elevated blood pressure.

**hypertrophy** The act of swelling or increasing in size, as with cells.

**Hypnosis** A trancelike state that allows people to become unusually responsive to suggestion.

**hyponatremia or water intoxication** Overconsumption of water, which leads to a dilution of sodium concentration in the blood, with potentially fatal results.

**hypothalamus** Area of the brain located near the pituitary gland; works in conjunction with the pituitary gland to control reproductive functions.

**hypothermia** Potentially fatal condition caused by abnormally low body core temperature.

**hysterectomy** Surgical removal of the uterus.

**ideal cardiovascular health (ICH)** The absence of clinical indicators of CVD and the presence of certain favorable behavioral and health factor metrics.

**identity theft** Stealing personal information and using it without permission.

**idiopathic** Of unknown cause.

**imagined rehearsal** Practicing, through mental imagery, to become better able to perform a task in actuality.

**immunocompetence** The ability of the immune system to respond to attack.

**immunocompromised** A condition in which the immune system becomes weakened and vulnerable to pathogens entering and gaining a foothold in the body.

**immunotherapy** Treatment strategies based on the concept of regulating the immune system,

as by administering antibodies or desensitization shots of allergens.

**impaired driving** Driving under the influence of alcohol or other drugs.

**in vitro fertilization (IVF)** Fertilization of an egg in a nutrient medium and subsequent transfer back to the mother's body.

**incomplete proteins** Proteins that lack one or more of the essential amino acids.

**incubation period** The time between exposure to a disease and the appearance of symptoms.

**infection** The state of pathogens being established in or on a host and causing disease.

**infertility** Inability to conceive after a year or more of trying.

**inflammatory bowel disease (IBD)** A group of disorders in which the intestines become inflamed.

**influenza** A common viral disease of the respiratory tract.

**informed consent** Acknowledgment that you have been told of the potential risks and benefits of a recommended test or treatment, understand what you have been told, and agree to the care.

**inhalants** Chemical vapors that are sniffed or inhaled to produce highs.

**inhalation** The introduction of drugs through the respiratory tract.

**inhibited sexual desire** Lack of sexual appetite or lack of interest and pleasure in sexual activity.

**inhibition** A drug interaction in which the effects of one drug are eliminated or reduced by the presence of another drug at the same receptor site.

**injection** The introduction of drugs into the body via a hypodermic needle.

**insomnia** A disorder characterized by difficulty in falling asleep quickly, frequent arousals during sleep, or early-morning awakening.

**insulin** Hormone secreted by the pancreas and required by body cells for the uptake and storage of glucose.

**insulin resistance** State in which body cells fail to respond to the effects of insulin; obesity increases the risk that cells will become insulin resistant.

**intact dilation and extraction (D&X)** Late-term abortion procedure in which the body of the fetus is extracted up to the head and then the contents of the cranium are aspirated.

**integrative medicine** The integration of complementary health approaches into conventional health care in a purposeful way.

**intended nationally determined contributions (INDCs)** Goals that individual countries said they would achieve in order to do their part in the Paris Agreement and reduce global emissions.

**intensity** As part of the FITT prescription, refers to how hard or how much effort is needed when a person exercises.

**intentional injuries** Injury, death, or psychological harm inflicted with the intent to harm.

**interest** A fee paid by the borrower of a loan.

**Internet addiction** Compulsive use of the computer, personal digital device, cell phone, or other forms of technology to access the Internet for activities such as e-mail, games, shopping, social networking, or blogging.

**intersexuality** Not exhibiting exclusively male or female sex characteristics; also known as disorders of sexual development (DSD).

**intervention** A planned confrontation with an alcoholic led by a professional counselor in which family members and/or friends try to get the alcoholic to face the reality of his or her problem and to seek help.

**intestate** Dying without a will.

**intimate connectedness** A relationship that makes you feel who you are is affirmed.

**intimate partner violence (IPV)** Describes physical, sexual, or psychological harm by a current or former partner or spouse.

**intimate relationships** Relationships with family members, friends, and romantic partners, characterized by behavioral interdependence, need fulfillment, emotional attachment, and emotional availability.

**intolerance** A type of interaction in which two or more drugs produce extremely uncomfortable reactions.

**intrauterine device (IUD)** A device, often T-shaped, that is inserted in the uterus to prevent pregnancy.

**intrauterine methods** Contraceptive methods that insert a device into the uterus to either introduce synthetic hormones or interfere with sperm movement or egg fertilization.

**ionizing radiation** Electromagnetic waves and particles having short wavelengths and energy high enough to ionize atoms.

**irritable bowel syndrome (IBS)** A functional bowel disorder caused by certain foods or stress that is characterized by nausea, pain, gas, or diarrhea.

**ischemia** Reduced oxygen supply to a body part or organ.

**jealousy** Aversive reaction evoked by a real or imagined relationship involving a person's partner and a third person.

**labia majora** "Outer lips," or folds of tissue covering the female sexual organs.

**labia minora** "Inner lips," or folds of tissue just inside the labia majora.

**leach** To dissolve and filter through soil.

**lead** Highly toxic metal found in emissions from lead smelters and processing plants; also sometimes found in pipes or paint in older buildings.

**learned behavioral tolerance** The ability of heavy drinkers to modify behavior so they appear to be sober even when they have high BAC levels.

**learned helplessness** Pattern of responding to situations by giving up because of repeated failure in the past.

**learned optimism** Teaching oneself to think positively.

**lesbian** Sexual orientation involving attraction of women to other women.

**leukoplakia** Condition characterized by leathery white patches inside the mouth, which is produced by contact with irritants in tobacco juice.

**libido** Sexual drive or desire.

**life expectancy** Expected number of years of life remaining at a given age, such as at birth.

**living will** A type of advance directive.

**locavore** A person who primarily eats food grown or produced locally.

**locus of control** The location, *external* (outside oneself) or *internal* (within oneself), that an individual perceives as the source and underlying cause of events in his or her life.

**loss of control** Inability to reliably predict whether a particular instance of involvement with the addictive substance or behavior will be healthy or damaging.

**low back pain (LBP)** Pain or discomfort in the lumbosacral region (lowest vertebrae) of the back.

**low sperm count** Sperm count below 20 million sperm per milliliter of semen.

**low-density lipoproteins (LDLs)** Compounds that facilitate the transport cholesterol in the blood to body cells.

**Lyme disease** Tick-borne disease whose symptoms may range from none, to a rash or bull's-eye lesion and flu-like symptoms, to chronic arthritis, blindness, and long-term disability

**lymphocyte** A type of white blood cell involved in the immune response.

**macrophage** A type of white blood cell that ingests foreign material.

**macular degeneration** Breakdown of the macula, the light-sensitive part of the retina responsible for sharp, direct vision.

**magnetic resonance imaging (MRI)** A device that uses magnetic fields, radio waves, and computers to generate an image of internal tissues of the body for diagnostic purposes without the use of radiation.

**mainstream smoke** Smoke that is drawn through tobacco while inhaling.

**major depression** Severe depressive disorder with physical effects such as sleep disturbance and exhaustion and mental effects such as the inability to concentrate; also called *clinical depression.*

**male condom** Single-use sheath of thin latex or other material designed to fit over an erect penis and to catch semen upon ejaculation.

**malignant** Very dangerous or harmful; refers to a cancerous tumor.

**malpractice** Improper or negligent treatment by a health practitioner that results in loss, injury, or harm to the patient.

**managed care** Type of health insurance plan based on coordination of care and cost-reduction strategies; emphasizes health education and preventive care.

**manipulative therapies** Treatments involving manipulation or movement of one or more body structures or the whole body.

**marijuana** Chopped leaves and flowers of *Cannabis indica* or *Cannabis sativa* plants (hemp); a psychoactive stimulant.

**massage therapy** Soft tissue manipulation by trained therapists for relaxation and healing.

**masturbation** Manual stimulation of genitals.

**measles** A viral disease that produces symptoms such as an itchy rash and a high fever.

**Medicaid** A federal–state matching funds program that provides health insurance to low-income people.

**medical abortion** Termination of a pregnancy during the first 9 weeks using hormonal medications that cause the embryo to be expelled from the uterus.

**medical model** A view of health in which health status focuses primarily on the individual and a biological or diseased-organ perspective.

**Medicare** A federal health insurance program that covers people over the age of 65, permanently disabled people, and people with end-stage kidney failure.

**meditation** A relaxation technique that involves deep breathing and concentration.

**melatonin** A hormone that affects sleep cycles, increasing drowsiness.

**menarche** The first menstrual period.

**meningitis** An infection of the meninges, the membranes that surround the brain and spinal cord.

**menopause** Permanent cessation of menstruation; generally occurs after age 45.

**mental health** The thinking part of psychological health; includes your values, attitudes, and beliefs.

**mental illnesses** Disorders that disrupt thinking, feeling, moods, and behaviors and that impair daily functioning.

**MET** A metabolic equivalent or resting level of energy expenditure $(3.5 \ ml \cdot kg^{-1} \cdot min^{-1})$

**metabolic syndrome (MetS)** A group of metabolic conditions occurring together that increases a person's risk of heart disease, stroke, and diabetes.

**metastasize** To spread from one area to different areas of the body.

**methicillin-resistant *Staphylococcus aureus* (MRSA)** Highly resistant form of staph infection that is growing in international prevalence.

**migraine** A type of headache characterized by debilitating symptoms that possibly results from alternating dilation and constriction of blood vessels.

**mindfulness** Practice of purposeful, nonjudgmental observation in which we are fully present in the moment.

**minerals** Inorganic, indestructible elements that aid physiological processes and build body structures.

**minority stress perspective** Theory positing that minority stress may be partially explained by disparities and the chronic stress inherent in populations where rejection, alienation, and hostility persist.

**miscarriage** Loss of the fetus before it is viable; also called *spontaneous abortion.*

**modeling** Learning specific behaviors by watching others perform them.

**monogamy** Exclusive sexual involvement with one partner.

**monosaccharides** One-molecule sugars; include fructose and glucose.

**mons pubis** Fatty tissue covering the pubic bone in females; in physically mature women, the mons is covered with coarse hair.

**morbidly obese** Having a body weight 100 percent or more above healthy recommended levels; in an adult, having a BMI of 40 or more.

**mortality** The proportion of deaths to population.

**motivation** A social, cognitive, and emotional force that directs human behavior.

**mourning** The culturally prescribed behavior patterns for the expression of grief.

**multidrug-resistant TB (MDR-TB)** Form of TB that is resistant to at least two of the best antibiotics available.

**mumps** A once common viral disease that is controllable by vaccination.

**municipal solid waste (MSW)** Solid waste such as durable and nondurable goods, containers and packaging, food waste, yard waste, and miscellaneous waste from residential, commercial, institutional, and industrial sources.

**muscle dysmorphia** Body image disorder in which men believe that their bodies are insufficiently lean or muscular.

**muscular endurance** A muscle's ability to exert force repeatedly without fatiguing or the ability to sustain a muscular contraction for a length of time.

**muscular strength** The amount of force that a muscle is capable of exerting in one contraction.

**mutant cells** Cells that differ in form, quality, or function from normal cells.

**myocardial infarction (MI; heart attack)** A blockage of normal blood supply to an area in the heart.

**mysophobia** (or *germophobia*) An obsessive fear of becoming infected with germs.

**narcolepsy** A neurological disorder that causes people to fall asleep involuntarily during the day.

**natural disaster** Any extreme environmental event that causes widespread destruction of land and/or property, injuries, and sometimes deaths.

**naturopathy (naturopathic medicine)** System of medicine in which practitioners work to support the body's innate healing mechanisms and use treatment approaches such as diet, exercise, and massage that are minimally invasive.

**negative consequences** Severe problems associated with addiction, such as physical damage, legal trouble, financial problems, academic failure, or family dissolution.

**neglect** Failure to provide a child's basic needs such as food, clothing, shelter, and medical care.

**neoplasm** A new growth of tissue that results from uncontrolled, abnormal cellular development and serves no physiological function.

**neurotransmitters** Biochemical messengers that bind to specific receptor sites on nerve cells.

**Nexplanon (Implanon)** A plastic capsule inserted in a woman's upper arm that releases a low dose of progestin to prevent pregnancy.

**nicotine** Primary stimulant chemical in tobacco products that is highly addictive.

**nicotine poisoning** Symptoms often experienced by beginning smokers, including dizziness, diarrhea, lightheadedness, rapid and erratic pulse, clammy skin, and nausea and vomiting.

**nicotine withdrawal** Symptoms including nausea, headaches, irritability, and intense tobacco cravings suffered by nicotine-addicted individuals who stop using tobacco.

**nocturia** Frequent urination at night caused by an overactive bladder.

**non-REM (NREM) sleep** A period of restful sleep dominated by slow brain waves; during non-REM sleep, rapid eye movement is rare.

**nonionizing radiation** Electromagnetic waves having relatively long wavelengths and enough energy to move atoms around or cause them to vibrate.

**nonpoint source pollutant** Pollutant that runs off or seeps into waterways from broad areas of land.

**nonverbal communication** Unwritten and unspoken messages, both intentional and unintentional.

**nuclear meltdown** Accident that results when the temperature in the core of a nuclear reactor increases enough to melt the nuclear fuel and breach the containment vessel.

**nurse practitioner (NP)** Nurse with advanced training obtained through either a master's degree program or a specialized nurse practitioner program.

**nurse** Health professional who provides patient care in a variety of settings.

**nutrients** The constituents of food that sustain humans physiologically: water, proteins, carbohydrates, fats, vitamins, and minerals.

**nutrition** The science that investigates the relationship between physiological function and the essential elements of foods eaten.

**NuvaRing** Soft, flexible ring inserted into the vagina that releases hormones similar to those in oral contraceptives; each ring is worn for 3 weeks.

**obesity** Having a body weight more than 20 percent above healthy recommended levels; in an adult, a BMI of 30 or more.

**obesogenic** Refers to environmental conditions that promote obesity, such as the availability of unhealthy foods, social and cultural norms that lead to high calorie consumption, and lack of physical activity.

**obsession** Excessive preoccupation with an addictive object or behavior.

**obsessive–compulsive disorder (OCD)** Form of anxiety disorder characterized by recurrent, unwanted thoughts and repetitive behaviors.

**oncogenes** Suspected cancer-causing genes present on chromosomes.

**one repetition maximum (1 RM)** The amount of weight or resistance that can be lifted or moved only once.

**open relationship** A relationship in which partners agree that sexual involvement can occur outside the relationship.

**ophthalmologist** Physician who specializes in the medical and surgical care of the eyes, including prescriptions for lenses.

**opioids** Drugs that induce sleep, relieve pain, and produce euphoria; includes derivatives of opium and synthetics with similar chemical properties; also called *narcotics.*

**opium** The parent drug of the opioids; made from the seedpod resin of the opium poppy.

**opportunistic infection** An infection that occurs when the immune system is vulnerable and the organism is able to gain a foothold in the body.

**optometrist** Eye specialist whose practice is limited to prescribing and fitting lenses to correct vision problems.

**oral contraceptives** Pills containing synthetic hormones that prevent ovulation by regulating hormones.

**oral ingestion** Intake of drugs through the mouth.

**organic** Grown without use of toxic and persistent pesticides, chemicals, or hormones.

**orthorexia nervosa** An eating disorder characterized by fixation on food quality and purity.

**osteoarthritis (OA)** Progressive deterioration of bones and joints that has been associated with the wear-and-tear theory of aging; also called *degenerative joint disease.*

**osteopath** General practitioner who receives training similar to a medical doctor's but with an emphasis on the skeletal and muscular systems; may use spinal manipulation as part of treatment.

**osteoporosis** A degenerative bone disorder characterized by increasingly porous bones.

**other specified feeding or eating disorder (OSFED)** Eating disorders that are a true psychiatric illness but that do not fit the strict diagnostic criteria for anorexia nervosa, bulimia nervosa, or binge-eating disorder.

**ovarian follicles** Areas within the ovary in which individual eggs develop.

**ovaries** Almond-sized organs that house developing eggs and produce hormones.

**overload** A condition in which a person feels overly pressured by demands.

**overuse injuries** Injuries that result from the cumulative effects of day-after-day stresses placed on tendons, muscles, and joints.

**overweight** Having a body weight more than 10 percent above healthy recommended levels; in an adult, having a BMI of 25 to 29.9.

**ovulation** The point of the menstrual cycle at which a mature egg ruptures through the ovarian wall.

**ovum** Single mature egg cell.

**palliative care** Any form of medical care focused on relieving the pain, symptoms, and stress of serious illness in order to improve the quality of life for patients and their families.

**palliative treatment** Those treatments designed to treat or ease symptoms but not cure the disease.

**pancreas** Organ that secretes digestive enzymes into the small intestine and hormones, including insulin, into the bloodstream.

**pandemic** Global epidemic of a disease.

**panic attack** Severe anxiety reaction in which a particular situation, often for unknown reasons, causes terror.

**Pap test** A procedure in which cells taken from the cervical region are examined for abnormal cellular activity.

**parasitic worms** The largest of the pathogens, most of which are more a nuisance than a threat.

**parasomnias** All of the abnormal things that disrupt sleep, not including some of the major problems such as sleep apnea.

**parasympathetic nervous system** Branch of the autonomic nervous system responsible for slowing systems stimulated by the stress response.

**passive euthanasia** The intentional withholding of treatment that would prolong life.

**pathogen** A disease-causing agent.

**pelvic inflammatory disease (PID)** Inflammation of the female genital tract that may cause scarring or blockage of the fallopian tubes, resulting in infertility.

**penis** Male organ through which urine and semen are expelled from the body.

**perceived exertion** The subjective perception of effort during exercise that can be used to monitor exercise intensity

**perfect-use failure rate** The number of pregnancies (per 100 users) likely to occur in the first year of use of a particular birth control method if the method is used consistently and correctly.

**perineum** Tissue that forms the "floor" of the pelvic region, found between the vulva and the anus.

**peripheral artery disease (PAD)** Atherosclerosis occurring in the lower extremities, such as in the feet, calves, or legs, or in the arms.

**permanent methods** Surgically altering a man's or woman's reproductive system to permanently prevent pregnancy.

**persistent depressive disorder (PDD)** Type of depression that is milder and harder to recognize than major depression; chronic; and often characterized by fatigue, pessimism, or a short temper. Also called *dysthymic disorder* or *dysthymia*.

**personal flotation device** A device worn to provide buoyancy and keep the wearer, conscious or unconscious, afloat with the nose and mouth out of the water; also known as a life jacket.

**personality disorder** Mental disorder characterized by inflexible patterns of thought and beliefs that lead to socially distressing behavior.

**pesticides** Chemicals that kill pests such as insects or rodents.

**phobia** Deep and persistent fear of a specific object, activity, or situation that results in a compelling desire to avoid the source of the fear.

**physical activity** Refers to all body movements produced by skeletal muscles, resulting in substantial increases in energy expenditure.

**physical fitness** A balance of health-related attributes that allows you to perform moderate to vigorous physical activities on a regular basis and complete daily physical tasks without undue fatigue.

**physician assistant (PA)** Health care practitioner trained to handle most routine care under the supervision of a physician.

**physiological dependence** The adaptive state that occurs with regular addictive behavior and results in withdrawal syndrome.

**phytochemicals** Naturally occurring non-nutrient plant chemicals believed to have beneficial properties.

**pituitary gland** Endocrine gland that controls the release of hormones from the gonads.

**placebo** Inactive substance used as a control in a clinical test to determine the effectiveness of a particular drug; the *placebo effect* occurs when patients given a placebo drug or treatment experience an improved state of health owing to the belief that they are receiving something that will be of benefit.

**placenta** Network of blood vessels connected to the umbilical cord that transports oxygen and nutrients to a developing fetus and carries away fetal wastes.

**plant sterols** Essential components of plant membranes that, when consumed in the diet, appear to help lower cholesterol levels.

**plaque** Buildup of deposits in the arteries.

**platelet adhesiveness** Stickiness of red blood cells associated with blood clots.

**pneumonia** Inflammatory disease of the lungs characterized by chronic cough, chest pain, chills, high fever, and fluid accumulation; may be caused by bacteria, viruses, fungi, chemicals, or other substances.

**point source pollutant** Pollutant that enters waterways at a specific location.

**poison** Any substance harmful to the body when ingested, inhaled, injected, or absorbed through the skin.

**pollutant** Substance that contaminates some aspect of the environment and causes potential harm to living organisms.

**polychlorinated biphenyls (PCBs)** Toxic chemicals that were once used as insulating materials in high-voltage electrical equipment.

**polydrug use** Use of multiple medications, vitamins, recreational drugs, or illicit drugs simultaneously.

**positive psychology** The scientific study of human strengths and virtues.

**positive reinforcement** Presenting something positive following a behavior that is being reinforced.

**postpartum depression** Mood disorder experienced by women who have given birth; involves depression, fatigue, and other symptoms and may last for weeks or months.

**posttraumatic stress disorder (PTSD)** Collection of symptoms that may occur as a delayed response to a traumatic event or series of events.

**power** Ability to make and implement decisions.

**prayer** Communication with a transcendent presence.

**preconception care** Medical care received prior to becoming pregnant that helps a woman assess and address potential health issues.

**prediabetes** Condition in which blood glucose levels are higher than normal, but not high enough to be classified as diabetes.

**preeclampsia** Pregnancy complication characterized by high blood pressure, protein in the urine, and edema.

**preexposure prophylaxis (PrEP) for HIV** A daily pill, taken by those having sex with someone with HIV or otherwise at high risk, to help prevent HIV infection.

**pregaming** Drinking heavily at home before going out to an event or other location.

**prehypertensive** Blood pressure is above normal, but not yet in the hypertensive range.

**prejudice** A negative evaluation of an entire group of people that is typically based on unfavorable and often wrong ideas about the group.

**premature ejaculation** Ejaculation that occurs prior to or almost immediately following penile penetration of the vagina; also known as *early ejaculation*.

**premenstrual dysphoric disorder (PMDD)** Group of symptoms similar to but more severe than PMS, including severe mood disturbances.

**premenstrual syndrome (PMS)** Mood changes and physical symptoms that occur in some women prior to menstruation.

**premium** Payment made to an insurance carrier, usually in monthly installments, that covers the cost of an insurance policy.

**primary aggression** Goal-directed, hostile self-assertion that is destructive in nature.

**primary care practitioner (PCP)** Medical practitioner who provides preventive care and treats routine ailments, gives general medical advice, and makes appropriate referrals when necessary.

**primary idiopathic hypersomnia** Excessive daytime sleepiness without narcolepsy or the associated features of other sleep disorders.

**principal** Either the original loan amount or the amount left outstanding on a loan, excluding interest.

**prion** A recently identified self-replicating, protein-based pathogen.

**process addictions** Behaviors such as disordered gambling, compulsive buying, compulsive Internet or technology use, work addiction, compulsive exercise, and sexual addiction that are known to be addictive because they are mood altering.

**procrastinate** To intentionally put off doing something.

**progesterone** Hormone secreted by the ovaries; helps the endometrium develop and helps maintain pregnancy.

**proof** Measure of the percentage of alcohol in a beverage; the proof is double the percentage of alcohol in the drink.

**prostaglandin** Hormone-like substance associated with muscle contraction and inflammation.

**prostate gland** Gland that secretes chemicals that help sperm fertilize an ovum and secretes neutralizing fluids into the semen.

**prostate-specific antigen (PSA)** An antigen found in prostate cancer patients.

**proteins** Large molecules made up of chains of amino acids; essential constituents of all body cells.

**protozoans** Microscopic single-celled organisms that can be pathogenic.

**psychoactive drugs** Drugs that affect brain chemistry and have the potential to alter mood or behavior.

**psychological hardiness** A personality trait characterized by control, commitment, and the embrace of challenge.

**psychological health** The mental, emotional, social, and spiritual dimensions of health.

**psychological resilience** The capacity to maintain or regain psychological well-being in the face of adversity, trauma, tragedy, threats, or significant sources of stress.

**psychoneuroimmunology (PNI)** The study of the interactions of behavioral, neural, and endocrine functions and the functioning of the body's immune system.

**puberty** Period of sexual maturation.

**pubic lice** Parasitic insects that can inhabit various body areas, especially the genitals.

**radiation-absorbed dose (rad)** Unit of measure of radiation exposure.

**radiotherapy** The use of radiation to kill cancerous cells.

**radon** Naturally occurring radioactive gas resulting from the decay of certain radioactive elements.

**rape** Sexual penetration without the victim's consent.

**rational suicide** The decision to kill oneself rather than endure constant pain and slow decay.

**reactive aggression** Hostile emotional reaction brought about by frustrating life experiences.

**receptor sites** Specialized areas of cells and organs where chemicals, enzymes, and other substances interact

**relapse** A return to a previous pattern of negative behavior after a period of time successfully avoiding that behavior.

**relational connectedness** Mutually rewarding face-to-face contacts.

**relative deprivation** The inability of lower-income groups to sustain the same lifestyle as higher-income groups in the same community, often resulting in feelings of anxiety and inferiority.

**REM sleep** A period of sleep characterized by brain-wave activity similar to that seen in wakefulness in which rapid eye movement and dreaming occur.

**remission** Meaning the cancer is responding to treatment and under control.

**repetitive motion disorders (RMDs)** Injuries to soft tissue, tendons, muscles, nerves, or joints due to the physical stress of repeated motions.

**resiliency** The ability to adapt to change and stressful events in healthy and flexible ways.

**resistant hypertension** A form of HBP that is difficult to control and may require three or more different classes of antihypertensive drugs to begin to control blood pressure.

**resting metabolic rate (RMR)** The energy expenditure of the body under BMR conditions plus other daily sedentary activities.

**restless legs syndrome (RLS)** A neurological disorder characterized by an overwhelming urge to move the legs when they are at rest.

**rheumatic heart disease** A heart disease caused by untreated streptococcal infection of the throat.

**rheumatoid arthritis (RA)** An autoimmune inflammatory joint disease.

**RICE** Acronym for the standard first-aid treatment for virtually all traumatic and overuse injuries: rest, ice, compression, and elevation.

**rickettsia** A small form of bacteria that live inside other living cells.

**risk behaviors** Actions that increase susceptibility to negative health outcomes.

**satiety** The feeling of fullness or satisfaction at the end of a meal.

**saturated fats** Fats that are unable to hold any more hydrogen in their chemical structure; derived mostly from animal sources; solid at room temperature.

**schizophrenia** Mental illness with biological origins characterized by irrational behavior, severe alterations of the senses, and often an inability to function in society.

**scrotum** External sac of tissue that encloses the testes.

**seasonal affective disorder (SAD)** Type of depression that occurs in the winter months, when sunlight levels are low.

**secondary sex characteristics** Characteristics associated with sex but not directly related to reproduction, such as vocal pitch, amount of body hair, breasts, and location of fat deposits.

**sedentary** Activity that expends no more than 1.5 times the resting energy level while seated or reclined.

**self-compassion** Treating yourself with as much understanding and care as you would a loved one.

**self-disclosure** Sharing feelings or personal information with others.

**self-efficacy** Describes a person's belief about whether he or she can successfully engage in and execute a specific behavior.

**self-esteem** One's realistic sense of self-respect or self-worth.

**self-injury** Intentionally causing injury to one's own body in an attempt to cope with overwhelming negative emotions; also called *self-mutilation, self-harm,* or *nonsuicidal self-injury (NSSI)*.

**self-nurturance** Developing individual potential through a balanced and realistic appreciation of self-worth and ability.

**self-talk** The customary manner of thinking and talking to yourself, which can affect your self-image.

**semen** Fluid containing sperm and nutrients that increase sperm viability and neutralize vaginal acid.

**seminal vesicles** Glandular ducts that secrete nutrients for the semen.

**serial monogamy** Series of monogamous sexual relationships.

**set point theory** Theory that a form of internal thermostat controls our weight and fights to maintain this weight around a narrowly set range.

**severe acute malnutrition** Lack of nutritious food that causes tissue wasting and stunted growth, impairs brain development, diminishes work capacity, and perpetuates poverty within communities.

**sexual addiction** Compulsive involvement in sexual activity.

**sexual assault** Any act in which one person is sexually intimate with another without that person's consent.

**sexual aversion disorder** Desire dysfunction characterized by sexual phobias and anxiety about sexual contact.

**sexual dysfunction** Problems associated with achieving sexual satisfaction.

**sexual fantasies** Sexually arousing thoughts and dreams.

**sexual harassment** Any form of unwanted sexual attention related to any condition of employment, education, or performance evaluation.

**sexual identity** Recognition of oneself as a sexual being; a composite of biological sex characteristics, gender identity, gender roles, and sexual orientation.

**sexual orientation** A person's enduring emotional, romantic, or sexual attraction to other persons.

**sexual performance anxiety** Sexual difficulties caused by anticipating some sort of problem during a sex act.

**sexual prejudice** Negative attitudes and hostile actions directed at those with a different sexual orientation.

**sexuality** Thoughts, feelings, and behaviors associated with being masculine or feminine, experiencing attraction, being in love, and being in relationships that include sexual intimacy.

**sexually transmitted infections (STIs)** Infectious diseases caused by pathogens transmitted through some form of sexual contact.

**shaping** Using a series of small steps to gradually achieve a particular goal.

**shift and persist** A strategy of reframing appraisals of current stressors and focusing on a meaningful future that protects a person from the negative effects of too much stress.

**sick building syndrome (SBS)** Describes a situation in which occupants of a building experience acute health effects linked to time spent there, but no specific illness or cause can be identified.

**sidestream smoke** Smoke from the burning end of a cigarette, pipe, or cigar or exhaled by smokers, commonly called *secondhand smoke.*

**simple carbohydrates** A carbohydrate made up of only one or two sugar molecules; also called *simple sugars.*

**simple rape** Rape by one person, usually known to the victim, that does not involve physical beating or use of a weapon.

**sinoatrial node (SA node)** Cluster of electric pulse–generating cells that serves as a natural pacemaker for the heart.

**situational inducement** Attempts to influence a behavior through situations and occasions that are structured to exert control over that behavior.

**sleep apnea** A disorder in which breathing is briefly and repeatedly interrupted during sleep.

**sleep debt** The difference between the number of hours of sleep an individual needed in a given time period and the number of hours he or she actually slept.

**sleep deprivation** A condition that occurs when sleep is insufficient.

**sleep disorders (somnipathy or dyssomnia)** Any medical disorders that have a negative effect on sleep patterns.

**sleep hygiene** The wide range of practices that can help you manage and create a systematic approach leading to normal, quality nighttime sleep and full daytime alertness.

**sleep inertia** A state characterized by cognitive impairment, grogginess, and disorientation that is experienced upon rising from short sleep or an overly long nap.

**sleep study** A clinical assessment of sleep in which the patient is monitored while spending the night in a sleep disorders center.

**smog** Brownish haze that is a form of pollution produced by the photochemical reaction of sunlight with hydrocarbons, nitrogen compounds, and other gases in vehicle exhaust.

**snuff** Powdered form of tobacco that is sniffed or absorbed through the mucous membranes in the nose or placed inside the cheek and sucked.

**social anxiety disorder** Phobia characterized by fear and avoidance of social situations; also called *social phobia.*

**social capital** Collective value of all the people in your social network and the likelihood of those people providing social support when you need it.

**social death** A seemingly irreversible situation in which a person is not treated like an active member of society.

**social health** Aspect of psychological health that includes interactions with others, ability to use social supports, and ability to adapt to various situations.

**social learning theory** Theory that people learn behaviors by watching role models—parents, caregivers, and significant others.

**social network** People you know who can provide social support when needed.

**social support** Network of people and services with whom you share ties and from whom you get support.

**social-cognitive model (SCM)** Model of behavior change emphasizing the role of social factors and thought processes (cognition) in behavior change.

**socialization** Process by which a society communicates behavioral expectations to its members.

**socioeconomic status (SES)** An individual or family's social and economic position in relation to others with regard to education, income, and occupation.

**somnolence** Drowsiness, sluggishness, and lack of mental alertness that can affect your daily performance and lead to life-threatening sleepiness while driving.

**spermatogenesis** The development of sperm.

**spermicide** Substance designed to kill sperm.

**spiritual community** A group of people who meet together for the purpose of enriching and expanding their spirituality.

**spiritual health** Aspect of psychological health that relates to having a sense of meaning and purpose to one's life, as well as a feeling of connection with others and with nature.

**spiritual intelligence (SI)** The ability to access higher meanings, values, abiding purposes, and unconscious aspects of the self; a characteristic that helps us find a moral and ethical path to guide us through life.

**spirituality** An individual's sense of peace, purpose, and connection to others and beliefs about the meaning of life.

**stalking** Willful, repeated, and malicious following, harassing, or threatening of another person.

**standard drink** Amount of any beverage that contains about 14 grams of pure alcohol.

**staphylococci** A group of round bacteria, usually found in clusters, that cause a variety of diseases in humans and other animals.

**starches** Polysaccharides that are the storage forms of glucose in plants.

**static stretching** Stretching techniques that slowly and gradually lengthen a muscle or group of muscles and their tendons.

**stereotactic radiosurgery** A type of radiation therapy that can be used to zap tumors; also known as gamma knife surgery.

**sterilization** Permanent fertility control achieved through surgical procedures.

**stigma** Negative perception about a group of people or a certain situation or condition.

**stillbirth** Death of a fetus after the 20th week of pregnancy but before delivery.

**stimulants** Drugs that increase activity of the central nervous system.

**Streptococcus** A round bacterium, usually found in chain formation.

**stress** A series of mental and physiological responses and adaptations to a real or perceived threat to one's well-being.

**stress inoculation** Stress-management technique in which a person consciously anticipates and prepares for potential stressors.

**stressor** A physical, social, or psychological event or condition that upsets homeostasis and produces a stress response.

**stroke** A condition occurring when the brain is damaged by disrupted blood supply; also called *cerebrovascular accident.*

**suction curettage** Abortion technique that uses gentle suction to remove fetal tissue from the uterus; also called vacuum aspiration or dilation and curettage (D&C).

**sudden cardiac death (SCD)** an abrupt, profound loss of heart function (cardiac arrest) that causes death either instantly or shortly after symptoms occur.

**sudden infant death syndrome (SIDS)** Sudden death of an infant under 1 year of age for no apparent reason.

**suicidal ideation** A desire to die and thoughts about suicide.

**super obese** Having a body weight higher than morbid obesity; in an adult, having a BMI of 50 or more.

**Superfund** Fund established under the Comprehensive Environmental Response, Compensation, and Liability Act to be used for cleaning up toxic waste dumps.

**suppositories** Mixtures of drugs in a waxy medium designed to melt at body temperature after being inserted into the anus or vagina.

**survivorship** Physical, psychological, emotional, and economic issues of cancer from diagnosis until the end of life.

**sustainable development** Development that meets the needs of the present without compromising the ability of future generations to meet their own needs.

**swine flu** A respiratory infection initially believed to be found primarily in pigs; also referred to as H1N1 or one of its variants.

**sympathetic nervous system** Branch of the autonomic nervous system responsible for stress arousal.

**sympathomimetics** Food substances that can produce stresslike physiological responses.

**synergism** Interaction of two or more drugs that produces more profound effects than would be expected if the drugs were taken separately; also called *potentiation*.

**syphilis** One of the most widespread bacterial STIs; characterized by distinct phases and potentially serious results.

**systolic blood pressure** The upper number in the fraction that measures blood pressure, indicating pressure on the walls of the arteries when the heart contracts.

**target heart rate** The heart rate range of aerobic exercise that leads to improved cardiorespiratory fitness (i.e., 64 to 96% of maximal heart rate).

**tar** Thick, brownish sludge condensed from particulate matter in smoked tobacco.

**temperature inversion** Weather condition that occurs when a layer of cool air is trapped under a layer of warmer air, preventing the air from circulating.

**teratogenic** Causing birth defects; may refer to drugs, environmental chemicals, radiation, or diseases.

**terrorism** Unlawful use of force or violence against persons or property to intimidate or coerce a government, civilian population, or any segment thereof in furtherance of political or social objectives.

**testes** Male sex organs that manufacture sperm and produce hormones.

**testosterone** Male sex hormone manufactured in the testes.

**tetrahydrocannabinol (THC)** The chemical name for the active ingredient in marijuana.

**thanatology** The study of death and dying.

**thrombolysis** Injection of an agent to dissolve clots and restore some blood flow, thereby reducing the amount of tissue that dies from ischemia.

**thrombus** A clot or blockage in the blood vessels.

**time** As part of the FITT prescription, refers to the duration of an exercise session.

**TNM staging system** A system for classifying cancer staging by assessing tumor size, nodal involvement, and degree of metastasis.

**tolerance** Phenomenon in which progressively larger doses of a drug or more intense involvement in a behavior is needed to produce the desired effects.

**toxic shock syndrome (TSS)** Rare, potentially life-threatening disease that occurs when specific bacterial toxins multiply and spread to the bloodstream, most commonly through improper use of tampons, diaphragms, or cervical caps.

**toxins** Poisonous substances produced by certain microorganisms that cause various diseases.

**toxoplasmosis** Disease caused by an organism found in cat feces that, when contracted by a pregnant woman, may result in stillbirth or birth defects.

**traditional Chinese medicine (TCM)** Ancient comprehensive system of healing that uses herbs, acupuncture, massage, and qigong to bring vital energy, *qi*, into balance and to remove blockages of *qi* that lead to disease.

**trans fats (*trans* fatty acids)** Fatty acids typically produced from the hydrogenation of polyunsaturated oils.

**transactional model of stress and coping** Theory proposed by psychologist Richard Lazarus, saying that our reaction to stress is about the interaction between perception, coping ability, and environment.

**transdermal** The introduction of drugs through the skin.

**transgender** Having a gender identity that does not match one's assigned biological sex.

**transient ischemic attacks (TIAs)** Brief interruption of the blood supply to the brain that causes only temporary impairment; often an indicator of impending major stroke.

**transtheoretical model** Model of behavior change that identifies six distinct stages people go through in altering behavior patterns; also called the *stages-of-change model*.

**traumatic injuries** Injuries that are accidental and occur suddenly.

**traumatic stress** A physiological and mental response that occurs for a prolonged period of time after a major accident, war, assault, natural disaster, or an event in which one may have been seriously hurt, killed, or witness to horrible things.

**trichomoniasis** Protozoan STI characterized by foamy, yellowish discharge and unpleasant odor.

**triglycerides** The most common lipids in our food supply and in the body; made up of glycerol and three fatty acid chains; commonly referred to as *fats*.

**trimester** A 3-month segment of pregnancy.

**triple marker screen (TMS)** Common maternal blood test that can be used to identify certain birth defects and genetic abnormalities in a fetus.

**tubal ligation** Sterilization of a woman that involves cutting and tying off or cauterizing the fallopian tubes.

**tuberculosis (TB)** A disease caused by bacterial infiltration of the respiratory system.

**tumor** A neoplasmic mass that grows more rapidly than surrounding tissue.

**type 1 diabetes** Form of diabetes mellitus in which the pancreas is not able to make insulin, and therefore blood glucose cannot enter the cells to be used for energy.

**type 2 diabetes** Form of diabetes mellitus in which the pancreas does not make enough insulin or the body is unable to use insulin correctly.

**type** As part of the FITT prescription, refers to what kind of exercises a person needs to do.

**typical-use failure rate** The number of pregnancies (per 100 users) likely to occur in the first year of use of a particular birth control method if the method's use is not consistent or always correct.

**ulcerative colitis** An inflammatory bowel disease that affects the mucous membranes of the large intestine and can lead to ulcers, erosion of the outer lining of the colon, and serious bleeding.

**ultrasonography (ultrasound)** Common prenatal test that uses sound waves to create a visual image of a developing fetus.

**underweight** Having a body weight more than 10 percent below healthy recommended levels; in an adult, having a BMI below 18.5.

**unintentional injuries** Injury, death, or psychological harm caused unintentionally or without premeditation.

**unsaturated fats** Fats that have regions not saturated with hydrogen; derived mostly from plants; liquid at room temperature.

**urethral opening** Opening through which urine is expelled.

**urinary incontinence** Inability to control urination.

**urinary tract infections (UTIs)** Infection, more common among women than men, of the urinary tract; causes include untreated STIs.

**uterus (womb)** Hollow, pear-shaped muscular organ whose function is to house a developing fetus.

**vaccination** Inoculation with killed or weakened pathogens or similar, less dangerous antigens, in order to prevent or lessen the effects of some disease.

**vagina** Muscular, tube-shaped organ in females that serves as a passageway connecting the vulva to the uterus.

**vaginal contraceptive film** A thin film infused with spermicidal gel that is inserted into the vagina so that it covers the cervix.

**vaginal intercourse** Insertion of the penis into the vagina.

**vaginismus** State in which the vaginal muscles contract so forcefully that penetaration cannot occur.

**values** Principles that influence our thoughts and emotions and guide the choices we make in our lives.

**variant sexual behavior** A sexual behavior that is not commonly practiced.

**vas deferens** Tube that transports sperm from the epididymis to the ejaculatory duct.

**vasectomy** Male sterilization procedure that involves cutting and tying off the vasa deferentia.

**vasocongestion** Engorgement of the genital organs with blood.

**vegetarian** A person who follows a diet that excludes some or all animal products.

**veins** Vessels that carry blood back to the heart from other regions of the body.

**ventricles** The heart's two lower chambers, which pump blood through the blood vessels.

**venules** Branches of the veins.

**very-low-calorie diets (VLCDs)** Diets with a daily caloric value of 400 to 700 calories.

**violence** Aggressive behaviors that produce injuries and can result in death.

**virulent** Strong enough to overcome host resistance and cause disease.

**viruses** Minute microbes consisting of DNA or RNA that invade a host cell and use the cell's resources to reproduce themselves.

**visualization** The creation of mental images to promote relaxation.

**vitamins** Essential organic compounds that promote metabolism, growth, and reproduction.

**vulva** External female genitalia.

**wellness** The achievement of the highest level of health possible in each of several dimensions.

**whole grains** Grains that retain the bran, germ, and endosperm, with only the husk removed.

**withdrawal** A series of temporary physical and biopsychosocial symptoms that occurs when an addict abruptly abstains from an addictive chemical or behavior.

**withdrawal (coitus interruptus)** Contraceptive method that involves withdrawing the penis from the vagina before ejaculation.

**work addiction** The compulsive use of work and the work persona to fulfill needs for intimacy, power, and success.

**Xulane** Patch that releases hormones similar to those in oral contraceptives; each patch is worn for 1 week.

**Yerkes-Dodson law of arousal** Theory suggesting that when arousal or stress increases, performance goes up to a point, after which performance declines.

**yo-yo diets** Cycles in which people diet and regain weight.

**yoga** System of physical and mental training involving controlled breathing, physical postures (*asanas*), meditation, chanting, and other practices believed to cultivate unity with the *Atman*, or spiritual life principle of the universe.

**zika virus** Emerging threat from bite of Aedes mosquito in U.S. and globally, particularly for pregnant women.

# REFERENCES

## Chapter 1

1. S. L. Murphy, K. D. Kochanek, J. Xu, and E. Arias. "Mortality in the United States, 2014," *NCHS Data Brief*, no. 229 (2015), Available at www.cdc.gov/nchs/data/databriefs/db229.pdf.

2. Centers for Disease Control and Prevention, "Achievements in Public Health, 1900–1999: Control of Infectious Diseases," *Morbidity and Mortality Weekly Report* 48, no. 29 (1999): 621–29, www.cdc.gov/mmwr/preview/mmwrhtml/mm4829a1.htm.

3. N. B. Johnson et al., "CDC National Health Report: Leading Causes of Morbidity and Mortality and Associated Behavioral Risk and Protective Factors—United States, 2005–2013," *Morbidity and Mortality Weekly Report* 63, no. 04 (2014): 3–27, www.cdc.gov/mmwr/preview/mmwrhtml/su6304a2.htm.

4. Organization for Economic Cooperation and Development, *Health at a Glance 2013: OECD Indicators*, 2013, doi: 10.1787/health_glance-2013-en.

5. U.S. Department of Health and Human Services (DHHS), "Health-Related Quality of Life & Well-Being," *Healthy People 2020* (Washington, DC: U.S. Government Printing Office), February 3, 2016, www.healthypeople.gov/2020/topics-objectives/topic/health-related-quality-of-life-well-being.

6. Centers for Disease Control and Prevention, "Adult Obesity Facts," September 21, 2015, http://www.cdc.gov/obesity/data/adult.html.

7. World Health Organization (WHO), "Constitution of the World Health Organization," *Chronicles of the World Health Organization* (Geneva: WHO, 1947), www.who.int/governance/eb/constitution/en/index.html.

8. R. Dubos, *So Human an Animal: How We Are Shaped by Surroundings and Events* (New York: Scribner, 1968), 15.

9. U.S. Department of Health and Human Services (DHHS), *Healthy People 2020*, 2016.

10. Centers for Disease Control and Prevention, "Chronic Disease Prevention and Health Promotion," December 2015, www.cdc.gov/chronicdisease/.

11. U.S. Burden of Disease Collaborators, "The State of US Health, 1990–2010: Burden of Diseases, Injuries, and Risk Factors," *Journal of the American Medical Association* 310, no. 6 (2013): 591–606; Centers for Disease Control and Prevention, "Alcohol Use and Health Fact Sheets," February 2016, www.cdc.gov/alcohol/fact-sheets/alcohol-use.htm; Centers for Disease Control and Prevention, "Smoking and Tobacco Use Fast Facts," December 2015, www.cdc.gov/tobacco/data_statistics/fact_sheets/fast_facts.

12. U.S. Burden of Disease Collaborators, "The State of US Health, 1990–2010," 2013.

13. Ibid.

14. CDC, "Alcohol Use and Health Fact Sheets," 2016.

15. CDC, "Smoking and Tobacco Use Fast Facts," December 2015, www.cdc.gov/tobacco/data_statistics/fact_sheets/fast_facts/index.htm#toll.

16. H. C. Gooding et al., "Optimal Lifestyle Components in Young Adulthood Are Associated with Maintaining the Ideal Cardiovascular Health Profile into Middle Age," *Journal of the American Heart Association* 4, no. 11 (2015): e002048.

17. R. A. Rudd, N. Aleshire, J. E. Zibbell, and R. M. Gladden, "Increases in Drug and Opioid Overdose Deaths—United States, 2000–2014," *Morbidity and Mortality Weekly Report* 64, no. 50 (2016): 1378–82.

18. Institute for Health Metrics and Evaluation, "U.S. County Profiles: Fairfax County, Virginia and McDowell County, West Virginia," Accessed March 2016, www.healthdata.org.

19. American College Health Association, *American College Health Association–National College Health Assessment II: Reference Group Executive Summary Spring 2015* (Linthicum, MD: American College Health Association, 2015), www.acha.org.

20. P. Pilkington, J. Powell, and A. Davis. "Evidence-Based Decision Making When Designing Environments for Physical Activity: The Role of Public Health," *Sports Medicine* (2016) [E-pub ahead of print].

21. M. J. Trowbridge and T. L. Schmid, "Built Environment and Physical Activity Promotion: Place-Based Obesity Prevention Strategies," *Journal of Law, Medicine and Ethics*, Weight of the Nation Supplement (Winter 2013): 46–51, Available at https://www.aslme.org/media/downloadable/files/links/j/l/jlme-41-4-supp_trowbridge.pdf.

22. S. Cummins, E. Flint, and S. A. Matthews, "New Neighborhood Grocery Store Increased Awareness of Food Access but Did Not Alter Dietary Habits or Obesity," *Health Affairs* 33, no. 2 (2014): 283–91.

23. A. M. Barry-Jester and B. Casselman, "33 Million Americans Still Don't Have Health Insurance," *FiveThirtyEight*, September 28, 2015, http://fivethirtyeight.com/features/33-million-americans-still-dont-have-health-insurance/.

24. Ibid.

25. The Commonwealth Fund, "Too High a Price: Out-of-Pocket Health Care Costs in the United States. Findings from the Commonwealth Fund Health Care Affordability Tracking Survey. September–October 2014," November 13, 2014, www.commonwealthfund.org/publications/issue-briefs/2014/nov/out-of-pocket-health-care-costs.

26. Ibid.

27. I. Rosenstock, "Historical Origins of the Health Belief Model," *Health Education Monographs* 2, no. 4 (1974): 328–35.

28. Bandura, A. "Human Agency in Social-Cognitive Theory," *American Psychologist* 44, no. 9 (September 1989): 1175–84.

29. P. J. Morgan et al. "Associations Between Program Outcomes and Adherence to Social Cognitive Theory Tasks: Process Evaluation of the SHED-IT Community Weight Loss Trial for Men," *International Journal of Behavioral Nutrition and Physical Activity* 11, no. 1 (2014): 89.

30. M. C. Snead et al., "Relationship between Social Cognitive Theory Constructs and Self-Reported Condom Use: Assessment of Behaviour in a Subgroup of the Safe in the City Trial," *BMJ Open* 4, no. 12 (2014): e006093.

31. J. O. Prochaska and C. C. DiClemente, "Stages and Processes of Self-Change of Smoking: Toward an Integrative Model of Change," *Journal of Consulting and Clinical Psychology* 51 (1983): 390–95.

32. National Institute on Drug Abuse, "Drugs, Brains, and Behavior: The Science of Addiction," July 2014, www.drugabuse.gov/publications/drugs-brains-behavior-science-addiction/treatment-recovery.

33. G. Goldzweig, I. Hasson-Ohayon, S. Alon, and E. Shalit, "Perceived Threat and Depression among Patients with Cancer: The Moderating Role of Health Locus of Control," *Psychology, Health, and Medicine* 21, no. 5 (2016): 601–7.

34. A. Ellis and M. Benard, *Clinical Application of Rational Emotive Therapy* (New York: Plenum Press, 1985).

35. National Institute on Drug Abuse, "Drugs, Brains, and Behavior," 2014.

36. American Cancer Society, "Staying Smoke-Free," February 6, 2014, www.cancer.org/healthy/stayawayfromtobacco/guideto quittingsmoking/guide-to-quitting-smoking-staying-smoke-free.

**Pulled Statistics:**

p. 3, A. M. Barry-Jester and B. Casselman, "33 Million Americans Still Don't Have Health Insurance," *FiveThirtyEight* (September 28, 2015), http://fivethirtyeight.com/features/33-million-americans-still-dont-have-health-insurance/.

p. 11, CDC, National Center for Health Statistics, "Life Expectancy," February 25, 2016, www.cdc.gov/nchs/fastats/life-expectancy.htm#.

# Chapter 2

1. K. Neff, *Self Compassion: The Proven Power of Being Kind to Yourself* (New York: HarperCollins, 2015).
2. A. H. Maslow, *Motivation and Personality,* 2nd ed. (New York: Harper and Row, 1970).
3. D. J. Anspaugh and G. Ezell, *Teaching Today's Health,* 10th ed. (Boston: Pearson, 2013).
4. Y. Yang et al., "Social Relationships and Physiological Determinants of Longevity Across the Lifespan," *Preeedings of the National Academy of Sciences of the United States of America* 113, no.3 (2016): 578–83; M. Ramsey and A. Gentzler, "An Upward Spiral: Bidirectional Associations Between Positive Affect and Positive Aspects of Close Relationships Across the Life Span," *Developmental Review* 36, (2015): 58–104.
5. D. *Melkasha*. Friendship and Happiness Across the Lifespan. 2015. Springer Publishing.
6. S. Straussner and C. Fewel. "Children of Parents Who Abuse Alcohol and Drugs," in A. Reupert, D. Mayberry and J. Licholson et al. (eds.) *Parentel Psychiatric Disorder: Distressed Parents and their Children.* Cambridge University Press. U.K.
7. S. Straussner and C. Fewel. "Children of Parents Who Abuse Acohol and Drugs," in A. Reupert, D. Mayberry and J. Licholson et al. (eds.) *Parentel Psychiatric Disorder: Distressed Parents and their Children.* Cambridge University Press. U.K.; W. Cheng, W. Ickes, and L. Verhofstadt, "How Is Family Support Related to Students' GPA Scores? A Longitudinal Study," *Higher Education* 64, no. 3 (2012): 399–420; L. Rice et al., "The Role of Social Support in Students' Perceived Abilities and Attitudes toward Math and Science," *Journal of Youth and Adolescence* 42, no. 7 (2013): 1028–40; J. Cullum et al., "Ignoring Norms with a Little Help from my Friends: Social Support Reduces Normative Influence on Drinking Behavior," *Journal of Social & Clinical Psychology* 32, no. 1 (2013): 17–33; J. Hirsch and A. Barton, "Positive Social Support, Negative Social Exchanges, and Suicidal Behavior in College Students," *Journal of American College Health* 59, no. 5 (2011): 393–98.
8. X. Wang et al., Social Support Moderates Stress Effect," 2014; W. Cheng, W. Ickes, and L. Verhofstadt, "How is Family Support Related to Students' GPA Scores? A Longitudinal Study," *Higher Education* 64, no. 3 (2012): 399–420; L. Rice et al., "The Role of Social Support in Students' Perceived Abilities and Attitudes toward Math and Science," *Journal of Youth and Adolescence* 42, no. 7 (2013): 1028–40; J. Cullum et al., "Ignoring Norms with a Little Help from my Friends: Social Support Reduces Normative Influence on Drinking Behavior," *Journal of Social & Clinical Psychology* 32, no. 1 (2013): 17–33.
9. M. Weijs-Perree et al. "Factors Influencing Social Satisfaction and Loneliness: A Path Analysis." *Journal of Transport Geography* 45 (2015): 24–31.
10. J. Cacioppo et al., "Loneliness Across Phylogeny and a Call for Comparative Studies and Animal Models," *Perspectives on Psychological Science* 10, no. 2 (2015): 202–12.
11. Ibid.
12. American College Health Association, *National College Health Assessment II: Reference Group Executive Summary, Spring 2015.*
13. National Cancer Institute, "Spirituality in Cancer Care (PDQ®)," Revised 2015, http://www.cancer.gov/about-cancer/coping/day-to-day/faith-and-spirituality/spirituality-pdq.
14. M. Seligman, *Helplessness: On Depression, Development, and Death* (New York: W. H. Freeman, 1975).
15. K. Huffman and C. A. Sanderson, *Real World Psychology* (Hoboken, NJ: Wiley, 2014).
16. P. Salovey and J. Mayer, "Emotional Intelligence," *Imagination, Cognition, and Personality* 9, no. 3 (1989): 185–211.
17. G. E. Gignac et al., "Emotional Intelligence as a Unique Predictor of Individual Differences in Humour Styles and Humour Appreciation," *Personality and Individual Differences* 56 (2014): 34–39.
18. HBR 10 Must Reads, *On Emotional Intelligence* (Boston: Harvard Business Review Press, 2015).
19. D. Goleman, R. Boyatzis, and A. McKee, *Primal Leadership: Unleashing the Power of Emotional Intelligence* (Boston: Harvard Business Review Press, 2013); I. Tuhovasky, *Emotional Intelligence: A Practical Guide to Making Friends with Your Emotions and Raising Your EQ* (Ian Tuhovasky, 2015).
20. D. Goleman, R. Boyatzis, and A. McKee, *Primal Leadership: Unleashing the Power of Emotional Intelligence* (Boston: Harvard Business Review Press, 2013).
21. Ibid.
22. M. Seligman et al., "White Paper: Positive Health and Heath Assets: Re-analysis of Longitudinal Datasets." *U Penn Positive Health* (2015), Available at https://ppc.sas.upenn.edu/sites/ppc.sas.upenn.edu/files/positivehealthassetspub.pdf.
23. Ibid.
24. M. Seligman, *Flourish: A Visionary New Understanding of Happiness and Well-Being* (New York: Free Press, 2011).
25. S. Donaldson et al., "Happiness, Excellence, and Optimal Human Functioning Revisited: Examining the Peer Reviewed Literature Linked to Positive Psychology," *Journal of Positive Psychology* 10, no. 3 (2015): 185–95.
26. M. Garaigordobil, "Predictor Variables of Happiness and Its Connection with Risk and Protective Factors for Health," *Frontiers in Psychology* 6 (2015): 1176.
27. Ibid.
28. Ibid.
29. P. de Souto Barreto and Y. Rolland, "Happiness and Unhappiness Have No Direct Effect on Mortality," *The Lancet* (2015).
30. E. Roysamb et al., "Well-Being: Heritable and Changeable," Stability of Happiness Theories and Evidence on Whether Happiness Can Change (San Diego: Academic Press, 2014): 9–35.
31. Mayo Clinic Staff, MayoClinic.com, "Mental Illness: Causes," October 2015, www.mayoclinic.org/diseases-conditions/mental-illness/basics/causes/con-20033813.
32. Ibid.
33. Substance Abuse and Mental Health Services Administration, "Results from the 2014 National Survey on Drug Use and Health: Mental Health Findings," NSDUH Series H-50, HHS Publication no. SMA 15-4927 (Rockville, MD: Substance Abuse and Mental Health Services Administration, 2015), Available at http://www.samhsa.gov/data/sites/default/files/NSDUH-FRR1-2014/NSDUH-FRR1-2014.pdf.
34. L. Szabo, "Cost of Not Caring: Nowhere to Go," *USA Today,* May 5, 2014, www.usatoday.com/story/news/nation/2014/05/12/mental-health-system-crisis/7746535/; T. Insel, "Director's Blog: Mental Health Awareness Month: By the Numbers," *National Institute of Mental Health,* May 15, 2015, http://www.nimh.nih.gov/about/director/2015/mental-health-awareness-month-by-the-numbers.shtml.
35. R. P. Gallagher, "National Survey of College Counseling 2014," *International Association of Counseling Services, Inc. Monograph Series* 9V (2014), Available at http://0201.nccdn.net/1_2/000/000/088/0b2/NCCCS2014_v2.pdf.
36. American College Health Association, *American College Health Association–National College Health Assessment II (ACHA–NCHA II): Reference Group Data Report Spring 2015* (Baltimore: American College Health Association, 2015), Available at http://www.acha-ncha.org/docs/NCHA-II_WEB_SPRING_2015_REFERENCE_GROUP_EXECUTIVE_SUMMARY.pdf.
37. Ibid.
38. Ibid.
39. U.S. National Library of Medicine, "Medline Plus: Mood Disorders," October 2014, https://www.nlm.nih.gov/medlineplus/mooddisorders.html.
40. American College Health Association, *American College Health Association–National College Health Assessment II (ACHA–NCHA II): Reference Group Data Report Spring 2015* (Baltimore: American College Health Association, 2015), Available at http://www.acha-ncha.org/docs/NCHA-II_WEB_SPRING_2015_REFERENCE_GROUP_EXECUTIVE_SUMMARY.pdf.
41. R. Uher, "Persistent Depressive Disorder, Dysthymia, and Chronic Depression: Update on Diagnosis, Treatment," *Psychiatric Times,* July 2014, www.psychiatrictimes.com/special-reports/persistent-depressive-disorder-dysthymia-and-chronic-depression/page/0/3.
42. Ibid.
43. American College Health Association, *American College Health Association–National College Health Assessment II (ACHA–NCHA II): Reference Group Data Report Spring 2015* (Baltimore: American College Health Association, 2015), Available at http://www.acha-ncha.org/docs/NCHA-II_WEB_SPRING_2015_REFERENCE_GROUP_EXECUTIVE_SUMMARY.pdf.

44. R. Uher, "Persistent Depressive Disorder, Systhymia and Chronic Depression: Update on Diagnosis, Treatment," *Psychiatric Times*, July 31, 2014, http://www.psychiatrictimes .com/special-reports/persistent-depressive-disorder-dysthymia-and-chronic-depression.

45. SAMHSA, "Mental Disorders: Bipolar and Related Disorders," October 27, 2015, www .samhsa.gov/disorders/mental.

46. WebMD, "Seasonal Depression (Seasonal Affective Disorder)," May 18, 2015 www .webmd.com/depression/guide/seasonal-affective-disorder.

47. Cleveland Clinic, "Seasonal Depression," Accessed February 2016, https://my.clevel andclinic.org/services/neurological_ institute/center-for-behavioral-health/ disease-conditions/hic-seasonal-depression.

48. Mayo Clinic Staff, MayoClinic.com, "Depression: Causes," 2015, www.mayoclinic.org/ diseases-conditions/depression/basics/causes/ con-20032977.

49. SAMSHA, "Mental Disorders: Anxiety Disorders," October 10, 2014, www.samhsa .gov/disorders/mental; R. Karg et al., "Past Year Mental Health Disorders among Adults in the U.S.," 2014.

50. American College Health Association, *American College Health Association–National College Health Assessment II (ACHA–NCHA II): Reference Group Data Report Spring 2015* (Baltimore: American College Health Association, 2015), Available at http:// www.acha-ncha.org/docs/NCHA-II_WEB_ SPRING_2015_REFERENCE_GROUP_ EXECUTIVE_SUMMARY.pdf.

51. National Institute of Mental Health, "Generalized Anxiety Disorder, GAD," Accessed February 2014, www.nimh.nih.gov/ health/publications/anxiety-disorders/ generalized-anxiety-disorder-gad.shtml.

52. American College Health Association, *American College Health Association–National College Health Assessment II (ACHA–NCHA II): Reference Group Data Report Spring 2015* (Baltimore: American College Health Association, 2015), Available at http://www.acha-ncha.org/docs/ NCHA-II_WEB_SPRING_2015_REFERENCE_ GROUP_EXECUTIVE_SUMMARY.pdf.

53. Mayo Clinic Staff, MayoClinic.com, "Panic Attacks and Panic Disorder: Symptoms," May 2015, www.mayoclinic.org/diseases-conditions/panic-attacks/basics/symptoms/ con-20020825.

54. Web MD, "Anxiety and Panic Disorders Health Center: Specific Phobias," February 24, 2016, www.webmd.com/anxiety-panic/specific-phobias; Web MD, "Anxiety and Panic Disorders Health Center: Specific Phobias," February 13, 2014, www.webmd.com/anxiety-panic/specific-phobias.

55. Ibid.

56. Ibid.

57. Mayo Clinic Staff, Mayo Clinic.com, "Generalized Anxiety Disorder: Causes," September 2014, www.mayoclinic.org/ diseases-conditions/generalized-anxiety-disorder/basics/causes/con-20024562.

58. Anxiety and Depression Association of America, "Facts and Statistics," September 2014, www.adaa.org/about-adaa/press-room/ facts-statistics.

59. National Institute of Mental Health, "Obsessive Compulsive Disorder," January 2016, http://www.nimh.nih.gov/health/ topics/obsessive-compulsive-disorder-ocd/ index.shtml.

60. Anxiety and Depression Association of America, "Facts and Statistics," September 2014, www.adaa.org/about-adaa/press-room/ facts-statistics.

61. Ibid; J. Gradus, "Epidemiology of PTSD," PTSD: National Center for PTSD," *U.S. Department of Veterans Affairs, National Center for PTSD,* February 23, 2016, http://www .ptsd.va.gov/professional/PTSD-overview/ epidemiological-facts-ptsd.asp.

62. National Institute of Mental Health, "Post-Traumatic Stress Disorder," February 2016, www.nimh.nih.gov/health/topics/ post-traumatic-stress-disorder-ptsd/index .shtml#part4.

63. J. Gradus, "Epidemiology of PTSD," *United States Department of Veterans Affairs, National Center for PTSD,* February 23, 2016, www.ptsd .va.gov/professional/PTSD-overview/ epidemiological-facts-ptsd.asp; S. Staggs, "Myths and Facts about PTSD," *PsychCentral*, February 2014, http://psychcentral.com/lib/ myths-and-facts-about-ptsd.

64. American Psychiatric Association, *Diagnostic and Statistical Manual of Mental Disorders,* 5th ed. (Washington, DC: American Psychiatric Association, 2013).

65. National Institutes of Health, "Any Personality Disorder," National Institute of Mental Health, Accessed February 2016, www.nimh.nih .gov/health/statistics/prevalence/any-personality-disorder.shtml; P. Tyrer, F. Reed, and M. Crawford, "Classification, Assessment Prevalence, and Effect of Personality Disorder," *The Lancet* 385, no. 9969 (2015): 717–26.

66. A.D.A.M. Medical Encyclopedia, "Antisocial Personality Disorder," PubMed Health (Bethesda, MD: U.S. National Library of Medicine, 2012).

67. Mayo Clinic Staff, MayoClinic.com, "Borderline Personality Disorder," July 2015, http:// www.mayoclinic.org/diseases-conditions/ borderline-personality-disorder/basics/ symptoms/con-20023204.

68. Mayo Clinic, "Borderline Personality Disorder," July 2015, www.mayoclinic.org/ diseases-conditions/borderline-personality-disorder/basics/definition/con-20023204.

69. National Institutes of Health, "Borderline Personality Disorder," National Institute of Mental Health, Accessed February 2016, http://www.nimh.nih.gov/health/topics/ borderline-personality-disorder/index.shtml.

70. Ibid.

71. National Institute of Mental Health, "Schizophrenia," February 2016, www.nimh.nih.gov/ health/topics/schizophrenia/index.shtml.

72. Ibid.

73. Ibid.

74. World Health Organization, "Preventing Suicide: A Global Imperative," 2014, Available at www.who.int/mental_health/suicide-prevention/world_report_2014/en/.

75. Ibid.

76. Ibid.

77. M. Heron, "Deaths: Leading Causes for 2010," *National Vital Statistics Reports* 62, no. 6 (2013), Available at http://www.cdc. gov/nchs/data/nvsr/nvsr62/nvsr62_06.pdf.

78. American College Health Association, *American College Health Association–National College Health Assessment II (ACHA–NCHA II): Reference Group Data Report Spring 2015* (Baltimore: American College Health Association, 2015), Available at http://www.acha-ncha.org/docs/ NCHA-II_WEB_SPRING_2015_REFERENCE_ GROUP_EXECUTIVE_SUMMARY.pdf.

79. Ibid.; Centers for Disease Control and Prevention, "Suicide Facts at a Glance 2015," Accessed February 2016, http://www.cdc .gov/violenceprevention/pdf/suicide-datasheet-a.pdf.

80. A. Haas et al., "Suicide Attempts Among Transgender and Gender Non-Conforming Adults: Findings of the National Transgender Discrimination Survey," American Foundation for Suicide Prevention, January 2014.

81. Ibid; E. Mereish, C. O'Clerigh, and J. Bradford, "Interrelationships between LGBT-Based Victimization, Suicide, and Substance Use Problems in a Diverse Sample of Sexual and Gender Minority Men and Women," *Psychology, Health & Medicine* 19, no. 1 (2014): 1–13

82. Centers for Disease Control and Prevention, "Suicide Facts at a Glance 2015," Accessed February 2016, http://www.cdc.gov/violence prevention/pdf/suicide-datasheet-a.pdf.

83. Ibid.

84. American Foundation for Suicide Prevention, "Warning Signs of Suicide," Accessed February 2016, www.afsp.org/preventing-suicide/risk-factors-and-warning-signs.

85. Ibid; Befrienders Worldwide, "The Warning Signs of Suicide," Accessed February 2016, http://www.befrienders.org/warning-signs.

86. Ibid; Befrienders Worldwide, "Helping a Suicidal Friend or Relative," Accessed February 2016, http://www.befrienders.org/helping-a-friend; and Befrienders Worldwide, "Suicidal Feelings," Accessed February 2016, http:// www.befrienders.org/suicidal-feelings.

87. Substance Abuse and Mental Health Services Administration, "Results from the 2014 National Survey on Drug Use and Health: Mental Health Findings," NSDUH Series H-50, HHS Publication no. SMA 15-4927 (Rockville, MD: Substance Abuse and Mental Health Services Administration, 2015), Available at http://www.samhsa.gov/data/ sites/default/files/NSDUH-FRR1-2014/ NSDUH-FRR1-2014.pdf.

88. MentalHealth.gov, "Mental Health Myths and Facts," Accessed February 2016, www .mentalhealth.gov/basics/myths-facts/.

89. A. Lasalvia et al., "Global Pattern of Experienced and Anticipated Discrimination Reported by People with Major Depressive

Disorder: A Cross-Sectional Survey," *The Lancet* 381, no. 9860 (2013): 55–62.

90. K. Huffman and C. A. Sanderson, *Real World Psychology* (Hoboken, NJ: Wiley, 2014).

91. Ibid.

92. Mayo Clinic, Cognitive Behavioral Therapy, February 2016, http://www.mayoclinic.org/tests-procedures/cognitive-behavioral-therapy/home/ovc-20186868.

93. Drug Watch, "FDA Warnings for Antidepressants," October 12, 2015, http://www.drugwatch.com/ssri/fda-warnings; R. Friedman, "Antidepressants' Black-Box Warning—10 Years Later," *New England Journal of Medicine* 371, no. 18 (2014): 1666–68.

**Pulled Statistics:**

p. 33, Centers for Disease Control and Prevention, "Suicide: Facts at a Glance, 2015," Accessed February 2016, Available at www.cdc.gov/violenceprevention/pdf/suicide-datasheet-a.pdf.

p. 43, D. Eisenberg et al., "Data from the Healthy Minds Network: The Economic Case for Student Mental Health Services," *Depression Center.org*, March 13, 2014, www.depressioncenter.org/docc/2014/pdf/eisenberg-lipson-economic-case-for-student-mental-health.pdf.

# Chapter 2A

1. K. Eagan et al., *The American Freshman: National Norms Fall 2014* (Los Angeles: Higher Education Research Institute, UCLA, 2014), Available at http://heri.ucla.edu/monographs/TheAmericanFreshman2014-Expanded.pdf.

2. Ibid.

3. H. G. Koenig, "Religion, Spirituality and Health: A Review and Update," *Advances in Mind–Body Medicine* 29, no. 3 (2015): 19–26.

4. K. Eagan et al., *The American Freshman*, 2014.

5. B. A. Alper, "Millennials Are Less Religious Than Older Americans, but Just as Spiritual," *Pew Research Center*, November 23, 2015, www.pewresearch.org/fact-tank/2015/11/23/millennials-are-less-religious-than-older-americans-but-just-as-spiritual/.

6. K. Eagan et al., *The American Freshman*, 2014.

7. B. L. Seaward, *Managing Stress: Principles and Strategies for Health and Well Being*, 7th ed. (Sudbury, MA: Jones and Bartlett, 2012).

8. American College Health Association. *American College Health Association–National College Health Assessment II: Reference Group Executive Summary Fall 2015* (Hanover, MD: American College Health Association, 2016).

9. DanahZohar.com, "Learn the Qs," Accessed January 2014, http://dzohar.com/?page_id=622.

10. C. Wigglesworth, "Spiritual Intelligence and Why It Matters," Deep Change, 2011, www.deepchange.com/SpiritualIntelligenceEmotionalIntelligence2011.pdf.

11. NIH, NCCIH, Research Results, accessed March 2015, https://nccih.nih.gov/research/results.

12. D. Fishbein et al., "Behavioral and Psychophysiological Effects of a Yoga Intervention on High-Risk Adolescents: A Randomized Control Trial," *Journal of Child and Family Studies* 25, no. 2 (2016): 518–29; L. Carim-Todd, S. H. Mitchell, and B. S. Oken, "Mind–Body Practices: An Alternative, Drug-Free Treatment for Smoking Cessation?: A Systematic Review of the Literature," *Drug and Alcohol Dependence* 132, no. 3 (2013): 399–410; H. Lu et al., "The Brain Structure Correlates of Individual Differences in Trait Mindfulness: A Voxel-Based Morphometry Study," *Neuroscience* 272 (2014): 21–8; H. Huang et al., "A Meta-Analysis of the Benefits of Mindfulness-Based Stress Reduction (MBSR) on Psychological Function Among Breast Cancer (BC) Survivors," *Breast Cancer*, Published online March 28, 2015 at http://link.springer.com/article/10.1007/s12282-015-0604-0#page-1.

13. National Cancer Institute (NCI), "Spirituality in Cancer Care," July 17, 2015, www.cancer.gov/cancertopics/pdq/supportivecare/spirituality/HealthProfessional/page1.

14. M. Mollica et al., "Spirituality is Associated with Better Prostate Cancer Treatment Decision Making Experiences," *Journal of Behavioral Medicine* 39, no. 1 (2016): 161–9.

15. P. Rajguru et al., "Use of Mindfulness Meditation in the Management of Chronic Pain: A Systematic Review of Randomized Controlled Trials," *American Journal of Lifestyle Medicine* 9, no 3 (2015): 176–84.

16. E. Singer, R. McElroy, and P. Muennig, "Social Capital and the Paradox of Poor but Healthy Groups in the United States," *Journal of Immigrant and Minority Health*, Published online 23 March 2016, doi 10.1007/s10903-016-0396-0.

17. C. Aldwin et al., "Differing Pathways between Religiousness, Spirituality, and Health: A Self-Regulation Perspective," *Psychology of Religion and Spirituality* 6, no. 1 (2014): 9–21.

18. H. Jim et al., "Religion, Spirituality, and Physical Health in Cancer Patients: A Meta-Analysis," *Cancer* 121, no. 21 (2015): 3760–8.

19. S. Hooker, K. Masters, and K. Carey, "Multidimensional Assessment of Religiousness/Spirituality and Health Behaviors in College Students," *International Journal for the Psychology of Religion* 24, no. 3 (2014): 228–40; V. Kress et al., "Spirituality/Religiosity, Life Satisfaction, and Life Meaning as Protective Factors for Nonsuicidal Self-Injury in College Students," *Journal of College Counseling* 18, no. 2 (2015): 160–74.

20. NCI, "Spirituality in Cancer Care," 2015.

21. A. Wachholtz and M. Rogoff, "The Relationship between Spirituality and Burnout among Medical Students," *Journal of Contemporary Medical Education* 1, no. 2 (2013): 83–91.

22. National Center for PTSD, "Spirituality and Trauma: Professionals Working Together," February 23, 2016, www.ptsd.va.gov/professional/provider-type/community/fs-spirituality.asp.

23. L. D'raven, L., N. Moliver, and D. Thompson, "Happiness Intervention Decreases Pain and Depression, Boosts Happiness Among Primary Care Patients," *Primary Health Care Research and Development* 16, no. 2 (2015): 114–26; J. C. Huffman et al., "Feasibility and Utility of Positive Psychology Exercises for Suicidal Inpatients," *General Hospital Psychiatry* 36, no. 1 (2014): 88–94.

24. B. A. Alper, "Millennials Are Less Religious Than Older Americans, but Just as Spiritual," *Pew Research Center*, November 23, 2015, www.pewresearch.org/fact-tank/2015/11/23/millennials-are-less-religious-than-older-americans-but-just-as-spiritual/.

25. Ibid.; NCCAM, "Prayer and Spirituality in Health: Ancient Practices, Modern Science," *CAM at the NIH: Focus on Complementary and Alternative Medicine* 12, no. 1 (2005), www.jpsych.com/pdfs/NCCAM%20-%20Prayer%20and%20Spirituality%20in%20Health.pdf; NCI, "Spirituality in Cancer Care," 2015.

26. A. Grecucci et al., "Mindful Emotion Regulation: Exploring the Neurocognitive Mechanisms behind Mindfulness," *BioMed Research International* 2015 (2015), Available at http://dx.doi.org/10.1155/2015/670724.

27. G. Desbordes et al., "Effects of Mindful-Attention and Compassion Meditation Training on Amygdala Response to Emotional Stimuli in an Ordinary, Non-meditative State," *Frontiers in Human Neuroscience* 6, no. 292 (2012), doi: 10.3389/fnhum.2012.00292.

28. National Center for Complementary and Integrative Health (NCCIH), "Research Spotlight: Meditation May Increase Empathy," Modified January 2012, https://nccih.nih.gov/research/results/spotlight/060608.htm.

29. G. Desbordes et al., "Effects of Mindful-Attention and Compassion Meditation," 2012.

30. F. Zeidan et al., "Neural Correlates of Mindfulness Meditation-Related Anxiety Relief," *Social Cognitive and Affective Neuroscience* 9, no. 6 (2014): 751–59, doi: 10.1093/scan/nst041; G. Desbordes et al., "Effects of Mindful-Attention," 2012; J. C. Ong et al., "A Randomized Controlled Trial of Mindfulness Meditation for Chronic Insomnia," *Sleep* 37, no. 9 (2013): 1553–63; NCCIH, "Research Spotlight," 2014.

31. S. Keng et al. "Effects of Mindfulness on Psychological Health: A Review of Empirical Studies," *Clinical Psychology Review* 31, no. 6 (2011): 1041–56; E. Hoge et al., "Randomized Controlled Trial of Mindfulness Meditation for Generalized Anxiety Disorder: Effects on Anxiety and Stress Reactivity," *Journal of Clinical Psychiatry* 74, no. 8 (2013): 786–92; S. Jedel et al., "A Randomized Controlled Trial of Mindfulness-Based Stress Reduction to Prevent Flare-Up in Patients with Inactive Ulcerative Colitis," *Digestion* 89, no. 2 (2014): 142–55. R. Baer, *Mindfulness-Based Treatment Approaches: Clinician's Guide to Evidence Base and Applications*, 2nd ed. (London: Elsevier, 2014).

32. W. Marchand, "Neural Mechanisms of Mindfulness and Meditation: Evidence from Neuroimaging Studies," *World Journal of Radiology* 6, no. 7 (2014): 471–79, doi: 10.4329/wjr.v6.i7.471.

33. S. Keng et al. "Effects of Mindfulness on Psychological Health," *Clinical Psychology Review* 31, no. 6 (2011); 1041–56; M. Spijkerman, W. Pots, and E. Bohlmeijer, "Effectiveness of Online Mindfulness-Based Interventions in Improving Mental Health: A Review and Meta-Analysis of Randomised Controlled Trials," *Clinical Psychology Review* 45 (2016): 102–14.

34. W. Marchand, "Neural Mechanisms of Mindfulness and Meditation," 2014; B. Holzel et al., "Neural Mechanisms of Symptom Improvements in Generalized Anxiety Disorder Following Mindfulness Training," *Neuroimage: Clinical* 2 (2013): 448–58; A. Taren et al., "Mindfulness Meditation Training Alters Stress-Related Amygdala Resting State Functional Connectivity: A Randomized Controlled Trial," *Social Cognitive and Affective Neuroscience* 10, no. 12 (2015): 1758–68.

35. A. Lucette et al., "Spirituality and Religiousness Are Associated with Fewer Depressive Symptoms in Individuals with Medical Conditions," *Psychosomatics* (2016), doi: 10.1016/j.psym.2016.03.005; University of Minnesota Center for Spirituality and Healing, "What Is Prayer?," August 2013, www.takingcharge.csh.umn.edu/explore-healing-practices/prayer.

36. L. Larkey et al., "Randomized Controlled Trial of Qigong/Tai Chi Easy on Cancer-Related Fatigue in Breast Cancer Survivors," *Annals of Behavioral Medicine* 49, no. 2 (2015): 165–76; American Tai Chi Association, "Psychiatric Expert: Tai Chi and Qigong Can Improve Mood in Older Adults," September 6, 2013, www.americantaichi.net/TaiChiQigong-ForHealthArticle.asp?cID=2&sID=10&article=chi_201309_1&subject=Mental Health.

37. G. Zheng et al., "Tai Chi and the Protection of Cognitive Ability," *American Journal of Preventive Medicine* 49, no. 1 (2015): 89–97; G. Zheng et al., "Effectiveness of Tai Chi on Physical and Psychological Health of College Students: Results of a Randomized Controlled Trial," *PLoS ONE* 10, no. 7 (2015): e0132605, doi:10.1371/journal.pone.0132605.

38. M. Rudd and J. Aakers, "How to Be Happy by Giving to Others," *Scientific American*, July 8, 2014, www.scientificamerican.com/article/how-to-be-happy-by-giving-to-others/.

39. F. Warneken and M. Tomasello, "The Roots of Human Altruism," *British Journal of Psychology* 100, no. 3 (2009): 455–71; C. Carter, *Raising Happiness: 10 Simple Steps for More Joyful Kids and Happier Parents* (New York: Ballantine, 2010); R. I. Dunbar et al., "Social Laughter Is Correlated with an Elevated Pain Threshold," *Proceedings of the Royal Society,* September 14, 2011, doi: 10.1098/rspb.2011.1373.39%.

**Pulled Statistics:**

p. 52, K. Eagan et al., *The American Freshman: National Norms Fall* 2014 (Los Angeles: Higher Education Research Institute, UCLA, 2014), available at http://heri.ucla.edu/monographs/TheAmericanFreshman2014-Expanded.pdf.

p. 55, Emily Esfahani Smith and Jennifer L. Aaker, "Millennial Searchers," *The New York Times Sunday Review*, November 13, 2013, Available at www.nytimes.com/2013/12/01/opinion/sunday/millennial-searchers.html?_r=0.

p. 59, H. Cramer et al., "Prevalence, Patterns, and Predictors of Yoga Use: Results of a US Nationally Representative Survey," *American Journal of Preventive Medicine* 50, no. 2 (2016): 230–35.

## Chapter 3

1. W. Lovallo, *Stress and Health: Biological and Psychological Interactions*, 3rd ed. (Los Angeles, CA: Sage, 2016).

2. American Psychological Association, "Stress in America: Paying with Our Health," February 2015, Available at https://www.apa.org/news/press/releases/stress/2014/stress-report.pdf.

3. C. Wallis, "Stress: Can We Cope?" *Time*, June 6, 1983, http://content.time.com/time/magazine/article/0,9171,950883,00.html.

4. American Psychological Association, "Stress in America," 2015; American Psychological Association, "Stress in America Annual Survey: Are Teens Adopting Adults' Stress Habits?" February 11, 2014, Available at www.apa.org/news/press/releases/2013/stress-report.pdf; S. Bethune, "Health-care Falls Short on Stress Management," *Monitor on Psychology* 44, no. 4 (2013): 22.

5. American Psychological Association, "A Stress Snapshot:Women Continue to Face an Uphill Battle with Stress," Accessed January 30, 2015, http://apa.org/news/press/releases/stress/2013/snapshot.aspx.

6. American Psychological Association, "Stress in America," 2015.

7. American Psychological Association, "Stress: The Different Kinds of Stress," Accessed February 2014, www.apa.org/helpcenter/stress-kinds.aspx.

8. B. L. Seaward, *Managing Stress: Principles and Strategies for Health and Well-Being*, 8th ed. (Sudbury, MA: Jones & Bartlett, 2013), 8; National Institute of Mental Health (NIMH), "Fact Sheet on Stress," Accessed January 2016, www.nimh.nih.gov/health/publications/stress/index.shtml/index.shtml.

9. H. Selye, "A Syndrome Produced by Diverse Nocuous Agents," *Nature* 138, no. 3479 (1936): 32; S. Szabo, T. Yvette, and A Somogyi, "The Legacy of Hans Selye and the Origins of Stress Research: A Retrospective 75 Years After His Landmark Brief 'Letter' to the Editor of *Nature*," *Stress* 15, no. 5 (2012): 472–78.

10. W. B. Cannon, *The Wisdom of the Body* (New York: Norton, 1932).

11. C. Fagundes and B. Way, "Early-Life Stress and Adult Inflammation," *Current Directions in Psychological Science* 23, no. 4 (2014): 277–83; J. Morey et al., "Current Directions in Stress and Human Immune Function," *Current Opinion in Psychology* 5 (2015): 13–17.

12. M. Dentato, "The Minority Stress Perspective," *American Psychological Association*, Accessed January 2016, www.apa.org/pi/aids/resources/exchange/2012/04/minority-stress.aspx.

13. R. Yerkes and J. Dodson, "The Relation of Strength of Stimulus to Rapidity of Habit-Formation," *Journal of Comparative Neurology and Psychology* 18, no. 5 (1908): 459–82.

14. C. Cardoso and M. A. Ellenbogen, "Tend-and-Befriend is a Beacon for Change in Stress Research: A Reply to Tops," *Psychoneuroendocrinology* 45 (2014): 212–13; J. Berger et al., "Cortisol Modulates Men's Affiliative Responses to Acute Social Stress," *Psychoneuroendocrinology* 63 (2016): 1–9.

15. Ibid.

16. A. Crum, P. Salovey, and S. Achor, "Rethinking Stress: The Role of Mindsets in Determining the Stress Response," *Journal of Personality and Social Psychology* 104, no. 4 (2013): 716–33.

17. P. Gianaros and T. Wager, "Brain–Body Pathways Linking Psychological Stress and Physical Health," *Current Directions in Psychological Science* 24, no. 4 (2015): 313–21; K. M. Scott et al., "Associations Between Lifetime Traumatic Events and Subsequent Chronic Physical Conditions: A Cross-National, Cross-Sectional Study," *PLoS ONE* 8, no. 11 (2013), e80573.

18. K. M. Scott et al., "Associations Between Lifetime Traumatic Events and Subsequent Chronic Physical Conditions," 2013.

19. Robert Scaer, *The Body Bears the Burden: Trauma, Dissociation, and Disease*, 3rd ed. (New York: Routledge, 2014).

20. A. Steptoe and M. Kivimaki, "Stress and Cardiovascular Disease: An Update on Current Knowledge," *Annual Review of Public Health* 34 (2013): 337–54; H. Maxime, J. Kuysie, and I. Bot, "Acute and Chronic Psychological Stress as Risk Factors for Cardiovascular Disease: Insights Gained from Epidemiological, Clinical, and Experimental Studies," *Brain, Behavior, and Immunity* 50, no. 11 (2015): 18–30.

21. N. Aggarwal et al., "Perceived Stress is Associated with Subclinical Cerebrovascular Disease in Older Adults," *American Journal of Geriatric Psychiatry* 22, no. 1 (2014): 53–62; A. Steptoe and M. Kivimaki, "Stress and Cardiovascular Disease: An Update on Current Knowledge," *Annual Review of Public Health* 34 (2013): 337–54; H. Maxime, J. Kuysie, and I. Bot, "Acute and Chronic Psychological Stress as Risk Factors for Cardiovascular Disease," 2015.

22. M. Kivimäki and I. Kawachi, "Work Stress as a Risk Factor for Cardiovascular Disease," *Current Cardiology Reports* 17, no. 9 (2015): 1–9; M. Skogstad et al., "Systematic Review of the Cardiovascular Effects of Occupational Noise," *Occupational Medicine* 66, no. 1 (2016): 10–16.

23. S. Garbarino and N. Magnavita, "Work Stress and Metabolic Syndrome in Police Officers: A Prospective Study," *PLoS ONE* 10, no. 12 (2015): e0144318; F. Bartoli et al., "Posttraumatic Stress Disorder and Risk of Obesity: Systematic Review and Meta-analysis," *Journal of Clinical Psychiatry* 76, no. 10 (2015): e1253–61.

24. Mayo Clinic, "Stress and Hair Loss: Are They Related?," January 2014, www.mayoclinic.com/health/stress-and-hair-loss/AN01442.

25. American Diabetes Association, "Stress and Diabetes," June 7, 2013, www.diabetes.org/living-with-diabetes/complications/mental-health/stress.html; J. Montane, L. Cadavez, and A. Novials, "Stress and the Inflammatory

Process: A Major Cause of Pancreatic Cell Death in Type 2 Diabetes," *Diabetes, Metabolic Syndrome, and Obesity* 7, no. 2 (2014): 25–34.

26. C. Lee et al., "*Journal of Aging and Health* 26 (2014): 952–68.

27. M. Virtanen et al., "Psychological Distress and Incidence of Type 2 Diabetes in High Risk and Low Risk Populations: The Whitehall II Cohort Study," *Diabetes Care* 37, no. 8 (2014): 2091–97.

28. National Digestive Diseases Information Clearinghouse (NDDIC), "Irritable Bowel Syndrome: How Does Stress Affect IBS?" Accessed January, 2016. http://digestive .niddk.nih.gov/ddiseases/pubs/ibs/#stress.

29. H. F. Herlong, "Digestive Disorders White Paper–2013," *Johns Hopkins Health Alerts*, 2013, www.johnshopkinshealthalerts.com.

30. E. Carlsson et al., "Psychological Stress in Children May Alter the Immune Response," *Journal of Immunology* 192, no. 5 (2014): 2071–81; J. Morey et al., "Current Directions in Stress and Human Immune Function," 2015.

31. F. Dhabhar, "Effects of Stress on Immune Function: The Good, the Bad, and the Beautiful," *Immunologic Research* 58, no. 2–3 (2014): 193–210; J. Morey et al., "Current Directions in Stress and Human Immune Function," 2015.

32. American College Health Association (ACHA), *American College Health Association–National College Health Assessment II (ACHA-NCHA II): Reference Group Data Report Spring, 2015* (Hanover, MD: American College Health Association, 2016).

33. Ibid.

34. Ibid.

35. O. T. Wolf et al., "Stress and Memory: A Selective Review on Recent Developments in the Understanding of Stress Hormone Effects on Memory and Their Clinical Relevance," *Journal of Neuroendocrinology* (2015), doi: 10.1111/jne.12353; R. M. Shansky and J. Lipps, "Stress-Induced Cognitive Dysfunction: Hormone–Neurotransmitter Interactions in the Prefrontal Cortex," *Neuroscience and Biobehavioral Reviews* 7 (2013): 123, Available at www.ncbi.nlm.nih .gov/pmc/articles/PMC3617365.

36. J. Oliver et al., "Impairments of the Spatial Working Memory and Attention Following Acute Psychosocial Stress," *Stress and Health* 31, no. 2 (2015): 115–23.

37. D. Baglietto-Vargas et al., "Short-term Modern Life-like Stress Exacerbates Aβ-Pathology and Synapse Loss in 3xTg-AD Mice," *Journal of Neurochemistry* 134, no. 5 (2015): 915–26; E. Marcello, F. Gardoni, and M. Di Luca, "Alzheimer's Disease and Modern Lifestyle: What is the Role of Stress?," *Journal of Neurochemistry* 134, no. 5 (2015): 795–98.

38. L. Mah, C. Szabuniewicz, and Alexandra J. Fiocco, "Can Anxiety Damage the Brain?" *Current Opinion in Psychiatry* 29, no. 1 (2016): 56–62; T. Frodi and V. O'Keane, "How Does the Brain Deal with Cumulative Stress?: A Review with Focus on Developmental Stress, HPA Axis Function and Hippocampal Struc-

ture in Humans," *Neurobiology of Disease* 52 (2013): 24–37.

39. American Psychological Association, "Stress in America," 2015.

40. S. Charles et al., "The Wear and Tear of Daily Stressors on Mental Health," *Psychological Science* 24, no. 5 (2013): 733–41; J. R. Piazza et al., "Affective Reactivity to Daily Stressors and Long-Term Risk of Reporting a Chronic Physical Health Condition," *Annals of Behavioral Medicine* 45, no. 1 (2013): 110–20; C. Aldwin et al., "Do Hassles Mediate between Life Events and Mortality in Older Men?: Longitudinal Findings from the VA Normative Aging Study," *Experimental Gerontology* 59 (2014): 74–80.

41. C. Aldwin et al., "Do Hassles Mediate between Life Events and Mortality?," 2014; S. O'Neill et al., "Affective Reactivity to Daily Interpersonal Stressors as a Prospective Predictor of Depressive Symptoms," *Journal of Social and Clinical Psychology* 23, no. 2 (2004): 172–94.

42. K. M. Krajnak, "Potential Contribution of Work-Related Psychosocial Stress to the Development of Cardiovascular Disease and Type II Diabetes: A Brief Review," *Environmental Health Insights* 8, Supplement 1 (2014): 41–45; N. Vurtanen, S. T. Nyberg, and G. D. Batty, "Perceived Job Insecurity as a Risk Factor for Incident Coronary Heart Disease: Systematic Review and Meta-Analysis," *British Medical Journal* 347 (2013): f4746; K. Toren et al., "A Longitudinal General Population-Based Study of Job Strain and Risk for Coronary Heart Disease and Stroke in Swedish Men," *British Medical Journal Open* 4, no. 3 (2014): e004355.

43. Jeffery Sparshott, "Congratulations, Class of 2015. You're the Most Indebted Ever (For Now)," *Wall Street Journal*, May 8, 2015, http:// blogs.wsj.com/economics/2015/05/08/ congratulations-class-of-2015-youre-the-most-indebted-ever-for-now/.

44. American College Health Association, *National College Health Assessment II: Reference Group Data Report Spring, 2015*, 2016.

45. S. Schwartz et al., "Acculturation and Well-Being Among College Students from Immigrant Families," *Journal of Clinical Psychology* 69, no. 4 (2013): 298–318; A. Pieterse et al., "An Exploratory Examination of the Associations Among Racial and Ethnic Discrimination, Racial Climate, and Trauma-Related Symptoms in a College Student Population," *Journal of Counseling Psychology* 57, no. 3 (2010): 255–63; A. McAleavey, L. Castonguay, and B. Locke, "Sexual Orientation Minorities in College Counseling: Prevalence, Distress, and Symptom Profiles," *Journal of College Counseling* 14, no. 2 (2011): 127–42.

46. American Psychological Association, "Stress in America," 2015; The Commonwealth Fund, "Comparative Survey of Minority Health," Accessed February 2016, www.common wealthfund.org.

47. K. Cokley et al., "An Examination of the Impact of Minority Status Stress and Imposter Feelings on the Mental Health of Diverse Ethnic Minority College Students," *Journal of*

*Multicultural Counseling and Development* 41, no. 2 (2013): 82–95; U.S. Department of Health and Human Services: Office of Minority Health, "Heart Disease and African Americans," January 28, 2016, http://minority health.hhs.gov/omh/browse.aspx?lvl=4& lvlid=19; American Heart Association, "Bridging the Gap: CVD Health Disparities," Accessed January 2016, www.heart.org.

48. American Psychological Association, "Stress in America," 2015; The Commonwealth Fund, "Comparative Survey of Minority Health," 2016; U.S. Department of Health and Human Services, Office of Minority Health, "Heart Disease and African Americans," January 28, 2016, http://minorityhealth.hhs.gov/omh/ browse.aspx?lvl=4&lvlid=19; American Heart Association, "Bridging the Gap: CVD Health Disparities," Accessed January 2016, www .heart.org.

49. K. N. Mossakowski, "Disadvantaged Family Background and Depression among Young Adults in the United States: The Roles of Chronic Stress and Self-esteem," *Stress and Health* 31, no. 1 (2015): 52–62; K. R. Conner et al., "Posttraumatic Stress Disorder and Suicide in 5.9 Million Individuals Receiving Care in the Veterans Health Administration Health System," *Journal of Affective Disorders* 166 (2014): 1–5; K. Brown, *Predictors of Suicide Ideation and the Moderating Effects of Suicide Attitudes*, Master's thesis, University of Ohio, 2011, http://etd.ohiolink.edu; J. Gomez, R. Miranda, and L Polanco, "Acculturative Stress, Perceived Discrimination and Vulnerability to Suicide Attempts Among Emerging Adults," *Journal of Youth and Adolescence* 40, no. 11 (2011): 1465–76.

50. B. L. Seaward, *Managing Stress*, 2013.

51. J. Twenge, *Generation Me–Revised and Updated: Why Today's Young Americans Are More Confident, Assertive, Entitled and More Miserable Than Ever* (New York, Simon & Schuster, 2014).

52. A. Peng, J. Schaubroeck, and J. Xie, "When Confidence Comes and Goes: How Variation in Self-Efficacy Moderates Stressor–Strain Relationships," *Journal of Occupational Health Psychology* 20, no. 3 (2015): 359–76; R. Fida et al., "'Yes I Can'": The Protective Role of Personal Self Efficacy in Hindering Counterproductive Work Activity Under Stressful Conditions," *Anxiety, Stress and Coping* 28, no 5 (2014): 479–99.

53. A. Peng, J. Schaubroeck, and J. Xie, "When Confidence Comes and Goes," 2015.

54. D. L. Merritt and W. Buboltz, "Academic Success in College: Socioeconomic Status and Parental Influence as Predictors of Outcome," *Open Journal of Social Sciences* 3, no. 5 (2015): 127; M. Komarraju and D. Nadler, "Self Efficacy and Academic Achievement: Who Do Implicit Beliefs, Goals and Effort Regulation Matter?," *Learning and Individual Differences* 25 (2013): 67–72.

55. P. N. von der Embse and S. Witmer, "High-Stakes Accountability: Student Anxiety and Large-Scale Testing," *Journal of Applied School Psychology* 30, no. 2 (2014): 132–56.

56. A. Zuffiano et al., "Academic Achievement: The Unique Contribution of Self Efficacy Beliefs in Self-Regulated Learning beyond Intelligence, Personality Traits and Self-esteem," *Learning and Individual Differences* 23 (2013): 158–62.

57. M. Friedman and R. H. Rosenman, *Type A Behavior and Your Heart* (New York: Knopf, 1974).

58. S.C. Kobasa, "Stressful Life Events, Personality, and Health: An Inquiry into Hardiness," *Journal of Personality and Social Psychology* 37, no. 1 (1979): 1–11.

59. R. Graber, F. Pichon, and E. Carubine, "Psychological Resilience: State of Knowledge and Future Research Agendas: Working Paper 425," October 2015, Available at http://www.odi.org/sites/odi.org.uk/files/odi-assets/publications-opinion-files/9872.pdf.

60. M. Sarkar and D. Fletcher, "Ordinary Magic, Extraordinary Performance: Psychological Resilience and Thriving in High Achievers," *Sport, Exercise, and Performance Psychology* 3, no. 1 (2014): 46.

61. A. Duckworth and J. J. Gross, "Self-Control and Grit Related but Separable Determinants of Success," *Current Directions in Psychological Science* 23, no. 5 (2014): 319–25.

62. A. Rosenberg et al., "Promoting Resilience in Stress Management: A Pilot Study of a Novel Resilience-Promoting Intervention for Adolescents and Young Adults with Serious Illness," *Journal of Pediatric Psychology* 40, no. 9 (2015): 992–9; J. Creswell and E. Lindsay, "How Does Mindfulness Training Affect Health?: A Mindfulness Stress Buffering Account," *Current Directions in Psychological Science* 23, no. 6 (2014): 401–07.

63. P. Pimple et al., "Association Between Anger and Mental Stress–Induced Myocardial Ischemia," *American Heart Journal* 169, no. 1 (2015): 115–21.

64. S. J. Kelly and M. Ismail, "Stress and Type 2 Diabetes: A Review of How Stress Contributes to the Development of Type 2 Diabetes," *Annual Review of Public Health* 36 (2015): 441–62.

65. G. Mate, *When the Body Says No: Understanding the Stress–Disease Connection* (Hoboken, NJ: Wiley, 2011).

66. J. Thayer et al., "Potential Biological Pathways Linking Type-D Personality and Poor Health: A Cross-Sectional Investigation," *Psychotherapy and Psychosomatics* 84 (2015); R. Garcia-Retamero et al., "On the Relationship Between Type-D Personality and Cardiovascular Health," *European Health Psychologist* 17, Supplement (2015): 707.

67. E. Chen, K. C. McLean, and G. E. Miller, "Shift-and-Persist Strategies: Associations with Socioeconomic Status and the Regulation of Inflammation Among Adolescents and Their Parents," *Psychosomatic Medicine* 77, no. 4 (2015): 371–82.

68. Higher Education Research Institute, "A Year of Change: First Year," Accessed January 30, 2015, www.heri.ucla.edu/infographics/YFCY-2014-Infographic.pdf; J. K. Eagen et al., *The American Freshman: National Norms Fall 2014–Expanded Edition* (Los Angeles, CA: Higher Education Research Institute, 2015), www.heri.ucla.edu/monographs/TheAmerican Freshman2014-Expanded.pdf

69. Higher Education Research Institute, "A Year of Change," 2015; K. Eagen, *The American Freshman*, 2015.

70. B. L. Seaward, *Managing Stress*, 2016.

71. Kristin Neff, "What Is Self Compassion?" Accessed February 2016, http://self-compassion.org.

72. J. Gu et al., "How Do Mindfulness-Based Cognitive Therapy and Mindfulness-Based Stress Reduction Improve Mental Health and Wellbeing?: A Systematic Review and Meta-analysis of Mediation Studies," *Clinical Psychology Review* 37 (2015): 1–12.

73. E. R. Stein and B. W. Smith, "Social Support Attenuates the Harmful Effects of Stress in Healthy Adult Women," *Social Science and Medicine* 146 (2015): 129–36.

74. N. Saha and A. C. Karpinski, "The Influence of Social Media on International Students' Global Life Satisfaction and Academic Performance," *Campus Support Services, Programs, and Policies for International Students* (2016): 57; J. Moskowitz et al., "A Positive Affect Intervention for People Experiencing Health-Related Stress: Development and Non-randomized Pilot Test," *Journal of Health Psychology* 17, no. 5 (2012): 676–92.

75. M. Panagioti et al., "Perceived Social Support Buffers the Impact of PTSD Symptoms on Suicidal Behavior: Implications into Suicide Resilience Research," *Comprehensive Psychiatry* 55, no. 1 (2014): 104–12.

76. B. L. Seaward, *Managing Stress,* 2016.

77. W. Lovallo, *Stress and Health: Biological and Psychological Interactions*, 3rd ed. (Thousand Oaks, CA: Sage, 2016); A. Lurie and K. Monahan, "Humor, Aging, and Life Review: Survival Through the Use of Humor," *Social Work in Mental Health* 13, no. 1 (2015): 82–91; C. Dormann, "Laughter as the Best Medicine: Exploring Humour-Mediated Health Applications," in *Distributed, Ambient, and Pervasive Interactions*, ed. N. Streitz (New York: Springer, 2015), 639–50.

78. W. Lovallo, *Stress and Health*, 2016; D. A. Girdano, D. E. Dusek, and G. S. Everly, *Controlling Stress and Tension*, 9th ed. (San Francisco: Benjamin Cummings, 2013), 375.

79. W. Lovallo, *Stress and Health*, 2016; M. A. Stults-Kolehmainen and R. Sinha, "The Effect of Stress on Physical Activity and Exercise," *Sports Medicine* 44, no. 1 (2014): 81–121; E. M. Jackson, "Stress Relief: The Role of Exercise in Stress Management," *ACSM Health and Fitness Journal* 17, no. 3 (2013): 14–19.

80. P. M. Gollwitzer and G. Oettingen, "Implementation Intentions," in *Encyclopedia of Behavioral Medicine* (Part 9), eds. M. Gellman and J. R. Turner (New York: Springer-Verlag, 2013), 1043–48; C. Stern et al., "Effects of Implementation Intention on Anxiety, Perceived Proximity and Motor Performance," *Personality and Social Psychology Bulletin* 39, no. 5 (2013): 623–35.

81. Yoga Journal and Yoga Alliance, "Yoga in America Study," January 2016, Available at http://media.yogajournal.com/wp-content/uploads/2016-Yoga-in-America-Study-Comprehensive-RESULTS.pdf.

82. Lau, Caren, Ruby Yu, and Jean Woo. "Effects of a 12-Week Hatha Yoga Intervention on Cardiorespiratory Endurance, Muscular Strength and Endurance, and Flexibility in Hong Kong Chinese Adults: A Controlled Clinical Trial." *Evidence-Based Complementary and Alternative Medicine* 2015 (2015), doi: 10.1155/2015/958727; M. E. Papp, et al., "Effects of High-Intensity Hatha Yoga on Cardiovascular Fitness, Adipocytokines, and Apolipoproteins in Healthy Students: A Randomized Controlled Study," *Journal of Alternative and Complementary Medicine* 22, no. 1(2016): 81–87; NIH Medline Plus, "What Yoga Can and Can't Do for You," December 2013, www.nlm.nih.gov/medlineplus/news/fullstory_143813.html.

83. P. E. Jeter et al., "Yoga as a Therapeutic Intervention: A Rearnoteliometric Analysis of Published Research Studies from 1967 to 2013," *Journal of Alternative and Complementary Medicine* 21, no. 10 (2015): 586–92; S. R. Steinhubl et al., "Cardiovascular and Nervous System Changes During Meditation," *Frontiers in Human Neuroscience* 9 (2015): 145; R. Jerath et al., "Self-Regulation of Breathing as a Primary Treatment for Anxiety," *Applied Psychophysiology and Biofeedback* 40, no. 2 (2015): 107–15.

84. S. R. Steinhubl et al., "Cardiovascular and Nervous System Changes During Meditation," 2015; R. D. Brook et al., "Beyond Medications and Diet: Alternative Approaches to Lowering Blood Pressure: A Scientific Statement from the American Heart Association," *Hypertension* 61, no. 6 (2013): 1360–83.

85. National Center for Complementary and Integrative Health, "Massage Therapy for Health Purposes: What You Need to Know," May 2015, http://nccam.nih.gov/health/massage/massageintroduction.htm.

**Pulled statistics:**

p. 65, American Psychological Association, "Stress in America," 2015.

p. 72, American Psychological Association, "Stress in America," 2015.

p. 78, American Psychological Association, "Stress in America," 2015.

p. 78, American Psychological Association, "Stress in America," 2015.

## Chapter 3A

1. B. Bosworth, G. Burtless, K. Zhang, "Later Retirement, Inequality in Old Age, and the Growing Gap in Longevity Between Rich and Poor," *Economic Studies at Brookings*, January 2016, Available at www.brookings.edu/~/media/Research/Files/Reports/2016/01/life-expectancy-gaps-promise-social-security/

BosworthBurtlessZhang_retirementine
qualitylongevity_012815.pdf; Institute for
Health Metrics and Evaluation, "U.S County
Profiles," Accessed March 17, 2016, www
.healthdata.org/us-county-profiles.

2. World Health Organization, "Social Determinants of Health: Key Concepts," *Commission on Social Determinants of Health, 2005–2008,* Accessed March 2016, www.who.int/social_determinants/thecommission/finalreport/key_concepts/en.

3. OECD, *How's Life? 2015: Measuring Well-being* (Paris: OECD Publishing, October 13, 2015). www.oecd.org/statistics/how-s-life-23089679.htm.

4. P. Jha et al., "Global Hazards of Tobacco and the Benefits of Smoking Cessation and Tobacco Taxes," *Cancer: Disease Control Priorities*, 3rd ed. (The World Bank, 2015), www.ncbi.nlm.nih.gov/books/NBK343639/.

5. Ibid.

6. A. Carlsson et al., "Financial Stress in Late Adulthood and Diverse Risks of Incident Cardiovascular Disease and All-Cause Mortality in Women and Men," *BMC Public Health* 14, no. 1 (2014): 17.

7. R. Pruchno, M. Wilson-Genderson, and A. K. Gupta, "Neighborhood Food Environment and Obesity in Community-Dwelling Older Adults: Individual and Neighborhood Effects," *Journal of Public Health* 104, no. 5 (2014): 924–9; D. Viola et al., "Overweight and Obesity: Can We Reconcile Evidence about Supermarkets and Fast Food Retailers for Public Health Policy?," *Journal of Public Health Policy* 34, no. 3 (2013): 424–38.

8. Centers for Disease Control and Prevention, "Food Deserts," Updated June 2013, www.cdc.gov/healthcommunication/toolstemplates/entertainmented/tips/fooddesert.html.

9. A. H. Gaglioti et al., "Access to Primary Care in US Counties Is Associated with Lower Obesity Rates," *Journal of the American Board of Family Medicine* 29, no. 2 (2016): 182–90.

10. American Cancer Society, "Cancer Facts and Figures 2016," Accessed March 2016, Available at www.cancer.org/research/cancerfactsstatistics/cancerfactsfigures2016/.

11. K. N. Dauner, N. A. Wilmot, and J. F. Schultz, "Investigating the Temporal Relationship Between Individual-Level Social Capital and Health in Fragile Families," *BMC Public Health* 15, no. 1 (2015): 1130.

12. S. B. Johnson, J. L. Riis, and K. G. Noble, "State of the Art Review: Poverty and the Developing Brain," *Pediatrics* (2016): pii:peds.2015-3075. [E-pub ahead of print.]

13. College Board, Trends in Higher Education, "Tuition and Fees and Room and Board over Time," Accessed March 2016, http://trends.collegeboard.org/college-pricing/figures-tables/tuition-fees-room-board-time.

14. College Board, Trends in Higher Education, "Average Estimated Undergraduate Budgets, 2015–2016," Accessed March 2016, http://trends.collegeboard.org/college-pricing/figures-tables/average-estimated-undergraduate-budgets-2015-16.

15. National Survey of Student Engagement, *NSSE Annual Results 2015: Engagement Insights: Survey Findings on the Quality of Undergraduate Education* (Bloomington: Indiana University Center for Postsecondary Research, 2015).

16. American College Health Association, *American College Health Association–National College Health Assessment II (ACHA-NACHA II): Undergraduate Students, Reference Group Data Report, Spring 2015* (Hanover, MD: American College Health Association, 2015).

17. K. Eagan et al., *The American Freshman: National Norms Fall 2015* (Los Angeles: Higher Education Research Institute, UCLA, 2016); Sallie Mae and Ipsos, *How America Pays for College 2015: A National Study*, Accessed March 2016, http://news.salliemae.com/files/doc_library/file/HowAmericaPaysforCollege-2015FNL.pdf.

18. K. Eagan et al., *The American Freshman*, 2016.

19. Ibid.

20. Sallie Mae and Ipsos, *How America Pays for College 2015*, 2016.

21. The White House, President Barack Obama, "Higher Education," Accessed March, 2016, https://www.whitehouse.gov/issues/education/higher-education.

22. Ibid.

23. Ibid.

24. Sallie Mae and Ipsos, *How America Pays for College 2015*, 2016.

25. National Center for Education Statistics, "Institutional Retention and Graduation Rates for Undergraduate Students," *The Condition of Education*, 2015 (NCES 2015-144), May 2015, https://nces.ed.gov/programs/coe/indicator_cva.asp.

26. National Center for Education Statistics, "Annual Earnings of Young Adults," *The Condition of Education 2015* (NCES 2015-0144), May 2015, http://nces.ed.gov/pubs2015/2015144.pdf.

27. American College Health Association, *American College Health Association–National College Health Assessment II (ACHA-NACHA II): Undergraduate Students, Reference Group Data Report, Spring 2015*.

28. F. R. Avilucea et al., "The Costs of Operative Complications for Ankle Fractures: A Case Control Study," *Advances in Orthopedics* 2014 (2014), http://dx.doi.org/10.1155/2014/709241.

29. K. M. Walsemann, "Sick of Our Loans: Student Borrowing and the Mental Health of Young Adults in the United States," *Social Science and Medicine* 124 (2015): 85–93.

30. Board of Governors of the Federal Reserve System, "Consumer Credit," March 7 2016. www.federalreserve.gov/releases/g19/current/.

31. NASDAQ, "Credit Card Debt Statistics," September 23, 2014, www.nasdaq.com/article/credit-card-debt-statistics-cm393820.

32. Federal Reserve Bank of New York, Research and Statistics Group, Microeconomic Studies, "Quarterly Report on Household Debt and Credit," November 2015, www.newyorkfed.org.

33. Ibid.

34. Credit Card Accountability Responsibility and Disclosure Act, *The CARD Act of 2009*, Pub.L. 111–24, 111th Cong. (2009). Full text available at www.gpo.gov.

35. Javelin Strategy & Research, "2015 Identity Fraud: Protecting Vulnerable Populations," March 2015, Available at https://www.javelinstrategy.com/coverage-area/2015-identity-fraud-protecting-vulnerable-populations.

36. Federal Trade Commission, Consumer Information, "Lost or Stolen Credit, ATM, and Debit Cards," August 2012, www.consumer.ftc.gov/articles/0213-lost-or-stolen-credit-atm-and-debit-cards.

37. J. Herron, "Survey: Student Loan Debt Forces Many to Put Life on Hold," *Bankrate Money Pulse Survey*, August 5, 2015. Available at www.bankrate.com/finance/consumer-index/money-pulse-0815.aspx.

**Pulled statistics:**

p. 97, Nerd Wallet, "American Household Credit Card Debt Statistics: 2015," December 2015, www.nerdwallet.com/blog/credit-card-data/average-credit-card-debthousehold.

p. 99, Javelin Strategy & Research, "The 2014 Identity Fraud Report: Card Data Breaches and Inadequate Consumer Password Habits Fuel Disturbing Fraud Trends," February 2014, www.javelinstrategy.com.

# Chapter 4

1. Centers for Disease Control and Prevention, "Insufficient Sleep Is A Public Health Problem," September 3, 2015, www.cdc.gov/features/dssleep/; Y. Liu et al., "Prevalence of Healthy Sleep Duration Among Adults—United States, 2014," *Mortality and Morbidity Weekly Report* 65, no. 6 (2016): 137–41.

2. Centers for Disease Control and Prevention, "Insufficient Sleep Is a Public Health Problem," September 3, 2015, www.cdc.gov/features/dssleep/; Y. Liu et al., "Prevalence of Healthy Sleep Duration Among Adults—United States, 2014," 2016.

3. National Sleep Foundation, "2013 International Bedroom Poll: Summary of Findings," Accessed February 2016, Available at https://sleepfoundation.org/sites/default/files/RPT495a.pdf.

4. Centers for Disease Control and Prevention, "Insufficient Sleep Is a Public Health Problem," 2015.

5. Centers for Disease Control and Prevention, "Insufficient Sleep Is a Public Health Problem," 2015; Y. Liu et al., "Prevalence of Healthy Sleep Duration among Adults—United States, 2014," 2016.

6. National Highway Traffic Safety Administration, "Research on Drowsy Driving," Accessed February 2016, www.nhtsa.gov/Driving+Safety/Drowsy+Driving.

7. Centers for Disease Control and Prevention, "Insufficient Sleep Is a Public Health Problem," 2015; National Highway Traffic

Safety Administration, "Research on Drowsy Driving," 2016.

8. *American College Health Association, American College Health Association–National College Health Assessment II (ACHA–NCHA II): Reference Group Data Report Spring 2015* (Hanover, MD: American College Health Association, 2016), Available at www.achancha.org/reports_ACHA-NCHAII.html.

9. S. Hershner and R. Chevin, "Causes and Consequences of Sleepiness Among College Students," *Nature and Science of Sleep* 6 (2014): 73–84; A. Wald et al., "Associations Between Healthy Lifestyle Behaviors and Academic Performance in U.S. Undergraduates: A Secondary Analysis of the American College Health Association's National College Health Assessment II," *American Journal of Health Promotion* 28, no. 5 (2014): 298–305; K. Ahrberg et al., "Interaction between Sleep Quality and Academic Performance," *Journal of Psychiatric Research* 46, no. 12 (2012): 1618–22.

10. *American College Health Association, American College Health Association–National College Health Assessment II (ACHA–NCHA II): Reference Group Data Report Spring 2015*, 2016.

11. S. Hershner and R. Chevin. "Causes and Consequences of Sleepiness Among College Students," 2014; A. Wald et al., "Associations Between Healthy Lifestyle Behaviors," 2014.

12. *American College Health Association, American College Health Association–National College Health Assessment II (ACHA–NCHA II): Reference Group Data Report Spring 2015*, 2016.

13. National Sleep Foundation, "Excessive Sleepiness," Accessed February 2016, http://sleepfoundation.org/sleep-disorders-problems/excessive-sleepiness.

14. Centers for Disease Control and Prevention, "Insufficient Sleep Is a Public Health Problem," 2015.

15. American Academy of Sleep Medicine, *The International Classification of Sleep Disorders: Diagnostic—Coding Manual*, 3rd ed. (Westchester, IL: American Academy of Sleep Medicine, 2015).

16. National Sleep Foundation, "Who's at Risk?," Accessed February 5, 2015, http://drowsydriving.org/about/whos-at-risk/; Harvard University, Radcliff Institute for Advanced Study, "Drowsy Driving," Accessed February 5, 2015, www.radcliffe.harvard.edu/news/radcliffe-magazine/drowsy-driving.

17. National Sleep Foundation, "Excessive Sleepiness and Industrial Accidents," Accessed March 2016, https://sleepfoundation.org/excessivesleepiness/content/the-relationship-between-sleep-and-industrial-accidents; S. Rajaratname et al., "Sleep Loss and Circadian Disruption in Shift Work: Health Burden and Management," *Medical Journal of Australia* 199, no. 8 (2013): 11–15.

18. Ibid.

19. National Sleep Foundation, "Who's at Risk?," 2016.

20. G. Hertz et al., "Sleep Dysfunction in Women," Medscape, 2014, http://emedicine.medscape.com/article/1189087-overview;

National Sleep Foundation, "Why are Women Sleepier Than Men?: What's Up with Sleepiness in Women?" Accessed February 2016, https://sleepfoundation.org/sleep-news/why-are-women-sleepier-men-whats-sleepiness-women.

21. Centers for Disease Control and Prevention, "Insufficient Sleep Is a Public Health Problem," 2015; K. Johnson et al., "Association of Sleep Habits with Accidents and Near Misses in U.S. Transportation Operators," *Journal of Occupational and Environmental Medicine/American College of Occupational and Environmental Medicine* 56, no. 5 (2014): 510–5; K. Ward et al. "Excessive Daytime Sleepiness Increases the Risk of Motor Vehicle Crash in Obstructive Sleep Apnea," *Journal of Clinical Sleep Medicine* 9, no. 10 (2013): 1013–21.

22. N. Rod et al., "The Joint Effect of Sleep Duration and Disturbed Sleep on Cause-Specific Mortality: Results from the Whitehall II Cohort Study," *PLoS ONE* 9, no. 4 (2014): e91965.

23. K. M. Orzech et al., "Sleep Patterns Are Associated with Common Illness in Adolescents," *Journal of Sleep Research* 23, no. 2 (2013): 133–42; A. Prather et al., "Behaviorally Assessed Sleep and Susceptibility to the Common Cold," *Sleep* 38, no. 9 (2015): 1353–59.

24. X. Yu et al., "TH17 Cell Differentiation Is Regulated by Circadian Clock," *Science* 342, no. 6159 (2013): 727–30; N. Labrecque and N. Cermakian, "Circadian Clocks in the Immune System," *Journal of Biological Rhythms* 30, no. 4 (2015): 277–90.

25. F. Heredia et al., "Self-Reported Sleep Duration, White Blood Cell Counts and Cytokine Profiles in European Adolescents: The Helena Study, " *Sleep Medicine* 15, no. 10 (2014): 1251–58.

26. R. Fukuoka et al., "Nocturnal Intermittent Hypoxia and Short Sleep Duration were Independently Associated with Elevated C-reactive Protein Level in Patients with Coronary Artery Disease," *Circulation* 132, Suppl. 3 (2015): A17077; S. Nakamura et al., "Impact of Sleep-Disordered Breathing and Efficacy of Positive Airway Pressure on Mortality in Patients with Chronic Heart Failure and Sleep-Disordered Breathing: A Meta-Analysis," *Clinical Research in Cardiology* 104, no. 3 (2015): 208–16.

27. A. Cooper et al., "Sleep Duration and Cardiometabolic Risk Factors Among Individuals with Type 2 Diabetes," *Sleep Medicine* 16, no. 1 (2015): 119–25; M. Kohasieh and A. Makaryus, "Sleep Deficiency and Sleep Deprivation Leading to CVD," *International Journal of Hypertension* 2015 (2015): 615681.

28. M. A. Miller and F. P. Cappuccio, "Biomarkers of Cardiovascular Risk in Sleep Deprived People." *Journal of Human Hypertension* 27 (2013): 583–8; A. Cooper et al., "Sleep Duration and Cardiometabolic Risk Factors Among Individuals with Type 2 Diabetes," 2015; F. Sofi et al., "Insomnia and Risk of Cardiovascular Disease: A Meta-Analysis," *European Journal of Preventive Cardiology* 21, no. 1 (2014): 51–67.

29. A. Cooper et al., "Sleep Duration and Cardiometabolic Risk Factors Among Individuals with Type 2 Diabetes," 2015; M. A. Miller et al., "Sustained Short Sleep and Risk of Obesity: Evidence in Children and Adults," in *Handbook of Obesity*, vol. 1, 3rd ed., eds. G. A. Bray and C. Bouchard (Boca Raton, FL: CRC Press, Taylor & Francis Group, 2014), 397–41; Q. Xiao et al., "A Large Prospective Investigation of Sleep Duration, Weight Change and Obesity in the NIH-AARP Diet and Health Study," *American Journal of Epidemiology* 178, no. 11 (2013): 1600–10.

30. M. A. Miller et al., "Sustained Short Sleep and Risk of Obesity," 2014; Q. Xiao et al., "A Large Prospective Investigation of Sleep Duration," 2013; National Sleep Foundation, "Obesity and Sleep," Accessed January 2016, www.sleepfoundation.org/article/sleep-topics/obesity-andsleep.

31. Z. Shan et al., "Sleep Duration and Risk of Type 2 Diabetes: A Meta-analysis of Prospective Studies," *Diabetes Care* 38, no. 3 (2015): 529–37; J. Ferrie et al., "Change in Sleep Duration and Type 2 Diabetes: The Whitehall II Study," *Diabetes Care* 38, no. 8 (2015): 1467–72; A. Cooper et al., "Sleep Duration and Cardiometabolic Risk Factors Among Individuals with type 2 Diabetes," 2015; C. L. Jackson et al., "Association between Sleep Duration and Diabetes in Black and White Adults," *Diabetes Care* 36, no. 11 (2013): 3557–65; American Diabetes Association, "Too Little Sleep Linked to Higher A1C," January 2014, www.diabetesforecast.org/2014/Jan/too-little-sleep-linked-to.html.

32. T. K. Jensen et al., "Association of Sleep Disturbances with Reduced Semen Quality: A Cross-Sectional Study Among 953 Healthy Young Danish Men," *American Journal of Epidemiology* 177, no. 10 (2013): 1027–37.

33. National Institutes of Health, "Information about Sleep," Accessed February 2016, http://science.education.nih.gov/supplements/nih3/sleep/guide/info-sleep.html; C. Peri, "What Lack of Sleep Does to Your Mind," WebMD, April 30, 2013, www.webmd.com/sleep-disorders/excessive-sleepiness-10/emotions-cognitive.

34. A. Chatburn et al., "Complex Associative Memory Processing and Sleep: A Systematic Review and Meta-Analysis of Behavioural Evidence and Underlying EEG Mechanisms." *Neuroscience and Biobehavioral Reviews* 47 (2014): 645–55; S. Hershner and R. Chervin, "Causes and Consequences of Sleepiness among College Students," 2014.

35. Ibid.; A. Gomes, J. Tavares, and M. Azevedo, "Sleep and Academic Performance in Undergraduates: A Multi-Measure, Multi-Predictor Approach," *Chronobiology International* 28, no. 9 (2011): 786–801; Yu-Chih Chiang, "The Effects of Sleep on Performance of Undergraduate Students Working in the Hospitality Industry as Compared to Those Who Are Not Working in the Industry," 2013, http://lib.dr.iastate.edu/cgi/viewcontent.cgi?article=4067&context=etd.

36. H. Fullagar et al., "Sleep and Athletic Performance: The Effects of Sleep Loss on Exercise Performance, and Physiological and Cognitive Responses to Exercise," *Sports Medicine* 45, no. 2 (2015): 161–86.

37. National Highway Traffic Safety Administration, "Research on Drowsy Driving," Accessed February 2016, www.nhtsa.gov/Driving+Safety/Drowsy+Driving; Centers for Disease Control and Prevention, "Drowsy Driving—19 States and the District of Columbia, 2009–2010," *Morbidity and Mortality Weekly Report* 61, no. 51 (2013): 1033–37; National Sleep Foundation, "Healthy Sleep Project Urges Parents to Teach Teens to Avoid Drowsy Driving," April 7, 2015, Available at www.sleepeducation.org/docs/default-document-library/healthy-sleep-teen-drowsy-driving.pdf.

38. National Sleep Foundation, "Depression and Sleep," Accessed February 2016, https://sleepfoundation.org/sleep-disorders-problems/depression-and-sleep.

39. National Institute of General Medical Sciences, "Circadian Rhythms Fact Sheet," Accessed February 5, 2015, www.nigms.nih.gov/Education/Pages/Factsheet_Circadian Rhythms.aspx.

40. A. Ramkisoengsing and J. Meijer, "Synchronization of Biological Clock Neurons by Light and Peripheral Feedback Systems Promotes Circadian Rhythms and Health," *Frontiers in Neurology* 6, no. 128 (2015): 128; M. Vitaterna, J. Takahashi, and F. Turek, "Overview of Circadian Rhythms," National Institute on Alcohol Abuse and Alcoholism, 2014, http://pubs.niaaa.nih.gov/publications/arh25-2/85-93.htm.

41. NIH, "Teacher's Guide–Information About Sleep," Accessed February 2016, http://science.education.nih.gov/supplements/nih3/sleep/guide/info-sleep.htm.

42. B. Rasch and J. Born, "About Sleep's Role in Memory," *Physiological Reviews* 93, no. 2 (2013): 681–766.

43. N. Watson et al., "Joint Consensus Statement of the American Academy of Sleep Medicine and Sleep Research Society on the Recommended Amount of Sleep for a Healthy Adult: Methodology and Discussion," *Journal of Clinical Sleep Medicine* 11, no. 8 (2015): 931–52; N. F. Watson et al., "Recommended Amount of Sleep for a Healthy Adult: A Joint Consensus Statement of the American Academy of Sleep Medicine and Sleep Research Society," *Sleep* 38, no. 6 (2015): 843–44.

44. Centers for Disease Control and Prevention, "Insufficient Sleep Is a Public Health Epidemic," 2014; C. Nugent and L. Black, "Sleep Duration, Quality of Sleep, and Use of Sleep Medication, by Sex and Family Type, 2013–2014," *NCHS Data Brief* 230 (2016); "Why Americans Can't Sleep," *Consumer Reports*, January 14, 2016, Available at www.consumerreports.org/sleep/why-americans-cant-sleep/.

45. NIH, "Teacher's Guide–Information About Sleep," 2016.

46. E. Mezick et al., "Sleep Duration and Cardiovascular Responses to Stress in Undergraduate Men," *Psychophysiology* 51, no. 1 (2014): 88–96.

47. A. Ramkisoengsing and J. Meijer, "Synchronization of Biological Clock Neurons by Light and Peripheral Feedback Systems Promotes Circadian Rhythms and Health," 2015.

48. N. Rod, M. Kumari, and T. Lange et al., "The Joint Effect of Sleep Duration and Disturbed Sleep on Cause-Specific Mortality: Results from the Whitehall II Cohort Study," *PLoS ONE* 9, no. 4 (2014): e91965; Q. Xiao et al., "A Large Prospective Investigation of Sleep Duration," 2013; C. L. Jackson et al., "Association Between Sleep Duration and Diabetes," 2013; F. Cappuccio et al., "Sleep Duration Predicts Cardiovascular Outcomes: A Systematic Review and Meta-analysis of Prospective Studies," *European Heart Journal* 32, no. 12 (2011): 1484–92.

49. A. Prather et al., "Behaviorally Assessed Sleep and Susceptibility to the Common Cold," *Sleep* 38, no. 9 (2015): 1353–59.

50. P. Slobodanka et al., "Effects of Recovery Sleep After One Work Week of Mild Sleep Restriction on Interleukin-6 and Cortisol Secretion and Daytime Sleepiness and Performance," *American Journal of Physiology-Endocrinology and Metabolism* 305, no. 7 (2013): E890–6.

51. Ibid.

52. Ying-Hu, Fu, "What Genes Tell Us About Sleep," TEDX Thatcher School Video Lecture Series, November 23, 2015.

53. Centers for Disease Control and Prevention, "Insufficient Sleep Is a Public Health Problem," 2015; A. Ramkisoengsing and J. Meijer, "Synchronization of Biological Clock Neurons by Light and Peripheral Feedback Systems Promotes Circadian Rhythms and Health," 2015.

54. Centers for Disease Control and Prevention, "Insufficient Sleep Is a Public Health Problem," 2015; A. Ramkisoengsing and J. Meijer, "Synchronization of Biological Clock Neurons by Light and Peripheral Feedback Systems Promotes Circadian Rhythms and Health," 2015.

55. Ibid.

56. Ibid.

57. National Sleep Foundation, "Caffeine and Sleep," Accessed February 2016, https://sleepfoundation.org/sleep-topics/caffeine-and-sleep; *American College Health Association–National College Health Assessment II (ACHA–NCHA II): Reference Group Data Report Spring 2015*, 2016.

58. National Sleep Foundation, "Insomnia," Accessed February 5, 2016, http://sleepfoundation.org/sleep-disorders-problems/insomnia.

59. Ibid.

60. Ibid.

61. Ibid.

62. Society of Behavioral Medicine, "Adult Insomnia," Accessed February 2016, www.behavioralsleep.org/index.php/sbsm/about-adult-sleep-disorders/adult-insomnia.

63. National Sleep Foundation, "Sleep Apnea and Sleep," Accessed March 2016, https://sleepfoundation.org/sleep-disorders-problems/sleep-related-breathing-disorders/obstructive-sleep-apnea.

64. Sleep Disorders Guide, "Sleep Apnea Statistics," Accessed January 2015, http://www.sleepdisordersguide.com/sleepapnea/sleep-apnea-statistics.html.

65. National Sleep Foundation, "Sleep Apnea and Sleep," 2016.

66. Ibid.

67. Ibid.

68. U.S. Food and Drug Administration, "Inspire Upper Airway Stimulation - P130008," January 11, 2016, www.fda.gov/MedicalDevices/ProductsandMedicalProcedures/DeviceApprovalsandClearances/Recently-ApprovedDevices/ucm398321.htm.

69. National Institute of Neurological Disorders and Stroke, "Restless Legs Syndrome Fact Sheet," July 27, 2015, www.ninds.nih.gov/disorders/restless_legs/detail_restless_legs.htm; How Sleep Works, "Sleep Disorders," Accessed March 2016, http://howsleepworks.com/disorders.html.

70. Ibid.

71. National Institute of Neurological Disorders and Stroke, "Narcolepsy Fact Sheet," updated January 5, 2015, www.ninds.nih.gov/disorders/narcolepsy/detail_narcolepsy.htm.

72. National Sleep Foundation, "Narcolepsy and Sleep," Accessed February, 2016, https://sleepfoundation.org/sleep-disorders-problems/narcolepsy-and-sleep.

73. National Sleep Foundation, "Sleep Hygiene," Accessed February 2016, https://sleepfoundation.org/ask-the-expert/sleep-hygiene.

74. NIH, "Brain Basics: Understanding Sleep," April 17, 2015, www.ninds.nih.gov/disorders/brain_basics?understand_sleep.htm; J. Levenson et al., "The Pathophysiology of Insomnia," *CHEST Journal* 147, no. 4 (2015): 1179–92.

75. National Sleep Foundation, "What You Breathe While You Sleep Can Affect How You Feel the Next Day," Accessed February 5, 2015, http://sleepfoundation.org/bedroom/smell.php.

76. Vanderbilt University Medical Center Reporter, "Take a Walk in the Sun to Ease Time Change Woes, Sleep Expert Says," October 30, 2014, http://news.vanderbilt.edu/2014/10/take-a-walk-in-the-sun-to-ease-time-change-woes-says-vanderbilt-sleep-expert/.

77. National Sleep Foundation, "Exercise and Sleep," Accessed February 2016, https://sleepfoundation.org/sleep-polls-data/sleep-in-america-poll/2013-exercise-and-sleep.

78. National Sleep Foundation, "Sleep Hygiene," 2016.

79. N. Olson, "Caffeine Consumption Habits and Perceptions Among University of New Hampshire Students," 2013, http://scholars.unh.edu/cgi/viewcontent.cgi?article=1102&context=honors; M. Drici et al., "Cardiac Safety of So-Called 'Energy Drinks,'" *European Heart Journal* 35 (2014); H. Whiteman, Medical News Today, "Rising Energy Drink

Consumption May Pose a Threat to Public Health, Says WHO," October 15, 2014, www.medicalnewstoday.com/articles/283929; J. J. Breda et al., "Energy Drink Consumption in Europe: A Review of the Risks, Adverse Health Effects and Policy Options," *Frontiers in Public Health* 2 (2014): 134.

80. National Sleep Foundation, "Sleep Hygiene," 2016.

81. M. Thakkar et al., "Alcohol Disrupts Sleep Homeostasis," *Alcohol* 49, no. 4 (2015): 299–310.

82. J. M. Trauer et al., "Cognitive Behavioral Therapy for Chronic Insomnia: A Systematic Review and Meta-analysis," *Annals of Internal Medicine* 163, no. 3 (2015): 191–204.

83. "Why Americans Can't Sleep," *Consumer Reports*, 2016.

84. Ibid.

85. Y. Chong et al., "Prescription Sleep Aid Use Among Adults: U.S. 2005–2010," *NCHS Data Brief* 127 (2013), Available at www.cdc.gov/nchs/data/databriefs/db127.htm#x2013;2010.

86. R. N. Hansen et al., "Sedative Hypnotic Medication Use and the Risk of Motor Vehicle Crash," *American Journal of Public Health* 105, no. 8 (2015): e64–e69; "The Problem with Sleeping Pills," *Consumer Reports*, January 5, 2016, Available at http://www.consumerreports.org/drugs/the-problem-with-sleeping-pills/.

**Pulled statistics:**

p. 105, NHTSA, "Research on Drowsy Driving," Accessed March 2016, www.nhtsa.gov/Driving+Safety/Drowsy+Driving.

## Chapter 5

1. Institute of Medicine, Food and Nutrition Board, *Dietary Reference Intakes for Water, Potassium, Sodium, Chloride, and Sulfate* (Washington, DC: National Academies Press, 2004).

2. A. E. Carroll, "No, You Do Not Have to Drink 8 Glasses of Water a Day," *New York Times*, August 24, 2015, www.nytimes.com/2015/08/25/upshot/no-you-do-not-have-to-drink-8-glasses-of-water-a-day.html?_r=0.

3. J. Mazziotta, "The Amount of Water You Actually Need Per Day," *Health*, September, 16, 2015, http://news.health.com/2015/09/16/the-amount-of-water-you-actually-need-per-day/?xid=time.

4. T. Hew-Butler et al., "Statement of the 3rd International Exercise-Associated Hyponatremia Consensus Development Conference, Carlsbad, California," *British Journal of Sports Medicine* 49, no. 22 (2015): 1432–46.

5. S. C. Killer, A. K. Blannin, and A. E. Jeukendrup, "No Evidence of Dehydration with Moderate Daily Coffee Intake: A Counterbalanced Cross-Over Study in a Free-Living Population," *PLoS ONE* 9, no. 1 (2014): e84154.

6. American College of Sports Medicine (ACSM), "Selecting and Effectively Using Hydration for Fitness," 2011, www.acsm.org/docs/brochures/selecting-and-effectively-using-hydration-for-fitness.pdf.

7. U.S. Department of Agriculture, What We Eat in America, NHANES 2011–2012," February 11, 2015, www.ars.usda.gov/SP2UserFiles/Place/80400530/pdf/1112/Table_1_NIN_GEN_11.pdf.

8. Food and Nutrition Board, Institute of Medicine, *Dietary Reference Intakes for Energy, Carbohydrate, Fiber, Fat, Fatty Acids, Cholesterol, Protein, and Amino Acids (Macronutrients)* (Washington, DC: National Academies Press, 2005), Available at www.nap.edu/openbook.php?isbn=0309085373.

9. Dietitians of Canada, the Academy of Nutrition and Dietetics, and the American College of Sports Medicine, "Nutrition and Athletic Performance: Position of Dietitians of Canada, the Academy of Nutrition and Dietetics, and the American College of Sports Medicine," February 2016, Available at https://www.dietitians.ca/Downloads/Public/noap-position-paper.aspx.

10. Institute of Medicine of the National Academies, "Dietary, Functional, and Total Fiber," *Dietary Reference Intakes for Energy, Carbohydrate, Fiber, Fat, Fatty Acids, Cholesterol, Protein, and Amino Acids* (Washington, DC: National Academies Press, 2005), 339–421, Available at www.nap.edu/openbook.php?isbn=0309085373.

11. J. DiNicolantonio, S. C. Lucan, and J. H. O'Keefe, "The Evidence for Saturated Fat and for Sugar Related to Coronary Heart Disease," *Progress in Cardiovascular Disease* (2015): pii: S0033-0620(15)30025-6. doi: 10.1016/j.pcad.2015.11.006. [Epub ahead of print]

12. Ibid.

13. A. Astrup, "A Changing View on Saturated Fatty Acids and Dairy: From Enemy to Friend," *American Journal of Clinical Nutrition* 100, no. 6 (2014): 1407–8.

14. U.S. Department of Health and Human Services and U.S. Department of Agriculture, *2015–2020 Dietary Guidelines for Americans*, 8th ed., December 2015, Available at http://health.gov/dietaryguidelines/2015/guidelines/.

15. C. E. Ramsden et al., "Use of Dietary Linoleic Acid for Secondary Prevention of Coronary Heart Disease and Death: Evaluation of Recovered Data from the Sydney Diet Heart Study and Updated Meta-Analysis," *British Medical Journal* 346 (2013): e8707; M.A. Leslie et al., "A Review of the Effect of Omega-3 Polyunsaturated Fatty Acids on Blood Triacylglycerol Levels in Normolipidemic and Borderline Hyperlipidemic Individuals," *Lipids in Health and Disease* 14, no. 1 (2015): 1.

16. W. Willet, "Dietary Fats and Coronary Heart Disease," *Journal of Internal Medicine* 272, no. 1 (2012): 13–24.

17. U.S. Food and Drug Administration, "Final Determination Regarding Partially Hydrogenated Oils (Removing *Trans* Fat)," June 16, 2015, www.fda.gov/Food/IngredientsPackagingLabeling/FoodAdditivesIngredients/ucm449162.htm.

18. Ibid.

19. Institute of Medicine of the National Academies, "Dietary, Functional, and Total Fiber," 2005.

20. H. J. Silver et al., "Consuming a Balanced High Fat Diet for 16 Weeks Improves Body Composition, Inflammation and Vascular Function Parameters in Obese Premenopausal Women," *Metabolism* 63, no. 4 (2014): 562–73; A. Trichpoulou et al., "Definitions and Potential Health Benefits of the Mediterranean Diet: Views from Experts Around the World," *BMC Medicine* 12, no. 1 (2014): 112.

21. H. R. Lieberman et al., "Patterns of Dietary Supplement Use Among College Sudents," *Clinical Nutrition* 34, no. 5 (2015): 976–85.

22. National Institutes of Health Office of Dietary Supplements, "Dietary Supplement Fact Sheet: Vitamin D," February 11, 2016, http://ods.od.nih.gov/factsheets/VitaminD-HealthProfessional.

23. Ibid.

24. Ibid.

25. Institute of Medicine, Food and Nutrition Board, *Dietary Reference Intakes for Water, Potassium, Sodium, Chloride, and Sulfate* (Washington, DC: National Academies Press, 2004).

26. U.S. Department of Health and Human Services and U.S. Department of Agriculture, *2015–2020 Dietary Guidelines for Americans*. 2015.

27. Ibid.

28. D. C. Bauer, "Calcium Supplements and Fracture Prevention," *New England Journal of Medicine* 369, no. 16 (2013): 1537–43, Available at www.aahs.org/medstaff/wp-content/uploads/CalciumSuppNEJM2013.pdf.

29. I. R. Reid, "Should We Prescribe Calcium Supplements for Osteoporosis Prevention?" *Journal of Bone Metabolism* 21, no. 1 (2014): 21–28.

30. S. A. McNaughton et al., "An Energy-Dense, Nutrient-Poor Dietary Pattern Is Inversely Associated with Bone Health in Women," *Journal of Nutrition* 141, no. 8 (2011): 1516–23.

31. World Health Organization, "Micronutrient Deficiencies: Iron Deficiency Anemia," Accessed February 2016, www.who.int/nutrition/topics/ida/en/index.html.

32. Food and Nutrition Board, Institute of Medicine, *Dietary Reference Intakes for Vitamin A, Vitamin K, Arsenic, Boron, Chromium, Copper, Iodine, Iron, Manganese, Molybdenum, Nickel, Silicon, Vanadium, and Zinc* (Washington, DC: National Academies Press, 2001).

33. R. Gozzelino and P. Arosio, "Iron Homeostasis in Health and Disease," *International Journal of Molecular Sciences* 17, no. 1 (2016): 130.

34. Academy of Nutrition and Dietetics, "Position of the Academy of Nutrition and Dietetics: Functional Foods," *Journal of the Academy of Nutrition and Dietetics*, 113 (2013): 1096–103.

35. Ibid.

36. J. Fiedor and K. Burda, "Potential Role of Carotenoids as Antioxidants in Human Health and Disease," *Nutrients* 6, no. 2 (2014): 466–88.

37. J. Harasym and R. Oledzki, "Effect of Fruit and Vegetable Antioxidants on Total Antioxidant

Capacity of Blood Plasma," *Nutrition* 30, no. 5 (2014): 511–17.

38. M. E. Obrenovich et al., "Antioxidants in Health, Disease, and Aging," *CNS & Neurological Disorders Drug Targets* 10, no. 2 (2011): 192–207; V. Ergin, R. E. Hariry, and C. Karasu, "Carbonyl Stress in Aging Process: Role of Vitamins and Phytochemicals as Redox Regulators," *Aging and Disease* 4, no. 5 (2013): 276–94.

39. H. Stutz, N. Bresgen, and P. M. Ecki, "Analytical Tools for the Analysis of Beta-Carotene And Its Degradation Products," *Free Radical Research* 49, no. 4 (2015): 650–80; M. J. Gostner et al., "The Good and Bad of Antioxidant Foods: An Immunological Perspective," *Food and Chemical Toxicology* 80 (2015): 72–79.

40. U.S. Department of Agriculture, "Food Availability (Per Capita) Data System," November 12, 2015, www.ers.usda.gov/data-products/food-availability-(per-capita)-data-system/.aspx#26715.

41. U.S. Department of Health and Human Services and U.S. Department of Agriculture, *2015–2020 Dietary Guidelines for Americans.* 2015.

42. U.S. Department of Agriculture, "Empty Calories: How Do I Count the Empty Calories I Eat?," September 30, 2015, www.choosemyplate.gov/how-do-i-count.

43. U.S. Food and Drug Administration, "Label Claims for Conventional Foods and Dietary Supplements," November 2014, www.fda.gov/Food/IngredientsPackagingLabeling/LabelingNutrition/ucm111447.htm.

44. The Vegetarian Resource Group, "How Often Do Americans Eat Vegetarian Meals? And How Many Adults in the U.S. Are Vegan?" May 29, 2015, www.vrg.org/blog/2015/05/29/how-often-do-americans-eat-vegetarian-meals-and-how-many-adults-in-the-u-s-are-vegetarian-2/.

45. Ibid.

46. Y. Yokoyama et al., "Vegetarian Diets and Blood Pressure: A Meta-Analysis," *Journal of the American Medical Association Internal Medicine* 174, no. 4 (2014): 577–87.

47. C. G. Lee et al., "Vegetarianism as a Protective Factor for Colorectal Adenoma and Advanced Adenoma in Asians," *Digestive Diseases and Science* 59, no. 5 (2014): 1025–35.

48. Council for Responsible Nutrition, "2015 CRN Consumer Survey on Dietary Supplements," October 23, 2015, www.crnusa.org/CRNPR15-CCSurvey102315.html.

49. Ibid.

50. Office of Dietary Supplements, "Frequently Asked Questions," July 2013, http://ods.od.nih.gov/Health_Information/ODS_Frequently_Asked_Questions.aspx#; V. A. Moyer, "Vitamin, Mineral, and Multivitamin Supplements for the Primary Prevention of Cardiovascular Disease and Cancer: U.S. Preventive Services Task Force Recommendation Statement," *Annals of Internal Medicine* 160, no. 8 (2014): 558–64.

51. M.J. Krantz et al., "Effects of Omega-3 Fatty Acids on Arterial Stiffness in Patients with Hypertension: A Randomized Pilot Study,"

*Journal of Negative Results in Biomedicine* 14, no. 1 (2015): 21.

52. New York State Office of the Attorney General, "Attorney General Schneiderman Asks Major Retailers to Halt Sales of Certain Herbal Supplements as DNA Tests Fail to Detect Plant Materials Listed on Majority of Products Tested," February 3, 2015, www.ag.ny.gov/press-release/ag-schneiderman-asks-major-retailers-halt-sales-certain-herbal-supplements-dna-tests.

53. U.S. Department of Health and Human Services, "Food Safety Modernization Act (FSMA)," November 2013, www.fda.gov/Food/GuidanceRegulation/FSMA/ucm304045.htm.

54. FDA, "'Natural' on Food Labeling," December 24, 2015, www.fda.gov/Food/GuidanceRegulation/GuidanceDocuments RegulatoryInformation/LabelingNutrition/ucm456090.htm.

55. Organic Trade Association, "Market Analysis: U.S. Organic Industry Survey, 2015," https://www.ota.com/resources/market-analysis.

56. Ibid.

57. C. Smith-Spangler et al., "Are Organic Foods Safer or Healthier Than Conventional Alternatives?: A Systematic Review," *Annals of Internal Medicine* 157, no. 5 (2012): 348–66; M. Barański et al., "Higher Antioxidant and Lower Cadmium Concentrations and Lower Incidence of Pesticide Residues in Organically Grown Crops: A Systematic Literature Review and Meta-Analyses," *British Journal of Nutrition* 112, no. 5 (2014): 794–811.

58. International Agency for Research on Cancer, "IARC Monographs Volume 112: Evaluation of Five Organophosphate Insecticides and Herbicides," March 20, 2015, Available at www.iarc.fr/en/media-centre/iarcnews/pdf/MonographVolume112.pdf.

59. U.S. Environmental Protection Agency, "Food and Pesticides," December 2015, www.epa.gov/safepestcontrol/food-and-pesticides.

60. J. L. Wood et al., "Microbiological Survey of Locally Grown Lettuce Sold at Farmers' Markets in Vancouver, British Columbia," *Journal of Food Protection* 78, no. 1 (2015): 203–08.

61. CDC, "Estimates of Food-Borne Illnesses in the United States," January 2014, www.cdc.gov/foodborneburden/index.html.

62. CDC, "Trends in Foodborne Illness in the United States, 2012," May 2014, www.cdc.gov/foodborneburden/trends-in-foodborne-illness.html.

63. CDC, "Listeria (Listeriosis)," January 2016, www.cdc.gov/listeria.

64. Ibid.

65. Ibid.

66. Ibid.

67. CDC, "About Botulism," July 26, 2012, http://www.cdc.gov/nczved/divisions/dfbmd/diseases/botulism/consumers.html=.

68. U.S. Government Accountability Office, "Improving Federal Oversight of Food Safety," February 11, 2015, Available at www.gao.gov/highrisk/revamping_food_safety/why_did_study#t=0.

69. M. Jay-Russell et al., "Exploration of the Impact of Application Intervals for the Use of Raw Animal Manure as a Soil Amendment, on Tomato Contamination," 2015, Available at www.wifss.ucdavis.edu/wp-content/uploads/2015/pdfs/OryangJayRussell PosterOFVMScienceaResearchConference_08_14.pdf.

70. CDC, "Surveillance for Foodborne Disease Outbreaks—United States, 1998–2008," *Morbidity and Mortality Weekly Report* 62, no. SS2 (2013), www.cdc.gov/foodsafety/fdoss/data/annual-summaries/mmwr-questions-and-answers-1998-2008.html.

71. U.S. Food and Drug Administration, "Food Irradiation: What You Need to Know," March 2014, www.fda.gov/Food/ResourcesForYou/Consumers/ucm261680.htm.

72. National Institute of Allergy and Infectious Diseases, "Food Allergy," January 2016, www.niaid.nih.gov/topics/foodallergy/Pages/default.aspx.

73. National Institute of Allergy and Infectious Diseases, "Anaphylaxis," April 2015, http://www.niaid.nih.gov/topics/anaphylaxis/Pages/default.aspx.

74. U.S. Food and Drug Administration, "Food Allergies: What You Need to Know," September 2015, www.fda.gov/food/resourcesforyou/consumers/ucm079311.htm.

75. National Institute of Diabetes and Digestive and Kidney Diseases, "Celiac Disease," June 2015, www.niddk.nih.gov/health-information/health-topics/digestive-diseases/celiac-disease/Pages/facts.aspx.

76. A. Fasano et al., "Non-Celiac Gluten Sensitivity," *Gastroenterology* 148, no. 6 (2015): 1195–204.

77. National Institute of Child Health and Human Development, "Lactose Intolerance," May 2014, https://www.nichd.nih.gov/health/topics/lactose/Pages/default.aspx.

78. W. Klumper and M Qaim, "A Meta-Analysis of the Impacts of Genetically Modified Crops," *PLoS ONE* 9, no. 11 (2014): e111629.

79. Union of Concerned Scientists, "Genetic Engineering Risks and Impacts," November 2013, www.ucsusa.org/food_and_agriculture/our-failing-food-system/genetic-engineering/risks-of-genetic-engineering.html.

80. Natural Resources Defense Council, "Alarming Decline in Monarch Population Justifies Immediate Action: NRDC Urges UN to Declare Mexican Butterfly Refuge 'in Danger,'" June 26, 2015, www.nrdc.org/media/2015/150626.asp.

81. Union of Concerned Scientists, "Genetic Engineering Risks and Impacts," November 2013, www.ucsusa.org/food_and_agriculture/our-failing-food-system/genetic-engineering/risks-of-genetic-engineering.html.

82. American Association for the Advancement of Science, "Statement by the AAAS Board of Directors on Labeling of Genetically Modified Foods," March 31, 2014, www.aaas.org/news/statement-aaas-board-directors-labeling-genetically-modified-foods; World Health Organization, "20 Questions on Genetically Modified Foods," Accessed

March 2014, www.who.int/foodsafety/ publications/biotech/20questions/en

**Pulled statistics:**

p. 135, M. W. Eich, "Healthiest Yogurts: How Much Sugar is in Your Favorite Yogurt?— Updated March 2016," *Margaret Wertheim, MS, RDN, Nutrition for Fertility*, Pregnancy, and Beyond, April 27, 2015, http:// margaretwertheimrd.com/healthiest-yogurts-how-much-added-sugar-is-in-your-favorite-yogurt/.

p. 141, *American College Health Association–National College Health Assessment II: Reference Group Executive Summary Spring 2015* (Hanover, MD: American College Health Association, 2015).

# Chapter 6

1. American College Health Association. *American College Health Association–National College Health Assessment II: Reference Group Executive Summary Fall 2015* (Hanover, MD: American College Health Association, 2016).

2. M. Ng et al., "Global, Regional, and National Prevalence of Overweight and Obesity in Children and Adults during 1980–2013: A Systematic Analysis for the Global Burden of Disease Study 2013," *The Lancet* 384, no. 9945 (2014): 766–81; C. L. Ogden et al., "Prevalence of Childhood and Adult Obesity in the United States, 2011–2012," *Journal of the American Medical Association* 311, no. 8 (2014): 806–14; C. L. Ogden et al., "Prevalence of Obesity Among Adults: United States, 2011–2012," *National Center for Health Statistics Data Brief* 131 (2013), www.cdc.gov/ nchs/data/databriefs/db131.htm.

3. CDC, National Center for Health Statistics, "Health, United States, 2014; Table 64, Healthy Weight, Overweight, and Obesity Among Adults Aged 20 and Over, by Selected Characteristics: United States, Selected Years 1988–1994 through 2009–2012," May 2015, Available at www.cdc.gov/nchs/hus/ contents2014.htm#064.

4. C. L. Ogden et al., "Prevalence of Obesity Among Adults," 2013.

5. C. L. Ogden et al., "Trends in Obesity Prevalence Among Children and Adolescents in the United States. 1988 through 2013–2014," *Journal of the American Medical Association* 315, no. 21 (2016): 2292–99, doi: 10.1001/ jama.2016.636; D. Mozaffarian et al., "Heart Disease and Stroke Statistics—2016 Update: A Report from the American Heart Association," *Circulation* 133, no. 4 (2016): 447–54.

6. D. Mozaffarian et al., "Heart Disease and Stroke Statistics." 2016.

7. K. M. Flegal et al., "Trends in Obesity Among Adults in the United States, 2005–2016." *Journal of the American Medical Association* 315, no. 21 (2016): 2284–91, doi:10.1001/ jama.2016.6458.

8. Ibid.

9. D. Mozaffarian et al., "Heart Disease and Stroke Statistics," 2016. Ibid.

10. Ibid.

11. Ibid.

12. World Health Organization (WHO), "Obesity and Overweight Fact Sheet," January 2015, www.who.int/mediacentre/factsheets/ fs311/en.

13. Ibid.; M. Ng et al., "Global, Regional, and National Prevalence of Overweight and Obesity in Children and Adults during 1980–2013," 2014.

14. K. M. Flegal et al., "Association of All-Cause Mortality with Overweight and Obesity Using Standard Body Mass Index Categories: A Systematic Review and Meta-Analysis," *Journal of the American Medical Association* 309, no. 1 (2013): 71–82.

15. M. Simmonds et al., "Predicting Adult Obesity from Childhood Obesity: A Systematic Review and Meta-Analysis," *Obesity Reviews* 17, no. 2 (2015): 95–107

16. American Diabetes Association, "Statistics about Diabetes," April 1, 2016, www.diabetes .org/diabetes-basics/statistics.

17. R. Mitchell et al., "Associations between Obesity and Overweight and Fall Risk, Health Status and Quality of Life in Older People," *Australian and New Zealand Journal of Public Health* 38, no. 1(2014): 13–18. 12152.

18. M. Gurnani, C. Birken, and J. Hamilton, "Childhood Obesity: Causes, Consequences, and Management," *Pediatric Clinics of North America* 62, no. 4 (2015): 821–40; J. Baidal et al., "Risk Factors for Childhood Obesity in the First 1,000 Days: A Systematic Review," *American Journal of Preventive Medicine* (2016), doi:10.1016/j.amepre.2016.11.012.

19. J. Buss et al., "Associations of Ghrelin with Eating Behaviors, Stress, Metabolic Factors, and Telomere Length Among Overweight and Obese Women: Preliminary Evidence of Attenuated Ghrelin Effects in Obesity," *Appetite* 76, no. 1 (2014): 84–94; R. Boswell and H. Kober, "Food Cue Reactivity and Craving Predict Eating and Weight Gain: A Meta-Analytic Review," *Obesity Reviews* 17, no. 2 (2015): 159–77.

20. C. Llewelyn and J. Wardle, "Behavioral Susceptibility to Obesity: Gene–Environment Interlay in the Development of Weight," *Physiology and Behavior* 152 (2015): 494–501.

21. Ibid.

22. Ibid.; L. Quan et al., "Association of Fat-Mass and Obesity-Associated Genet FTO rs9939609 Polymorphism with the Risk of Obesity Among Children and Adolescents: A Meta-Analysis," *European Review for Medical and Pharmacological Sciences* 19, no. 4 (2015): 614–23.

23. M. Khatib et al., "Effect of Ghrelin on Regulation of Growth Hormone Release: A Review," *The Health Agenda* 2, no. 1 (2014), Available at www.healthagenda.net/wp-content/uploads/ 2013/11/Effect-of-ghrelin-on-regulation-of-growth-hormone-release-A-review.pdf; T. Sato et al., "Physiological Roles of Ghrelin on Obesity," *Obesity Research and Clinical Practice* 8, no. 5 (2014): e405–13; Healthy Children.org, "Organic Causes of weight Gain and Obesity," November 21, 2015, Available at https://www.healthychildren.org/

English/health-issues/conditions/obesity/ Pages/Organic-Causes-of-Weight-Gain-and-Obesity.aspx.

24. H. Feng et al., "Review: The Role of Leptin in Obesity and the Potential for Leptin Replacement Therapy," *Endocrine* 44, no. 1 (2013): 33–9; C. Llewelyn and J. Wardle, "Behavioral Susceptibility to Obesity," 2015.

25. C. Llewelyn and J. Wardle, "Behavioral Susceptibility to Obesity," 2015; M. Graff, J. S. Ngwa, and T. Workalemahu, "Genome-Wide Analysis of BMI in Adolescents and Young Adults Reveals Additional Insight into the Effects of Genetic Loci over the Life Course," *Human Molecular Genetics* 22, no. 17 (2013): 3597–607.

26. E. Horn et al., "Behavioral and Environmental Modification of the Genetic Influence on BMI: A Twin Study," *Behavior Genetics* 45, no. 4 (2015): 409–26.

27. D. Sellayah, F. Cagampang, and R. Cox, "On the Evolutionary Origins of Obesity: A New Hypothesis," *Endocrinology* 155, no. 5 (2014): 1573–88; J. R. Speakman et al., "Evolutionary Perspectives on the Obesity Epidemic: Adaptive, Maladaptive, and Neutral Viewpoints," *Annual Review of Nutrition* 33 (2013): 289–317.

28. M. Reinhart et al., "A Human Thrifty Phenotype Associated with Less Weight Loss During Caloric Restriction," *Diabetes* 64, no. 8 (2015): 2859–67.

29. A. Tremblay et al., "Adaptive Thermogenesis Can Make a Difference in the Ability of Obese Individuals to Lose Body Weight," *International Journal of Obesity* 37 (2013): 759–64.

30. L. K. Mahan and S. Escott-Stump, *Krause's Food, Nutrition, and Diet Therapy,* 13th ed. (New York: W. B. Saunders, 2012).

31. USDA Economic Research Service, "Food Availability (per capita) Data System," November 2015, www.ers.usda.gov/data-products/food-availability-(per-capita)-data-system.aspx.

32. Ibid.

33. CDC, "Early Release of Selected Estimates Based on Data From the January–September 2015 National Health Interview Survey," February 23, 2016, www.cdc.gov/nchs/nhis/ releases/released201602.htm#7.

34. Ibid.

35. M. Wang, L. Pbert, and S. Lemon, "Influence of Family, Friend and Co-worker Social Support and Social Undermining on Weight Gain Prevention Adults," *Obesity* 22, no. 9 (2014): 1973–80.

36. J. Kolodziejczyk et al., "Influence of Specific Individual and Environmental Variables on the Relationship between Body Mass Index and Health-Related Quality of Life in Overweight and Obese Adolescents," *Quality of Life Research* 24, no. 1 (2015): 251–61.

37. CDC, "About Adult BMI," May 15, 2015, www.cdc.gov/healthyweight/assessing/bmi/ adult_bmi/index.html.

38. Ibid.

39. Ibid.

40. J. I. Mechanick et al., "Clinical Practice Guidelines for the Perioperative Nutritional, Metabolic and Nonsurgical Support of the Bariatric Surgery Patient—2013 Update,"

References | **R-13**

*Endocrine Practice* 19, no. 2 (2013): e1–36, www.aace.com/files/publish-ahead-of-print-final-version.pdf.

41. K. M. Flegal. "Trends in Obesity Among Adults in the United States, 2005–2016," *Journal of the American Medical Association* 315, no. 21 (2016):2284–91; CDC, "Obesity Prevalence Maps," September 11, 2015, www.cdc.gov/obesity/data/prevalence-maps.html.

42. American Heart Association, "Body Composition Tests," February 25, 2016. www.heart.org/HEARTORG/GettingHealthy/NutritionCenter/Body-Composition-Tests_UCM_305883_Article.jsp; S. J. Mooney, A. Baecker, and A. G. Rundel, "Comparison of Anthropometric and Body Composition Measures as Predictors of Components of the Metabolic Syndrome in the Clinical Setting," *Obesity Research and Clinical Practice* 7, no. 1 (2013): e55–e66.

43. C. L. Ogden et al., "Prevalence of Childhood and Adult Obesity in the United States," 2014; National Center for Health Statistics, "Health, United States, 2014" Hyattsville, MD; U.S. Department of Health and Human Services, 2015, Available at http://www.cdc.gov/nchs/data/hus/hus14.pdf.

44. B. Major et al., "The Ironic Effects of Weight Stigma," *Journal of Experimental Social Psychology* 51 (2014): 74–80; S. A. Mustillo, K. Budd, and K. Hendrix, "Obesity, Labeling, and Psychological Distress in Late-Childhood and Adolescent Black and White Girls: The Distal Effects of Stigma," *Social Psychology Quarterly* 76, no. 3 (2013): 268–89.

45. L. Goh et al., "Anthropometric Measurements of General and Central Obesity and the Prediction of Cardiovascular Disease Risk in Women: A Cross-Sectional Study," *BMJ Open* 4, (2014): e004138.

46. National Heart, Lung, and Blood Institute, "Classification of Overweight and Obesity by BMI, Waist Circumference and Associated Disease Risks," Accessed March 2016, www.nhlbi.nih.gov/health/public/heart/obesity/lose_wt/bmi_dis.htm.

47. University of Maryland Medical Center, Rush University, "Waist to Hip Ratio," February 7, 2016, http://umm.edu/health/medical/reports/images/waisttohip-ratio.

48. P. Brambilla et al., "Waist Circumference-to-Height Ratio Predicts Adiposity Better than Body Mass Index in Children and Adolescents," *International Journal of Obesity* 37, no. 7 (2013): 943–46.

49. A. Saltiel, "New Therapeutic Approaches for the Treatment of Obesity," *Science Translational Medicine* 8, no. 323 (2016): 323rv2; J. Domecq et al., "Drugs Commonly Associated with Weight Change: A Systematic Review and Meta-Analysis," *Journal of Clinical Endocrinology and Metabolism* 100, no. 2 (2015): 363–70.

50. C. E. Weber et al., "Obesity and Trends in Malpractice Claims for Physicians and Surgeons," *Surgery* 154, no. 2 (2013): 299–304.

51. Mayo Clinic, "Gastric Bypass Surgery: Risks," January 2016, www.mayoclinic.org/tests-procedures/bariatric-surgery/basics/risks/prc-20019138.

52. John's Hopkins Health Library, "BPD/DS Weight-Loss Surgery," March 2014, www.hopkinsmedicine.org/healthlibrary/test_procedures/gastroenterology/bpdds_weight-loss_surgery_135,64.

53. I. Lanza, "Enhancing the Metabolic Benefits of Bariatric Surgery: Tipping the Scales with Exercise," *Diabetes* 64, no. 11 (2015): 3656–58. J. Yu et al., "The Long Term Effects of Bariatric Surgery for Type 2 Diabetes: Systematic Review and Meta-Analysis of Randomized and Non-randomized Evidence," *Obesity Surgery* 25, no. 1 (2015): 143–58.

**Pulled Statistics:**

p. 155, American College Health Association. *American College Health Association–National College Health Assessment II: Reference Group* Executive Summary Fall 2015 (Hanover, MD: American College Health Association, 2016).

p. 158, S. Vikraman et al., "Caloric Intake from Fast Food Among Children and Adolescents in the U.S. 2011–2012," *NCHS Data Brief* No. 213 (2015), www.cdc.gov.

p. 161, Centers for Disease Control and Prevention, National Health Statistics, "Obesity and Overweight," February 25, 2016, www.cdc.gov/nchs/Fastats/obesity-overweight.htm; CDC, "Health, United States, 2014," Accessed April 2016, Available at http://www.cdc.gov/nchs/data/hus/hus14.pdf#059.

## Chapter 6A

1. M. Dahl, "Stop Obsessing: Women Spend 2 Weeks a Year on Their Appearance, TODAY Survey Shows" *Today,* February 24, 2014, http://www.today.com/health/stop-obsessing-women-spend-2-weeks-year-their-appearance-today-2D12104866.

2. Ibid.

3. M. Bucchianeri et al., "Body Dissatisfaction from Adolescence to Young Adulthood: Findings from a 10-Year Longitudinal Study," *Body Image* 10, no. 1 (2013): 1–7.

4. National Eating Disorders Association (NEDA), "What is Body Image?," Accessed February 2016, https://www.nationaleatingdisorders.org/what-body-image.

5. Common Sense Media, "Children, Teens, Media, and Body Image," January 21, 2015, Available at https://www.commonsensemedia.org/research/children-teens-media-and-body-image.

6. A. Conason, "Is Facebook Making Us Hate Our Bodies?," *Psychology Today,* June 9, 2015, https://www.psychologytoday.com/blog/eating-mindfully/201506/is-facebook-making-us-hate-our-bodies.

7. R. Williams, "The Body Image and Eating Disorder Tsunami," *Psychology Today,* May 18, 2015, https://www.psychologytoday.com/blog/wired-success/201505/the-body-image-and-eating-disorder-tsunami.

8. K. Schreiber, "Promoting a Thin and Ultra-Athletic Physique Has Unforeseen Consequences," *Psychology Today,* September 1, 2015, https://www.psychologytoday.com/articles/201509/mind-your-body-body-conscious.

9. Centers for Disease Control and Prevention, "FASTSTATS: Obesity and Overweight," February 25, 2016, www.cdc.gov/nchs/fastats/obesity-overweight.htm.

10. Fathers: L. Choate, July 3, 2015, "Dads: What's Your Impact on Your Daughter's Body Image?," *Psychology Today,* https://www.psychologytoday.com/blog/girls-women-and-wellness/201507/dads-whats-your-impact-your-daughters-body-image Mothers: L. Choate, June 29, 2015, "Moms: What Will Your Body Image Legacy Be?," *Psychology Today,* https://www.psychologytoday.com/blog/girls-women-and-wellness/201506/moms-what-will-your-body-image-legacy-be?collection=1076687.

11. Ibid.

12. R. Puhl et al., "Cross-National Perspectives About Weight-Based Bullying in Youth: Nature, Extent and Remedies," *Pediatric Obesity* (2015), doi: 10.1111/ijpo.12051.

13. L. Rakhkovskaya et al., "Sociocultural and Identity Predictors of Body Dissatisfaction in Ethnically Diverse College Women," *Body Image* 16 (2016): 32–40.

14. Mayo Clinic, "Body Dysmorphic Disorder," May 2013, http://www.mayoclinic.org/diseases-conditions/body-dysmorphic-disorder/basics/causes/con-20029953.

15. S. Rossell et al., "Can Understanding the Neurobiology of Body Dysmorphic Disorder (BDD) Inform Treatment?," *Australasian Psychiatry* 23, no. 4 (2015), doi: 10.1177/1039856215591327.

16. K. Phillips et al., "A Preliminary Candidate Gene Study in Body Dysmorphic Disorder," *Journal of Obsessive–Compulsive Related Disorders* 6 (2015): 72–6.

17. Ibid.

18. Body Image Health, "The Model for Healthy Body Image and Weight," Accessed February 2016, http://bodyimagehealth.org/model-for-healthy-body-image.

19. I. Ahmed et al., "Body Dysmorphic Disorder," *Medscape Reference,* August 2014, http://emedicine.medscape.com/article/291182-overview.

20. Mayo Clinic Staff, "Body Dysmorphic Disorder," 2013; KidsHealth, "Body Dysmorphic Disorder," February 2016, http://kidshealth.org/parent/emotions/feelings/bdd.html.

21. Ibid.

22. I. Ahmed et al., "Body Dysmorphic Disorder," 2014.

23. C. Gottlieb, "Disordered Eating or Eating Disorder: What's the Difference?" *Psychology Today,* February 23, 2014, https://www.psychologytoday.com/blog/contemporary-psychoanalysis-in-action/201402/disordered-eating-or-eating-disorder-what-s-the.

24. American Psychiatric Association, *Diagnostic and Statistical Manual of Mental Disorders,* 5th ed. (Washington, DC: American Psychiatric Association, 2013).

25. National Eating Disorders Association, "Get the Facts on Eating Disorders," Accessed February 2016, www.nationaleatingdisorders.org/get-facts-eating-disorders.

26. D. A. Gagne et al., "Eating Disorder Symptoms and Weight and Shape Concerns in a Large Web-Based Convenience Sample of Women Ages 50 and Above: Results of the Gender and Body Image (GABI) Study," *International Journal of Eating Disorders* 45, no. 7 (2012): 832–44.

27. American College Health Association, *National College Health Assessment II: Undergraduates Reference Group Executive Summary Spring 2015* (Hanover, MD: American College Health Association, 2015), Available at www.acha-ncha.org/reports_ACHA-NCHAII.html.

28. National Collegiate Athletic Association (NCAA), "Disordered Eating in Student-Athletes: Understanding the Basics and What We Can Do About It," Accessed February 2016, http://www.ncaa.org/health-and-safety/nutrition-and-performance/disordered-eating-student-athletes-understanding-basics.

29. Alliance for Eating Disorder Awareness, "What Are Eating Disorders?," Accessed February 2016, http://www.allianceforeatingdisorders.com/portal/what-are-eating-disorders#.VrKmr5MrKRt.

30. Ibid.

31. National Eating Disorders Association, "Anorexia Nervosa," Accessed February 2016, www.nationaleatingdisorders.org/anorexia-nervosa.

32. S. A. Swanson et al., "Prevalence and Correlates of Eating Disorders in Adolescents: Results from the National Comorbidity Survey Replication Adolescent Supplement," *Archives of General Psychiatry* 68, no. 7 (2011): 714–23.

33. American Psychiatric Association, 2013.

34. A. R. Smith, T. E. Joiner, and D. R. Dodd, "Examining Implicit Attitudes Toward Emaciation and Thinness in Anorexia Nervosa," *International Journal of Eating Disorders* 47, no. 2 (2013): 138–47; R. N. Carey, N. Donaghue, and P. Broderick, "Concern Among Australian Adolescent Girls: The Role of Body Comparisons with Models and Peers," *Body Image* 11, no. 1 (2014): 81–4.

35. A.D.A.M. Medical Encyclopedia, U.S. National Library of Medicine, "Anorexia Nervosa," March 10, 2014, https://www.nlm.nih.gov/medlineplus/ency/article/000362.htm; B. Suchan et al., "Reduced Connectivity between the Left Fusiform Body Area and the Extrastriate Body Area in Anorexia Nervosa Is Associated with Body Image Distortion," *Behavioural Brain Research* 241 (2013): 80–5.

36. R. Kessler et al., "The Prevalence and Correlates of Binge Eating Disorder in the World Health Organization World Mental Health Surveys," *Biological Psychiatry* 73, no. 9 (2013): 904–14.

37. American Psychiatric Association, 2013.

38. National Institute of Mental Health, "Eating Disorders," February 2016, www.nimh.nih.gov/health/topics/eating-disorders/index.shtml.

39. T. A. Oberndorfer et al., "Altered Insula Response to Sweet Taste Processing After Recovery from Anorexia and Bulimia Nervosa," *American Journal of Psychiatry* 170, no. 10 (2013): 1143–51.

40. Mayo Clinic, "Binge-Eating Disorder," February 9, 2016, http://www.mayoclinic.org/diseases-conditions/binge-eating-disorder/basics/definition/con-20033155.

41. R. Kessler et al., "The Prevalence and Correlates of Binge Eating Disorder," 2013.

42. American Psychiatric Association, 2013.

43. Ibid.

44. National Eating Disorders Collaboration, "What is OSFED?" April 24, 2015, http://www.nedc.com.au/osfed.

45. T. Insel, "Director's Blog: Spotlight on Eating Disorders," National Institute of Mental Health, February 24, 2012, http://www.nimh.nih.gov/about/director/2012/spotlight-on-eating-disorders.shtml#i; Mirasol Eating Disorder Recovery Centers, "Eating Disorder Statistics," Accessed March 2016, http://www.mirasol.net/learning-center/eating-disorder-statistics.php.

46. M. Smith, L. Robinson, and J. Segal, "Helping Someone with an Eating Disorder," *Helpguide.org*, February 2016, http://www.helpguide.org/articles/eating-disorders/helping-someone-with-an-eating-disorder.htm.

47. National Eating Disorder Association, "Find Help and Support," Accessed February 2016, www.nationaleatingdisorders.org/find-help-support.

48. B. Cook, "Exercise Addiction and Compulsive Exercising: Relationship to Eating Disorders, Substance Use Disorders, and Addictive Disorders," in *Eating Disorders, Addictions and Substance Use Disorders* (New York: Springer, 2014): 127–44.

49. J. J. Waldron, "When Building Muscle Turns into Muscle Dysmorphia," Association for Sport Applied Psychology, Accessed February 2016, www.appliedsportpsych.org/resource-center/health-fitness-resources/when-building-muscle-turns-into-muscle-dysmorphia.

50. A. Foster, "Muscle Dysmorphia: Could It Be Classified as an Addiction to Body Image?," *Journal of Behavioral Addictions* 4, no. 1 (2015): 1–5; J. J. Waldron, "When Building Muscle Turns into Muscle Dysmorphia," 2016.

51. J. J. Waldron, "When Building Muscle Turns into Muscle Dysmorphia," 2016.

52. Ibid.

53. L. M. Gottschlich et al., "Female Athlete Triad," December 17, 2014, http://emedicine.medscape.com/article/89260-overview.

54. National Collegiate Athletic Association, "2014 Female Athlete Triad Consensus Statement on Guidelines for Treatment and Return to Play," Accessed March 2016, Available at: http://www.ncaa.org/health-and-safety/nutrition-and-performance/2014-female-athlete-triad-consensus-statement-guidelines.

55. L. Bacon, *Health at Every Size: The Surprising Truth About Your Weight* (Dallas, TX: BenBella Books, 2010).

**Pulled statistics:**

p. 180, American College Health Association, *National College Health Assessment II: Undergraduates Reference Group Executive Summary Spring 2015* (Hanover, MD: American College Health Association, 2015), Available at www.acha-ncha.org/reports_ACHA-NCHAII.html.

## Chapter 7

1. H. Hausenblas and R. E. Rhodes, *Exercise Psychology, Physical Activity and Sedentary Behavior* (Burlington, MA: Jones & Bartlett, 2017).

2. World Health Organization, "Physical Activity and Adults," Accessed May 2016, www.who.int/dietphysicalactivity/factsheet_adults/en/.

3. Centers for Disease Control and Prevention (CDC), "Nutrition, Physical Activity an Obesity: Data, Trends, and Maps," June 20, 2015, www.cdc.gov/nccdphp/DNPAO/index.html.

4. Ibid.

5. Ibid.

6. C. Bouchard, S. N. Blair, and P. Katzmarzyk, "Less Sitting, More Physical Activity, or Higher Fitness?," *Mayo Clinic Proceedings* 90, no. 11 (2015): 1–8; A. Biswas et al., "Sedentary Time and Its Association with Risk for Disease Incidence, Mortality, and Hospitalization in Adults," *Annals of Internal Medicine* 162, no. 2 (2015): 123–32.

7. H. Hausenblas and R. E. Rhodes, *Exercise Psychology, Physical Activity and Sedentary Behavior*, 2017.

8. Ibid.

9. American College Health Association, *American College Health Association–National College Health Assessment II (ACHA-NCHA II): Reference Group Executive Summary, Fall 2015* (Hanover, MD: American College Health Association, 2016), Available at www.acha-ncha.org/docs/NCHA-II%20FALL%202015%20REFERENCE%20GROUP%20EXECUTIVE%20SUMMARY.pdf.

10. C. Bouchard, S. N. Blair, and P. T. Katzmarzyk, "Less Sitting, More Physical Activity, or Higher Fitness?," 2015.

11. L. R. S. M. Cart, "Letter to the Editor: Standardized Use of the Terms 'Sedentary' and 'Sedentary Behaviours'," *Applied Physiology, Nutrition and Metabolism* 37 (2012): 540–2.

12. L. F. M. Rezende et al., "All-Cause Mortality Attributable Risk to Sitting Time Analysis of 54 Countries Worldwide," *American Journal of Preventive Medicine* (2016): e1–e11, doi:10.1016/jamepre.2016.01.022.

13. Ibid.

14. Ibid.

15. L. R. S. M. Cart, "Letter to the Editor," 2012.

16. N. Owen et al., "Too Much Sitting: The Population-Health Science of Sedentary Behavior," *Exercise and Sport Science Reviews* 38, no. 3 (2010): 105–13.

17. C. Bouchard, S. N. Blair, and P. Katzmarzyk, "Less Sitting, More Physical Activity, or Higher Fitness?," 2015; A. Biswas et al., "Sedentary Time and Its Association with Risk for Disease Incidence, Mortality, and Hospitalization in Adults," 2015.

18. A. Biswas et al., "Sedentary Time and Its Association with Risk for Disease Incidence, Mortality, and Hospitalization in Adults," 2015.

19. S. Plowman and D. Smith, *Exercise Physiology for Health, Fitness, and Performance,* 4th ed. (Philadelphia: Lippincott Williams & Wilkins, 2014).

20. M. Böejesson, A. Onerup, S. Lundqvist, and B. Dahlöf, "Physical Activity and Exercise Lower Blood Pressure in Individuals with Hypertension: Narrative Review of 27 RTCs," *British Journal of Sports Medicine* 50, no. 6 (2016): 356–61.

21. D. J. Elmer et al., "Inflammatory, Lipid and Body Composition Response to Interval Training or Moderate Aerobic Training," *European Journal of Applied Physiology* 116 (2016): 601–9; B. B. Gibbs et al., "Six-Month Changes in Ideal Cardiovascular Health vs. Framingham 10-Year Coronary Heart Disease Risk Among Adults Enrolled in a Weight Loss Intervention," *Preventive Medicine* 86 (2016): 123–9; American Heart Association, "About Cholesterol," Updated April 21, 2014, www.heart.org.

22. D. J. Elmer et al., "Inflammatory, Lipid and Body Composition Response to Interval Training or Moderate Aerobic Training," 2016; B. B. Gibbs et al., "Six-Month Changes in Ideal Cardiovascular Health vs. Framingham 10-Year Coronary Heart Disease Risk Among Adults Enrolled in a Weight Loss Intervention," 2016.

23. D. T. Lackland and J. H. Voeks, "Metabolic Syndrome and Hypertension: Regular Exercise as Part of Lifestyle Management," *Current Hypertension Reports* 16, no. 11 (2014): 1–7; P. R. P. Nunes, et al., "Effects of Resistance Training on Muscular Strength and Indicators of Abdominal Adiposity, Metabolic Risk, and Inflammation in Postmenopausal: Controlled and Randomized Clinical Trial of Efficacy or Training Volume," *Age* 38, no. 2 (2016): 1–13.

24. Ibid.

25. D. T. Lackland and J. H. Voeks, "Metabolic Syndrome and Hypertension," 2014.

26. J. Henson et al., "Sedentary Behavior as a New Behavioural Target in the Prevention and Treatment of Type 2 Diabetes," *Diabetes Metabolism Research and Reviews* 32, Suppl. 1 (2016): 213–20; L. Pai et al., "The Effectiveness of Regular Leisure-Time Physical Activities on Long-Term Glycemic Control in People with Type 2 Diabetes: A Systemic Review and Meta-Analysis," *Diabetes Research and Clinical Practice* 113 (2016): 77–85.

27. E. M. Balk et al., "Combined Diet and Physical Activity Promotion Programs to Prevent Type 2 Diabetes Among Persons at Increased Risk: A Systematic Review for the Community Preventive Task Force," *Annals of Internal Medicine* 163, no. 6 (2015): 437–51; M. J. Armstrong and R. J. Sigal, "Exercise Is Medicine: Key Concepts in Discussing Physical Activity with Patients Who Have Type 2 Diabetes," *Canadian Journal of Diabetes* 39 (2015): s129–s133.

28. Ibid.

29. J. Erdrich et al.,"Proportion of Colon Cancer Attributable to Lifestyle in a Cohort of US Women," *Cancer, Causes and Control* (2015), doi: 10.1007/s10552-015-0619-z; M. Harvie, A. Howell, and D. Evans, "Can Diet and Lifestyle Prevent Breast Cancer: What is the Evidence?" *ASCO Educational Book* 35 (2015): e66–73, doi: 10.14694/EdBook_AM.2015.35.e66.

30. American Cancer Society, "Diet and Physical Activity: What's the Cancer Connection?," February 5, 2016, www.cancer.org/cancer/cancercauses/dietandphysicalactivity/diet-and-physical-activity.

31. Ibid.; F. Canches-Gomas et al., "Physical Inactivity and Low Fitness Deserve More Attention to Alter Cancer Risk and Prognosis," *Cancer Prevention Research* 8 (2015): 105–10; D. Schmid and M. Leitzman, "Association between Physical Activity and Mortality among Breast Cancer and Colorectal Cancer Survivors: A Systematic Review and Meta-Analysis," *Annals of Oncology* 25, no. 7 (2014): 1293–1311, doi: 10.1093/annonc/mdu012; D. Brenner et al., "Physical Activity After Breast Cancer: Effect on Survival and Patient-Reported Outcomes," *Current Breast Cancer Reports* 6 (2014): 193–201.

32. L. F. M. Rezende et al., "All-Cause Mortality Attributable Risk to Sitting Time Analysis of 54 Countries Worldwide," 2016; A. Biswas et al., "Sedentary Time and Its Association with Risk for Disease Incidence, Mortality, and Hospitalization in Adults," 2015.

33. A. D. Hagstrom et al., "The Effects of Resistance Training on Markers of Immune Function and Inflammation in Previously Sedentary Women Recovering from Breast Cancer: A Randomized Controlled Trial," *Breast Cancer Research and Treatment* 155, no. 3 (2016): 471–82; J. Schmidt et al., "A 3-Week Multimodal Intervention Involving High-Intensity Interval Training Female Cancer Survivors: A Randomized Controlled Trial," *Physiological Reports* 4, no. 3 (2016), doi: 10.14814phy2.12693.

34. R. Hirschey et al., "Exploration of Exercise Outcome Expectations among Breast Cancer Survivors," *Cancer Nursing* (2016).

35. C. M. Weaver et al., "National Osteoporosis Foundation's Position Statement on Peak Bone Mass Development and Lifestyle Factors: A Systematic Review and Implementation Recommendations," *Osteoporosis International* 27, no. 4 (2016): 1281–1386.

36. Ibid.

37. Ibid.; K. G. Greenway, J. W. Walkley, and P. A. Rich. "Relationships Between Self-Reported Lifetime Physical Activity, Estimates of Current Physical Fitness, and a BMD in Adult Post-Menopausal Women," *Archives of Osteoporosis* 10, no. 1 (2015): 1–13.

38. J. Xu et al., "Effects of Exercise on Bone Status in Female Subjects, from Young Girls to Postmenopausal Women: An Overview of Systematic Reviews and Meta-Analyses," *Sports Medicine* (2016); M. A. Strope et al., "Physical Activity-Assessed Bone Loading During Adolescence and Young Adulthood is Positively Associated with Adult Bone Mineral Density in Men," *American Journal of Men's Health* 9, no. 6 (2014): 442–50.

39. R. Rizzoli, C. A. Abraham, and M. L. Brandi, "Nutrition and Bone Health: Turning Knowledge and Beliefs in Healthy Behavior," *Current Medical Research and Opinion* 30, no. 1 (2014): 131–41.

40. H. J. Pownall et al., "Changes in Body Composition over Eight Years in a Randomized Trial of a Lifestyle Intervention: The Look AHEAD Study," *Obesity* 23, no. 3 (2015): 565–72; L. Montessi et al., "Long-Term Weight Loss Maintenance for Obesity: A Multidisciplinary Approach," *Diabetes, Metabolic Syndrome and Obesity: Targets and Therapy* 9 (2016): 37–46.

41. L. Montessi et al., "Long-Term Weight Loss Maintenance for Obesity," 2016.

42. D. M. Steinberg et al., "Weighing Every Day Matters: Daily Weighing Improves Weight Loss and Adoption of Weight Control Behaviors," *Journal of the Academy of Nutrition and Dietetics* 115, no. 4 (2015): 511–8.

43. Ibid.

44. J. G. Thomas et al., "Weight-Loss Maintenance for 10 Years in the National Weight Control Registry," *American Journal of Preventive Medicine* 46, no. 1 (2014): 17–23.

45. The National Weight Control Registry, "The National Weight Control Registry," Accessed April 2016, www.nwcr.ws/default.htm.

46. The National Weight Control Registry, "NWCR Facts," Accessed April 2016, www.nwcr.ws/Research/default.htm.

47. L. G. Ogden et al., "Dietary Habits and Weight Maintenance Success in High versus Low Exercisers in the National Weight Control Registry," *Journal of Physical Activity and Health* 11, no. 8 (2014): 1540–48.

48. B. K. Greer et al., "EPOC Comparison Between Isocaloric Bouts of Steady-State Aerobic, Intermittent Aerobic, and Resistance Training," *Research Quarterly for Exercise and Sport* 86, no. 2 (2015): 190–5.

49. J. E. Turner, "Is Immunosenescence Influenced by Our Lifetime 'Dose' of Exercise?," *Biogerontology* 17, no. 3 (2016): 581–602.

50. G. J. Koelwyn et al., "Exercise in Regulation of Inflammation-Immune Axis Function in Cancer Initiation and Progression," *Oncology,* December 15, 2015, www.cancernetwork.com/oncology-journal/exercise-regulation-inflammation-immune-axis-function-cancer-initiation-and-progression; N. Sallam and I. Laher, "Exercise Modulates Oxidative Stress and Inflammation in Aging and Cardiovascular Disease," *Oxidative Medicine and Cellular Longevity* (2016), doi: 10.1155/2016/7239639.

51. J. E. Turner, "Is Immunosenescence Influenced by Our Lifetime 'Dose' of Exercise?," 2016.

52. Ibid.

53. C. Jin et al., "Exhaustive Submaximal Endurance and Resistance Exercises Induce Temporary Immunosuppression via Physical and Oxidative Stress," *Journal of Exercise Rehabilitation* 11, no. 4 (2015): 198–203.

54. American College Health Association, *American College Health Association–National College Health Assessment II*, 2016.

55. J. D. de Vries et al., "Exercise as an Intervention to Reduce Study-Related Fatigue Among University Students: A Two-Arm Parallel Randomized Controlled Trial," *PLoS ONE* 11, no. 3 (2016): e0152137.

56. Ibid.

57. F. B. Schuch et al., "Exercise as a Treatment for Depression: A Meta-Analysis Adjusting for Publication Bias," *Journal of Psychiatric Research* 77 (2016): 42–51.

58. Ibid.

59. Ibid.

60. C. Huang et al., "Cardiovascular Reactivity, Stress, and Physical Activity," *Frontiers in Physiology* 4 (2013): 1–13, doi: 10.3389/fphys.201300314.

61. J. Richards et al., "Don't Worry, Be Happy: Cross-Sectional Associations Between Physical Activity and Happiness in 15 European Countries," *BMC Public Health* 15, no. 1 (2015): 1.

62. H. Hausenblas and R. E. Rhodes, *Exercise Psychology, Physical Activity and Sedentary Behavior*, 2017.

63. Ibid.

64. J. W. de Greeff et al., "Physical Fitness and Academic Performance in Primary School Children with and Without a Social Disadvantage," *Health Education Research* 29, no. 5 (2014): 853–60.

65. S. Covell et al., "Physical Activity Level and Future Risks of Mild Cognitive Impairment or Dementia: A Critically Appraised Topic," *Neurologist* 19, no. 3 (2015): 89–91; C. P. Bezold et al., "The Effects Changes in Physical Fitness on Academic Performance Among New York City Youth," *Journal of Adolescent Health* 55, no. 6 (2014): 774–81.

66. J. D. de Vries et al., "Exercise as an Intervention to Reduce Study-Related Fatigue Among University Students," 2016; D. Bellar et al., "Exercise and Academic Performance among Nursing and Kinesiology Students at US Colleges," *Journal of Education and Health Promotion* 3, no. 1 (2014): 48–52.

67. J. D. de Vries et al., "Exercise as an Intervention to Reduce Study-Related Fatigue Among University Students," 2016.

68. D. Bellar et al., "Exercise and Academic Performance among Nursing and Kinesiology Students at US Colleges," 2014.

69. A. N. Slade and S. M. Kies, "The Relationship Between Academic Performance and Recreation Use Among First-Year Medical Students," *Medical Education Online* 20 (2015), doi: 10.3404/meo.v20.25105.

70. Ibid.

71. M. Daly, D. McMinn, and J. Allan, "A Bidirectional Relationship Between Physical Activity and Executive Function in Older Adults," *Frontiers in Human Neuroscience* 8 (2014): 1–9.

72. J. Hu et al., "Exercise Improves Cognitive Function in Aging Patients," *International Journal of Clinical and Experimental Medicine* 7, no. 10 (2014): 3144–9.

73. M. Beckett et al., "A Meta-Analysis of Prospective Studies in the Role of Physical Activity and the Prevention of Alzheimer's Disease in Older Adults," *BMC Geriatrics* 15, no. 9 (2015), doi: 10.10.1186/s12877-015-0007-2.

74. C. Bouchard, S. N. Blair, and P. Katzmarzyk, "Less Sitting, More Physical Activity, or Higher Fitness?," 2015.

75. Ibid.; L. F. M. Rezende et al., "All-Cause Mortality Attributable Risk to Sitting Time Analysis of 54 Countries Worldwide," 2016.

76. D. Dunlop et al., "Sedentary Time in US Older Adults Associated with Disability in Activities of Daily Living Independent of Physical Activity," *Journal of Physical Activity and Health* 12, no. 1 (2015): 93–101.

77. T. Deliens, "Determinants of Physical Activity and Sedentary Behaviour in University Students: A Qualitative Study Using Focus Group Discussions," *BMC Public Health* 15, no. 1 (2015): 1.

78. Ibid.

79. Ibid.

80. American College of Sports Medicine, *A SM's Guidelines for Exercise Testing and Prescription*, 9th ed. (Baltimore, MD: Lippincott Williams & Wilkins, 2014).

81. Ibid.

82. Ibid.

83. Ibid.

84. American College of Sports Medicine, *ACSM's Resource Manual for Guidelines for Exercise Testing and Prescription* (Philadelphia: Lippincott Williams & Wilkins, 2014).

85. D. G. Behm et al., "Acute Effects of Muscle Stretching on Physical Performance, Range of Motion, and Injury Incidence in Healthy Adults: A Systematic Review," *Applied Physiology, Nutrition, and Metabolism* 41, no. 1 (2016): 1–11; J. Natour et al., "Pilates Improves Pain Function and Quality of Life in Patients with Chronic Low Back Pain: A Randomized Controlled Trial," *Clinical Rehabilitation* 29, no. 1 (2015): 59–68.

86. Ibid.

87. M. Pahor et al., "Effect of Structured Physical Activity on Prevention of Major Mobility Disability in Older Adults: The LIFE Study Randomized Clinical Trial," *Journal of the American Medical Association* 311, no. 23 (2014): 2387–96.

88. American College of Sports Medicine, *Guidelines for Exercise Testing and Prescription*, 2014.

89. Ibid.

90. D. G. Behm et al., "Acute Effects of Muscle Stretching on Physical Performance, Range of Motion, and Injury Incidence in Healthy Adults," 2016.

91. Ibid.

92. Ibid.

93. D. G. Behm and J. C. Colao Sanchez, "Instability Resistance Training Across the Exercise Continuum," *Sports Health: A Multidisciplinary Approach* 5, no. 6 (2013): 500–3.

94. Ibid.

95. M N. Sawka et al., "American College of Sports Medicine Position Stand: Exercise and Fluid Replacement," *Medicine and Science in Sports and Exercise* 39, no. 2 (2007): 377–90.

96. Ibid.

97. J. Potter and B. Fuller, "The Effectiveness of Chocolate Milk as a Post-Climbing Recovery Aid," *Journal of Sports Medicine and Physical Fitness* 55, no. 12 (2015): 1438–44.

98. P. Beeson, "Plantar Faciopathy: Revisiting the Risk Factors," *Foot and Ankle Surgery* 20, no. 3 (2014): 160–5.

99. American Academy of Ophthalmology, "Eye Health in Sports and Recreation," March 2016, www.aao.org/eye-health/tips-prevention/injuries-sports.

100. Ibid.

101. Bicycle Helmet Safety Institute, "Helmet-Related Statistics from Many Sources," January 2016, www.helmets.org/stats.htm.

102. American College Health Association, *National College Health Assessment II: Reference Group Data Report, Fall 2015*, 2016.

103. Bicycle Helmet Safety Institute, "Helmet-Related Statistics from Many Sources," 2014.

104. American College of Sports Medicine, *ACSM's Guidelines for Exercise Testing and Prescription*, 2014.

105. Mayo Clinic, "Hypothermia: Definition," June 18, 2014, www.mayoclinic.org/diseases-conditions/hypothermia/basics/definition/con-20020453.

106. American College of Sports Medicine, *ACSM's Guidelines for Exercise Testing and Prescription*, 2014.

107. American Council on Exercise, "Exercising in the Cold," Accessed April 2016, www.acefitness.org/acefit/healthy_living_fit_facts_content.aspx?itemid=2619.

**Pulled statistics:**

p. 191, Centers for Disease Control and Prevention, Division of Nutrition, Physical Activity and Obesity, "How Much Physical Activity Do Adults Need?" *Physical Activity for Everyone*, June 2015, www.cdc.gov/phsicalactivity/basics/adults/index.htm.

p. 198, Centers for Disease Control and Prevention (CDC), "Nutrition, Physical Activity an Obesity: Data, Trends, and Maps," June 20, 2015, www.cdc.gov/nccdphp/DNPAO/index.html.

## Chapter 8

1. J. Holt-Lunstad et al., "Loneliness and Social Isolation as Risk Factors for Mortality: A Meta-Analytic Review," *Perspectives on Psychological Science* 10, no. 2 (2015): 227–37.

2. J. T. Cacioppo, Rewarding Social Connections Promote Successful Aging, American Association for the Advancement of Science Annual Meeting, Chicago, Illinois, 2016.

3. J. Holt-Lunstad et al., "Loneliness and Social Isolation as Risk Factors for Mortality," 2015.

4. J. T. Cacioppo and B. Patrick, *Loneliness: Human Nature and the Need for Social Connection* (New York: W. W. Norton, 2008).

5. J. Holt-Lunstad et al., "Loneliness and Social Isolation as Risk Factors for Mortality," 2015; J. L. Kohn and S. L. Averett, "The Effect of Relationship Status on Health with Dynamic Health and Persistent Relationships," *Journal of Health Economics* 36 (2014): 69–83.

6. J. Holt-Lunstad, T. Smith, and J. Layton, "Social Relationships and Mortality Risk: A Meta-Analytic Review," *PLoS Medicine* 7, no. 7 (2010): e1000316; L. C. Hawkley and John P. Capitanio, "Perceived Social Isolation, Evolutionary Fitness and Health Outcomes: A Lifespan Approach," *Philosophical Transactions of the Royal Society B* 370, no. 1669 (2015): 20140114.

7. J. Holt-Lunstad, T. Smith, and J. Layton, "Social Relationships and Mortality Risk," 2010.

8. Y. C. Yang et al., "Social Relationships and Physiological Determinants of Longevity across the Human Life Span," *Proceedings of the National Academy of Sciences* 113, no. 3 (2016): 578–83.

9. E. Robinson, J. Thomas, P. Aveyard, and S. Higgs, "What Everyone Else is Eating: A Systematic Review and Meta-Analysis of the Effect of Informational Eating Norms on Eating Behavior," *Journal of the Academy of Nutrition and Dietetics* 114, no. 3 (2014) 414–29.

10. J. Holt-Lunstad and B. N. Uchino, "Social Support and Health," in K. Glanz, B. K. Rimer, and K. Viswanath, *Health Behavior and Health Education: Theory, Research, and Practice*, 5th ed. (San Francisco, CA: Jossey-Bass, 2015).

11. S. Schnall, K. D. Harber, J. K. Stefanucci, and D. R. Proffitt, "Social Support and the Perception of Geographical Slant," *Journal of Experimental Social Psychology*, 44, no. 5 (2008): 1246–55.

12. K. Hampton, L. S. Goulet, L. Rainie, and K. Purcell, "Social Networking Sites and Our Lives," *Pew Internet and American Life Project*, June 16, 2011, Available at www.pewinternet .org/files/old-media//Files/Reports/2011/ PIP%20-%20Social%20networking%20 sites%20and%20our%20lives.pdf.

13. L. F. Berkman, I. Kawachi, and M. Glymour, eds., *Social Epidemiology* (New York: Oxford University Press, 2014).

14. J. T. Cacioppo and B. Patrick, *Loneliness*, 2008.

15. K. Hampton, L. S. Goulet, L. Rainie, et al., "Social Networking Sites and Our Lives," 2011.

16. J. T. Cacioppo and B. Patrick, *Loneliness*, 2008.

17. M. T. Frías, A. Brassard, and P. R. Shaver, "Childhood Sexual Abuse and Attachment Insecurities as Predictors of Women's Own and Perceived-Partner Extradyadic Involvement," *Child Abuse and Neglect* 38, no. 9 (2014): 1450–58; A. Lowell, K. Renk, and A. H. Adgate, "The Role of Attachment in the Relationship Between Child Maltreatment and Later Emotional and Behavioral Functioning," *Child Abuse and Neglect* 38, no. 9 (2014): 1436–49

18. R. Sternberg, "A Triangular Theory of Love," *Psychological Review* 93 (1986): 119–35.

19. R. Sternberg, *Cupid's Arrow: The Course of Love through Time* (New York: Cambridge University Press, 1998).

20. H. Fisher, *Anatomy of Love: A Natural History of Mating, Marriage, and Why We Stray* (New York: W. W. Norton, 2016).

21. Ibid.

22. L. Festinger, S. Schachter, and K. Back, *Social Pressures in Informal Groups: A Study of Human Factors in Housing* (Stanford, CA: Stanford University Press, 1950); R. L. Crooks and K. Baur, *Our Sexuality*, 13th ed. (Boston, MA: Cengage Learning, 2016).

23. R. L. Crooks and K. Baur, *Our Sexuality*, 2016.

24. Ibid.

25. C. Finkenauer and A. Buyukcan-Tetik, "To Know You Is to Feel Intimate with You: Felt Knowledge is Rooted in Disclosure, Solicitation, and Intimacy," *Family Science* 6, no. 1 (2015): 109–18; C. R. Rogers, "Interpersonal Relationship: The Core of Guidance," in *Person to Person: The Problem of Being Human,* eds. C. R. Rogers and B. Stevens (Lafayette, CA: Real People Press, 1967).

26. B. Hurn and B. Tomalin, *Cross-Cultural Communication: Theory and Practice* (London: Palgrave-Macmillan, 2013).

27. Ibid.

28. Ibid.

29. J. Wood, *Interpersonal Communication: Everyday Encounters,* 8th ed. (Boston, MA: Woodsworth Publishing, 2015).

30. Ibid.

31. M. Gendon et al., "Perceptions of Emotion from Facial Expressions Are Not Culturally Universal: Evidence from a Remote Culture," *Emotion* 14, no. 2 (2014): 251–62.

32. K. Hampton, L. S. Goulet, L. Rainie, and K. Purcell, "Social Networking Sites and Our Lives," 2011.

33. Ibid.

34. Ibid.

35. Ibid.

36. Ibid.

37. Ibid.

38. Ibid.

39. E. C. Tandoc, P. Ferrucci, and M. Duffy, "Facebook Use, Envy, and Depression Among College Students: Is Facebooking Depressing?," *Computers in Human Behavior* 43, (2015): 139–46; M. N. Steers, R. E. Wickham, and L. K. Acitelli, "Seeing Everyone Else's Highlight Reels: How Facebook Usage Is Linked to Depressive Symptoms," *Journal of Social and Clinical Psychology* 33, no. 8, (2014): 701–31.

40. Ibid.

41. K. M. Hertlein and K. Ancheta, "Advantages and Disadvantages of Technology in Relationships: Findings from an Open-Ended Survey," *The Qualitative Report* 19, no. 22 (2014): 1–11.

42. Y. T. Uhls et al., "Five Days at Outdoor Education Camp Without Screens Improves Preteen Skills with Nonverbal Emotion Cues," *Computers in Human Behavior* 39, (2014): 387–92.

43. T. Worley, "Exploring the Association between Relational Uncertainty, Jealousy About Partner's Friendships, and Jealousy Expression in Dating Relationships," *Communication Studies* 65, no. 4 (2014): 370–88; B. D. L. Zandbergen and S. G. Brown, "Culture and Gender Differences in Romantic Jealousy," *Personality and Individual Differences* 72 (2015): 122–7.

44. United States Department of Labor, Bureau of Labor Statistics, "American Time Use Survey Summary–2014 Results," June 24, 2015, http://www.bls.gov/news.release/atus .nr0.htm.

45. The Gottman Institute, "Research FAQs," Accessed March 6, 2016, https://www .gottman.com/about/research/faq/.

46. G. F. Kelly, *Sexuality Today*, 11th ed. (New York, NY: McGraw-Hill, 2014).

47. F. Newport and J. Wilke, "Most in U.S. Want Marriage, but Its Importance Has Dropped," *Gallup*, August 2, 2013, www.gallup.com/ poll/163802/marriage-importance-dropped .aspx.

48. W. Wang and K. Parker, "Record Share of Americans Have Never Married," Pew Research Center, September 24, 2014, http:// www.pewsocialtrends.org/2014/09/24/ record-share-of-americans-have-never- married/.

49. G. Livingston, "Four-in-Ten Couples Are Saying 'I Do' Again," Pew Research Center, November 14, 2014, www.pewsocialtrends .org/2014/11/14/four-in-ten-couples-are- saying-i-do-again/.

50. U.S. Census Bureau, "Families and Living Arrangements: 2015, Table MS-2 Estimated Median Age at First Marriage, by Sex: 1890 to the Present," www.census.gov/hhes/families/ data/marital.html.

51. S. Kennedy and S. Ruggles, "Breaking Up Is Hard to Count: The Rise of Divorce in the United States, 1980–2010," *Demography* 51, no. 2 (2014): 587–98.

52. K. Heller, "The Myth of the High Rate of Divorce," *Psych Central*, April 2, 2014, http:// psychcentral.com/lib/2012/the-myth-of-the- high-rate-of-divorce.

53. C. C. Miller, "The Divorce Surge Is Over, but the Myth Lives On," *New York Times*, December 2, 2014, www.nytimes.com/ 2014/12/02/upshot/the-divorce-surge-is- over-but-the-myth-lives-on.html.

54. Ibid.

55. A. J. Cherlin, "Multiple Partners, but One at a Time," *New York Times* Blog, May 21, 2013.

56. R. G. Watt et al., "Social Relationships and Health Related Behaviors Among Older US Adults," *BMC Public Health* 14, no. 1 (2014): 533; G. E. Miller and Y. Pylypchuk, "Marital Status, Spousal Characteristics, and the Use of Preventive Care," *Journal of Family and Economic Issues* 35, no. 3 (2014): 323–38.

57. C. C. Miller, "Study Finds More Reasons to Get and Stay Married," *New York Times*, January 8, 2015, www.nytimes.com/2015/ 01/08/upshot/study-finds-more-reasons-to- get-and-stay-married.html?rref=upshot&abt =0002&abg=0&_r=2.

58. R. G. Watt et al., "Social Relationships and Health Related Behaviors Among Older US Adults," *BMC Public Health* 14, no. 1 (2014); G. E. Miller and Y. Pylypchuk, "Marital Status, Spousal Characteristics, and the Use of Preventive Care," *Journal of Family and Economic Issues* 35, no. 3 (2014): 323–38.

59. Ibid.

60. Ibid.

61. U.S. Census Bureau, "America's Families and Living Arrangements: 2014: Adults, Table A1"

https://www.census.gov/hhes/families/data/cps2014A.html.

62. U.S. Department of Health and Human Services, Division of Vital Statistics, "First Premarital Cohabitation in the United States: 2006–2010 National Survey of Family Growth," *National Health Statistics Report* 64 (2013), Available at www.cdc.gov/nchs/data/nhsr/nhsr064.pdf; U.S. Department of Health and Human Services, Center for Health Statistics, "Key Statistics from the National Survey of Family Growth," April 20, 2015, www.cdc.gov/nchs/nsfg/key_statistics/c.htm.

63. Ibid.

64. A. Kuperberg, "Age at Co-Residence, Premarital Cohabitation and Marriage Dissolution: 1985–2009," *Journal of Marriage and Family,* 76 no. 2 (2014): 352–69.

65. U.S. Department of Health and Human Services, Division of Vital Statistics, "First Premarital Cohabitation in the United States," 2013; U.S. Department of Health and Human Services, Center for Health Statistics, "Key Statistics from the National Survey of Family Growth," 2015.

66. U.S. Census Bureau, "Characteristics of Same-Sex Households: 2014," Accessed March 2016, www.census.gov/hhes/samesex/; D. Cohn, "How Many Same-Sex Couples in the U.S.," Pew Research Center, June 24, 2015, www.pewresearch.org/fact-tank/2015/06/24/how-many-same-sex-married-couples-in-the-u-s-maybe-170000/.

67. Obergefell v. Hodges 576 U.S. 1-103 (2015).

68. Ibid.

69. Ibid.

70. A. Blinder and T. Lewin, "Clerk in Kentucky Chooses Jail Over Deal on Same-Sex Marriage," September 3, 2015, www.nytimes.com/2015/09/04/us/kim-davis-same-sex-marriage.html?_r=0; K. Calamur, "In Some States, Defiance of Supreme Court's Same-Sex Ruling," June 29, 2015, www.npr.org/sections/thetwo-way/2015/06/29/418600672/in-some-states-defiance-over-supreme-courts-same-sex-marriage-ruling.

71. U.S. Census Bureau, "America's Families and Living Arrangements: 2014: Adults, Table A1," 2016.

72. A. Krueger, "9 Reasons to Love Being Single," *Forbes*, February 14, 2014, www.forbes.com/sites/alysonkrueger/2014/02/14/9-reasons-to-love-being-single/#53ae926818bb; S. Dembling, "What if Staying Single Weren't Stigmatized?," *Psychology Today*, January 9, 2014, https://www.psychologytoday.com/blog/the-introverts-corner/201401/what-if-staying-single-werent-stigmatized.

73. A. Krueger, "9 Reasons to Love Being Single," 2014.

74. F. Newport and J. Wilke, "Desire for Children Still Norm in the U.S.," Gallup, September 25, 2013, www.gallup.com/poll/164618/desire-children-norm.aspx.

75. U.S. Census, "Families and Living Arrangements, Table C9. Children/1 by Presence and Type of Parent(s), Race, and Hispanic Origin/2: 2014," Accessed May 2016, www.census.gov/hhes/families/data/cps2014C.html.

**Pulled statistics:**

p. 227, A. Smith, "15% of American Adults Have Used Online Dating Sites or Mobile Dating Apps," Pew Research, 2016, www.pewinternet.org/2016/02/11/15-percent-of-american-adults-have-used-online-dating-sites-or-mobile-dating-apps/.

p. 234, K. Parker, W. Wang, and M. Rohol, "Record Share of Americans Have Never Married," Pew Research, 2014, www.pewsocialtrends.org/files/2014/09/2014-09-24_never-Married-Americans.pdf.

# Chapter 9

1. E. Schroeder and J. Kuriansky (Eds), *Sexuality education: Past, present, and future*, Vol 1 (Westport, CT: Praeger, 2015).

2. C. E. Bruess and E. Schroeder, *Sexuality Education: Theory and Practice*, 6th ed. (Burlington, MA: Jones and Bartlett, 2014).

3. Ibid.

4. I. A. Hughes et al., "Consensus Statement on Management of Intersex Disorders," *Archives of Disease in Childhood* 91, no. 7 (2006): 554–63.

5. J. S. Greenberg, C. E. Bruess, and S. B. Oswalt, *Exploring the Dimensions of Human Sexuality,* 5th ed. (Burlington, MA: Jones and Bartlett, 2014).

6. W. J. Chambliss and D. S. Eglitis, *Discover Sociology,* 2nd ed. (Los Angeles: Sage Publications, 2015).

7. Ibid.

8. Human Rights Campaign, "Sexual Orientation and Gender Identity Definitions," Accessed May 2016, http://www.hrc.org/resources/sexual-orientation-and-gender-identity-terminology-and-definitions.

9. Ibid.

10. GLAAD, "GLAAD Media Reference Guide—Transgender Issues," Accessed May 2016, http://www.glaad.org/reference/transgender.

11. GLAAD, "GLAAD Media Reference Guide—Terms to Avoid," Accessed May 2016, http://www.glaad.org/reference/offensive.

12. M. Rosario and E. Schrimshaw, "Theories and Etiologies of Sexual Orientation," *APA Handbook of Sexuality and Psychology* 1 (2014): 555–96.

13. J. McCarthy, "Satisfaction with Acceptance of Gay People Plateaus at 53%," *Gallup*, January 22, 2015, http://www.gallup.com/poll/181235/satisfaction-acceptance-gay-people-plateaus.aspx?g_source=homosexuality&g_medium=search&g_campaign=tiles.

14. G. M. Herek, "Beyond 'Homophobia': Thinking More Clearly About Stigma, Prejudice, and Sexual Orientation," *American Journal of Orthopsychiatry* 85, no. 5S (2015): S29–S37.

15. Federal Bureau of Investigation, "Bias Breakdown," November 16, 2015, https://www.fbi.gov/news/stories/2015/november/latest-hate-crime-statistics-available.

16. S. M. Cabrera et al., "Age of Thelarche and Menarche in Contemporary U.S. Females: A Cross-Sectional Analysis," *Journal of Pediatric Endocrinology and Metabolism* 27, nos. 1–2 (2014): 47–51.

17. J. S. Greenberg, C. E. Bruess, and S. B. Oswalt, *Exploring the Dimensions of Human Sexuality,* 5th ed. (Burlington, MA: Jones and Bartlett, 2014).

18. M. K. Cocker et al., "Sexual Dimorphisms in the Associations of BMI and Body Fat with Indices of Pubertal Development in Girls and Boys," *Journal of Clinical Endocrinology and Metabolism* 99, no. 8 (2014): E1519–29.

19. D. F. Maron, "Early Puberty: Causes and Effects," *Scientific American*, May 1, 2015, http://www.scientificamerican.com/article/early-puberty-causes-and-effects/.

20. Womenshealth.gov, "Premenstrual Syndrome (PMS) Fact Sheet," December 23, 2014, http://womenshealth.gov/publications/our-publications/fact-sheet/premenstrual-syndrome.html#e.

21. Ibid.

22. Ibid.

23. Ibid.

24. Mayo Clinic Staff, "Diseases and Conditions: Menstrual Cramps," May 8, 2014, www.mayoclinic.org/diseases-conditions/menstrual-cramps/basics/definition/con-20025447.

25. WebMD, "Understanding Toxic Shock Syndrome," March 4, 2015, http://www.webmd.com/women/guide/understanding-toxic-shock-syndrome-basics?page=2.

26. MedlinePlus, "Menopause," May 6, 2016, https://www.nlm.nih.gov/medlineplus/menopause.html.

27. Ibid.

28. Ibid.

29. Ibid.

30. Ibid.; H. Levine, "Is Hormone Replacement Therapy Making a Comeback?," *Consumer Reports*, May 15, 2016, http://www.consumerreports.org/women-s-health/is-hormone-replacement-therapy-making-a-comeback/.

31. H. Hu, et al., "Racial Differences in Age-Related Variations of Testosterone Levels Among U.S. Males: Potential Implications for Prostate Cancer and Personalized Medication," *Journal of Racial and Ethnic Health Disparities* 2, no. 1 (2015): 69–76.

32. Mayo Clinic Staff, "Male Menopause: Myth or Reality?," June 3, 2014, www.mayoclinic.org/healthy-living/mens-health/in-depth/male-menopause/art-20048056.

33. Ibid.

34. Ibid.

35. Mayo Clinic Staff, "Testosterone Therapy: Potential Benefits and Risks as You Age," Mayo Clinic, April 1, 2015, http://www.mayoclinic.org/healthy-lifestyle/sexual-health/in-depth/testosterone-therapy/art-20045728.

36. C. Clark, "Brain Sex in Men and Women—From Arousal to Orgasm," BrainBlogger, May 20, 2014, http://brainblogger.com/2014/05/20/brain-sex-in-men-and-women-from-arousal-to-orgasm/.

37. National Institute on Aging, "Sexuality in Later Life," December 22, 2015, https://www.nia.nih.gov/health/publication/sexuality-later-life.

38. Ibid.; WebMD, "Common Physical Changes in Men," November 14, 2014, http://www.webmd.com/healthy-aging/guide/sexuality-and-physical-changes-with-aging-common-physical-changes-in-men.

39. National Institute on Aging, "Sexuality in Later Life," December 22, 2015, https://www.nia.nih.gov/health/publication/sexuality-later-life.

40. K. Cherney and K. Watson, "Managing Antidepressant Sexual Side Effects," March 3, 2016, www.healthline.com/health/erectile-dysfunction/antidepressant-sexual-side-effects#Overview1.

41. Mayo Clinic, "Female Sexual Dysfunction," March 5, 2016, http://www.mayoclinic.org/diseases-conditions/female-sexual-dysfunction/basics/treatment/con-20027721.

42. Mayo Clinic, "Erectile Dysfunction," May 27, 2015, www.mayoclinic.org/diseases-conditions/erectile-dysfunction/basics/definition/con-20034244.

43. Ibid.

44. National Kidney and Urological Diseases Information Clearinghouse, "Erectile Dysfunction," November 2015, http://kidney.niddk.nih.gov/KUDiseases/pubs/ED/index.aspx.

45. Ibid.

46. Ibid.

47. Medscape, "Premature Ejaculation," March 15, 2016, http://emedicine.medscape.com/article/435884-overview.

48. International Society for Sexual Medicine, "What Causes Female Orgasmic Disorder (FOD)?" Accessed May 29, 2016, http://www.issm.info/education-for-all/sexual-health-qa/what-causes-female-orgasmic-disorder-fod.

49. International Society for Sexual Medicine, "How is Female Orgasmic Disorder (FOD) Treated?," Accessed May 29, 2016, http://www.issm.info/education-for-all/sexual-health-qa/how-is-female-orgasmic-disorder-fod-treated.

50. Ibid.

51. Ibid.

52. Ibid.

53. Women's Health Rehab and Supply, "What Causes Vaginismus?," Accessed May 29, 2016, https://www.vaginismus.com/vaginismus causes/.

54. J. P. Wincze and R. B. Weisberg. *Sexual Dysfunction: A Guide for Assessment and Treatment* (New York: Guilford Press, 2015).

55. D. G. Duryea, N. G. Calleja, and D. A. MacDonald, "Nonmedical Use of Prescription Drugs by College Students with Minority Sexual Orientations," *Journal of College Student Psychotherapy* 29, no. 2 (2015): 147–59.

56. T. M. Hall, S. Shoptaw, and C. J. Reback, "Sometimes Poppers Are Not Poppers: Huffing as an Emergent Health Concern Among MSM Substance Users," *Journal of Gay and Lesbian Mental Health* 19, no. 1 (2015): 118–21; T. Kofler, et al. "Use of Poppers (Amyl Nitrite): Unpleasant Side Effects in a Brothel," *European Journal of Case Reports in Internal Medicine* 1, no. 1 (2014): doi: 10.12890/2014_000139.

57. Rape, Abuse, and Incest National Network, "Drug-Facilitated Sexual Assault," Accessed May 2016, https://rainn.org/get-information/types-of-sexual-assault/drug-facilitated-assault.

58. Ibid.

59. E. Brown, S. Hendrix, and S. Svrluga, "Drinking Is Central to College Culture and to Sexual Assaults," *Washington Post*, June 14, 2015, https://www.washingtonpost.com/local/education/beer-pong-body-shots-keg-stands-alcohol-central-to-college-and-assault/2015/06/14/7430e13c-04bb-11e5-a428-c984eb077d4e_story.html.

60. G. F. Kelly, *Sexuality Today*, 11th ed. (New York: McGraw-Hill, 2014).

61. W. Maltz, "The CERTS Model for Health Sex," Healthysex.com, Accessed May 2016, http://healthysex.com/healthy-sexuality/part-one-understanding/the-certs-model-for-healthy-sex/.

62. R.L. Crooks and K. Baur, *Our Sexuality*, 13th ed. (Wadsworth Publishing: Belmont, CA, 2016).

63. American College Health Association, *American College Health Association–National College Health Assessment II (ACHA-NCHA II) Reference Group Data Report, Fall 2015* (Hanover, MD: American College Health Association, 2015), Available at http://www.acha-ncha.org/docs/NCHA-II%20FALL%202015%20REFERENCE%20GROUP%20DATA%20REPORT.pdf.

64. M. Castleman, "Adult Toys: Both Women and Men Increasingly Love Them," *Psychology Today*, January 1, 2015, https://www.psychologytoday.com/blog/all-about-sex/201501/adult-toys-both-women-and-men-increasingly-love-them.

65. Good Vibrations, "How to Care and Clean your Sex Toys," Accessed May 2016, http://www.goodvibes.com/s/content/c/Sex-Toy-Material-Cleaning.

66. American College Health Association, *National College Health Assessment II: Reference Group Data Report, Fall 2015*, 2015.

67. Ibid.

68. Ibid.

69. SIECUS, "Life Behaviors of a Sexually Healthy Adult," Accessed May 2016, www.siecus.org.

70. R. Anderson, "Seven Reasons You Should Have More Sex," *Psychology Today*, February 27, 2016, https://www.psychologytoday.com/blog/the-mating-game/201602/7-reasons-why-you-should-have-more-sex; P. Rogers, "The Health Benefits of Sex," Healthline, July 21, 2014, http://www.healthline.com/health/healthy-sex-health-benefits#Overview1;

71. J. Rider et al., "Ejaculation Frequency and Risk of Prostate Cancer: Updated Results from the Health Professionals Follow-Up Study," *Journal of Urology* 193, no. 4 (2015).

**Pulled statistics:**

p. 243, Data from American College Health Association, *American College Health Association—National College Health Assessment II (ACHA-NCHA II) Reference Group Data Report Fall 2015* (Baltimore: American College Health Association, 2015).

p. 251, Data from American College Health Association, *American College Health Association—National College Health Assessment II (ACHA-NCHA II) Reference Group Data Report Fall 2015* (Baltimore: American College Health Association, 2015).

## Chapter 10

1. M. Lino, "Expenditures on Children by Families, 2013," *U.S. Department of Agriculture, Center for Nutrition Policy and Promotion, Miscellaneous Publication No. 1528-2013 (2014)*, Available at www.cnpp.usda.gov/ExpendituresonChildrenbyFamilies.

2. Truven Health Analytics, "The Cost of Having a Baby in the United States," January 2013, Available at http://transform.childbirthconnection.org/wp-content/uploads/2013/01/Cost-of-Having-a-Baby1.pdf.

3. T. J. Mathews and B. E. Hamilton, *"First Births to Older Women Continue to Rise,"* NCHS Data Brief 152 (2014): 1–8, www.cdc.gov/nchs/data/databriefs/db152.pdf.

4. B. E. Hamilton et al., "Births: Final Data for 2014," *National Vital Statistics Report* 64, no. 12 (2015), Available at http://www.cdc.gov/nchs/data/nvsr/nvsr64/nvsr64_12.pdf.

5. American Pregnancy Association, "Miscarriage," Updated August 2015, http://americanpregnancy.org/pregnancycomplications/miscarriage.html.

6. Committee on Gynecologic Practice of American College of Obstetricians and Gynecologists, "Female Age-Related Fertility Decline," *Committee Opinion* 589 (2014), Available at http://www.acog.org/Resources-And-Publications/Committee-Opinions/Committee-on-Gynecologic-Practice/Female-Age-Related-Fertility-Decline.

7. Centers for Disease Control and Prevention (CDC), "Preconception Health and Health Care: Women," January 2015, www.cdc.gov/preconception/women.html.

8. Ibid.

9. Ibid.; S. M. Schrader and K. L. Marlow, "Assessing the Reproductive Health of Men with Occupational Exposures," *Asian Journal of Andrology* 16, no. 1 (2014): 23–30.

10. B. M. D'Onofrio et al., "Paternal Age at Childbearing and Offspring Psychiatric and Academic Morbidity," *Journal of the American Medical Association Psychiatry* 71, no. 4 (2014): 432–38.

11. Planned Parenthood, "Pregnancy Tests," Accessed April 2015, https://www.plannedparenthood.org/learn/pregnancy/pregnancy-test.

12. American Congress of Obstetricians and Gynecologists, "ACOG Committee Opinion no. 548: Weight Gain During Pregnancy," *Obstetrics and Gynecology* 121, no. 1 (2013): 210–2, doi: 10.1097/01.AOG.0000425668.87506.4c.

13. Ibid.

14. Ibid.

15. The American Congress of Obstetricians and Gynecologists, "FAQ: Tobacco, Alcohol, Drugs, and Pregnancy," December 2013,

www.acog.org/~/media/For%20Patients/faq170.pdf?dmc=1&ts=20140516T2242271513.

16. Ibid.; National Center for Chronic Disease Prevention and Health Promotion, "Tobacco Use and Pregnancy," September 2015, www.cdc.gov/Reproductivehealth/TobaccoUse Pregnancy/index.htm.

17. CDC, "Facts about Cleft Lip and Cleft Palate," November 2015, www.cdc.gov/ncbddd/birthdefects/cleftlip.html.

18. CDC, "Zika Virus: Zika and Pregnancy," January 2016, http://www.cdc.gov/zika/pregnancy/question-answers.html.

19. B. E. Hamilton et al., "Births: Final Data for 2014," *National Vital Statistics Report* 64, no. 12 (2015), Available at http://www.cdc.gov/nchs/data/nvsr/nvsr64/nvsr64_12.pdf.

20. J. Christensen, "Why So Many C-Sections Have Medical Groups Concerned," *CNN*, May 8, 2014, www.cnn.com/2014/05/08/health/c-section-report.

21. Mayo Clinic, "Preeclampsia," July 3, 2014, http://www.mayoclinic.org/diseases-conditions/preeclampsia/basics/definition/con-20031644.

22. E. Puscheck et al., "Early Pregnancy Loss," *Medscape Reference: Drugs, Diseases & Procedures*, Updated November 15, 2015, http://reference.medscape.com/article/266317-overview.

23. Mayo Clinic, "Rh Factor Blood Test," June 23, 2015, http://www.mayoclinic.org/tests-procedures/rh-factor/basics/definition/prc-20013476.

24. Ibid.

25. Ibid.

26. Ibid.

27. V. P. Sepilian et al., "Ectopic Pregnancy," *Medscape Reference*, Updated November 2015, http://emedicine.medscape.com/article/2041923-overview.

28. What to Expect, "Stillbirth," Accessed March 2016, www.whattoexpect.com/pregnancy/pregnancy-health/complications/stillbirth.aspx.

29. K. L. Wisner et al., "Onset Timing, Thoughts of Self-harm, and Diagnoses in Postpartum Women with Screen-Positive Depression Findings," *JAMA Psychiatry* 70, no. 5 (2013): 1–9, doi:10.1001/jamapsychiatry.2013.87.

30. Ibid.

31. American Academy of Pediatrics, "Policy Statement: Breastfeeding and the Use of Human Milk," *Pediatrics* 129, no. 3 (2012): 496.

32. American Academy of Pediatrics, "Benefits of Breastfeeding for Mom," Updated November 2015, www.healthychildren.org/English/ages-stages/baby/breastfeeding/pages/Benefits-of-Breastfeeding-for-Mom.aspx.

33. CDC, "Sudden Unexpected Infant Death and Sudden Infant Death Syndrome," January 2016, www.cdc.gov/sids.

34. Ibid.

35. Ibid.

36. March of Dimes, "Low Birthweight," October 2014, http://www.marchofdimes.org/complications/low-birthweight.aspx.

37. CDC, "Infertility FAQs," Reproductive Health, April 2016, www.cdc.gov/reproductivehealth/Infertility/.

38. MayoClinic.com, "Infertility: Causes," July 2014, www.mayoclinic.com/health/infertility/DS00310/DSECTION=causes.

39. U.S. Department of Health and Human Services, "Polycystic Ovary Syndrome (PCOS) Fact Sheet," December 2014, www.womenshealth.gov/publications/our-publications/fact-sheet/polycystic-ovary-syndrome.html.

40. B. Kumbak, E. Oral, and O. Bukulmez, "Female Obesity and Assisted Reproductive Technologies," *Seminars in Reproductive Medicine* 30, no. 6 (2012): 507–16, doi: 10.1055/s-0032-1328879.

41. CDC, "Pelvic Inflammatory Disease CDC Fact Sheet," Sexually Transmitted Diseases, February 2016, www.cdc.gov/std/PID/STDFact-PID.htm.

42. CDC, "Infertility: FAQs," April 2016, www.cdc.gov/reproductivehealth/Infertility/index.htm#4.

43. National Infertility Association, "The Semen Analysis," Accessed May 2016, http://www.resolve.org/about-infertility/male-workup/the-semen-analysis.html.

44. Ibid.; Mayo Clinic Staff, "Low Sperm Count," July 2015, www.mayoclinic.org/diseases-conditions/low-sperm-count/basics/causes/con-20033441.

45. CDC, "Infertility: FAQs," April 2016, www.cdc.gov/reproductivehealth/Infertility/index.htm#4.

46. Ibid.

47. WebMD Medical Reference, "Fertility Drugs," June 2015, www.webmd.com/infertility-and-reproduction/guide/fertility-drugs.

48. American Society for Reproductive Medicine, "Fertility Drugs and the Risk for Multiple Births," Accessed March 2016, www.asrm.org/uploadedFiles/ASRM_Content/Resources/Patient_Resources/Fact_Sheets_and_Info_Booklets/fertilitydrugs_multiple births.pdf.

49. WebMD, "Using a Surrogate Mother, What You Need to Know," September 2015, www.webmd.com/infertility-and-reproduction/guide/using-surrogate-mother.

50. R. M. Kreider and D. A. Loftquist, "Adopted Children and Stepchildren: 2010," *U.S. Census Bureau*, April 2014, Available at www.census.gov/content/dam/Census/library/publications/2014/demo/p20-572.pdf.

51. Intercountry Adoption, U.S. Department of State, "FY 2013 Annual Report on Intercountry Adoption," March 2014, http://travel.state.gov/content/dam/aa/pdfs/fy2013_annual_report.pdf.

52. Adoption.com, "Adoption Costs," Accessed March 2016, http://costs.adoption.com.

53. American College Health Association, *American College Health Association—National College Health Assessment III (ACHA-NCHA III): Reference Group Data Report, Fall 2015* (Hanover, MD: American College Health Association, 2015), Available at http://www.acha-ncha.org/reports_ACHA-NCHAIIc.html.

54. L. B. Finer and M. R. Zolna, "Shifts in Intended and Unintended Pregnancies in the United States, 2001–2008," *American Journal of Public Health* 104, no. S1 (2014): S44–S48.

55. J. Trussell, "Contraceptive Efficacy," in *Contraceptive Technology*, 20th rev. ed., eds. R. A. Hatcher et al. (New York: Ardent Media, 2011).

56. World Health Organization, "Nonoxynol-9 Ineffective in Preventing HIV Infection," Accessed March 2016, www.who.int/mediacentre/news/notes/release55/en.

57. J. Trussell, "Contraceptive Efficacy," 2011.

58. Ibid.

59. Ibid.

60. Mayo Clinic Staff, "Risks: Spermicide," January 2016, http://www.mayoclinic.org/tests-procedures/spermicide/details/risks/cmc-20168563; World Health Organization, "Nonoxynol-9 Ineffective in Preventing HIV Infection," Accessed March 2016, www.who.int/mediacentre/news/notes/release55/en.

61. Ibid.

62. J. Trussell, "Contraceptive Efficacy," 2011.

63. Ibid.

64. Ibid.

65. Ibid.

66. Ibid.

67. Ibid.

68. American College Health Association, *American College Health Association—National College Health Assessment III (ACHA-NCHA III): Reference Group Data Report, Fall 2015* (Hanover, MD: American College Health Association, 2015), Available at http://www.acha-ncha.org/reports_ACHA-NCHAIIc.html.

69. J. Trussell, "Contraceptive Efficacy," 2011.

70. Ibid.

71. Ibid.

72. Ibid.

73. Ibid.

74. Ibid.

75. Association of Reproductive Health Professionals, "Combined Hormonal Contraception," June 2014, http://www.arhp.org/Publications-and-Resources/Quick-Reference-Guide-for-Clinicians/choosing/Combined-Hormonal-Contraception.

76. O. Lidegaard, "The Risk of Arterial Thrombosis Increases with the Use of Combined Oral Contraceptives," *Evidence Based Medicine* 21, no. 1 (2016): 38; X. Zhenlin, et al. "Current Use of Oral Contraceptives and the Risk of First-Ever Ischemic Stroke: A Meta-analysis of Observational Studies," *Thrombosis Research* 136, no. 1 (2015): 52–60.

77. J. Trussell, "Contraceptive Efficacy," 2011.

78. E. G. Raymond, "Progestin-Only Pills," in *Contraceptive Technology*, 20th rev. ed., eds. R. A. Hatcher et al. (New York: Ardent Media, 2011).

79. Janssen Pharmaceuticals, "OrthoEvra," September 2014, http://www.janssen.com/us/sites/www_janssen_com_usa/files/products-documents/ortho_evra_pi_039836-150904.pdf; Drugs.com, "Xulane," February 2016, www.drugs.com/mtm/xulane_transdermal.html.

80. J. Trussell, "Contraceptive Efficacy," 2011.

81. Drugs.com, "Xulane," December 2015, http://www.drugs.com/pro/xulane.html.

82. U.S. Food and Drug Administration, "Drug Safety Labeling Changes," October 2015, http://www.fda.gov/Safety/MedWatch/SafetyInformation/ucm211821.htm.

83. J. Trussell, "Contraceptive Efficacy," 2011.

84. Ibid.

85. Pfizer, "Depo-subQ Provera U.S. Patient Product Information," January 2015, http://www.pfizer.com/products/product-detail/depo_subq_provera_104.

86. J. Trussell, "Contraceptive Efficacy," 2011.

87. Merck & Co., Inc., "Nexplanon," Accessed March 2016, www.nexplanon.com/en/consumer/.

88. K. Daniels et al., "Current Contraceptive Use and Variation by Selected Characteristics Among Women Aged 15–44: United States, 2011–2013," *National Health Statistics Reports* 86 (2015): 1–15.

89. The American Congress of Obstetricians and Gynecologists, "ACOG Committee Opinion-Adolescents and Long-Acting Reversible Contraception: Implants and Intrauterine Devices," Number 539, October 2012, www.acog.org/Resources_And_Publications/Committee_Opinions/Committee_on_Adolescent_Health_Care/Adolescents_and_Long-Acting_Reversible_Contraception.

90. J. Trussell, "Contraceptive Efficacy," 2011.

91. American College Health Association, *National College Health Assessment III: Reference Group Data Report Fall 2015*, 2015.

92. J. Trussell, "Contraceptive Efficacy," 2011.

93. American College Health Association, *National College Health Assessment III: Reference Group Data Report Spring 2015*, 2015.

94. J. Trussell, "Contraceptive Efficacy," 2011.

95. K. Daniels, J. Daugherty, and J. Jones, "Current Contraceptive Status among Women Aged 15–44: United States 2011–2013," *National Health Statistics Data Brief*, no. 173 (Hyattsville, MD: National Center for Health Statistics, 2014).

96. U.S. Food and Drug Administration, "Medical Devices, FDA Activities," March 4, 2016, http://www.fda.gov/MedicalDevices/ProductsandMedicalProcedures/ImplantsandProsthetics/EssurePermanentBirthControl/ucm452254.htm.

97. J. Trussell, "Contraceptive Efficacy," 2011.

98. Ibid.

99. Office of Population Research & Association of Reproductive Health Professionals, The Emergency Contraception Website, "Answers to Frequently Asked Questions About Effectiveness," Updated March 2016, http://ec.princeton.edu/questions/eceffect.html.

100. American College Health Association, *National College Health Assessment II: Undergraduate Students Reference Group Data Fall 2015*, 2015.

101. Guttmacher Institute, "Fact Sheet: Induced Abortion in the United States," March 2016, www.guttmacher.org/fact-sheet/induced-abortion-united-states.

102. American Psychological Association (APA), Task Force on Mental Health and Abortion, *Report of the Task Force on Mental Health and Abortion* (Washington, DC: American Psychological Association, 2008), Available at www.apa.org/pi/wpo/mental-health-abortion-report.pdf.

103. *Roe v. Wade*, 410 U.S. 113 (1973).

104. L. Saad, "Abortion," *Gallup Politics*, Blog, January 22, 2013, www.gallup.com/poll/160058/majority-americans-support-roe-wade-decision.aspx.

105. E. N. Brown, "U.S. Passed 47 New Anti-Abortion Laws in 2015," December 2015, http://reason.com/blog/2015/12/30/anti-abortion-laws-passed-in-2015.

106. APA, *Report of the Task Force*, 2008; J. R. Steinberg, C. E. McCulloch, and N. E. Adler, "Abortion and Mental Health: Findings from the National Comorbidity Survey-Replication," *Obstetrics & Gynecology* 123, no. 2 (2014): 263–70.

107. Ibid.

108. Ibid.

109. Guttmacher Institute, "Fact Sheet: Induced Abortion in the United States," March 2016.

110. Ibid.

111. Ibid.

112. Ibid.

113. Planned Parenthood, "The Abortion Pill," March 2016, https://www.plannedparenthood.org/learn/abortion/the-abortion-pill.

114. K. Cleland et al., "Significant Adverse Events and Outcomes After Medical Abortion," *Obstetrics and Gynecology* 121, no. 1 (2013): 166–171.

115. K. Cleland et al., "Significant Adverse Events and Outcomes After Medical Abortion," 2013.

**Pulled statistics:**

p. 275, Source: American College Health Association, *American College Health Association—National College Health Assessment III (ACHA-NCHA III): Reference Group Data Report, Fall 2015* (Hanover, MD: American College Health Association, 2015), Available at www.achancha.org/reports_ACHA_NCHAII.htm.

p. 00, Gallup, "U.S. Still Split on Abortion: 47% Pro-Choice, 46% Pro-Life," 2014, www.gallup.com/poll/170249/split-abortion-pro-choice-pro-life.aspx.

## Chapter 10A

1. M. Potenza, "Perspective: Behavioral Addictions Matter," *Nature* 522, Suppl. 62 (2015): doi: 10.1038/522S62a; S. S. Alavi et al., "Behavioral Addiction versus Substance Addiction: Correspondence of Psychiatric and Psychological Views," *International Journal of Preventive Medicine* 3, no. 4 (2012): 290–4.

2. N. Volkow et al., "Neurobiologic Advances from the Brain Disease Model of Addiction," *New England Journal of Medicine* 374, no. 4 (2016): 363–71.

3. Ibid.; National Institute on Drug Abuse, "Drugs, Brains, and Behavior: The Science of Addiction," August 2014, www.nida.nih.gov/scienceofaddiction.

4. American Society of Addiction Medicine, "Definition of Addiction," April 2011, www.asam.org/for-the-public/definition-of-addiction.

5. M. J. Burns et al., "Delirium Tremens (DTs)," *Medscape*, April 14, 2015, http://emedicine.medscape.com/article/166032-overview#a0156.

6. J. Kinney, *Loosening the Grip: A Handbook of Alcohol Information*, 11th ed. (Boston: McGraw-Hill, 2014), 179.

7. National Institute on Drug Abuse, "Drugs, Brains, and Behavior: The Science of Addiction," August 2014, www.drugabuse.gov/publications/science-addiction Howard J. Edenberg, "Genes Contributing to the Development of Alcoholism," *Alcohol Research: Current Reviews* 34, no. 3 (2012): 336–8.

8. National Institute on Drug Abuse, "Drugs, Brains, and Behavior: The Science of Addiction," August 2014, www.drugabuse.gov/publications/science-addiction.

9. J. Kinney, *Loosening the Grip*, 2014, 106.

10. Ibid.

11. Ibid.

12. National Institute on Drug Abuse, National Institutes of Health, U.S. Department of Health and Human Services, *Drugs, Brains, and Behavior: The Science of Addiction*, NIH Publication No. 07-5605 (Bethesda, MD: National Institute on Drug Abuse, Revised 2014), Available at www.nida.nih.gov/scienceofaddiction.

13. National Council on Problem Gambling, "March Madness and Gambling: Have the Conversation," March 9, 2016, Available at https://images.production.membersuite.com/7339289f-0004-c76f-a8b9-0b3842784d72/20987/7339289f-001c-c537-bd2e-0b3b1fb1a928; American Psychiatric Association, *Diagnostic and Statistical Manual of Mental Disorders*, 5th ed. (Arlington, VA: American Psychiatric Publishing, 2013), p. 585.

14. American Psychiatric Association, 2013, p. 585.

15. D. Nutt et al., "The Dopamine Theory of Addiction: 40 Years of Highs and Lows," *Nature Reviews Neuroscience* 16, no. 5 (2015): 305–12.

16. Elements Behavioral Health, "Internet, Gambling Addicts Also Suffer From Withdrawal," Accessed March 2016, https://www.elementsbehavioralhealth.com/behavioral-process-addictions/internet-gambling-addicts-also-suffer-from-withdrawal/.

17. National Council on Gambling, "Comments on SAMHSA's Leading Change 2.0: Advancing the Behavioral Health of the Nation 2015-2018," August 18, 2014, http://www.ncpgambling.org/wp-content/uploads/2014/08/NCPG-Comments-on-SAMHSA-Leading-Change-2.0-Advancing-the-Behavioral-Health-of-the-Nation-2015-2018.pdf.

18. Ibid.

19. D. W. Black et al., "A Direct, Controlled, Blind Family Study of DSM-IV Pathological Gambling." *Journal of Clinical Psychiatry* 75,

no. 3 (2014): 215–21; American Psychiatric Association, 2013, p. 589.

20. D. V. Rinker, et al., "Racial and Ethnic Differences in Problem Gambling among College Students," *Journal of Gambling Studies* 32, no. 2 (2015): 581–90; National Center for Responsible Gambling, "Fact Sheet: Gambling on College Campuses," Accessed February 2016, http://www.collegegambling.org/just-facts/gambling-college-campuses.

21. Ibid.

22. Ibid.

23. A. Muller et al., "Compulsive Buying," *American Journal on Addictions* 24, no. 2 (2015): 132–7

24. Ibid.; H. Hatfield, "Shopping Spree or Addiction?" *WebMD*, 2014, www.webmd.com/mental-health/features/shopping-spree-addiction.

25. Ibid.

26. A. Weinsten et al., "A Study Investigating the Association between Compulsive Buying with Measure of Anxiety and Obsessive-Compulsive Behavior Among Internet Shoppers," *Comprehensive Psychiatry* 57 (2015): 46–50; P. Trotzke et al., "Pathological Buying Online as a Specific Form of Internet Addiction: A Model-Based Experimental Investigation," *PLoS ONE* 10, no. 10 (2015): e0140296; K. Deryshire et al., "Problematic Internet Use and Associated Risks in a College Sample," *Comprehensive Psychiatry* 54, no. 5 (2013): 415–22.

27. A. Harvanko et al., "Prevalence and Characteristics of Compulsive Buying in College Students," *Psychiatry Research* 210, no. 3 (2013): 1079–85.

28. Ibid.

29. Ibid.

30. A. Perrin and M. Duggan, "Americans' Internet Access: 2000–2015," Pew Research Center, June 26, 2015, http://www.pewinternet.org/2015/06/26/americans-internet-access-2000-2015/.

31. A. Perrin, "One-Fifth of Americans Report Going Online 'Almost Constantly'," *Pew Research Center*, December 8, 2015, http://www.pewresearch.org/fact-tank/2015/12/08/one-fifth-of-americans-report-going-online-almost-constantly/.

32. Ibid.

33. Ibid.

34. A. Perrin, "Social Media Usage: 2005–2015," *Pew Research Center*, October 8, 2015 http://www.pewinternet.org/2015/10/08/social-networking-usage-2005-2015/.

35. Ibid.

36. Ibid.

37. Net Addiction, "FAQs," Accessed March 2016, http://netaddiction.com/faqs/; H. Pontes, D. Kuss, and M. Griffiths, "Clinical Psychology of Internet Addiction: A Review of its Conceptualization, Prevalence, Neuronal Processes, and Implications for Treatment," *Neuroscience and Neuroeconomics* 4 (2015): 11–23.

38. W. Li et al., "Characteristics of Internet Addiction: Pathological Internet Use in U.S. University Students: A Qualitative-Method

Investigation," *PLoS ONE* 10, no. 2 (2015): e0117372.

39. American College Health Association, *American College Health Association—National College Health Assessment II: Reference Group Data Report Spring 2015* (Baltimore. MD: American College Health Association, 2015).

40. EDUCAUSEreviewOnline, "Exploring Students' Mobile Learning Practices in Higher Education," October 7, 2013, www.educause.edu/ero/article/exploring-students-mobile-learning-practices-higher-education.

41. re:fuel, "Tech-Savvy College Students Are Gathering Gadgets, Saying Yes to Showrooming and Rejecting Second Screening," June 13, 2013, https://globenewswire.com/news-release/2013/06/13/554002/10036312/en/Tech-Savvy-College-Students-Are-Gathering-Gadgets-Saying-Yes-to-Showrooming-and-Rejecting-Second-Screening.html.

42. Ibid.

43. Wordpress.com, "How Much Time Do College Students Spend with Technology?" June 2013, www.researchresults.wordpress.com/2013/06/28/how-much-time-do-college-students-spend-with-technology.

44. S. Sussman, "Workaholism: A Review," *Journal of Addiction Research and Therapy* 10, no. 6 (2012): 4120, www.ncbi.nlm.nih.gov/pmc/articles/PMC3835604.

45. Ibid.

46. Ibid.

47. M. Clark, et al., "All Work and No Play?: A Meta-analytic Examination of the Correlates and Outcomes of Workaholism," *Journal of Management* (February 28, 2014): 1–38, http://jom.sagepub.com/content/early/2014/02/28/0149206314522301.full.pdf+html.

48. L. Kravina, et al., "Work Alcoholism and Work Engagement in the Family: The Relationship Between Parents and Children as a Risk Factor," *European Journal of Work and Organizational Psychology* (September 17, 2013).

49. M. Clark, et al., "All Work and No Play?: A Meta-Analytic Examination of the Correlates and Outcomes of Workaholism," *Journal of Management* (February 28, 2014): 1–38, http://jom.sagepub.com/content/early/2014/02/28/0149206314522301.full.pdf+html.

50. A. Szabo, et al., "Methodological and Conceptual Limitations in Exercise Addiction Research," *Yale Journal of Biology and Medicine* 88, no. 3 (2015): 303–8; A. Weinstein and Y. Weinstein, "Exercise Addiction: Diagnosis, Bio-psychological Mechanisms, and Treatment Issues," *Current Pharmaceutical Design* 20, no. 25 (2014): 4062–69.

51. R. Weiss, "Hypersexuality: Symptoms of Sexual Addiction," *Psych Central,* March 2016, http://psychcentral.com/lib/hypersexuality-symptoms-of-sexual-addiction.

52. Ibid.

53. N. Volkow et al., "Neurobiologic Advances from the Brain Disease Model of Addiction," *New England Journal of Medicine* 374, no. 4 (2016): 363–71.

54. National Institute on Drug Abuse, "Trends and Statistics: The Cost of Substance Abuse,"

August 2015, https://www.drugabuse.gov/related-topics/trends-statistics.

**Pulled statistics:**

p. 306, Center for Personal Finance Editors, "Tough Times Series: It Was Such a Bargain: Help for Compulsive Shoppers," 2014, http://hffo.cuna.org/12433/article/353/html.

p. 307, "Our Addiction to Technology Trumps Caffeine, Chocolate, and Alcohol," Technology: The Business and Culture of Our Digital Lives (blog), *Los Angeles Times*, August 11, 2011, http://latimesblogs.latimes.com/technology/2011/08/technology-addiction-chocolate-caffeine.html.

## Chapter 11

1. T. Naimi et al., "Confounding and Studies of 'Moderate' Alcohol Consumption: The Case of Drinking Frequency and Implications for Low Risk Drinking Guidelines," *Addiction* 108, no. 9 (2013): 1534–43;

2. Ibid.

3. National Center for Health Statistics, "Summary Health Statistics for U.S. Adults: National Health Interview Survey, 2012," *Vital and Health Statistics* 10, no. 260 (2014): 34.

4. Ibid.

5. Ibid.

6. Ibid.

7. Ibid.

8. Centers for Disease Control and Prevention, "Fact Sheets: Binge Drinking," October 2015, http://www.cdc.gov/alcohol/fact-sheets/binge-drinking.htm.

9. Ibid.

10. Ibid.

11. Ibid.

12. Ibid.

13. Health Essential, "Alcohol May Cause You to Develop Irregular Heart Beat," October 30, 2014, https://health.clevelandclinic.org/2014/10/alcohol-may-cause-irregular-heartbeat/.

14. National Institute on Alcohol Abuse and Alcoholism, "Alcohol's Effects on the Body," Accessed May 4, 2016, http://niaaa.nih.gov/alcohol-health/alcohols-effects-body.

15. Blowfish for Hangovers, "How it Works," Accessed May 2016, http://forhangovers.com/pages/about.

16. Centers for Disease Control and Prevention, "Unintentional Drowning: Get the Facts," April 28, 2016, http://www.cdc.gov/HomeandRecreationalSafety/Water-Safety/waterinjuries-factsheet.html.

17. Ibid.

18. Mental Health America, "Suicide," June 18, 2016, http://www.mentalhealthamerica.net/suicide.

19. K. Conner, et al., "Alcohol and Suicidal Behavior: What is Known and What Can Be Done," *American Journal of Preventive Medicine* 47, no. 3 (2014): S204–8.

20. N. Barnett, et al., "Description and Predictors of Positive and Negative Alcohol-Related Consequences in the First Year of College," *Journal of Studies on Alcohol and Drugs* 75, no.1 (2014): 103–14.

21. American College Health Association, *American College Health Association—National College Health Assessment II: Reference Group Executive Summary Fall 2015* (Hanover, MD: American College Health Association, 2016), http://www.acha-ncha.org/docs/NCHA-II%20FALL%202015%20REFERENCE%20GROUP%20EXECUTIVE%20SUMMARY.pdf.

22. N. Barnett, et al., 2014.

23. *Washington Post*, "Poll: One in Five Women Say They Have Been Sexually Assaulted in College," June 12, 2015, https://www.washingtonpost.com/graphics/local/sexual-assault-poll/.

24. Ibid.

25. Ibid.

26. Ibid

27. Ibid

28. R. Rettner, "Cheers?: Counting the Calories in Alcoholic Drinks," *Livescience,* December 7, 2015, http://www.livescience.com/52990-alcohol-calories-weight-loss-be-healthy.html.

29. Centers for Disease Control and Prevention, "Alcohol Poisoning Deaths," January 6, 2015, http://www.cdc.gov/vitalsigns/alcohol-poisoning-deaths/index.html.

30. Ibid.

31. L. Squeglia, et al., "Brain Development in Heavy Drinking Adolescents," *American Journal of Psychiatry* 172, no. 6 (2015): 531–42.

32. Ibid.

33. J. H. O'Keefe et al., "Alcohol and Cardiovascular Health: The Dose Makes the Poison . . . or the Remedy," *Mayo Clinic Proceedings* 89, No. 3 (2014): 382–93; A. Artero et al., "The Impact of Moderate Wine Consumption on Health," *Maturitas* 80, no. 1 (2015): 3–13.

34. The American Heart Association, "Alcohol and Heart Health," 2015, www.heart.org.

35. Ibid.

36. Ibid.

37. Ibid.

38. NTP (National Toxicology Program). 2014. *Report on Carcinogens, Thirteenth Edition.* Research Triangle Park, NC: U.S. Department of Health and Human Services, Public Health Service. http://ntp.niehs.nih.gov/pubhealth/roc/roc13/.

39. Y. Cao, et al., "Light to Moderate Intake of Alcohol, Drinking Patterns, and Risk of Cancer: Results from Two Prospective US Cohort Studies," *British Medical Journal* 351 (2015): h4238.

40. Ibid.

41. Ibid.

42. I. Romieu et al., "Alcohol Intake and Breast Cancer in the European Prospective Investigation into Cancer and Nutrition," *International Journal of Cancer* 137, no. 8 (2015): 1921–30.

43. Ibid.

44. M. Thakkar, "Alcohol Disrupts Sleep Homeostasis," *Alcohol* 49, no. 4 (2015): 299–310.

45. G. Szabo and R. Saha, "Alcohol's Effect on Host Defense," *Alcohol Research: Current Reviews* 37, no. 2 (2015): 159.

46. Ibid.

47. Ibid.

48. SAMSHA, "Protect Your Unborn Baby," Accessed January 2016, http://www.samhsa.gov/sites/default/files/programs_campaigns/fasd/fasd-infographic.pdf.

49. Centers for Disease Control and Prevention, "Fetal Alcohol Spectrum Disorders (FASDs): Alcohol Use during Pregnancy," April 17, 2014, www.cdc.gov/ncbddd/fasd/alcohol-use.html.

50. Ibid.

51. Centers for Disease Control and Prevention, "Fetal Alcohol Spectrum Disorders (FASDs): Data and Statistics," Updated November 17, 2015, www.cdc.gov/ncbddd/fasd/data.html.

52. Fetal Alcohol Spectrum Disorders (FASD) Center for Excellence, "What Is FASD?," March 2014, www.Fasdcenter.samhsa.gov.

53. Centers for Disease Control and Prevention, 2015.

54. Ibid.

55. American College Health Association, *National College Health Assessment II: Reference Group Executive Summary Fall 2015, 2016.*

56. Ibid.

57. Substance Abuse and Mental Health Services Administration, "Results from the 2014 National Survey on Drug Use and Health: Summary of National Findings 2014," July 2015, www.samhsa.gov.

58. U.S. Department of Health and Human Services, National Institute on Alcohol Abuse and Alcoholism, "Moderate and Binge Drinking," Accessed May 2016, http://www.niaaa.nih.gov/alcohol-health/overview-alcohol-consumption/moderate-binge-drinking.

59. American College Health Association, *National College Health Assessment II: Reference Group Data Report, Fall 2015, 2016.*

60. Ibid.

61. C. Foster et al., "National College Health Assessment Measuring Negative Alcohol-Related Consequences among College Students," *American Journal of Public Health Research* 2, no. 1 (2014): 1–5.

62. S. Onyper et al., "Class Start Times, Sleep and Academic Performance in College: A Path Analysis," *Chronobiology* 29, no. 3 (2012): 318–35; S. Kenney et al., "Global Sleep Quality as a Moderator of Alcohol Consumption and Consequences in College Students," *Addictive Behaviors* 37, no. 4 (2012): 507–12.

63. American College Health Association, *National College Health Assessment II: Reference Group Data Report, Fall 2015, 2016.*

64. A. White and R. Hingson, "The Burden of Alcohol Use: Excessive Alcohol Consumption and Related Consequences among College Students," *Alcohol Research: Current Reviews* 35, no. 2 (2014): 201.

65. Ibid.

66. L. Varvil-Weld et al., "Parents' and Students' Reports of Parenting: Which Are More Reliably Associated with College Student Drinking?," *Addictive Behaviors* 38, no. 3 (2013): 1699–1703.

67. L. D. Johnston, *Monitoring the Future National Survey Results on Drug Use, 1975–2015: Volume II, College Students and Adults Ages 19–50* (Ann Arbor: Institute for Social Research, University of Michigan, 2016), Available at http://www.monitoringthefuture.org/pubs/monographs/mtf-overview2015.pdf.

68. Ibid.

69. J. W. LaBrie et al., "Are They All the Same?: An Exploratory, Categorical Analysis of Drinking Game Types," *Addictive Behaviors* 38, no. 5 (2013): 2133–9; N. P. Barnett et al., "Predictors and Consequences of Pregaming Using Day and Week-Level Measures," *Psychology of Addictive Behaviors* 27, no. 4 (2013): 921.

70. B. Zamboanga et al., "Knowing Where They're Going: Destination-Specific Pregaming Behaviors in a Multiethnic Sample of College Students," *Journal of Clinical Psychology* 69, no. 4 (2013): 383–96.

71. J. W. LaBrie et al., 2013; N. P. Barnett et al., 2013.

72. J. Alfonso et al., "Do Drinking Games Matter?: An Examination by Game Type and Gender in a Mandated Student Sample," *American Journal of Drug and Alcohol Abuse* 39, no. 5 (2013): 312–9; J. W. LaBrie et al., "Are They All the Same?," 2013.

73. N. P. Barnett et al., 2013.

74. Ibid.

75. R. Martin et al., "Hazardous Drinking and Weight-Conscious Drinking Behaviors in a Sample of College Students and College Student Athletes," *Substance Abuse* (2016). doi: 10.1080/08897077.2016.1142922.

76. M. Eisenberg and C. Fitz, "'Drunkorexia': Exploring the Who and Why of a Disturbing Trend in College Students' Eating and Drinking Behaviors," *American Journal of College Health* 62, no. 8 (2014): 570–7.

77. Ibid.

78. Ibid.

79. J. Leasure et al., "Exercise and Alcohol Consumption: What We Know, What We Need to Know, and Why It Is Important," *Frontiers in Psychiatry* (2015): 6. doi: 10.3389/fpsyt.2015.00156; D. Conroy et al., "Daily Physical Activity and Alcohol Use across the Adult Lifespan," *Health Psychology* 34, no. 6 (2015): 653–60.

80. J. Stogner et al., "Innovative Alcohol Use: Assessing the Prevalence of Alcohol without Liquid and Other Non-Oral Routes of Alcohol Administration," *Drug and Alcohol Dependence* 142, no. 1 (2014): 74–8.

81. M. Miguez, "The Need of Widening the Lens of Alcohol Research, but Sharpening the Focus on Type of Alcohol Beverage," *Journal of Alcoholism and Drug Dependence* (2014). doi: 10.4172/2329-6488.1000e112.

82. American College Health Association, *National College Health Assessment II: Reference Group Data Report, Fall 2015, 2016.*

83. G. DiFulvio, et al., "Effectiveness of the Brief Alcohol and Screening Intervention for College Students (BASICS) Program for Mandated Students," *Journal of American College Health* 60, no. 4 (2012): 269–80.

84. National Social Norms Institute, "Case Studies: Alcohol," Accessed 2014, www.socialnorms.org/CaseStudies/alcohol.php.

85. Centers for Disease Control and Prevention, "Ten Leading Causes of Death by Age

Group," February 2016, www.cdc.gov/injury/wisqars/leadingcauses.html.

86. Centers for Disease Control and Prevention (CDC), "Impaired Driving: Get the Facts," April 15, 2016, http://www.cdc.gov/motorvehiclesafety/impaired_driving/impaired-drv_factsheet.html.

87. Ibid.

88. Centers for Disease Control and Prevention (CDC), "Vital Signs: Drinking and Driving," 2013.

89. American College Health Association, *National College Health Assessment II: Reference Group Data Report, Fall 2015,* 2016.

90. Insurance Institute for Highway Safety, "Alcohol-Impaired Driving 2014," February 2016, http://www.iihs.org/iihs/topics/t/alcohol-impaired-driving/fatalityfacts/alcohol-impaired-driving/2014.

91. Ibid.

92. Ibid.

93. Ibid.

94. K. Keyes et al., "The Role of Race/Ethnicity in Alcohol-Attributable Injury in the United States," *Epidemiologic Reviews* 34, no. 1 (2012): 89–102.

95. Ibid.

96. T. Zaploski et al., "Less Drinking, yet More Problems: Understanding African American Drinking and Related Problems," *Psychological Bulletin* 140, no. 1 (2013): 188–223.

97. National Institute on Alcohol Abuse and Alcoholism, "Alcohol and the Hispanic Community," July 2013, http://pubs.niaaa.nih.gov/publications/HispanicFact/hispanicFact.htm.

98. Ibid.

99. Ibid.

100. Ibid.

101. Ibid.

102. Substance Abuse and Mental Health Services Administration, Results from the 2013 National Survey on Drug Use and Health: Summary of National Findings (NSDUH Series H-48, HHS Publication No. [SMA] 14-4863) (Rockville, MD: Substance Abuse and Mental Health Services Administration, 2014).

103. J. Otto et al., "Association of the ALDHA1*2 Promoter Polymorphism with Alcohol Phenotyptes in Young Adults with or without ALDH2*2," *Alcoholism Clinical and Experimental Research* 37, no. 1 (2013): 164–9.

104. Medline Plus, "Alcoholism and Alcohol Abuse," March 2015, www.nlm.nih.gov/medlineplus/ency/article/000944.htm.

105. National Institute on Alcohol Abuse and Alcoholism, "College Drinking," December 2015, http://pubs.niaaa.nih.gov/publications/CollegeFactSheet/CollegeFactSheet.pdf.

106. K. Beck et al., "Social Contexts of Drinking and Subsequent Alcohol Use Disorder among College Students," *American Journal of Alcohol Abuse* 39, no. 1 (2012): 38–43.

107. A. Arria, "College Student Success: The Impact of Health Concerns and Substance Abuse," Lecture presented at NASPA Alcohol and Mental Health Conference (Fort Worth, TX: January 19, 2013).

108. S. Gupta, "Are You a Functioning Alcoholic?" *Everyday Health*, April 25, 2016, http://www.everydayhealth.com/news/are-you-someone-you-know-functional-alcoholic/.

109. M. Waldron et al., "Parental Separation and Early Substance Involvement: Results from Children of Alcoholic and Cannabis Twins," *Drug and Alcohol Dependence* 134 (2014): 78–84.

110. M. Schuckit, "A Brief History of Research on the Genetics of Alcohol and Other Drug Use Disorders," *Journal of Studies on Alcohol and Drugs* 75, Suppl. 17 (2014): 59–67.

111. Ibid.

112. B. Taub, "Here's What Happens to Alcoholics' Brains When They Quit Drinking," *IFLScience*. March 3, 2016, http://www.iflscience.com/brain/what-happens-alcoholics-brains-when-they-quit-drinking.

113. Centers for Disease Control and Prevention, Fact Sheet, "Excessive Alcohol Use and Risks to Women's Health," November 19, 2014, www.cdc.gov/alcohol/fact-sheets/womens-health.htm.

114. National Association for Children of Alcoholics, "National Association for Children of Alcoholics Network Newsletter," Summer 2015, http://www.nacoa.org/pdfs/Network%20Summer%202015.pdf.

115. Centers for Disease Control and Prevention, "Excessive Drinking is Draining the U.S. Economy," January 12, 2016, www.cdc.gov/features/CostsOfDrinking.

116. Ibid.

117. Ibid.

118. Ibid.

119. U.S. Department of Health and Human Services, "Report to Congress on the Prevention and Reduction of Underage Drinking," *Substance Abuse and Mental Health Services* Vol. 1 (December 2015), Available at www.stopalcoholabuse.gov/media/ReportToCongress/2015/report_main/2015_RTC_Volume_I.pdf.

120. Ibid.

121. National Institute on Alcohol Abuse and Alcoholism, "Alcohol Facts and Statistics," January 2016, http://www.niaaa.nih.gov/alcohol-health/overview-alcohol-consumption/alcohol-facts-and-statistics.

122. S. Finn, "Alcohol Consumption, Dependence, and Treatment Barriers: Perceptions among Nontreatment Seekers with Alcohol Dependence," *Substance Use and Misuse* 49 no. 6 (2014): 762–9.

123. A. Laudet et al., "Collegiate Recovery Community Programs: What Do We Know and What Do We Need to Know?" *Journal of Social Work Practice in the Addictions* 14 (2014): 84–100; A. Laudet et al., "Characteristics of Students Participating in Collegiate Recovery Programs: A National Survey," *Journal of Substance Abuse Treatment* 51 (2014): 38–46.

124. O. Manejwala, "How Often Do Long-Term Sober Alcoholics and Addicts Relapse?" *Psychology Today*, February 13, 2014, https://www.psychologytoday.com/blog/craving/201402/how-often-do-long-term-sober-alcoholics-and-addicts-relapse.

**Pulled statistics:**

p. 320, A. Laudet et al., "In College and in Recovery: Reasons for Joining a Collegiate Recovery Program," *Journal of American College Health* 64, no. 3 (2016): 250.

p. 326, American College Health Association, *American College Health Association—National College Health Assessment II (ACHA-NCHA II) Reference Group Data Report Fall 2015* (Linthicum, MD: American College Health Association, 2016).

## Chapter 12

1. U.S. Department of Health and Human Services, *The Health Consequences of Smoking—50 Years of Progress: A Report of the Surgeon General* (Atlanta, GA: U.S. Department of Health and Human Services, Centers for Disease Control and Prevention, National Center for Chronic Disease Prevention and Health Promotion, Office on Smoking and Health, 2014), Available at: www.surgeongeneral.gov/library/reports/50-years-of-progress/exec-summary.pdf.

2. Ibid.

3. Substance Abuse and Mental Health Services Administration, Results from the 2013 National Survey on Drug Use and Health: Summary of National Findings, NSDUH Series H-48, HHS Publication No. (SMA) 14-4863 (Rockville, MD: Substance Abuse and Mental Health Services Administration, 2014).

4. Centers for Disease Control and Prevention, "Current Cigarette Smoking Among Adults—United States, 2005–2014," *Morbidity and Mortality Weekly Report* 64, no. 44 (2015): 1233–40.

5. Center for Behavioral Health Statistics and Quality. (2015). *Behavioral Health Trends in the United States: Results from the 2014 National Survey on Drug Use and Health* (HHS Publication No. SMA 15-4927, NSDUH Series H-50), Available at http://www.samsha.gov/data/.

6. Centers for Disease Control and Prevention, "Current Cigarette Smoking Among Adults—United States, 2005–2014," 2015.

7. National Institute on Drug Abuse, "Drug Facts: Cigarettes and Other Tobacco Products," August 2015, https://www.drugabuse.gov/publications/drugfacts/cigarettes-other-tobacco-products.

8. Campaign for Tobacco-Free Kids, "The Path to Tobacco Addiction Starts at Very Young Ages," December 21, 2015, https://www.tobaccofreekids.org/research/factsheets/pdf/0127.pdf.

9. U.S. Department of Health and Human Services, *The Health Consequences of Smoking—50 Years of Progress,* 2014.

10. Campaign for Tobacco-Free Kids, "Toll of Tobacco in the United States of America," March 8, 2016, www.tobaccofreekids.org/research/factsheets/pdf/0072.pdf?utm_source=factsheets_finder&utm_medium=link&utm_campaign=analytics.

11. Ibid.

12. Ibid.

13. American Cancer Society, "Cancer Facts & Figures 2016," Accessed April 2016, www.cancer.org/research/cancerfactsstatistics/cancerfactsfigures2016.

14. Centers for Disease Control and Prevention, "Current Cigarette Smoking Among Adults—United States 2005–2014," 2015.

15. Centers for Disease Control and Prevention, "Smoking and Tobacco Use: Fast Facts," February 2016, www.cdc.gov/tobacco/data_statistics/fact_sheets/fast_facts.

16. U.S. Department of Health and Human Services, "Let's Make the Next Generation Tobacco Free," July 2015, Available at http://www.surgeongeneral.gov/library/reports/50-years-of-progress/consumer-guide.pdf.

17. A. Loukola et al., "Genetics and Smoking," *Current Addiction Reports* 1, no. 1 (2014): 75–82; C. Amos, M. Spitz, and P. Cinciripini, "Chipping Away at the Genetics of Smoking Behavior," *Nature Genetics* 42, no. 5 (2010): 366–8.

18. U.S. Department of Health and Human Services, "Let's Make the Next Generation Tobacco Free," 2015.

19. D. Mays et al., "Parental Smoking Exposure and Adolescent Smoking Trajectories," *Pediatrics* 133, no. 6 (2014): 983–91; C. Lakon et al., "A Dynamic Model of Adolescent Friendship Networks, Parental Influences, and Smoking," *Journal of Youth and Adolescence* 44, no. 9 (2015): 1667–1786.

20. A. Annamalai, et al., "Smoking Use and Cessation Among People with Serious Mental Illness," *Yale Journal of Biology and Medicine* 88, no 3 (2015): 271–7.

21. Ibid.; SAMHSA-HRSA Center for Integrated Health Solutions, "Tobacco Cessation," Accessed April 2016, http://www.integration.samhsa.gov/health-wellness/wellness-strategies/tobacco-cessation-2.

22. Centers for Disease Control and Prevention, "Stress and Smoking," March 15, 2015, http://www.cdc.gov/tobacco/campaign/tips/quit-smoking/guide/stress-and-smoking.html.

23. J. Rosa and P. Aloise-Young, "A Qualitative Study of Smoker Identity among College Student Smokers," *Substance Use and Misuse* 15, no. 2 (2015): 1510–7, doi: 10.3109/10826084.2015.1018549.

24. Ibid.

25. Campaign for Tobacco-Free Kids, "Toll of Tobacco in the United States of America," 2016.

26. U.S. Department of Health and Human Services, *The Health Consequences of Smoking—50 Years of Progress,* 2014.

27. Campaign for Tobacco-Free Kids, "Toll of Tobacco in the United States of America," 2016.

28. American College Health Association, *American College Health Association–National College Health Assessment II: Reference Group Data Report, Spring 2015* (Baltimore: American College Health Association, 2015), Available from www.achancha.org/reports_ACHA-NCHAII.html.

29. Ibid.

30. Ibid.

31. L. D. Johnston et al., "Monitoring the Future National Survey Results on Drug Use, 1975–2014: Volume 2, College Students and Adults Ages 19–55" (Ann Arbor: Institute for Social Research, University of Michigan, 2015), Available at http://www.monitoringthefuture.org/pubs/monographs/mtf-vol2_2014.pdf.

32. Ibid.

33. L. D. Johnston et al., "Monitoring the Future National Survey Results on Drug Use, 1975–2014," 2015.

34. J. Rosa and P. Aloise-Young, "A Qualitative Study of Smoker Identity Among College Student Smokers," 2015.

35. Ibid.; E. Leas et al., "Smokers Who Report Smoking but Do Not Consider Themselves Smokers: A Phenomenon in Need of Further Attention," *Tobacco Control* (2014), doi: 10.1136/tobaccocontrol-2013-051400.

36. American Cancer Society, "Light Smoking as Risky as a Pack a Day?," January 2013, http://blogs.cancer.org/expertvoices/2013/01/02/light-smoking-as-risky-as-a-pack-a-day/.

37. Stop Smoking, "Smoking and Birth Control Pills Are Not Made for Each Other!" Accessed March 6, 2016, www.stop-smoking-updates.com/quitsmoking/smoking-factsheet/facts/smoking-and-birth-control-pills-are-not-made-for-each-other.htm.

38. U.S. Department of Health and Human Services, *The Health Consequences of Smoking—50 Years of Progress,* 2014.

39. Ibid.

40. *Diagnostic and Statistical Manual of Mental Disorders, Fifth Edition* (Washington, DC: American Psychiatric Association, 2013).

41. Ibid.

42. S. Zhu et al., "Four Hundred and Sixty Brands of E-Cigarettes and Counting: Implications for Product Regulation," *Tobacco Control* 23, Suppl. 3 (2014): iii3–iii9.

43. American College Health Association, *American College Health Association–National College Health Assessment II: Reference Group Data Report, Spring 2015,* 2015.

44. A. Littlefield et al., "Electronic Cigarette Use among College Students: Links to Gender, Race/Ethnicity, Smoking and Heavy Drinking," *Journal of American College Health* 63, no. 8 (2015): 523–9.

45. American Cancer Society, "Cancer Facts & Figures 2016." 2016.

46. National Cancer Institute, "Cigar Smoking and Cancer," Accessed March 13, 2016, http://www.cancer.gov/about-cancer/causes-prevention/risk/tobacco/cigars-fact-sheet.

47. American Cancer Society, "Cancer Facts & Figures 2016," 2016.

48. National Cancer Institute, "Cigar Smoking and Cancer."

49. American Cancer Society, "Questions About Smoking, Tobacco, and Health," February 2014, Available at https://www.mtyhd.org/QI/wp-content/uploads/2015/06/Smoking-FAQ.pdf.

50. Centers for Disease Control and Prevention, "Smoking and Tobacco Use: Bidis and Kreteks,"

November 9, 2015, www.cdc.gov/tobacco/data_statistics/fact_sheets/tobacco_industry/bidis_kreteks.

51. Ibid.

52. Campaign for Tobacco Free Kids, "Smokeless Tobacco in the United States," 2016.

53. Campaign for Tobacco Free Kids, "Toll of Tobacco in the United States of America," 2016.

54. National Cancer Institute, "Lung Cancer Prevention," February 2016, www.cancer.gov/cancertopics/pdq/prevention/lung/HealthProfessional/page2.

55. American Cancer Society, "Cancer Facts & Figures 2016," 2016.

56. American Cancer Society, "What Are Oral Cavity and Oropharyngeal Cancers?," January 2016, www.cancer.org/cancer/oralcavityandoropharyngealcancer/detailedguide/oral-cavity-and-oropharyngeal-cancer-what-is-oral-cavity-cancer.

57. American Cancer Society, "Cancer Facts & Figures 2016," 2016.

58. Ibid.

59. American Heart Association, *Heart Disease and Stroke Statistics—2016 Update* (Dallas, TX: American Heart Association, 2016), Available at http://circ.ahajournals.org/content/early/2015/12/16/CIR.0000000000000350.long.

60. Ibid.

61. Ibid.

62. Ibid.

63. American Lung Association, "Benefits of Quitting," Accessed March 2016, http://www.lung.org/stop-smoking/i-want-to-quit/benefits-of-quitting.html.

64. U.S. Department of Health and Human Services, *The Health Consequences of Smoking—50 Years of Progress*, 2014.

65. American Lung Association, "Lung Health Diseases: What Causes COPD," Accessed April 2016, http://www.lung.org/lung-health-and-diseases/lung-disease-lookup/copd/symptoms-causes-risk-factors/what-causes-copd.html.

66. C. B. Harte et al., "Association between Cigarette Smoking and Erectile Tumescence: The Mediating Role of Heart Rate Variability," *International Journal of Impotence Research* 25, no. 4 (2013): 155–9, doi: 10.1038/ijir.2012.43.

67. Centers for Disease Control and Prevention, "Tobacco Use and Pregnancy," September 2015, www.cdc.gov/reproductivehealth/TobaccoUsePregnancy.

68. Ibid.

69. American Academy of Periodontology, "Gum Disease Risk Factors," Accessed April 2014, www.perio.org/consumer/risk-factors; Centers for Disease Control and Prevention, "Smoking, Gum Disease, and Tooth Loss," September 2015, http://www.cdc.gov/tobacco/campaign/tips/diseases/periodontal-gum-disease.html.

70. S. Karama et al., "Cigarette Smoking and Thinning of the Brain's Cortex," *Molecular Psychiatry* 20 (2015): 778–85; I. Moreno-Gonzalez, et al., "Smoking Exacerbates

Amyloid Pathology in a Mouse Model of Alzheimer's Disease," *Nature Communications* 4 (2013), www.nature.com/ncomms/journal/v4/n2/abs/ncomms2494.html.

71. Centers for Disease Control and Prevention, "Smoking and Tobacco Use Facts: Second-hand Smoke," February 2016, www.cdc.gov/tobacco/data_statistics/fact_sheets/secondhand_smoke/general_facts.

72. American Nonsmokers' Rights Foundation, "Overview List–How Many Smoke-Free Laws," April 4, 2016, www.no-smoke.org/pdf/mediaordlist.pdf.

73. Ibid.

74. Ibid.

75. American Lung Association, "Health Effects of Secondhand Smoke," Accessed April 2016, http://www.lung.org/stop-smoking/smoking-facts/health-effects-of-secondhand-smoke.html.

76. American Nonsmokers' Rights Foundation, "Overview List–How Many Smoke-Free Laws," 2016.

77. U.S. Department of Health and Human Services, "Let's Make the Next Generation Tobacco Free," 2015; National Cancer Institute, "Harms of Cigarette Smoking and Health Benefits of Quitting," December 2014, http://www.cancer.gov/about-cancer/causes-prevention/risk/tobacco/cessation-fact-sheet#q3.

78. Centers for Disease Control and Prevention, "Health Effects of Secondhand Smoke Fact Sheet," February 2016, http://www.cdc.gov/tobacco/data_statistics/fact_sheets/secondhand_smoke/health_effects/index.htm.

79. American Lung Association, "Health Effects of Secondhand Smoke," 2016.

80. Ibid.

81. U.S. Department of Health and Human Services, "Environmental Tobacco Smoke Exposure in Children Aged 3–19 Years With and Without Asthma in the United States, 1999–2010. *NCHS Data Brief* No. 126 (2013).

82. L. Pagani, "Environmental Tobacco Smoke Exposure and Brain Development: The Case of Attention Deficit/Hyperactivity Disorder," *Neuroscience and Biobehavioral Reviews* 44 (2014): 195–205.

83. U.S. Department of Health and Human Services, *The Health Consequences of Smoking—50 Years of Progress*, 2014.

84. Ibid.

85. Tobacco-Free Kids, "1998 State Tobacco Settlement 17 Years Later," December 2015, http://www.tobaccofreekids.org/microsites/statereport2016/.

86. *Family Smoking Prevention and Tobacco Control Act of 2009*, HR 1256, 111th Congress of the United States of America, Available at www.govtrack.us/congress/billtext.xpd?bill=h111-1256.

87. Centers for Disease Control and Prevention, "Tobacco Use: Smoking Cessation," February 2016, www.cdc.gov/tobacco/data_statistics/fact_sheets/cessation/quitting/index.htm#quitting.

88. American Lung Association, "Benefits of Quitting," Accessed April 2016, www.lung.org/stop-smoking/i-want-to-quit/benefits-of-quitting.html; Centers for Disease Control and Prevention, "Quitting Smoking," Smoking and Tobacco Use, February 2016, www.cdc.gov/tobacco/data_statistics/fact_sheets/cessation/quitting/index.htm?utm_source=feedburner&utm_medium=feed&utm_campaign=Feed%3A+CdcSmokingAndTobaccoUseFactSheets+%28CDC+-+Smoking+and+Tobacco+Use+-+Fact+Sheets%29.

89. Ibid.

90. Ibid.

91. Ibid.

92. H. Holmes, "What a Pack of Cigarettes Costs Now, State by State," *The Awl*, August 28, 2015, www.theawl.com/2015/08/what-a-pack-of-cigarettes-costs-in-every-state.

93. American Cancer Society, "Guide to Quitting Smoking: A Word About Success Rates for Quitting Smoking," February 2014, www.cancer.org/Healthy/StayAwayfromTobacco/GuidetoQuittingSmoking/guide-to-quitting-smoking-success-rates.

94. Drugs.com, "Nicotine Patch," Accessed March 2016, http://www.drugs.com/price-guide/nicotine.

95. Drugs.com, "Nicotine Patch," 2016.

96. U.S. Food and Drug Administration, "FDA 101: Smoking Cessation Products," February 2016, http://www.fda.gov/ForConsumers/ConsumerUpdates/ucm198176.htm.

**Pulled statistics:**

p. 337, The Tobacco Atlas, "Smoking's Death Toll," Accessed April 2016, http://www.tobaccoatlas.org/topic/smokings-death-toll/.

p. 342, Americans for Nonsmokers Rights, "Colleges and Universities," April 4, 2016, http://no-smoke.org/goingsmokefree.php?id=447.

## Chapter 13

1. Center for Behavioral Health Statistics and Quality, "Behavioral Health Trends in the United States: Results from the 2014 National Survey on Drug Use and Health," HHS Publication No. SMA 15-4927, NSDUH Series H-50 (2015), Retrieved from http://www.samhsa.gov/data.

2. L. D. Johnston et al., *Monitoring the Future National Results on Drug Use 1975-2015 Overview, Key Findings on Adolescent Drug Use* (Ann Arbor: Institute for Social Research, University of Michigan, 2016).

3. Ibid.

4. National Institute of Drug Abuse, "Drug Facts: Nationwide Trends," June 2015, www.drugabuse.gov/publications/drugfacts/nationwide-trends.

5. National Institute on Drug Abuse, "Trends and Statistics," August 2015, https://www.drugabuse.gov/related-topics/trends-statistics.

6. E. Kantor et al., "Trends in Prescription Drug Use among Adults in the United States from 1999–2012," *Journal of the American Medical Association* 314, no. 17 (2015): 1818–30.

7. Ibid.

8. Consumer Health Care Products Association, "Statistics on OTC Use," Accessed May 2016, http://www.chpa.org/MarketStats.aspx.

9. U.S. National Library of Medicine, "Over-the-Counter Medicines," April 21, 2016, https://www.nlm.nih.gov/medlineplus/overthecountermedicines.html.

10. L. D. Johnston et al., *Monitoring the Future National Results on Drug Use*, 2016.

11. Erowid, The DXM Vault, Accessed June 2016, www.erowid.org.

12. U.S. Food and Drug Administration, "Legal Requirements for the Sale and Purchase of Drug Products Containing Pseudoephedrine, Ephedrine, and Phenylpropanolamine," May 19, 2016, http://www.fda.gov/Drugs/DrugSafety/InformationbyDrugClass/ucm072423.htm.

13. Center for Behavioral Health Statistics and Quality, "Behavioral Health Trends in the United States: Results from the 2014 National Survey on Drug Use and Health," 2015.

14. Ibid.

15. Ibid.

16. L. D. Johnston et al., *Monitoring the Future National Results on Drug Use*, 2016.

17. Centers for Disease Control and Prevention, "Understanding the Epidemic," March 2016, http://www.cdc.gov/drugoverdose/epidemic/.

18. American College Health Association, *American College Health Association–National College Health Assessment Fall 2015 Reference Group Executive Summary*, 2016, Available at http://www.acha-ncha.org/docs/NCHA-II_WEB_SPRING_2015_REFERENCE_GROUP_EXECUTIVE_SUMMARY.pdf.

19. American College Health Association, *American College Health Association—National College Health Assessment* Fall 2015 Reference Group Data Report, 2016, Available at http://www.acha-ncha.org/docs/NCHA-II%20FALL%202015%20REFERENCE%20GROUP%20DATA%20REPORT.pdf.

20. Ibid.

21. Higher Education Center for Alcohol and Drug Misuse Prevention and Recovery, "College Prescription Drug Study," Accessed June 2016, Available at http://hecaod.osu.edu/wp-content/uploads/2015/10/CPDS-Key-Findings-Report-1.pdf.

22. Ibid.

23. Center for Behavioral Health Statistics and Quality, "Behavioral Health Trends in the United States: Results from the 2014 National Survey on Drug Use and Health," 2015.

24. Ibid.

25. L. D. Johnston et al., *Monitoring the Future National Results on Drug Use*, 2016.

26. A. Arria, et al., "Drug Use Patterns and Continuous Enrollment in College: Results from a Longitudinal Study," *Journal of Studies on Alcohol and Drugs* 74 (2013): 71–83.

27. A. Arria et al., "Drug Use Patterns in Young Adulthood and Post-College Employment," *Drug and Alcohol Dependence* 127, no. 1–3 (2013): 23–30.

28. Higher Education Center for Alcohol and Drug Misuse Prevention and Recovery, "College Prescription Drug Study," Accessed June 2016, Available at http://hecaod.osu.edu/wp-content/uploads/2015/10/CPDS-Key-Findings-Report-1.pdf.

29. Center for Behavioral Health Statistics and Quality, "Behavioral Health Trends in the United States: Results from the 2014 National Survey on Drug Use and Health," 2015.

30. American College Health Association, *American College Health Association–National College Health Assessment Fall 2015 Reference Group Executive Summary, 2016.*

31. Addiction Center, "Drinking and Drug Abuse in Greek Life," February 15, 2015, www.addictioncenter.com/college/drinking-drug-abuse-greek-life/.

32. Ibid.

33. Addiction Center, "College Drug Abuse," Accessed June 2016, https://www.addictioncenter.com/college/.

34. Center for Behavioral Health Statistics and Quality, "Behavioral Health Trends in the United States: Results from the 2014 National Survey on Drug Use and Health," 2015.

35. L. D. Johnston et al., *Monitoring the Future National Results on Drug Use,* 2016.

36. Medscape, "Methamphetamine Use Triples Parkinson's Risk," *Multispecialty,* 2014 http://www.medscape.com/viewarticle/837025.

37. NIH, National Institute on Drug Abuse, "DrugFacts: Methamphetamine," September 2013, www.drugabuse.gov/publications/research-reports/methamphetamine/what-are-long-term-effects-methamphetamine-abuse.

38. Ibid.

39. NIH, National Institute on Drug Abuse, "What are Synthetic Cathinones?," January 2016, https://www.drugabuse.gov/publications/drugfacts/synthetic-cathinones-bath-salts.

40. Ibid.

41. Ibid.

42. Ibid.

43. Ibid.

44. D. C. Mitchell et al., "Beverage Caffeine Intakes in the U.S.," *Food and Chemical Toxicology* 63 (2014): 136–42.

45. Ibid.

46. Ibid.

47. Caffeineinformer, "20 Harmful Effects of Caffeine," April 1, 2016, http://www.caffeineinformer.com/harmful-effects-of-caffeine.

48. Caffeineinformer, "23 Possible Caffeine Health Benefits" April 1, 2016, http://www.caffeineinformer.com/harmful-effects-of-caffeine.

49. National Institute on Drug Abuse, "DrugFacts: Marijuana," March 2016, https://www.drugabuse.gov/publications/drugfacts/marijuana.

50. Center for Behavioral Health Statistics and Quality, "Behavioral Health Trends in the United States: Results from the 2014 National Survey on Drug Use and Health," 2015.

51. L. D. Johnston et al., *Monitoring the Future National Results on Drug Use,* 2016.

52. The 420 Times, "10 of the Most Popular Strains of Marijuana," July 24, 2015, http://the420times.com/2015/07/10-of-the-most-popular-marijuana-strains/.

53. Leaf Science, "A Beginner's Guide to Marijuana Edibles," October 27, 2015, http://www.leafscience.com/2015/10/27/beginners-guide-marijuana-edibles/.

54. Ibid.

55. National Institute on Drug Abuse, "Drug Facts: Marijuana," 2016.

56. National Institutes of Health, "Marijuana," March 2016, https://www.drugabuse.gov/sites/default/files/marijuanadrugfacts_march_2016.pdf.

57. Ibid.

58. Ibid.

59. AAA, "Fatal Road Crashes Involving Marijuana Double After State Legalizes Drugs," May 10, 2016, https://www.oregon.aaa.com/2016/05/fatal-road-crashes-involving-marijuana-double-after-state-legalizes-drug/.

60. Ibid.

61. Ibid.

62. Ibid.

63. American Lung Association, "Marijuana and Lung Health," March 23, 2015, http://www.lung.org/stop-smoking/smoking-facts/marijuana-and-lung-health.html.

64. National Institute on Drug Abuse, "Drug Facts: Marijuana," 2016.

65. G. Schauer, "Toking, Vaping, and Eating for Health or Fun," *American Journal of Preventive Medicine* 50, no. 1 (2016): 108.

66. D. Tashkin, "How Beneficial is Vaping Cannabis to Respiratory Health Compared to Smoking?" *Addiction* 110, no. 11 (2015): 1706–7.

67. National Institute on Drug Abuse, "Drug Facts: Marijuana," 2016.

68. C. Blanco et al., "Cannabis Use and Risk of Psychiatric Disorders," *JAMA Psychiatry* 73, no. 4 (2016): 388–95.

69. Ibid.

70. L. Degenhardt et al., "The Persistence of the Association between Adolescent Cannabis Use and Common Mental Disorders into Young Adulthood," *Addiction* 108, no. 1 (2013): 124–33.

71. American Academy of Pediatrics, "Marijuana Legalization," March 2016, https://www.aap.org/en-us/advocacy-and-policy/state-advocacy/Documents/Marijuana%20Legalization.pdf.

72. Ibid.

73. Ibid.

74. V. Wlassoff, "The Dope on Pot—How Marijuana Affects Sleep and Dreams," *BrainBlogger* April 2015, http://brainblogger.com/2015/04/03/the-dope-on-pot-how-marijuana-affects-sleep-and-dreams/.

75. National Institute on Drug Abuse, Marijuana: Facts for Teens, May 2015, www.drugabuse.gov/publications/marijuana-facts-teens; Science Daily, "Marijuana Use Prior to Pregnancy Doubles Risk of Premature Birth," July 17, 2012, www.sciencedaily.com.

76. National Institute on Drug Abuse (NIDA), "Drug Facts: Synthetic Cannabinoids," November 2015, https://www.drugabuse.gov/publications/drugfacts/synthetic-cannabinoids.

77. L. D. Johnston et al., *Monitoring the Future National Survey Results on Drug Use,* 2016.

78. K. L. Egan, et al., "K2 and Spice Use Among a Cohort of College Students in the Southeast Region of the USA," *American Journal of Drug and Alcohol Abuse,* 41 no. 4 (2015): 317–22.

79. L. D. Johnston et al., *Monitoring the Future National Survey Results on Drug Use,* 2016.

80. National Institute on Drug Abuse (NIDA), "Drug Facts: Synthetic Cannabinoids," 2015.

81. Ibid.

82. Ibid.

83. Substance Abuse and Mental Health Services Administration, "Not for Human Consumption: Spice and Bath Salts," March 3, 2015, http://newsletter.samhsa.gov/2015/03/03/not-for-human-consumption-spice-and-bath-salts/.

84. NIDA, "What are CNS Depressants?" 2014, https://www.drugabuse.gov/publications/research-reports/prescription-drugs/cns-depressants/what-are-cns-depressants.

85. Ibid.

86. WebMD, "Barbiturate Abuse Overview, 2016, http://www.webmd.com/mental-health/addiction/barbiturate-abuse.

87. The Partnership at Drugfree.org, "GHB," Accessed June 2016, www.drugfree.org/drug-guide/ghb.

88. NIDA, "What are Opioids?" 2014, https://www.drugabuse.gov/publications/research-reports/prescription-drugs/opioids/what-are-opioids.

89. NIDA, "Drug Facts: Heroin," 2014, https://www.drugabuse.gov/publications/drugfacts/heroin.

90. Center for Behavioral Health Statistics and Quality, "Behavioral Health Trends in the United States: Results from the 2014 National Survey on Drug Use and Health," 2015; Healthline, "Prescription Drugs are Leading to Heroin Addiction," February, 2016. http://www.healthline.com/health-news/prescription-drugs-lead-to-addiction.

91. Centers for Disease Control and Prevention, "Increases in Drug and Opioid Overdose Deaths—United States, 2000–2014," *Morbidity and Mortality Weekly* 64, no. 50 (2016): 1378–82.

92. Ibid.; National Institute on Drug Abuse, "Prescription Opiod Use is a Risk Factor for Heroin Use," December, 2015, https://www.drugabuse.gov/publications/research-reports/relationship-between-prescription-drug-heroin-abuse/prescription-opioid-use-risk-factor-heroin-use.

93. Ibid.; Healthline. "Prescription Drugs are Leading to Heroin Addiction." February, 2016, http://www.healthline.com/health-news/prescription-drugs-lead-to-addiction.

94. Centers for Disease Control and Prevention, "Vital Signs: Demographic and Substance Use Trends Among Heroin Users—United States 2002–2013," *Morbidity and Mortality Weekly* 64, no. 26 (2015): 719–25; T. Cicero, "The Changing Face of Heroin Use in the United States: A Retrospective Analysis of the Past 50 Years," *Journal of the American Medical Association* 71, no. 7 (2014): 821–26.

95. NIDA, "Drug Facts: Heroin," 2014.

96. Center for Behavioral Health Statistics and Quality, "Behavioral Health Trends in the United States: Results from the 2014 National Survey on Drug Use and Health," 2015.

97. L. D. Johnston et al., *Monitoring the Future National Survey Results on Drug Use,* 2016.

98. NIDA, "Common Hallucinogens and Dissociative Drugs," 2015, https://www.drugabuse.gov/publications/research-reports/hallucinogens-dissociative-drugs/what-are-dissociative-drugs.

99. NIDA, "Hallucinogens," 2016, https://www.drugabuse.gov/publications/drugfacts/hallucinogens.

100. Ibid.

101. NIDA, "What is MDMA?" 2016, https://www.drugabuse.gov/publications/drugfacts/mdma-ecstasymolly.

102. National Institute on Drug Abuse, "DrugFacts: MDMA (Ecstasy/Molly)," February 2016, https://www.drugabuse.gov/publications/drugfacts/mdma-ecstasymolly.

103. Ibid.

104. Drugs.com "PCP (Phencyclidine)," http://www.drugs.com/illicit/pcp.html.

105. Ibid.

106. Drugs.com, "Mescaline," 2016, http://www.drugs.com/illicit/mescaline.html.

107. NIDA "Hallucinogens," 2016.

108. NIDA "Commonly Used Club Drugs," 2016, https://www.drugabuse.gov/drugs-abuse/commonly-abused-drugs-charts#ketamine; Drugs.com, "Ketamine," 2016, http://www.drugs.com/cdi/ketamine.html.

109. National Institute on Drug Abuse, "DrugFacts: Hallucinogens," January 2016, www.drugabuse.gov/publications/drugfacts/hallucinogens.

110. Ibid.

111. Ibid.

112. Ibid.

113. Partnership for Drug-Free Kids, "Inhalants," 2016, http://www.drugfree.org/drug-guide/inhalants.

114. Ibid.

115. Drugs.com "Amyl Nitrite," 2016, http://www.drugs.com/cons/amyl-nitrite-inhalation-oral-nebulization.html.

116. J. van Amsterdam et al., "Recreational Nitrous Oxide Use: Prevalence and Risks," *Regulatory Toxicology and Pharmacology* 73, no. 3 (2015) 790–6.

117. A. Moyaya, M. Fawal, and R. Estes, "Performance-Enhancing Substances in Sports: A Review of the Literature," *Sports Medicine* 45, no. 4 (2015): 517–31.

118. National Collegiate Athletic Association, "NCAA National Study of Substance Use Habits of College Student Athletes—Final Report 2014," August 2014, www.ncaa.org/sites/default/files/Substance%20Use%20Final%20Report_FINAL.pdf.

119. National Collegiate Athletic Association, 2014.

120. National Collegiate Athletic Association, "Substance Use: National Study of Substance Use Trends among NCAA College Student-Athletes," 2012, www.ncaapublications.com/productdownloads/SAHS09.pdf.

121. H. G. Pope et al., "The Lifetime Prevalence of Anabolic-Androgenic Steroid Use and Dependence in Americans: Current Best Estimates," *American Journal on Addictions* 23, no. 4 (2014): 371–7.

122. American College Health Association, *American College Health Association-National College Health Assessment-Reference Group, Spring 2015,* 2016, http://www.acha-ncha.org/docs/NCHA-II%20FALL%202015%20REFERENCE%20GROUP%20DATA%20REPORT.pdf.

123. National Institute on Drug Abuse, "What Are Anabolic Steroids," 2016, https://www.drugabuse.gov/publications/drugfacts/anabolic-steroids.

124. Ibid.

125. Association Against Steroid Use, "Legal Ramifications of Steroid Use," http://www.steroidabuse.com/legal-ramifications-of-steroid-abuse.html.

126. Substance Abuse and Mental Health Services Administration, "Results from the 2014 National Survey," 2015.

127. Alcoholic Anonymous "Over 80 Years of Growth," 2016, http://www.aa.org/pages/en_US/aa-timeline/to/1; Rehabs.com "AA Success Rates," 2016, http://luxury.rehabs.com/12-step-programs/aa-success-rates/.

128. National Institute on Drug Abuse, "Dr. Thomas Kosten Q & A: Vaccines to Treat Addiction," 2015, https://www.drugabuse.gov/news-events/nida-notes/2015/06/dr-thomas-kosten-q-vaccines-to-treat-addiction.

129. A. Sifferlin, "Why You've Never Heard of the Vaccine for Heroin Addiction," *Time* (2015), http://time.com/3654784/why-youve-never-heard-of-the-vaccine-for-heroin-addiction/.

130. SAMSHA, "Naltrexone," 2016, http://www.samhsa.gov/medication-assisted-treatment/treatment/naltrexone.

131. A. Laudet et al., "In College and in Recovery: Reasons for Joining a Collegiate Recovery Program," *Journal of American College Health* 64, no. 3 (2016): 242–50.

132. Ibid.

133. Ibid.

134. Association for Recovery in Higher Education, "Kennesaw State University: About the Program," 2016, http://collegiaterecovery.org/portfolio_post/kennesaw-state-university/; Kennesaw State University, "Center for Young Adult Addiction and Recovery," accessed May 2016 http://www.kennesaw.edu/studentsuccessservices/crc/.

135. Texas Tech University, "The Center for Collegiate Recovery Communities at Texas Tech University," Accessed May 2016, www.depts.ttu.edu/hs/csa.

136. Office of National Drug Control Policy, "How Illicit Drug Use Affects Business and the Economy," *Executive Office of the President,* Accessed June 2016, www.whitehouse.gov/ondcp/ondcp-fact-sheets/how-illicit-drug-use-affects-business-and-the-economy.

137. Ibid.

138. Center for Behavioral Health Statistics and Quality, "Behavioral Health Trends in the United States: Results from the 2014 National Survey on Drug Use and Health," 2015.

139. National Council on Alcoholism and Drug Dependence, "Drugs and Alcohol in the Workplace," April 26, 2015, https://ncadd.org/about-addiction/addiction-update/drugs-and-alcohol-in-the-workplace.

140. Substance Abuse and Mental Health Services Administration, "Substance Use and Substance Use Disorder by Industry," April 26, 2015, http://www.samhsa.gov/data/sites/default/files/report_1959/ShortReport-1959.html.

141. Pew Research Center, "America's New Drug Policy Landscape," April 2, 2014, http://www.people-press.org/2014/04/02/americas-new-drug-policy-landscape/; SAMSHA, "Prevention of Substance Abuse and Mental Illness," 2016, http://www.samhsa.gov/prevention.

142. D. Wesley, "Losing Effort: The United States' War on Drugs," Accessed May 12, 2016, http://visualeconomics.creditloan.com/losing-effort-the-united-states-war-on-drugs/.

143. Ibid.

144. Ibid.

**Pulled statistics:**

p. 359, Center for Behavioral Health Statistics and Quality, "Behavioral Health Trends in the United States: Results from the 2014 National Survey on Drug Use and Health," HHS Publication No. SMA 15-4927, NSDUH Series H-50 (2015), Retrieved from http://www.samhsa.gov/data.

p. 371, Center for Behavioral Health Statistics and Quality, "Behavioral Health Trends in the United States: Results from the 2014 National Survey on Drug Use and Health," HHS Publication No. SMA 15-4927, NSDUH Series H-50 (2015), Retrieved from http://www.samhsa.gov/data.

p. 374, Center for Behavioral Health Statistics and Quality, "Behavioral Health Trends in the United States: Results from the 2014 National Survey on Drug Use and Health," HHS Publication No. SMA 15-4927, NSDUH Series H-50 (2015), Retrieved from http://www.samhsa.gov/data.

## Chapter 14

1. WHO, "Zika Virus and Complications," April 7, 2016. http://www.who.int/emergencies/zika-virus/en/.

2. M. Day et al., "Surveillance of Zoonotic Infectious Disease Transmitted by Small Companion Animals," *Emerging Infectious Diseases* (2012), wwwnc.cdc.gov/eid/article/18/12/12-0664_article.

3. WHO, "Fact Sheet: World Malaria Report 2015," December 9, 2015, http://www

.who.int/malaria/media/world-malaria-report-2015/en/.

4. CDC, "Chikungunya Virus: 2015 Provisional Date for United States," January 12, 2016, http://www.cdc.gov/chikungunya/geo/united-states-2015.html.

5. WHO, "Dengue Control," Accessed April 2016, http://www.who.int/denguecontrol/en/; Centers for Disease Control and Prevention, "Dengue," January 19, 2016, www.cdc.gov/Dengue/.

6. Ibid.

7. E. Hoberg and D. Brooks, "Evolution in Action: Climate Change, Biodiversity Dynamics and Emerging Infectious Disease," *Philosophical Transactions of the Royal Society of London B: Biological Sciences* 370, no. 1665 (2015), doi: 10.1098/rstb.2013.0553; S. Altizer et al., "Climate Change and Infectious Diseases: From Evidence to a Predictive Framework," *Science* 341, no. 6145 (2013): 514–9; WHO, "Climate Change and Infectious Disease," May 2015, www.who.int/globalchange/publications/climatechangechap6.pdf; C. Heffernan, "Climate Change and Infectious Disease: Time for a New Normal?" *Lancet Infectious Diseases* 15, no. 2 (2015): 143–6.

8. Agency for Toxic Substances and Disease Registry (ATSDR), "Health Effects of Chemical Exposure," Accessed March 2016, Available at http://www.atsdr.cdc.gov/emes/public/docs/Health%20Effects%20of%20Chemical%20Exposure%20FS.pdf.

9. NIH, National Institute of Allergy and Infectious Diseases, "Autoimmune Diseases," January 5, 2016, http://www.niaid.nih.gov/topics/autoimmune/Pages/default.aspx.

10. American Autoimmune Related Diseases Association, "Autoimmune Statistics," 2014, http://www.aarda.org/autoimmune-information/autoimmune-statistics/; National Institute of Arthritis and Musculoskeletal and Skin Diseases, "Understanding Autoimmune Diseases," October 2012, Available at http://www.niams.nih.gov/Health_Info/Autoimmune/.

11. Centers for Disease Control and Prevention (CDC), "Birth–18 years and 'Catch-Up' Immunization Schedules," March 29, 2016, www.cdc.gov/vaccines/schedules/hcp/child-adolescent.html.

12. CDC, "Antibiotic/Antimicrobial Resistance," March 2, 2016, http://www.cdc.gov/drugresistance/.

13. Pew Charitable Trust, "Variation in Outpatient Antibiotic Prescribing in the United States," November 2015, Available at http://www.pewtrusts.org/~/media/assets/2015/11/variation-in-outpatient-antibiotic-prescribing-in-the-us_fs_final.pdf?la=en.

14. CDC, "HAI Data and Stats," March 2, 2016, www.cdc.gov/HAI/surveillance/; S. Magill et al., "Multistate Point-Prevalence Survey of Health Care–Associated Infections," *New England Journal of Medicine* 370, no. 13 (2014): 1198–208.

15. Ibid.

16. Ibid.

17. CDC, "General Information about MRSA in the Community," March 24, 2016, www.cdc.gov/mrsa/community/index.html.

18. Centers for Disease Control and Prevention-Newsroom, "Nearly Half a Million Americans Suffered from *Clostridium difficile* Infections in a Single Year," February 2015, www.cdc.gov/media/releases/2015/p0225-clostridium-difficile.html.

19. CDC, "Group B Strep (GBS) Prevention in Newborns," June 1, 2014, http://www.cdc.gov/groupbstrep/about/prevention.html.

20. WHO, "Global Health Observatory (GHO) Data: Meningococcal Meningitis," Accessed March 28, 2016, http://www.who.int/gho/epidemic_diseases/meningitis/en/; CDC, "Meningococcal Disease: Surveillance," August 5, 2015, http://www.cdc.gov/meningococcal/surveillance/index.html.

21. Ibid.

22. Ibid.

23. WHO, "Media Centre: Tuberculosis," March 2016, www.who.int/mediacentre/factsheets/fs104/en/.

24. CDC, "Tuberculosis (TB): Data and Statistics," September 2015, www.cdc.gov/tb/statistics/.

25. Ibid.

26. Ibid.

27. CDC, "New Treatment Regimen for Latent Tuberculosis Infection," March 11, 2014, http://www.cdc.gov/tb/topic/treatment/12dose_video.htm; ScienceDaily, "Curcumin May Help Overcome Drug-Resistant Tuberculosis," March 25, 2016, www.sciencedaily.com/releases/2016/03/160325093704.htm.

28. Ibid.

29. Consumer Reports, "Mosquito Repellents That Best Protect Against Zika," March 18, 2016, http://www.consumerreports.org/insect-repellents/mosquito-repellents-that-best-protect-against-zika/.

30. CDC, "Common Colds: Protect Yourself and Others," February 2016, www.cdc.gov/features/rhinoviruses/.

31. Ibid.

32. Web MD, "Cold, Flu, & Cough Health Center: What's Causing My Cold?," January 2015, www.webmd.com/cold-and-flu/cold-guide/common_cold_causes; CDC, "Common Colds: Protect Yourself and Others," February 2016, http://www.cdc.gov/features/rhinoviruses/.

33. CDC, "2015–2016 Flu Season," February 25, 2016, http://www.cdc.gov/flu/about/season/upcoming.htm; CDC, "Estimating Seasonal Influenza-Associated Deaths in the United States: CDC Study Confirms Variability of Flu," March 18, 2015, http://www.cdc.gov/flu/about/disease/us_flu-related_deaths.htm.

34. CDC, "Influenza (Flu): Seasonal Influenza Q&A," September 18, 2015, http://www.cdc.gov/flu/about/qa/disease.htm.

35. CDC, "Selecting the Viruses in the Seasonal Influenza (Flu) Vaccine," October 20, 2015, www.cdc.gov/flu/about/season/vaccine-selection.htm.

36. CDC, "Seasonal Influenza Vaccine & Total Doses Distributed," March 15, 2016, http://www.cdc.gov/flu/professionals/vaccination/vaccinesupply.htm.

37. CDC, "ACIP Votes Down Use of LAIV for 2016–2017 Flu Season," June 2016, http://www.cdc.gov/media/releases/2016/s0622-laiv-flu.html.

38. T. V. Murphy, "Progress Toward Eliminating Hepatitis A Disease in the United States," *Morbidity and Mortality Weekly Report Supplements* 65, no. 1 (2016): 29–41; CDC, "Viral Hepatitis: Hepatitis A Questions and Answers for Health Professionals," May 31, 2015, http://www.cdc.gov/hepatitis/hav/havfaq.htm#general.

39. CDC, "Viral Hepatitis Surveillance-United States-2013," 2015; WHO, "Hepatitis B," July 2015, http://www.who.int/mediacentre/factsheets/fs204/en/.

40. E. Aspinall et al., "Are Needle and Syringe Programmes Associated with a Reduction in HIV Transmission among People Who Inject Drugs: A Systematic Review and Meta-analysis," *International Journal of Epidemiology*, 43, no. 1 (2014): 235–48; A. Dutta et al., "Key Harm Reduction Interventions and Their Impact on Reduction of Risky Behavior and HIV Incidence Among People Who Inject Drugs in Low-Income and Middle-Income Countries," *Current Opinion HIV AIDS* 7, no. 4 (2012): 362–8.

41. CDC, "Viral Hepatitis Surveillance, United States, Disease Burden from Viral Hepatitis A, B, and C in the United States–2013," May 2015, www.cdc.gov/hepatitis/Statistics/index.htm.

42. Ibid.

43. CDC, "Hepatitis C FAQs for the Public," January 8, 2016, http://www.cdc.gov/hepatitis/hcv/cfaq.htm#cFAQ21; CDC, "Viral Hepatitis Surveillance, United States, Disease Burden from Viral Hepatitis A, B, and C," 2015.

44. CDC, "Hepatitis C FAQs for the Public," April 2015.

45. Ibid.

46. Ibid.

47. N. Afdhal et al., "Ledipasvir and Sofosbuvir for Previously Treated HCV Genotype 1 Infection," *New England Journal of Medicine* 370, no. 16 (2014): 1483–93.

48. R. Seither et al., "Vaccination Coverage among Children in Kindergarten–United States 2013-2014 School Year," *Morbidity and Mortality Weekly Report* 63, no. 41 (2014): 913–20; California Department of Public Health, "Vaccine Preventable Disease Surveillance in California–Annual Report–2013," 2014, www.cdph.ca.gov/programs/immunize/Documents/VPD-Disease Summary2013.pdf.

49. CDC, "West Nile Virus Disease Cases and Presumptive Viremic Blood Donors by State – United States, 2015," January 12, 2016, http://www.cdc.gov/westnile/statsmaps/preliminarymapsdata/histatedate.html.

50. WHO, "Cumulative Number of Confirmed Human Cases for Avian Influenza A(H5N1) Reported to WHO," February 25, 2016, http://www.who.int/influenza/human_

animal_interface/H5N1_cumulative_table_
archives/en.

51. Ibid.

52. CDC, "The 2009 H1N1 Pandemic," August
2010, www.cdc.gov/h1n1flu/cdcresponse.htm.

**Pulled statistics:**

p. 392, WHO, "Global Tuberculosis Report, 2015,"
Accessed April 2016, Available at http://www
.who.int/tb/publications/global_report/
gtbr2015_executive_summary.pdf?ua=1.

p. 398, American Autoimmune-Related Disease
Association, "Autoimmune Disease in
Women," Accessed March 28, 2016, http://
www.aarda.org/autoimmune-information/
autoimmune-disease-in-women/

## Chapter 15

1. Centers for Disease Control and Prevention,
"College Health and Safety," August 2015,
http://www.cdc.gov/family/college/.

2. CDC, "Fact Sheet–Reported STDs in the
United States," November 2015, http://
www.cdc.gov/std/stats14/std-trends-508.pdf;
United States Department of Health and
Human Services, Office of Adolescent
Health, "Sexually Transmitted Diseases,"
February 2016, http://www.hhs.gov/ash/
oah/adolescent-health-topics/reproductive-
health/stds.html; CDC, "2014 Sexually
Transmitted Disease Surveillance," February
2016, Available at www.cdc.gov/std/stats14.

3. CDC, "Reported Cases of Sexually Transmitted Diseases on the Rise in United States,"
November 17, 2015, http://www.cdc.gov/
nchhstp/newsroom/2015/std-surveillance-
report-press-release.html.

4. Ibid.; CDC, "2014 Sexually Transmitted
Disease Surveillance," February 2016,
Available at www.cdc.gov/std/stats14.

5. CDC, "STDs in Adolescents and Young
Adults," December 2014, www.cdc.gov/std/
stats13/adol.htm.

6. Ibid.

7. United States Department of Health and
Human Services. Office of Adolescent Health.
"Sexually Transmitted Diseases. May, 2016.
http://www.hhs.gov/ash/oah/adolescent-
health-topics/reproductive-health/stds.html.

8. American College Health Association,
*American College Health Association—National
College Health Assessment II (ACHA-NCHA II)
Reference Group Executive Summary, Fall 2015*
(Hanover, MD: American College Health
Association, 2016), Available at www.acha-
ncha.org.

9. Ibid.

10. T. Wray et al., "Daily Co-Occurrence of
Alcohol Use and High Risk Sexual Behavior
among Heterosexual, heavy Drinking
Emergency Department Patients," *Drug and
Alcohol Dependence* 152 (2015): 109–15.

11. CDC, "CDC Fact Sheet: Chlamydia
(Detailed)," May 2016, http://www.cdc.gov/
std/chlamydia/stdfact-chlamydia-detailed
.htm.

12. Ibid.

13. Ibid.

14. MedlinePlus, "Pelvic Inflammatory Disease
(PID)," Updated September 2015, www.nlm
.nih.gov/medlineplus/ency/article/000888
.htm; Mayo Clinic Staff, "Urinary Tract
Infection: Risk Factors," July 23, 2015, http://
www.mayoclinic.org/diseases-conditions/
urinary-tract-infection/basics/risk-factors/
con-20037892.

15. CDC, "CDC Fact Sheet: Gonorrhea
(Detailed)," May 2016, http://www.cdc.gov/
std/gonorrhea/stdfact-gonorrhea.htm.

16. Ibid.

17. Ibid.

18. CDC, "CDC Fact Sheet: Syphilis (Detailed),"
May 2016, http://www.cdc.gov/std/syphilis/
stdfact-syphilis.htm.

19. Ibid.

20. Ibid.

21. Ibid.

22. CDC, "CDC Fact Sheet: Genital Herpes
(Detailed)," May 2016. textbfwww.cdc.gov/
std/herpes/stdfact-herpes.htm.

23. American Sexual Health Association,
"Herpes: Fast Facts," Accessed February 2016,
www.ashasexualhealth.org/stdsstis/herpes/
fast-facts-and-faqs/.

24. Ibid.

25. Ibid.

26. Ibid.

27. CDC, "CDC Fact Sheet: Genital HPV
Infection," February 2016, www.cdc.gov/std/
HPV/STDFact-HPV.htm.

28. Ibid.

29. Ibid.

30. CDC, "Cervical Cancer," October 2015,
http://www.cdc.gov/cancer/cervical/.

31. CDC, "What is HPV?," December 2015,
http://www.cdc.gov/hpv/parents/whatishpv
.html; CDC, "What Should I Know About
Screening?," March 2014, www.cdc.gov/
cancer/cervical/basic_info/screening.htm;
CDC, "Cervical Cancer," October 2015,
http://www.cdc.gov/cancer/cervical/.

32. American Cancer Society, "Cancer Facts &
Figures 2016" (Atlanta, GA: American Cancer
Society, 2016), Available at http://www
.cancer.org/acs/groups/content/@research/
documents/document/acspc-047079.pdf.

33. CDC, "Human Papillomavirus (HPV) and
Oropharyngeal Cancer–Fact Sheet," February
2016, http://www.cdc.gov/std/hpv/stdfact-
hpvandoropharyngealcancer.htm.

34. Ibid.

35. Ibid.

36. CDC, "Trichomoniasis: CDC Fact Sheet,"
November 2015, www.cdc.gov/std/
trichomonas/stdfact-trichomoniasis.htm.

37. Ibid.

38. WHO, "Global HIV/AIDS Observatory Data,"
Accessed March 2016, http://www.who.int/
gho/hiv/en/.

39. UNAIDS, "Fact Sheet, 2016," Accessed July
2016, Available at http://www.unaids.org/en/
resources/fact-sheet.

40. Ibid.

41. Ibid.

42. Ibid.

43. CDC, "HIV in the United States," September
2015, http://www.cdc.gov/hiv/statistics/

overview/ataglance.html; CDC, "Today's
HIV/AIDS Epidemic," February 2016,
Available at http://www.cdc.gov/nchhstp/
newsroom/docs/factsheets/todaysepidemic-
508.pdf.

44. Ibid.

45. Ibid.

46. CDC, "Today's HIV/AIDS Epidemic," 2016.

47. CDC, "HIV among Women," March 2016,
www.cdc.gov/HIV/risk/gender/women/facts/
index.html.

48. WHO, "Mother to Child Transmission of HIV,"
July 2015, www.who.int/hiv/topics/mtct/en.

49. Ibid.

50. Pharmaceutical Research and Manufacturers
of America, "Medicine in Development: 2014
Report," May 2015, www.phrma.org/sites/
default/files/pdf/2014-meds-in-dev-hiv-
aids.pdf.

51. Ibid.

52. Ibid.

53. CDC, "Clinical Prevention Guidelines–2015
STD Treatment Guidelines," June 2015, http://
www.cdc.gov/std/tg2015/clinical.htm.

54. Ibid.

**Pulled statistics:**

p. 411, U.S. Department of Health and Human
Services, Office of Adolescent Health, "Sexually Transmitted Diseases: Did You Know?"
February 23, 2016, http://www.hhs.gov/ash/
oah/adolescent-health-topics/reproductive-
health/stds.html.

p. 417, CDC, "HIV in the United States: At a
Glance," September 2015, http://www.cdc
.gov/hiv/statistics/overview/ataglance.html.

## Chapter 16

1. N. Allen et al., "Blood Pressure Trajectories in
Early Adulthood and Subclinical Atheroscle-
rosis in Middle Age," *Journal of the American
Medical Association* 311, no. 5 (2014): 490–7.

2. H. Ning et al., "Status of Cardiovascular
Health in US Children Up to 11 Years of Age.
The National Health and Nutrition Examination Surveys 2003–2010," *Circulation: Cardiovascular Quality and Outcomes* 8, no. 2 (2015):
164–71; L. Hayman and S. Camhi, "Ideal
Cardiovascular Health in Adolescence is
Associated with Reduced Risks of Hypertension, Metabolic Syndrome, and High
Cholesterol," *Evidence Based Nursing* 16, no. 1
(2013): 24–5.

3. K. Liu et al., "Can Antihypertensive Treat-
ment Restore the Risk of Cardiovascular
Disease to Ideal Levels?: The Coronary Artery
Risk Development in Young Adults (CARDIA)
Study and the Multi-Ethnic Study of Ath-
erosclerosis (MESA)," *Journal of the American
Heart Association* 4, no. 9 (2015): e002275;
N. Allen et al., "Blood Pressure Trajectories in
Early Adulthood and Subclinical Atheroscle-
rosis in Middle Age," 2014.

4. D. Mozaffarian et al., "Heart Disease and
Stroke Statistics—2016 Update: A Report
From the American Heart Association,"
*Circulation* 133, no. 4 (2016): e38–e360.

5. Ibid.

6. C. Greenwell, "Heart Disease and Stroke Cost America Nearly $1 Billion a Day in Medical Costs, Lost Productivity," *CDC Foundation*, April 29, 2015, http://www.cdcfoundation.org/pr/2015/heart-disease-and-stroke-cost-america-nearly-1-billion-day-medical-costs-lost-productivity.

7. Ibid.

8. D. Mozaffarian et al., "Heart Disease and Stroke Statistics," 2016.

9. Ibid.

10. American Heart Association, "Cardiovascular Health," April 2015, www.heart.org/idc/groups/heart-public/@wcm/@sop/@smd/documents/downloadable/ucm_462014.pdf; D. M. Lloyd-Jones et al., "Defining and Setting National Goals for Cardiovascular Health Promotion and Disease Reduction: The AHA's Strategic Impact Goal through 2020 and Beyond," *Circulation* 121 (2010): e14–e31.

11. D. Mozaffarian et al., "Heart Disease and Stroke Statistics," 2016; D. M. Lloyd-Jones et al., "Defining and Setting National Goals for Cardiovascular Health Promotion and Disease Reduction," 2010.

12. D. Mozaffarian et al., "Heart Disease and Stroke Statistics," 2016.

13. Ibid.

14. Ibid.

15. Ibid.

16. Cleveland Clinic, "Sudden Cardiac Death," Accessed May 2016, http://my.clevelandclinic.org/services/heart/disorders/arrhythmia/sudden-cardiac-death.

17. CDC, "Women and Heart Disease Fact Sheet," November 30, 2015, http://www.cdc.gov/dhdsp/data_statistics/fact_sheets/fs_women_heart.htm.

18. Ibid.

19. CDC, "Men and Heart Disease Fact Sheet," November 30, 2015, http://www.cdc.gov/dhdsp/data_statistics/fact_sheets/fs_men_heart.htm.

20. World Health Organization, "Cardiovascular Disease (CVD)-Key Facts," January 2015, http://www.who.int/mediacentre/factsheets/fs317/en/.

21. Ibid.

22. American Heart Association, "Why Blood Pressure Matters," August 2014, www.heart.org/HEARTORG/Conditions/HighBloodPressure/WhyBloodPressureMatters/Why-Blood-Pressure-Matters_UCM_002051_Article.jsp.

23. D. Mozaffarian et al., "Heart Disease and Stroke Statistics," 2016.

24. Ibid.

25. Ibid.

26. Ibid.

27. Ibid.

28. L. Rutten-Jacobs et al., "Cardiovascular Disease Is the Main Cause of Long-Term Excess Mortality after Ischemic Stroke in Young Adults," *Hypertension* 65, no. 3 (2015): 670–5.

29. D. Mozaffarian et al., "Heart Disease and Stroke Statistics," 2016.

30. Ibid.

31. Centers for Disease Control and Prevention, "High Blood Pressure Facts," February 19, 2015, www.cdc.gov/bloodpressure/facts.htm.

32. D. Mozaffarian et al., "Heart Disease and Stroke Statistics," 2016.

33. Ibid.; American Heart Association, "About Peripheral Artery Disease," March 23, 2016, www.heart.org/HEARTORG/Conditions/More/PeripheralArteryDisease/About-Peripheral-Artery-Disease-PAD_UCM_301301_Article.jsp.

34. D. Mozaffarian et al., "Heart Disease and Stroke Statistics," 2016; American Heart Association, "About Peripheral Artery Disease," March 23, 2016. www.heart.org/HEARTORG/Conditions/More/PeripheralArteryDisease/About-Peripheral-Artery-Disease-PAD_UCM_301301_Article.jsp.

35. Ibid.

36. D. Mozaffarian et al., "Heart Disease and Stroke Statistics," 2016.

37. Ibid.

38. Ibid.

39. Ibid.; American Heart Association, "Angina (Chest Pain)," April 18, 2016, www.heart.org/HEARTORG/Conditions/HeartAttack/SymptomsDiagnosisofHeartAttack/Angina-Chest-Pain_UCM_450308_Article.jsp; American Heart Association, "Angina in Women Can Be Different Than Men," April 18, 2016, http://www.heart.org/HEARTORG/Conditions/HeartAttack/WarningSignsofaHeartAttack/Angina-in-Women-Can-Be-Different-Than-Men_UCM_448902_Article.jsp#.VzJHJmQrIfE

40. D. Mozaffarian et al., "Heart Disease and Stroke Statistics," 2016.

41. American Heart Association, "Causes of Heart Failure." April 2015. http://www.heart.org/HEARTORG/Conditions/HeartFailure/CausesAndRisksForHeartFailure/Causes-of-Heart-Failure_UCM_477643_Article.jsp#.V6Iyaj9TF2Z.

42. Ibid.

43. Ibid.

44. Ibid.

45. Ibid.

46. CDC, "Cerebrovascular Disease or Stroke," April 27, 2016, http://www.cdc.gov/nchs/fastats/stroke.htm.

47. D. Ingram and J. Montresor-Lopez, "Differences in Stroke Mortality, Adults Aged 45 and Over: United States 2010–2013," *NCHS Data Brief* 207, July 2015, Available at http://www.cdc.gov/nchs/data/databriefs/db207.pdf; D. Mozaffarian et al., "Heart Disease and Stroke Statistics," 2016.

48. D. W. J. Dipple, "Chances of Good Outcomes after Stroke Reduced by Delay in Restoring Blood Flow," *JAMA* Network Journals, December 21, 2015, http://media.jamanetwork.com/news-item/chances-of-good-outcome-after-stroke-reduced-by-delays-in-restoring-blood-flow/.

49. M. Goyal et al., "Recent Endovascular Trials: Implications for Radiology Departments, Radiology Residency, and Neuro-radiology Fellowship Training at Comprehensive Stroke Centers," *Radiology* 278, no. 3 (2016): 642–5.

50. N. E. Synhaeve et al., "Poor Long-Term Functional Outcome After Stroke among Adults Aged 18 to 50 Years Follow-Up of Transient Ischemic Attack and Stroke Patients and Unelucidated Risk Factor Evaluation (FUTURE) Study," *Stroke* 45, no. 4 (2014): 1157–60.

51. C. J. L. Murray et al., "The State of US Health, 1990–2010 Burden of Diseases, Injuries, and Risk Factors," *Journal of the American Medical Association* 310, no. 6 (2013): 591–608.

52. D. Mozaffarian et al., "Heart Disease and Stroke Statistics," 2016; A. Noortie, "Ischaemic Stroke in Young Adults: Risk Factors and Long-term Consequences," *Nature Reviews Neurology* 10, no. 6 (2014): 315–25; Y. Yano et al., "Isolated Systolic Hypertension in Young and Middle-Aged Adults and 31-year Risk for Cardiovascular Mortality," *Journal of the American College of Cardiology* 65, no. 4 (2015): 327–33

53. L. Nelson et al., "Hypertension and Inflammation in Alzheimer's Disease: Close Partners in Disease Development and Progression!," *Journal of Alzheimer's Disease* 41, no. 2 (2014): 331–43.

54. M. Baumgart et al., "Summary of Evidence on Modifiable Risk Factors for Cognitive Decline and Dementia: A Population-Based Perspective," *Alzheimer's and Dementia* 11, no. 6 (2016): 718–26.

55. Ibid.

56. Ibid.

57. M. Aguilar et al., "Prevalence of the Metabolic Syndrome in the United States, 2003–2012," *Journal of the American Medical Association* 313, no. 19 (2015): 1973–4.

58. Ibid.

59. D. Mozaffarian et al., "Heart Disease and Stroke Statistics," 2016; S. Grundy et al., "Definition of Metabolic Syndrome. Report of the National Heart, Lung, and Blood Institute/American Heart Association Conference on Scientific Issues Related to Definition," *Circulation* 109, no. 2 (2011): 433–8.

60. N. Allen et al., "Blood Pressure Trajectories in Early Adulthood and Subclinical Atherosclerosis in Middle Age," 2014; Y. Yano et al., "Isolated Systolic Hypertension in Young and Middle-Aged Adults and 31-Year Risk for cardiovascular Mortality," 2015; P. Chu et al., "Comparative Effectiveness of Personalized Lifestyle Management Strategies for Cardiovascular Disease Risk Reduction," *Journal of the American Heart Association* 5, no. 3 (2016): e002737.

61. D. Mozaffarian et al., "Heart Disease and Stroke Statistics," 2016.

62. Ibid.

63. Ibid.

64. Ibid.; National Cancer Institute, "Fact Sheet: Harms of Cigarette Smoking and Health Benefits of Quitting," December, 2014, http://www.cancer.gov/about-cancer/causes-prevention/risk/tobacco/cessation-fact-sheet.

65. D. Mozaffarian et al., "Heart Disease and Stroke Statistics," 2016; National Cancer Institute, "Fact Sheet: Harms of Cigarette Smoking and Health Benefits of Quitting,"

December, 2014, http://www.cancer.gov/about-cancer/causes-prevention/risk/tobacco/cessation-fact-sheet.

66. Ibid.

67. U.S. Department of Health and Human Services and U.S. Department of Agriculture, *2015–2020 Dietary Guidelines for Americans.* 8th Edition, December 2015, Available at http://health.gov/dietaryguidelines/2015/guidelines/.

68. Ibid.

69. Ibid.

70. Ibid.

71. AHA, "Guidelines Resource Center," March 2016, http://www.heart.org/HEARTORG/Conditions/Understanding-the-New-Guidelines_UCM_458155_Article.jsp#.VyaPNfkrKUk.

72. G. Qiuping et al., "Prescription Cholesterol-Lowering Medication Use in Adults Aged 40 and Over: United States 2003–2012," *NCHS Data Brief*, No. 177 (Hyattsville, MD: National Center for Health Statistics USDHHS, 2015); D. Mozaffarian et al., "Heart Disease and Stroke Statistics," 2016.

73. Ibid.

74. D. Keene et al., "Effect on Cardiovascular Risk of High Density Lipoprotein Targeted Drug Treatments Niacin, Fibrates, and CETP Inhibitors: Meta-analysis of Randomised Controlled Trials Including 117,411 Patients," *British Medical Journal* 349 (2014): g4379, doi: http://dx.doi.org/10.1136/bmj.g4379.

75. N. J. Stone et al., "2013 ACC/AHA Guidelines on the Treatment of Blood Cholesterol to Reduce Atherosclerotic Cardiovascular Risk in Adults," *Circulation* 63, no. 25, pt. B (2014): 2889–934.

76. Bernard M. F. M., et al. "Minimal Intensity Physical Activity (Standing and Walking) of Longer Duration Improves Insulin Action and Plasma Lipids More than Shorter Periods of Moderate to Vigorous Exercise (Cycling) in Sedentary Subjects When Energy Expenditure Is Comparable," *PLoS ONE* 8, no. 2 (2013): e55542, doi: 10.1371/journal.pone.0055542; AHA, "Recommendations for Physical Activity in Adults," July 2016, http://www.heart.org/HEARTORG/HealthyLiving/PhysicalActivity/FitnessBasics/American-Heart-Association-Recommendations-for-Physical-Activity-in-Adults_UCM_307976_Article.jsp#.V6JAGz9TF2Y.

77. D. Mozaffarian et al., "Heart Disease and Stroke Statistics," 2016.

78. Ibid.

79. AHA, "Shaking the Salt Habit," April 8, 2016, http://www.heart.org/HEARTORG/Conditions/HighBloodPressure/PreventionTreatmentofHighBloodPressure/Shaking-the-Salt-Habit_UCM_303241_Article.jsp#.VyePYfkrKUk.

80. S. Wood and R. Valentino, "The Brain Norepinephrine System, Stress and Cardiovascular Vulnerability," *Neuroscience and Biobehavioral Reviews* (2016), doi: 10.1016/j.neurobiorev.2016.04.018; N. Batelaan et al., "Anxiety and New Onset of Cardiovascular Disease: Critical Review and Meta-Analysis,"

*British Journal of Psychiatry* 208, no. 3 (2016): 223–31.

81. Ibid.

82. D. Mozaffarian et al., "Heart Disease and Stroke Statistics," 2016.

83. Ibid.; T Huang and F. Hu, "Gene–Environmental Interactions and Obesity: Recent Developments and Future Directions," *BMC Medical Genomics* 8, Suppl. 1 (2015): S2;

84. D. Mozaffarian et al., "Heart Disease and Stroke Statistics," 2016.

85. Ibid.

86. P. Ridker, "A Test in Context: High Sensitivity C-Reactive Protein," *Journal of the American College of Cardiology* 67, no. 6 (2016): 712–23; M. Jimenez et al., "Association Between High Sensitivity C-Reactive Protein and Total Stroke by Hypertensive Stroke Among Men," *Journal of the American Heart Association* 4, no. 9 (2015): e002013.

87. "The PLAC Test: Predicting Heart Attack Risk in People with No Symptoms." *Scientific American-Health After 50*, 27, no. 2 (2015): 1–2.

88. R. Chowdhury et al., "Association of Dietary, Circulating, and Supplement Fatty Acids with Coronary Risk: A Systematic Review and Meta Analysis," *Annals of Internal Medicine* 160, no. 6 (2014): 398–406, doi: 10.7326?M13-1788.

89. American Heart Association, "Fish and Omega 3 Fatty Acids," June 15, 2015, www.heart.org/HEARTORG/General/Fish-and-Omega-3-Fatty-Acids_UCM_303248_Article.jsp.

90. Ibid.

91. D. Wald, J. Morris, and N. Wald, "Reconciling the Evidence on Serum Homocysteine and Ischemic Heart Disease: A Meta-analysis," *PLoS ONE* 6, no. 2 (2011): e16473; P. Ganguly and S. Alam, "Role of Homocysteine in the Development of CVD," *Nutrition Journal* 14, no. 1 (2015):1.

92. American Heart Association, "Homocysteine, Folic Acid, and Cardiovascular Disease," March 18, 2014, www.heart.org.

93. U.S. Preventive Services Task Force, "Understanding Task Force Recommendations: Aspirin Use for the Primary Prevention of Cardiovascular Disease and Colorectal Cancer," April 2016, http://www.uspreventiveservicestaskforce.org/Home/GetFile/11/218/aspr-cvccrc-finalrsfact/pdf; FDA, "Can an Aspirin a Day Help Prevent a Heart Attack?," February 22, 2016, www.fda.gov/For Consumers/ConsumerUpdates/ucm390539.htm.

94. American Heart Association, "Prevention and Treatment of Heart Attack," February 10, 2016, http://www.heart.org/HEARTORG/Conditions/HeartAttack/PreventionTreatmentofHeartAttack/Prevention-and-Treatment-of-Heart-Attack_UCM_002042_Article.jsp#.VzJaa2QrIfE.

95. D. Mozaffarian et al., "Heart Disease and Stroke Statistics," 2016.

**Pulled statistics:**

p. 424, C. Greenwell, "Heart Disease and Stroke Cost America Nearly $1 Billion a Day in

Medical Costs, Lost Productivity," *CDC Foundation*, April 29, 2015, http://www.cdcfoundation.org/pr/2015/heart-disease-and-stroke-cost-america-nearly-1-billion-day-medical-costs-lost-productivity.

p. 426, D. Mozaffarian, et al. "Heart Disease and Stroke Statistics—2016 Update: A Report from the American Heart Association," 2016.

## Chapter 16A

1. American College Health Association, *American College Health Association-National College Health Assessment II: Reference Group Executive Summary Fall 2015* (Hanover, MD: American College Health, 2016); H. Cheng et al., "The Health Consequences of Obesity in Young Adulthood," *Current Obesity Reports* 5, no. 1 (2016): 30–7.

2. E. Gregg et al., "Changes in Diabetes Complications in the United States, 1990–2010," *New England Journal of Medicine* 370, no. 16 (2014): 1514–23.

3. NCD Risk Factor Collaboration (NCD-RisC), "Worldwide Trends in Diabetes Since 1980: A Pooled Analysis of 751 Population-Based Studies with 4.4 Million Participants," *The Lancet* 387 (2016): 1513–30.

4. Centers for Disease Control and Prevention, "Long Term Trends in Diabetes in the United States," April 2016, https://www.cdc.gov/diabetes/statistics/slides/long_term_trends.pdf.

5. Centers for Disease Control and Prevention, "National Diabetes Statistics Report, 2014," May 2015, www.cdc.gov/diabetes/pubs/statsreport14/national-diabetes-report-web.pdf; Centers for Disease Control and Prevention, "Early Release of Selected Estimates Based on Data from the National Health Interview Survey–January to June, 2014," May 2015, www.cdc.gov/nchs/data/nhis/earlyrelease/earlyrelease201412.pdf.

6. Centers for Disease Control and Prevention, "National Diabetes Statistics Report, 2014," May 2015.

7. Centers for Disease Control and Prevention, National Center for Health Statistics, "Summary Health Statistics for U.S. Adults: National Health Interview Survey, 2014," October 19, 2015, Available at http://ftp.cdc.gov/pub/Health_Statistics/NCHS/NHIS/SHS/2014_SHS_Table_A-4.pdf.

8. T. Dall et al., "The Economic Burden of Elevated Blood Glucose Levels in 2012: Diagnosed and Undiagnosed Diabetes, Gestational Diabetes Mellitus, and Prediabetes," *Diabetes Care* 37, no. 12 (2014): 3172–79.

9. Endocrine Society, "Endocrine Facts and Figures: Diabetes," Accessed June 2016, http://endocrinefacts.org/health-conditions/diabetes-2/.

10. T. Dall et al., "The Economic Burden of Elevated Blood Glucose Levels in 2012," 2014.

11. American Diabetes Association, "Diabetes Basics: Type 1," Accessed May, 2016, www.diabetes.org/diabetes-basics/type-1.

12. American Diabetes Association, "Genetics of Diabetes," Accessed May 2016, http://www

.diabetes.org/diabetes-basics/genetics of diabetes.html.

13. Ibid.

14. Centers for Disease Control and Prevention, "National Diabetes Statistics Report, 2014," May 2015; V. Lyssenko and M. Laakso, "Genetic Screening for the Risk of Type 2 Diabetes," *Diabetes Care* 36, Suppl. 2 (2013): S120–S126.

15. V. Lyssenko and M. Laakso, "Genetic Screening for the Risk of Type 2 Diabetes," 2013.

16. Ibid.

17. Ibid.

18. T. Huang et al., "Genetic Predisposition to Central Obesity and Risk of Type 2 Diabetes: two Independent Cohort Studies," *Diabetes Care* 38, no. 7 (2015): 1306–11.

19. American Diabetes Association, "Statistics About Diabetes," April 1, 2016, http://www.diabetes.org/diabetes-basics/statistics.

20. Centers for Disease Control and Prevention, "National Diabetes Statistics Report, 2014," May 2015.

21. R. Hamman et al., "The SEARCH for Diabetes in Youth Study: Rationale, Findings, and Future Directions," *Diabetes Care* 37, no. 12 (2014): 3336–44.

22. D. J. Pettitt et al., "Prevalence of Diabetes in U.S. Youth in 2009: The SEARCH for Diabetes in Youth Study," *Diabetes Care* 37, no. 2 (2014): 402–8.

23. American Diabetes Association, "Genetics of Diabetes," May 20, 2014, http://www.diabetes.org/diabetes-basics/genetics-of-diabetes.html; K. Colclough et al., "Clinical Utility Gene Card: Maturity-Onset Diabetes of the Young," *European Journal of Human Genetics* 22, no. 9 (2014), doi: 10.1038/ejhg.2014.14.

24. F. He et al., "Abdominal Obesity and Metabolic Syndrome Burden in Adolescents—Penn State Children Cohort Study," *Journal of Clinical Densitometry* 18, no. 1 (2015): 30–6; T. Huang et al., "Genetic Predisposition to Central Obesity and Risk of Type 2 Diabetes," 2015.

25. Ibid.

26. P. L. Capers et al., "A Systematic Review and Meta-analysis of Randomized Controlled Trials of the Impact of Sleep Duration on Adiposity and Components of Energy Balance," *Obesity Reviews* 16, no. 9 (2015): 771–82; L. Bromley et al., "Sleep Restriction Decreases the Physical Activity of Adults at Risk for Type 2 Diabetes," *Sleep* 35, no. 7 (2012): 977–84.

27. Z. Shan et al., "Sleep Duration and Risk of Type 2 Diabetes: A Meta-analysis of Prospective Studies," *Diabetes Care* 38, no. 3 (2015): 529–37; H. C. Hung et al., "The Association between Self-Reported Sleep Quality and Metabolic Syndrome," *PLoS ONE* 8, no. 1 (2013): e54304, doi: 10.1371/journal.pone.0054304.

28. S. Kelly and M. Ismail, "Stress and Type 2 Diabetes: A Review of How Stress Contributes to the Development of Type 2 Diabetes," *Annual Review of Public Health* 36 (2015): 441–62.

29. Ibid.

30. Centers for Disease Control and Prevention (CDC), "National Diabetes Statistics Report, 2014"; CDC, "Prediabetes: Could It Be You?," 2014, www.cdc.gov/diabetes/pubs/statsreport14/prediabetes-infographic.pdf.

31. N. Yahia et al., "Assessment of College Students' Awareness and Knowledge about Conditions Relevant to Metabolic Syndrome," *Diabetology and Metabolic Syndrome* 6, no. 1 (2014): 111; J. Stack et al., "Factors Associated with Diabetes Risk in South Texas College Students," *International Journal of Exercise Science: Conference Proceedings* 7, no. 2 (2014): 2; A. Lima et al., "Risk Factors for Type 2 Diabetes Mellitus in College Students: Association with Sociodemographic Variables," *Revista latino-americana de enfermagem* 22, no. 3 (2014): 484–90; C. Hao et al., "Prevalence and Risk Factors of Diabetes and Impaired Fasting Glucose among University Applicants in Eastern China: Findings from a Population-Based Study," *Diabetic Medicine* 31, no. 10 (2014): 1194–98.

32. American Heart Association, "About Metabolic Syndrome," May 14, 2014, http://www.heart.org/HEARTORG/Conditions/More/MetabolicSyndrome/About-Metabolic-Syndrome_UCM_301920_Article.jsp#.V0z5w_z2aUk.

33. Ibid.

34. National Heart Lung and Blood Institute, "Who is at Risk for Metabolic Syndrome?," November 2015, http://www.nhlbi.nih.gov/health/health-topics/topics/ms/atrisk.

35. M. Aguilar et al., "Prevalence of the Metabolic Syndrome in the United States, 2003–2012," *Journal of the American Medical Association* 313, no. 19 (2015): 1973–4.

36. Ibid.

37. CDC, "Prediabetes: Could It Be You?," 2014.

38. Centers for Disease Control, "Awareness of Prediabetes—United States, 2005–2010," March 2013, www.cdc.gov.

39. Z. Zou et al., "Influence of Primary Intervention of Exercise on Obese Type 2 Diabetes Mellitus: A Meta-analysis Review," *Primary Care Diabetes* 10, no. 3 (2016): 186–201.

40. American Diabetes Association, "What Is Gestational Diabetes?," June 2014, www.diabetes.org/diabetes-basics/gestational/what-is-gestational-diabetes.html.

41. Ibid.; C. G. Chodick et al., "The Risk of Overt Diabetes Mellitus among Women with Gestational Diabetes: A Population-Based Study," *Diabetic Medicine* 27, no. 7 (2010): 779–85; E. Noctor and F. Dunne, "Type 2 Diabetes After Gestational Diabetes: The Influence of Changing Diagnostic Criteria," *World Journal of Diabetes* 6, no. 2 (2015): 234–44.

42. Ibid.

43. National Healthy Mothers, Healthy Babies Coalition, "The Lasting Impact of Gestational Diabetes on Mother and Children," May 2015, www.hmhb.org/virtual-library/interviews-with-experts/gestational-diabetes.

44. Mayo Clinic, "Gestational Diabetes Complications," April 25, 2014, http://www.mayoclinic.org/diseases-conditions/gestational-diabetes/basics/complications/con-20014854.

45. Centers for Disease Control and Prevention, "National Diabetes Statistics Report, 2014," May 2015; American Diabetes Association, "Living with Diabetes: Complications," May 2014, www.diabetes.org/living-with-diabetes/complications/; K. Weinspach et al., "Level of Information about the Relationship between Diabetes Mellitus and Periodontitis—Results from a Nationwide Diabetes Information Program," *European Journal of Medical Research* 18, no. 1 (2013): 6, doi: 10.1186/2047-783X-18-6.

46. National Kidney Foundation, "Fast Facts," May 2016. www.kidney.org/news/newsroom/factsheets/FastFacts.cfm; United States Renal Disease Data System, "Annual Data Report, 2015," (Bethesda, MD: 2015), Available at https://www.usrds.org/adr.aspx.

47. Ibid.

48. Centers for Disease Control and Prevention. "National Diabetes Statistics Report, 2014," May 2015.

49. Ibid.

50. Prevent Blindness America, "Diabetic Retinopathy Prevalence by Age," May 2014, www.visionproblemsus.org/diabetic-retinopathy/diabetic-retinopathy-by-age.html.

51. American Diabetes Association, "Diabetes and Oral Health Problems," October 2014, www.diabetes.org/living-with-diabetes/treatment-and-care/oral-health-and-hygiene/diabetes-and-oral-health.html.

52. Ibid.

53. American Diabetes Association, "Standards of Medical Care in diabetes—2016: Summary of Revisions," *Diabetes Care* 39, Suppl. 1 (2016): S4–S5.

54. American Diabetes Association, "Diagnosing Diabetes and Learning about Prediabetes," June 9, 2015, www.diabetes.org/diabetes-basics/diagnosis; American Diabetes Association, "Diabetes Pro-Toolkit #3: All about Prediabetes," Accessed May 2016, Available at http://professional2.diabetes.org/content/PML/All_About_Prediabetes_24dee6ff-cbf0-4a55-80b7-9d5d29de0bd7/All_About_Prediabetes.pdf.

55. Diabetes Prevention Program Research Group, "Reduction in the Incidence of Type 2 Diabetes with Lifestyle Intervention or Metformin," *New England Journal of Medicine* 345 (2002): 393–403.

56. Linus Pauling Institute, "Glycemic Index and Glycemic Load," Accessed May 2016, http://lpi.oregonstate.edu/infocenter/foods/grains/gigl.html.

57. American Diabetes Association, "Grains and Starchy Vegetables," February 2014, http://www.diabetes.org/food-and-fitness/food/what-can-i-eat/making-healthy-food-choices/grains-and-starchy-vegetables.html; A. Chanson-Rolle et al., "Systematic Review and Meta-analysis of Human Studies to Support a Quantitative Recommendation for Whole Grain Intake in Relation to Type 2 Diabetes," *PLoS ONE* 10, no. 6 (2015): e0131377.

58. S. Bhupathiraju et al., "Glycemic Index, Glycemic Load and Risk of Type 2 Diabetes: Results from 3 Large US Cohorts and an Updated Meta-Analysis," *Circulation* 129, Suppl. 1 (2014): AP140–AP140 A. Olubukola, P. English, and J. Pinkney, "Systematic Review and Meta-Analysis of Different Dietary Approaches to the Management of Type 2 Diabetes," *American Journal of Clinical Nutrition* 97, no. 3 (2013): 505–16.

59. A. Wallin et al., "Fish Consumption and Frying of Fish in Relation to Type 2 Diabetes Incidence: A Prospective Cohort Study of Swedish Men," *European Journal of Nutrition* (2015): 1–10; Y. Kim, P. Xun, and K. He, "Fish Consumption, Long-Chain Omega-3 Polyunsaturated Fatty Acid Intake and Risk of Metabolic Syndrome: A Meta-analysis," *Nutrients* 7, no. 4 (2015): 2085–2100.

60. Ibid.

61. A. Wallin et al., "Fish Consumption and Frying of Fish in Relation to Type 2 Diabetes Incidence," 2015; C. Jeppesen, K. Schiller, and M. Schultze, "Omega-3 and Omega-6 Fatty Acids and Type 2 Diabetes," *Current Diabetes Reports* 13, no. 2 (2013): 279–88.

62. American Diabetes Association, "What We Recommend," May 19, 2015, www.diabetes.org/food-and-fitness/fitness/types-of-activity/what-we-recommend.html; National Diabetes Information Clearing House, "Diabetes Prevention Program," September 2013, http://diabetes.niddk.nih.gov/dm/pubs/preventionprogram/index.aspx.

63. American Diabetes Association, "Your Weight Loss Plan," March 2014, http://www.diabetes.org/food-and-fitness/weight-loss/getting-started/your-weight-loss-plan.html; U. Hostalek, M. Gwilt, and S. Hildeman, "Therapeutic Use of Metformin in Prediabetes and Diabetes Prevention," *Drugs* 75, no. 10 (2015): 1071–94.

64. J. Yu et al., "The Long Term Effects of Bariatric Surgery for Type 2 Diabetes: Systematic Review and Meta-analysis of Randomized and Non Randomized Evidence," *Obesity Surgery* 25, no. 1 (2015): 143–55.; S. R. Kashyap et al., "Metabolic Effects of Bariatric Surgery in Patients with Moderate Obesity and Type 2 Diabetes," *Diabetes Care* 36, no. 8 (2013): 2175–82.

65. P. R. Schauer et al., "Bariatric Surgery versus Intensive Medical Therapy for Diabetes–3 Year Outcomes," *New England Journal of Medicine* 370 (2014): 2002–13.

66. M. Jenson et al., "2013 AHA/ACC/TOS Guideline for the Management of Overweight and Obesity in Adults: A Report of the American College of Cardiology/American Heart Association Task Force on Practice Guidelines and The Obesity Society," *Circulation* 25, Suppl. 2 (2014): S139–40.

67. Medtronic, "Medtronic Gains Approval of First Artificial Pancreas Device System with Threshold Suspend Automation," September 2013, http://newsroom.medtronic.com/phoenix.zhtml?c=251324&p=irol-newsArticle&id=1859361.

68. A. Haider et al., "Comparison of Dual-Hormone Artificial Pancreas, Single-Hormone Artificial Pancreas, and Conventional Insulin Pump Therapy for Glycemic Control in Patients with Type 1 Diabetes: An Open-Label Randomised Controlled Crossover Trial," *The Lancet: Diabetes and Endocrinology* 3, no. 1 (2015): 17–25.

**Pulled statistics:**

p. 450, American Diabetes Association, "Genetics of Diabetes," June 2014, http://www.diabetes.org/diabetes-basics/genetics-of-diabetes.html?referrer=https://www.google.com/#sthash.LrF6iRNb.dpuf.

p. 454, J. Salas-Salvado et al., "Protective Effects of the Mediterranean Diet on Type 2 Diabetes and Metabolic Syndrome," *Journal of Nutrition* 146, no. 4 (2016): 920S–927S.

# Chapter 17

1. Adolescents and Young Adults with Cancer," May 2016, http://www.cancer.gov/types/aya.

2. D. Mozaffarian et al., "Heart Disease and Stroke Statistics—2016 Update: A Report from the American Heart Association," *Circulation* 133, no. 1 (2016): e38–e60.

3. American Cancer Society, *Cancer Facts & Figures 2016* (Atlanta, GA: American Cancer Society, 2016), Available at http://www.cancer.org/acs/groups/content/@research/documents/document/acspc-047079.pdf.

4. Ibid.

5. Ibid.

6. Ibid.

7. Ibid.

8. Ibid.

9. Ibid.

10. Ibid.

11. Ibid.

12. American Cancer Society, *Cancer Facts & Figures 2016*. Atlanta, GA: American Cancer Society, 2015, Available at http://www.cancer.org/acs/groups/content/@editorial/documents/document/acspc-044552.pdf.

13. American Cancer Society, *Cancer Facts & Figures 2016* (Atlanta, GA: American Cancer Society, 2016), Available at http://www.cancer.org/acs/groups/content/@research/documents/document/acspc-047079.pdf.

14. Ibid.

15. Ibid.

16. Ibid.; Centers for Disease Control and Prevention, "Smoking and Cancer," April 2015, www.cdc.gov/tobacco/data_statistics/sgr/50th-anniversary/pdfs/fs_smoking_cancer_508.pdf.

17. U.S. Department of Health and Human Services, "The Health Consequences of Smoking: 50 Years of Progress: A Report of the Surgeon General" (Atlanta, GA: U.S. Department of Health and Human Services, Centers for Disease Control and Prevention, National Center for Chronic Disease Prevention and Health Promotion, Office on Smoking and Health, 2014).

18. American Cancer Society, "Cancer Facts and Figures," 2016.

19. World Health Organization, "Report on the Global Tobacco Epidemic, 2015," July 7, 2015, Available at www.who.int/tobacco/global_report/2015/en.

20. Cancer Research UK, "Worldwide Cancer," May 2015, http://publications.cancerresearchuk.org/downloads/Product/CS_KF_WORLDWIDE.pdf.

21. V. Bagnardi et al., "Alcohol Consumption and Site-Specific Cancer Risk: A Comprehensive Dose-Response Meta-Analysis," *British Journal of Cancer* 112, no. 3 (2015): 580–93.

22. S. Y. Park et al., "Alcohol Consumption and Breast Cancer Risk Among Women from Five Ethnic Groups with Light to Moderate Intake: The Multiethnic Cohort Study," *International Journal of Cancer* 134, no. 6 (2014): 1504–10; Y. Cao et al, "Light to Moderate Intake of Alcohol, Drinking Patterns, and Risk of Cancer: Results from Two Prospective US Cohort Studies," *British Medical Journal* 351 (2015): h4238.

23. CDC, "Fact Sheet—Alcohol Use and Your Health," February 29, 2016, http://www.cdc.gov/alcohol/fact-sheets/alcohol-use.htm; CDC, "Fact Sheets—Excessive Alcohol Use and Risks to Men's Health," March 7, 2016, http://www.cdc.gov/alcohol/fact-sheets/mens-health.htm; National Cancer Institute, "Alcohol and Cancer Risk Sheet," June 24, 2013, www.cancer.gov/cancertopics/factsheet/Risk/alcohol.

24. American Cancer Society, "Cancer Facts and Figures," 2016.

25. Ibid.; D. Aune et al., "Anthropometric Factors and Endometrial Cancer Risk: A Systematic Review and Dose–Response Meta-Analysis of Prospective Studies," *Annals of Oncology* 26, no. 8 (2015): 1635–48.

26. N. Keum et al., "Adult Weight Gain and Adiposity-Related Cancers: A Dose–Response Meta-Analysis of Prospective Observational Studies," *Journal of the National Cancer Institute* 107, no. 2 (2015): djv088.

27. European Association for the Study of Obesity, "Higher BMI, Waist Circumference Are Associated with Increased Risk of Aggressive Prostate Cancer," *ScienceDaily*, Accessed June 13, 2016, www.sciencedaily.com/releases/2016/06/160602121838.htm.

28. Ibid.

29. American Cancer Society, "Does Body Weight Affect Cancer Risks?," February 5, 2016, http://www.cancer.org/cancer/cancercauses/dietandphysicalactivity/bodyweightandcancerrisk/body-weight-and-cancer-risk-effects.

30. Ibid.

31. Ibid.

32. Ibid.

33. K. Heikkila et al., "Work Stress and Risk of Cancer: Meta-Analysis of 5700 Incident Cancer Events in 116,000 European Men and Women," *British Medical Journal* 346 (2013): 1165, doi: 10.1136/bmj.1165.

34. American Cancer Society, "Family Cancer Syndromes," June 25, 2014, www.cancer.org/cancer/cancercauses/geneticsandcancer/heredity-and-cancer.

35. Ibid.

36. American Cancer Society, "Breast Cancer Overview: Do We Know What Causes Breast Cancer?," May 4, 2016, www.cancer.org/Cancer/BreastCancer/DetailedGuide/breast-cancer-what-causes; American Cancer Society, "Cancer Facts and Figures," 2016.

37. American Cancer Society, "Cancer Facts and Figures for Hispanic/Latinos, 2012–2014," Accessed May 2014, www.cancer.org/acs/groups/content/@epidemiologysurveilance/documents/document/acspc-034778.pdf; M. Banegas et al., "The Risk of Developing Invasive Breast Cancer in Hispanic Women," *Cancer* 119, no. 7 (2013): 1373–80.

38. Y. Guo et al., "Association between C-Reactive Protein and Risk of Cancer: A Meta-Analysis of Prospective Cohort Studies," *Asian Pacific Journal of Cancer Prevention* 14 (2013), doi: http://dx.doi.org/10.7314/APJCP.2013.14.1.243.

39. D. Baumeister et al., "Childhood Trauma and Adulthood Inflammation: A Meta-Analysis of Peripheral C-Reactive Protein, Interleukin-6 and Tumour Necrosis Factor-α," *Molecular Psychiatry* 21 (2016): 642–9.

40. R. Francescone, V. Hou, and S. Grivennikov, "Microbiome, Inflammation, and Cancer," *Cancer Journal* 20, no. 3 (2014): 181–9.

41. Ibid.

42. Crohn's and Colitis Foundation of America, "Bringing to Light the Risk of Colorectal Cancer among Crohn's & Ulcerative Colitis Patients," Accessed June 2016, http://www.ccfa.org/resources/risk-of-colorectal-cancer.html; S. Sebastian et al., "Colorectal Cancer in Inflammatory Bowel Disease: Results of the 3rd ECCO Pathogenesis Scientific Workshop(I)," *Journal of Crohn's and Coilitis* 8, no. 1 (2014): 5–18.

43. National Cancer Institute, "Fact Sheet—Cell Phones and Cancer Risk," May 27, 2016. www.cancer.gov/cancertopics/factsheet/Risk/cellphones.

44. American Cancer Society, "Can Infections Cause Cancer?," September 24, 2014, www.cancer.org/Cancer/CancerCauses/OtherCarcinogens/InfectiousAgents/InfectiousAgentsandCancer/infectious-agents-and-cancer-intro.

45. Ibid.

46. Centers for Disease Control and Prevention, "Put Vaccination on Your Back to School List," August 5, 2015, https://www.cdc.gov/features/hpvvaccine.

47. Ibid.; American Cancer Society, "Cancer Facts and Figures," 2016; National Cancer Institute, "Fact Sheet–HPV and Cancer," February 19, 2015, www.cancer.gov/cancertopics/factsheet/Risk/HPV.

48. American Cancer Society, "Cancer Facts and Figures," 2016.

49. Ibid.

50. American Cancer Society, "Infections That Can Lead to Cancer," May 2014, www.cancer.org/cancer/cancercauses/othercarcinogens/infectiousagents/infectiousagentsandcancer/infectious-agents-and-cancer-toc.

51. American Cancer Society, "Cancer Facts and Figures," 2016.

52. Ibid.

53. American Lung Association, "Lung Cancer Fact Sheet," Accessed June 2016, http://www.lung.org/lung-health-and-diseases/lung-disease-lookup/lung-cancer/learn-about-lung-cancer/lung-cancer-fact-sheet.html.

54. American Cancer Society, "Why Non-Smokers Get Lung Cancer," October 30, 2015, http://www.cancer.org/cancer/news/features/why-lung-cancer-strikes-nonsmokers.

55. Ibid.

56. American Cancer Society, "Cancer Facts and Figures," 2016.

57. Ibid.

58. Ibid.

59. American Cancer Society, "Benefits of Quitting Over Time," November 13, 2105, http://www.cancer.org/healthy/stayawayfromtobacco/benefits-of-quitting-smoking-over-time.

60. American Cancer Society, "Cancer Facts and Figures," 2016.

61. Ibid.

62. Ibid.

63. Ibid.

64. Ibid.

65. American Cancer Society, "Breast MRI (Magnetic Resonance Imaging)," April 25, 2016, http://www.cancer.org/treatment/understandingyourdiagnosis/examsandtestdescriptions/mammogramsandotherbreastimagingprocedures/mammograms-and-other-breast-imaging-procedures-breast-m-r-i.

66. Ibid.

67. U.S. Preventive Services Task Force, "Breast Cancer: Screening, November 2009," December 30, 2013, http://www.uspreventiveservicestaskforce.org/Page/Document/RecommendationStatementFinal/breast-cancer-screening.

68. American Cancer Society, "Cancer Facts and Figures," 2016.

69. Ibid.

70. Ibid.

71. Ibid.

72. Susan G. Komen for the Cure, "Genetic Testing for BRCA1 and BRCA2 Gene," February 4, 2016, ww5.komen.org/BreastCancer/GeneMutationsampGeneticTesting.html.

73. I. Lahart et al., "Physical Activity, Risk of Death and Recurrence in Breast Cancer Survivors: A Systematic Review and Meta-analysis of Epidemiological Studies," *Acta Oncologica* 54, no. 5 (2015): 635–54, doi: 10.3109/0284186X.2014.998275; Y. Wu, D. Zhang, and S. Kang, "Physical Activity and Risk of Breast Cancer: A Meta-Analysis of Prospective Studies," *Breast Cancer Research and Treatment* 137, no. 3 (2013): 869–82.

74. Y. Wu et al., "Meta-Analysis of Studies on Breast Cancer Risk and Diet in Chinese Women," *International Journal of Clinical and Experimental Medicine* 8, no. 11 (2015): 73–85.

75. American Cancer Society, "Colorectal Cancer Facts and Figures, 2014–2016," Accessed June 2016, www.cancer.org/acs/groups/content/documents/document/acspc-042280.pdf; American Cancer Society, "Cancer Facts and Figures," 2016.

76. American Cancer Society, "Colorectal Cancer Facts and Figures, 2014–2016," Accessed June 2016, www.cancer.org/acs/groups/content/documents/document/acspc-042280.pdf; American Cancer Society, "Cancer Facts and Figures," 2016.

77. American Cancer Society, "Cancer Facts and Figures," 2016.

78. Ibid.

79. Ibid.

80. Ibid.

81. Ibid.

82. Ibid.

83. Ibid.

84. National Cancer Institute, "Colorectal Cancer Prevention," February 5, 2016, www.cancer.gov/cancertopics/pdq/prevention/colorectal/Patient/page3#_139.

85. American Cancer Society, "Cancer Facts and Figures," 2015.

86. Ibid.

87. Ibid.

88. Ibid.

89. Skin Cancer Foundation, "Skin Cancer Facts," June 8, 2016, www.skincancer.org/skin-cancer-information/skin-cancer-facts.

90. UCSF School of Medicine, "Melanoma," May 4, 2007, http://www.dermatology.ucsf.edu/skincancer/general/types/melanoma.aspx.

91. C. Heckman et al., "Psychiatric and Addictive Symptoms of Young Adult Female Indoor Tanners," *American Journal of Health Promotion* 28, no. 3 (2014): 168–74.

92. American Cancer Society, "Cancer Facts and Figures," 2016.

93. Ibid.

94. Ibid.

95. Ibid.

96. Ibid.

97. Ibid.

98. Ibid.

99. Ibid.

100. Ibid.

101. Ibid.

102. Ibid.

103. K. Zu, et al. "Dietary Lycopene, Angiogenesis, and Prostate Cancer: A Prospective Study in the Prostate-Specific Antigen Era," *Journal of the National Cancer Institute* 106, no. 2 (2014): 1093–97.

104. American Cancer Society, "Cancer Facts and Figures," 2016.

105. Ibid.

106. Ibid.

107. Ibid.

108. Ibid.

109. Ibid.

110. Ibid.

111. Ibid.

112. National Cancer Institute, "Uterine Cancer," Accessed June 2016, www.cancer.gov/cancertopics/types/endometrial.

113. National Institute of Health, National Cancer Institute, "SEER Stat Fact Sheets: Testis Cancer,"

February 2016, http://seer.cancer.gov/statfacts/html/testis.html.

114. Ibid.

115. American Cancer Society, "Testicular Cancer," February 12, 2016, www.cancer.org/cancer/testicularcancer/detailedguide/testicular-cancer-risk-factors; American Cancer Society, "What Are the Key Statistics About Testicular Cancer?" February 12, 2016, http://www.cancer.org/cancer/testicularcancer/detailedguide/testicular-cancer-key-statistics.

116. Ibid.

117. American Cancer Society, "Cancer Facts and Figures," 2016.

118. Ibid.

119. Ibid.

120. Ibid.

121. Ibid.

122. Ibid.

123. Ibid.

124. Ibid.

125. Centers for Disease Control and Prevention, "Cancer Survivors—United States, 2007," January 16, 2013, Available at http://www.cdc.gov/cancer/dcpc/research/articles/pdf/articlesummary_cancersurvivors.pdf; National Cancer Survivors Day Foundation, "Cancer Survivorship Issues," Accessed June 2016, http://www.ncsd.org/cancer-survivorship-issues.

126. National Cancer Institute, "Dictionary of Cancer Terms," Accessed June 2016, www.cancer.gov/dictionary.

**Pulled statistics:**

p. 465, American Cancer Society, "Cancer Facts & Figures," 2016, Available at http://www.cancer.org/research/cancerfactsstatistics/cancerfactsfigures2016/.

p. 468, American Cancer Society, "Colorectal Cancer Facts and Figures, 2014–2016," Accessed June 2016, www.cancer.org/acs/groups/content/documents/document/acspc-042280.pdf.

## Chapter 18

1. Centers for Disease Control and Prevention, "Chronic Disease Prevention and Health Promotion," May 24, 2016, http://www.cdc.gov/chronicdisease/.

2. A. Chatterjee et al., "Checkup Time. Chronic Disease and Wellness in America: Measuring the Economic Burden in a Changing Nation," *The Milken Institute*, January 2014, Available at http://assets1b.milkeninstitute.org/assets/Publication/ResearchReport/PDF/Checkup-Time-Chronic-Disease-and-Wellness-in-America.pdf.

3. Ibid.

4. American Lung Association, "How Lungs Work," Accessed June 2016, http://www.lung.org/lung-health-and-diseases/how-lungs-work/.

5. American Lung Association, "Estimated Prevalence and Incidence of Lung Disease," May 2014, www.lung.org/finding-cures/our-research/trend-reports/estimated-prevalence.pdf; Centers for Disease Control and Prevention, "Leading Causes of Death," April 27, 2016, www.cdc.gov/nchs/fastats/leading-causes-of-death.htm.

6. National Center for Health Statistics. "FastStats, Chronic Obstructive Pulmonary Disease (COPD) Includes: Chronic Bronchitis and Emphysema, July, 2016. www.cdc.gov/nchs/fastats/copd.htm.

7. Ibid.

8. Centers for Disease Control and Prevention, "Chronic Obstructive Pulmonary Disease (COPD) Includes: Chronic Bronchitis and Emphysema- Summary Health Statistics Tables for U.S. Adults: National Health Interview Survey. 2014-Table A-2," April 2016, Available at http://ftp.cdc.gov/pub/Health_Statistics/NCHS/NHIS/SHS/2014_SHS_Table_A-2.pdf.

9. Centers for Disease Control and Prevention, "Chronic Obstructive Pulmonary Disease (COPD) Includes: Chronic Bronchitis and Emphysema- Summary Health Statistics Tables for U.S. Adults: National Health Interview Survey. 2014-Table A-2," April 2016, Available at http://ftp.cdc.gov/pub/Health_Statistics/NCHS/NHIS/SHS/2014_SHS_Table_A-2.pdf.

10. Ibid.

11. Ibid.

12. National Center for Health Statistics, "Faststats: Asthma," February 2016, www.cdc.gov/nchs/fastats/asthma.htm.

13. Ibid; Centers for Disease Control and Prevention, "Data, Statistics and Surveillance: Asthma Surveillance Data," March 2016, www.cdc.gov/asthma/asthmadata.htm.

14. Asthma and Allergy Foundation of America, "What Causes or Triggers Asthma?" September 2015, www.aafa.org/page/asthma-triggers-causes.

15. Ibid.

16. Ibid; D. Morales et al. "NSAIDexacerbated Respiratory Disease: A Metaanalysis Evaluating Prevalence, Mean Provocative Dose of Aspirin and Increased Asthma Morbidity," *Allergy* 70, no. 7 (2015): 828–835; WebMD, "Aspirin and Other Drugs That Trigger Asthma," Accessed June 2016, www.webmd.com/asthma/guide/medications-trigger-asthma.

17. Centers for Disease Control and Prevention, "FastStats: Asthma," February 2016, www.cdc.gov/nchs/fastats/asthma.htm.

18. Centers for Disease Control and Prevention, "Data, Statistics and Surveillance: Asthma Surveillance Data," March 2016, www.cdc.gov/asthma/asthmadata.htm.

19. National Institute of Allergy and Infectious Diseases, "Allergic Diseases," May 2016, www.niaid.nih.gov/topics/allergicdiseases/Pages/default.aspx.

20. American Academy of Allergy, Asthma, and Immunology, "Allergy Statistics," Accessed June 2016, www.aaaai.org/about-the-aaaai/newsroom/allergy-statistics.aspx.

21. Ibid.

22. Ibid.

23. American College Health Association. *American College Health Association-National College Health Assessment II: Reference Group Executive Summary Fall 2015.* (Hanover, MD: American College Health Association; 2016).

24. Ibid.

25. Ibid; Centers for Disease Control and Prevention, "Allergies and Hay Fever," February 2016: www.cdc.gov/nchs/fastats/allergies.htm.

26. Centers for Disease Control and Prevention, "Allergies and Hay Fever," February, 2016; www.cdc.gov/nchs/fastats/allergies.htm Food Allergy Research and Statistics, "Facts and Statistics," Accessed June 2016, www.foodallergy.org/facts-and-stats.

27. Ibid.

28. National Institute of Allergies and Infectious Diseases, , "Food Allergy, May 2016, www.niaid.nih.gov/topics/foodallergy/Pages/default.aspx.

29. National Library of Medicine.- Medline Plus, "Neurological Diseases," April 2016, www.nlm.nih.gov/medlineplus/neurologicdiseases.html.

30. R. Burch et al., "The Prevalence and Burden of Migraine and Severe Headache in the United States: Updated Statistics from Government Health Surveillance Studies," *Headache: The Journal of Head and Face Pain* 55, no. 1 (2015): 21–34, doi: 10.1111/head.12482.

31. Cleveland Clinic, "Overview of Headaches in Adults," Accessed June 2016, http://my.clevelandclinic.org/health/diseases_conditions/hic_Overview_of_Headaches_in_Adults.

32. Ibid.

33. Ibid.

34. Cleveland Clinic. "Tension-Headaches (also called 'stress' headaches). 2016. http://my.clevelandclinic.org/health/diseases_conditions/hic.

35. Ibid.

36. Ibid.

37. R. Burch et al., "The Prevalence and Burden of Migraine and Severe Headache in the United States," *Headache: The Journal of Head and Face Pain* 55, no. 1 (2015): 21–34; National Institute of Neurological Disorders and Stroke, "NINDS Migraine Information Page," November 3, 2015, www.ninds.nih.gov/disorders/migraine/migraine.htm; American Migraine Foundation, "Types of Headache-Migraine," Accessed June 2016, https://americanmigrainefoundation.org/living-with-migraines/types-of-headachemigraine.

38. American Migraine Foundation, "Types of Headache-Migraine," Accessed June 2016, https://americanmigrainefoundation.org/living-with-migraines/types-of-headache migraine.

39. R. Burch et al., "The Prevalence and Burden of Migraine and Severe Headache in the United States," *Headache: The Journal of Head and Face Pain* 55, no. 1 (2015): 21–34; National Institute of Neurological Disorders and Stroke, "NINDS Migraine Information Page," November 3, 2015, www.ninds.nih.gov/disorders/migraine/migraine.htm; American Migraine

Foundation, "Types of Headache-Migraine," Accessed June 2016, https://americanmigrainefoundation.org/living-with-migraines/types-of-headachemigraine.

40. National Institute of Neurological Disorders and Stroke, NINDS Migraine Information Page," 2015.

41. Ibid.

42. American Migraine Foundation, "Types of Headache-Migraine," 2016.

43. American Migraine Foundation. "Cluster Headaches," Accessed June 2016, https://americanmigrainefoundation.org/living-with-migraines/types-of-headachemigraine/cluster-headaches/.

44. American Migraine Foundation. "Cluster Headaches," Accessed June 2016, https://americanmigrainefoundation.org/living-with-migraines/types-of-headachemigraine/cluster-headaches/; American Migraine Foundation, "Types of Headache-Migraine," 2016.

45. American Migraine Foundation. "Cluster Headaches," Accessed June 2016, https://americanmigrainefoundation.org/living-with-migraines/types-of-headachemigraine/cluster-headaches/; American Migraine Foundation, "Types of Headache-Migraine," 2016.

46. Centers for Disease Control and Prevention, "Epilepsy Fast Facts," February 2016, www.cdc.gov/epilepsy/basics/fast_facts.htm; Lundbeck Foundation, "Epilepsy," March 2014, https://lundbeck.com/global/brain-disorders/disease-areas/other-diseases/epilepsy.

47. National Digestive Diseases Information Clearinghouse, "Digestive Diseases Statistics for the United States," November 2014, www.niddk.nih.gov/health-information/health-statistics/Pages/digestive-diseases-statistics-for-the-united-states.aspx.

48. Centers for Disease Control and Prevention, "Epidemiology of the IBD," March 2015, www.cdc.gov/ibd/ibd-epidemiology.htm; M. Basson et al., "Ulcerative Colitis," *Medscape*, November 18, 2015, http://emedicine.medscape.com/article/183084-overview.

49. Centers for Disease Control and Prevention, "Epidemiology of the IBD," March 2015, www.cdc.gov/ibd/ibd-epidemiology.htm; M. Basson et al., "Ulcerative Colitis," *Medscape*, November 18, 2015, http://emedicine.medscape.com/article/183084-overview.

50. Centers for Disease Control and Prevention, "Epidemiology of the IBD," March 2015, www.cdc.gov/ibd/ibd-epidemiology.htm; M. Basson et al., "Ulcerative Colitis," *Medscape*, November 18, 2015, http://emedicine.medscape.com/article/183084-overview; Crohn's and Colitis Foundation of American, "What Is Ulcerative Colitis?" Accessed June 2016, http://www.ccfa.org/what-are-crohns-and-colitis/what-is-ulcerative-colitis/.

51. Crohn's and Colitis Foundation of American, "What Is Ulcerative Colitis?" Accessed June 2016, http://www.ccfa.org/what-are-crohns-and-colitis/what-is-ulcerative-colitis/.

52. Centers for Disease Control and Prevention, "Epidemiology of the IBD," March 2015, http://www.cdc.gov/ibd/ibd-epidemiology.htm; M. Basson et al., "Ulcerative Colitis," *Medscape*, November 18, 2015, http://emedicine.medscape.com/article/183084-overview; Crohn's and Colitis Foundation of American, "What Is Ulcerative Colitis?" Accessed June 2016, http://www.ccfa.org/what-are-crohns-and-colitis/what-is-ulcerative-colitis/

53. Centers for Disease Control and Prevention, "Epidemiology of the IBD," March 2015, http://www.cdc.gov/ibd/ibd-epidemiology.htm; M. Basson et al., "Ulcerative Colitis," *Medscape*, November 18, 2015, http://emedicine.medscape.com/article/183084-overview; Crohn's and Colitis Foundation of American, "What Is Ulcerative Colitis?" Accessed June 2016, http://www.ccfa.org/what-are-crohns-and-colitis/what-is-ulcerative-colitis/; Herlong, H. F. *Digestive Disorders. The Johns Hopkins White Papers.* Baltimore, MD: Johns Hopkins Medicine, 2013.

54. Crohn's and Colitis Foundation of American, "What is Ulcerative Colitis?" Accessed June 2016, http://www.ccfa.org/what-are-crohns-and-colitis/what-is-ulcerative-colitis/.

55. Ibid.

56. Crohn's and Colitis Foundation of American. "What Is Crohn's disease?" Accessed June, 2016. http://www.ccfa.org/what-are-crohns-and-colitis/what-is-crohns-disease/.

57. Ibid.

58. Centers for Disease Control and Prevention, "Inflammatory Bowel Disease (IBD)," September 2014, www.cdc.gov/ibd.

59. National Institute of Diabetes and Digestive and Kidney Diseases. "Definition and Facts for Irritable Bowel Syndrome," February 23, 2015, www.niddk.nih.gov/health-information/health-topics/digestive-diseases/irritable-bowel-syndrome/Pages/definition-facts.aspx

60. National Institute of Diabetes and Digestive and Kidney Diseases. "Definition and Facts for Irritable Bowel Syndrome," February 23, 2015, www.niddk.nih.gov/health-information/health-topics/digestive-diseases/irritable-bowel-syndrome/Pages/definition-facts.aspx; Herlong, H. F. *Digestive Disorders. The Johns Hopkins White Papers.* Baltimore, MD: Johns Hopkins Medicine, 2013.

61. National Institute of Diabetes and Digestive and Kidney Diseases. "Definition and Facts for Irritable Bowel Syndrome," February 23, 2015, www.niddk.nih.gov/health-information/health-topics/digestive-diseases/irritable-bowel-syndrome/Pages/definition-facts.aspx; Herlong, H. F. *Digestive Disorders. The Johns Hopkins White Papers.* Baltimore, MD: Johns Hopkins Medicine, 2013.

62. Centers for Disease Control, "Data and Statistics, Arthritis," April 14, 2016, www.cdc.gov/arthritis/data_statistics.

63. Centers for Disease Control, "National Arthritis Statistics: Future Burden of Arthritis," April, 2016, www.cdc.gov/arthritis/data_statistics/national-statistics.html#Future Arthritis Burden.

64. Ibid.

65. Centers for Disease Control, "National Arthritis Statistics: Future Arthritis Burden," April 14, 2016, www.cdc.gov/arthritis/data_statistics/national-statistics.html#Future ArthritisBurden; Arthritis Foundation, "Arthritis Facts," June 2015, www.arthritis.org/about-arthritis/understanding-arthritis/arthritis-statistics-facts.php.

66. National Institute of Arthritis and Musculoskeletal and Skin Disease, "Hand-out on Health: Osteoarthritis," April 2015, http://www.niams.nih.gov/health_info/osteoarthritis/.

67. Centers for Disease Control, "National Arthritis Statistics: Future Arthritis Burden," April 14, 2016, www.cdc.gov/arthritis/data_statistics/national-statistics.html#Future ArthritisBurden; Arthritis Foundation, "What Is Rheumatoid Arthritis?" Accessed June 2016, http://www.arthritis.org/about-arthritis/types/rheumatoid-arthritis/what-is-rheumatoid-arthritis.php016

68. Centers for Disease Control, "National Arthritis Statistics: Future Arthritis Burden," April 14, 2016, www.cdc.gov/arthritis/data_statistics/national-statistics.html#Future ArthritisBurden; Arthritis Foundation, "What Is Rheumatoid Arthritis?" Accessed June 2016, http://www.arthritis.org/about-arthritis/types/rheumatoid-arthritis/what-is-rheumatoid-arthritis.php016.

69. Arthritis Foundation, "What Is Rheumatoid Arthritis?" Accessed June 2016. http://www.arthritis.org/about-arthritis/types/rheumatoid-arthritis/what-is-rheumatoid-arthritis.php.

70. International Osteoporosis Foundation, "Epidemiology," Accessed June 2016, www.iofbonehealth.org/epidemiology.

71. Ibid.

72. D. Hoy et al., "The Global Burden of Low Back Pain: Estimates from the Global Burden of Disease 2010 Study," *Annals of Rheumatic Disease* 73 (2014): 968–74.

73. National Information Institute of Neurological Disorders and Stroke, "NINDS Back Pain Information Page," November 2015, www.ninds.nih.gov/disorders/backpain/backpain.htm.

74. Ibid.

75. A. Searle et al., "Exercise Interventions for the Treatment of Chronic Low Back Pain: A Systematic Review and Meta-analysis of Randomized, Controlled Trials," *Clinical Rehabilitation* 29, no. 12(2015):1155-1167.

76. National Institute of Neurological Disorders and Stroke, "Low Back Pain Fact Sheet," NIH Publication no. 03-5161, Updated November 2015, www.ninds.nih.gov/disorders/backpain/detail_backpain.htm.

77. I. Calvo-Munos, A. Gomes-Conesa, and J. Sanches-Meca, "Prevalence of Low Back Pain in Children and Adolescents: A Meta-Analysis," *Pediatrics* 13, no. 14 (2013), www.biomedcentral.com/1471-2431/13/14

78. Centers for Disease Control and Prevention, National Institute of Neurological Disorders, "NINDS Repetitive Motion Disorders Information Page," July 2013, www.ninds.nih.gov/disorders/repetitive_motion/repetitive_motion.htm.

**Pulled statistics:**

p. 483, A. Chatterjee et al., "Checkup Time. Chronic Disease and Wellness in America-Measuring the Economic Burden in a Changing Nation," The Milken Institute, 2014, http://assets1b.milkeninstitute.org/assets/Publication/ResearchReport/PDF/Checkup-Time-Chronic-Disease-and-Wellness-in-America.pdf.

p. 495, H. F. Herlong, *Digestive Disorders, The Johns Hopkins White Papers* (Baltimore: Johns Hopkins Medicine, 2013).

# Chapter 19

1. T. C. Clarke, B. W. Ward, G. Freeman, and J. S. Schiller, "Early release of selected estimates Based on Data from the January–September 2015 National Health Interview Survey," *National Center for Health Statistics*, February 2016, http://www.cdc.gov/nchs/data/nhis/earlyrelease/earlyrelease201602.pdf

2. M. A. Hillen et al., "How Can Communication by Oncologists Enhance Patients' Trust? An Experimental Study," *Annals of Oncology* 25, no. 4 (2014): 896–901; D. D. Quigley et al., "Specialties Differ in Which Aspects of Doctor Communication Predict Overall Physician ratings," *Journal of General Internal Medicine* 29, no. 3 (2014): 447–454.

3. The Joint Commission, "About the Joint Commission," 2016, www.jointcommission.org.

4. J. James, "A New, Evidence-Based Estimate of Patient Harms Associated with Hospital Care," *Journal of Patient Safety* 9, no. 3 (2013): 122–28.

5. Consumer Health, "Patient Rights: Informed Consent," March 2015, http://www.emedicinehealth.com/patient_rights/article_em.htm

6. Cochrane Review, "Industry Sponsorship and Research Outcome." January 2013, Available at http://community-archive.cochrane.org/features/industry-sponsorship-and-research-outcome.

7. Centers for Disease Control and Prevention, "Therapeutic Drug Use," April 27, 2016, www.cdc.gov/nchs/fastats/drug-use-therapeutic.htm.

8. Ibid.

9. L. Gallelli et al., "Safety and Efficacy of Generic Drugs with Respect to Brand Formulation," *Journal of Pharmacology and Pharmacotherapeutics* 4, Supplement 1 (2013): S110–14.

10. National Center for Complementary and Integrative Health, "Complementary, Alternative, or Integrative Health: What's in a Name?," April 2016, www.nccih.nih.gov/health/integrative-health.

11. L. Gallelli et al., "Safety and Efficacy of Generic Drugs with Respect to Brand Formulation," *Journal of Pharmacology and Pharmacotherapeutics* 4, Supplement 1 (2013): S110–14.

12. Ibid.

13. T. C. Clarke et al., "Trends in the Use of Complementary Health Approaches among Adults: United States, 2002–2012," National Health Statistics Reports, no. 79 (Hyattsville, MD: National Center for Health Statistics), February 2015. Available at www.cdc.gov/nchs/data/nhsr/nhsr079.pdf.

14. Ibid.

15. National Center for Complementary and Integrative Health, "Traditional Chinese Medicine: In Depth," April 2016, https://nccih.nih.gov/health/whatiscam/chinesemed.htm.

16. Ibid.

17. National Center for Complementary and Integrative Health, "Ayurvedic Medicine: In Depth," April, 2016, http://nccih.nih.gov/health/ayurveda/introduction.htm.

18. Ibid.

19. Ibid.

20. National Center for Complementary and Integrative Health, "Homeopathy," April 2016, http://nccih.nih.gov/health/homeopathy.

21. Ibid.

22. National Center for Complementary and Integrative Health, "Naturopathy," February 2016, https://nccih.nih.gov/health/naturopathy.

23. Ibid.

24. National Center for Complementary and Integrative Health, "Complementary, Alternative, or Integrative Health: What's in a Name?," April, 2016. www.nccih.nih.gov/health/integrative-health.

25. American Chiropractic Association, "Facts About Chiropractic," Accessed April 2016, http://www.acatoday.org/News-Publications/News/Facts-About-Chiropractic.

26. National Center for Complementary and Integrative Health, "Spinal Manipulation," April, 2016, https://nccih.nih.gov/health/spinalmanipulation.

27. American Chiropractic Association, "Facts About Chiropractic," Accessed April 2016.

28. National Center for Complementary and Integrative Health, "Massage Therapy for Health Purposes," April 2016, https://nccih.nih.gov/health/massage/massageintroduction.htm

29. Ibid.

30. Ibid.

31. Bureau of Labor Statistics, U.S. Department of Labor, "Massage Therapists," *Occupational Outlook Handbook, 2016–2017 Edition,* December 2015, http://www.bls.gov/ooh/healthcare/massage-therapists.htm.

32. National Center for Complementary and Integrative Health, "Acupuncture: In Depth," March 2016, https://nccih.nih.gov/health/acupuncture/introduction.

33. Ibid; R. S. Hinman et al., "Acupuncture for Chronic Knee Pain. A Randomized Clinical Trial," *Journal of the American Medical Association* 312, no. 13 (2014): 1313–22.

34. A. J. Vickers and K. Linde, "Acupuncture for Chronic Pain," *Journal of the American Medical Association* 311, no. 9 (2014): 955–56.

35. National Center for Complementary and Integrative Health, "Acupuncture: In Depth," March 16, 2016, https://nccih.nih.gov/health/acupuncture/introduction#hed2.

36. G. A. Kelley and K. S. Kelley, "Meditative Movement Therapies and Health-Related Quality-of-Life in Adults: A Systematic Review of Meta-Analyses," *PLoS ONE* 10, no. 6 (2015): e0129181, doi: 10.1371/journal.pone.0129181

37. R. Hammerschlag, B. L. Marx, and M. Alckin, "Nontouch Biofield Therapy: A Systematic Review of Human Randomized Controlled Trials Reporting Use of Only Nonphysical Contact Treatment," *Journal of Alternative and Complementary Medicine* 20, no. 12 (2014): 881–92, doi: 10.1089/acm.2014.0017.

38. U.S. Food and Drug Administration, "'Natural' on Food Labeling," May 2016, www.fda.gov/Food/GuidanceRegulation/GuidanceDocumentsRegulatoryInformation/LabelingNutrition/ucm456090.htm.

39. U.S. Pharmacopoeial Convention, "USP Verified Dietary Supplements," Accessed May 2016, http://www.usp.org/usp-verification-services/usp-verified-dietary-supplements.

40. U.S. Food and Drug Administration, "Pink Bikini and Shorts on the Beach Dietary Supplements by Lucy's Weight Loss System: Recall—Undeclared Drug Ingredient," January 2016, http://www.fda.gov/Safety/MedWatch/SafetyInformation/SafetyAlertsforHumanMedicalProducts/ucm484002.htm.

41. National Center for Complementary and Integrative Health, "Using Dietary Supplements Wisely," May 2016, https://nccih.nih.gov/health/supplements/wiseuse.htm.

42. U.S. Centers for Medicare and Medicaid Services, "The Fee for Not Having Health Insurance," Accessed May 2016, https://www.healthcare.gov/fees/fee-for-not-being-covered/.

43. MedlinePlus, "Managed Care," January 2016, https://www.nlm.nih.gov/medlineplus/managedcare.html.

44. Kaiser Family Foundation, "Total HMO Enrollment, July 2015," April 2016, http://kff.org/other/state-indicator/total-hmo-enrollment/

45. U.S. Centers for Medicare and Medicaid Services, "National Health Expenditure Projections 2014–2024," July 2015, www.cms.gov/Research-Statistics-Data-and-Systems/Statistics-Trends-and-Reports/NationalHealthExpendData/Downloads/Proj2014.pdf.

46. National Committee to Preserve Social Security and Medicare, "Fast Facts About Medicare," March 2016, www.ncpssm.org/Medicare.

47. Ibid.

48. J. Paradise, "Medicaid Moving Forward," *The Henry J. Kaiser Family Foundation*, March 9,

2015, http://kff.org/health-reform/issue-brief/medicaid-moving-forward/.

49. U.S. Department of Health & Human Services, "2016 Poverty Guidelines," January 2016, https://aspe.hhs.gov/poverty-guide lines.

50. U.S. Department of Health & Human Services, "The Affordable Care Act Is Work-ing," June 2015, http://www.hhs.gov/healthcare/facts-and-features/fact-sheets/aca-is-working/index.html

51. U.S. Centers for Medicare and Medicaid Services, "Children's Health Insurance Pro-gram," July 2015, www.medicaid.gov/chip/chip-program-information.html

52. National Conference of State Legislators, "Health Insurance: Premiums and Increases," April 2016, www.ncsl.org/issues-research/health/health-insurance-premiums.aspx.

53. T. C. Clarke, B. W. Ward, G. Freeman, and J. S. Schiller, "Early Release of Selected Estimates Based on Data from the January-September 2015 National Health Interview Survey," *National Center for Health Statistics*, February 2016, http://www.cdc.gov/nchs/data/nhis/earlyrelease/earlyrelease201602.pdf.

54. Ibid.

55. American College Health Association, *American College Health Association–National College Health Assessment II: Reference Group Executive Summary. Spring 2015* (Hanover, MD: American College Health Association, 2015).

56. Bureau of Labor Statistics, U.S. Department of Labor, "Physicians and Surgeons," *Occupational Outlook Handbook, 2016-2017 Edition*, December 2015, www.bls.gov/ooh/healthcare/physicians-and-surgeons.htm

57. American Hospital Association, "Fast Facts on U.S. Hospitals," January 2016, www.aha.org/research/rc/stat-studies/fast-facts.shtml.

58. O. W. Brawley, *How We Do Harm: A Doctor Breaks Ranks about Being Sick in America* (New York: St. Martin's Press, 2011).

59. U.S. Centers for Medicare and Medicaid Services, "National Health Expenditure Projections 2015–2025," July 2016.

60. Ibid.

61. U.S. Centers for Medicare and Medicaid Services, "The 80/20 Rule: How Insurers Spend Your Health Insurance Premiums," February 2013, https://www.cms.gov/CCIIO/Resources/Files/Downloads/mlr-report-02-15-2013.pdf.

62. L. S. Dafny, "Evaluating the Impact of Health Insurance Industry Consolidation: Learning from Experience," *The Commonwealth Fund*, November 20, 2015, http://www.commonwealthfund.org/publications/issue-briefs/2015/nov/evaluating-insurance-industry-consolidation.

63. Ibid.

64. Central Intelligence Agency, "Country Comparison: Life Expectancy at Birth, 2015 Estimates," *CIA World Factbook*, April 2016, https://www.cia.gov/library/publications/the-world-factbook/rankorder/2102rank.html.

65. Ibid.

66. Central Intelligence Agency, "Country Comparison: Infant Mortality Rate, 2015 Estimates," *CIA World Factbook*, April 2016, https://www.cia.gov/library/publications/the-world-factbook/rankorder/2091rank.html.

67. Department of Health and Human Services, "The National Quality Strategy: Fact Sheet," September 2014, http://www.ahrq.gov/workingforquality/nqs/nqsfactsheet.htm.

68. T. C. Clarke, B. W. Ward, G. Freeman, and J. S. Schiller, "Early Release of Selected Estimates Based on Data from the January-September 2015 National Health Interview Survey," February 2016.

**Pulled statistics:**

p. 504, U. S. Centers for Disease Control and Prevention, "Hospital Utilization," February 2016, www.cdc.gov/nchs/fastats/hospital.htm.

p. 513, T. C. Clarke et al., "Trends in the Use of Complementary Health Approaches among Adults: United States, 2002–2012," *National Health Statistics Reports*, no. 79 (Hyattsville, MD: National Center for Health Statistics), February 2015. Available at www.cdc.gov/nchs/data/nhsr/nhsr079.pdf.

p. 523, J. James, "New Evidence-Based Estimates of Patient Harms Associated with Hospital Care," *Journal of Patient Safety* 9, no. 3 (2013): 122–8.

# Chapter 20

1. Voltaire, "Semiramis," V.1, trans. by J. K. Hoyt, in *The Cyclopaedia of Practical Quotations*, 1896. New York: Funk & Wagnalls Company.

2. World Health Organization, *World Report on Violence and Health* (Geneva: World Health Organization, 2002), Available at www.who.int/violence_injury_prevention/violence/world_report/en.

3. Ibid.

4. Centers for Disease Control and Prevention, "Deaths, Percent of Total Deaths, and Death Rates for the 15 Leading Causes of Death: United States and Each State, 1999–2014," June 1, 2016, http://www.cdc.gov/nchs/nvss/mortality/lcwk1.htm.

5. WHO, "Youth Violence: The Health Sector Role in Prevention and Response," 2015, http://www.who.int/violence_injury_prevention/violence/youth/yv_infographic_small.pdf?ua=1; World Health Organization, "Violence Prevention—The Evidence," 2010, http://apps.who.int/iris/bitstream/10665/77936/1/9789241500845_eng.pdf.

6. U.S. Department of Justice, Federal Bureau of Investigation, *Crime in the United States, Preliminary Semiannual Uniform Crime Report for January–June 2015*, 2015, https://www.fbi.gov/about-us/cjis/ucr/crime-in-the-u.s/2015/preliminary-semiannual-uniform-crime-report-januaryjune-2015/tables/table-3.

7. L. Langton and J. Truman, "Criminal Victimization-2014," Bureau of Justice Statistics, August 27, 2015, http://www.bjs.gov/index.cfm?ty=pbdetail&iid=5366.

8. C. Barnett-Ryan, L. Langton, M. Planty, "The Nation's Two Crime Measures," September 18, 2014, *Bureau of Justice Statistics,* www.bjs.gov/index.cfm?ty=pbdetail&iid=5112; Bureau of Justice Statistics, "Reporting Crimes to Police," February 11, 2015, www.bjs.gov/index.cfm?ty=tp&tid=96.

9. U.S. Department of Justice, Federal Bureau of Investigation, *Crime in the United States, Preliminary Semiannual Uniform Crime Report for January–June 2015*, 2015, https://www.fbi.gov/about-us/cjis/ucr/crime-in-the-u.s/2015/preliminary-semiannual-uniform-crime-report-januaryjune-2015/tables/table-3.

10. L. Langton and J. Truman, "Criminal Victimization-2014," Bureau of Justice Statistics, August 27, 2015, http://www.bjs.gov/index.cfm?ty=pbdetail&iid=5366.

11. Ibid.

12. American College Health Association, *American College Health Association—National College Health Assessment II: Reference Group Data Report, Fall, 2015* (Baltimore, MD: American College Health Association, 2016)

13. Ibid.

14. Ibid.

15. National Criminal Justice Reference Service, "Section 6: Statistical Overviews," *NCVRW Resource Guide*, 2014, http://ovc.ncjrs.gov/ncvrw2014/pdf/StatisticalOverviews.pdf.

16. Center for Public Integrity, "Sexual Assault on Campus: A Frustrating Search for Justice," Updated February 2013, www.public integrity.org/accountability/education/sexual-assault-campus.

17. World Health Organization Violence Prevention Alliance, "The Ecological Frame-work," Accessed June 2016, www.who.int/violenceprevention/approach/ecology/en/index.html; Centers for Disease Control and Prevention, National Center for Injury Prevention and Control, "Understanding School Violence: Fact Sheet—2015," Accessed June 2016, http://www.cdc.gov/violence prevention/pdf/School_Violence_Fact_Sheet-a.pdf.

18. R. Felner and M. DeVries, "Poverty in Child-hood and Adolescence: A Transactional-Ecological Approach to Understanding and Enhancing Resilience in Contexts of Disad-vantage and Developmental Risks," in *Hand-book of Resilience in Children* (2013): 105–126, New York: Springer; American Psychological Association, "Violence and Socioeconomic Status," Accessed June 2014, www.apa.org/pi/ses/resources/publications/factsheet-violence.aspx.

19. World Health Organization Violence Prevention Alliance, "The Ecological Frame-work," Accessed June 2014, www.who.int/violenceprevention/approach/ecology/en/index.html; L. Kiss et al., "Gender-based Violence and Socioeconomic Inequalities: Does Living in More Deprived Neighbor-hoods Increase Women's Risk of Intimate Partner Violence?," *Social Science and Medicine* 74, no. 8 (2012): 1172–79.

20. M. L. Hunt, A. W. Hughey, and M. G. Burke, "Stress and Violence in the Workplace and on Campus: A Growing Problem for Business, Industry and Academia," *Industry and Higher Education* 26, no. 1 (2012): 43–51.

21. T. Dishion, "A Developmental Model of Aggression and Violence: Microsocial and Macrosocial Dynamic within an Ecological Framework," *Handbook of Developmental Psychology* (Springer US, 2014): 449–65. New York.

22. K. Makin-Byrd and K. L. Bierman, "Individual and Family Predictors of the Perpetration of Dating Violence and Victimization in Late Adolescence," *Journal of Youth Adolescence* 42, no. 4 (2013): 536–50, doi: 10.1007/s10964-012-9810-7; J. H. Derzon, "The Correspondence of Family Features with Problem, Aggressive, Criminal and Violent Behaviors: A Meta-Analysis," *Journal of Experimental Criminology* 6, no. 3 (2010): 263–92, doi: 10.1007/s11292-010-9098-0; C. Cook et al., "Predictors of Bullying and Victimization in Childhood and Adolescence: A Meta-Analytic Investigation," *School Psychology Quarterly* 25, no. 2 (2010): 65–83.

23. R. Puff and J. Segher, *The Everything Guide to Anger Management: Proven Techniques to Understand and Control Anger* (Adams Media, Inc. A Division of F. and W. Media, 2014). Avon, MA.

24. N. Fernandez-Castillo and B. Cormand, "Aggressive Behavior in Humans: Genes and Pathways Identified through Association Studies," *American Journal of Medical Genetics Part B: Neuropsychiatric Genetics* 171(2016): 676–696; P. Asherson and B. Cormand, "The Genetics of Aggression: Where are We Now?" *American Journal of Medical Genetics Part B: Neuropsychiatric Genetics* 171, no. 5 (2016): 559–561; D. Boisvert and J. Vaske, "Genetic Theories of Criminal Behavior," *The Encyclopedia of Criminology and Criminal Justice* (2014): 1–6, Boston, MA: Wiley-Blackwell.

25. S. Swearer and S. Hymel, "Understanding the Psychology of Bullying: Moving toward a Social-ecological Diathesis–stress Model," *American Psychologist* 70, no. 4(2015): 344–353; M. Nielsen et al., "Post-traumatic Stress Disorder as a Consequence of Bullying at Work and at School: A Literature Review and Meta-analysis," *Aggression and Violent Behavior* 21(2015):17–24. Doi:10.1016/j.avb.2015.01.001.)

26. S. Swearer and S. Hymel, "Understanding the Psychology of Bullying: Moving Toward a Social-Ecological Diatheses-Stress model," *American Psychologist* 70, no. 4 (2015): 344; W. Gunter and B. Newby, "From Bullied to Deviant: The Victim-Offender-Overlap among Bullying Victims," *Youth Violence and Juvenile Justice* 13, no. 1(2015): 3–17

27. C. Crane, et al., "The Proximal Effects of Acute Alcohol Consumption on Male-to-Female Aggression: A Meta-analytic Review of the Experimental Literature," *Trauma, Violence, & Abuse.* (2015): 1524838015584374. [Epub ahead of print]; S. Valdebenito, M. Ttofi, and M. Eisner, "Prevalence Rates of Drug Use Among School Bullies and Victims: A Systematic Review and Meta-analysis of Cross-Sectional studies," *Aggression and Violent Behavior* 23 (2015): 137–146; K. M Devries et al., "Intimate Partner Violence Victimization and Alcohol Consumption in Women: A Systematic Review and Meta-Analysis," *Addiction* 109 (2014): 379–91, doi: 10.1111/add.12393; A. Sanderlund et al. "The Association Between Sports Participation, Alcohol Use and Aggression and Violence: A Systematic Review," *Journal of Science and Medicine in Sport* 17, no. 1 (2014): 2–7.

28. C. Cunradi, "Discrepant Patterns of Heavy Drinking, Marijuana Use, and Smoking and Intimate Partner Violence: Results From the California Community Health Study of Couples," *Journal of Drug Education* 45, no. 2 (2015): 73–95.

29. Ibid.

30. A. Sanderlund et al., "The Association Between Sports Participation, Alcohol Use and Aggression and Violence: A Systematic Review," *Journal of Science and Medicine in Sport* 17, no. 1 (2014): 2–7.

31. C. Love et al., "Understanding the Connection between Suicide and Substance Abuse: What the Research Tells Us," SAMHSA Webinar Series, September 11, 2014, http://captus.samhsa.gov/sites/default/files/capt_resource/webcast_suicide_and_substance_abuse_part_1_sept_11_2014_final.pdf.

32. C. Ferguson, "Does Media Violence Predict Societal Violence? It Depends on What you Look at and When?" *Journal of Communication* 65, no. 1(2015):E1-E22; W. Gunter and K. Daley, "Causal or Spurious? Using Propensity Score Matching to Detangle the Relationship between Violent Video Games and Violent Behavior," *Computers in Human Behavior* 4, no. 28 (2012): 1348–55.

33. T. Greitemeyer and D. Mugge, "Video Games Do Affect Social Outcomes: A Meta-Analytic Review of the Effects of Violent and Prosocial Video Game Play," *Personality and Social Psychology Bulletin* 40, no. 5 (2014): 578–89.

34. C. J. Ferguson et al, "Not Worth the Fuss After All? Cross-Sectional and Prospective Data on Violent Video Game Influences on Aggression, Visuospatial Cognition and Mathematics Ability in a Sample of Youth," *Journal of Youth and Adolescence* 42, no. 1 (2013): 109–22.

35. R. A. Ramos et al., "Comfortably Numb or Just Yet Another Movie? Media Violence Exposure Does NOT Reduce Viewer Empathy for Victims of Real Violence Among Primarily Hispanic Viewers," *Psychology of Popular Media Culture* 2, no. 1 (2013): 2–10.

36. ChildStats.Gov, "America's Children in Brief: Key National Indicators of Well-Being, 2012," Accessed June 2014, http://childstats.gov/pdf/ac2012/ac_12.pdf.

37. Centers for Disease Control and Prevention, "Youth Violence: Definitions," March 2016, www.cdc.gov/violenceprevention/youth violence/definitions.html; L. L. Dahlberg and E. G. Krug, "Violence: A Global Public Health Problem," in *World Report on Violence and Health* (Geneva: World Health Organization, 2002), 1–21.

38. Centers for Disease Control and Prevention, "Health, United States, 2015," April 2016, http://www.cdc.gov/nchs/data/hus/hus15.pdf

39. U. S. Department of Justice, Federal Bureau of Investigation, "Crime in the United States, 2014: Expanded Homicide Data, Table 10," Accessed July 2016, Available at https://www.fbi.gov/about-us/cjis/ucr/crime-in-the-u.s/2014/crime-in-the-u.s.-2014/offenses-known-to-law-enforcement/expanded-homicide;

40. Ibid.

41. Centers for Disease Control and Prevention, "Health, United States, 2015," April 2016, http://www.cdc.gov/nchs/data/hus/hus15.pdf

42. Bureau of Justice Statistics. "Hate Crime," February 11, 2016, http://www.bjs.gov/index.cfm?ty=tp&tid=37#summary.

43. Federal Bureau of Investigation, "Latest Hate Crime Statistics Available," November 16, 2015, https://www.fbi.gov/news/stories/2015/november/latest-hate-crime-statistics-available.

44. Ibid.

45. Bureau of Justice Statistics, "Hate Crime Victimization-2004-2012-Statistical Tables," February 2014, www.bjs.gov/index.cfm?ty=pbdetail&iid=4883.

46. Ibid.

47. Centers for Disease Control and Prevention-Injury Prevention and Control, "The National Intimate Partner and Sexual Violence Survey," May 2015, http://www.cdc.gov/violenceprevention/nisvs/index.html.

48. American Psychological Association, "Intimate Partner Violence—Facts and Resources," Accessed June 2016, http://www.apa.org/topics/violence/partner.aspx.

49. Ibid.

50. Centers for Disease Control and Prevention-Injury Prevention and Control, "The National Intimate Partner and Sexual Violence Survey," May 2015, http://www.cdc.gov/violenceprevention/nisvs/index.html.

51. American Psychological Association, "Intimate Partner Violence—Facts and Resources," Accessed June 2016, http://www.apa.org/topics/violence/partner.aspx.

52. Ibid.

53. L. Walker, *The Battered Woman* (New York: Harper and Row, 1979).

54. L. Walker, *The Battered Woman Syndrome*, 3rd ed. (New York: Springer, 2009).

55. M. Breiding et al., "Intimate Partner Violence Surveillance: Uniform Definitions and Recommended Data Elements, Version 2.0," Center for Disease Control and Prevention, 2015, Available at http://www.cdc.gov/violenceprevention/pdf/intimatepartner violence.pdf; American Psychological Association, "Intimate Partner Violence—Facts and Resources," Accessed June 2016, http://www.apa.org/topics/violence/partner.aspx.

56. Centers for Disease Control and Prevention, "Understanding Intimate Partner Violence Fact Sheet," 2014, Available at https://www.cdc.gov/violenceprevention/pdf/ipv-factsheet.pdf; M. Breiding et al., "Intimate Partner Violence Surveillance: Uniform Definitions and Recommended Data Elements,

56. Version 2.0," Center for Disease Control and Prevention, 2015, Available at http://www.cdc.gov/violenceprevention/pdf/intimate-partnerviolence.pdf.

57. Centers for Disease Control and Prevention, "Understanding Intimate Partner Violence Fact Sheet," 2014, Available at https://www.cdc.gov/violenceprevention/pdf/ipv-factsheet.pdf; M. Breiding et al., "Intimate Partner Violence Surveillance: Uniform Definitions and Recommended Data Elements, Version 2.0," Center for Disease Control and Prevention, 2015, Available at http://www.cdc.gov/violenceprevention/pdf/intimatepartnerviolence.pdf.

58. Centers for Disease Control and Prevention, "Understanding Intimate Partner Violence Fact Sheet," 2014, Available at https://www.cdc.gov/violenceprevention/pdf/ipv-factsheet.pdf; M. Breiding et al., "Intimate Partner Violence Surveillance: Uniform Definitions and Recommended Data Elements, Version 2.0," Center for Disease Control and Prevention, 2015, Available at http://www.cdc.gov/violenceprevention/pdf/intimatepartnerviolence.pdf.

59. Child Welfare Information Gateway. (2013). *What Is Child Abuse and Neglect? Recognizing the Signs and Symptoms.* Washington, DC: U.S. Department of Health and Human Services, Children's Bureau.

60. Childhelp, "Child Abuse Statistics and Facts," Accessed July 2016, www.childhelp.org/child-abuse-statistics.

61. Ibid.

62. Centers for Disease Control and Prevention, "Understanding Elder Abuse, Fact Sheet 2016," Accessed July 2016, https://www.cdc.gov/violenceprevention/pdf/em-factsheet-a.pdf.

63. I. Quellet-Morin, et al., "Intimate Partner Violence and New Onset Depression: A Longitudinal Study of Women's Childhood and Adult Histories of Abuse," *Depression and Anxiety* 32, no. 5 (2015): 316–324.

64. Federal Bureau of Investigation. "Preliminary Semiannual Uniform Crime Report. Data Declaration," 2015, https://www.fbi.gov/about-us/cjis/ucr/crime-in-the-u.s/2015/preliminary-semiannual-uniform-crime-report-januaryjune-2015/tables/table-3/table_3_january_to_june_2015_percent_change_for_consecutive_years.xls/@@template-layout-view?override-view=data-declaration.

65. M. Breiding et al., "Prevalence and Characteristics of Sexual Violence, Stalking, and Intimate Partner Violence Victimization—National Intimate Partner and Sexual Violence Survey, United States, 2011," *Morbidity and Mortality Weekly Report* 63, no. SS08 (2014): 1–18, Available at www.cdc.gov/mmwr/preview/mmwrhtml/ss6308a1.htm?s_cid=ss6308a1_e.

66. Ibid.

67. White House Task Force to Protect Students from Sexual Assault, *Not Alone: First Report of White House Task Force to Protect Students from Sexual Assault,* April 2014, www.whitehouse.gov/sites/default/files/docs/report_0.pdf.

68. The Federal Register, "The Daily Journal of the United States Government: Violence Against Women Act," October 20, 2014, Available at https://www.federalregister.gov/articles/2014/10/20/2014-24284/violence-against-women-act#print_view.

69. National Criminal Justice Reference Service, "School and Campus Crime," *Resource Guide*, Accessed June 2014, www.victimsofcrime.org/docs/ncvrw2013/2013ncvrw_stats_school.pdf?sfvrsn=0.

70. N. Anderson, "These Campuses Have the Most Reports of Rape," *The Washington Post*, June 7, 2016, https://www.washingtonpost.com/news/grade-point/wp/2016/06/07/these-colleges-have-the-most-reports-of-rape/.

71. White House Task Force to Protect Students from Sexual Assault, "Not Alone," 2014.

72. A. Jackson, "State Contexts and the Criminalization of Marital Rape Across the United States," *Social Science Research* 51 (2015): 290–306.

73. National Children's Alliance, "CAC Statistics," Accessed June 2016. http://www.nationalchildrensalliance.org/cac-statistics.

74. The Children's Assessment Center, "Child Sexual Abuse Facts," Accessed June 2016, http://cachouston.org/child-sexual-abuse-facts/; RAIN. Child Sexual Abuse. Accessed June, 2016. https://www.rainn.org/articles/child-sexual-abuse; Childhelp, "Child Abuse in America—2014," Accessed June, 2016; U.S. Department of Health and Human Services, Children's Bureau, "Child Maltreatment," 2013, www.acf.hhs.gov/sites/default/files/cb/cm2012.pdf.

75. The Children's Assessment Center, "Child Sexual Abuse Facts," Accessed June 2016, http://cachouston.org/child-sexual-abuse-facts/; RAIN. Child Sexual Abuse. Accessed June, 2016. https://www.rainn.org/articles/child-sexual-abuse; Childhelp, "Child Abuse in America—2014," Accessed June, 2016; U.S. Department of Health and Human Services, Children's Bureau, "Child Maltreatment," 2013, www.acf.hhs.gov/sites/default/files/cb/cm2012.pdf.

76. M. Bouroughs, et al., "Complexity of Childhood Sexual Abuse: Predictors of Current Post-Traumatic Stress Disorder, Mood Disorders, Substance Use, and Sexual Risk Behavior Among Adult Men Who Have Sex with Men," *Archives of Sexual Behavior* 44, no. 7 (2015): 1891–1902; Childhelp, "Child Abuse in America—2014," Accessed June, 2016; T. Hilberg, C. Hamilton-Giachrtsis, and L. Dixon, "Review of Meta-Analyses on the Association Between Child Sexual Abuse and Adult Mental Health Difficulties: A Systematic Approach," *Trauma, Violence, & Abuse* 12, no. 1 (2011): 38–49.

77. Childhelp, "Child Abuse in America—2014," Accessed June, 2016

78. Oregon State University, Sexual Harassment and Sexual Violence, Accessed June 2016, http://eoa.oregonstate.edu/sexual-harassment-and-violence-policy.

79. Centers for Disease Control, "Sexual Violence, Stalking, and Intimate Partner Violence Widespread in the US," NISVS 2010 Summary Report, Press Release, December 2011.

80. National Criminal Justice Reference Service (NCVRW), "Crime Victimization in the United States: Statistical Overviews," in *NCVRW Resource Guide-2012*, June 2014, www.ncjrs.gov/ovc_archives/ncvrw/2012/pdf/StatisticalOverviews.pdf.

81. Centers for Disease Control and Prevention, "Sexual Violence, Stalking, and Intimate Partner Violence Widespread in the US," 2011; National Criminal Justice Reference Service (NCVRW), "Crime Victimization in the United States: Statistical Overviews," in *NCVRW Resource Guide—2012*, Accessed June 2014, Available at www.ncjrs.gov/ovc_archives/ncvrw/2012/pdf/Statistical-Overviews.pdf.

82. M. Breiding et al., "Prevalence and Characteristics of Sexual Violence, Stalking, and Intimate Partner Violence Victimization," 2014.

83. Centers for Disease Control and Prevention, "Sexual Violence, Stalking, and Intimate Partner Violence Widespread in the US," 2011; NCVRW "Crime Victimization in the United States," 2014.

84. Stopbullying.gov, "Facts About Bullying," October 14, 2014, http://www.stopbullying.gov./news/media/facts#listing.

85. E. Lund and S. Ross, "Bullying Perpetration, Victimization, and Demographic Differences in College Students: A Review of the Literature," *Trauma, Violence, & Abuse* (2016): 1524838015620818.

86. FBI, "National Gang Report, 2015," 2015, Available at https://www.fbi.gov/stats-services/publications/national-gang-report-2015.pdf; U.S. Department of Justice, "Juvenile Justice Fact Sheet—Highlights of the 2012 National Youth Gang Survey," December 2014, www.ojjdp.gov/pubs/248025.pdf; Federal Bureau of Investigation, "2013 National Gang Threat Assessment-Emerging Trends," February 2015, www.fbi.gov/stats-services/publications/national-gang-report-2013.

87. FBI, "2013 National Gang Threat Assessment," 2015.

88. Violence Prevention Institute, "Why People Join Gangs and What You Can Do," Accessed June 2016, http://www.violenceprevention-institute.com/youngpeople.html.

89. U.S. Code of Federal Regulations, Title 28CFR0.85.

**Pulled statistics:**

p. 537, K. Carey et al., "Incapacitated and Forcible Rape of College Women: Prevalence across the First Year," *Journal of Adolescent Health* 56, no. 6 (2015): 678–80.

p. 539, Bureau of Justice Statistics, "Female Victims of Sexual Violence, 1994–2010," Revised May 31, 2016, Available at http://www.bjs.gov/content/pub/pdf/fvsv9410.pdf.

## Chapter 20A

1. Centers for Disease Control and Prevention, "The 10 Leading Causes of Death in the United States by Age2014. 2015. Leading

Causes of Death by Age Group, United States–2014 https://www.cdc.gov/injury/wisqars/pdf/leading_causes_of_death_by_age_group_2014-a.pdf.

2. Centers for Disease Control and Prevention, "10 Leading Causes of Death by Age Group, United States–2014," February 25, 2016, Available at http://www.cdc.gov/injury/wisqars/leadingcauses.html.

3. Ibid.

4. Centers for Disease Control and Prevention, "10 Leading Causes of Injury Deaths by Age Group Highlighting Unintentional Injury Deaths, United States, 2014," February 25, 2016, Available at www.cdc.gov/injury/wisqars/leadingcauses.html.

5. Ibid.

6. NHTSA, "The Fatality Analysis Reporting System (FARS) and the National Automotive Sampling System (NASS) General Estimates System (GES)," Data Webinar, January 15, 2015, www.nrd.nhtsa.dot.gov.

7. National Highway Traffic Safety Administration, "Traffic Safety Facts, 2014 Data: Alcohol-Impaired Driving," December 2015, www.nrd.nhtsa.dot.gov/Pubs/812231.pdf

8. Ibid.

9. Ibid.

10. National Institute on Drug Abuse, "Drug Facts: Drugged Driving," Revised June 2016, www.drugabuse.gov/publications/drugfacts/drugged-driving.

11. Ibid.

12. S. Salomonsen-Sautel et al., "Trends in Fatal Motor Vehicle Crashes Before and After Marijuana Commercialized in Colorado," *Drug and Alcohol Dependence* 140 (2014): 137–44.

13. National Institute on Drug Abuse, "Drug Facts: Drugged Driving," Revised June 2016, www.drugabuse.gov/publications/drugfacts/drugged-driving.

14. Centers for Disease Control and Prevention, "Drowsy Driving: Asleep at the Wheel," November 5, 2015, www.cdc.gov/features/dsDrowsyDriving.

15. Centers for Disease Control and Prevention, "Distracted Driving," March 7, 2016, www.cdc.gov/motorvehiclesafety/distracted_driving/.

16. Ibid.

17. Ibid.

18. Ibid.

19. United States Department of Transportation, "Distraction.gov: State Laws," Accessed May 2015, www.distraction.gov/stats-research-laws/state-laws.html.

20. National Highway Traffic Safety Administration, "Aggressive Driving," Accessed June 2016, www.nhtsa.gov/Aggressive.

21. C.M. Richard et al., "Motivations for Speeding: Volume 1: Summary Report," National Highway Traffic Safety Administration, available at www.nhtsa.gov.

22. Ibid.

23. National Highway Traffic Safety Administration, "Quick Facts 2014," March 2016, Available at http://www-nrd.nhtsa.dot.gov/Pubs/812234.pdf.

24. Centers for Disease Control and Prevention, "Policy Impact: Seat Belts," Updated January 2014, www.cdc.gov/Motorvehiclesafety/seatbeltbrief.

25. National Highway Traffic Safety Administration, "Traffic Safety Facts: 2014 Data," March 2016, www-nrd.nhtsa.dot.gov/Pubs/812246.pdf.

26. National Highway Traffic Safety Administration, "Quick Facts 2014," March 2016, Available at http://www-nrd.nhtsa.dot.gov/Pubs/812234.pdf.

27. Insurance Institute for Highway Safety, "Vehicle Size and Weight," March 2016, www.iihs.org/iihs/topics/t/vehicle-size-and-weight/qanda.

28. Ibid.

29. Insurance Institute for Highway Safety, "Motorcycles and ATVs," February 2016, www.iihs.org/iihs/topics/t/motorcycles/fatalityfacts/motorcycles.

30. National Highway Traffic Safety Administration, "Traffic Safety Facts: 2014 Data," 2016.

31. Ibid.

32. National Highway Traffic Safety Administration, "Quick Facts 2014," March 2016, Available at http://www-nrd.nhtsa.dot.gov/Pubs/812234.pdf.

33. Ibid.

34. Insurance Institute for Highway Safety, "Motorcycle Helmet Use," May 2016, http://www.iihs.org/iihs/topics/laws/helmetuse.

35. National Highway Traffic Safety Administration, *Traffic Safety Facts 2014 Data,* 2016.

36. National Highway Traffic Safety Administration, "Bicyclists and Other Cyclists," May 2015, www-nrd.nhtsa.dot.gov/Pubs/812151.pdf.

37. Insurance Institute for Highway Safety, "Pedestrians and bicyclists," February 2016, http://www.iihs.org/iihs/topics/t/pedestrians-and-bicyclists/fatalityfacts/bicycles.

38. Consumer Product Safety Commission, "CPSC Fact Sheet: Skateboarding Safety," CPSC Publication 93 (2012), Available at www.cpsc.gov/PageFiles/122356/093.pdf.

39. T. Waters, "2015 Skateboarding Fatalities," April 17, 2016, Skaters for Public Skateparks, http://www.skatepark.org/park-development/2016/04/2015-skateboarding-fatalities/.

40. Consumer Product Safety Commission, "CPSC Fact Sheet: Skateboarding Safety," CPSC Publication 93 (2012).

41. National Ski Areas Association, "Fatality Fact Sheet," October 15, 2015, www.nsaa.org/media/254886/Fatality_Fact_Sheet_10_15_2015.pdf.

42. National Ski Areas Association, "Fatality Fact Sheet," October 15, 2015, www.nsaa.org/media/254886/Fatality_Fact_Sheet_10_15_2015.pdf.

43. National Ski Areas Association, "Fatality Fact Sheet," October 15, 2015, www.nsaa.org/media/254886/Fatality_Fact_Sheet_10_15_2015.pdf.

44. College of Optometrists, "Look After Your Eyes: Skiing," Accessed May 2016, http://lookafteryoureyes.org/eye-care/sun-and-sunshine/skiing.

45. Centers for Disease Control and Prevention, "10 Leading Causes of Injury Deaths by Age Group Highlighting Unintentional Injury Deaths, United States, 2014," February 25, 2016, Available at www.cdc.gov/injury/wisqars/leadingcauses.html.

46. Ibid; Centers for Disease Control and Prevention, "Unintentional Drowning: Get the Facts," April 28, 2016, www.cdc.gov/HomeandRecreationalSafety/Water-Safety/waterinjuries-factsheet.html.

47. Centers for Disease Control and Prevention, "Unintentional Drowning: Get the Facts," April 28, 2016, www.cdc.gov/HomeandRecreationalSafety/Water-Safety/waterinjuries-factsheet.html.

48. Ibid.

49. U. S. Coast Guard, "Coast Guard News: U.S. Coast Guard Releases 2014 Recreational Boating Statistics Report," May 13, 2015, http://www.uscgnews.com/go/doc/4007/2504554/US-Coast-Guard-releases-2014-Recreational-Boating-Statistics-Report.

50. Ibid.

51. Ibid.

52. U. S. Coast Guard, "Boating Safety Resource Center: BUI Initiatives," April 2014, www.uscgboating.org/recreational-boaters/boating-under-the-influence.php.

53. American Boating Association, "Boating Safety—It Could Mean Your Life," 2015, www.americanboating.org/safety.asp.

54. Y. Tu and D. V. Granados, "2014 Fireworks Annual Report," U.S. Consumer Product Safety Commission, June 2015, www.cpsc.gov.

55. National Council on Fireworks Safety, "Key Fireworks Safety Information," Accessed May 2016, www.fireworksafety.com.

56. Centers for Disease Control and Prevention, "Opioid Overdose," March 16, 2016, www.cdc.gov/drugoverdose/; Centers for Disease Control and Prevention, "10 Leading Causes of Injury Deaths by Age Group Highlighting Unintentional Injury Deaths, United States, 2014," February 25, 2016, Available at www.cdc.gov/injury/wisqars/leadingcauses.html.

57. J. B. Mowry et al., "2014 Annual Report of the American Association of Poison Control Centers' National Poison Data System (NPDS): 32nd Annual Report," *Clinical Toxicology* 53, no. 10 (2015): 962–1147, doi: 10.3109/15563650.2015.1102927.

58. American Association of Poison Control Centers, "Prevention," February 2015, www.aapcc.org/prevention

59. Centers for Disease Control and Prevention, "10 Leading Causes of Injury Deaths by Age Group Highlighting Unintentional Injury Deaths, United States, 2014," February 25, 2016, Available at www.cdc.gov/injury/wisqars/leadingcauses.html.

60. Centers for Disease Control and Prevention, "Important Facts About Falls," January 20, 2016, www.cdc.gov/homeandrecreationalsafety/falls/adultfalls.html.

61. U.S. Fire Administration, "U.S. Fire Deaths, Fire Death Rates, and Risks of Dying in a Fire," April 27, 2016, www.usfa.fema.gov/data/statistics/fire_death_rates.html.

62. U.S. Fire Administration, "Campus Fire Fatalities in Residential Buildings (2000–2015)," November 2015, https://www.usfa.fema.gov/downloads/pdf/publications/campus_fire_fatalities_report.pdf.

63. U.S. Fire Administration, "Campus Fire Fatalities in Residential Buildings (2000–2015)," November 2015, https://www.usfa.fema.gov/downloads/pdf/publications/campus_fire_fatalities_report.pdf.

64. Ibid.

65. American Heart Association, "Hands-Only CPR," Accessed May 2016, http://handsonlycpr.org.

66. National Institute on Deafness and Other Communication Disorders (NIDCD), "Quick Statistics About Hearing" May 19, 2016, www.nidcd.nih.gov/health/statistics/quick-statistics-hearing.

67. Ibid.

68. J. A. G. Balanay and G. D. Kearney, "Attitudes Toward Noise, Perceived Hearing Symptoms, and Reported Use of Hearing Protection Among College Students: Influence of Youth Culture," *Noise and Health* 17, no. 19 (2015): 394–405.

69. K. Hannah et al., "Evaluation of the Olivocochlear Efferent Reflex Strength in the Susceptibility to Temporary Hearing Deterioration After Music Adults," *Noise and Health* 16, no. 69 (2014): 108–15, doi: 10.4103/1463-1741.132094.

70. U. S. Bureau of Labor Statistics, "2014 Census of Fatal Occupational Injuries Summary," April 21, 2016, www.bls.gov/iif/oshwc/cfoi/cftb0286.pdf.

71. U. S. Bureau of Labor Statistics, "2014 Census of Fatal Occupational Injuries Summary," April 21, 2016, www.bls.gov/iif/oshwc/cfoi/cftb0286.pdf.

72. U. S. Bureau of Labor Statistics, "2014 Census of Fatal Occupational Injuries Summary," April 21, 2016, www.bls.gov/iif/oshwc/cfoi/cftb0286.pdf.

73. National Institute of Neurological Disorders and Stroke, "Low Back Pain Fact Sheet," November 3, 2015, www.ninds.nih.gov/disorders/backpain/detail_backpain.htm.

74. American College Health Association, *American College Health Association—National College Health Assessment: Reference Group Executive Summary*, Spring, 2015. (Baltimore, MD: American College Health Association, 2015.) www.acha-ncha.org.

75. Department of Homeland Security, "Build a Kit," Accessed June 2016, https://www.ready.gov/build-a-kit; CDC, "Emergency Preparedness and Reponse: Gather Emergency Supplies," January 14, 2016, https://emergency.cdc.gov/.

**Pulled statistics:**

p. 550, Centers for Disease Control and Prevention, "Drug Overdose Deaths Hit Record Numbers in 2014," December 18, 2015, http://www.cdc.gov/media/releases/2015/p1218-drug-overdose.html.

p. 552, American College Health Association, *American College Health Association–National College Health Assessment II: Reference Group Executive Summary Spring 2015* (Hanover, MD: American College Health Association, 2015).

## Chapter 21

1. World Wildlife Fund, "Living Planet Index," July 2015, wwf.panda.org/about_our_earth/all_publications/living_planet_report/living_planet_index2.

2. Mead, M. *Male and Female: A Study of Sexes in a Changing World*. (1950). London: Gollancz.

3. P. Gerland et al., "World Population Stabilization Unlikely This Century," *Science* 346, no. 6206 (2014): 231–37; Worldwatch Institute, "U.N. Raises 'Low' Population Projections for 2050," updated July 7, 2016., www.worlwatch.org/node/6038.

4. United Nations, Department of Economic and Social Affairs, Population Division (2015). World Population Prospects: The 2015 Revision, Key Findings and Advance Tables. Working Paper No. ESA/P/WP.241. *Available at* https://esa.un.org/unpd/wpp/publications/files/key_findings_wpp_2015.pdf.

5. United Nations Environmental Programme, "Rate of Environmental Damage Increasing Across the Planet but There Is Still Time to Reverse Worst Impacts if Governments Act Now, UNEP Assessment Says," May 19, 2016, www.unep.org/newscentre/Default.aspx?DocumentID=27074&ArticleID=36180&l=en

6. Population Reference Bureau, "World Population Data Sheet," 2015, http://www.prb.org/pdf15/2015-world-population-data-sheet_eng.pdf; Population Reference Bureau, "2014 World Population Data Sheet, 2014: The Decline in U.S. Fertility," Accessed July 2016, www.prb.org/Publications/Datasheets/2014/2014-world-population-data-sheet/us-fertility-decline-factsheet.aspx.

7. Central Intelligence Agency, *The World Factbook: Country Comparison: Total Fertility Rate*, Accessed July 2014, https://www.cia.gov/library/publications/the-world-factbook/rankorder/2127rank.html.

8. U.S. Census Bureau, Population Division, "International Database Country Rankings," Accessed July 2016, http://sasweb.ssd.census.gov/idb/ranks.html.

9. United States Census Bureau, "U.S. and World Population Clock," July 2016, http://www.census.gov/popclock.

10. Ibid; Global Footprint Network, "Key Findings of the National Footprint Accounts, 2016 Edition," June 8, 2016., http://www.footprintnetwork.org/en/index.php/GFN/page/footprint_data_and_results.

11. World Wildlife Fund, "Living Planet Index," 2015.

12. United Nations, *UNEP Yearbook: Emerging Issues in our Global Environment, 2014*, 2015, http://www.unep.org/yearbook/2014/.

13. G. Ceballos et al., "Accelerated Modern Human-induced Species Losses: Entering the Sixth Mass Extinction," *Science Advances* 1, no. 5 (2015): e1400253, doi: 10.1126/sciadv.1400253.

14. The IUCN Red List of Threatened Species, "IUCN Red List Status: Mammals," June 2015, www.iucnredlist.org/initiatives/mammals/analysis/red-list-status.

15. Ibid.

16. G. Whillemyer et al., "Illegal Killing for Ivory Drives Global Decline in African Elephants," *Proceedings of the National Academy of Sciences* 111, no. 36 (2014): 13117–121; W. Ripple, et al., "Collapse of the World's Largest Herbivores," *Science Advances* 1, no. 4 (2015): e1400103.

17. The IUCN Red List of Threatened Species, "IUCN Red List Status: Amphibians," 2014.

18. United Nations, *Global Environment Outlook*, Accessed July, 2016, http://www.unep.org/geo/.

19. United Nations, "UNEP Yearbook, 2014," 2015.

20. Ibid.

21. United Nations, *UNEP Yearbook: Emerging Issues in our Global Environment, 2014*, 2015, http://www.unep.org/yearbook/2014/.

22. United Nations Environmental Program, "Towards a Green Economy: Pathways to Sustainable Development and Poverty Eradication," June 2011, www.unep.org/greeneconomy/greeneconomyreport/tabid/29846/default.aspx; V. Christenson et al., "A Century of Fish Biomass Decline in the Ocean," *Marine Ecology Program Series* 512 (2014): 155–166, doi: 10.3354/meps10946.

23. Ibid.

24. Institute for Energy Research, "China: World's Largest Energy Consumer and Greenhouse Gas Emitter," May 20, 2015, http://instituteforenergyresearch.org/analysis/china-worlds-largest-energy-consumer-and-greenhouse-gas-emitter/.

25. U.S. Energy Information Administration, "Today in Energy-International Energy Outlook-2016." June, http://www.eia.gov/forecasts/ieo/.

26. U.S. Environmental Protection Agency, "Air Enforcement," December, 2015. https://www.epa.gov/enforcement/air-enforcement.

27. U.S. Environmental Protection Agency, "Overview of Greenhouse Gases: Carbon Dioxide Emissions," May 26, 2016, https://www3.epa.gov/climatechange/ghgemissions/gases/co2.html.

28. Ibid.

29. S. M. Platt et al., "Two-Stroke Scooters Are a Dominant Source of Air Pollution in Many Cities," *Nature Communications* 5 (2014), doi:10.1038/ncomms4749. (Epub ahead of print.)

30. Environmental Protection Agency, "Air Trends," February 23, 2016, https://www3.epa.gov/airtrends/; American Lung Association, "State of the Air-2016," Accessed July 2016, http://www.lung.org/assets/documents/healthy-air/state-of-the-air/sota-2016-full.pdf.

31. American Lung Association, "State of the Air-2016," Accessed July 2016, http://www.lung.org/assets/documents/healthy-air/state-of-the-air/sota-2016-full.pdf.

32. Ibid.

33. U.S. Environmental Protection Agency, "Acid Rain," May 2016, https://www.epa.gov/acidrain.

34. Ibid.; A. Soos, "Acid Rain Change," *Environmental News Network*, 2013, www.enn.com.

35. U.S. Environmental Protection Agency, "Effects of Acid Rain," March 31, 2016. https://www.epa.gov/acidrain/effects-acid-rain.

36. U.S. Environmental Protection Agency, "An Introduction to Indoor Air Quality," March 16, 2016, https://www.epa.gov/indoor-air-quality-iaq/introduction-indoor-air-quality.

37. Ibid.

38. Ibid.

39. American Nonsmoker's Rights Foundation, "Smokefree Lists, Maps and Data," July 1, 2016, http://www.no-smoke.org/going smokefree.php?id=519.

40. U.S. Environmental Protection Agency, "Radon," May 17, 2016. https://www.epa.gov/radon.

41. U.S. Environmental Protection Agency, "Health Risk of Radon," June 21, 2016, https://www.epa.gov/radon/health-risk-radon.

42. Centers for Disease Control and Prevention, "Lead," June 2016, www.cdc.gov/nceh/lead/; Centers for Disease Control and Prevention, "Blood Lead Levels in Children Aged 1–5 Years—United States, 1999–2010," *Morbidity and Mortality Weekly Report* 62, no. 13 (2013): 245–48, Available at www.cdc.gov.

43. U.S. Department of Housing and Urban Development, "Making Homes Healthier for Families," Accessed July 2016, http://portal.hud.gov/hudportal/HUD?src=/program_offices/healthy_homes/healthyhomes.

44. National Center for Environmental Health, "Mold: Basic Facts," May 2014, www.cdc.gov/mold/faqs.htm#affect.

45. The Environmental Illness Resource, "Sick Building Syndrome," May 5, 2016. http://www.ei-resource.org/illness-information/related-conditions/sick-building-syndrome/.

46. T. Stafford, "Indoor Air Quality and Academic Performance," Accessed June 2014, http://research.economics.unsw.edu.au/RePEc/papers/2013-25.pdf.

47. U.S. Environmental Protection Agency, "Evidence from Scientific Literature About Improved Academic Performance," November 2015, https://www.epa.gov/iaq-schools/evidence-scientific-literature-about-improved-academic-performance.

48. U.S. Environmental Protection Agency, "Overview of Greenhouse Gases: Emissions and Trends: Carbon Dioxide," 2014; U.S. Global Change Research Group, "Climate Change Impacts in the United States," May 2014, Available at http://nca2014.global change.gov/downloads/report; National Aeronautics and Space Administration, "Ozone Hole Watch," July 2016, http://ozonewatch.gsfc.nasa.gov.

49. American Association for the Advancement of Science, "What We Know: The Reality, Risks, and Response to Climate Change," Accessed July 2016, Available at http://whatweknow.aaas.org/wp-content/uploads/2014/07/whatweknow_website.pdf; J. Cook, et al. "Consensus on Consensus: A Synthesis of Consensus Estimates on Human-caused Global Warming," *Environmental Research Letters* 11, no. 4 (2016): 048002.

50. U.S. Global Research Program, "Understand Climate Change," Accessed July 2016, http://www.globalchange.gov/climate-change; American Association for the Advancement of Science, "What We Know: The Reality, Risks, and Response to Climate Change," Accessed July 2016, Available at http://whatweknow.aaas.org/wp-content/uploads/2014/07/whatweknow_website.pdf; J. Cook, et al. "Consensus on Consensus: A Synthesis of Consensus Estimates on Human-caused Global Warming," *Environmental Research Letters* 11, no. 4 (2016): 048002.

51. American Association for the Advancement of Science, "What We Know: The Reality, Risks, and Response to Climate Change," Accessed July 2016, Available at http://whatweknow.aaas.org/wp-content/uploads/2014/07/whatweknow_website.pdf.

52. U.S. Global Change Research Group, "Climate Change Impacts in the United States," May 2014, Available at http://nca2014.global change.gov/downloads/report; NASA, "Climate Change: How Do We Know?," Accessed July 2016, http://climate.nasa.gov/evidence/; U.S. Global Change Research Program, "The Impacts of Climate Change on Human Health in the United States: A Scientific Assessment," April 2016, https://health2016.globalchange.gov.

53. Environmental Protection Agency, "Climate Change Facts: Answers to Common Questions," February 2016, https://www3.epa.gov/climatechange/basics/facts.html; The National Academy of Sciences, "Attribution of Extreme Weather Events in the Context of Climate Change," 2016, https://nas-sites.org/americasclimatechoices/other-reports-on-climate-change/2016-2/attribution-of-extreme-weather-events-in-the-context-of-climate-change; Environmental Protection Agency, "Climate Change Facts: Answers to Common Questions," February 23, 2016, https://www3.epa.gov/climatechange/basics/facts.html; The National Academy of Sciences, "Attributions of Extreme Weather Events in the Context of Climate Change," 2016. https://nas-sites.org/americasclimate choices/other-reports-on-climate-change/2016-2/attribution-of-extreme-weather-events-in-the-context-of-climate-change/.

54. NASA, "Global Climate Change" Accessed July 2016, http://climate.nasa.gov/; Environmental Protection Agency, "Climate Change Facts: Answers to Common Questions," 2016; J. Olivier et al., "Trends in Global $CO_2$ Emissions—2015 Report," 2015, http://edgar.jrc.ec.europa.eu/news_docs/jrc-2015-trends-in-global-co2-emissions-2015-report-98184.pdf; NASA, "Global Climate Change: A Blanket Around the Earth," Accessed July 2016, http://climate.nasa.gov/causes/; NOAA, "Greenhouse Gases," Accessed July 2016, https://www.ncdc.noaa.gov/monitoring-references/faq/greenhouse-gases.php.

55. J. Cook, et al. "Consensus on Consensus: A Synthesis of Consensus Estimates on Human-Caused Global Warming," *Environmental Research Letters* 11, no. 4 (2016): 048002; NASA, "Global Climate Change," 2016.

56. J. Cook, et al. "Consensus on Consensus: A Synthesis of Consensus Estimates on Human-Caused Global Warming," *Environmental Research Letters* 11, no. 4 (2016): 048002; NASA, "Global Climate Change," 2016; J. Olivier et al., "Trends in Global $CO_2$ Emissions—2015 Report," 2015. http://edgar.jrc.ec.europa.eu/news_docs/jrc-2015-trends-in-global-co2-emissions-2015-report-98184.pdf.

57. J. C. L. Olivier et al., "Trends in Global $CO_2$ Emissions—2015 Report," 2015; Environmental Protection Agency, "National Greenhouse Gas Emissions Data," April 2014, www.epa.gov/climatechange/ghgemissions/usinventoryreport.html.

58. J. C. L. Olivier et al., "Trends in Global $CO_2$ Emissions—2015 Report," 2015; Environmental Protection Agency, "National Greenhouse Gas Emissions Data," April 2014, www.epa.gov/climatechange/ghgemissions/usinventoryreport.html.

59. United Nations. "The Future We Want—Sustainable Development, 2012, https://sustainabledevelopment.un.org/future wewant.html..

60. D. Vine, Center for Climate and Energy Solutions, "Achieving the United States' Intended National Determined Contributions," April 2016, http://www.c2es.org/docUploads/achieving-us-indc.pdf

61. Ibid.

62. J. C. L. Olivier et al., "Trends in Global $CO_2$ Emissions–2015 Report," 2015.

63. Ibid.

64. Ibid.

65. Ibid.

66. International Renewable Energy Agency, "Letting in the Light: How Solar Photovoltaics Will Revolutionise the Electricity System," Accessed July 2016, http://www.irena.org/menu/index.aspx?mnu=Subcat&PriMenuID=36&CAtID=141&SubcatID=2735.

67. Solar Energy Industries Association (SEIA), "Solar Industry Data," Accessed July 2016, http://www.seia.org/research-resources/solar-industry-data.

68. Ibid.

69. Conserve Energy Future. "What Are Alternative Energy Sources?" Accessed July, 2016. http://www.conserve-energy-future.com/AlternativeEnergySources.php

70. Ibid.

71. Environmental Defense Fund, "Cap and Trade—How Cap and Trade Works, 2015, www.edf.org/climate/how-cap-and-trade-works.

72. OSU Sustainability Initiative. "Eco 2 Go Reusable Food container Program" 2016. http://uhds.oregonstate.edu/dining/sustainability-initiative.

73. The Water Information Program, "Water Facts," June 2015, www.waterinfo.org/resources/water-facts.

74. Ibid.

75. Ibid.

76. Ibid.

77. Pacific Institute, "Water Use Trends in the United States," April 2015, http://pacinst.org/wp-content/uploads/sites/21/2015/04/Water-Use-Trends-Report.pdf.

78. Ibid; United States Geological Survey. "Water Questions & Answers. How Much Water Does the Average Person Use at Home per Day?" May 2016, http://water.usgs.gov/edu/qa-home-percapita.html.

79. Pacific Institute, "Water Use Trends in the United States," April 2015, http://pacinst.org/wp-content/uploads/sites/21/2015/04/Water-Use-Trends-Report.pdf.

80. The Water Information Program, "Water Facts," June 2015, www.waterinfo.org/resources/water-facts.

81. Director of National Intelligence, "Worldwide Threat Assessment of the Intelligence Community," January 9, 2014, www.dni.gov/files/documents/Intelligence%20Reports/2014%20WWTA%20%20SFR_SSCI_29_Jan.pdf.

82. The Milken Institute Global Conference, "Solving the Global Water Challenge," May 3, 2016 http://www.milkeninstitute.org/events/conferences/global-conference/2016/panel-detail/6175; World Economic Forum, "Global Agenda Council on Water Security 2012–2014," June 2015, www3.weforum.org/docs/GAC/2013/Connect/WEF_GAC_Water_Security_2012-2014_Connect.pdf; Water Information Program. "Water Facts," 2015.

83. Director of National Intelligence, "Global Water Security," 2012; World Economic Forum, "Global Agenda Council on Water Security 2012–2014," 2014.

84. U.S. Geological Survey, "National Water Quality Assessment Program" June 2015, http://water.usgs.gov/nawqa;.

85. M. Kostich, A. Batt, and J. Lazorcheck, "Concentrations of Prioritized Pharmaceuticals in Effluents from 50 Large Wastewater Treatment Plants in the U.S. and Implications for Risk Estimation," *Environmental Pollution* 184 (2014): 354–59.

86. J. Donn, et al, "Pharmaceuticals Found in Drinking Water, Affecting Wildlife and Maybe Humans," *Associated Press*, Accessed July 2016, http://hosted.ap.org/specials/interactives/pharmawater_site/day1_01.html.

87. M. Kostich, A. Batt, and J. Lazorcheck, "Concentrations of Prioritized Pharmaceuticals in Effluents from 50 Large Wastewater Treatment Plants in the U.S. and Implications for Risk Estimation," *Environmental Pollution* 184 (2014): 354–59.

88. Environmental Protection Agency, Office of Underground Storage Tanks, "Underground Storage Tanks- 2015," June 2016, https://www.epa.gov/ust.

89. Ibid.

90. Ibid.

91. Environmental Protection Agency, "Natural Gas Extraction: Hydraulic Fracturing," April 27, 2016, https://www.epa.gov/hydraulicfracturing.

92. Agency for Toxic Substances and Disease Registry (ATSDR), "Toxic Substances Portal: Polychlorinated Biphenyls (PCBs)," August 2014, http://www.atsdr.cdc.gov/toxfaqs/tf.asp?id=140&tid=26.

93. U.S. Environmental Protection Agency, "Pesticides," July 6, 2016, https://www.epa.gov/pesticides.

94. U.S. Environmental Protection Agency, "Advancing Sustainable Materials Management 2013 Fact Sheet—Assessing Trends in Material Generation, Recycling and Disposal in the United States," June 2015, www.epa.gov/epawaste/nonhaz/municipal/pubs/2013_advncng_smm_fs.pdf.

95. Ibid.

96. Ibid.

97. U.S. Environmental Protection Agency, "Superfund: Superfund National Accomplishments Summary, Fiscal Year 2015," May, 2016, www.epa.gov/superfund/accomp/pdfs/FY_2013_SF_EOY_accomp_sum_FINAL.pdf.

98. U.S. Environmental Protection Agency, "Hazardous Waste," June 2015, www.epa.gov/osw/basic-hazard.htm; U.S. Environmental Protection Agency, "Household Hazardous Waste," March 10, 2016, http://www.epa.gov/osw/conserve/materials/hhw.htm.

99. U.S. Nuclear Regulatory Commission, "Radiation Basics," 2014, www.nrc.gov/about-nrc/radiation/health-effects/radiation-basics.html.

100. Ibid.

101. National Council on Radiation Protection and Measurements, "NCRP Report No. 160 Section 1 Pie Chart," 2010, http://ncrponline.org/publications/reports/ncrp-report-160-pie-charts/.

102. International Atomic Energy Agency, "IAEA Issues Projections for Nuclear Power from 2020–2050," November 2, 2015, www.iaea.org/newscenter/news/iaea-issues-projections-nuclear-power-2020-2050; U.S. Energy Information Administration, "Independent Statistics and Analysis," 2012.

103. R. Balmforth, "Factbox: Key Facts on Chernobyl Nuclear Accident," Reuters, March 15, 2011, www.reuters.com/article/2011/03/15/uk-nuclear-chernobyl-facts-idUSTRE72E69R20110315.

104. M. Penny and M. Selden, "The Severity of the Fukushima Daiichi Nuclear Disaster: Comparing Chernobyl and Fukushima," *Global Research*, 2011, www.globalresearch.ca/PrintArticle.php?articleId=24949.

**Pulled statistics:**

p. 563, Population Reference Bureau, "2015 World Population Data Sheet," 2015, http://www.prb.org/pdf13/2013-population-data-sheet_eng.pdf.

p. 578, U.S. Environmental Protection Agency, "Advancing Sustainable Materials Management, 2013 Fact Sheet," June 2015, Available at https://www.epa.gov/sites/production/files/2015-09/documents/2013_advncng_smm_fs.pdf.

# Chapter 22

1. J. C. Cavanaugh and F. Blanchard-Fields, *Adult Development and Aging*, 7th ed. (Belmont, CA: Wadsworth, Cengage Learning, 2014); S. Hillier and G. Barrow, *Aging, the Individual, and Society*, 10th ed. (Belmont, CA: Wadsworth, Cengage Learning, 2014).

2. National Institute on Aging, "Biology of Aging," January 22, 2015, Available at www.nia.nih.gov/health/publication/biology-aging/preface; S. Krauss, "Fulfillment at Any Age," *Psychology Today*, June 23, 2012, www.psychologytoday.com/blog/fulfillment-any-age/201206/what-s-your-true-age.

3. A. Harmell et al. "Resilience-Building Intervention for Successful and Positive Aging." In H. Lavretsky, et al. Complementary and Integrative Therapies for Mental Health and Aging. Oxford University Press. 2016; S. Krauss, "Fulfillment at Any Age," *Psychology Today*, June 23, 2012, www.psychologytoday.com/blog/fulfillment-any-age/201206/what-s-your-true-age.

4. Central Intelligence Agency, *The World Factbook. Country Comparisons: Life Expectancy at Birth,* 2014, www.cia.gov/library/publications/the-world-factbook/rankorder/2102rank.html.

5. U.S. Department of Health and Human Services, "Profile of Older Americans: 2015," Accessed June 2016, http://www.aoa.acl.gov/aging_statistics/profile/2015/3.aspx.

6. Ibid.

7. U.S. Department of Health and Human Services, "Projected Future Growth of the Older Population," *Administration on Aging, (2014).* http://www.aoa.acl.gov/Aging_Statistics/future_growth/future_growth.aspx.

8. U.S. Department of Health and Human Services, "Profile of Older Americans: 2015," Accessed June 2016, http://www.aoa.acl.gov/aging_statistics/profile/2015/3.aspx.

9. Ibid.

10. Ibid.

11. Ibid.

12. Genworth, "Compare Long-Term Care Costs Across the United States," February 2015, www.genworth.com/corporate/about-genworth/industry-expertise/cost-of-care.html

13. Ibid; U.S. Department of Health and Human Services, "Profile of Older Americans: 2015," Accessed June 2016, http://www.aoa.acl.gov/aging_statistics/profile/2015/3.aspx.

14. M. Stibich, "Wear and Tear Theory of Aging," *Verywell*, March 3, 2016, https://www.verywell.com/wear-and-tear-theory-of-aging-2224235.

15. N. W. Shock, "Aging," *Encyclopaedia Britannica* May 12, 2016, http://www.britannica.com/science/aging-life-process.

16. Ibid.

17. Ibid.

18. Administration on Aging, "A Profile of Older Americans," 2014.

19. International Osteoporosis Foundation, "Epidemiology," Accessed June 2016, https://www.iofbonehealth.org/epidemiology.

20. Centers for Disease Control and Prevention, "Arthritis-Related Statistics," April 2016, www.cdc.gov/arthritis/data_statistics/arthritis_related_stats.htm

21. U.S. National Library of Medicine, "Aging Changes in the Face," October 2014, https://www.nlm.nih.gov/medlineplus/ency/article/004004.htm.

22. J. Weinstein et al., "The Aging Kidney," *NIH-Advanced Chronic Kidney Disease* 17, no. 4 (2011): 302–307; Merck Manual Consumer Version, "Effects of Aging on Urinary Tract," June 2015, www.merck manuals.com.

23. Ibid.

24. Mayo Clinic, "Urinary Incontinence: Causes," August 7, 2014, http://www.mayoclinic.org/diseases-conditions/urinary-incontinence/basics/causes/.

25. Mayo Clinic, "Urinary Incontinence: Treatments and Drugs," August 7, 2014, http://www.mayoclinic.org/diseases-conditions/urinary-incontinence/basics/treatment/con-20037883.

26. U.S. National Library of Medicine, "Aging Changes in the Heart and Blood Vessels," September 2014, https://www.nlm.nih.gov/medlineplus/ency/article/004006.htm.

27. U.S. National Library of Medicine, "Aging Changes in the Lungs, October 2014, https://www.nlm.nih.gov/medlineplus/ency/article/004011.htm.

28. P. Roland et al., "Presbycusis," *Medscape*, November 24, 2015, http://reference.medscape.com/article/855989-overview#a6.

29. T. E. Howe et al., "Exercise for Improving Balance in Older People," *Cochrane Database of Systematic Reviews* (2012), www.cochrane.org/CD004963/MUSKINJ_exercise-for-improving-balance-in-older-people.

30. Medline Plus, "Aging Changes in the Senses," 2014, https://www.nlm.nih.gov/medlineplus/ency/article/004013.htm.

31. Ibid.

32. Ibid.

33. L. Stein, "Sex and Seniors: The 70-Year Itch," *HealthDay,* January 20, 2016 https://consumer.healthday.com/encyclopedia/aging-1/misc-aging-news-10/sex-and-seniors-the-70-year-itch-647575.html; M. N. Lochlainne et al., "Sexual Activity and Aging," *Journal of American Medical Directors Association* 14, no. 8 (2013): 565–72.

34. Benjamin Rose, "Sexually Transmitted Diseases in Older Adults, Accessed June 2016, http://www.benrose.org/Resources/article-stds-older-adults.cfm.

35. M. Smith et al., "Age-Related Memory Loss: What's Normal, What's Not and When to Seek Help," HelpGuide.Org, Accessed June 2016, http://www.helpguide.org/articles/memory/age-related-memory-loss.htm.

36. S. Hayes et al., "Physical Activity is Positively Associated with Episodic Memory in Aging," *Journal of the International Neuropsychological Society* 21, no. 10 (2015): 780–790.

37. M. Smith et al., "Age-Related Memory Loss: What's Normal, What's Not and When to Seek Help," HelpGuide.Org, Accessed June 2016, http://www.helpguide.org/articles/memory/age-related-memory-loss.htm.

38. Alzheimer's Association, "Quick Facts: Prevalence," 2016, http://www.alz.org/facts/#prevalence

39. Ibid.

40. Ibid.

41. Ibid.

42. Ibid.

43. Ibid.

44. Ibid.

45. Ibid.

46. Centers for Disease Control and Prevention, "Depression Is Not a Normal Part of Growing Older," March 2015, http://www.cdc.gov/aging/mentalhealth/depression.htm.

47. Centers for Disease Control and Prevention, "Important Facts About Falls," January 2016, http://www.cdc.gov/homeandrecreational safety/falls/adultfalls.html.

48. H.A. Bischoff-Ferrari, "Monthly High Dose Vitamin D Treatment for Prevention of Functional Decline," *JAMA Internal Medicine* 176, no. 2 (2016): doi:10.1001/jamainternmed.2015.7148.

49. I. Young Kim et al., "Quantity of Dietary Protein Intake, but Not Pattern of Intake, Affects Net Protein Balance Primarily Through Differences in Protein Synthesis in Older Adults," *American Journal of Physiology Endocrinology and Metabolism* 308, no. 1 (2015): E21–E28.

50. (L. Stein, "Seniors and Alcohol Abuse," *Health Day* (2016). https://consumer.healthday.com/encyclopedia/aging-1/misc-aging-news-10/seniors-and-alcohol-abuse-646138.html.

51. National Council on Alcoholism and Drug Dependence, "Alcohol, Drug Dependence and Seniors, June 2015, https://www.ncadd.org/about-addiction/seniors/alcohol-drug-dependence-and-seniors.

52. Centers for Disease Control and Prevention, "Health, United States, 2013," June 2016, Available at www.cdc.gov/nchs/hus.htm.

53. Substance Abuse and Mental Health Services Administration, "Specific Populations and Prescription Drug Misuse and Abuse," October 2015, http://www.samhsa.gov/prescription-drug-misuse-abuse/specific-populations.

54. National Institute on Drug Abuse, "Prescription Drug Abuse," November 2014, https://www.drugabuse.gov/publications/research-reports/prescription-drugs/trends-in-prescription-drug-abuse/older-adults.

55. Ibid.

56. Substance Abuse and Mental Health Services Administration, "Specific Populations and Prescription Drug Misuse and Abuse," October 2015, http://www.samhsa.gov/prescription-drug-misuse-abuse/specific-populations.

57. R. Powell, "Millennials' New Retirement Number? $1.8 million (or more!)," March 29, 2016, http://www.usatoday.com/story/money/columnist/powell/2016/03/29/millennials-new-retirement-number-18-million-more/81329246/.

58. Ibid.

59. U.S. Department of Health and Human Services, "Health, United States, 2015," 2015 http://www.cdc.gov/nchs/data/hus/hus15.pdf#014.

60. By permission. From *Merriam-Webster's Collegiate® Dictionary*, 11th Edition © 2014 by Merriam-Webster, Inc., Available at www.Merriam-Webster.com

61. President's Commission on the Uniform Determination of Death, *Defining Death: Medical, Ethical and Legal Issues in the Determination of Death* (Washington, DC: U.S. Government Printing Office, 1981).

62. Ad Hoc Committee of the Harvard Medical School to Examine the Definition of Brain Death, "A Definition of Irreversible Coma," *Journal of the American Medical Association* 205 (1968): 377.

63. Elisabeth Kübler-Ross, *On Death and Dying* (New York: Scribner, 2014).

64. M. K. Shear, "Complicated Grief," *The New England Journal of Medicine* 372, no. 2 (2015): 153–160.

65. R. Perper, "Worden's Four Tasks of Grieving," *Therapy Changes,* May 26, 2015, http://therapychanges.com/blog/2015/05/review-wordens-four-tasks-of-grieving/.

66. Kidshealth.org.nz, "Helping Your Child After Their Sister, Brother or Cousin Has Died," Accessed June 2016, http://www.kidshealth.org.nz/helping-your-child-after-their-sister-brother-or-cousin-has-died; Dr. Christina Hibbert, "Siblings & Grief: 10 Things Everyone Should Know" Accessed June 2016, http://www.drchristinahibbert.com/dealing-with-grief/siblings-grief-10-things-everyone-should-know/.

67. Dr. Christina Hibbert, "Siblings & Grief: 10 Things Everyone Should Know" Accessed June 2016, http://www.drchristinahibbert.com/dealing-with-grief/siblings-grief-10-things-everyone-should-know/.

68. National Institute on Aging, "Health and Aging, Advance Care Planning," March 10, 2016, https://www.nia.nih.gov/health/publication/advance-care-planning.

69. Aging with Dignity, "Five Wishes," 2016, www.agingwithdignity.org.

70. National Hospice and Palliative Care Organization, "NHPCO Facts and Figures: Hospice Care in America, 2014 Edition," 2014, www.nhpco.org.

71. U.S. National Library of Medicine, "Organ Donation," September 22, 2015, https://www.nlm.nih.gov/medlineplus/organdonation.html.

72. U.S. Department of Health and Human Services, "The Need Is Real," June 2015, www.organdonor.gov/about/data.html.

**Pulled statistics:**

p. 589, U.S. Dept. of Health and Human Services, Administration on Aging, "A Profile of Older Americans: 2015," 2016, http://www.aoa.acl.gov/Aging_Statistics/Profile/2015/14.aspx.

p. 594, U.S. Dept. of Health and Human Services, Administration on Aging, "A Profile of Older Americans: 2015," 2015, http://www.aoa.acl.gov/Aging_Statistics/Profile/2015/3.aspx.

# PHOTO CREDITS

**Chapter 1** Chapter Opener: Image Source/Getty Images; 1.1: Bennett/Getty Images; 4: Sports Studio Photos/Contributor/Getty Images; 5: Ryan Garza/Detroit Free Press/ZUMA Press/Newscom; 1.2: AGE Fotostock; 6: Maridav/Fotolia; 1.4: Michaeljung/Fotolia; 1.6 (bottom left): Web Photographer/Getty Images; 1.6 (bottom right): Grantly Lynch/UK Stock Images Ltd/Alamy; 1.6 (top left): Stray_Cat/Getty Images; 1.6 (top right): Yeko Photo Studio/Shutterstock; 9: Arthur Tilley/Stockbyte/Getty Images; 11: Karl Weatherly/Getty Images; 12: Photographee.eu/Fotolia; 13: Oliveromg/Shutterstock; 1.7: Wavebreakmedia/Shutterstock; 15: SuperStock/Alamy Stock Photo; 16: Wavebreakmedia/Shutterstock; 18: Manley099/E+/Getty Images; 19: Steve Lindridge/Alamy.

**Chapter 2** Chapter Opener: Swissmediavision/Getty Images; 2.2 (left): Getty Images; 2.2 (right): Terry Vine/Getty Images; 28: Pascal Broze/AGE Fotostock; 31: Corbis; 33: laszlolorik/Fotolia; 35: Don Victorio/Shutterstock; 36: Stockbyte/Getty Images; 37: Altanaka/Shutterstock; 38: iStock/Getty Images; 39: Pavel L/Shutterstock; 40: Science Source; 41: Bubbles Photolibrary/Alamy Stock Photo; 42: G.Binuya/Everett Collection; 45: Endostock/Fotolia; 46: David H.Seymour/Shutterstock.

**Focus On: Cultivating Your Spiritual Health** Chapter Opener: John Lund/Drew Kelly/Brand X Pictures/Getty Images; 52: Armands Pharyos/Alamy Stock Photo; 53: Jim West/Alamy Stock Photo; 54: Anne-Marie Palmer/Alamy Stock Photo; 55: Rick Gomez/Corbis/Getty Images; Figure 2: Wolfilser/Fotolia; 57: Jiang Hongyan/Shutterstock; 58: PhotoAlto sas/Alamy Stock Photo; 59: Blend Images/Alamy Stock Photo; 60: Blend Images/Alamy Stock Photo; 60: BRD/Fotolia.

**Chapter 3** Chapter Opener: Hero Images/Getty Images; 65: Jupiter Images/Getty Images; 3.3: Oliver Furrer/Alamy Stock Photo; 3.4: iStock/Getty Images; 69: Boyarkina Marina/Fotolia; 70: Artpose Adam Borkowski/Shutterstock; 70: Matt Benoit/Shutterstock; 71: Pavel L Photo and Video/Shutterstock; 71: Photodisc/Getty Images; 3.5: Radius Images/Corbis; 73: Antoniodiaz/Shutterstock; 74: Chad Baker/Jason Reed/Ryan McVay/Getty Images; 75: Shahrul Azman/Shutterstock; 76: Kate_sept2004/Getty Images; 78: Pressmaster/Shutterstock; 80: Dmitriy Shironosov/123rf.com; 81: Asia Images Group Pte Ltd/Alamy Stock Photo; 82: DEX Image/Getty Images; 83: Elliott Kaufman/Corbis/Getty Images; 3.6: Dorling Kindersley Limited; 3.7: John Dowland/Getty Images; 86: Photographee.eu/Fotolia.

**Focus On: Improving Your Financial Health** Chapter Opener: Hero Images/Getty Images; 92: Jack Frog/Shutterstock; 92: Robert Nickelsberg/News/Getty Images; 94: Wavebreakmedia/Shutterstock; 95: Michael Jung/Shutterstock; 96: karandaev/Fotolia; 97: RosaIreneBetancourt 2/Alamy Stock Photo; 98: Wirojsid/Fotolia; 100: Steve Stock/Alamy Stock Photo.

**Chapter 4** Chapter Opener: Valentinrussanov/Getty Images; 4.1: Getty Images; 104: Kamal Shahi/EPA/Newscom; 107: Spauln/E+/Getty Images; 4.2: Pressmaster/Shutterstock; 110: Philippe Garo/Science Source; 4.5: E+/Leadinglights/Getty Images; 112: ImageBroker/Alamy Stock Photo; 115: Getty Images; 116: RubberBall/Alamy Stock Photo.

**Chapter 5** Chapter Opener: Peathegee Inc/Blend Images/Getty Images; 5.1: Web Photographer/Getty Images; 124: Nick Haslam/Alamy Stock Photo; 5.2: Pearson Education, Inc.; 126: Andrew Gentry/Fotolia; 128: David R. Frazier Photolibrary, Inc./Alamy Stock Photo; 129: Marek/Fotolia; 131: Suzifoo/Getty Images; 132: Innervisionpro/123rf.com; 133: Matka Wariatka/Getty Images; 5.5.1: JRB/Fotolia; 5.5.2: Chris Bence/Shutterstock; 5.5.3: Edward Westmacott/Getty Images; 5.5.4: Stargazer/Shutterstock; 5.5.5: Hurst Photo/Shutterstock; 134: Al Freni/Getty Images; 136: Voyagerix/Fotolia; 139: Clarke Canfield/Associated Press; 140: Brian Hagiwara/Getty Images; 140: Shutterstock; 141: Rolf Bruderer/Blend Images/Getty Images; 144: Subbotina Anna/Fotolia; 146: MorePixels/Getty Images; 147: ChameleonsEye/Shutterstock.

**Chapter 6** Chapter Opener: Michael DeYoung/Blend Images/Getty Images; 6.2: Big Cheese Photo LLC/Alamy Stock Photo; 157: Bikeriderlondon/Shutterstock; 157: Brian Kersey/UPI/Newscom; 158: Ariel Skelley/Blend/Glow Images; 159: Brand X Pictures/Stockbyte/Getty Images; 160: Image Source/Getty Images; 162: Imagine China/Newscom; 6.5.1: David Madison/Getty Images; 6.5.2: Marcin Ciesielski/Sylwia Cisek/Alamy; 6.5.3: May/Science Source; 6.5.4: Phanie/Science Source; 6.5.5: COSMED USA, Inc; 164: Yuri Arcurs/iStock/Getty Images; 6.7 (left): EPF/Alamy Stock Photo; 6.7 (right): Image Source/Getty Images; 166: Sullivan/Corbis/Getty Images; 169: UpperCut Images/Alamy Stock Photo; 172: Byron Purvis/AdMedia/Newscom.

**Focus On: Enhancing Your Body Image** Chapter Opener: Yukmin/Asia Images/Getty Images; 177 (left): Everett Collection Inc/Alamy Stock Photo; 177 (right): Sarah Edwards/WENN Ltd/Alamy Stock Photo; Figure 1 (left): Custom Medical Stock Photo/Alamy Stock Photo; Figure 1 (right): Sakala/Shutterstock; 179: Brand X Pictures/Stockbyte/Getty Images Plus/Getty Images; 181: Eric Wells/LatitudeStock/Alamy Stock Photo; Figure 2 (left): Brand X Pictures/Stockbyte/Getty Images; Figure 2 (right): Li Kim Goh/E+/Getty Images; Figure 4: Vladimirfloyd/Fotolia; Figure 5: Mike Watson/Moodboard/Getty Images Plus/Corbis/Getty Images; 185: Creatista/Shutterstock; Figure 6: Photodisc/Getty Images.

**Chapter 7** Chapter Opener: Christopher Futcher/E+/Getty Images; 190: Fuse/Corbis/Getty Images; 7.1: Miroslav Georgijevic/Vetta/Getty Images; Table 7.2.1: Mile Atanasov/123RF; Table 7.2.2: Stephen VanHorn/Alamy Stock Photo; Table 7.2.3: PaulMaguire/iStock/Getty Images; Table 7.2.4: Stephen VanHorn/Alamy Stock Photo; Table 7.2.5: GVictoria/Shutterstock; Table 7.2.6: Rod Ferris/Shutterstock; Table 7.2.7: Deymos.HR/Shutterstock; Table 7.2.8: Kirsty Pargeter/iStock/Getty Images Plus/Getty Images; Table 7.2.9: Enderbirer/iStock / Getty Images Plus; Table 7.2.10: Ali Ender Birer/Shutterstock; Table 7.2.11: Dandanian/E+/Getty Images; 195: Flashon Studio/Shutterstock; 196: Jupiter Images/Creatas/Getty Images Plus; 7.3.1: Teo Lannie/PhotoAlto Agency/Getty Images; 7.3.2: Pearson Education, Inc.; 7.3.3: Photodisc/Getty Images; 7.3.4: Graham Mitchell/SuperStock; 7.3.5: Toxawww/iStock/Getty Images; 198: John Fryer/Alamy Stock Photo; 200: Ludmila Smite/Fotolia; 201: Microgen/123RF; 7.4.1: Dan Dalton/Digital Vision/Getty Images; 7.4.2: MIXA/Getty Images; 7.4.3: Ganiel Grill/Alamy Stock Photo; 203: Rolf Adlercreutz/Alamy Stock Photo; 7.6a: Pearson Education, Inc.; 7.6b: Karl Weatherly/Photodisc/Getty Images; 204: Kathy Willens/AP Images; 205: Ammentorp/Alamy Stock Photo; 206: AntonioDiaz/Fotolia; Table 7.4.1: Radu Razvan/Shutterstock; Table 7.4.2, Table 7.4.3: Pearson Education, Inc.; 208: Wavebreakmedia Ltd/Wavebreak Media/Getty Images; 7.7: Pearson Education, Inc.; 209: Radius Images/Getty Images; 211: Juice Images/Alamy Stock Photo; 7.8: Windu/Shutterstock; 214: Dennis Welsh/UpperCut Images/AGE Fotostock; 215: Praisaeng/Shutterstock.

**Chapter 8** Chapter Opener: Andersen Ross/Brand X Pictures/Getty Images; 219: Photo Library/Getty Images; 220: Jetta Productions/Blend Images/Getty Images; 224: Blue Jean Images/Getty Images; 225: mangostock/Shutterstock; 226: Cathy Yeulet/Stock Photo/123rf.com; 227: Zero Creatives/Cultura/AGE Fotostock; 230: Eric Audras//Brand X Pictures/Getty Images; 231: Michaeljung/Shutterstock; 232: PhotoAlto/John Dowland/Getty Images; 234: Purestock/Getty Images; 235 (left): Ryan McVay/Photodisc/Getty Images; 235 (right): Monkey Business Images/Shutterstock.

**Chapter 9** Chapter Opener: Lucia Lambriex/DigitalVision/Getty Images; 241: Picture Net/Corbis; 242: Everett Collection Inc/Alamy Stock Photo; 248: Nam Fook Voon/AGE Fotostock; 252: Frederic Cirou/Photo Alto/Alamy; 253: Banana Stock/Getty Images; 254: Jessmine/Fotolia; 255: Ozgur Donmaz/Getty Images; 256: Dragon Images/Shutterstock; 257: Jon Kopaloff/Contributor/FilmMagic/Getty Images; 258: iStock/Alamy Stock Photo.

**Chapter 10** Chapter Opener: Hero Images/Getty Images; 10.2: KidStock/Getty Images; 10.3a: Claude Edelman/Science Source; 10.3b: Petit Format/Science Source; 10.3c: Petit Format/Nestle/Science Source; 268: Blend Images/Fotolia; 272: Plush Studios/Getty Images; 273: Donna Coleman/Getty Images; 275: David J. Green - lifestyle themes/Alamy Stock Photo; 278: Fuse/Corbis/Getty Images; 10.7: Keith Brofsky/Photodisc/Getty Images; 10.8: Debi Treloar/Jules Selmes/Dorling Kindersley Limited; 281: FemCap; 282: Peter Ardito/Getty Images; 283: Image Point Fr/Shutterstock; 284: Tomasz Trojanowski/Fotolia; 285: BSIP SA/Alamy Stock Photo; 286: Saturn Stills/Science Source; 289 (top): Image Source/Getty Images; 289 (bottom): Pearson Education, Inc.

**Focus On: Recognizing and Avoiding Addiction** Chapter Opener: Vm/E+/Getty Images; 300: Allstar Picture Library/Alamy; 301: Auremar/Fotolia; 303: Freefly/Fotolia; 304: John Howard/Digital Vision/Getty Images; 305: Alamy Stock Photo; 306: Juice Images/Alamy Stock Photo; Figure 3: Clover/Alamy Stock Photo; 309: Image Source/AGE Fotostock;

**Chapter 11** Chapter Opener: Andresr/E+/Getty Images; 315: Goodshoot/Getty Images; 316: Patrick T. Fallon/Bloomberg/Getty Images; 11.4: Photo Library/

# INDEX

## A

A1C/glycosylated hemoglobin test (HbA1C), 454
*ABCDE* rule for melanoma, 470
Abortion, 292–293
  emotional aspects, 294
  medical, 295
  political debate about, 293–294
  surgical, 294–295
"Abortion pill" *See* Medical abortions
Abstinence
  in addiction recovery, 309–310
    definition, 309
  avoidance of intercourse
    contraceptive method, 286
    definition, 255
Academic performance, impediments to, 2*f*
Acceptable macronutrient distribution ranges (AMDRs), 121
Accessory glands (male), 248
Accountability, in caring for self, 221
Acid deposition, 568
Acid rain, 567
Acid reflux *See* Gastroesophageal reflux disease (GERD)
Acquaintance rape, 537
Acquired immune deficiency syndrome (AIDS) *See* HIV/AIDS
Action step in improving health behavior, 19
  countering, 19
  journal, 20
  positive reinforcement, 20
  relapse management, 20
  self-talk change, 19–20
  situational inducement, 19
  visualization, 19
Active listening, 226
Active transportation, 201
Acupressure, 514, 514*f*
Acupuncture, 514, 514*f*
Acute alcohol intoxication *See* Alcohol poisoning
Acute stress, definition, 65
Adaptability, as dimension of health, 6
Adaptive response, definition, 66
Addiction, 300
  as a form of operant conditioning, 300
  common characteristics, 300
  costs, 309
  development, 301
  impact on family/friends, 301
  multiple, 308–309
  physiology, 301–302

and "pleasure circuit" in the brain, 359
recovery, 309
  intervention, 309
  relapse, 310
  steps, 310
  treatment, 309–310
  treatment program search criteria, 310
risk factors, 303*f*
*See also* Alcohol use disorder (AUD); Biopsychosocial model
  of (physiological) addiction; Codependence; Enablers;
  Smoking
Addictive behaviors (process addictions), 304
  compulsive buying disorder, 305–306
  compulsive sexual behavior, 308
  exercise addiction, 308
  gambling disorder, 304–305
  technology addictions, 306–307
  work addiction, 307–308
Adequate intakes (AIs), 121
Adiposity, 154
Adoption, 274
Adrenaline (epinephrine), definition, 66
Adrenocorticotropic hormone (ACTH), in alarm phase
  of GAS, 67
Adult-onset diabetes *See* Type 2 diabetes
Advance directive, 601
Aerobic capacity (power), definition, 198
Aerobic exercise, definition, 198
Aggravated rape, 537
Aggregate nutrient density index (ANDI), 139
Aging, 587–588
  definition, 587
  health issues, 589–590
    ethical and moral considerations, 590
    health care costs, 589
    housing/living arrangements, 589–590, 590*f*
  healthy (strategies for)
    avoid alcohol/drug use, 596
    eating for longevity, 595–596
    enrich spiritual side, 596
    financial planning, 596
    improve fitness, 594–595, 595*t*
    social relationships, 596
  physical and mental changes, 591, 591*f*
    bones and joints, 591–592
    dementias and Alzheimer's disease, 593–594
    depression, 37, 594
    head and face, 592
    heart and lungs, 592

Masturbation, 255–256
Maturity and lifespan, 31
Mayer, John, 30
Measles and mumps, 402
Medicaid, 521
Medical abortions, 295
Medical model of health, 5
Medical practices linked to cancer, 465
Medicare, 519
    supplement plans, 519, 521
Medication *See* Drugs/medications
Meditation
    benefits, 57
    and brain scans, 58
    breath, 58
    candle, 59
    color, 59
    definition, 57, 85
    mantra, 58
    process, 57–58
    for stress reduction, 85–86
Meditative movement practices, 59–60
Melatonin
    and blue light exposure, 114
    definition, 108
    and pineal body, 108*f*
    as sleep aid, 116
Menarche, definition, 245
Meningitis, 398
Menopause, 247
Menstrual cycle *See* Female sexual/reproductive anatomy/
    physiology
Mental health
    definition, 27
    improvement with physical activity, 196–197
    and neurological functioning/sleep deprivation
        effects, 107
    professionals, 44–46, 45*t*
    threats to college students, 33–34, 34*f*
Mental illnesses, 33
    seeking professional help, 43
    and smoking, 339
    stigmas, 43–44
    treatments/costs, 44
    *See also* Disorders common among college students;
        Eating disorders
Mental work (to reduce stress), 78
    journaling, 78
    self-compassion in self-talk/-thought, 78–79
Menthol cigarettes, 342
Meridian channels, 514, 514*f*
Mescaline, 376
Mesolimbic dopamine circuit ("pleasure circuit"), 359
MET (metabolic equivalent), definition, 192
Metabolic syndrome (MetS), quick risk profile, 194, 433–434
Metabolism
    adaptive thermogenesis, 157
    basal metabolic rate (BMR), 156

exercise metabolic rate (EMR), 157
    metabolic rates, 156–157
    resting metabolic rate (RMR), 157
    thrifty/spendthrift metabolism, 156
    and weight, 156
Metastasize, definition, 460
Methicillin-resistant Staphylococcus aureus
        (MRSA), 397
Millennials, increase in obesity/type 2 diabetes, 446
Mind and body practices, 513
    chiropractic medicine, 513
    massage therapy, 513
    movement therapies, 513–514
Mind-body connection, 31–33
    and human health and wellness, 55–56
Mindfulness, 52*f*, 56–57
    definition, 56
    essential qualities of, 57*f*
Minerals, 131
    calcium, 131–132, 132*f*
    definition, 131
    guide, 131*t*
    iron, 132
    sodium, 131, 132
Minority populations
    and disparities in health, 9
    the minority stress perspective, 68
    and stress, 74–75
Mirena (IUD), 285, 286*f*
Miscarriage, 271
Modeling, 18
Modeling industry, changes to body image issues, 179
Mold, and indoor pollution, 570–571
Money
    and access to resources, 92, 92*f*
    and stress, 91–92
Monogamy, definition, 233
Monosaccharides, definition, 125
Monounsaturated fatty acids (MUFAs), 127
Mons pubis, 244, 244*f*
Mood
    disorders, 34, 36–38
    and rate of alcohol absorption, 315
"Morbidly obese" classification, 161
"Morning-after pills" (emergency contraception pills/
        ECPs), 289
Mortality, definition, 3
Motor tasks, and sleep, 107
Motor vehicle injuries, 550–553
Mourning, 598
Movement therapies, 513–514
MRSA (Methicillin-resistant Staphylococcus aureus), 397
Multiple sclerosis, 494*t*
Municipal solid waste (MSW), 578–579
Muscle dysmorphia, definition, 186
Muscular endurance, definition, 198
Muscular resistance methods, 207*t*
Muscular strength, definition, 198

# BEHAVIOR CHANGE CONTRACT

Complete the Assess Yourself questionnaire. After reviewing your results and considering the various factors that influence your decisions, choose a health behavior that you would like to change, starting this quarter or semester. Sign the contract at the bottom to affirm your commitment to making a healthy change and ask a friend to witness it.

My behavior change will be:

_____

My long-term goal for this behavior change is:

_____

These are three obstacles to change (things that I am currently doing or situations that contribute this behavior to make it harder to change):

     1. _____

     2. _____

     3. _____

The strategies I will use to overcome these obstacles are:

     1. _____

     2. _____

     3. _____

Resources I will use to help me change this behavior include:

     a friend/partner/relative: _____

     a school-based resource: _____

     a community-based resource: _____

     a book or reputable website: _____

In order to make my goal more attainable, I have devised these short-term goals.

| short-term goal | target date | reward |
|---|---|---|
| short-term goal | target date | reward |
| short-term goal | target date | reward |

When I make the long-term behavior change described above, my reward will be:

_____ target date _____

I intend to make the behavior change described above. I will use the strategies and rewards to achieve the goals that will contribute to a healthy behavior change.

Signed: _____    Witness: _____